Microbiology

and infection control

for health professionals

I dedicate this book to my wife Cathie, and my parents Phillip and Phyllis, for their support and encouragement

Gary Lee

For my daughters, Karin, Christine and Gen

Penny Bishop

Microbiology and infection control for health professionals

GARY LEE
PENNY BISHOP

PRENTICE HALL

Sydney New York Toronto Mexico New Delhi London Tokyo Singapore Rio de Janeiro

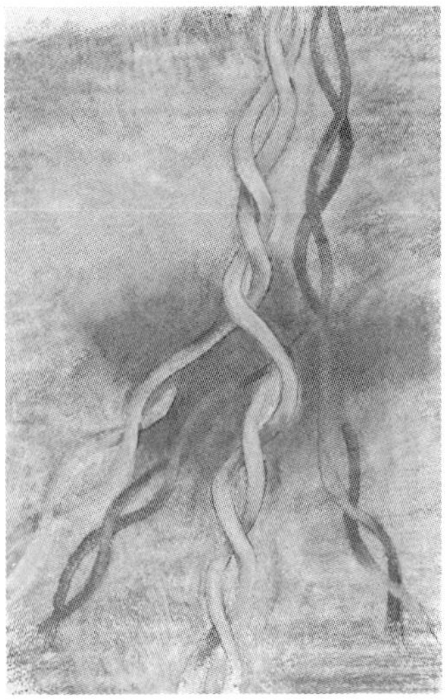

The illustration on the cover is an elegant artistic impression of a DNA molecule which symbolises the movement of microbiology into the twenty-first century. Molecular techniques of DNA analysis are increasingly being used to identify organisms which are difficult to grow in the laboratory, replacing, or adding to, traditional methods of microbial identification. The use of PCR, electrophoresis and DNA probes allows for the rapid detection of the presence of even small amounts of the DNA or RNA of a particular organism. In epidemiological studies, DNA typing can determine the source of the organism responsible for the outbreak of an infection.

Acquisitions Editor: Mark Burgess
Production Editor: Loretta Barnard
Production Manager: David Weston
Editorial Assistant: Christine Richardson
Copy Editor: Jo Rudd
Cover illustration and design and text design: Ramsay Macfarlane
Illustrations: Lorenzo Lucia, Tech View Studios
Indexer: Pamela Johnson
Typeset by Keyboard Wizards Pty Ltd, Allambie Heights, NSW

Printed in Singapore by Kyodo Printing Co. Ltd

1 2 3 4 5 98 97

ISBN 0 7248 0843 3

Disclaimer: All possible care has been taken to trace ownership of all copyright material included and to make full acknowledgement for its use. Any information that will enable the publisher to rectify any error or omission in subsequent editions is welcome.

National Library of Australia
Cataloguing-in-Publication Data

Lee, Gary Mark.
Microbiology and infection control for health professionals.

Includes bibliographical references and index.
ISBN 0 7248 0843 3.

1. Medical microbiology. I. Bishop, Penny. II. Title. IV.

616.01

Prentice Hall of Australia Pty Ltd, *Sydney*
Prentice Hall, Inc., *Englewood Cliffs, New Jersey*
Prentice Hall Canada, Inc., *Toronto*
Prentice Hall Hispanoamericana, *SA, Mexico*
Prentice Hall of India Private Ltd, *New Delhi*
Prentice Hall International, Inc., *London*
Prentice Hall of Japan, Inc., *Tokyo*
Prentice Hall of Southeast Asia Pte Ltd, *Singapore*
Editora Prentice Hall do Brasil Ltda, *Rio de Janeiro*

PRENTICE HALL

A division of Simon & Schuster

contents in brief

contents

preface

The last ten years has seen dramatic changes in tertiary education in Australia. The original decision to move from hospital-based nursing training programs to full-time Diploma courses in Colleges of Advanced Education was superseded by the Federal Labor Government's decision to abolish the two-tier system of tertiary education and amalgamate the colleges into new or existing universities. As a result of these changes, students in nursing and other health professions sciences now undertake a degree program to prepare them for work in hospitals and other health facilities. These changes have required the development of new curricula and created a demand for textbooks which cater specifically for the needs of health professionals.

The role of the health professional in today's society is complex, and the level of knowledge and skill required to work effectively is very high. Changing patterns of health care, new technologies, the emergence of new pathogens and increasing concerns about the incidence of hospital-acquired infections, all highlight the need for health professionals to have a thorough understanding of the microorganisms responsible for infectious diseases, the way they are spread, and methods for the prevention and control of infection.

The incidence and spread of infectious diseases in different parts of Australia are affected by socioeconomic conditions as well as geographical considerations. There is a wide variation in climatic conditions, in the distribution of insect vectors and also in people's access to health services. Because Australia is geographically isolated from the rest of the world, it is free of some of the diseases which are prevalent in other countries. However, increasing world travel creates opportunities for these diseases to spread to Australia. So health professionals need to have a knowledge of the kinds of diseases which they may encounter.

Nurses are now regularly confronted with a range of situations requiring knowledge and skills in infection control: for example, the care and treatment of patients with blood-borne illnesses such as AIDS and hepatitis B and C; the risk of transmission of serious diseases by needlestick injuries; and the progressive development of strains of microorganisms resistant to antibiotics. Advances in technology and methods of treatment mean that many patients who would have died in previous years, now survive. As a result, hospitals contain a large number of acutely ill patients who are highly susceptible to infection.

In this book, we have attempted to present a comprehensive text on the subject of microbiology and infection control, suitable for use by students in nursing and other health professions. The format is similar to other microbiology texts, but there is an emphasis on Australian data throughout the book.

We believe that health professionals need a thorough understanding of microbiology in order to provide safe, effective health care. This book provides basic information with applications to clinical situations wherever possible.

Bearing in mind that microbiology is presented in different ways in different health science courses, and that the time allocated for its inclusion in nursing programs also varies from one institution to another, the book is designed so that the information can be accessed in a number of ways. It can be used at different levels depending on the science background of the students and the number of hours available for the course. The content has been arranged so that educators can use the book according to the way they prefer to teach the course. For example, the major groups of microorganisms could be covered, followed by applications to transmission and control. Alternatively, the nature of infectious diseases could be covered using the 'body systems' approach and then relating it to transmission and prevention. The content of the book is selected specifically for health professionals and many of the chapters can be used for self-directed learning activities.

There are 21 chapters, divided into four units. The first unit contains basic information about the different types of microorganisms (bacteria, viruses, fungi and parasites) and the types of diseases they cause. It includes the historical background to our current knowledge of medical microbiology, an overview of microbial metabolism and a description of the techniques of microscopy.

The second unit deals with general host-microbe relationships. A description of types of infection and disease is followed by a discussion of the ways in which microbes gain access to, and exit from, the human body. General principles of epidemiology and the value of epidemiological studies are presented. The balance between pathogenic mechanisms and host defence mechanisms is discussed. This unit also includes a description of the non-specific and specific immune defences of the human body. Special emphasis is placed on the increasing occurrence of opportunistic infections in immunodeficient patients and the relevance of this to nursing practice.

The third unit is specifically designed for nurses and allied health professionals in Australia and New Zealand and includes methods of disease prevention and control. It covers principles of sterilisation and disinfection and provides information on current recommended procedures. Antimicrobial agents and their use are described and the problems associated with the development of resistant organisms are discussed. A chapter on hospital-acquired infections details the incidence of infection in Australian hospitals, describes methods of infection control and refers to the Australian guidelines for the control of transmission of infectious diseases. A unique feature of this unit is Chapter 14, 'Issues in Public Health', which addresses topics of particular interest to Australian students in the health professions. These include primary health care, notifiable diseases, community health services, Australian immunisation schedules and infectious diseases in remote areas of Australia. There is also a description of the health scene in New Zealand, including a comparison of the health of different ethnic groups.

The fourth unit is intended as a reference section and uses the 'body systems' approach to give a detailed description of individual diseases. It includes a chapter on methods of specimen collection and techniques for identification of particular pathogens. The major diseases which affect each body system are described, together with relevant data on their incidence in Australia, where applicable.

Microbiology and infection control for health professionals is intended to provide a comprehensive guide to microbiology and infectious diseases, suitable for students in nursing and other health professions. Many of the overseas texts currently available are designed for general college courses in the United States and do not focus specifically on the needs of health professionals. The central theme throughout the book is the relevance of microbiology to patient care. Wherever possible, the emphasis is placed on Australian data, the incidence of diseases in Australia, and NH&MRC guidelines for infection control practices. Where applicable New Zealand data is also included.

Features

The Spotlight boxes found throughout the text, deal with incidents or events that are of general interest.

Case study boxes are also included in the text to highlight clinical issues and to provide a focus for questions designed to test student understanding.

Each chapter has an introductory list of focus questions, a chapter summary and questions at two levels: revision and 'test your understanding'. Each chapter ends with a list of material for further reading.

The book contains a comprehensive glossary and is fully indexed. Extensive use is made of diagrams and colour figures to illustrate the text. We hope that readers will find this book a valuable addition to their professional libraries.

Penny Bishop
Gary Lee

Acknowledgments

The authors would like to thank their many colleagues who convinced them of the need for a new text and encouraged them to write it. Our thanks also go to Joy Whitton, Loretta Barnard, David Weston and the other members of the editorial and production team at Prentice Hall.

We are grateful to our colleagues who so willingly and carefully reviewed the individual chapters:

Dr Richard Benn
Royal Prince Alfred Hospital, Sydney.

Dr Ross Bradbury
Concord Repatriation Hospital, Sydney.

Dr C Shu Chan
Carillon Ave, Newtown, Sydney.

Professor Yvonne Cossart
Department of Infectious Diseases,
University of Sydney.

Ms Ilze Dalins
Department of Microbiology, University of Sydney.

Dr Ian Denham
Sexual Health Centre, Melbourne.

Dr Sharyn Errington
Northern Territory University, Darwin.

Mr Glen Funnell
Concord Repatriation Hospital, Sydney.

Dr Edward Hettiaratchi
Faculty of Health Sciences, University of Sydney.

Dr Bernie Hudson
Royal North Shore Hospital, Sydney.

Dr Tom Jeavons
Department of Chemistry, Monash University.

Dr Vicki Krause
Northern Territory Department of Health and Community Services, Darwin.

Professor Adrian Lee
Department of Microbiology and Immunology, University of New South Wales.

Mr David Muir
Royal North Shore Hospital, Sydney.

about the authors

Penny Bishop
M Sc, Ph D,
MASM

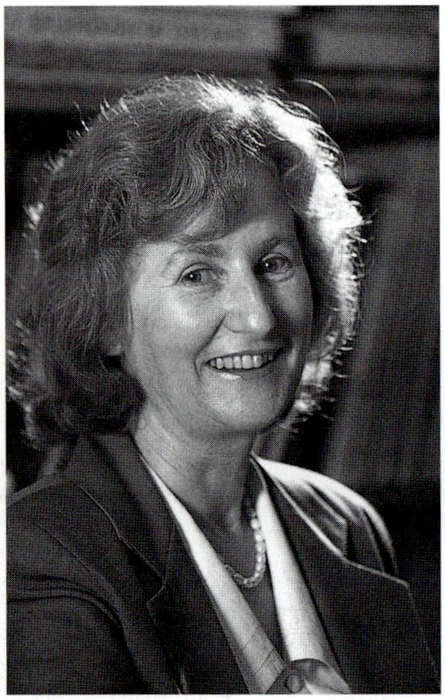

ANDREW TAYLOR

Penny Bishop has been teaching science in nursing programs since 1985 when the training of nurses was moved from hospital-based programs into the tertiary arena. She is currently a senior lecturer in the Department of Life Sciences in the Faculty of Nursing at the University of Sydney, where she is involved in the development and integration of science courses into the nursing curriculum. Her main area of teaching is microbiology and infection control for pre- and post-registration nursing students, and she has an ongoing interest in identifying factors which affect student performance in science subjects at a tertiary level.

Penny Bishop graduated with honours in Biochemistry from the University of Sydney and then worked at the Children's Medical Research Foundation, Sydney, where she obtained her M Sc for research on blood disorders. She continued her research career abroad, working in the Department of Bacteriology and Immunology at Harvard Medical School, and at the Karolinska Institute in Stockholm.

Dr Bishop obtained her Ph D from the University of Sydney for studies on the biochemical properties of bacterial cell membranes. She has a number of research publications in microbiology and molecular biology to her credit, and she has taught across a wide range of courses in the faculties of Science and Medicine at the University of Sydney and the University of New South Wales.

Dr Bishop is a member of the Australian Society for Microbiology (MASM), the Australian Society for Biochemistry and Molecular Biology (ASBMB) and COSINE. She is on the Infectious Diseases Committee of the University of Sydney and has also served as an external adviser for the science curriculum in nursing courses at other universities. Her current research interst is the relationship between nursing knowledge, nursing practice and the epidemiology of hospital-acquired infections.

Gary Lee
B Sc, Ph D,
MBA, MASM

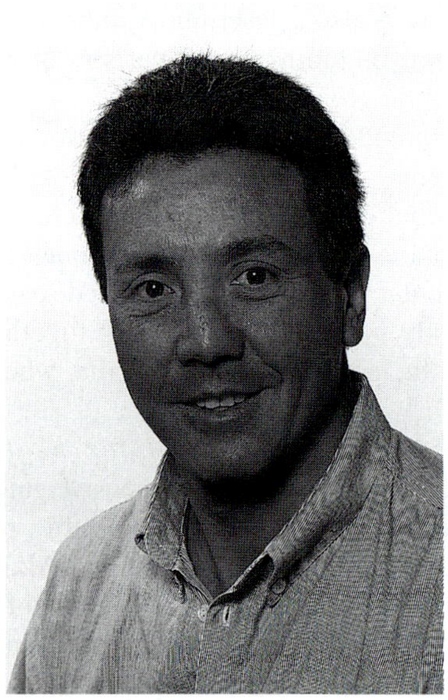

DAVID ROBINSON

Gary Lee is a lecturer in the Department of Biomedical Sciences, Faculty of Health Sciences at the University of Sydney. Since 1980 he has been teaching microbiology, immunology, physiology and pathophysiology at tertiary level in a broad range of health professional courses including nursing, medical radiation technology, occupational therapy and physiotherapy. He has also had several years' experience in diagnostic pathology laboratories, particularly those specialising in microbiology, haemotology, blood banking and serology.

Dr Lee received his B Sc in microbiology and immunology from the University of New South Wales, and obtained his Ph D for his work on infection and immunity to salmonella typhimurium. He completed an MBA at the University of Central Queensland.

Dr Lee is a member of the Australian Society for Microbiology and the Education Special Interest Group of the Society. He is also a member of COSINE, an Australasia-wide group that organises conferences on Science in Nurse Education. His research interests focus on infection control in hospitals, student assessment, and the development of interactive, multimedia learning packages and self-directed learning packages to enhance student learning.

From 1995–1997, Dr Lee was Associate Dean and Chair of the Faculty of Health Sciences Undergraduate Studies Committee, which enabled him to use and further develop his broad-ranging interest and understanding of student learning and assessment.

unit I

fundamental microbiology

chapter 1

history and scope of microbiology

Chapter focus

- *What have been the major discoveries in microbiology in the last 100 years?*
- *How have these discoveries contributed to the prevention and treatment of infectious diseases?*
- *What are the major problems posed by infectious diseases in the world today?*
- *How are microorganisms classified?*
- *What are the major groups of microorganisms that cause disease in humans?*

Microorganisms (or microbes) are organisms too small to be seen with the naked eye. The science of microbiology is the study of microorganisms, their properties, classification, growth requirements, method of reproduction and distribution in nature. These organisms range in size from tiny viruses to larger bacteria, protozoa, algae, fungi and some of the microscopic worms (helminths). They are present everywhere in our environment, in our homes, on our bodies, on the things we touch and on the food we eat. They are important for human survival on Earth, playing an essential role in many processes that maintain life. In nature, microorganisms carry out a number of important functions. They are responsible for the decomposition of organic matter and the recycling of nutrients that help to maintain the balance of chemicals in the soil. Special nitrogen-fixing bacteria live symbiotically with certain plants, absorbing nitrogen from the air and converting it into compounds which can be used by the plant for growth. Some algae are capable of photosynthesis, using energy from the sun to convert carbon dioxide in the air into carbohydrate. Marine microorganisms form the basis of the food chain in lakes, rivers and oceans. One of the most important groups of microorganisms is called **normal flora**, the microbes that reside on the human body.

As well as their role in nature, microorganisms are of benefit to humans in many other ways. Certain microorganisms are used in the manufacture of food and various pharmaceuticals and drugs, and in other industrial processes. They are a valuable tool for scientific research, and their use in laboratory experiments has been fundamental to many of the breakthrough discoveries made in biochemistry and molecular biology, such as the understanding of metabolic pathways and the discovery of the genetic code.

The science of microbiology includes the study of the relationship that exists between microorganisms and their environment (which may include a human host). In many circumstances this interaction is beneficial but, if the balance between microbe and nature is disturbed, a situation can arise where microbial growth becomes uncontrolled and the microorganisms cause disease. Some micro-organisms cause disease in plants, while others infect animals and/or humans. Very few of the thousands of different microorganisms actually cause disease although, up until the last 50 years, infectious diseases were a major cause of illness and death throughout the world.

The main focus of this book is on medical microbiology, the study of the microbes that cause disease (**pathogens**), the diseases they produce in humans and the way in which they are spread. Infectious diseases have a great impact on human lives and an understanding of this topic is essential for all health professionals.

History of Infectious Diseases

Our understanding of the relationship between microorganisms and infectious diseases dates back only to the late 19th century. Before that time, people viewed infectious diseases and epidemics with fear and superstition. Voyages of exploration throughout the world in the 16th and 17th centuries led to the development of trade routes that were responsible for carrying, not only goods, but also diseases from one part of the world to another. Travellers from the East brought diseases such as plague and cholera to Europe, where they were easily spread in the crowded, unsanitary and unhygienic conditions that existed in many cities. People thought that infections were spread in 'miasmas', or bad air, and blamed travellers for bringing disease. In Italy, travellers were isolated for 40 days to prevent the spread of plague—the Italian word for 40 is the origin of our word 'quarantine'.

Although various practices were followed to prevent the spread of diseases, they were not particularly effective because people had no real knowledge of the cause of the infection. During the last 100 years, there has been a dramatic increase in knowledge and understanding of the microbial causes of infection and with it has come an improvement in our ability to deal with outbreaks of disease. These changes are illustrated by the events surrounding an outbreak of plague in India in 1994, recounted in the Spotlight box on page 5.

We now know that plague is caused by the bacterium *Yersinia pestis*, which is carried by fleas found on rats or other rodents. When the rat dies from plague, the flea seeks an alternative host, which may be a human or another warm-blooded animal. The bacteria are injected into the bloodstream of the host and infect the lymph nodes, causing swelling, inflammation and haemorrhage, the 'black buboes' of bubonic plague. The organism may spread from the lymph glands to its preferred site in the lungs, where it results in pneumonic plague. From there, the bacteria are discharged in mucous secretions and spread directly from person to person in aerosol droplets. Unless

SPOTLIGHT
A MODERN EPIDEMIC

In early September, 1994, newspaper headlines throughout the world announced an 'Outbreak of Plague in India'. People conjured up visions of the Middle Ages, the Black Death, plagues of rats and piles of dead bodies. In India, there was fear and panic as people tried to flee from the city of Surat where the outbreak was centred. Health authorities closed all public places in Surat and trains were ordered not to stop in the city. International agencies advised travellers not to visit India unless strictly necessary. Airline companies announced a variety of precautions aimed at preventing the spread of the disease. What made the situation even more serious was that the outbreak was mainly of the pneumonic variety—that is, the disease could be spread directly from person to person via respiratory secretions. In this form of plague, death can occur within a couple of days. (This is in contrast to the bubonic form of plague which requires transmission via the bite of an infected flea from a diseased rat, and takes up to six days for the disease to develop.) The Indian people had good reason to panic. In the first half of this century, over 10 million people in India died from plague.

Plague is one of the oldest diseases known to mankind and its cyclical occurrence is well documented historically. The Black Death of 1348 is estimated to have killed half the population of Europe. From the 14th to the 17th century, plague was entrenched in Europe, the last two epidemics occurring in Milan in 1630 and London in 1665. After the 17th century, plague seemed to disappear from Europe. However, in 1894, a new cycle began with an epidemic in Hong Kong which spread through Asia to Europe, England, Africa, North and South America, and Australia and New Zealand. This was the epidemic that caused the 10 million deaths described above.

The epidemic in India in 1994 lasted only 2–3 months. The outbreak involved 1400 cases of bubonic plague and 3700 of pneumonic. There were only 56 confirmed deaths and the disease did not spread to the other major Indian cities. By the end of October, no further cases were being reported.

treatment is available, death occurs due to pneumonia, septicaemia and shock followed by collapse of all body functions. Fortunately, the organism is sensitive to antibiotics, including tetracycline, cephalosporin and streptomycin. The use of these drugs to treat the victims of plague in India, together with a massive campaign to clean up the town, was largely responsible for containing the outbreak of plague.

It must be pointed out, however, that, although there was so much publicity about the epidemic of plague in India, it was not an isolated event. During the period 1978–92, 14 856 cases of plague and 1451 deaths were notified in 21 different countries. In six of these countries (Brazil, Madagascar, Myanmar, Tanzania, Vietnam and the United States), cases were reported almost every year. The disease persists because there are more than 200 species of rats, and other rodents which act as reservoirs for the organism. Jackrabbits, mice and squirrels in California carry plague, and occasionally the disease finds its way via squirrels or domestic animals into the human population. Although there were some cases of plague in Australia from the epidemic that swept Asia early this century, Australia and New Zealand are free of plague, largely because the disease did not find a home among the wild animal population. Plague is a dramatic example of how an infectious disease that once caused millions of deaths and spread uncontrollably is now contained and can be treated. This has been achieved through of the contribution of a number of scientists and doctors over the last 100 years. Some are listed in Table 1.1.

TABLE 1.1
SCIENTIFIC DISCOVERIES

YEAR	SCIENTIST	DISCOVERY
1665	Robert Hooke	Light microscope
1673	Anton van Leeuwenhoek	Lens-observed microbes
1796	Edward Jenner	Smallpox vaccine
1840	Ignaz Semmelweis	Childbirth fever
1854	John Snow	Epidemiology of cholera
1857	Louis Pasteur	Fermentation
1861	Louis Pasteur	Disproved spontaneous generation
1864	Louis Pasteur	Pasteurisation
1867	Joseph Lister	Use of disinfectants in surgery
1876	Robert Koch	Discovery of anthrax germ theory of disease
1880	Louis Pasteur	Immunisation for cholera
1884	Elie Metchnikoff	Phagocytosis
1884	Hans Christian Gram	Gram staining method
1898	Ross, Grassi	Malaria—mosquitoes
1900	Walter Reed	Yellow fever—mosquitoes
1910	Paul Ehrlich	Sulpha drugs
1928	Fleming, Chain, Florey	Penicillin
1953	Watson and Crick	Structure of DNA

'SEEING IS BELIEVING'

Until the 17th century there were no instruments that could magnify sufficiently to make microorganisms visible to the human eye. The first person to use lenses for magnification was Robert Hooke, who built a simple compound microscope and was able to observe the structure of a thin layer of cork. He used the term 'cells' to describe the orderly arrangement of units that he saw. The Dutchman Anton van Leeuwenhoek was the first person to observe microoorganisms (or 'animalcules' as he called them) suspended in a drop of pond water in front of a carefully ground hand lens. His paper to the Royal Society in 1673 showed pictures of small creatures which look very like the familiar bacteria observed in laboratories today.

SPONTANEOUS GENERATION VERSUS BIOGENESIS

In the second half of the 19th century, there was considerable discussion among scientists as to the origin of living matter. One theory was that living cells could arise from non living matter, the theory of **spontaneous generation**. This theory arose from the observation that food left out in the air was soon found to contain millions of microscopic organisms. Other scientists contended that life could only arise from pre-existing living cells, the theory of **biogenesis**.

The arguments for each point of view became quite heated but the debate was finally settled by Louis Pasteur who, with a series of ingenious experiments, demonstrated the presence of microorganisms in air and in liquids. Figure 1.1 describes Pasteur's experiment.

Pasteur demonstrated that microorganisms are present in and on all kinds of non-living matter—solids, liquids and air. He went on to show that organisms can be destroyed by heat and that methods can be developed to prevent microbes from gaining access to the solutions that have been heat-treated. The knowledge that there are microorganisms everywhere in the environment and that, given the right conditions of temperature, water and nutrients, they can reproduce and multiply, is of great significance for both medical and laboratory procedures.

FIGURE 1.1
PASTEUR'S EXPERIMENT

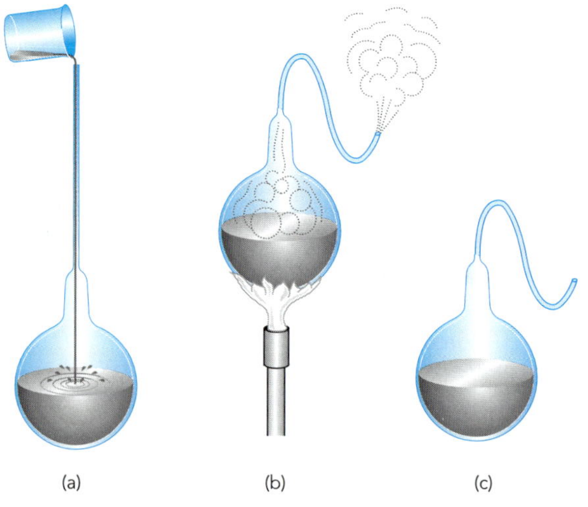

In order to disprove the theory of spontaneous generation, Pasteur devised the following experiment. He poured nutrient broth into a flask with a long thin neck, then heated the neck and bent it into an S-curve, a 'swan-necked' flask. He then boiled the broth in the flask, thus killing all the bacteria present in the flask, and expelling all the air. On cooling, air re-entered the flask, but the bacteria were trapped in the S-bend in the tube. Even after a long period of time no growth of microorganism occurred in the flask, showing that new cells could only arise from pre-existing living cells.

During the second half of the 19th century, a number of scientists and doctors were working on a variety of medical and scientific problems in different parts of Europe. They each contributed ideas and observations which together formed a picture of how microorganisms survive, reproduce and cause disease. Some of the discoveries they made were due to economic pressures and had a commercial basis. For example, in France, wine merchants were concerned because sometimes the wine they made turned sour when stored or shipped. Pasteur, from his work on the growth of microorganisms in liquid cultures, showed that the conversion of sugar to alcohol in the absence of air (a process called **fermentation**) was due to the activity of small organisms called yeasts. The presence of other organisms (bacteria) caused further reactions and led to souring of the wine. He showed that the undesirable organisms could be destroyed by heating the wine to 56°C for 30 minutes (a procedure now called pasteurisation), thus preventing the souring of the wine while still retaining its quality. This method was later extended to treat milk in order to remove undesirable organisms, some of which caused souring of the milk and others that were responsible for diseases such as tuberculosis. The observation that microorganisms were linked to food spoilage provided a basis for the concept that they might also be responsible for the production of disease.

In the 19th century, people had little, if any, knowledge about the cause of infections or how they were spread. In Europe, the Hungarian physician Ignaz Semmelweis was concerned at the high incidence of puerperal (childbirth) fever. He thought it might be due to the transfer of an 'infectious agent' from one patient to the next by the midwives. He also observed that many doctors were in the habit of going from patient to patient, or from an autopsy to attend a delivery, without washing their hands. He instituted methods of handwashing in chlorinated solutions for all physicians and nurses. Although there was a significant reduction in infections, his ideas were largely ridiculed by his colleagues. His abrasive personality led to his dismissal, he spent some time in an asylum and, ironically, is said to have died from a bacterial infection.

At about the same time, an American, Oliver Wendell Holmes, also noticed that women suffered fewer infections when they gave birth at home rather than in hospital, and concluded that the infection was carried from person to person on the hands of midwives and doctors.

In England, a surgeon named Joseph Lister had heard of Pasteur's work on bacterial fermentation. He wondered if the incidence of infections, such as gangrene, in surgical wounds might be reduced if microbes were prevented from gaining access to the wounds. He knew that phenol (carbolic acid) could kill bacteria so he began to treat surgical wounds with carbolic acid and developed procedures for surgery that were quickly adopted by other surgeons. These included boiling the instruments, soaking linen and bandages in carbolic acid, and spraying a fine mist of the disinfectant into the air during surgery. Carbolic acid is quite corrosive and its use must have caused severe pain and discomfort, but the incidence of postsurgical infections (and deaths) was dramatically reduced.

THE GERM THEORY OF DISEASE

The stage was set for the next important discovery—that bacteria are responsible for many infectious diseases. In the middle of the 19th century in Europe, the disease anthrax was killing large numbers of cattle. Both Pasteur and a German microbiologist, Robert Koch, were trying to find the cause of the disease. Koch examined a sample of blood from an animal that had died from anthrax and observed rod-shaped cells (bacilli) under the microscope. He transferred a drop of blood to a flask of nutrient broth in the laboratory, allowed the bacteria to multiply, and then injected the bacteria into otherwise healthy animals. The animals developed anthrax and died. (See Figure 1.2.) Koch then isolated the same bacteria from the blood of the dead animals. Based on these results, Koch proposed the **germ theory of disease**, which states that each infectious disease is caused by a particular microorganism.

He developed an experimental procedure which is referred to as **Koch's Postulates**, that outlined a set of principles to be followed in order to determine whether an organism was the causative agent of a particular disease. The organism had to be isolated from the diseased patient, grown in culture away from the patient, and then produce the same disease when introduced into a susceptible host. It was further required that the same organism could then be isolated from the second patient. (See Figure 1.2.) These principles were eagerly adopted by other scientists and during the next 30 years were used successfully to isolate and identify the causative organisms of most of the then known diseases of bacterial origin. (See Table 1.2.) To a large extent these principles are still valid today, although they require some modification in light of our current understanding of the nature of infections. They are discussed further in Chapter 7.

The methods developed by Koch were applicable only to diseases caused by bacteria. Viruses, which can replicate only inside living cells, and cannot be seen under a light microscope, could not be isolated and identified in this way, so the viral nature of some diseases was not established until much later.

Another important contribution made by Koch was the development of a technique for growing bacteria on plates of nutrient medium, solidified with agar. The method consists of streaking out a sample containing bacteria on the surface of an agar plate, incubating the plate overnight and then removing the isolated colonies that arise from a single bacterial cell. This technique is

FIGURE 1.2
KOCH'S EXPERIMENT SHOWING THAT ANTHRAX IS CAUSED BY A PARTICULAR BACTERIUM

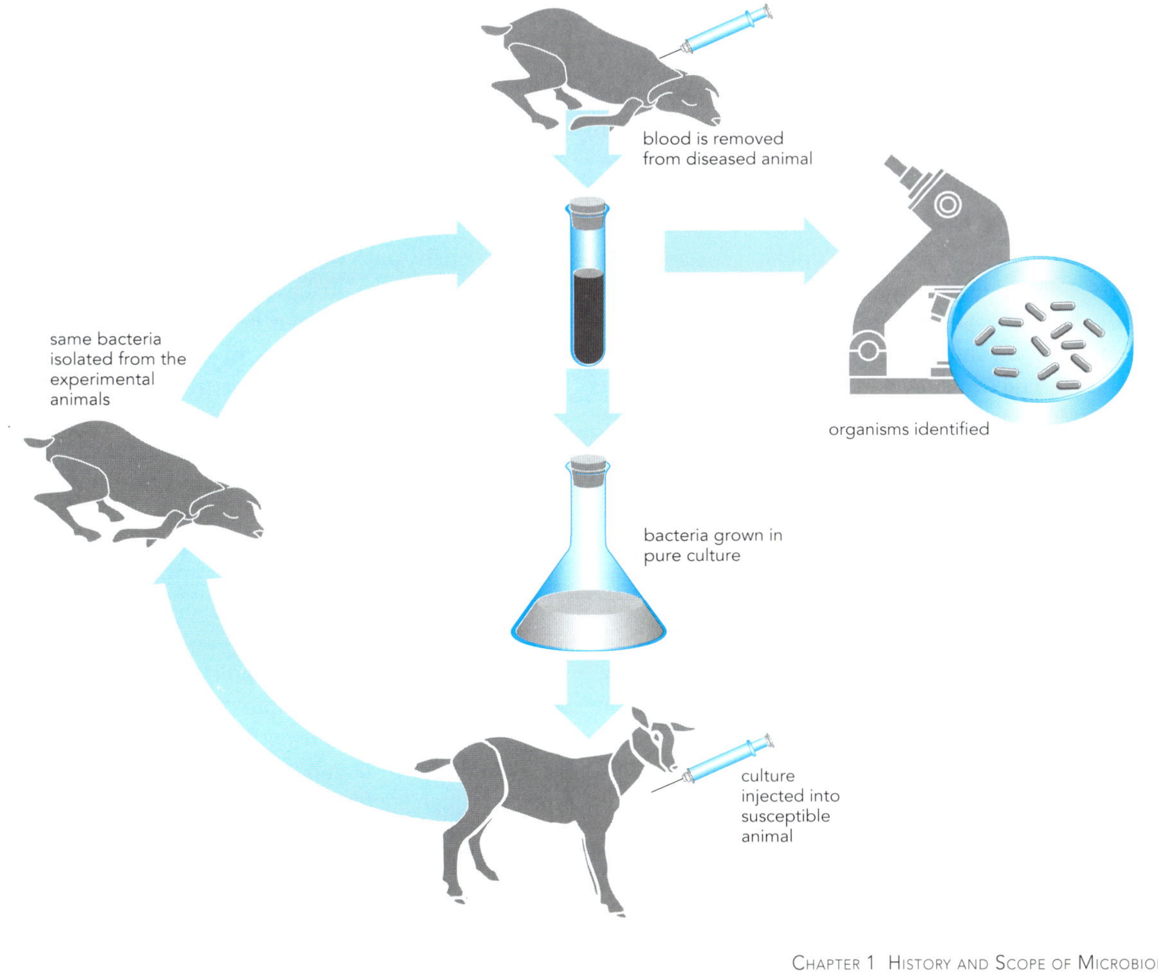

TABLE 1.2
IDENTIFICATION OF BACTERIA RESPONSIBLE FOR DISEASE

DATE	DISEASE	ORGANISM	SCIENTIST
1876	Anthrax	*Bacillus anthracis*	Koch
1878	Infection	*Staphylococcus*	Koch
1879	Leprosy	*Mycobacterium leprae*	Hansen
1880	Gonorrhoea	*Neisseria gonorrhoea*	Neisser
1880	Typhoid	*Salmonella typhii*	Eberth
1880	Pneumonia	*Pneumococcus*	Pasteur, Sternberg
1882	Tuberculosis	*Mycobacterium tuberculosis*	Koch
1883	Cholera	*Vibrio cholerae*	Koch
1883	Diphtheria	*Corynebacterium diphtheria*	Klebs
1885	Cystitis	*Escherichia coli*	Escherich
1885	Tetanus	*Clostridium tetani*	Nicolaier
1886	Pneumonia	*Streptococcus pneumoniae*	Fraenkel
1887	Meningitis	*Neisseria meningitidis*	Weichselbaum
1887	Brucellosis	*Brucella melitensis*	Bruce
1889	Tetanus	*Clostridium tetani*	Kitasato
1892	Gangrene	*Clostridium perfringens*	Welch, Nutall
1894	Plague	*Yersinia pestis*	Roux, Kitasato
1897	Botulism	*Clostridium botulinum*	van Ermengem
1898	Dysentery	*Shigella dysenteriae*	Shiga
1905	Syphilis	*Treponema pallidum*	Schaudinn, Hofmann
1906	Whooping cough	*Bordetella pertussis*	Bordet, Gengo

still the basis for the isolation and identification of bacteria in diagnostic microbiology laboratories. (See Chapter 4.)

INSECTS AS CARRIERS OF DISEASE

A further important discovery that occurred about this time was that diseases could be spread by insects. Two important diseases that were shown to be carried by mosquitoes were malaria and yellow fever. Scientists in several countries had been studying malaria, which was originally thought to be acquired by drinking contaminated water. By 1895, due mainly to the work of the French doctor Charles Laveran, the protozoan that causes malaria had been identified and the different forms of the parasite in the human body had been described. However there was no agreement on how the infection was acquired or transmitted from person to person.

In 1898, the work of the English army physician Ronald Ross in India, and Giovanni Grassi in Italy, finally demonstrated that the malaria parasite was spread by a particular type of mosquito, the Anopheles mosquito. There were many arguments about these findings and not until many years later was it accepted that control of mosquitoes was the most effective way to limit the spread of malaria. However, the implementation of mosquito eradication programs has not been successful and malaria, which is endemic in many parts of the world, is still responsible for at least one million deaths each year.

In 1900, during the building of the Panama Canal, many workers died from the haemorrhagic disease, yellow fever. It was shown by the US army surgeon, Walter Reed, that this disease is transmitted by mosquitoes. Although the viral nature of the disease was not known at the time, the discovery was important, as it was the first time that the transmission of a viral disease by an insect was recorded. Drainage of the swamps and a spraying program successfully eliminated mosquitoes from the area, dramatically reducing the incidence of the disease and allowing the completion of the canal.

TREATMENT AND PREVENTION

By the early part of the 20th century the causative organisms of many diseases had been identified, and in many cases it was known how they were spread from person to person. The work of Semmelweis and Lister had introduced the concept of transmission by human hands or contaminated instruments. Insects had also been implicated as carriers (vectors) of disease. However, effective methods for the treatment and prevention of infectious diseases had not yet been developed. To a large extent, treatment for infectious diseases was merely supportive, using procedures that relieved the symptoms but did not cure the disease or prevent its transmission.

The worldwide influenza epidemic of 1917–18 killed 21 million people, more than three times the number of deaths that occurred during World War I. Scientists such as Paul Ehrlich began the search for a drug, 'a magic bullet', which could destroy pathogens in the human body without harming the patient. This resulted in the discovery of the first chemotherapeutic agent, salvarsan, which was active against *Treponema pallidum*, the bacterium responsible for syphilis. The discovery of sulpha drugs followed and then the discovery of penicillin by ALEXANDER FLEMING in 1928. Penicillin was developed as a therapeutic agent World War II by HOWARD FLOREY and ERNST CHAIN. Since then, many other antimicrobial drugs have been isolated and synthesised. (See Chapter 12.)

IMMUNOLOGY

The work of other scientists expanded our knowledge of the disease process and the way in which the body responds to invasion by foreign organisms. As far back as 1796, EDWARD JENNER observed that milkmaids who suffered from cowpox, a relatively mild disease that produced pustular lesions similar to smallpox, appeared to be immune to smallpox. He tested his theory by inoculating a child with material taken from a cowpox lesion and subsequently exposing him to smallpox (see Figure 1.3). The child appeared to be immune. This procedure laid the basis for our modern methods of vaccination (named after the pox virus *Vaccinia*). At that time, the viral nature of the disease was not known. Almost 100 years later, Pasteur was experimenting with chicken cholera and accidentally used an old culture of the bacteria to inject some chickens. They did not become sick and were subsequently shown to be immune when exposed to a fresh culture. Pasteur realised that he had found an 'attenuated' or weakened strain of the pathogen which was able to protect the chickens against the virulent (disease-causing) strain in the same way as Jenner's cowpox had protected against smallpox. This concept was carried further by Pasteur when he developed a weakened strain of anthrax which provided protection against that disease.

A number of scientists attempted to produce effective vaccines by treating infectious organisms in various ways. Some of these were successful, but others—such as the tuberculin preparation against *Mycobacterium tuberculosis* developed by Koch—had disastrous consequences. Several of Koch's patients developed tuberculosis and the vaccine was discredited. Many modern vaccines consist of attenuated strains of viruses and are particularly effective because they mimic the disease, producing an immune response, without any symptoms of the disease (see Chapter 9). Others consist of killed microorganisms or fragments of bacteria or viruses which are able to provoke an immune response without producing symptoms of disease (see Chapter 9). Vaccination is the main method of prevention for viral diseases as there are few effective antiviral drugs that do not also damage the host cells (see Chapters 5 and 12).

Although these early scientists had some success in producing vaccines, they had little understanding of how the immune system functions. In the late 19th century many scientists believed that immunity was due to the presence of special components in the blood. The Russian zoologist ELIE METCHNIKOFF discovered that certain blood cells could ingest microbes. He called these cells **phagocytes**, meaning 'cell-eating'. We now know that phagocytes play an important role in the non-specific defences of the body. However, an understanding of the specific immune response, whereby the body produces antibodies specifically against the invading organism, and memory cells to maintain immunity, did not come until many years later. Ironically, the discovery in the 1980s of the AIDS virus, which specifically attacks the lymphocytes of the immune system, has generated a huge amount of research and contributed significantly to our knowledge of the functioning of the immune system.

FIGURE 1.3
JENNER INOCULATING A CHILD

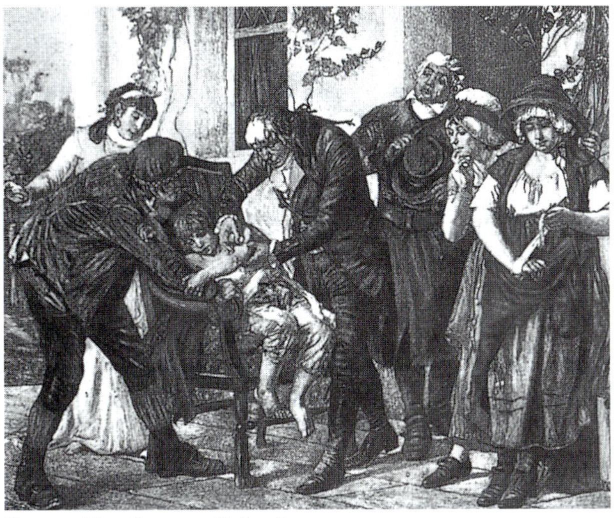

Source: The Granger Collection.

SUCCESS STORIES

During the last 100 years, the microorganisms responsible for most infectious diseases have been isolated and identified. In many cases, antimicrobial drugs have been discovered that can effectively treat or cure the disease. The control of the plague outbreak in India in 1994 is one such success story (see p. 5). Many infections can now be prevented by the administration of a vaccine. The vaccination campaign against smallpox has led to the worldwide eradication of this disease. Polio, which once crippled thousands of people annually, has been almost eradicated from Western countries. Improvements in hygiene and sanitation in the developed world have dramatically reduced the mortality rates from infectious diseases.

In the last 50 years there has been a rapid expansion of knowledge in the fields of virology, immunology and molecular biology. Specialised techniques using sophisticated equipment have enabled scientists to carry out research in these areas. We now understand the basis of inheritance at a molecular level, how information can be carried from one generation to the next and translated into functional cell components. It is possible to isolate and grow viruses in cell culture in the laboratory and to examine them using an electron microscope. Techniques developed for use in molecular biology have enabled the production of genetically engineered compounds such as hormones and vaccines that are of benefit to humans (see Chapter 4). Microorganisms can be identified by their genetic material, the nucleic acid DNA, using specific DNA probes to distinguished between closely related strains.

THE FUTURE

In the developed world, however, the earlier successes are now being clouded by the emergence of new diseases and resistant microorganisms. Diseases that had almost been eradicated, such as tuberculosis, have re-emerged, often in a form exhibiting multi-resistance to existing antimicrobial drugs. The human immunodeficiency virus, HIV, which is responsible for AIDS, appeared in the 1980s, attacking the immune system, destroying the T cells and leaving the patient susceptible to opportunistic infections. So far there is no effective treatment available and no prospect of a vaccine.

There are increasing numbers of people whose immune system is compromised to some extent, either from a disease such as AIDS, illnesses such as cancer, or the use of immunosuppressive drugs after transplant operations. They are particularly vulnerable to a range of otherwise harmless microorganisms. They also act as reservoirs for some of the more serious pathogens (e.g. multi-drug-resistant tuberculosis in AIDS patients).

In hospitals, strains of bacteria resistant to commonly used antimicrobial drugs are an increasing problem (see Chapter 12). Bacterial infections that were once easily treated with these drugs are now caused by resistant strains and are becoming increasingly life-threatening. In some tropical areas, strains of malaria have developed which are resistant to the usual antimalarial compounds, chloroquine and primaquine. Malaria poses a significant threat to travellers and residents in these areas.

Although vaccines are available for many diseases, there is widespread complacency in developed countries and many people do not have their children immunised. As a result, epidemics of diseases such as measles, diphtheria and whooping cough still occur, even in Australia, where all these vaccines are freely available. In undeveloped regions, people are still suffering and dying from infectious diseases such as gastroenteritis, measles and polio, which, given better hygiene and medical treatment, would not occur. Poverty, lack of education and lack of government finance for effective medical programs are largely to blame.

There are still very few antiviral drugs available. Several viruses have been identified that persist in the human body in a latent form, able to be reactivated if the immune system is depressed. Others, such as hepatitis B or hepatitis C, persist in a chronic, infective carrier state. Some of the viruses that persist in the body have been linked to diseases such as chronic fatigue syndrome (CFS). A large number of CFS sufferers show evidence of previous exposure to viruses such as Epstein-Barr (EB), cytomegalovirus (CMV), coxsacksie B virus, human herpes virus 6 (HHV6) and human T cell lymphotropic virus 1 (HTLV1). There is still very little understanding of how persistent viral infections affect the immune system.

NEW VIRAL DISEASES

In 1995 an outbreak of Ebola virus in Zaire made headlines. Ebola is a deadly haemorrhagic virus which attacks every tissue and organ in the body, causing death in most patients within a few days. The patient is highly infectious and the virus is spread by contact with infected blood or other body fluids. Since the patient is bleeding from the skin and body orifices, it is very easy for the virus to spread, especially in the unhygienic conditions that prevail in undeveloped countries. This was the third outbreak of this virus in recent years. It was eventually contained and did not spread outside the country, probably because the serious nature of the disease prevented people from travelling. Scientists believe that the Ebola virus is always present (endemic) in the wild rodent population but only crosses into the human population when the two come into contact.

There are other viruses that behave in this way—that is, cross the species barrier and infect both humans and animals. They include those responsible for Lassa fever and Marburg fever and the group of viruses known as hantaviruses. Like the Ebola virus, hantaviruses are haemorrhagic and associated with rodents. An outbreak of disease with influenza-like symptoms leading to death by respiratory failure occurred on an Indian reservation in New Mexico in 1993 and was found to be caused by a hantavirus. Epidemiologists linked the outbreak to a recent plague of deer mice. Most of these viruses are maintained in nature in a rodent reservoir. Humans acquire the diseases by direct contact with the animals or with virus shed in urine or saliva.

In September 1994, in Queensland, there was an outbreak of a pneumonia-like disease among the racehorses in a Brisbane stable. Fourteen horses died and their trainer also contracted the disease and died (see Spotlight box, p. 172). A previously unknown virus, an equine morbillivirus, was isolated from both the trainer and horses, and antibodies to the virus were found in the blood of a strapper who had also cared for the sick horses. In October 1995 there was a report of the death of another person who had assisted at the autopsy of a horse that had died in Mackay in August 1994. He also had antibodies to morbillivirus. There is serious concern that this is another example of a virus able to cross the species barrier.

As humans penetrate into unsettled areas and disturb the natural environment, it seems they are at risk of being exposed to previously unrecognised microbes. Sometimes, these are organisms that would not otherwise have come into contact with humans. Sometimes, the changes that humans make to the environment create more favourable conditions for the animal reservoir or insect vector of the organism. For example, planting of grain crops can encourage the rodents that carry some of the viruses described above. Irrigation may establish breeding grounds for mosquitoes or sandflies that transmit diseases.

Sometimes, our modern lifestyle facilitates the spread of an organism. For example, in some regions, virulent strains of cholera can be found in coastal waters. When this water is used as ballast for shipping, it may be discharged in harbours or rivers in other parts of the world. The virulent cholera bacteria are thus spread, contaminate the water and enter the food chain. Another example is the widespread use of air conditioning systems which have been blamed for spreading organisms around a building. They have also been linked to the occurrence of pneumonia caused by the organism *Legionella pneumophila*, which is spread in the fine aerosol vapour associated with water-cooled air conditioning units.

The history of infectious diseases is also the history of exploration and the spread of disease by travellers carrying organisms around the world. In the early days of settlement in Australia, infections such as influenza, measles and smallpox had a devastating effect on the Aboriginal population, who had never been exposed to these diseases before and therefore had no immunity. As an island continent, Australia has been for many years free of diseases that are endemic in other parts of the world (e.g. plague, rabies). Our isolation and stringent quarantine regulations combined to prevent these diseases from entering the country or becoming established in animal reservoirs. However, travel, complacency, lack of compliance with health regulations and the emergence of resistant strains of organisms are rapidly creating a situation where no area can be considered free of a particular infectious disease.

For the health professional, or the student of microbiology, a knowledge of the transmission and control of microorganisms, as well as methods for the prevention and treatment of infection, is essential.

Classification of Living Organisms

In the 20th century, techniques and instruments have been developed that have enabled scientists to study the different life forms. Early scientific observations were confined to a description of the **morphology** (external appearance) of living organisms and of the signs and symptoms of infectious diseases. The development of the microscope revealed the world of cells and cell structure and it became accepted that all living matter is made up of cells, 'the basic unit of life'. Some organisms consist of only one cell, some are made up of many similar cells. Complex or higher organisms are made up of many parts or organs differentiated into various types of cells according to the function they perform.

FIGURE 1.4
FIVE-KINGDOM CLASSIFICATION

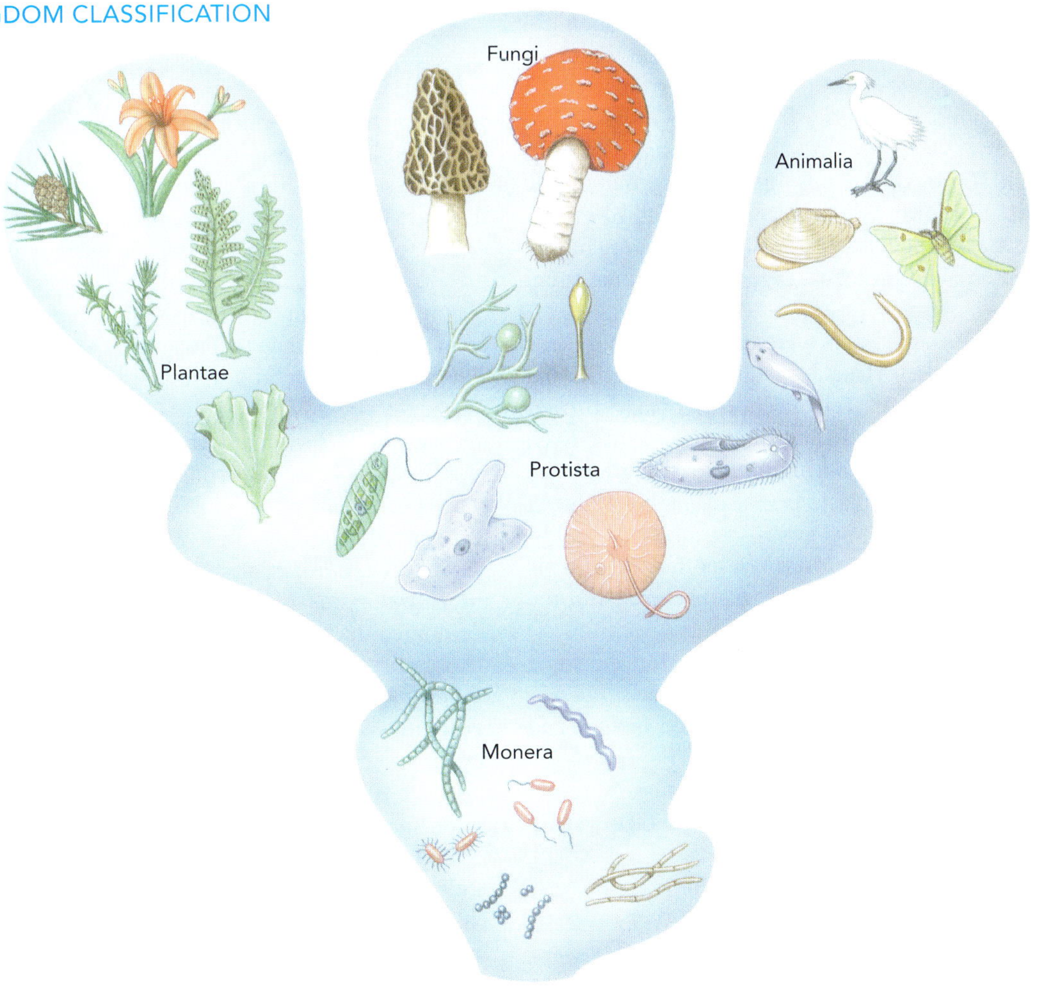

Improvements in microscopes enabled scientists to study the 'invisible' organisms—that is, those too small to be seen with the naked eye. They were able to show that certain of these microscopic creatures are responsible for the infectious diseases of higher organisms and to develop methods to identify these microorganisms and control and treat the diseases they cause. It is important to realise, however, that very few microorganisms actually cause disease. Most of them are harmless, some are essential for life and some are used in the manufacture of products that are of benefit to humans.

As scientists looked for a pattern in the complex world of living organisms, they felt the need to develop a system of classification. The classification of living organisms is a kind of shorthand used to describe groups of organisms which:

- have characteristics in common,
- have developed in certain ways,
- have certain growth requirements, or
- are found in certain locations.

The first attempt to group different life forms was made in the 1700s by the Swedish botanist Carl Linnaeus, who divided all living organisms into two kingdoms: plants and animals. He then devised a careful naming system for each species within the kingdoms, a system still widely used today.

As knowledge increased, it became apparent that the Linnaean system did not allow for the strange organisms that were visible only with a microscope and which did not really fit into the description of either plant or animal. Nor did it allow for 'plants' such as fungi which could not convert the energy from photosynthesis into food. In 1866, the German scientist Ernst Haeckel divided all living organisms into three groups—the **Animalia** and **Plantae** of Linnaeus, and a third group, the **Protista**. Protista consisted of single-celled organisms such as bacteria and protozoa, together with some fungi and algae.

As more microorganisms were discovered, and more was learnt about their structure, habitats and nutritional requirements, scientists felt the need to make further refinements to this classification; so, in 1969, R.H. Whittaker proposed a **five-kingdom classification** (see Figure 1.4). This system places organisms in the following groups:

1. **Monera**, or **Procaryota**—single-celled organisms comprising the **eubacteria**, or true bacteria, and the **archaebacteria**, or ancient bacteria.
2. **Protista**—including slime moulds, protozoa and some algae.
3. **Fungi**—single-celled yeasts, multicellular moulds and mushrooms.
4. **Plantae**—some algae together with mosses, ferns, gymnosperms (conifers) and angiosperms (flowering plants).
5. **Animalia**—invertebrates (worms), arthropods (insects) and vertebrates.

This five-kingdom classification is used today as a convenient way of grouping living organisms. Some difference of opinion still exists among scientists as to the precise location of all the different types of organisms but, in general, the scheme provides a useful method of classification. For the microbiologist, the divisions of Procaryota, Protista and Fungi are especially relevant as they contain most of the important disease-causing microorganisms. An advantage of this classification is that it places all bacteria in a single kingdom, the Monera, or Procaryotes. Other unicellular microorganisms are placed in the kingdom Protista, and fungi have a kingdom of their own.

The five-kingdom classification is based on microscopic observations of morphology and on the method of reproduction. Recent developments in techniques of molecular biology have allowed scientists to compare the DNA and ribosomal RNA from different cells. This has resulted in the description of the archaebacteria as a group distinct from the true bacteria (eubacteria). Based on ribosomal RNA studies, Woese has proposed that the archaebacteria should be grouped in a kingdom of their own as the most primitive of all organisms, the eubacteria should form a second kingdom, and all other organisms should form a third kingdom, the Eucaryotes. It may be that, in the future, further revisions of the system of classification may be required. For the present the five-kingdom system of classification is more useful for the medical microbiologist.

NAMING OF MICROORGANISMS

Linnaeus proposed that each group of organisms should be placed into a **genus** (plural: genera) the name of which is always spelt with a capital letter. Within the genera there are different **species** which have discrete but related characteristics. A species can be further divided into different **strains** that exhibit specific properties. For example, under the Linnaean system a bacterium would be named *Escherichia* (genus) *coli* (species), K12 (strain). The names assigned to organisms may reflect the place where the organism is found (e.g. coli = of the colon), the name of the researcher who first described the organism (e.g. Escherich) or sometimes the disease the bacterium causes (e.g. tetani) or its shape (e.g. bacillus, meaning rod-shaped).

A further refinement in the classification of microorganisms has come with the development of serological techniques that differentiate between strains of organisms on the basis of their antigenic properties or **serotypes** (i.e. the unique structure of the chemical molecules on the outside of the cell). Recently, the development of nucleic acid probes has enabled some organisms (viruses in particular) to be classified and named according to their DNA type.

In the higher kingdoms of plants and animals, the genera are grouped into families, orders, classes and phyla. These are required to classify the huge diversity of plants and animals, but are of less importance in the microbial world.

TABLE 1.3
CHARACTERISTICS OF PROCARYOTIC AND EUCARYOTIC CELLS

CHARACTERISTIC	PROCARYOTIC	EUCARYOTIC
Size	0.4 to 2.0 μm diameter	5 to 100 μm diameter
Cell wall	Always present	Bounded by wall or membrane
Nucleus	No defined region	Contains DNA, bounded by double membrane
Genetic material	One circular chromosome of double stranded DNA; plasmids in some cells of chromosomes	Double strand of DNA associated with proteins (histones) to form pairs; DNA also present in mitochondria and chloroplasts
Sub-cellular organelles	Absent	Present—include mitochondria, chloroplasts, Golgi apparatus, lysosomes, endoplasmic reticulum
Motility	Some are motile, use flagella	Some are motile, e.g. protozoa; most are non-motile
Plasma membrane	Present—selectively permeable	Present—contains sterols; selectively permeable
Cytoplasm	Contains all enzymes and chemicals; no defined structures	Has cytoskeleton, exhibits streaming moving of cytoplasmic fluid)
Endoplasmic reticulum	Absent	Present
Ribosomes	Present, smaller 70S	Present, larger 80S
Reproduction	mainly asexual binary fission	Sexual or asexual

Procaryotic and Eucaryotic Cells

The basic structural and functional unit of life is the cell. All cells contain a complex mixture of chemicals, consisting of proteins, lipids, nucleic acids and carbohydrates suspended in a watery fluid called cytoplasm, which is enclosed by the cell membrane and sometimes a cell wall. Microscopic observation of cells reveals that there are two distinct types of cells—**procaryotic** and **eucaryotic**. The development of the electron microscope has enabled the fine structure of cells to be examined in detail (see Chapter 3).

Table 1.3 summarises the principle characteristics of procaryotic and eucaryotic cells.

PROCARYOTES

Procaryotic organisms are unicellular and appear to have a very simple structure. They do not have a defined nucleus or any other discrete **organelles** visible in the cytoplasm. The members of the procaryotic kingdom make up a very large heterogeneous group but they are all classified as bacteria. There are two main groups of bacteria:

1. The largest group comprises the **eubacteria**, or true bacteria, and also contains a small subgroup of bacteria capable of photosynthesis, the **cyanobacteria** (formerly called blue-green algae).
2. The other, much smaller, group comprises the **archaebacteria**. These bacteria are thought to be of ancient origin and are able to live in extreme conditions of temperature and osmotic pressure.

The thousands of species of bacteria are differentiated by many factors, including shape (morphology), nutritional requirements, biochemical properties and their chemical composition. The classification and identification of bacteria will be described in more detail in Chapter 4.

Structure of procaryotic cells

Figure 1.5 is a schematic diagram of a typical procaryotic (bacterial) cell. Almost all procaryotic cells are bounded by a **cell wall**, a complex semi-rigid structure which is responsible for the shape of the cell. The cell wall is located outside the plasma membrane and protects the membrane and the internal parts of the cell from changes in the external environment such as a change in the osmotic pressure. The **plasma**, or **cytoplasmic membrane**, is a semi-permeable membrane that lies underneath the cell wall and controls the passage of chemicals in and out of the cell. When examined by electron microscopy, the **cytoplasm** of procaryotic cells appears as a granular mass with no clearly defined regions. The cytoplasm is mainly water and contains enzymes, nutrients and chemicals. The nuclear area of the cell contains its genetic information,

FIGURE 1.5
SCHEMATIC DIAGRAM OF A PROCARYOTIC CELL

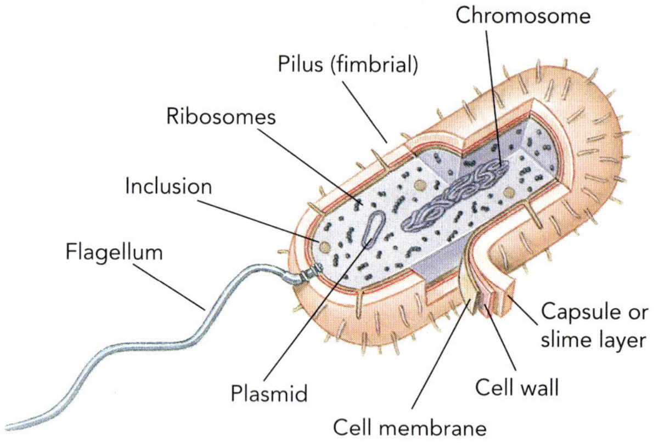

DNA, which in most bacteria consists of a single circular chromosome. **Ribosomes**, which are the site of protein synthesis, appear as round particles in the cytoplasm. There are also present various '**inclusions**'—deposits of reserve nutrients such as starch—which appear as large masses under the electron microscope. Some bacteria have **flagella** for motility. **Pili** and **fimbriae** are useful for attachment of the cell to surfaces or to other cells. Many bacteria have a layer external to the cell wall called variously the **capsule**, **slime layer** or **glycocalyx**.

EUCARYOTES

Eucaryotic organisms include all organisms other than the bacteria. They comprise single-celled organisms; the protozoa, yeasts and unicellular algae; multicellular organisms such as other algae and fungi; and the complex differentiated higher plants and animals. Microscopic examination reveals that eucaryotic cells are larger and structurally more complex than procaryotic cells. They contain a defined nucleus, as well as other membrane-bound **organelles** which are specialised structures responsible for carrying out specific functions.

Structure of eucaryotic cells

Figure 1.6 is a schematic diagram of a eucaryotic cell. Not all cells contain all types of organelles. For example, only plant cells capable of photosynthetic activity contain chloroplasts. The most characteristic eucaryotic organelle is the **nucleus**. This is frequently the largest organelle in the cell and is easily visible under the light microscope. It contains most of the cellular DNA. (Some DNA is also found in the mitochondria and chloroplasts.) The nucleus is surrounded by a double membrane, the **nuclear membrane** or envelope. Pores in the membrane allow the passage of substances in and out of the nucleus. Within the nucleus are found one or more spherical bodies called **nucleoli** (singular: nucleolus) which are the site of synthesis of ribosomal RNA. The DNA in the nucleus is combined with proteins called **histones** to form **chromosomes**.

Centrioles are located in the cytoplasm near the nucleus and are important in eucaryotic cell division.

The **endoplasmic reticulum** is a system of membranes located within the cytoplasm and connected to both the plasma membrane and the nuclear membranes. It forms a network of tubes on which are located the ribosomes—the site of protein synthesis. The endoplasmic reticulum provides a surface area for chemical reactions and the membranes control transport of molecules within the cell.

The **ribosomes** of eucaryotic cells are larger and slightly more dense than the ribosomes of procaryotic cells. They are described as '80S', which refers to their size and density, compared with 70S for procaryotic cells. In both procaryotic and eucaryotic cells, ribosomes are the site of protein synthesis. The messenger RNA attaches to the ribosomes to provide a structure where amino acids can be incorporated and joined to form proteins (see Chapter 4).

The **Golgi complex** is another membranous structure found in the cytoplasm. It consists of a series of flattened sacs or vesicles and is responsible for the secretion of certain proteins, such as enzymes and hormones.

Mitochondria (singular: mitochondrion) are found in the cytoplasm of eucaryotic cells. They consist of a double membrane structure, the inner one arranged in a series of folds called **cristae**. The structure of the mitochondria make it possible for enzyme reactions that are closely linked to be carried out in series. These include the energy-producing reactions involved in the metabolism of glucose and the production of ATP via the electron transport chain. Mitochondria are often called the 'powerhouses' of the cell as they are the main site of ATP production (see Chapter 2).

Chloroplasts are complex structures consisting of stacks of membranes (grana), and are found in photosynthetic algae and green plants. The chloroplast contains the pigment **chlorophyll** and the enzymes necessary to trap light energy and use it for synthesis of glucose during **photosynthesis**.

Lysosomes are small organelles, bounded by a single membrane and found mainly in animal cells. They consist of a sac containing strong digestive enzymes and appear to be important in breaking down foreign material and microorganisms that have been ingested by the cell. Human white blood cells (phagocytes) contain large numbers of lysosomes.

REPRODUCTION IN PROCARYOTIC AND EUCARYOTIC CELLS

Procaryotic cells mainly reproduce asexually by a process called **binary fission**: that is, the cell splits into two daughter cells with properties identical to those of the original cell.

Reproduction in eucaryotic cells can be sexual or asexual. **Asexual reproduction** occurs in protozoa and some algae and in normal cell division during growth of higher organisms. In this process, termed **mitosis**, the chromosomes replicate and two daughter nuclei are formed in a complex but organised process. The new nuclei move

FIGURE 1.6
SCHEMATIC DIAGRAM OF A EUCARYOTIC CELL

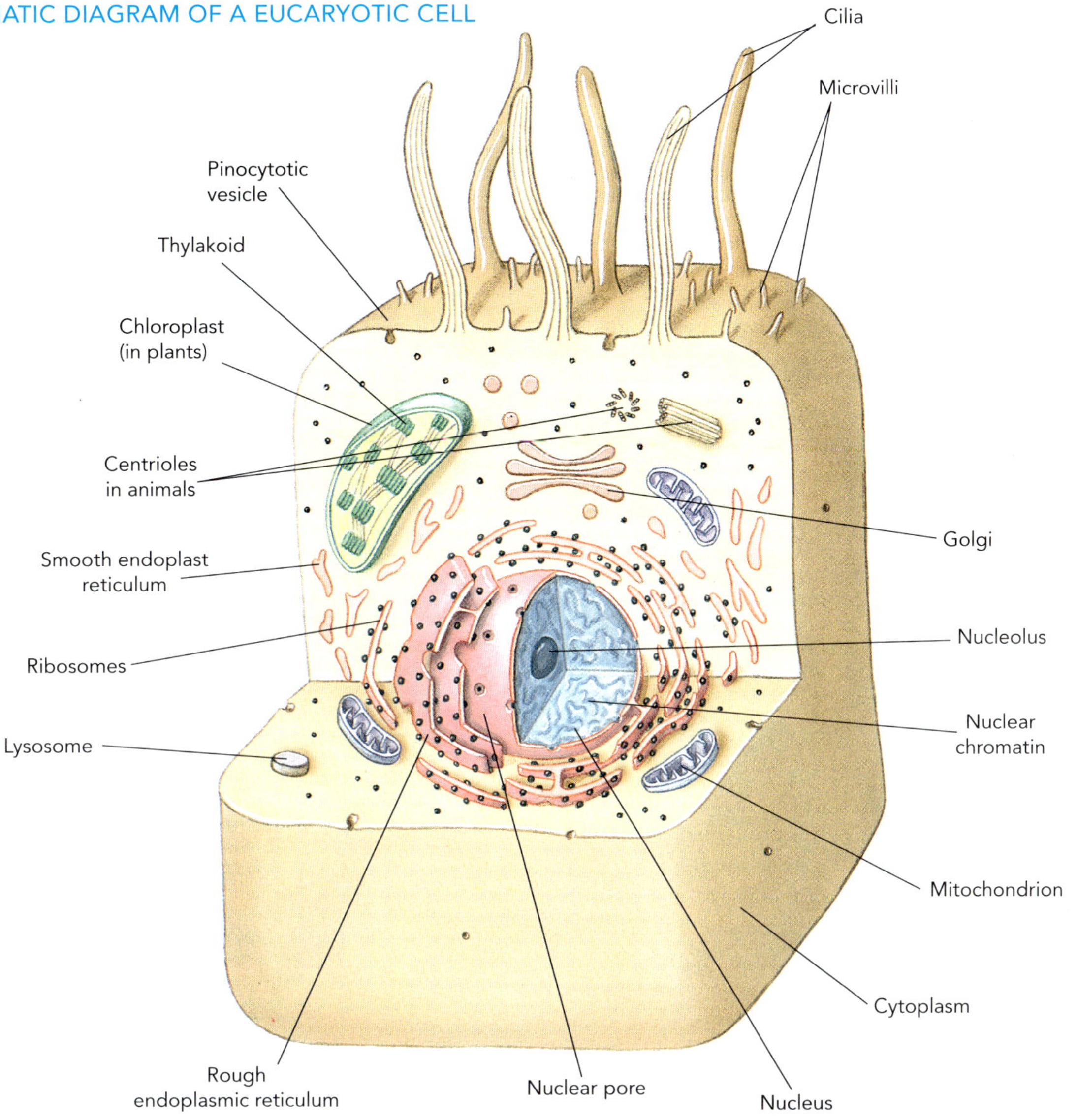

to opposite ends of the cell and the cell then splits into two identical daughter cells with identical sets of chromosomes. Sexual reproduction in eucaryotic organisms involves the formation of gametes by the parent cells. Fusion of the gametes produces a new cell which has received half its genetic material (chromosomes) from each parent. The new cell therefore has some, but not all, characteristics of each parent. The cell division process involved in gamete production is termed **meiosis**. Meiotic division and fusion of gametes is then followed by mitosis. Sexual reproduction allows for mixing of genetic material (i.e. characteristics) to occur and produces genetic diversity in the offspring.

Overview of the Microbial World

The major groups of organisms that are of medical importance are the viruses, bacteria, protozoa and fungi, and the microscopic stages of some multicellular parasites. These organisms vary in size from the viruses, (the smallest of which are about 20 nm or 0.02 μm) to the microscopic stages of some of the helminths (which are up to 400 μm in diameter and almost visible to the naked eye). It is generally considered that the limit of resolution of the human eye (the smallest unit that can be discerned without magnification) is about the diameter of a human hair (75 μm).

Figure 1.7 illustrates the relative sizes of some of these organisms. The distinctive properties of each group of organisms will be discussed in later chapters, together with descriptions of the types of diseases for which they are responsible. A brief overview of the various groups of organisms is presented here.

VIRUSES

According to the classification systems described above, viruses are not considered to be living cells because they are unable to reproduce or carry out any metabolic reactions on their own. However, viruses are very important pathogens and, together with bacteria, are the cause of many serious infectious diseases.

FIGURE 1.7
RELATIVE SIZE OF MICROORGANISMS

Range of electron microscope	0.01 µm – 0.3 µm	Poliovirius .02 µm
Range of light microscope	1 µm – 100 µm	chlamydiae 1.0 µm rickettsiae 1.0 µm coccus 1.0 µm bacillus 1-5 µm yeast 5-15 µm red blood cell 8 µm protozoa 5-100µm fungal spores 3-20 µm
Range of human eye	100 µm(0.1 mm)	louse 1mm

structure of virus particles. Electron microscopy has revealed that viruses exist in a huge range of sizes and shapes. Many have quite a regular shape and in some cases can be induced to crystallise from a pure preparation. The major shapes are (1) icosahedral, a regular 20-sided particle, (2) helical and (3) complex.

They range in size from the tiny polio virus which is only 20 nm (0.02 µm), to the large vaccinia (smallpox) virus which is 300 nm (0.3 µm). However, the largest viruses are still considerably smaller than even the smallest bacteria, which are about 1 µm in length.

Viruses are structurally very simple, consisting of a core of nucleic acid surrounded by protein and sometimes an envelope of glycoprotein. The core is made of only one type of nucleic acid, **RNA** or **DNA**, which contains the genetic information for the virus. The RNA or DNA may be single-stranded or double-stranded. The nucleic acid is enclosed in a layer of protein, the **capsid**, made up of protein units called **capsomeres** (see Figure 1.8). When infection of a host cell occurs, the virus first attaches to a specific receptor site on the surface of the target host cell. The viral nucleic acid directs the synthesis of new viral particles using the synthetic pathways and enzymes of the host cell. Completed viral particles, called **virions**, are released, usually causing the host cell to burst. The virions can then infect neighbouring cells. Some viruses have an envelope surrounding the capsid. The envelope is derived from part of the membrane of the host cell and is attached to the new viral particle when it is released from the host cell by budding. The envelope often has glycoprotein 'spikes' which help attach the virus to the target host cell.

Prions are unusual virus-like particles which appear to consist only of protein without any nucleic acid or other genetic material. This type of infective agent is considered to be responsible for diseases known as **spongiform encephalopathies**, such as **Creutzfeldt-Jakob disease (CJD)**, **scrapie** (a 'slow' viral disease of sheep), and bovine spongiform encephalopathy or 'mad cow disease'. Prions seem to be almost impossible to destroy by the usual methods of sterilisation and disinfection and are a cause for concern because of recent cases of apparent CJD transmission by the use of human growth hormone preparations in Australia and the ingestion of contaminated beef in Britain. (See Spotlight box, Chapter 5, p. 94).

FIGURE 1.8
SCHEMATIC DIAGRAM OF A VIRUS

(a) Naked virus

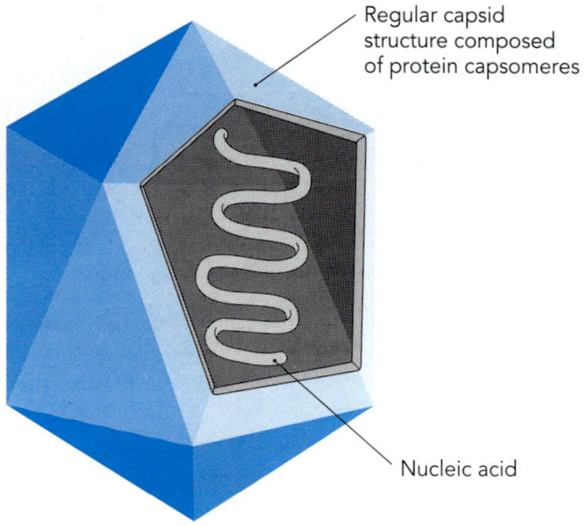

(b) Enveloped virus

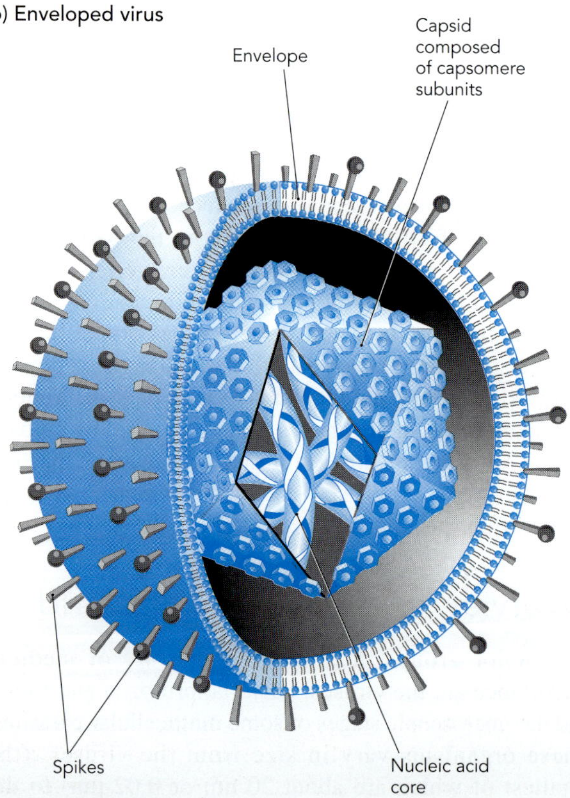

BACTERIA

There are many thousands of different species of bacteria living in our environment. Relatively few bacteria actually cause disease, but there are some pathogenic strains that can have serious effects on humans. Because bacteria are free-living and can be seen under an ordinary light microscope, they have been extensively studied. Even so, occasionally a previously unrecognised species will emerge as the cause of a disease—for example, *Legionella pneumophila,* the agent of **Legionnaires' disease**. (See Spotlight box, Chapter 8, p. 168).

All bacteria are procaryotic; that is, they are simple, unicellular organisms with no defined nucleus or subcellular organelles. They are freeliving in the environment, absorbing nutrients, and are capable of carrying out all the metabolic reactions necessary for growth and reproduction. Bacteria can multiply very rapidly. Under optimum conditions, a cell of *Escherichia coli* can reproduce itself in 20 minutes, which means that a single cell can give rise to about 1 million cells in 7–8 hours.

Most bacteria occur in one of three common shapes: spherical, rod-shaped or spiral. Their characteristic shape is important for their classification and identification. Spherical bacteria or, **cocci** (singular: **coccus**), are about 0.5–2.0 μm in diameter and may occur as single units, double units (**diplococci**), chains (**streptococci**) or clusters (**staphylococci**). The rod-shaped bacteria, or **bacilli** (singular: **bacillus**), vary in size. Some are quite small, 1–2 μm in length, while other bacilli may be 1–2 μm in diameter and up to 15 μm in length. Spiral-shaped bacteria belong to one of three groups—**spirochaetes**, **spirilla** (singular: **spirillum**) or **vibrio**. Spirochaetes, such as *Treponema pallidum*, the causative agent of **syphilis**, have a distinctive corkscrew appearance and axial filaments for motility. The spirilla usually lack axial filaments and instead use flagella for movement (e.g. *Helicobacter pylori*, an organism implicated in gastric ulcers). The third type of spiral, the **vibrio**, resembles a comma: that is, the cell is not a complete spiral, The best known example is *Vibrio cholerae*, the causative agent of cholera (see Figure 1.9).

Bacteria are remarkably adaptable and can grow in a variety of environmental conditions. While some organisms are very fastidious, many bacteria can use a wide range of nutrients and adapt to growth at different temperatures and oxygen levels.

Chlamydiae and **rickettsiae** are classified as bacteria even though they do not have all the characteristics described above. They usually reproduce inside a living cell and cannot be grown on an agar plate in the laboratory. However, they can be stained with conventional bacterial stains and are sensitive to antibacterial drugs. They are the cause of a number of important diseases.

ALGAE

Algae (singular: alga) are mainly aquatic organisms, occurring in freshwater ponds and streams as well as salt water. Many are unicellular, others consist of a chain of cells forming a filament. The large seaweeds are macroscopic algae. All algae contain chlorophyll, located in chloroplasts, and can carry out photosynthesis. Many are green but some contain other pigments that give them a red or brown colour.

Algae do not usually cause infections in humans. However, some species of dinoflagellates (unicellular plankton), such as *Gonyaulax*, produce **neurotoxins**. When these algae are eaten by shellfish, the toxin is concentrated in the fish and can cause poisoning if the shellfish is eaten by humans. These dinoflagellates are red in colour and when in high concentration in the sea produce a 'red tide'. Health authorities usually prohibit the harvesting of shellfish for human consumption during a red tide. Food poisoning associated with toxic shellfish occurs frequently along the coast of the North Island of New Zealand. Another alga, *Gambierdiscus toxicus*, is responsible for the production of a similar toxin, **ciguatera**, which is often found in fish in the South Pacific Ocean and the Caribbean.

Algae play an important role as part of the food chain, and seaweeds are a source of food in some countries. The gelling agent agar, which is used to prepare bacterial culture plates, is extracted from the red alga, *Gelidium*. Algae carry out photosynthesis, converting atmospheric carbon dioxide into carbohydrate and releasing oxygen (see Chapter 2). Algae thrive in the upper layers of water where there is plenty of light, often causing a green 'scum' to form. Heavy growth of algae (**algal bloom**) often indicates sewage pollution in rivers and waterways as algae thrive on the high concentrations of organic material and phosphates that exist in sewage or waste. When these blooms die and decompose, they severely deplete the water of oxygen, and this can result in the death of the fish population. True algae should be distinguished from the '**blue-green algae**', which can pollute inland waterways and produce a toxin that can affect animals who drink the water. Blue-green algae are really bacteria and are more correctly called **cyanobacteria**.

Some algae live in a symbiotic association with other organisms, the photosynthetic activity of the algae providing carbohydrate nutrients for the host. For example, algae are responsible for the bright blue/green colour of the 'lip' of the giant clam found on coral reefs. Lichens seen on rocks and decaying wood are combinations of algae and fungi.

PROTOZOA

Protozoa (singular: **protozoan**) are unicellular eucaryotic organisms that lack a cell wall. They are much larger than bacteria and have visible organelles. Most of them are found in aquatic environments. They are usually colourless and are distinguished from algae because they do not contain chlorophyll. Protozoa ingest their food, either by surrounding the food with a portion of their cell membrane and engulfing it, or by swallowing it through a specialised structure or 'mouth'. Very few protozoa are pathogenic, but there are some important species that cause serious diseases (see Chapter 6).

FIGURE 1.9
DIVERSITY OF BACTERIAL MORPHOLOGY
Fluorescent antibody labelling reveals (a) large rod-shaped cells of *Legionella pneumophila*; (b) tiny cells of *Chlamydia trachomatis* shown as intracellular clusters and as free particles released when the host cell ruptures; (c) negative stain of *Helicobacter pylori*.

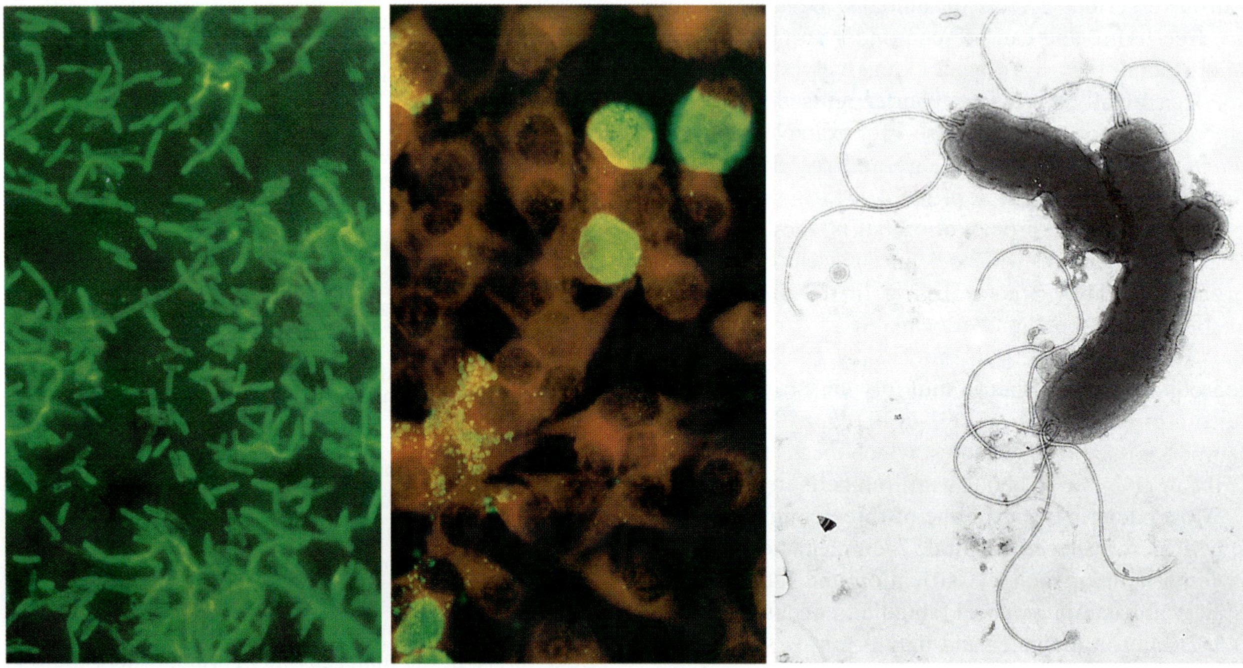

(a) (b) (c)

Protozoa are classified by the way they move. **Amoebae** move by flowing: the cell membrane stretches out to form pseudopods (false feet) and the cytoplasm flows into them. Flagellates have flagella which act like tails and allow the organisms to swim. The ciliates have cilia, tiny hair-like appendages which propel the cell with a wave-like motion. **Sporozoans** are non-motile protozoa. Many of them are carried by insect vectors and cause serious diseases (e.g. members of the genus *Plasmodium*, which causes malaria).

FUNGI

Fungi are a large, diverse group of eucaryotic organisms, ranging from microscopic yeast cells to large complex structures such as mushrooms. They are unicellular or multicellular and have a thick cell wall. Many fungi are beneficial to humans. They play an important role in the decomposition of organic matter and some species are a source of antibiotics. Yeasts are important in the food industry for making bread, wine and beer. The large fleshy mushrooms are a source of food.

Although many fungi are responsible for infections of plants, very few are pathogenic to humans. The fungi that cause human disease belong to two main groups: (1) the **yeasts** and (2) the **filamentous fungi**. Yeasts are unicellular and reproduce by budding. Filamentous fungi grow as long branching cells or filaments, called **hyphae**. These hyphae grow together to form a mat, or **mycelium**. Asexual reproduction occurs by the formation of **aerial hyphae**, on which **sporangia** or **spore sacs** are formed (see Figure 1.11). When the spores are released, they may be blown around on wind currents and inhaled, often causing severe lung infections. Most fungal infections are cutaneous, affecting only the upper layers of the skin or mucosa, and do not cause severe illness. However some fungal infections can become systemic, spreading throughout the body and causing life-threatening conditions.

Fungal infections (**mycoses**) are described in Chapter 6.

FIGURE 1.10
SCHEMATIC PROTOZOAN
Diagram showing cellular organelles of a typical ciliated protozoan (e.g. *Paramecium*).

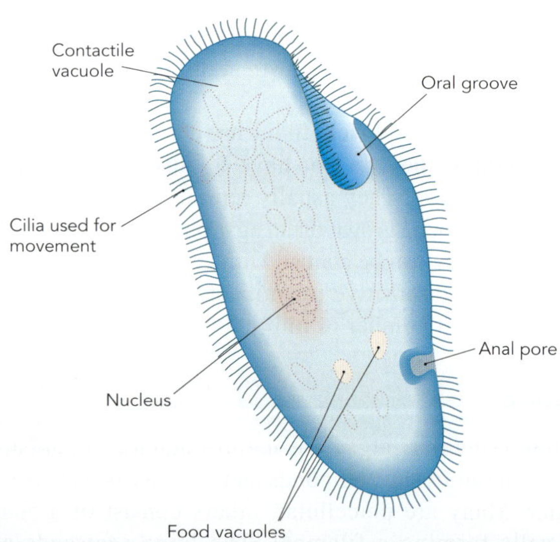

FIGURE 1.11
STRUCTURE OF FUNGI

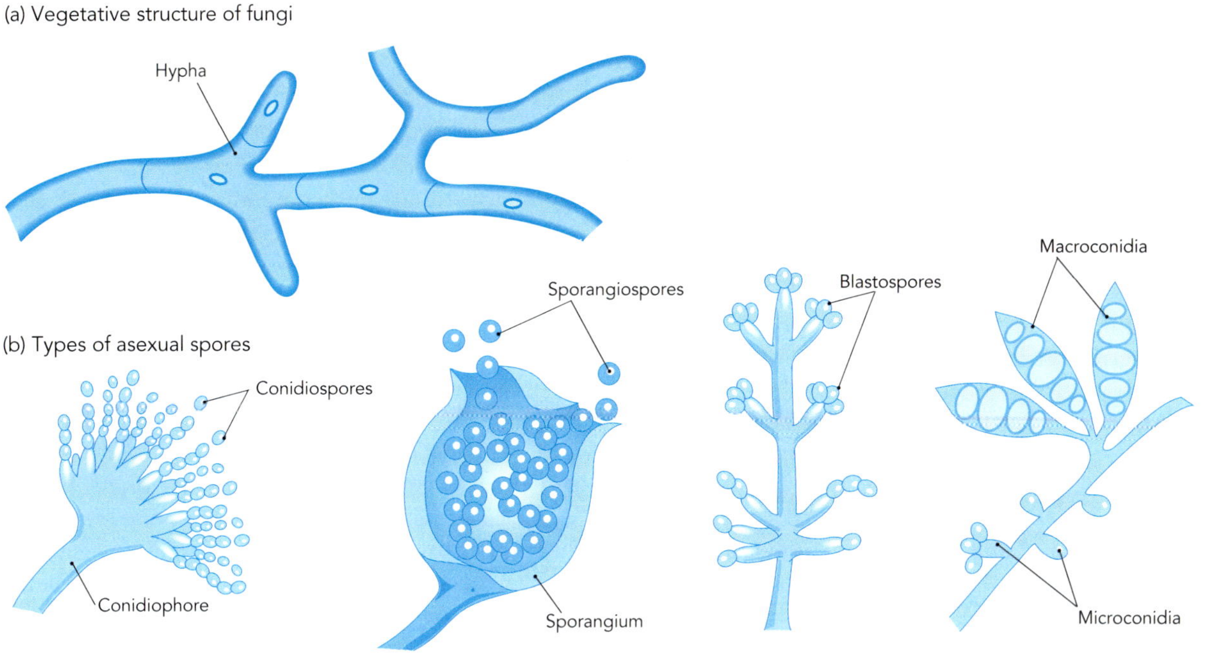

MICROSCOPIC PARASITES

Some worms have a microscopic stage in their life cycle, so infections caused by these parasites are usually classed as microbial diseases. Parasitic worms belong to the group called **helminths**. They include the **flatworms** (**tapeworms** and **flukes**) and **roundworms**. Infection of humans may occur in a number of ways—ingestion of the larvae or eggs, injection of the parasite by a blood-sucking insect, or the direct penetration of the skin by the larval stage of the parasite.

Helminth infections are most common in developing countries and transmission is influenced by socioeconomic conditions, general hygiene and other lifestyle factors.

Summary

- Microorganisms are present everywhere and play an essential role in many processes that maintain life. Very few microorganisms actually cause disease.

HISTORY OF INFECTIOUS DISEASES

- In the past, travellers spread diseases from the East to Europe.
- During the last 100 years, there has been a dramatic increase in knowledge and understanding of the microbial causes of infection.
- The development of suitable magnifying instruments was necessary in order to see microorganisms.
- Pasteur disproved the theory of spontaneous generation and showed that microorganisms were responsible for food spoilage.
- Scientists such as Semmelweis and Lister showed transmission of infection could be prevented.
- Robert Koch proposed the germ theory of disease and other scientists then isolated and identified the causative organisms of most of the then known diseases of bacterial origin.
- Work on malaria and yellow fever showed that some diseases are transmitted by mosquitoes.
- The search for drugs to treat infectious diseases led to the synthesis of sulpha drugs and the discovery of antibiotics.

IMMUNOLOGY

- Edward Jenner used cowpox to prevent infection by smallpox; this laid the basis for modern vaccination programs.
- Some diseases have been eradicated (smallpox), are preventable (polio) or are controllable (plague).
- Research in immunology and molecular biology has increased our understanding of how infectious diseases affect the body and can be treated.

THE FUTURE

- The successful treatment of infectious diseases in the future is threatened by the emergence of new and resistant organisms.

CLASSIFICATION OF LIVING ORGANISMS

- Classification is the grouping together of organisms that have characteristics in common.
- Carl Linnaeus divided living organisms into two kingdoms: plants and animals.
- R.H. Whittaker proposed a five-kingdom classification which places all bacteria in a single kingdom, the Monera or Procaryotes. Other unicellular microorganisms are classified as Protista, and fungi have a kingdom of their own. The other two kingdoms are Plantae and Animalia.
- Microorganisms are named according to their genus, species, strain, and can also be classified according to their serological properties or DNA type.

PROCARYOTIC AND EUCARYOTIC CELLS

- All cells can be described as either procaryotic or eucaryotic.
- Procaryotic organisms are unicellular with a simple structure consisting of a cell wall located outside the plasma membrane. Some bacteria have additional structures such an envelope, flagella, pili or fimbriae.
- The cytoplasm contains enzymes, nutrients, chemicals, ribosomes and a nuclear area containing a single circular chromosome.
- Eucaryotic organisms comprise all organisms other than the bacteria.
- The most characteristic eucaryotic organelle is the nucleus which is surrounded by the nuclear membrane. Other structures include the endoplasmic reticulum, on which are the ribosomes and other subcellular organelles such as the Golgi complex, mitochondria, lysosomes in animal cells, and chloroplasts in plant cells.

REPRODUCTION IN PROCARYOTIC AND EUCARYOTIC CELLS

- Procaryotic cells reproduce asexually by binary fission.
- Reproduction in eucaryotic cells can be sexual or asexual. Asexual reproduction is termed mitosis.
- Sexual reproduction in eucaryotic organisms involves the formation of gametes by meiosis, followed by mitosis. Sexual reproduction allows for mixing of genetic material and produces genetic diversity in the offspring.

OVERVIEW OF THE MICROBIAL WORLD

- The major groups of organisms of medical importance are viruses, bacteria, protozoa and fungi, and the microscopic stages of some multicellular parasites.

VIRUSES

- Viruses cause infection in animal, plant and bacterial cells and are quite specific for the cell type they attack.
- Viruses consist of a core of RNA or DNA surrounded by protein, and sometimes an envelope of glycoprotein.
- Viruses are very small and can only reproduce inside a cell they have infected.

BACTERIA

- All bacteria are procaryotic and live freely in the environment.
- They occur in one of three common shapes: spherical, rod-shaped or spiral.
- Bacteria multiply very rapidly, a single cell giving rise to about 1 million cells in 7–8 hours.

ALGAE

- Algae are mainly aquatic organisms occurring in both fresh and salt water.
- All algae contain chlorophyll and can carry out photosynthesis.
- Algae do not usually cause infections in humans, but some species produce neurotoxins which can concentrate in fish or shellfish and cause poisoning when eaten by humans.

PROTOZOA

- Protozoa are unicellular eucaryotic organisms, enclosed in a membrane, and contain visible organelles.
- They live mainly in water and ingest their food by engulfing it or by swallowing it through a specialised structure or 'mouth'.
- Some species of protozoa are the cause of serious diseases.

FUNGI

- Fungi are unicellular or multicellular and have a thick cell wall.
- They are important in the decomposition of organic matter and are important in the food industry; some species are a source of antibiotics.
- Very few fungi are pathogenic to humans.

MICROSCOPIC PARASITES

- Some worms (tapeworms, flukes and roundworms) have a microscopic stage in their life cycle, so infections with these parasites are usually classed as microbial diseases.
- Helminth infections are most common in developing countries.

Study Questions

1. Name the scientist responsible for proposing the germ theory of disease.
2. Describe some of the contributions made to microbiology by Louis Pasteur.
3. How is plague spread?
4. What is meant by the theory of spontaneous generation?
5. What contribution did Semmelweis make to our understanding of disease transmission?
6. How are malaria and yellow fever transmitted?
7. Who discovered penicillin?
8. What is the origin of the word 'vaccination'?
9. What are the major differences between a eucaryotic and a procaryotic cell?
10. What is the five-kingdom classification of living organisms?
11. How are bacteria named?
12. Which organisms belong to the procaryotic kingdom?
13. In eucaryotic cells, what is the function of the mitochondria?
14. Describe the basic structure of a virus.
15. What are the three basic shapes of bacterial cells?
16. How do algae differ from protozoa and fungi?
17. How are protozoa classified?
18. What kind of organism is the cause of malaria?
19. What are fungal infections called?
20. Who was the first person to use chemical disinfectants in surgery?

Test Your Understanding

1. Why are outbreaks of plague not as serious in the 1990s as in earlier times?
2. How has modern travel contributed to the spread of infectious diseases?
3. What is meant by an 'attenuated' strain of a microorganism? How are they used?
4. What are some of the major successes in the treatment and control of infectious diseases?
5. What are the main problems in infectious diseases confronting medicine today?
6. What methods are used to assign an organism to a particular classification?
7. How do viruses differ from other microorganisms?

FURTHER READING

Cumpston, J.H.L., *Health and Disease in Australia. A History*, Canberra: Australian Government Publishing Service, 1989.

Fenner, F. (ed.) *History of Microbiology in Australia*, Curtin ACT: Australian Society for Microbiology, 1990.

Kraut, A.M., *Silent Travellers, Germs, Genes and the 'Immigrant Menace'*, New York: Basic Books, 1994.

chapter 2

metabolic processes in microbial cells

Chapter focus

- *How does the structure of biological compounds relate to their function?*
- *What is the function of enzymes?*
- *What are the principal pathways of energy production in microorganisms?*
- *What is the relationship between the breakdown and synthesis of different biological molecules?*
- *What metabolic processes carried out by microorganisms are of use to humans?*

All living cells are continually undergoing processes of replication, breakdown, synthesis and repair. The overall term used to describe these processes is **metabolism** and refers to all the different reactions that must occur in order for a cell to grow and reproduce. The pathways of metabolism are remarkably similar in all living cells. The differences that do occur usually reflect the availability of nutrients or the need for a cell to provide for a specific function. This may be secretion, storage, structural support, energy for movement, or reproduction. Our knowledge of many of the metabolic processes that occur in human cells has been derived from research on the major pathways that also occur in microbial cells.

Catabolism is the process of breakdown of complex molecules, usually with the release of energy. **Anabolism** refers to the synthesis of new or replacement molecules. This is an energy-requiring process. A **metabolic pathway** is a series of reactions in the process of metabolism.

The basic concepts of metabolism do not require an extensive knowledge of chemistry. Many students are unnecessarily deterred from attempting to study the biochemistry of cells as they do not see its relevance to their work as health professionals. However, a knowledge of the processes that occur in all living cells will enable the students to understand the chemistry underlying many of the phenomena which they observe every day. For example:

- how food provides energy for growth and repair;
- how cells reproduce and die;
- how drugs work;
- why some microorganisms are killed or inhibited by antibiotics and others are not;
- how we can control disease;
- how we can identify microorganisms by biochemical tests.

This chapter on metabolism assumes a basic knowledge of atoms and molecules, of ionic and covalent bonds and some carbon chemistry. The metabolic pathways are described using diagrams, words and simple chemical formulae. Students can therefore study the reactions at a level suitable to their chemistry background.

Structure of Biological Molecules

All living matter is made up of a number of complex molecules containing the elements carbon, hydrogen, oxygen, nitrogen, phosphorus and sulphur, with lesser (trace) amounts of other elements. The way in which these elements are arranged determines the structure and unique function of each molecule. The most important element is carbon, a small atom with four electrons in its outer shell, capable of forming four covalent bonds. Compounds containing carbon are called **organic compounds**. When carbon combines with other atoms it forms a molecule with a particular shape (**stereospecificity**). (See Figure 2.1.) It is this configuration of atoms in the molecules of compounds containing carbon that gives rise to the enormous diversity we observe in biological molecules; it is also responsible for the specific shape and function of these molecules.

Another property conferred on biological molecules containing carbon is **stereoisomerism**. Because the carbon atom is linked to four other atoms, it often forms compounds which, although they have the same formula (composition), do not have the same structural configuration; they are mirror images and cannot be superimposed on each other (see Figure 2.2). This is can be likened to a pair of gloves, where the right-hand glove cannot be substituted for the left because it has a different configuration.

FIGURE 2.1
STRUCTURE OF CARBON-CONTAINING COMPOUNDS
A carbon atom with four single bonds has this shape because of the direction of the bonds. The tetrahedral molecule of methane, CH_4, shown here contains carbon bonded to four hydrogen atoms.

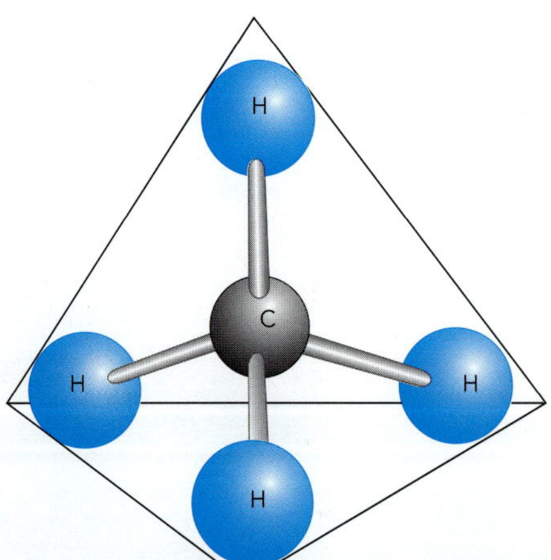

FIGURE 2.2
STEREOISOMERISM
Models of the L- and D- forms of an amino acid are mirror images and cannot be superimposed, just like the right- and left-hand gloves illustrated.

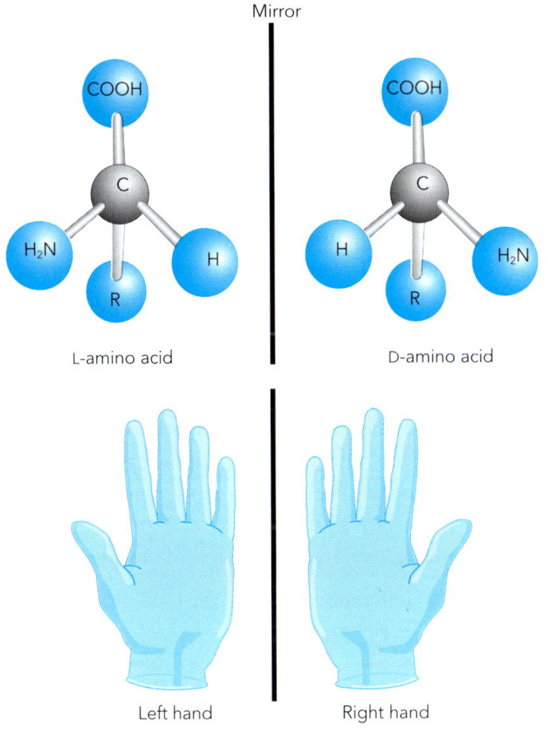

SPECIFICITY

One of the most fascinating things about biological molecules is their *specificity*—that is, the ability of a particular structure in a molecule to recognise and fit together with a complementary structure in another molecule. You may have experienced the frustration of having different pieces of electrical equipment that do not fit together; for example, having the wrong lead for a machine, or a plug and socket that do not 'match'. A similar situation occurs in living cells. Biological molecules contain particular chemical groups in unique structures that confer certain properties on the molecules, and the way in which these molecules interact forms the basis for the regulation of all life processes. If the structures of two molecules are compatible, then those molecules can combine and interact, in the same way that an electric plug will fit into a compatible socket (see Figure 2.3). To take this analogy further, sometimes an 'adaptor' is needed to join two pieces of equipment together. In biochemical terms this adaptor molecule is called a **cofactor** or **coenzyme**.

The specific interaction between two compatible biological molecules determines which reactions can take place. It explains the unique mechanism of many important processes, such as DNA replication, enzyme reactions, antigen-antibody interactions and the specificity of viral attack.

Energy Production in Biological Systems

The basic metabolic process of life is the production of energy for use in other cellular processes. Initially, all energy comes from the sun, the radiant energy being trapped by the chlorophyll in green plants. In a process known as **photosynthesis**, the basic molecules of carbon dioxide (from the air) and water are converted to a simple carbohydrate molecule, glucose (containing six carbon atoms), In the process, oxygen is released. The removal of carbon dioxide from the atmosphere and the release of oxygen enables the survival of oxygen-requiring organisms such as humans, other animals and many microorganisms.

$$\underset{\text{carbon dioxide}}{6\,CO_2} + \underset{\text{water}}{6\,H_2O} + \text{energy (from sun)} \xrightarrow{\text{Photosynthesis}} \underset{\text{glucose}}{C_6H_{12}O_6} + \underset{\text{oxygen}}{6\,O_2}$$

FIGURE 2.3
SPECIFICITY
The need for biological molecules to be the right shape in order to interact with each other is illustrated by these different electrical plugs and sockets.

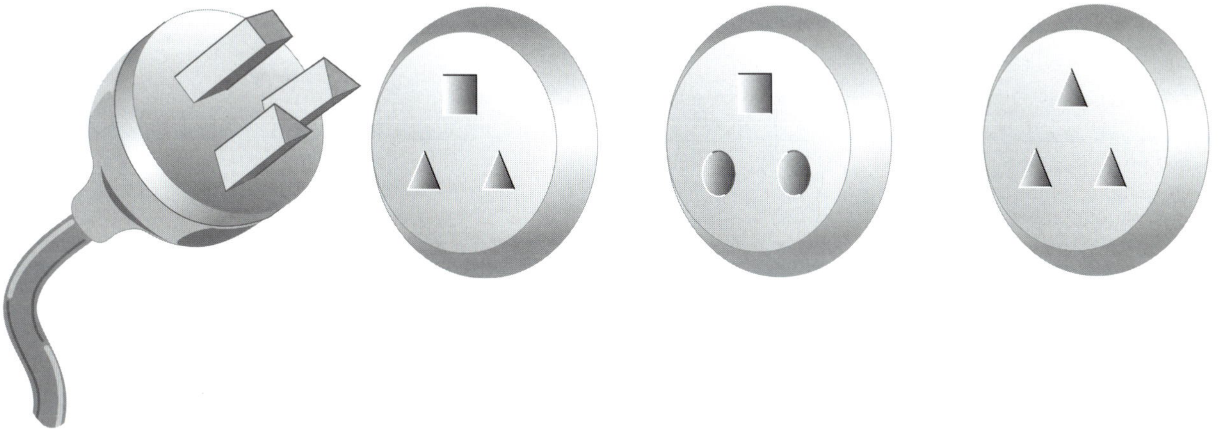

The energy from the sun that is trapped and used to produce glucose is released when a molecule of glucose is broken down during metabolism. This complex process is called **oxidation**, or **respiration**, and consists of a number of interrelated biochemical pathways, including those of **glycolysis, fermentation** and **aerobic respiration.** Reactions that occur in the presence of oxygen are termed **aerobic**; those that occur in the absence of oxygen are **anaerobic.** Many of these reactions require the involvement of various cofactors as well as enzymes, and result in the production of energy which is captured by the synthesis of a small molecule called **adenosine triphosphate (ATP)**. ATP is termed an 'energy-rich storage molecule' because breakdown of ATP releases energy for use in other reactions in the cell.

In animal cells (e.g. muscle cells) under aerobic conditions, glucose is completely broken down in a series of steps to form carbon dioxide and water, with the release of considerable amounts of energy. The overall reaction can be described as follows:

It is obvious that this is the reverse process to photosynthesis.

There are many other reactions that may take place, depending on the needs of the cell and the availability of oxygen. The reactions described in this chapter are mainly those of importance in microbial cells.

The energy released during the breakdown of the glucose molecule in living cells is used to form ATP, adenosine triphosphate. This small, soluble biological energy-storage molecule can move around the cell to provide energy for other reactions the cell may carry out. It consists of a molecule of the purine base, adenine, joined to the pentose sugar, ribose, and then to three phosphate groups. Each of these phosphate groups has a different 'bond energy', that is, the amount of energy required to form or break the bond. The third phosphate bond, the 'triphosphate', is very labile; that is, it is readily broken with the release of a large amount of energy. It also requires a large amount of energy to form it. The triphosphate bond is therefore referred to as a 'high-energy bond'. The base-ribose unit is called a **nucleoside,** and the base-ribose-phosphate is a **nucleotide**. ATP is also one of the building blocks of the nucleic acids, RNA and DNA. (See Figure 2.4.)

$C_6H_{12}0_6 + 6\ 0_2$	Respiration	$6\ C0_2 + 6\ H_20$	+	energy
glucose + oxygen	⟶	carbon dioxide and water	+	energy

FIGURE 2.4
STRUCTURE OF ATP
ATP is composed of the purine base, adenine, the sugar, ribose, and three phosphate groups. The addition of the third phosphate group to ADP requires a large amount of energy which is released when the bond is broken.

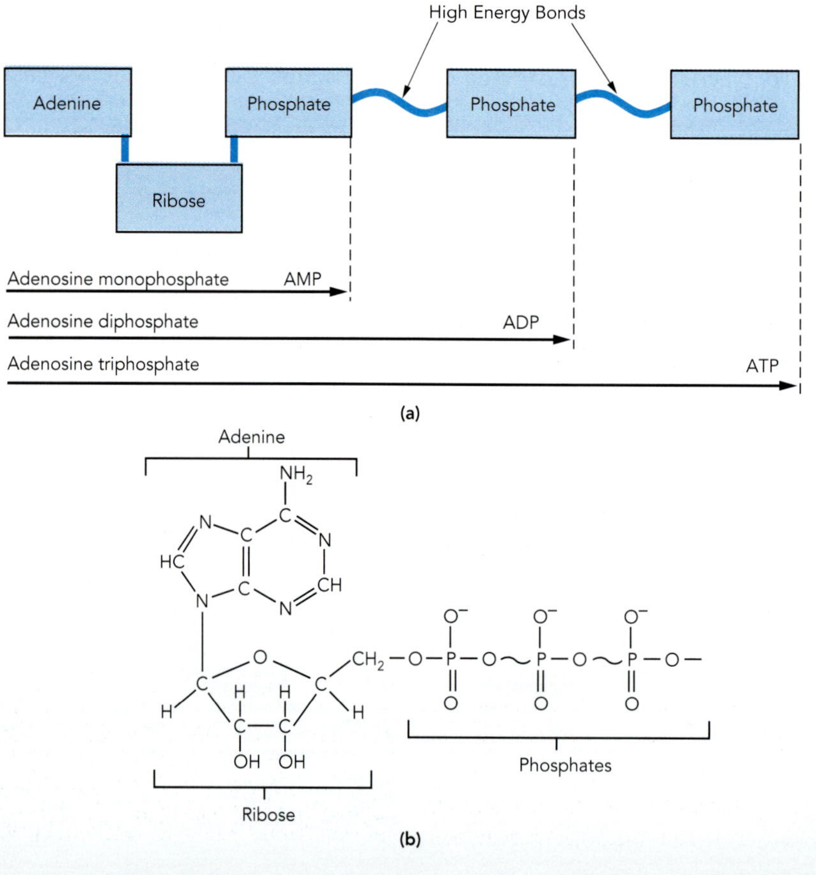

The conversion of ATP to ADP (adenosine diphosphate) releases energy. The phosphate is usually transferred to a recipient molecule which then becomes 'energy-rich' or 'activated'. For example:

glucose + ATP → glucose-6-phosphate + ADP

The 'activated' glucose molecule (glucose-6-phosphate) is now ready to participate in other cellular reactions.

The processes that occur in living cells can be likened to those in a complex piece of machinery. Fuel (in the form of nutrients) is broken down (oxidised, metabolised) to provide energy to carry out the functions of the machine. Manufactured engines, however, waste a lot of energy as heat, whereas living cells are highly efficient and use sophisticated energy-capturing systems such as ATP and other complex molecules.

ENERGY REQUIREMENTS OF MICROBIAL CELLS

Microbial cells require energy to carry out a wide range of activities necessary for their growth and reproduction. Some of these include:

- the synthesis of lipids, carbohydrates and different types of proteins;
- the formation of the various structural components of the cell;
- the repair and maintenance of the cellular environment;
- the accumulation and storage of nutrients and the disposal of waste products;
- the active transport of substances into and out of the cell;
- the movement of flagella and cilia.

Enzymes and Chemical Reactions

A **catalyst** can be defined as a substance that speeds up a chemical reaction by lowering the activation energy required for the reaction to take place. It takes part in the reaction but is itself unchanged.

What is **activation energy**?

The simplest definition is that it is the amount of energy required to make a reaction occur. For example, if two substances such as hydrogen and oxygen are mixed, a reaction will not occur at a measurable rate. However, if some energy is applied (in the form of a spark or heat), the reaction occurs very rapidly. The necessary input of energy is called the activation energy. In industry, the amount of energy in the form of heat that needs to be added is often very great, but the addition of a catalyst (e.g. a metal) will allow the reaction to occur with a much lower energy input. In other words, *the catalyst lowers the activation energy*.

In biological systems the addition of large amounts of heat would destroy the cellular proteins so an alternative way of providing the necessary energy has to be found. **Enzymes** act as biological catalysts by lowering the amount of energy (activation energy) required to get a reaction started. This is why enzymes are sometimes described as 'speeding up a chemical reaction' (see Figure 2.5).

Enzymes enable reactions to occur that might not otherwise happen; they give the reaction a 'push' so that it acquires a momentum of its own. They do this by providing a surface or site on which the reaction can take place, thereby allowing the reactant molecules to be held in close proximity to each other and increasing the efficiency of their interaction. All this is done at a temperature compatible with the normal activities of the cell.

Enzymes are proteins, produced in cells in response to the metabolic requirements of the cell. The genetic information needed for the synthesis of each particular enzyme is coded for in the DNA of the cell, together with information that enables the cell to synthesise all its other protein requirements (see Chapter 4). The name of the enzyme is usually derived from the **substrate** it uses and the type of reaction that occurs. Most enzyme names end in *-ase*. For example, lactic dehydrogenase is an enzyme that removes hydrogen from lactic acid.

STRUCTURE OF ENZYMES

Enzymes are proteins, and are therefore made up of chains of amino acids (see Figure 2.17 p. 36). Each enzyme has its own unique sequence of amino acids and is folded in a certain way to give it a specific shape. Within this shape there is a particular location or area on the molecule called the **active site**. This site is rather like an electrical socket. It allows the attachment of a correspondingly shaped molecule or **substrate**. Once attached, this substrate can be modified or split; that is, it undergoes a metabolic reaction. It is then released and another substrate molecule takes its place and the reaction continues. (See Figure 2.6.)

FIGURE 2.5
ACTIVATION ENERGY
A chemical reaction cannot take place unless a certain amount of activation energy is available to start it. Enzymes lower the amount of activation energy needed to initiate a reaction. They thus make it possible for biologically important reactions to occur at the relatively low temperatures that living organisms can tolerate.

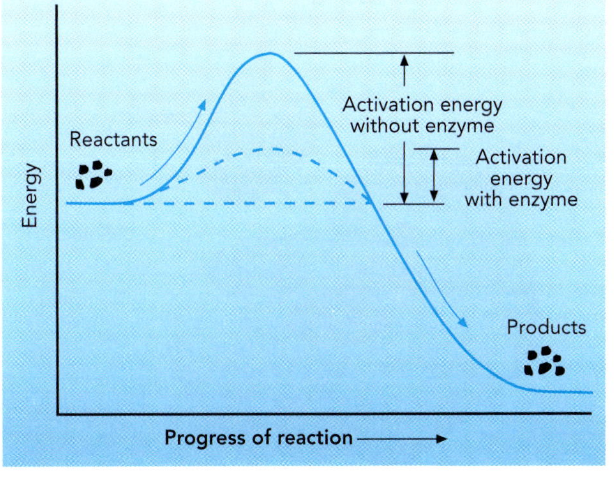

FIGURE 2.6
ENZYME-SUBSTRATE COMPLEX

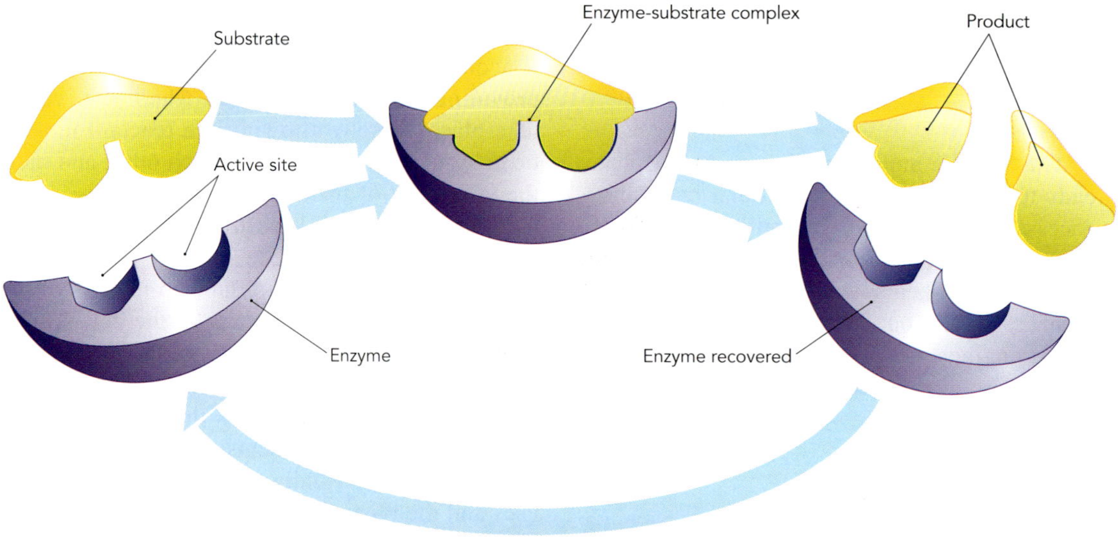

There are hundreds of different enzymes in each cell. Every reaction that occurs in a living cell is controlled by a specific enzyme. Each enzyme has an active site specific for the shape of a particular substrate. Some enzymes contain both a protein and a non-protein component. The non-protein part, called a **cofactor** or **prosthetic group**, is necessary for enzyme activity. If the cofactor is an organic molecule, it is called a **coenzyme.** These coenzymes fit into the active site like an adaptor (see Figure 2.7). Some coenzymes can be synthesised by the cell. Others must be obtained from the food supply and are considered **essential nutrients** or **vitamins**. Some enzymes require the presence of divalent metal ions as co-factors for activity, such as magnesium Mg^{++}, calcium Ca^{++}, manganese Mn^{++} or zinc Zn^{++}.

Bacteria are often able to synthesise all the coenzymes they require, whereas animals need to receive them in their diet (e.g. folic acid). These differences can be exploited when developing drugs to selectively inhibit the infecting bacteria without harming the host (human) cells. This topic is discussed further in Chapter 12.

FIGURE 2.7
COMPONENTS OF AN ENZYME
Many enzymes require both the protein portion of the enzyme as well as a cofactor (non-protein) portion for activity. Cofactors may be metal ions or organic molecules called coenzymes.

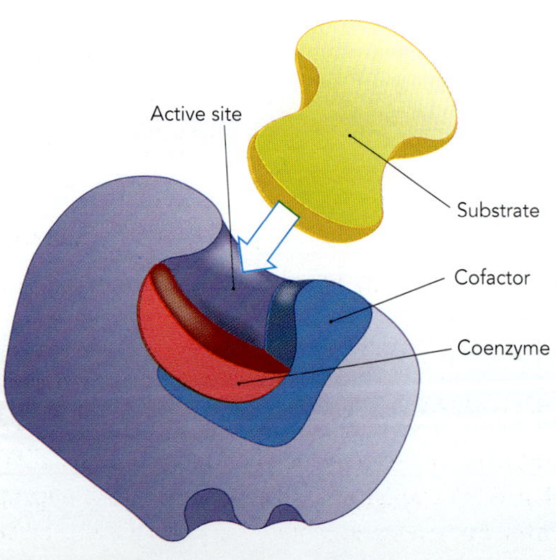

FACTORS INFLUENCING ENZYME ACTIVITY

As mentioned before, enzymes usually react preferentially with a particular substrate. Sometimes, however, they may bind to a closely related compound or **analogue**. When a compound with a structure similar to the substrate binds reversibly or irreversibly to the active site and prevents the real substrate reaching the enzyme, the activity of the enzyme is inhibited, or an inactive product is formed (see Figure 2.8).

Enzymes have been found to act optimally at certain pH values and salt (ionic) concentrations. This is because a change in pH or ionic concentration may alter the charge on the protein molecule and therefore its shape. If the shape of the active site is altered, the substrate may not be able to attach.

It is important to remember all these factors when considering the metabolic reactions described below. Environmental factors can also influence the metabolic reactions that occur in cells. In general, microorganisms have shown themselves to be particularly adaptable to changes in their environment and can utilise a range of nutrients depending on what is available.

Biochemical Pathways of Energy Production

We now consider in more detail the structure of the biological molecules that make up living cells—carbohydrates, lipids and proteins—and briefly describe the metabolic pathways involved in their synthesis and breakdown.

FIGURE 2.8
COMPETITIVE INHIBITION

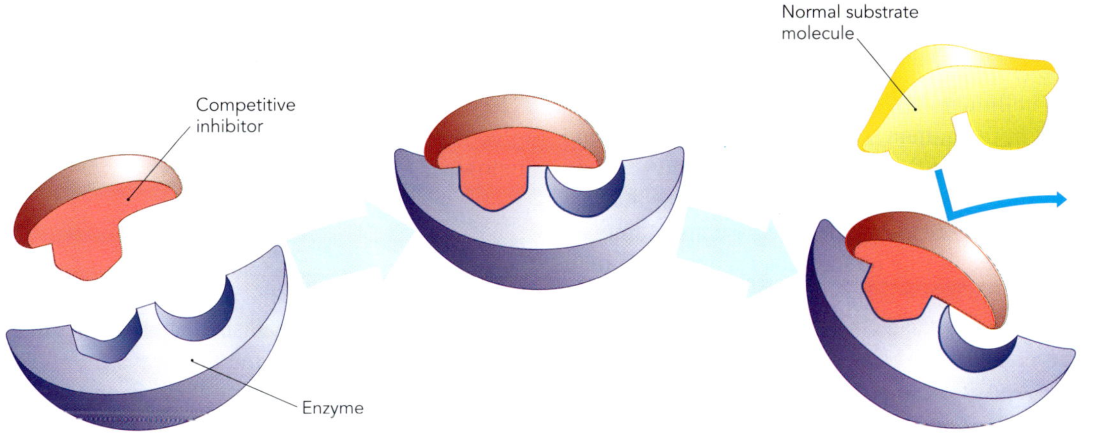

FIGURE 2.9
ISOMERS OF GLUCOSE
Different isomers of the 6-carbon sugar, glucose, may have the hydroxyl group at each carbon number in a different orientation. Fructose has a ketone group at carbon atom 2.

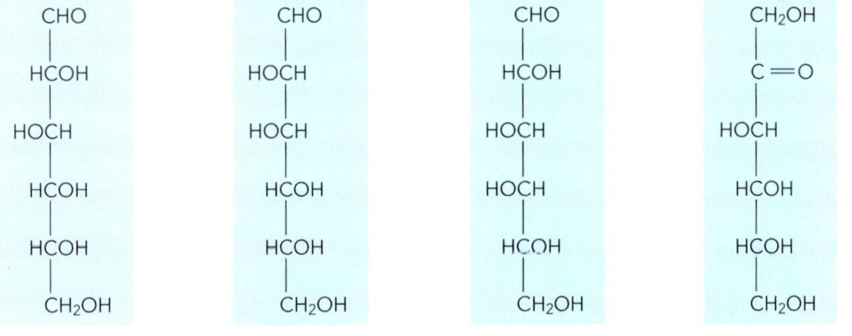

D(+)-Glucose D(+)-Mannose D(+)-Galactose D(–)-Fructose

STRUCTURE OF CARBOHYDRATES

Carbohydrates (sugars) are a group of compounds composed primarily of carbon, hydrogen and oxygen. The most common sugar unit is glucose. Glucose is a **hexose**, a 6-carbon compound containing six hydroxyl (OH) groups. Because of the stereoisomerism of the carbon atom, these hydroxyl groups can be arranged in different ways, giving rise to different **isomers** of glucose. Some of these are illustrated in Figure 2.9. In the cell, the molecule exists in a ring form with a three-dimensional shape (see Figure 2.10).

The most abundant sugars are the 6-carbon sugars described above, but another important group—the **pentoses**—contain five carbon atoms. The most important sugars in this group are **ribose** and **deoxyribose**, which occur in nucleic acids.

Monosaccharides, disaccharides and polysaccharides

Sugars are found in nature as single units (**monosaccharides**), double units (**disaccharides**) or polymers (**polysaccharides**). The monosaccharides include the hexoses and pentoses described above. Disaccharides and polysaccharides are made up of basic hexose units joined together. The way in which they are linked (i.e. the direction of the bond) determines the shape of the molecule. It is referred to as an α- or ß-linkage.

FIGURE 2.10
RING STRUCTURE OF GLUCOSE
Sugars exist in biological molecules in a three-dimensional ring form.

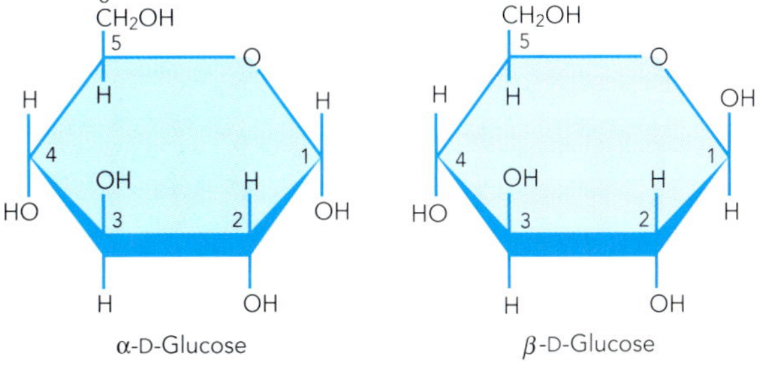

α-D-Glucose β-D-Glucose

BREAKDOWN OF CARBOHYDRATES

The ability of an organism to metabolise different saccharides depends on the presence of the appropriate enzymes. For example, human saliva contains the enzyme, amylase, which can break the α-linkages found between the glucose units in starch (Figure 2.11(b)). However, humans are not able to synthesise the enzyme which breaks the 1-4ß linkage that occurs between the glucose molecules in cellulose (Figure 2.11(c)), and so they are unable to metabolise cellulose. Cellulose therefore acts as fibre or roughage in the human diet and aids in digestion and formation of faeces without providing any energy. Many microorganisms, however, produce an enzyme which can break this bond and release single glucose units. Ruminant animals such as cows rely on the bacteria present in their stomachs to break down cellulose, which is the primary polysaccharide in grass and other fibrous plants. The ability of soil microorganisms to break down cellulose is important for the decomposition of plant organic matter.

Starch, with its branched structure, is mainly a storage carbohydrate. It can be utilised by many organisms, including humans, as a source of energy. Enzymes in the mouth (salivary amylase) and small intestine (pancreatic amylase) break it down to the disaccharide, maltose, for digestion and absorption. Most microorganisms use carbohydrates as their primary source of energy. They are broken down by various reactions to single glucose units, which then enter the pathways described below.

BREAKDOWN OF GLUCOSE

We shall now consider the principle pathways of glucose catabolism in micro-organisms. Sugars other than glucose can also be utilised but the pathways involved will not be described here. The first stage in the breakdown of glucose is called **glycolysis**, or the **Embden-Meyerhof pathway** (see Figure 2.12). It consists of 10 reactions,

FIGURE 2.11
STRUCTURE OF CARBOHYDRATES
(a) Two monosaccharides are joined to form a disaccharide by the removal of water and the formation of glycosidic bond; (b) Polysaccharides such as starch are formed by the linking of many monosaccharides in long chains;
(c) Structure of cellulose, 1-4β linkage gives rise to a straight chain polymer which cannot be broken down by human enzymes.

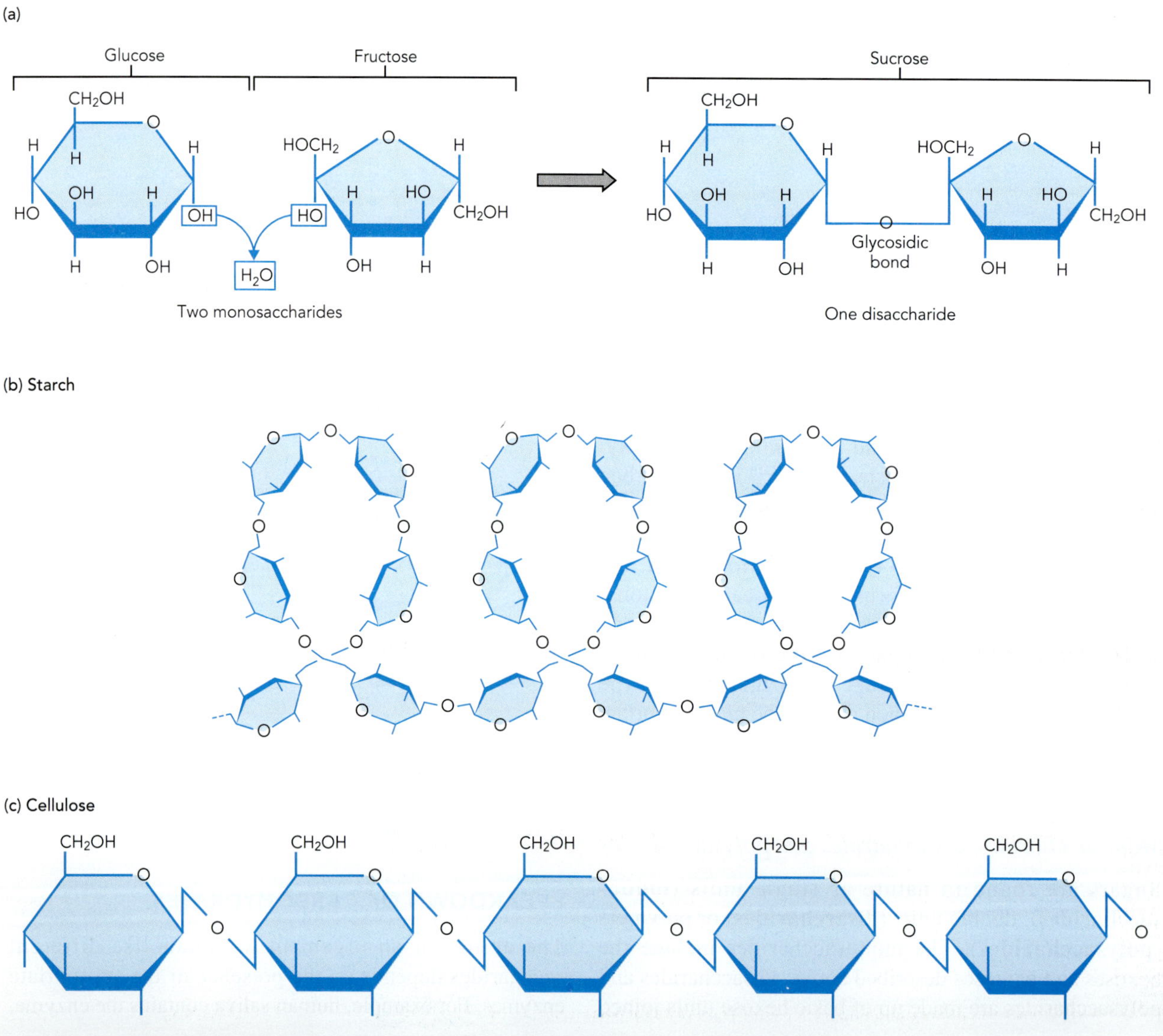

FIGURE 2.12

EMBDEN-MEYERHOF PATHWAY OF GLYCOLYSIS

One molecule of glucose gives rise to two molecules of pyruvic acid with the overall yield of two molecules of ATP.

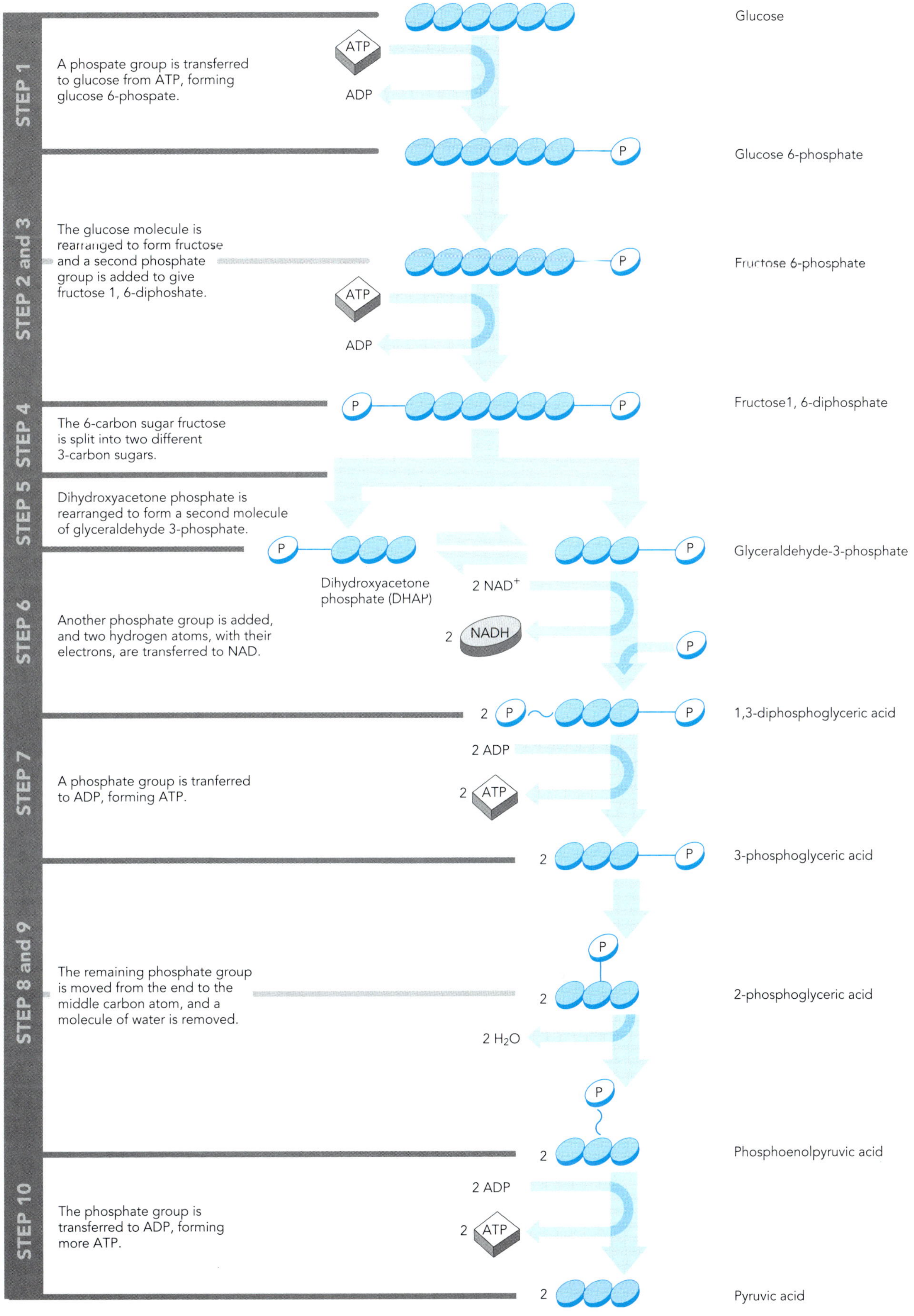

each catalysed by a different enzyme, and is essentially the same in all living cells, plant, animal or microbial. It occurs under aerobic or anaerobic conditions. During this process, each molecule of glucose (C_6) is broken down to form two molecules of **pyruvic acid** (C_3), yielding only a small amount of energy.

Pyruvic acid is an important intermediate, which can be further metabolised, either aerobically or anaerobically. Anaerobic metabolism is also called **fermentation** and results in only a low yield of energy (see below). Under aerobic conditions, **respiration** occurs, in which pyruvic acid is first converted to **acetyl CoA**, which then undergoes a series of reactions known as the **Krebs cycle** or **tricarboxylic acid (TCA) cycle**. This cycle leads to the formation of carbon dioxide and water, and large amounts of energy are released and stored as ATP. Acetyl CoA is a central intermediate which also occurs in the metabolism of lipids and proteins.

A number of other sugars, including fructose, can enter the glycolytic pathway and be converted to pyruvic acid. Under anaerobic conditions, pyruvic acid undergoes fermentation, but when oxygen is present, respiration occurs with the formation of large amounts of energy.

Fermentation of pyruvic acid

Fermentation is the term used to describe catabolic reactions that occur in the absence of oxygen and give rise to a number of useful products. In microorganisms a number of different fermentative pathways may be followed (see Figure 2.13).

No single organism has all the enzymes required for all these pathways. In fact, most organisms use only one pathway. This is a useful property for microbiologists as organisms can often be characterised by the end products they release into the environment from fermentation reactions. Conversely, pure cultures of specific microorganisms can be added to a particular substrate to produce a desired product. Many of the products of microbial fermentation are of great use to humans. For example, yeast (*Saccharomyces*) is added to grape juice to produce alcohol in winemaking; yeast is also added to bread to produce carbon dioxide which causes the bread to rise; lactobacilli are added to various milk products to induce 'souring' during the production of cheese and yoghurt. These processes are described in more detail later in this chapter (see Table 2.1, p. 40). Fermentation processes do not use atmospheric oxygen and do not produce large amounts of energy.

Respiration

Organisms that are capable of respiration oxidise pyruvic acid (three carbon atoms) to **acetyl CoA** (two carbon atoms), which then enters the Krebs or tricarboxylic acid (TCA) cycle (Figure 2.14). The TCA cycle provides a

FIGURE 2.13
MAJOR PATHWAYS OF FERMENTATION
Different microorganisms use characteristic fermentative pathways. The products of fermentation can be used to aid in identification of the microorganism.

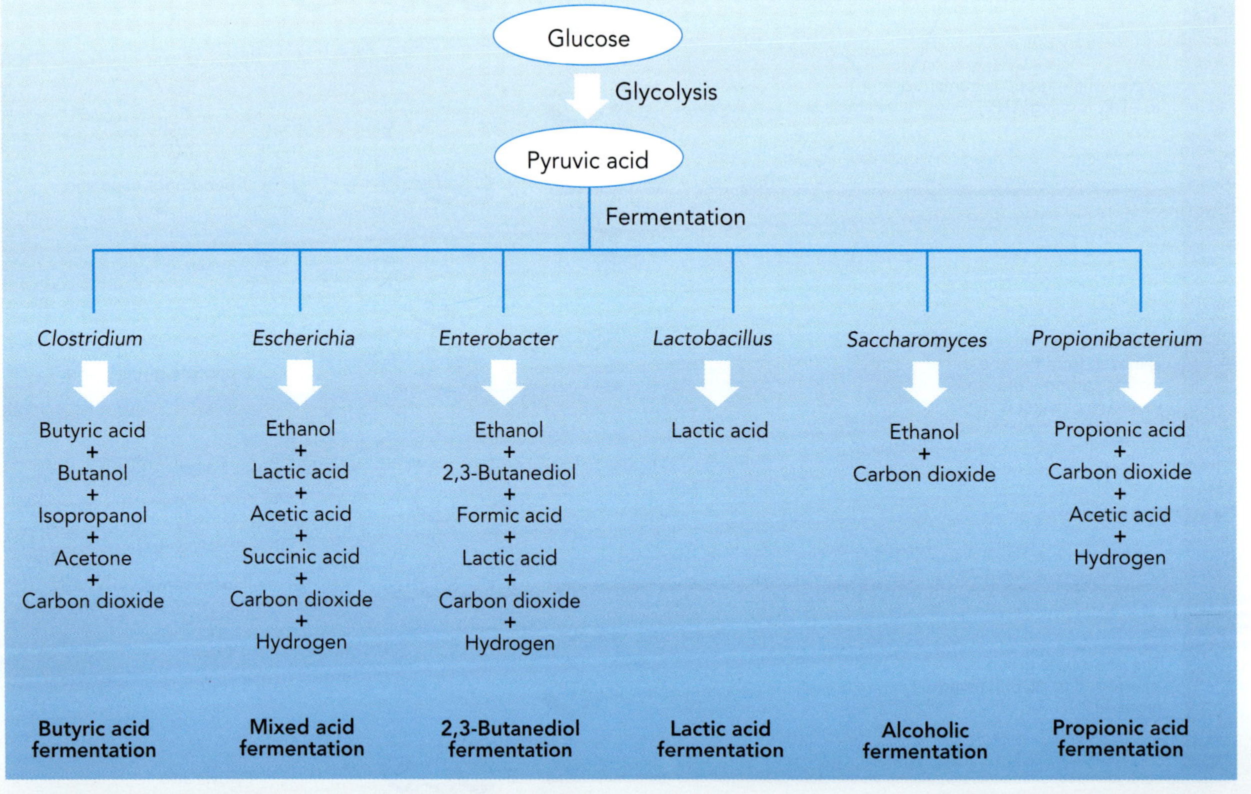

FIGURE 2.14

THE REACTIONS OF THE TCA CYCLE

Pyruvic acid from glycolysis is converted to the 2-carbon intermediate acetyl CoA which enters the cycle. Each turn of the cycle results in the release of two molecules of CO_2. ATP is produced by substrate level phosphorylation and by oxidative phosphorylation via the electron transport chain.

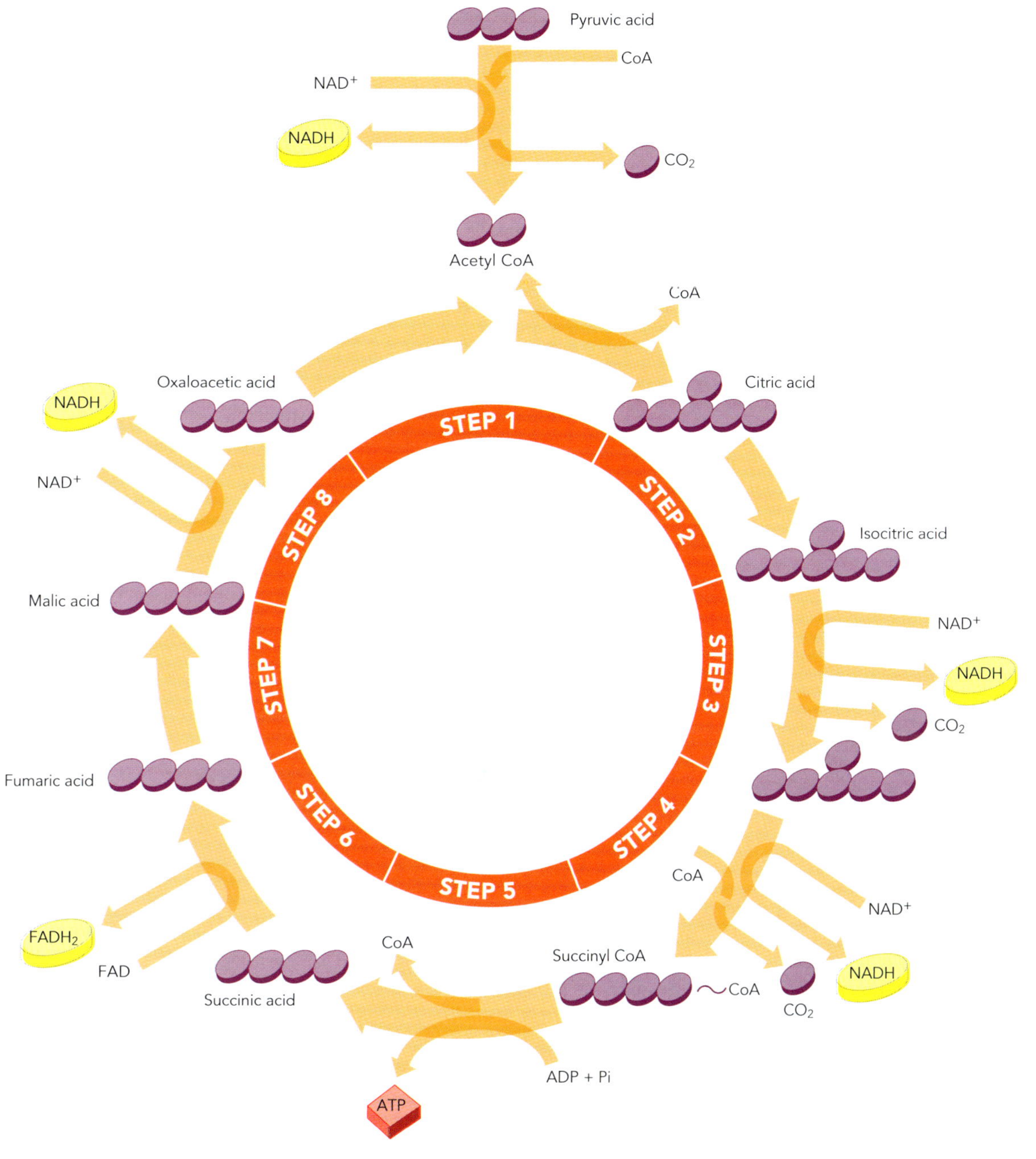

mechanism whereby molecules of acetyl CoA continuously enter the cycle and are broken down to carbon dioxide (CO_2) and water with the release of large amounts of energy in the form of ATP. The intermediate steps require the transfer of hydrogen (H) atoms to the coenzyme nicotinamide dinucleotide (NAD^+) to form NADH. NADH is part of the electron transport chain which is used to convert the energy from these reactions into ATP. This is discussed in detail below. The TCA cycle also provides intermediate compounds which link into pathways involved in the synthesis of lipids, proteins and nucleic acids (see Figure. 2.18).

Summary of glucose oxidation

The overall process of the aerobic oxidation of one molecule of glucose can be written:

$$\begin{array}{ccccccc} C_6H_{12}O_6 & + & 6\,O_2 & \rightarrow & 6\,CO_2 & + & 6\,H_2O \\ \text{glucose} & + & \text{oxygen} & \rightarrow & \text{carbon dioxide} & + & \text{water} \end{array}$$

The energy equation can be written:

$$\begin{array}{ccccc} 38\text{ ADP} & + & 38\text{ Pi} & \rightarrow & 38\text{ ATP} \\ \text{adenosine diphosphate} & + & \text{inorganic phosphate} & \rightarrow & \text{adenosine triphosphate} \end{array}$$

It can be seen that a supply of inorganic phosphate (Pi) is necessary for these reactions to occur. Phosphate, an essential nutrient, is used in fertilisers and is added as a water softener to laundry detergents. The release of this phosphate into our waterways promotes the growth of microorganisms, especially algae and cyanobacteria, which foul the water and produce toxins.

Oxidative phosphorylation and the electron transport chain

The description above is an outline of the major pathways involved in the breakdown of glucose. In the presence of oxygen, pyruvic acid is oxidised via the TCA cycle with the release of large amounts of energy. The cell uses a process called **oxidative phosphorylation** to capture this energy in the storage molecule ATP. The process involves the transfer of electrons from the reduced co-enzyme, NADH, along a series of specialised carrier molecules, to the final electron acceptor, molecular oxygen. This is known as the **electron transport chain**. It is a complex system comprising a series of steps in which each oxidation reaction is linked to a reduction reaction, that is, the energy released from one reaction is immediately used to carry out another reaction and to synthesise ATP.

Anaerobic respiration

Some microorganisms use inorganic substances as the final electron acceptor instead of oxygen. For example, some species of *Pseudomonas* and *Bacillus* can use the nitrate ion (NO_3^-) as the acceptor, forming nitrite (NO_2), nitric oxide (NO) or nitrogen gas. Others use sulphate or carbonate. The amount of ATP formed is not usually as great as that produced when molecular oxygen is the final electron acceptor, but is quite significant.

The metabolic reactions described above are for glucose, which is the primary source of energy in most cells. However, lipids and proteins can also be broken down with the release of energy and the formation of small molecules (building blocks) that can be used in other cellular processes.

STRUCTURE OF LIPIDS

Fats, or triglycerides, are lipids consisting of glycerol and long chain fatty acids. **Glycerol** is a 3-carbon compound containing three hydroxyl (OH) groups. **Fatty acids** are long chains of carbon and hydrogen (usually 16 or 18 carbon atoms in length) with a single carboxyl (COOH) group at one end. Triglycerides consist of a glycerol molecule combined with three long chain fatty acids joined by ester linkages (see Figure 2.15).

Another important group of lipid molecules are the **phospholipids**. These consist of glycerol esterified with two long chain fatty acids. The third position is occupied by a phosphate group which can also be joined to another side chain. Phospholipids are an integral component of all cell membranes (see Chapter 4).

The fatty acids in the phospholipid molecules give a particular structure to the membrane and the polar (hydrophilic) phosphate group allows the molecule to be oriented in such a way as to be able to carry out its unique membrane function.

Catabolism of lipids

Triglycerides are readily broken down by enzymes called **lipases** which split the fatty acids off from the glycerol molecule. The glycerol can be converted to dihydroxyacetone phosphate, an intermediate in glycolysis (see step 5, Figure 2.12). The fatty acids are broken down by ß-oxidation into 2-carbon units of acetyl CoA which enter the TCA cycle. The metabolism of fats therefore yields large amounts of energy.

STRUCTURE OF PROTEINS

Proteins consist of chains of amino acids arranged in a specific sequence. There are 20 different naturally occurring amino acids which serve as the building blocks of proteins. Amino acids are a group of organic molecules which all contain an amino (NH_2) group and a carboxyl (COOH) group attached to various side chain groups (usually designated R). The differences in the side chain groups confer different properties on the amino acids. For

FIGURE 2.15
STRUCTURE OF TRIGLYCERIDES

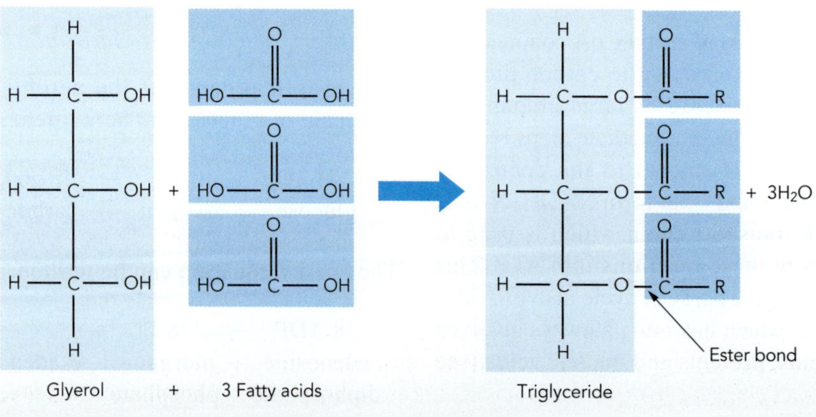

FIGURE 2.16
STRUCTURES OF THE 20 NATURALLY OCCURRING AMINO ACIDS
The nature of the R side chain confers special properties on the amino acid molecule.

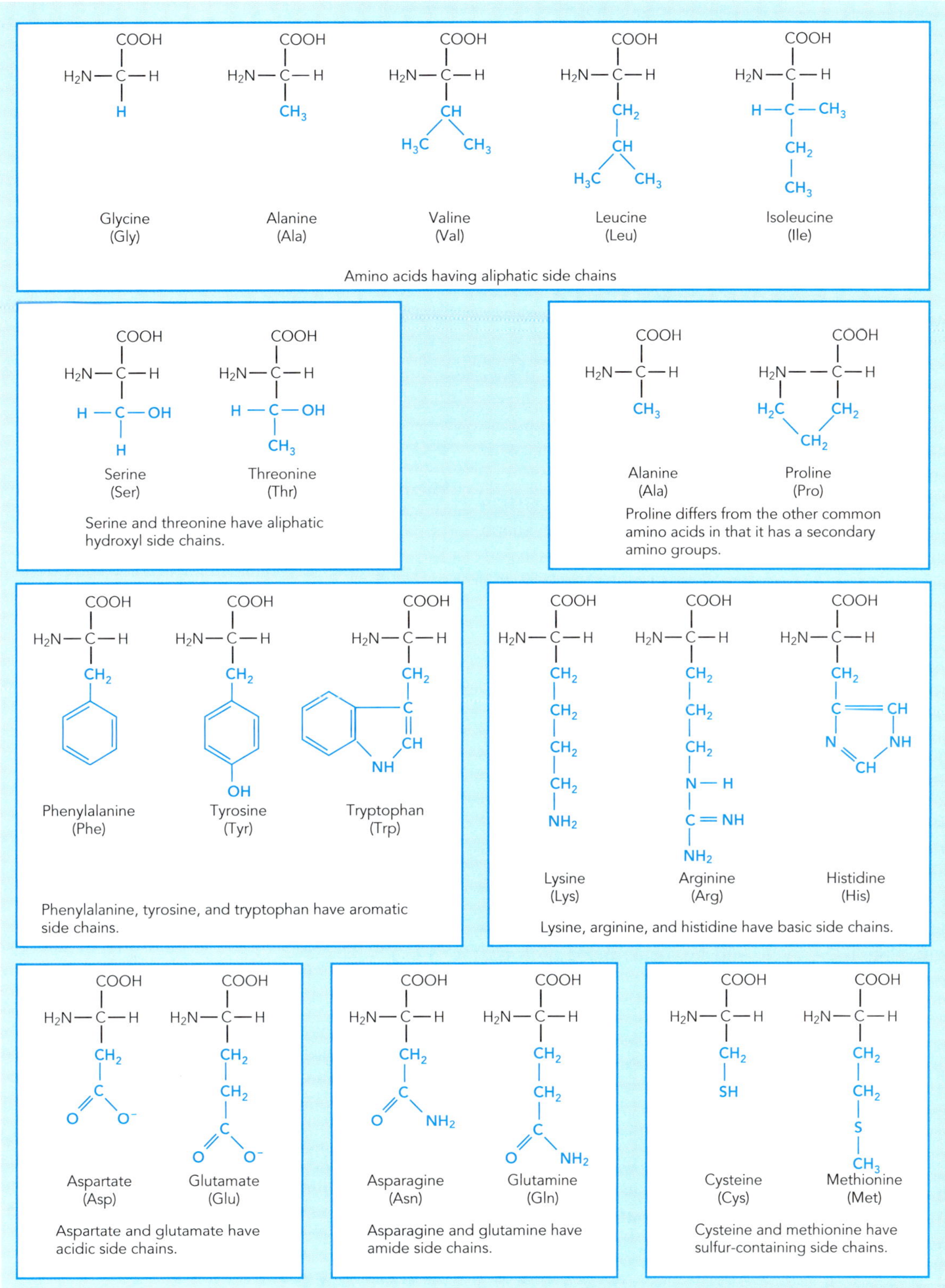

example glutamic acid has a carboxyl group in its side chain, so is quite acidic, lysine has an amino group so is basic; cysteine has a sulphydryl (SH) group, so is capable of forming disulphide bridges (S-S) within the protein molecule. The structures of the 20 naturally occurring amino acids are shown in Figure 2.16.

When two amino acids join together, they do so through the amino and carboxyl groups of adjacent acids, with the removal of one molecule of water, to form a peptide bond (Figure 2.17). Short sequences of amino acids joined together are frequently referred to as **peptides**, longer ones are called **polypeptides**. Proteins are long polypeptide

FIGURE 2.17

SYNTHESIS OF A PEPTIDE BOND

Two amino acids join together to form a dipeptide. Water is eliminated from adjacent molecules to form the peptide bond

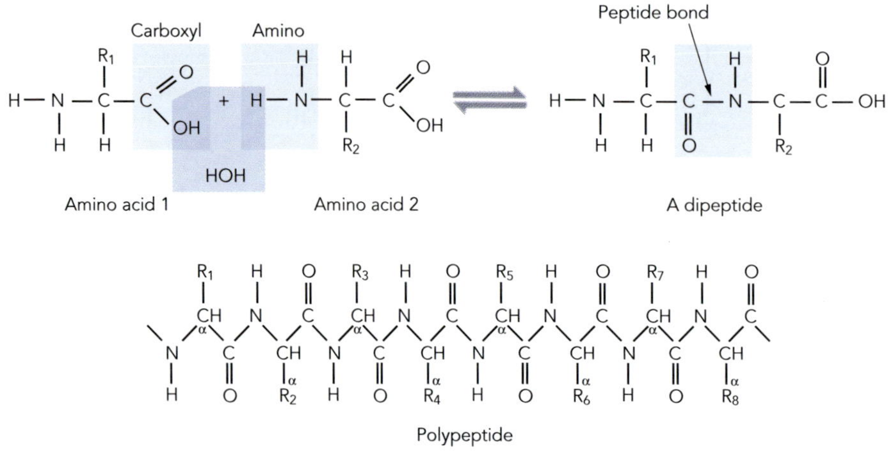

chains, folded and cross-linked to form compounds with a specific molecular structure.

The nature of the side chains of the amino acids affects the overall structure of the protein chains. The size, shape and charge of each amino acid determines the ability of the protein to fold, form hydrogen bonds between the chains and assume a particular conformation and activity. When this conformation is disrupted, the proteins are said to be 'denatured' and their function or enzyme activity may be lost.

Breakdown of proteins

Proteins are broken down in most bacterial cells by proteolytic enzymes (called proteases or peptidases) to form smaller peptide fragments or single amino acids. The amino acids are reused for protein synthesis or are metabolised further. The removal of the amino group by a deamination reaction gives rise to compounds which can enter the TCA cycle and be metabolised with the formation of ATP.

Anabolism—Biosynthesis of Cellular Components

The energy released in the reactions described above is used by the cell in a number of different ways. ATP is needed for the synthesis of the chemical components of the cell: carbohydrates, lipopolysaccharides, RNA and DNA, structural proteins and enzymes, the cell wall, and the phospholipids of the cell membrane. ATP combines with the small building blocks of these complex macromolecules and activates them so that they have sufficient energy to enter their respective biosynthetic pathways. Energy is also needed for the movement of flagella and cilia and for active transport of substances into and out of the cell.

BIOSYNTHESIS OF CARBOHYDRATES

Microorganisms utilise different pathways for the synthesis of carbohydrates depending on the availability of nutrients and the particular needs of the organism.

Autotrophs are organisms which can use carbon dioxide as their primary source of carbon; that is, they can live without access to complex molecules. They are able to use energy from the sun during photosynthesis to synthesise glucose from carbon dioxide with the release of oxygen. These organisms include photosynthetic bacteria (cyanobacteria, green sulphur and purple sulphur bacteria), algae and green plants.

Heterotrophs, which include most bacteria, fungi and protozoa, must be provided with a source of organic carbon in their environment in order to synthesise glucose and larger polysaccharides. The intermediates in the TCA cycle, or other breakdown products from lipid or protein metabolism, can be a suitable source. Depending on the needs of the cell and the availability of energy in the form of ATP, various biosynthetic pathways are utilised which are the reverse of (or parallel to) those described for the breakdown of carbohydrates. However, some microorganisms have strict nutritional requirements that will be described in Chapter 4.

One important complex polysaccharide molecule that is synthesised only by procaryotic cells is **peptidoglycan**, a compound that provides strength and rigidity to bacterial cell walls. Peptidoglycan is a complex molecule containing sugar, lipid and peptide moieties (see Chapter 4).

BIOSYNTHESIS OF LIPIDS

Bacteria are also capable of synthesising lipids, usually by the formation of long chain fatty acids from units of acetyl CoA derived from carbohydrate metabolism. The fatty acids are condensed with a molecule of glycerol to form triglycerides.

FIGURE 2.18
INTERRELATIONSHIP OF METABOLIC PATHWAYS
Bacteria are able to synthesise all their cellular requirements when supplied with a simple carbon source, nitrogen (ammonia) and inorganic salts.

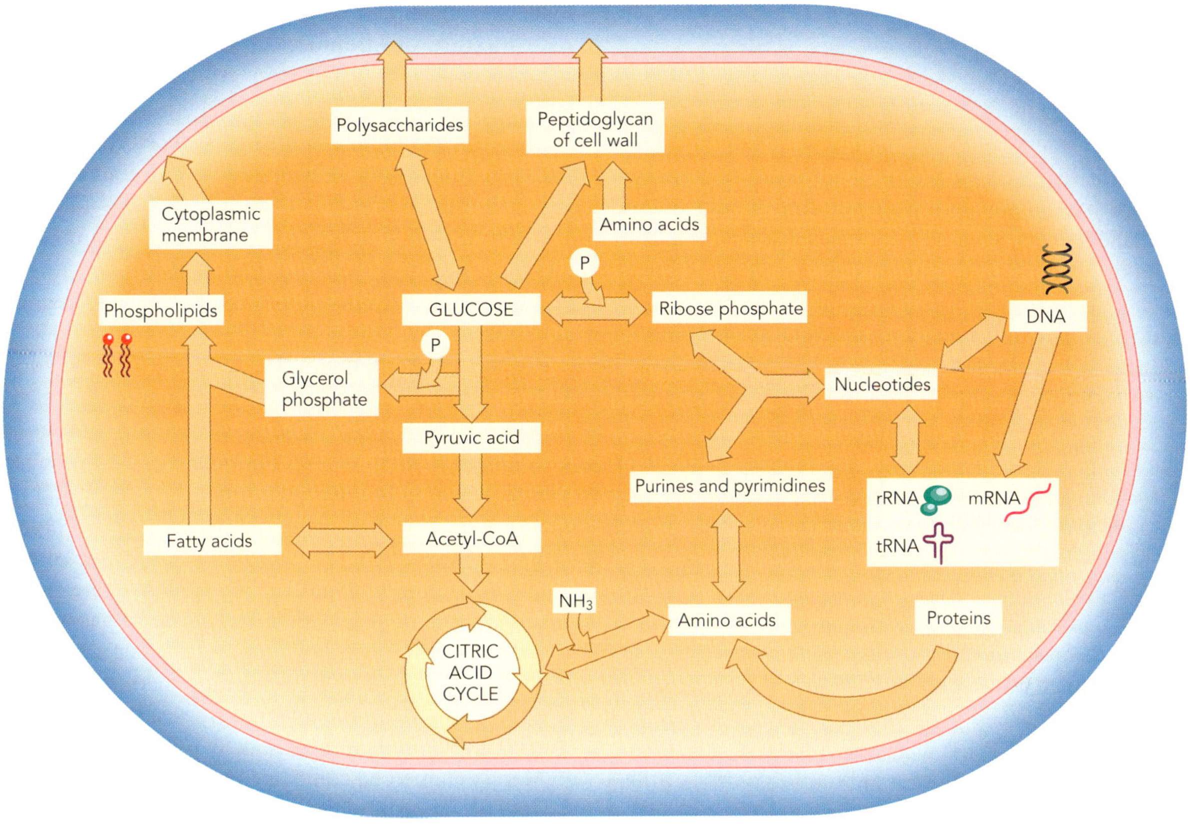

BIOSYNTHESIS OF AMINO ACIDS

Amino acids are required for the synthesis of proteins. Amino acids also serve as precursors for the purine and pyrimidine bases which are the building blocks of the nucleic acids RNA and DNA (see Chapter 4). Amino acids are synthesised in microbial cells by the incorporation of nitrogen as an amino group into various intermediates in the TCA cycle. The nitrogen may be supplied in the form of ammonium salts (NH_4^+) nitrates (NO_3), or be derived from nitrogen in the atmosphere. Some bacteria are capable of using atmospheric nitrogen to form nitrogenous compounds in a process called **nitrogen fixation**.

BIOSYNTHESIS OF PROTEINS

The biosynthesis of proteins is under the direction of the genetic material of the cell, the DNA. It requires the participation of RNA and other nucleotides and will be described in detail in Chapter 4.

Interrelationship of Metabolic Pathways

Microorganisms show great diversity in their nutritional requirements (see Chapter 4). These differences reflect their biosynthetic abilities. For example, some microorganisms can synthesise all their cellular requirements from simple organic or inorganic compounds. Others require more complex molecules such as sugars, amino acids, and vitamins or cofactors. Some mutant strains may have an absolute requirement for a particular compound (e.g. a fatty acid or amino acid). Figure 2.18 illustrates the interrelationship between the pathways which the bacterial cell can utilise to synthesise all its cellular components. It is beyond the scope of this text to examine all these pathways in detail, but it is important to remember that most microorganisms of medical importance are heterotrophic—

FIGURE 2.19
MANNITOL-FERMENTATION TEST
Growth on mannitol salt agar distinguishes different species of staphylococci. *Staphylococcus aureus* ferments mannitol, producing acid which turns the indicator in the medium to yellow. *Staphylococcus epidermidis* does not produce a colour change.

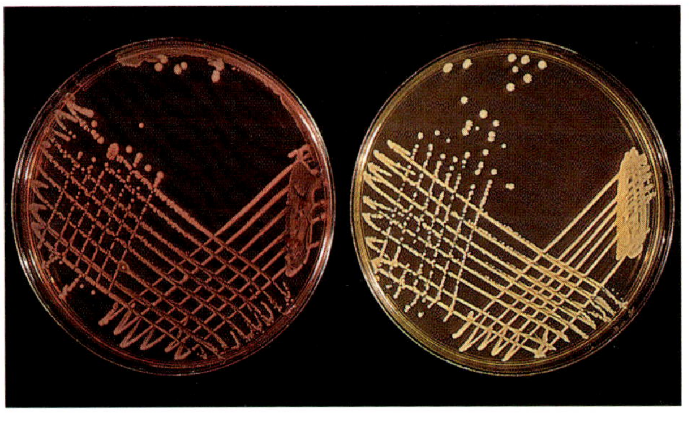

that is, they use complex carbon-containing molecules as their primary nutritional source. This property is useful for the identification and control of potential pathogens.

Practical Applications of Microbial Processes

The metabolic pathways described in this chapter represent only a small fraction of the reactions carried out by living cells. These reactions are controlled by specific enzymes produced by cells according to the information which is contained in their genes. In animal cells, the production of a set of enzymes by a cell is usually fixed, and reflects the function of that cell. If the required enzymes are not produced or are produced in the wrong amount, the workings of the cell are greatly affected. The measurement of the amount of enzyme produced by a cell can be used to diagnose whether a cell is functioning normally. For example, in humans, liver function tests measure the levels of different enzymes that may be altered when the liver is damaged by diseases such as hepatitis or cirrhosis.

In the microbial world, bacteria in particular show a wide diversity in the enzymes they are capable of producing, and this property has been used to advantage by scientists and microbiologists. Many bacteria are able to adapt the metabolic pathways they use to the nutrients available. Mostly, they prefer to use glucose and produce large amounts of ATP, but when provided with alternative carbon sources they are often able to break them down and use them for growth. The metabolic pathways employed are often a reflection of the environment in which the organism is generally found—for example, the sulphur bacteria occur in hot springs and use sulphur compounds as electron acceptors.

The metabolic abilities of specific microorganisms are used by scientists in a number of areas including diagnostic microbiology, industry, in scientific research and in genetic engineering. The ability of microorganisms to break down large biological molecules is of importance in the environment.

DIAGNOSTIC MICROBIOLOGY

The ability (or lack of it) to grow under different environmental conditions is used by microbiologists to differentiate between species of organisms that may appear morphologically identical. This is the principle behind the selective and differential media used in a diagnostic microbiology laboratory. These media are described in more detail in Chapter 4, but a brief introduction is appropriate here to show how an understanding of metabolic pathways helps to identify different pathogens.

A **selective medium** is one to which chemical compounds have been added to prevent the growth of certain microorganisms, but not others. The 'compound' is often something as simple as a high salt concentration. A **differential medium** is one to which some sort of indicator, usually a dye, has been added. This allows the clinical microbiologist to differentiate between various chemical reactions carried out during growth.

Sometimes the medium may be both differential and selective at the same time. For example mannitol salt agar (MS agar) can be used to aid in the identification of a mixture of streptococci and different species of staphylococci. Staphylococci grow readily in the high salt concentration whereas the growth of streptococci is inhibited. *Staphylococcus aureus* produces enzymes which utilise mannitol (a sugar alcohol) and convert it to an acid that turns the pink indicator dye to yellow. *Staphylococcus epidermidis*, which appears similar under the microscope to *Staphylococcus aureus* does not metabolise mannitol, so there is no acid production and no colour change in the medium (see Figure 2.19).

A battery of different tests is used in the microbiology laboratory to help identify a particular microorganism and many of these involve the measurement of an enzyme reaction. In effect, these tests detect the presence or absence of enzymes required for catabolic reactions similar to the ones described above and thus indicate the kind of organism which is present. The change in dye colour measures pH changes occurring as a result of the ability of the organism to ferment different sugars. Production of gases such as carbon dioxide or hydrogen can also be seen by the appearance of bubbles in the culture medium. Hydrogen sulphide production is detected by reacting it with iron (ferric) compounds—as well as by its offensive smell!

Many commercial companies market diagnostic kits for the identification of microorganisms. These kits test for the presence of several different enzymes in a single specimen. Some of these reagents are very sensitive and can give a positive diagnosis when only a small amount of specimen is available. This topic is discussed further in Chapter 15.

INDUSTRIAL APPLICATIONS OF MICROBIAL METABOLISM

In industry, microorganisms are used in three main ways: as live microbial cells, for the preparation of purified enzymes, and as a source of primary or secondary metabolites.

1. Live microbial cells are used in a number of processes. For example, yeasts which are unicellular fungi, are widely used in the food industry. Fermentation of sugar by yeast under anaerobic conditions produces alcohol and carbon dioxide. Some examples follow:
   - Wine is made from fermented grape juice. Wild yeast cells are found on grapes in nature. In practice, the wine they produce is of variable quality, so most winemakers add a pure culture of the yeast, *Saccharomyces ellipsoideus*, and control the fermentation by the amount of oxygen present. An understanding of metabolism can be used to achieve the desired product. When oxygen is low or absent, yeast fermentation produces mainly alcohol. When oxygen is available, carbon dioxide is also formed. When the alcohol concentration reaches 12–14% the yeast cells die. Champagne is made by a

secondary fermentation. Yeast and sugar are added to still wine in a sealed bottle. The carbon dioxide produced cannot escape and remains as bubbles in the champagne.

- Beer is also a product of yeast fermentation. Instead of grapes, grains such as barley are used to make an extract or 'malt'. Hops are added for flavour. Special strains of yeast, *Saccharomyces carlsbergensis* or *Saccharomyces cerevisiae* are used.
- The leavening of bread also relies on the properties of the yeast cell. When added to the dough, yeast produces alcohol and carbon dioxide gas. The carbon dioxide causes the bread to rise. When the bread is baked, the alcohol and carbon dioxide are driven off, leaving the distinctive holes in the bread. Sour dough bread is made by adding cultures of lactic acid bacteria to the dough to produce the distinctive 'sour' taste.

Lactic acid bacteria produce lactic acid from the fermentation of glucose and are responsible for the 'souring' of milk to produce cheese, yoghurt, buttermilk and other products. Various other bacteria and some fungi can be added to produce the intermediate compounds which impart a distinctive appearance and flavour to cheeses (e.g. different strains of the mould *Penicillium* are used for blue cheeses and camembert).

Cultures of the nitrogen fixing bacteria *Rhizobium* are frequently inoculated on to leguminous plant seeds in order to encourage the formation of root nodules where nitrogen fixation can take place.

Mushrooms are cultivated for food.

2. Microorganisms are used as a source of enzymes which are used industrially. Some chemical reactions are difficult to carry out by non-enzymic means. You will recall from earlier in this chapter that enzymes allow chemical reactions to occur more efficiently by lowering the activation energy—often giving a much higher yield of product for a lower cost. Specific enzyme proteins can be extracted from large scale preparations of microorganisms, purified and used in the commercial production of a particular substance. Examples are protein-digesting enzymes (proteases in laundry detergents) and glucose isomerase, which converts glucose to fructose for use in the confectionery industry. Another useful enzyme is penicillin acylase which is used in the manufacture of semi-synthetic penicillins.
3. The products of microbial metabolism are of major importance. They are of two kinds: the **primary metabolites**—that is, those products formed in the major pathways of fermentation; and the **secondary metabolites**, which are usually formed when the cell culture has ceased to grow rapidly and has entered the stationary phase.

Primary metabolites

Many organic chemicals are produced by microorganisms in the metabolic reactions outlined in this chapter. These compounds can often be obtained in sufficient yields to be of use commercially. We shall describe briefly some important metabolites here.

- Citric acid, an intermediate in the TCA cycle, is widely used as a flavouring in foods and beverages.
- Sorbose, produced when the bacterium *Acetobacter* oxidises sorbitol, is used to make ascorbic acid (Vitamin C).
- Acetic acid (vinegar) is a product of the oxidation of alcohol (one of the products of fermentation) by members of the genera *Acetobacter* and *Gluconobacter*. Sometimes the *Acetobacter* are an accidental contaminant of food and cause acid production or 'souring'. Vinegar can be produced commercially from the alcohol present in wine or any other product of alcoholic fermentation. Vinegar is used to preserve (pickle) food as most harmful bacteria cannot tolerate acid conditions.
- Vitamins and growth factors are used as food supplements for humans and in animal feeds. Most vitamins are made commercially by chemical synthesis, but a few are too complex and so are produced by microbial fermentation. These include Vitamin B12 and riboflavin. Amino acids are also produced by microbial means. Although these are relatively simple compounds, chemical synthesis usually results in the formation of a mixture of the D- and L- stereoisomers (see p. 25). Naturally occurring amino acids are only the L- form. Using microorganisms to produce the L-amino acid means that a pure product can be obtained. Some useful amino acids are:
  - glutamic acid, or monosodium glutamate, MSG, used as a flavour enhancer;
  - phenylalanine and aspartic acid, which are components of the sweetener aspartame;
  - lysine, an essential amino acid for humans, is produced as a food supplement.

Some uses for products of microbial fermentation are listed in Table 2.1.

Secondary metabolites

Secondary metabolites are an interesting group of metabolites produced by microorganisms. Each compound is usually produced by relatively few organisms and does not appear to be essential for growth or reproduction. The formation of these metabolites is very dependent on growth conditions. It is possible to select for specific strains of an organism in order to enhance the yield of the desired metabolite. The most important group are the **antibiotics**.

As agents for the treatment of infectious diseases, antibiotics have had an enormous impact on the practice of medicine since the first commercial development of penicillin in the 1940s. Over 5,000 antibiotic substances have been described, but most of them are too toxic for human use. Most commercially useful antibiotics are produced by filamentous fungi and bacteria of the actinomyces group (see Table 2.2).

TABLE 2.1
SOME USEFUL FERMENTATION REACTIONS

PRODUCT	USES	SUBSTRATE	MICROORGANISM
Lactic acid	Cheese, yoghurt Sauerkraut	Milk Cabbage	*Lactobacillus* spp.
Propionic acid and carbon dioxide	Swiss cheese	Milk	*Propionibacterium*
Ethanol	Beer	Malt extract	*Saccharomyces cerevisiae* (yeast)
	Wine	Grape juice	*Saccharomyces* ellipsoideus (yeast)
	Fuel	Agricultural waste	*Saccharomyces* cerevisiae
Acetic acid	Vinegar	Ethanol	*Acetobacter* (bacterium)
Glycerol	Industry/Food Pharmaceutical	Molasses	*Saccharomyces cerevisiae*
Citric acid	Flavouring	Molasses	*Aspergillus* (fungus)
Sorbose	Vitamin C	Sorbitol	*Acetobacter*

TABLE 2.2
COMMERCIAL PRODUCTION OF ANTIBIOTICS

ANTIBIOTIC	MICROORGANISM	TYPE
Penicillin	*Penicillium chrysogenum*	Fungus
Cephalosporin	*Cephalosporium* spp.	Fungus
Bacitracin	*Bacillus subtilis*	Bacterium
Polymixin B	*Bacillus polymyxa*	Bacterium
Cycloheximide	*Streptomyces griseus*	Actinomycete
Streptomycin	*Streptomyces griseus*	Actinomycete
Erythromycin	*Streptomyces erythreus*	Actinomycete
Aminoglycosides	*Streptomyces* spp.	Actinomycete
Tetracycline	*Streptomyces rimosus*	Actinomycete

MICROORGANISMS AS TOOLS IN SCIENTIFIC RESEARCH

The metabolic processes that occur in microorganisms are very similar to those occurring in the cells of higher organisms. In fact, much of the scientific knowledge about cellular metabolism was derived from laboratory research using bacteria. Bacteria are easy to grow in large numbers on a defined medium (that is, controlled nutrients and growth conditions). They provide the research worker with a uniform population of cells, making it easier to interpret results. The simple genetic material (the DNA is all on one circular chromosome) provided the ideal system for early genetic mapping experiments. The techniques and knowledge obtained from this 'simple' system have now been adapted for use in more ambitious projects such as mapping of the DNA of the human genome. A knowledge of the processes of DNA replication in bacteria provided the scientist with a tool for manipulating the genetic information in cells—**genetic engineering**.

GENETIC ENGINEERING

A very important use for microorganisms in recent years has been the production of specific compounds for medical use by the process of genetic engineering. Scientists have developed methods of inserting genetic information into microbial cells in such a way as to direct the microbe to synthesise large amounts of a desired compound. Examples of genetic engineering include production of human insulin, human growth hormone, and some vaccines. Genetic engineering will be described in more detail in Chapter 4.

ENVIRONMENTAL USES FOR MICROORGANISMS

Decomposition

The catabolic reactions carried out by many microorganisms are essential for the decomposition of organic matter such as plant material and sewage. The enzymes produced by the microorganisms break down complex carbohydrates and other biological compounds using the pathways described above, and releasing small organic molecules into the soil. These molecules are a source of nutrients for growing plants.

Hydrocarbon metabolism

Hydrocarbons are organic compounds containing only hydrogen and carbon, and are usually insoluble in water. Some examples are oil and petroleum. Very few microorganisms can utilise hydrocarbons for growth. Exceptions are some strains of *Pseudomonas*, *Nocardia*, *Mycobacterium* and some yeasts and moulds. The chemical breakdown of hydrocarbons requires oxygen and is a fairly slow process. In 1989, microorganisms were used to help disperse the oil spill resulting from the *Exxon Valdez* disaster. Cultures of *Pseudomonas* were dumped on the oil. Usually, the hydrocarbon metabolism would proceed too slowly to be of use, but the addition of other nutritional requirements, nitrogen and phosphate, speeded up the metabolism and growth of the bacteria so that the oil was broken down and dispersed.

Summary

- Metabolism is the overall term used to describe the chemical reactions of breakdown (catabolism), synthesis (anabolism) and repair that occur in living cells.

STRUCTURE OF BIOLOGICAL MOLECULES

- Living matter is made up of complex molecules containing the elements carbon, hydrogen, oxygen, nitrogen, phosphorus, sulphur and other trace elements.
- Organic compounds are compounds containing carbon; they exhibit stereoisomerism by forming four covalent bonds with other atoms.
- The arrangement of atoms within a molecule determines its shape and function.
- The particular structure of biological molecules enables them to combine with complementary molecules. This is termed 'specificity'.

ENERGY PRODUCTION IN BIOLOGICAL SYSTEMS

- Photosynthesis uses energy from the sun to convert carbon dioxide and water to glucose.
- Cells break down glucose and release energy by the processes of glycolysis, fermentation and respiration.
- ATP is a small biological energy-storage molecule.
- Breaking the bond of the terminal phosphate group of ATP releases large amounts of energy, used by the cell for essential processes.

ENZYMES AND CHEMICAL REACTIONS

- Enzymes are proteins which act as biological catalysts to lower the activation energy of a reaction.
- The production of enzymes is under the control of the DNA of the cell.
- Enzymes have a particular shape, containing an active site which is specific for the substrate; some require a cofactor for activity.

BIOCHEMICAL PATHWAYS OF ENERGY PRODUCTION

STRUCTURE OF CARBOHYDRATES

- Carbohydrates (sugars) are organic compounds made up of carbon, hydrogen and oxygen.
- The most common sugars are hexoses and pentoses; they may exist as monosaccharides, disaccharides or polysaccharides.
- Energy is produced from the oxidation of carbohydrates by a process of glycolysis followed by either fermentation or respiration.
- Fermentation occurs anaerobically and results in the formation of a number of useful products, depending on the microorganism.
- Respiration via the Krebs (TCA) cycle occurs in the presence of oxygen with the formation of carbon dioxide, water and large amounts of energy which is stored as ATP.

STRUCTURE OF LIPIDS

- Fats, or triglycerides, are composed of glycerol and long chain fatty acids.

STRUCTURE OF PROTEINS

- There are 20 different naturally occurring amino acids.
- Proteins consist of chains of amino acids joined by peptide bonds in a specific sequence and folded into a particular shape.
- Proteins are broken down by proteolytic enzymes to amino acids which can take part in other reactions or in the synthesis of new proteins.

ANABOLISM—BIOSYNTHESIS OF CELLULAR COMPONENTS

- Autotrophs are organisms that use carbon dioxide to synthesise glucose.
- Heterotrophs require a source of organic carbon to synthesise cellular components.
- Bacteria synthesise lipids from acetyl CoA and glycerol.
- Amino acids are synthesised by incorporation of nitrogen from nitrates or ammonia into the intermediates of the TCA cycle.
- Some bacteria can use atmospheric nitrogen to synthesise nitrates and ammonia.
- Proteins are formed in a complex series of reactions, directed by the nucleic acids, DNA and RNA.

INTERRELATIONSHIP OF METABOLIC PATHWAYS

- Microorganisms can use many different interrelated metabolic pathways to synthesise cellular requirements.

PRACTICAL APPLICATIONS OF MICROBIAL PROCESSES

- Many of the reactions carried out by microorganisms are of benefit to humans.
- Biochemical reactions are used to identify bacteria.
- Microorganisms and their products are used in the food industry.
- Genetic engineering involves the use of microorganisms to produce compounds for human use.
- Microbial metabolism is important for the decomposition of sewage and other organic matter.

Study Questions

1. What is meant by metabolism?
2. What are the major types of elements in biological molecules?
3. What name is given to compounds containing carbon?
4. (a) What name is given to the process of which carbon dioxide from the air is converted to glucose?
   (b) What type of microorganism can carry out this process?
5. How do microbial cells obtain energy for their synthetic reactions?
6. What is meant by a 'biological catalyst'?
7. What is meant by the 'active site' of an enzyme?
8. Give two examples of each of the naturally occurring monosaccharides, disaccharides and polysaccharides.
9. What is the final product in glycolysis?
10. Which compound is the key intermediate that links different metabolic pathways?
11. Give three examples of fermentative processes that are of use to humans.
12. How do microorganisms contribute to the recycling of nutrients to the environment?

Test Your Understanding

1. Give three examples of specificity in biological systems.
2. Explain how the properties of the carbon atom contribute to the shape and function of biological molecules.
3. Explain how the energy released in the oxidation of glucose via the TCA cycle is converted into ATP.
4. How can the biochemical properties of microorganisms be used to aid in their identification?

FURTHER READING

Conn, E.E., P.K.Stumpf, G.Bruenning & R.H. Doi, *Outlines of Biochemistry*, 5th edn, New York: Jon Wiley & Sons Inc., 1987. (An overview of biochemistry with emphasis on structure and metabolism.)

Dawes, I. W. & I.W. Sutherland, *Microbial Physiology*, 2nd edn, Blackwell Scientific Publications, Oxford, England, 1992. (A comprehensive text covering microbial energy production and growth, biosynthesis and metabolic regulation.)

Selinger, B., *Chemistry in the Market Place*, Marrickville: Harcourt Brace Jovanovich, 1988. (A practical text giving the chemical background to the phenomena we observe in everyday life.)

Stryer, L., *Biochemestry*, 4th edn, New York: Freeman, 1995. (A classic biochemistry text dealing with structure—function relationships as well as all metabolic pathways.)

chapter 3

microscopy and staining

Chapter focus

- *What is the value of microscopy in medical microbiology?*
- *What types of microscopes and microscopic techniques are commonly used in medical microbiology?*
- *What techniques are used for the preparation of material for microscopic examination?*
- *What is the value of the Gram stain in microbiology?*

One of the major discoveries that gave birth to the field of microbiology was the development of instruments that could magnify, so that objects too small to be seen with the naked eye could be visualised. Robert Hooke in 1665, using an instrument with two sets of lenses (a crude compound microscope), was the first person to describe cells as life's smallest structural units. In the early 1670s Anton van Leeuwenhoek used a simple magnifying lens to observe microbes he called 'animalcules' in rainwater, and was possibly the first person to observe microorganisms. Since then, lenses and lens systems have been so extensively developed that we now have compound light microscopes (microscopes using visible light and multiple lenses) that can achieve magnifications hundreds of times greater than that of van Leeuwenhoek's. The development of electron microscopes in the 1930s enabled magnifications of a further hundred times greater to be achieved.

Another major advance in microbiology was the development of stains which colour the normally colourless microbial cells, or specific structures in them, and enable them to be seen more readily under a microscope. The major types of microscopes, their use and the common types of staining procedures are described in this chapter.

Microscopes

There are three types of microscopes used for the visualisation and examination of microorganisms. The **compound light microscope** uses visible light to illuminate the specimen. This is the most common type of microscope used in diagnostic microbiology laboratories because it is powerful enough to enable the observation of all types of microbes, except for viruses. For the observation of viruses and small structures of other microbes, much greater magnification is needed, and this can be achieved with a **transmission electron microscope**. A special type of electron microscope, called a **scanning electron microscope**, provides a dramatic three-dimensional image of a specimen, at very high magnifications. Electron microscopes are highly specialised, expensive pieces of equipment, and are therefore found in research institutes and some virus laboratories, but not in routine diagnostic laboratories.

THE COMPOUND LIGHT MICROSCOPE

The light microscope consists of a series of lenses (see Figure 3.1(a)). The condenser lens focuses the rays of light from the lamp onto the specimen. The light passes through the specimen and is directed by the condenser into the objective lens, which is the first of the magnifying lenses. A number of objective lenses are mounted on a revolving nosepiece that allows the desired lens to be

FIGURE 3.1
A COMPARISON OF THE LENS SYSTEMS OF (a) A COMPOUND LIGHT MICROSCOPE AND (b) AN ELECTRON MICROSCOPE

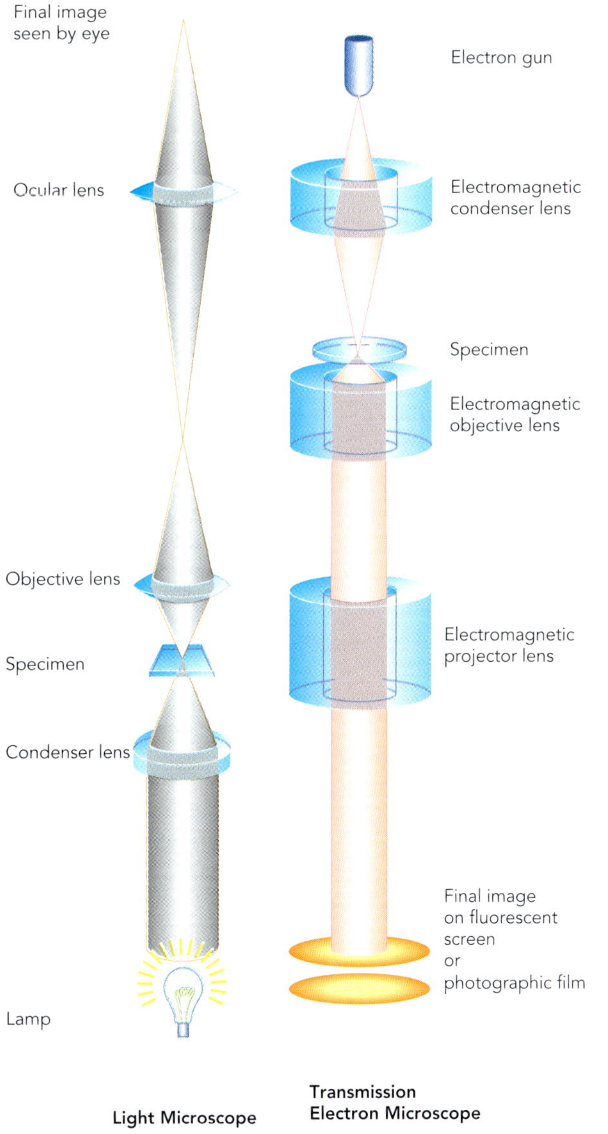

selected and clicked into place. The objectives offer different magnifications—the usual combination is a 10 X (10 times), 40 X (40 times) and 100 X (100 times). They are referred to, respectively, as the low power, high power, and oil immersion objectives. The oil immersion objective is specially designed to be used with oil (actually immersed in a drop of it), to prevent excessive dispersion of the light and maximal collection by the objective lens. From the objective, the light passes through a tube containing a series of prisms to the eyepiece (ocular) lens, which magnifies the image by a further 10 or 20 times. The operator observes the specimen by looking into the eyepiece. The total magnification achievable in a standard compound light microscope is the product of the magnifications of the objective and eyepiece lenses, and is therefore 100 X, 400 X or 1000 X (with a 10 X eyepiece), depending on which objective lens is used.

The specimen for observation is usually mounted on a glass slide which is placed on the stage of the microscope. The use of coarse and fine focusing brings the specimen into focus for the eye. The condenser focusing knob is used to ensure proper focusing of the light onto the specimen. The amount of light (brightness) can be controlled by diaphragms, usually on the condenser lens and lamp.

Apart from magnification, the other main requirement of a high performance microscope is resolution (or resolving power). This is, the ability of the microscope to distinguish, as separate, two objects that are close together—that is, to distinguish fine detail—and provide a sharp, clear image. Resolution is related to the wavelength of light, and the maximum resolution of a microscope using white light is about 0.2 μm. That is, any objects that are closer to each other than 0.2 μm will appear to be joined. The highest useful magnification achievable with a light microscope is limited by this resolution, and is therefore about 2000 times. In contrast, the resolving power of the human eye is about 100 μm.

The use of a direct light source to fully illuminate the specimen is called **bright-field microscopy**. It is also possible to use the compound light microscope in other ways, such as in dark-field microscopy, phase-contrast microscopy and fluorescence microscopy. These techniques allow microorganisms to be observed in different ways, and provide a means of observing the special properties of some organisms.

Dark-field microscopy

Dark-field microscopy involves the use of a special condenser that blocks light from entering the objective lens unless it is reflected off objects in the specimen. In this form of microscopy, objects in the specimen appear bright against a dark background. It is particularly useful for the visualisation of bacteria that are not readily seen or identified by conventional staining and microscopic methods. For example, *Treponema pallidum*, the causative agent of syphilis, can be seen in appropriate specimens as a spiral-shaped organism that moves with a corkscrew-type action (see Figure 3.2). This organism is too thin to be readily seen using standard microscope methods.

FIGURE 3.2
DARK FIELD MICROGRAPH OF *TREPONEMA PALLIDUM*

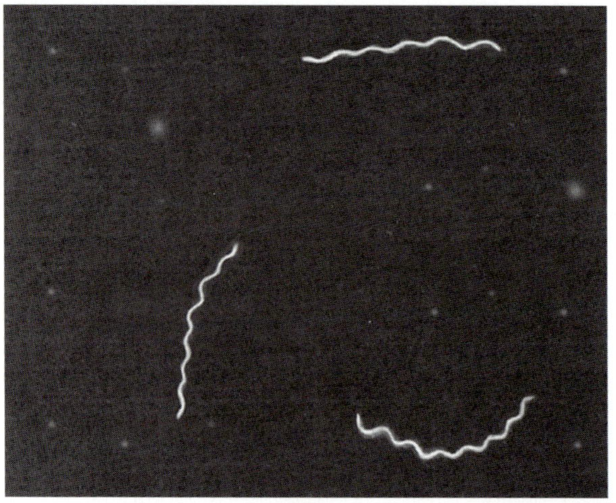

Since staining is not required, living organisms can be observed using this method.

Fluorescence microscopy

Fluorescence microscopy is based on the principle that certain compounds absorb invisible light of short wavelengths and give off visible light of longer wavelengths. Brilliant shades of yellow, orange or green are seen against a dark background. Ultraviolet light has a short wavelength and is used as the light source instead of white light. Some microorganisms naturally fluoresce, but most have to be coated with fluorescent dyes (e.g. fluorescein, rhodamine, acridine) in order to be seen in a fluorescence microscope.

The major application of this method is the fluorescent antibody (or immunofluorescence) technique. **Antibodies** are protein molecules present in serum, produced by the body to defend itself against foreign microorganisms (see Chapter 9). These antibodies react specifically with the microbes against which they are produced. In the fluorescent antibody technique, antibodies to a particular organism are collected and purified, and then a fluorescent dye is attached to them. If a patient is suspected of suffering from disease caused by that particular organism, the diagnosis can be confirmed by collecting an appropriate specimen, treating it with fluorescent antibodies, and examining it microscopically. If the suspected organism is present, it will readily be seen as a brightly fluorescing object when observed microscopically (see Figure 3.3). This technique is particularly useful for the visualisation and rapid identification of organisms that are otherwise difficult to detect in clinical specimens, such as *Legionella pneumophila* (Legionnaires' disease), *Mycobacterium tuberculosis* (tuberculosis) and *Treponema pallidum* (syphilis), as well as viruses, which can only be grown in cell culture.

THE TRANSMISSION ELECTRON MICROSCOPE

The electron microscope is able to achieve much greater resolution (and magnification) than light microscopes because it uses rays of electrons to visualise the specimen.

FIGURE 3.3
FLUORESCENT ANTIBODY STAIN
Showing different morphologies of *Giardia* (larger) and *Cryptosporidium.*

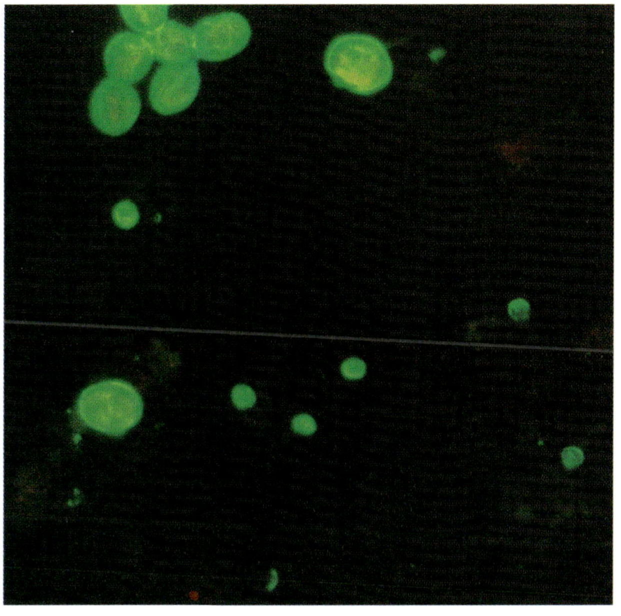

These have a much shorter wavelength than white light (about 100 000 times shorter). Because the wavelength is so short, magnifications of more than 100 000 times can be achieved that will resolve minute structures as small as 0.001 μm (1 nm), the size of some viral structures.

Instead of a light source, the electron microscope has an electron gun which emits a finely focused beam of electrons. The electrons are directed at the specimen, which is an ultra-thin section of the material fixed to a grid. The specimen has to be thin enough (20–100 nm) to allow the electrons to pass through it, and it must be specially treated with stains, usually salts of heavy metals such as lead, osmium, tungsten or uranium. These stains scatter electrons well and increase the contrast between structures. The electrons pass through the specimen and then through electromagnetic lenses (see Figure 3.1(b)) which magnify the degree of scatter of the electrons. Finally, the electrons are focused by another electromagnetic lens onto a fluorescent screen. An image of the specimen is then visible on this screen. For a permanent record of the observation, or for prolonged examination, the electrons can be directed onto a photographic plate to produce a photograph called an **electron micrograph** (see Figure 3.4). Note that there is no natural colour in a specimen examined by an electron microscope, but sometimes micrographs are artificially coloured. The colour in an electron micrograph does not necessarily bear any relationship to the real colour of the object in the specimen.

The components of the electron microscope are contained within a sealed vacuum chamber, to prevent scattering of electrons by dust and other particles in air, which can cause distortion of the image (see Figure 3.5). The basic principles of electron microscopy are similar to those of light microscopy, except that the former utilises

FIGURE 3.4
ELECTRON MICROGRAPH
A photograph taken from an image produced in an electron microscope. This micrograph shows *Helicobacter* (spiral-shaped organism) in a gastric crypt.

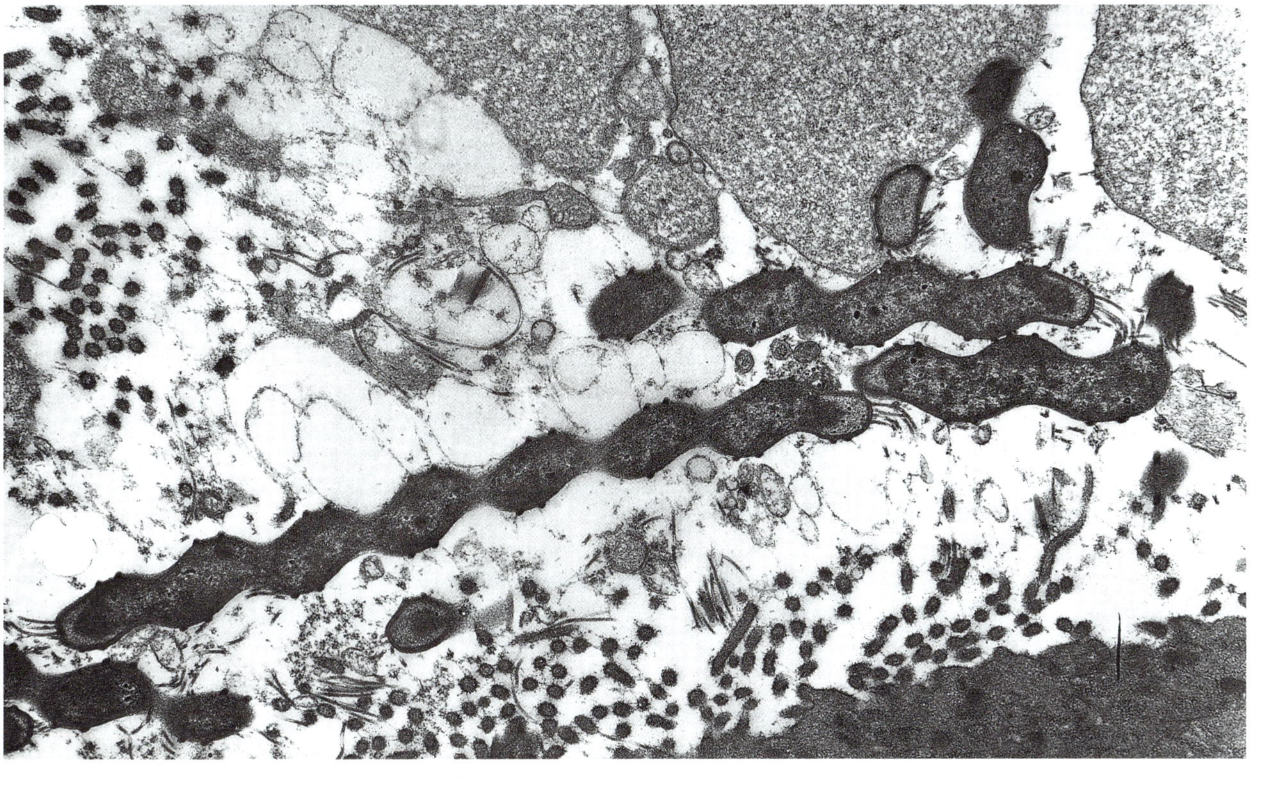

FIGURE 3.5
AN ELECTRON MICROSCOPE

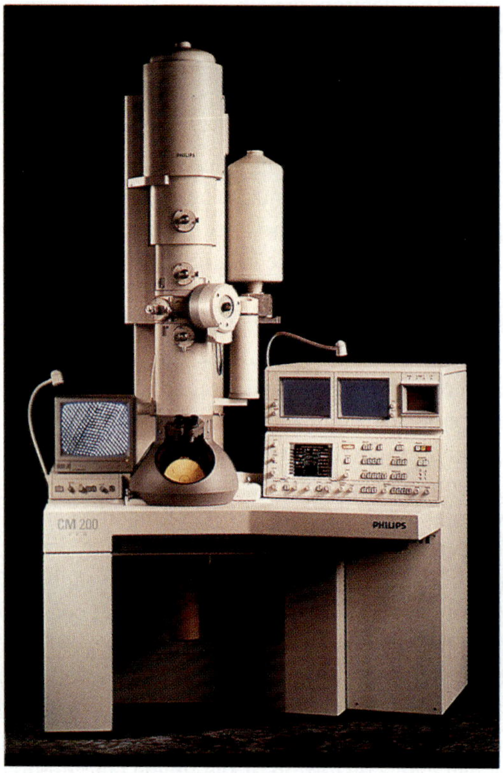

electrons and electromagnets to focus them, where the latter uses white light and glass lenses.

The main advantage of transmission electron microscopy is the high resolution and magnification that can be achieved. However, it also has distinct disadvantages resulting from the severe treatments (fixing, dehydrating and staining) that the specimen must be subjected to when it is being prepared for electron microscopy. These treatments mean that living cells cannot be examined, and that alteration or distortion of cell structures may occur. Sometimes, new structures may even be created, and these artefacts (not real cell structures) are an ever-present concern in the interpretation of electron micrographs.

THE SCANNING ELECTRON MICROSCOPE

The scanning electron microscope is a development of the electron microscope that produces three-dimensional images of objects with high resolution and magnification. In the scanning electron microscope the beam of electrons is directed at the specimen which has first been coated with a thin film of a heavy metal, such as platinum. The whole specimen is showered with electrons, which are deflected from the specimen at different angles and collected by a sophisticated detector that scans back and forth. As for the transmission microscope, the image is produced on a viewing screen or photographic plate.

The scanning electron microscope enables the three-dimensional structure of objects to be visualised and examined, as shown in Figure 3.6. Magnifications of up to 10 000 X can be achieved with this microscope.

Preparation of Specimens for Light Microscopy

Two methods are generally used for the observation of microorganisms with the light microscope: wet preparations and fixed, stained preparations. Living bacteria, yeasts and protozoa can be observed directly in a light microscope by suspending the organisms in a drop of fluid. This is called a **wet preparation**. However, most microorganisms are colourless, so they are usually stained (coloured) prior to microscopic examination. **Staining** provides a greater contrast between the microorganisms and the background.

WET PREPARATIONS

Microorganisms can be observed in the living state when suspended in fluid, placed on a microscope slide, and observed with the light microscope. Using a wet preparation, characteristics of microorganisms, such as their ability to move or their cellular arrangements (e.g. clusters or chains of bacteria) can be observed. Better contrast can be obtained in some situations with the use of weak stains, such as dilute methylene blue. Wet preparations are generally used for the examination of fungi and protozoa, which are large enough to be readily seen using this method. The India ink stain, a black suspension of carbon particles, is used specifically to examine and identify cells of the pathogenic yeast *Cryptococcus neoformans*. These cells have a thick capsule which excludes the stain and shows up in this procedure as a clear structure around the cell against a black background. Wet preparations are also useful for the direct observation of urine and cerebrospinal fluid specimens, in which the presence of host cells, especially red and white cells, can be readily determined. Wet preparations are also used when dark-field or phase-contrast microscopy techniques are being used.

FIXED, STAINED PREPARATIONS

Bacteria can be seen more readily in a light microscope when they are stained. Staining can also help to visualise some internal structures (e.g. spores), and to identify and separate different bacteria. Before staining, the bacteria must be fixed (or attached) to a microscope slide to prevent them being washed away by the liquid stains. A fixed and stained preparation can be kept for future reference or long-term study.

To fix a specimen to a glass slide, a thin film of the material is spread over a portion of a glass slide. The film can be made in a number of ways; for example, by suspending a colony of bacterial growth from a culture plate in a small drop of tap water; or by wiping a swab, taken from a patient, over the surface of a slide. This smear of material is allowed to air dry completely. It is then fixed to the slide by gently heating the underside of the slide by passing it several times through the flame of a Bunsen burner. The stain(s) are then applied and after an appropriate time washed off with water.

FIGURE 3.6

SCANNING ELECTRON MICROGRAPH

A scanning electron micrograph of marine bacteria with a polysaccharide secretion. This micrograph was originally stored on computer, and is therefore, a computer image of the original micrograph.

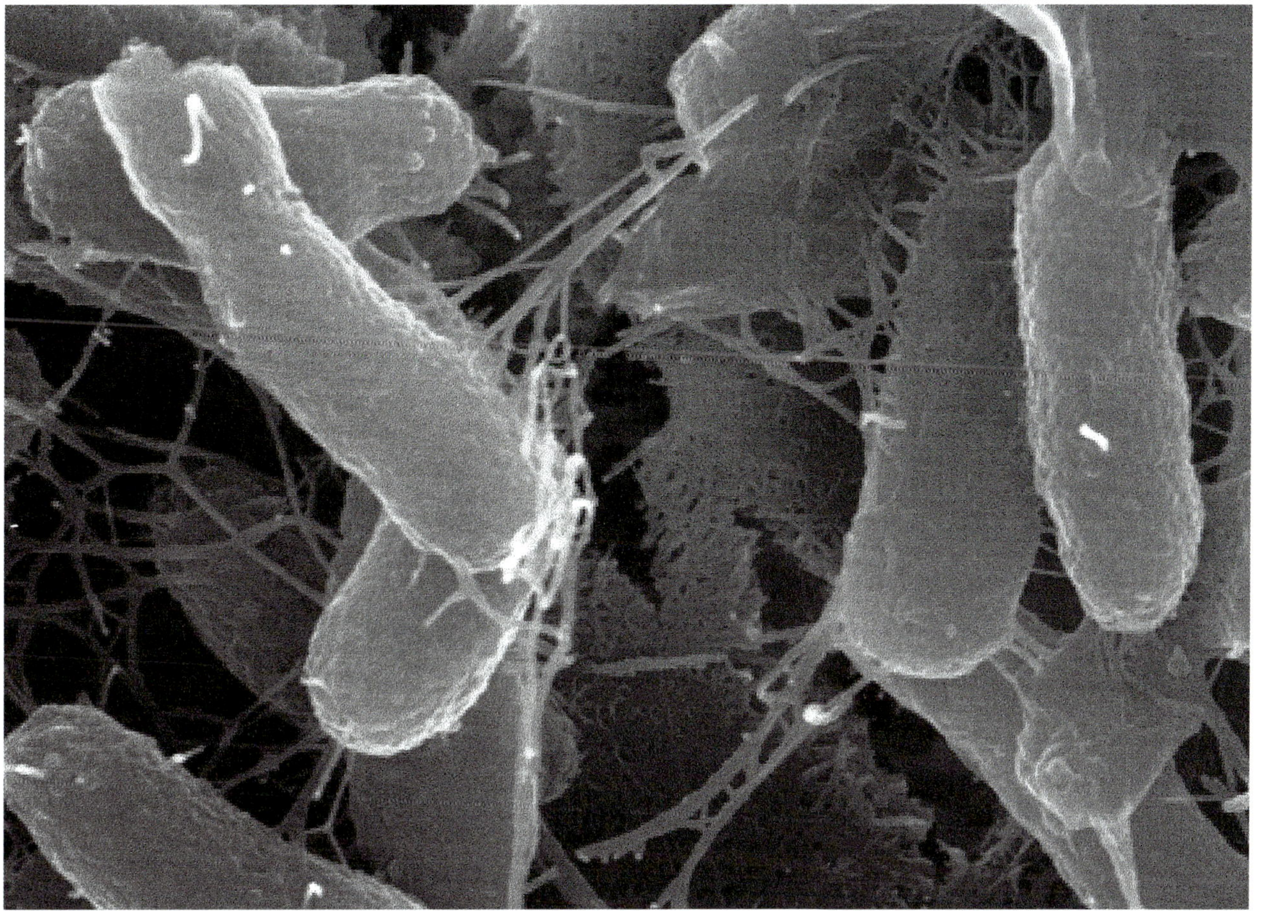

FIGURE 3.7

THE GRAM STAIN PROCEDURE

(1) A heat fixed smear of bacteria on a glass microscope slide is treated with crystal violet, then rinsed in water. (2) The smear is treated with iodine and then rinsed with water. (3) The smear is then briefly treated with ethanol or acetone and rinsed with water. (4) The smear is finally treated with safranin, rinsed with water and dried. Gram-positive bacteria are purple coloured. Gram-negative bacteria have a pink/red or orange colour.

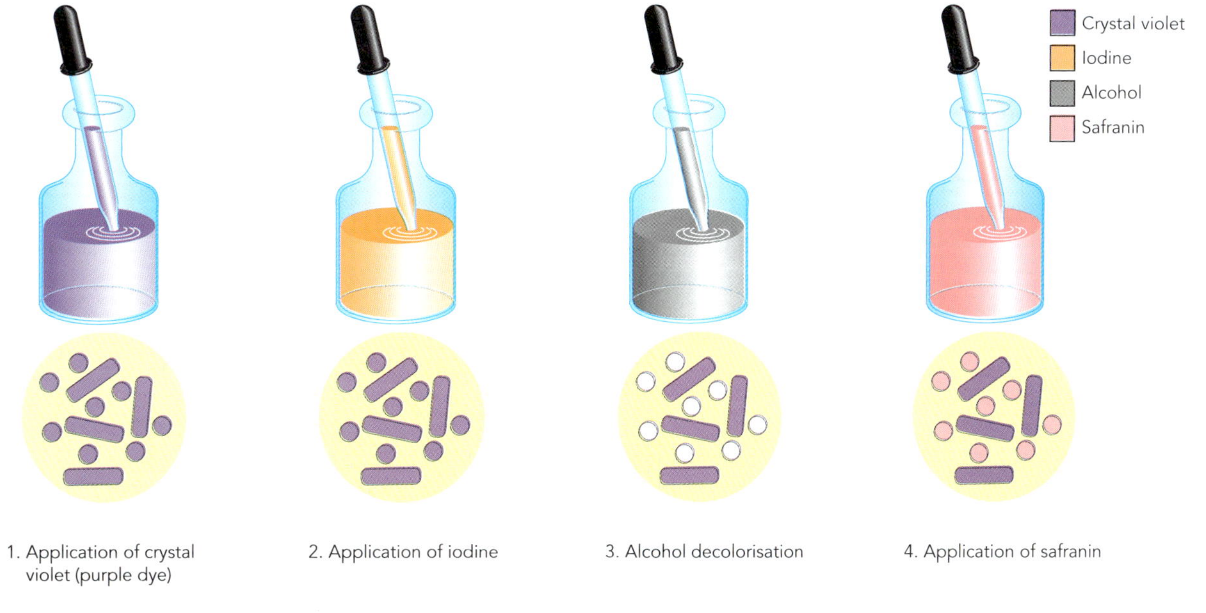

Various stains are used in the microbiology laboratory to examine bacteria, or certain structures within them, but the **Gram stain** is undoubtedly the most useful and important staining procedure used. Developed in 1884 by the Danish bacteriologist Hans Christian Gram, it has become the standard procedure for staining bacteria because it divides almost all bacteria into two groups, and serves as the first step in classifying and identifying bacteria. Bacteria stain as Gram-positive or Gram-negative, depending on the composition of their cell wall (see Chapter 4). The Gram staining reaction is characteristic for each species.

The Gram staining procedure involves the application of several solutions to a fixed smear of bacteria (see Figure 3.7).

1. The slide is first covered with a solution of a purple due, usually crystal violet. After a short time (approximately 30 seconds) the dye is washed off with water, leaving the bacterial cells purple-coloured.
2. The smear is next treated with an iodine solution, which acts as a mordant; that is, it fixes the purple due firmly in the cells. After the iodine is washed off all cells are still coloured a dark purple.
3. The smear is then treated briefly (a few seconds) with an alcohol or alcohol-acetone solution, followed quickly by a water rinse. This decolourises some cells by removing the purple dye from them. In this critical stage, Gram-positive bacteria retain the purple dye, but Gram-negative bacteria lose it, becoming colourless.
4. The final treatment (or counterstain) is with a red/pink dye, usually safranin or methyl red. This is necessary because the Gram-negative bacteria, which have lost their colour (stain), would not be visible under the microscope. The cells that retained the purple dye in step 3 remain purple. The safranin is washed off after a short time (approximately 30 seconds) and the slide is then gently blotted dry and is ready for microscopic examination.

As shown in Figure 3.7, after Gram staining bacterial cells are either a dark violet or purple colour (Gram-positive) or a pink/red or orange colour (Gram-negative), and can be readily seen in the light microscope. The Gram stain is thus termed a differential stain. In Gram-stained smears of clinical specimens (e.g. swabs, cerebrospinal fluid), bacteria as well as host cells, especially polymorphonuclear leucocytes (white cells or pus cells) can be observed, if present. A direct Gram stain of a clinical specimen can be performed within minutes of receiving the specimen in the laboratory. After microscopic examination of the stained smear, a presumptive diagnosis can be made in some circumstances. For example, in bacterial meningitis, the observation of bacterial cells and pus cells in a Gram stain of cerebrospinal fluid can sometimes give a good indication of the possible causative agent.

Several other stains are used by microbiologists for specific purposes. The **Ziehl-Neelsen** or **acid-fast stain** is an important one because it is used to identify bacteria belonging to the genus *Mycobacterium*, such as *M. tuberculosis* and *M. leprae*, the causative agents of tuberculosis and leprosy, respectively.

Mycobacteria have a waxy substance in their cell wall which prevents them from being stained using Gram's method. The acid-fast stain is a multi-step procedure which stains the mycobacteria a red colour, and all other bacteria and material another colour, usually blue (see Figure 3.8). It is useful for the detection of mycobacteria in sputum specimens from patients with pulmonary tuberculosis.

Other bacterial stains include the spore stain and flagella stain, used to highlight spores and flagella for easier recognition.

Stains are one of the more important techniques used by microbiologists to aid in the visualisation, classification and identification of bacteria. The Gram stain is particularly important because it is usually the first step in the identification of bacteria. Preliminary microbiology laboratory report forms often provide results of Gram stains performed directly on clinical specimens. Although other more intricate and sensitive techniques are being developed for the detection of microorganisms in clinical specimens (e.g. the polymerase chain reaction and DNA probes—see Chapter 15), the ability to visualise the Gram reaction, shape and arrangement of bacterial cells is still very important in diagnostic medical microbiology.

FIGURE 3.8
A ZIEHL-NEELSEN STAIN
The mycobacteria are stained a red colour against a blue background.

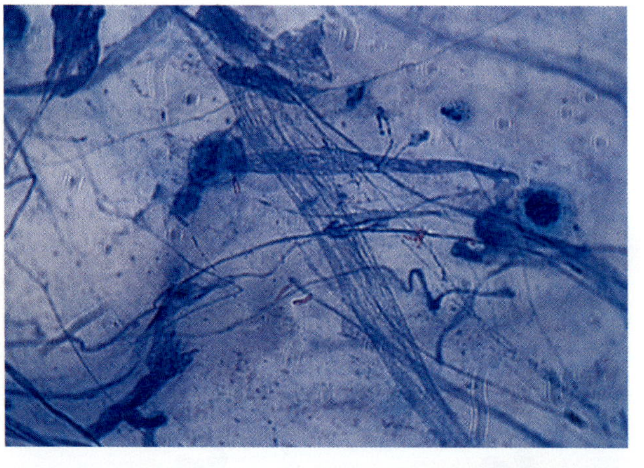

Summary

- One of the main discoveries that gave birth to the field of microbiology was the development of magnifying instruments.
- Another major advance in microbiology was the development of stains to colour the normally colourless microbial cells.

MICROSCOPES

THE COMPOUND LIGHT MICROSCOPE

- The light microscope consists of a series of lenses.
- The condenser lens focuses the rays of light from the lamp onto the specimen.
- The light passes through the specimen and is directed by the condenser into the objective lens, the first of the magnifying lenses.
- A number of objective lenses mounted on a revolving nosepiece provide different magnifications.
- From the objective lens, the light passes through a series of prisms to the eyepiece lens, which further magnifies the image.
- The maximum magnification achievable in a standard compound light microscope is about 1000–2000 times.
- The specimen for observation is usually mounted on a glass slide which is placed on the stage of the microscope.
- Apart from magnification, the other major requirement of a microscope is resolution—the ability of the microscope to separate two objects that are close together (i.e. to distinguish fine detail). Resolution is related to the wavelength of light.
- Dark-field microscopy involves the use of a special condenser that blocks light from entering the objective lens, so that objects in the specimen appear bright against a dark background.
- Fluorescence microscopy is based on the principle that certain compounds absorb invisible light of short wavelengths and give off visible light of longer wavelengths.
- The major application of fluorescence microscopy is the fluorescent antibody (immunofluorescence) technique.

THE TRANSMISSION ELECTRON MICROSCOPE

- The electron microscope is able to achieve much greater resolution (and magnification) than light microscopes because it uses rays of electrons, which have a much shorter wavelength than white light.
- Magnifications of more than 100 000 times can be achieved.
- The specimen must be specially treated with stains, usually salts of heavy metals to scatter the electrons and increase the contrast between structures.
- The electrons pass through the specimen and then through electromagnetic lensES, which magnify the degree of scatter of the electrons.
- The electrons are focused by an electromagnetic lens onto a fluorescent screen to produce an image of the specimen.
- The electrons can be directed onto a photographic plate to produce a photograph called an electron micrograph.
- The major disadvantages of transmission electron microscopy are that living cells cannot be examined and that alteration or distortion of cell structures may occur.

THE SCANNING ELECTRON MICROSCOPE

- The scanning electron microscope is a development of the electron microscope. It produces three-dimensional images of objects at magnifications of up to 10 000 times.

PREPARATION OF SPECIMENS FOR LIGHT MICROSCOPY

- Living bacteria, yeasts and protozoa can be observed directly in a light microscope by suspending the organisms in a drop of fluid. This is called a wet preparation.
- Wet preparations are also useful for the direct observation of body fluid specimens, in which the presence of host cells, especially red and white cells, can be readily determined.
- Most microorganisms are colourless, so they are usually stained prior to microscopic examination.
- The Gram stain is the most useful and important staining procedure used in the microbiology laboratory because it divides almost all bacteria into two groups, thus serving as the first step in classifying and identifying bacteria.
- In the Gram staining procedure bacteria stain as Gram-positive (purple) or Gram-negative (pink/red or orange), depending on the composition of their cell wall.
- The Gram staining reaction is characteristic for each species.
- A direct Gram stain of a clinical specimen can be performed within minutes of receiving the specimen in the laboratory, and in some circumstances, a presumptive diagnosis can be made.

Study Questions

1. Why are microscopes required for the study of microorganisms?
2. Which are the magnification lenses in a compound light microscope?
3. What is the function of the condenser lens in the light microscope?
4. What is meant by the term 'resolution' in microscopy?
5. What is the maximum useful magnification achievable with a light microscope?
6. What is fluorescence microscopy?
7. How is the fluorescent antibody technique used to aid the diagnosis of infectious diseases?
8. Why is an electron microscope able to achieve much greater magnifications than a light microscope?
9. What are the magnifying lenses in an electron microscope?
10. What is an electron micrograph?
11. What are the main disadvantages of electron microscopy?
12. What is the main feature of a scanning electron microscope?
13. Why are preparations of microorganisms usually stained before they are examined with a light microscope?
14. Why is the Gram stain so important in microbiology?
15. What is the acid-fast stain and what is it used for?

Test Your Understanding

1. Compare the resolving power of the human eye with that of a compound light microscope.
2. Describe the essential differences between a light microscope and an electron microscope.
3. Describe the essential differences between the images obtained with a transmission electron microscope and those obtained with a scanning electron microscope.
4. Explain how the different Gram staining reactions relate to differences in the cell wall structure of bacteria.
5. Explain how the Gram stain can be used to achieve a rapid presumptive diagnosis of some infectious diseases.

FURTHER READING

Balows, A., W.J. Hausler, K.L. Herrmann, H.D. Isenberg and H.J. Shadomy (eds), *Manual of Clinical Microbiology,* 5th edn, Washington DC: American Society of Microbiology, 1991. (Has chapters on microscopy and staining techniques.)

chapter 4

bacteria

Chapter focus

- *What are the major properties of bacterial cells?*
- *What are the major growth requirements and phases of growth of bacteria?*
- *How are bacteria classified?*
- *What are the major groups of medically important bacteria?*
- *How does the genetic composition of a cell determine its properties?*
- *How has the discovery of the process of DNA recombination contributed to advances in biotechnology?*

The largest group of microorganisms are the **procaryotes** or **bacteria** (see Figure 4.1). They are responsible for many skin and wound infections in the human body, and are the causative agents of various defined disease syndromes. However, most bacteria are harmless and, in fact, many are beneficial to humans. The thousands of species of bacteria are differentiated by size, shape, morphology, staining characteristics, nutritional requirements, and biochemical activities. In this chapter we examine in detail the properties of bacteria, and the complex process of classifying bacteria.

Size, Shape and Appearance of Bacterial Cells

Bacteria vary significantly in their **morphology**, that is, their appearance. They range in size from 0.2 μm to 1 μm in diameter and 1 μm to 10 μm in length. There are three basic shapes of cells: spherical, rod-shaped and spiral (see Figure 4.2). Sometimes, groups of cells remain together after cell division to form clusters or chains. Some bacteria are motile; that is, they are capable of movement, possessing one or more extracellular appendages called **flagella** (singular: **flagellum**) which enable them to swim.

A spherical or round bacterium is called a **coccus** (plural: **cocci**). This is typically a small cell and may occur singly, in pairs (**diplococcus**), in clusters (**staphylococcus**) or chains (**streptococcus**). Frequently, the grouping of the cocci is reflected in the naming of the organism. Hence *Streptococcus pyogenes* is an organism with a cellular arrangement consisting of chains of cocci.

A rod-shaped or cylindrical bacterium is called a **bacillus** (plural: **bacilli**) (see Figure 4.3). Most bacilli appear as single cells, but a few are joined end to end to form **diplobacilli** or **streptobacilli**. Some form palisades (e.g. species of *Corynebacterium*). Some bacilli form endospores—a very resistant form of the cell which is able to withstand adverse environmental conditions. These are described in more detail later in the chapter.

Spiral bacteria may have one of three shapes. The **spirochaetes** have a corkscrew-like appearance and a strong axial filament running the length of the cell. Rotation of this filament propels the cell along. **Spirilla** (singular: **spirillum**) are not as tightly coiled and move by means of a flagellum, a propeller-like tail. **Vibrios** are slightly curved rod-shaped cells, resembling a comma or incomplete spiral. (See Figure 4.4.)

Most species of bacteria always grow in their characteristic shape and this can be a useful means of identification. However, the actual size of the cell can be influenced by the availability of nutrients in the medium. A few bacteria occur in more than one shape (e.g. some species of *Rhizobium* and *Corynebacterium*), which makes identification more difficult. These bacteria are termed **pleomorphic** (*pleo* = many).

FIGURE 4.1
DIAGRAM OF A TYPICAL PROCARYOTIC CELL

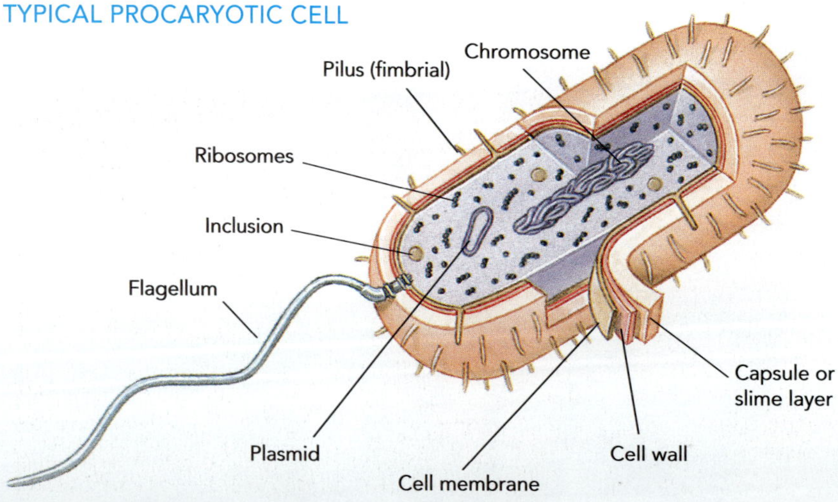

FIGURE 4.2
REPRESENTATIVE BACTERIAL SHAPES (MORPHOLOGY)

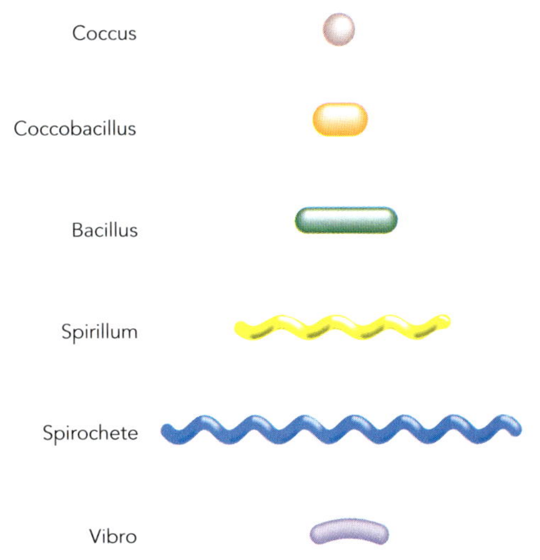

FIGURE 4.3
(a) SPHERICAL AND (b) ROD-SHAPED BACTERIA

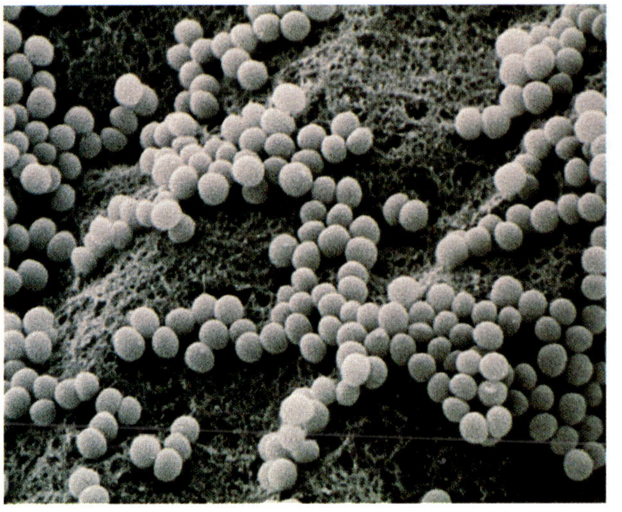
(a)

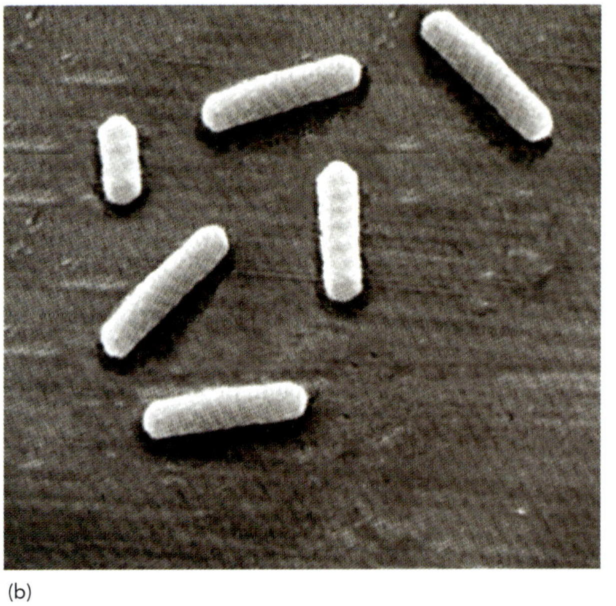
(b)

Structure of Bacteria

CELL WALL

The most characteristic structure of bacteria is their cell wall (see Figure 4.6). It is a semi-rigid structure present in almost all bacteria and is responsible for determining the shape of the cell as well as some of its staining properties. It also provides mechanical support so that the cell does not burst when exposed to conditions of osmotic pressure that allow movement of water into the cell. Bacterial cell walls contain varying amounts of different macromolecules, which bestow certain characteristics on the cell. One of the major components is a complex substance called **peptidoglycan**, which consists of repeating units of a disaccharide molecule containing two glucose derivatives, N-acetylglucosamine and N-acetylmuramic acid. The disaccharide molecules are cross-linked by an interbridge of four or five amino acids to form a complex rigid network (see Figure 4.5).

FIGURE 4.4
SPIRAL BACTERIA

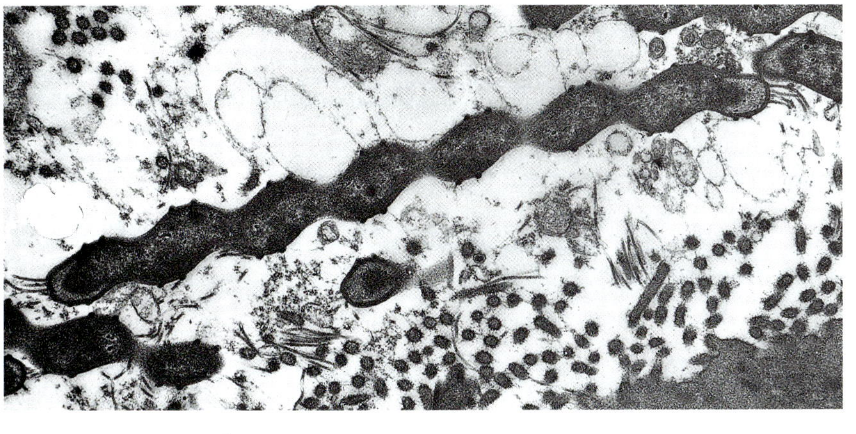

FIGURE 4.5
PEPTIDOGLYCAN, A MAJOR COMPONENT OF GRAM-POSITIVE CELL WALLS

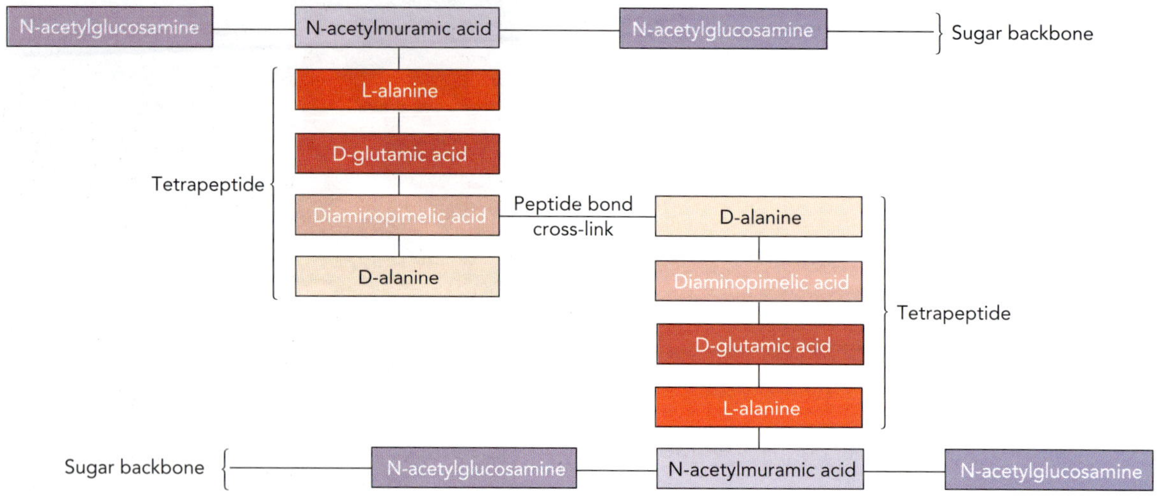

Three dimensional structure of peptidoglycan.

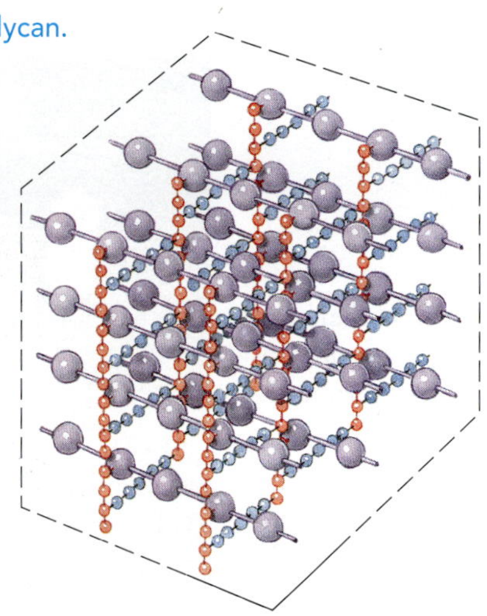

The composition of the cell wall differs between bacteria and so is useful for classification. Nearly all bacteria can be placed in one of two groups, Gram-negative or Gram-positive, based on the composition of the wall.

Structure of Gram-positive cell walls

Cells classified as Gram-positive have a defined cell wall structure which determines their reaction in the staining procedure developed by the Danish microbiologist Hans Christian Gram (see Chapter 3). The main component of Gram-positive cell walls is a thick layer of peptidoglycan. Attached to the peptidoglycan are other complex polysaccharides called **teichoic acids**. These teichoic acids have a strong negative charge which appears to influence the passage of materials in and out of the cell and provides a large part of the antigenic specificity of the cell (see Chapter 9).

Structure of Gram-negative cell walls

The group of bacteria classified as Gram-negative have a more complex outer structure than the Gram-positives (see Figure 4.6). The cell wall consists of a thin layer of peptidoglycan covered by an outer membrane containing **lipopolysaccharides**, **lipoproteins** and **phospholipids**. The outer membrane has several functions. It provides a barrier to the entry of various substances (e.g. some antibiotics) into the cell and also prevents the entry of certain enzymes that break down the cell wall (e.g. **lysozyme**). The lipopolysaccharide component, called the O-polysaccharide or O-antigen, has a distinctive structure in each strain of bacteria. This is useful in serological tests to distinguish between different strains of bacteria (see Chapter 15). The lipid portion known as **lipid A** is an **endotoxin**. It is responsible for some of the toxic effects (such as fever and shock) that occur when certain Gram-negative bacteria containing lipid A infect the human body (see Chapter 10).

Acid-fast bacteria

Not all bacteria can be grouped as either Gram-negative or Gram-positive. Some bacteria (e.g. the mycobacteria) have an outer layer composed of peptidoglycan similar to the Gram-positive wall, but covered by a thick waxy layer that interferes with the Gram-stain procedure. The presence of mycobacteria (e.g. the causative agent of

FIGURE 4.6
DIAGRAMMATIC REPRESENTATION OF BACTERIAL CELL WALLS

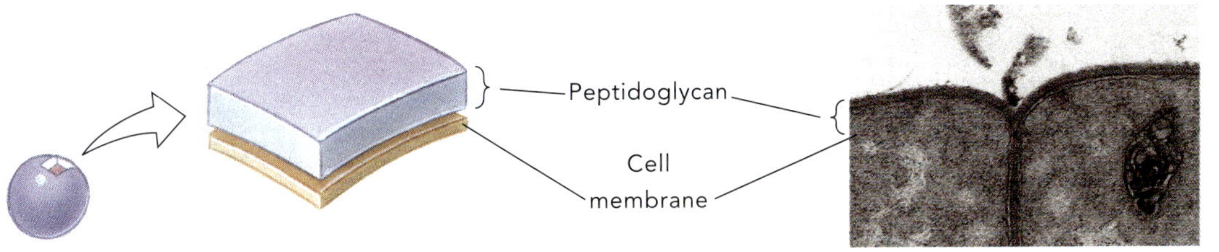

(a) Gram-positive bacteria

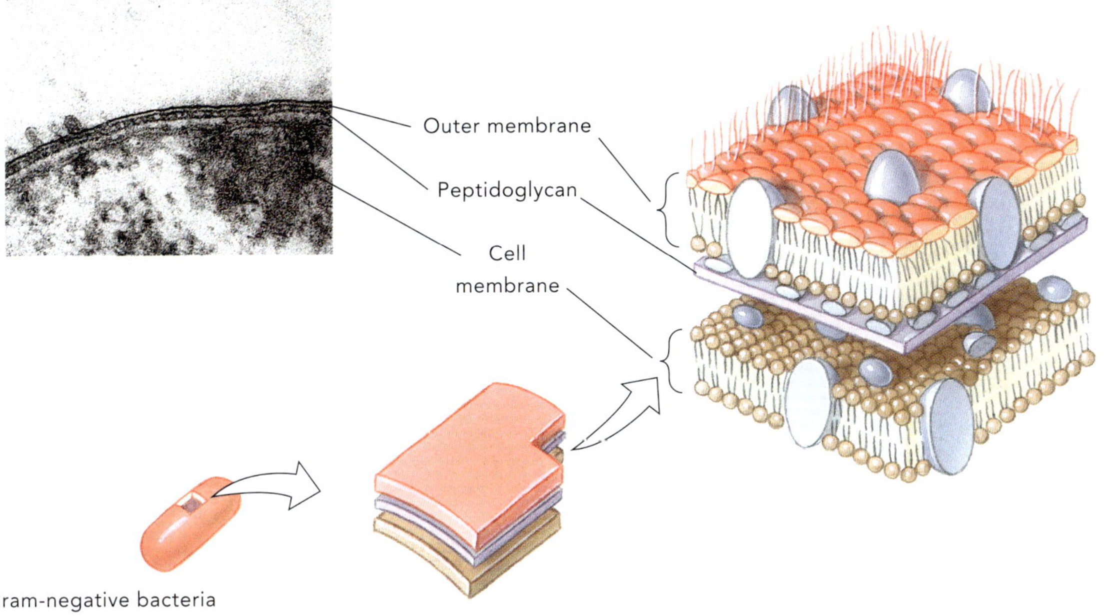

(b) Gram-negative bacteria

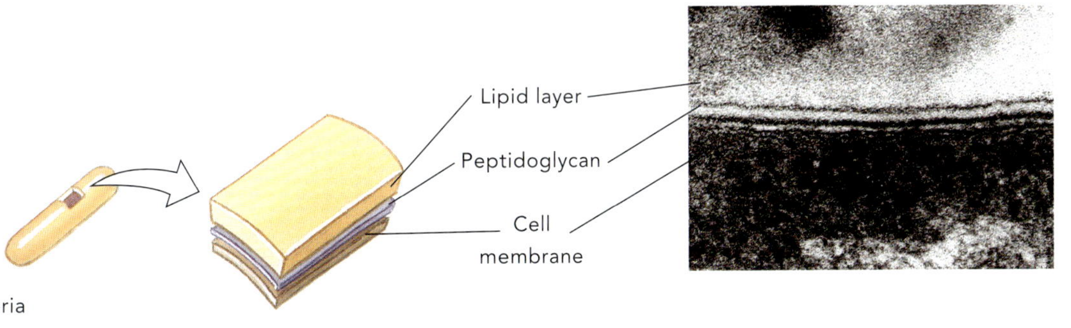

(c) Acid-fast bacteria

tuberculosis, *Mycobacterium tuberculosis*) is usually detected in sputum or lung biopsies by using the **Ziehl-Neelsen acid-fast stain** (see Chapter 3). Mycobacteria are often referred to as 'acid fast bacilli'.

Damage to the cell wall

An intact cell wall is important to the structural integrity of the bacterial cell and to its ability to survive in the environment. Thus the bacterial cell is particularly vulnerable to substances that destroy or damage the wall. Among these substances is the enzyme **lysozyme**, which occurs in egg white as well as in human tears and saliva. Lysozyme exerts an antibacterial role by breaking the bonds in the peptidoglycan layer in the walls of Gram-positive bacteria, thus destroying the cell walls. When the wall is destroyed, the cell is left surrounded by only the plasma membrane. This structure is called a **protoplast**

FIGURE 4.7
THE FLUID MOSAIC MODEL OF MEMBRANE STRUCTURE

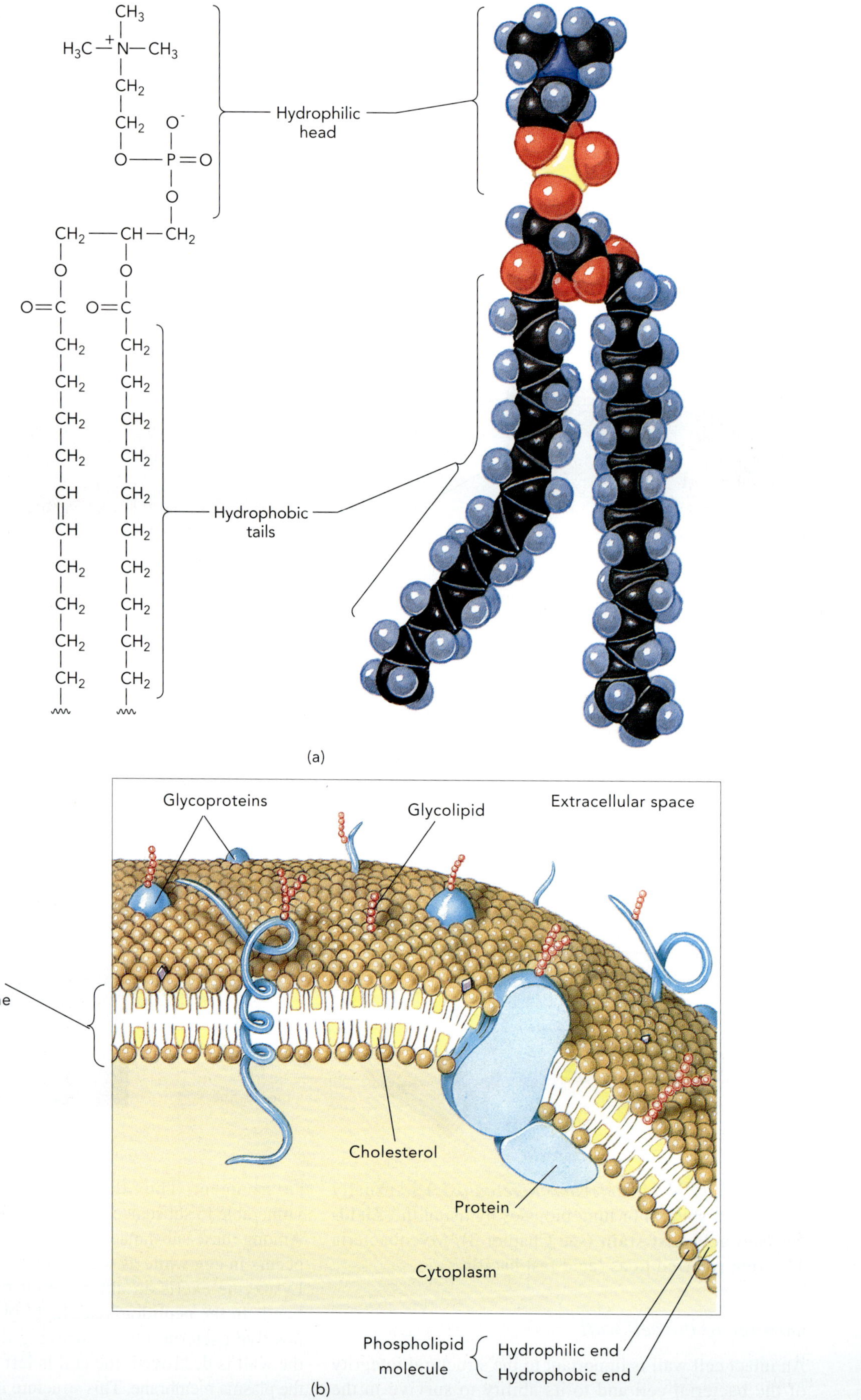

and is very vulnerable to damage by osmotic pressure. Lysozyme does not have such a dramatic effect on the cell walls of Gram-negative bacteria because it is unable to penetrate the outer cell membrane and therefore cannot destroy the peptidoglycan layer.

Certain antibiotics specifically target the cell wall. **Penicillin** exerts its effect by inhibiting the formation of the cross-linking amino acid interbridges during the synthesis of peptidoglycan in rapidly growing cells (see Figure 4.5). For this reason, rapidly multiplying Gram-positive bacteria are particularly susceptible to the action of penicillin. Gram-negative organisms are not as easily affected because their outer membrane interferes with the entry of penicillin to the cell. Some of the semi-synthetic penicillins, which are able to penetrate the outer membrane, are more effective against Gram-negative organisms (see Chapter 12).

CELL MEMBRANE

All bacterial cells have a **cell membrane** or **plasma membrane**, which lies just underneath the cell wall. Bacterial membranes have a structure that is essentially similar to the membranes of all other living cells. It consists of a double layer of phospholipid molecules (a **phospholipid bilayer**) with an irregular arrangement of proteins embedded in the lipid layers. Bacterial cell membranes consist only of proteins and phospholipids whereas eucaryotic cell membranes also contain sterols and carbohydrates that bestow additional properties on the eucaryotic membrane. The structure of the membrane is uniquely suited to its function in the cell. When examined under the electron microscope, it appears as a double layer. It is now generally accepted that this double layer consists of phospholipid molecules arranged in a particular orientation.

Phospholipids are compounds consisting of a molecule of glycerol esterified with two long chain fatty acids (see Chapter 2). Fatty acids are long hydrocarbon chains that are **non-polar** (i.e. do not have any charged groups) and so are insoluble in water. They are therefore described as **hydrophobic**, or 'water-hating'. The phosphate group, which is attached to the third hydroxyl group of the glycerol molecule, is **polar** (i.e. charged) and is usually joined to another charged molecule such as ethanolamine or choline, or another molecule of **glycerol**. This part of the phospholipid molecule is termed **hydrophilic** ('water-loving'). Phospholipids therefore have two distinct regions—a polar, water-soluble, hydrophilic 'head' and a non-polar hydrophobic 'tail' (see Figure 4.7(a)).

In the cell membrane, two layers of phospholipids are arranged so that the polar, hydrophilic 'heads' are oriented towards the 'outside' water environment, while the non-polar fatty acid 'tails' are oriented towards the hydrophobic interior of the membrane. Embedded in the phospholipid bilayer are protein molecules which carry out various functions. This widely accepted model of membrane structure was proposed by Singer and Nicholson and is usually called the Singer-Nicholson model or **fluid-mosaic model**. The term 'fluid-mosaic' describes the major characteristics of this membrane structure. The structure is quite fluid, the degree of fluidity being determined by the nature of the fatty acids it contains. Within the lipid matrix, lipid and protein molecules are able to move sideways (see Figure 4.7(b)).

Movement of substances in and out of the cell

The main function of the plasma membrane is to act as a selectively permeable barrier for the cell. Many water-soluble compounds cannot penetrate the non-polar hydrophobic interior of the membrane. They must be assisted across the membrane by proteins acting as carriers and forming pores or channels that allow the passage of selected substances into and out of the cell. This is often termed **facilitated diffusion** and does not require the expenditure of energy. It allows the movement of a substance across a membrane from an area of high concentration to an area of low concentration. This enables the cell to absorb the nutrients and substances it requires for growth and to rid itself of waste products.

Active transport occurs when a substance is transported in or out of a cell *against* a concentration gradient; that is, there is a higher concentration of the substance on one side of the membrane. This usually requires the expenditure of energy. Specialised protein molecules called **transport proteins** carry the substance through the membrane.

Osmosis

Osmosis is the passage of a solvent (usually water) from one side of a membrane to another. Usually, the cell membrane allows unrestricted movement of small molecules such as water, oxygen and carbon dioxide. The water molecules move from an area of 'high' water concentration (i.e. a dilute solution) to an area of 'low' water concentration (e.g. a more concentrated solution inside the cell). **Osmotic pressure** is the pressure required to prevent the flow of water molecules across a selectively permeable membrane.

Unlike human cells, which use homeostatic mechanisms to maintain a constant environment, bacterial cells can be subjected to different kinds of solutions in their environment. This may create differences in the osmotic pressure exerted on the cell. If the overall concentration of salts and ions (solutes) in the solution outside the cell is the same as inside, the solution is said to be **isotonic** (and water enters and leaves the cell at the same rate). If the solute concentration is higher outside the cell than inside, the solution is said to be **hypertonic**. Water leaves the cell and the cell dehydrates. If the solute concentration is lower outside than inside (e.g. as in distilled water), the solution is said to be **hypotonic**. Water passes through the membrane into the cell and the cell may burst. The rigid cell wall plays an important part in protecting bacteria from the effect of variations in osmotic pressure.

Other functions of the bacterial cell membranes

Procaryotic cells lack other cellular membranes, so the plasma membrane in bacteria is the site of additional functions that are performed by the organelles in eucaryotic cells. These include:

- synthesis of cell wall components;
- cellular respiration and synthesis of ATP; and
- the secretion of proteins and enzymes, which are released from the cell as extracellular enzymes or toxins.

The membrane is a vital part of the cell and as such is very susceptible to damage. Many antimicrobial compounds exert their effect by disrupting the structure of the membrane. These include disinfectants, such as alcohol and the quaternary ammonium compounds, and the polymyxin group of antibiotics.

INTERNAL STRUCTURES OF BACTERIAL CELLS

The **cytoplasm** of bacterial cells is about 80% water and contains the proteins, carbohydrates, lipids and salts that are essential for the activities of the cell. The nuclear area of the cell contains a single circular chromosome, consisting of a double strand of DNA which carries the genetic information necessary for the structure and function of the cell. Bacteria often carry one or more extra pieces of DNA, small circular structures called **plasmids.** Plasmids vary in size and replicate independently of the main chromosomal DNA. They appear to carry information that is not essential for the growth of the cell. such as genes for resistance to antibiotics or the production of toxins. Other plasmids carry the gene for the production of the sex **pili**, which are involved in the transfer of genetic information from one bacterium to another during conjugation. The transfer of genetic information by plasmids is used by scientists in the process of genetic engineering, described later in this chapter.

Ribosomes are small granular particles, consisting of two subunits, each containing protein and ribonucleic acid (RNA). Ribosomes of procaryotic cells are designated **70S** which refers to their rate of sedimentation when subjected to ultracentrifugation. They are slightly smaller and less dense than the ribosomes of eucaryotic organisms which are designated **80S**. Ribosomes are the site of protein synthesis in the cell. Messenger RNA (mRNA) attaches to the ribosomes to provide a site for the incorporation of amino acids into the growing peptide chain. Groups of ribosomes attached to messenger RNA are called **polyribosomes**.

Electron micrographs of bacterial cells usually have a granular appearance, with some areas appearing to be denser than others. The granules, or **inclusions**, can be identified by staining with simple dyes such as methylene blue or iodine. These inclusions are usually polymers of cellular material and act as storage for the cell. For example, **volutin** is a polymer of phosphate molecules. Polymers of glucose, such as **glycogen** or **starch**, are also frequently present. Occasionally, cells contain **vesicles** or **vacuoles**. These are usually filled with gas to give the cell buoyancy.

EXTERNAL STRUCTURES OF BACTERIAL CELLS

Glycocalyx

Some bacteria are surrounded by the **glycocalyx**, a sticky, polysaccharide-containing layer which is secreted onto their cell surface. Depending on its structure and function it is referred to as a **capsule** or **slime layer**.

Bacterial capsules are composed of polysaccharide and/or polypeptide molecules. They are usually synthesised inside the cell and excreted to the cell surface where they form an organised gelatinous layer firmly attached to the cell wall. An important function of the capsule is to help the bacterium adhere to host cell surfaces. The capsule possesses specific molecules which bind to complementary receptor molecules on the surface of the susceptible animal cell.

The capsule also has a protective function, allowing the bacterial cell to avoid phagocytosis, apparently because the phagocyte is unable to attach to the bacterial cell surface. The capsule is therefore considered to contribute to the **virulence** (degree of pathogenicity) of the organism. For example, encapsulated strains of *Streptococcus pneumoniae* are highly virulent whereas strains that lack a capsule are unable to produce disease symptoms.

The composition of the capsule is determined by the particular strain of bacteria in which it is found. The oral bacterium, *Streptococcus mutans*, forms a capsule containing glucan, a polymer of glucose, which is a major component of dental plaque. It helps bacteria to adhere to the tooth surface and cause dental decay.

Slime layers are composed of glycoproteins and polysaccharides and usually exist as a loosely attached, less defined structure than capsules.

Flagella

Many bacteria are motile, that is, capable of movement in a water environment. The most common way in which procaryotic cells move is by means of **flagella** (singular: **flagellum**), thin, rigid filaments that are usually many times longer than the cell itself. Some bacteria have only one flagellum located at one end of the cell; others have two, one at each end of the cell (see Figure 4.8). A few bacteria have numerous flagella, located all over the cell. Flagella consist of protein subunits arranged in a complex structure. They are attached to the cell membrane and wall of the bacterium by a structure called a **basal body**, a series of concentric protein rings which allow the flagellum to rotate. Movement of the bacterium is achieved by rotation of the flagella with a propellor-like motion, a process requiring energy in the form of ATP. Motile bacteria appear to respond to a stimulus in their environment and swim towards it. This phenomenon is called **chemotaxis**.

Pili and fimbriae

Pili (singular: pilus) and fimbriae (singular: fimbria) appear as hair-like appendages on the outside of Gram-negative bacterial cells. Each has a distinct function. The thicker

FIGURE 4.8
BACTERIUM WITH NUMEROUS FLAGELLA
Proteus vulgaris

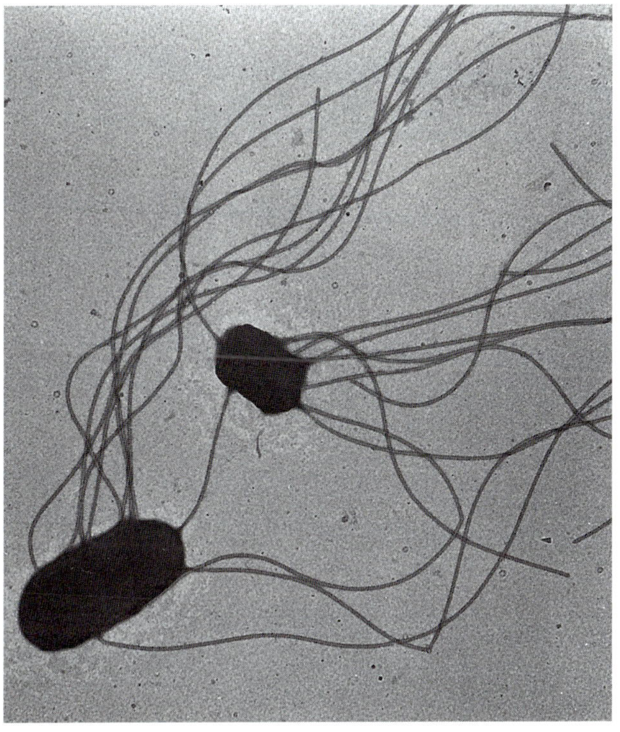

sex **pili** (1 to 10 per cell) are located on the surface of the cell; they are involved in the joining together of bacterial cells to allow transfer of the genetic material, DNA, from one cell to another during conjugation (see p. 81). There are several thousand **fimbriae** per cell (sometimes called attachment pili). They are thinner than pili and concerned mainly with the attachment of the bacteria to the surface of mucosal cells, so that the organism can adhere to the host cell and colonise it. Thus the presence of fimbriae contributes to the pathogenicity of the organism. For example, strains of *Neisseria gonorrhoea* that lack fimbriae are not as capable of causing disease as strains that have fimbriae to help attach the organism to the mucosal cells lining the host genital tract.

ENDOSPORES

When environmental conditions are unfavourable, certain Gram-positive bacilli are able to form endospores. Bacterial sporulation does not occur when cells are growing rapidly, but only when growth ceases due to the exhaustion of essential nutrients. An **endospore** is a specialised type of resting cell which is formed inside the bacterial cell membrane. It is surrounded by a **spore coat**, consisting of thick layers of peptidoglycan and protein (see Figure 4.9).

The endospore develops inside the bacterial cell membrane and can be located by special staining procedures (see Chapter 3). The spore has a lower water content than vegetative cells and does not carry out metabolic reactions. It does, however, contain the cellular nucleic acid and various other enzymes and substances that are essential if spore germination is to occur when conditions become favourable. When the spore is placed in a favourable medium, water enters, germination occurs and the vegetative cell that is produced resumes normal growth and metabolism. Endospore formation is *not* a method of reproduction. One bacterial cell gives rise to only one endospore, which then germinates into a single cell again. It is, however, a very important method of survival for certain species of bacteria and has important clinical significance. Bacterial endospores have been shown to survive in the soil for many years. The spores of *Bacillus anthracis*—the organism responsible for anthrax, a disease that affects humans as well as cattle—were found more than 20 years later at a site where diseased animals had been buried.

Many of the Gram-positive bacteria that form endospores are important pathogens. These include members of the genus *Clostridium*—*Clostridium perfringens* (food poisoning and gas gangrene), *Clostridium tetani* (tetanus) and *Clostridium botulinum* (botulism). Endospores survive conditions that kill most bacteria, such as boiling for up to five hours, freezing, desiccation (drying out) and exposure to chemicals and radiation. In the food industry, spores may survive the normal cooking process and cause food poisoning. An example is *Clostridium perfringens*, which is common in the environment.

Spores of *Clostridium* may be ingested in food, germinate in the intestine and produce symptoms of gastroenteritis (stomach cramps and diarrhoea) about 12 hours later. This organism is also the cause of gas gangrene. If wounds are contaminated with *Cl. perfringens*, either from the environment or from unsterilised medical equipment, gangrene may develop.

Clostridium botulinum spores are widespread in nature and may sometimes be found in preserved or canned foods that have not been adequately sterilised. The organism grows in the food under anaerobic conditions, producing a powerful neurotoxin (poison).

Clostridium tetani is a common inhabitant of the large intestine of humans and animals. Tetanus spores are frequently found in faeces or in soil where manure is spread. When introduced into deep puncture wounds, the spores germinate, grow anaerobically and produce the tetanus toxin responsible for spasms, paralysis and death. A vaccine is available against tetanus.

Knowledge of the existence of highly resistant forms of bacteria is important for the development of adequate methods of sterilisation and disinfection. Bacterial endospores are highly resistant to heat, partly because of their comparatively low water content. A temperature of 121°C for 15 minutes in an autoclave is required to kill endospores. In addition, the complex nature of the spore coat makes them highly resistant to most germicides.

Bacterial Growth

Growth is usually defined as an increase in size. However, when microbiologists speak about bacterial growth, they are usually referring to an increase in numbers of bacterial cells. This may appear confusing until it is realised that

FIGURE 4.9
VEGETATIVE AND SPORULATIVE CYCLES IN BACTERIA

(a)

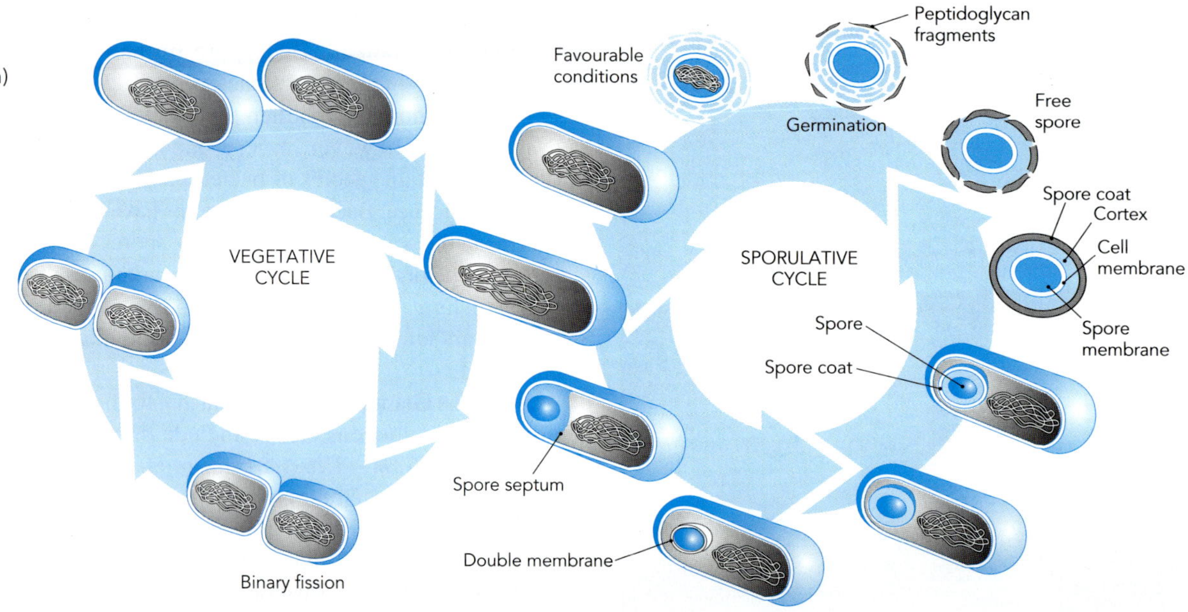

(b) Diagrammatic representation of a bacterial endospore showing protective layers.

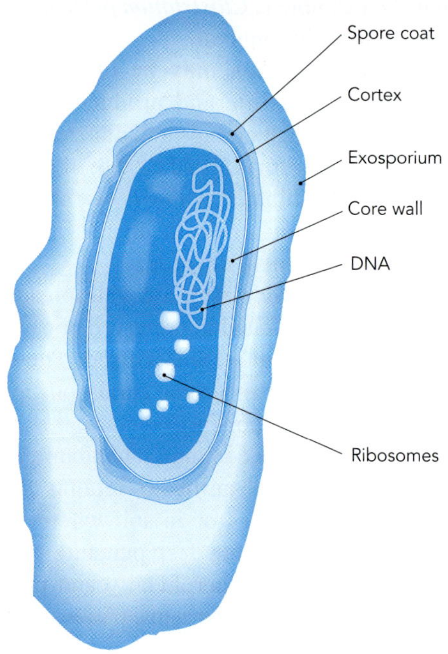

bacteria do not increase in size very much during their life span. As soon as a bacterial cell has approximately doubled in size, it divides to form two identical daughter cells. Bacterial growth is therefore defined as *an increase in cell numbers*.

Cells use the energy derived from the metabolic breakdown of nutrients to produce new cellular components. In most bacteria, as the cell elongates, the genetic information contained in the chromosome is duplicated and one new chromosome moves to each end of the cell. The membrane and cell wall begin to grow inwards at a point about half way along the cell, until a septum forms. The cell then splits, forming two new cells that contain identical components to the parent cell. This whole process is called **binary fission** (Figure 4.10). The two daughter cells are identical; they are both completely new cells—not one old cell and one new cell. The time taken for the cell to reproduce itself is called the **generation time**; this can vary enormously, depending on the type of organism and the environmental conditions. Under favourable conditions, some bacteria can reproduce in 20 minutes. Important clinical species, such as *Escherichia coli*, can reproduce at this rate. This means that a single cell can give rise to over one million cells in 8–10 hours. Other species (e.g. *Mycobacteria* and some anaerobic organisms) are very slow-growing and may take up to 12 hours to reproduce even when conditions are optimal (see Table 4.1).

FIGURE 4.10
BINARY FISSION IN A BACTERIUM

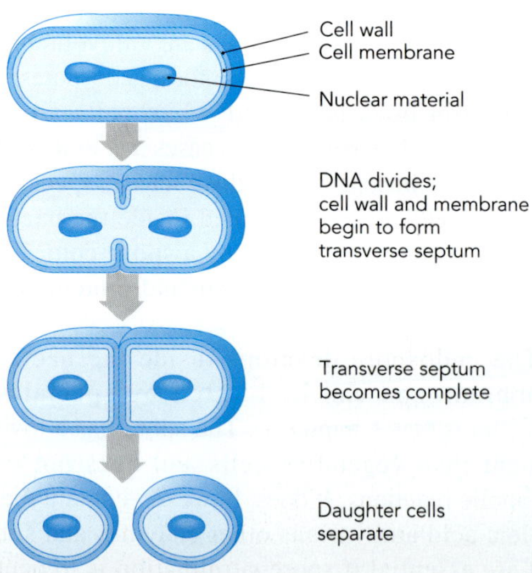

TABLE 4.1
BACTERIAL GROWTH

TIME (HOURS)	NUMBER OF CELLS
0	1
0.5	2
1	4
1.5	8
2	16
2.5	32
3	64
3.5	128
4	256
4.5	512
5	1024
5.5	2048
6	4096
6.5	8192
7	16 384
7.5	32 768
8	65 536
8.5	131 072
9	262 144
9.5	524 288
10	1048 376

The time required to culture and identify an organism from a clinical specimen depends very much on the growth rate. Many bacteria can be grown successfully overnight (18 hours), but some bacteria take days or even weeks. It is important to be aware of differences in growth rate when trying to identify a specimen in the laboratory. Cultures must be incubated for long enough to enable cells to grow and be identified, otherwise the presence of a pathogen may be missed. Specimens obtained from patients or the environment typically contain a mixture of bacteria. Individual kinds of bacteria can be isolated from a mixed culture by streaking the sample out on an agar plate until single colonies are obtained (see Chapter 15).

Requirements for Growth

The rate at which bacteria reproduce is determined by both physical and chemical factors in their environment. Physical aspects include temperature, pH, osmotic pressure and the presence of oxygen. Chemical or nutritional factors include availability of water, a suitable carbon source, nitrogen, phosphorus, sulphur and other trace elements and minerals. Some bacteria have an absolute requirement for a particular compound or growth factor. Overall, bacteria can grow in a wide range of environments, but each species has its own set of optimal conditions that allow it to achieve maximum growth rate. For most human pathogenic bacteria, the conditions are very similar to those found in the human body.

PHYSICAL FACTORS

Temperature

Most bacteria will grow at the environmental temperatures usually encountered in temperate zones, 10°C to 39°C, but each will have a minimum, maximum and optimum temperature. Organisms that grow at moderate temperatures are called **mesophiles**. Those that thrive in low temperatures are called **psychrophiles** (cold-loving) and those that like high temperatures are termed **thermophiles** (heat-loving). Figure 4.11 shows the growth curves for these bacteria at different temperatures.

The most common method of preserving food is refrigeration. The rate of growth of most bacteria is greatly reduced by the temperature in a domestic refrigerator (4°C). However, some bacteria will survive long periods

FIGURE 4.11
EFFECT OF TEMPERATURE ON RATE OF BACTERIAL GROWTH
Comparison of the growth rates of typical psychophilic, mesophylic and thermophilic organisms. There is some overlap of ranges at which these organisms can survive, but rates of growth are much lower at the extreme ends of the ranges. (Redrawn with permission, from Black, Jacquelyn G., *Microbiology: Principles and Applications*, 2nd edn., Englewood Cliffs, N.J.: Prentice-Hall Inc., 1992.

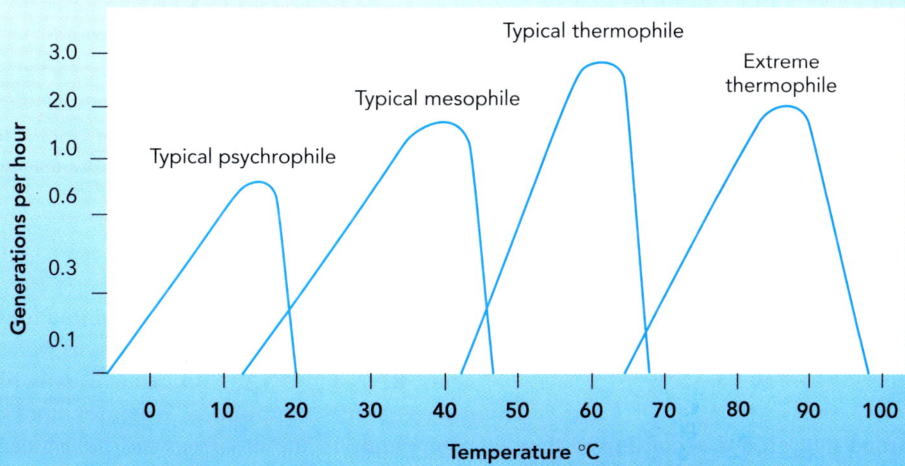

of storage in the cold and even withstand freezing. Thus, although food spoilage is greatly reduced at low temperatures, it is not completely prevented and food may still be contaminated by any pathogens that were present before refrigeration.

Pathogenic bacteria usually have an optimum growth temperature similar to the human body (i.e. 37°C) and so clinical diagnostic laboratories routinely incubate most cultures close to that temperature.

pH

The level of acidity or alkalinity of the culture medium (pH) is very important for bacterial growth. For most bacteria, the pH optimum, at which maximum growth occurs, is close to neutral, that is, pH 7. Most bacteria do not grow at all above pH 8 or below pH 6. Some bacteria produce organic acids during metabolism, causing a drop in pH that inhibits further growth. An important group of bacteria which can tolerate acid conditions belong to the genus *Lactobacillus*. The lactic acid group of bacteria produces lactic acid by fermentation of lactose and is responsible for the souring of milk to make products such as yoghurt. These bacteria can only tolerate moderate levels of acid (i.e. pH 4) so when the pH drops below 4 the culture stops growing. This is an excellent method of preservation of milk products—spoilage is inhibited because most other bacteria cannot tolerate even mildly acid conditions.

Water and osmotic pressure

Water is essential for bacterial growth. Bacterial cells are at least 80% water and growth will only occur in a moist environment. The composition of its water environment will affect the bacterial cell, which obtains all its nutrients from its surroundings. The dissolved substances exert osmotic pressure on the bacterial cell, which will be able to reproduce optimally if the growth medium is isotonic (see p. 63). This means that, if a bacterial cell is placed in a hypotonic solution such as distilled water, water moves into the cell which swells up and becomes turgid. Normally, the cell would burst, but the rigid structure of the bacterial cell wall exerts an opposing pressure and prevents cell **lysis**. However, if the cell is placed in a hypertonic solution—that is, a solution with a higher salt concentration (osmotic pressure) than the bacterial cytoplasm—water tends to move out of the bacterial cell into the surrounding medium, causing the cell membrane to shrink away from the wall. This greatly slows down or inhibits growth. This phenomenon is useful in food preservation. High concentrations of salt or sugar (hypertonicity) in foodstuffs prevent the growth of bacteria and subsequent food spoilage. Some examples are salted or cured meat and fish, jams and fruit syrups.

Oxygen

Bacteria can be divided into groups according to their requirement for molecular oxygen for growth. Organisms that use oxygen are called **aerobes**. Those that *require* oxygen for growth are called **obligate aerobes**. Some bacteria have developed the ability to grow in the presence or absence of oxygen and these are called **facultative anaerobes**. They carry on aerobic metabolism when oxygen is present but change to anaerobic pathways when oxygen is limited. Many of these organisms are found in the human intestine.

Bacteria that grow in the absence of oxygen are called **anaerobes**. Some of them are termed **obligate anaerobes** because they are not only inhibited, but destroyed, in the presence of oxygen. These obligate anaerobes are killed by a special form of oxygen called a **free radical** or **superoxide** (O_2^-), which is a compound formed in most cells during aerobic oxidation, but usually destroyed by two enzymes—**superoxide dismutase** and **catalase**. Obligate anaerobes lack these enzymes and the cells are killed by the toxic effect of the free radicals.

Two pathogenic organisms that are sensitive to oxygen are *Clostridium tetani* (tetanus) and *Clostridium perfringens* (gas gangrene). Tetanus and gangrene are infections that occur in deep puncture wounds or necrotic tissue where oxygen is absent. Both infections are sometimes treated by placing the patient in a hyperbaric oxygen chamber. Tissues are saturated with oxygen in an attempt to kill the causative organisms. Obligate aerobes such as *Mycobacteria tuberculosis* are often found as pathogens in areas of high oxygen tension, such as the lungs.

The oxygen requirement of pathogenic organisms is an important factor to consider when collecting specimens for laboratory diagnosis. Even a short exposure to oxygen (10 minutes) is sufficient to kill some anaerobes. Special techniques have been developed to collect and transport sensitive organisms (see Chapter 15).

NUTRITIONAL REQUIREMENTS

Water

Bacteria grow best in an environment which is saturated with water. Although many bacteria can survive dry conditions, they require water to reproduce.

Carbon

The essential element in all living cells is carbon. Most bacteria need to be supplied with a suitable simple organic carbon compound in the medium. The bacteria break down these carbon compounds to smaller molecules which they use to synthesise their own cellular requirements. A few bacteria are **autotrophic** and are able to use carbon dioxide from the air as their sole carbon source.

Nitrogen

Nitrogen is an essential element required for the synthesis of enzymes and other cellular proteins as well as the nucleic acids, RNA and DNA. Nitrogen is usually obtained from nitrogenous compounds, nitrates and ammonium compounds in the environment, but some bacteria are capable of 'fixing' nitrogen from the air—that is, converting gaseous nitrogen into compounds such as nitrates which can be utilised by plants for growth.

Phosphorus

Phosphorus is needed for nucleotides, the nucleic acids RNA and DNA, the energy storage molecule, ATP, and for the structural phospholipids of the cell membrane.

Sulphur

Sulphur is an essential component of some amino acids, and of the sulphur-containing vitamin, **biotin**. The sulphur-containing amino acids form disulphide linkages between different parts of polypeptide chains and contribute to the folding of the chains into the correct secondary and tertiary protein structure.

Trace elements

Many microorganisms require trace amounts of minerals in order to grow. Often these elements are needed as cofactors in specific enzyme reactions (e.g. magnesium). They may be components of essential compounds, such as iron (Fe) in the cytochromes of the electron transport chain, or cobalt (Co) in the cofactor cyanocobalamine (vitamin B12).

Organic growth factors

Most bacteria can synthesise all their cellular requirements from a variety of nutritional sources. A few have requirements for specific organic compounds which must be added to the medium for growth to occur. These may be vitamins, which act as coenzymes. Often the requirement will be for a specific amino acid that the bacterium is unable to synthesise for itself, but is essential for the formation of protein. This inability may be inherent in the species, or it may be the result of a mutation which has given rise to a particular strain of bacteria that has lost the ability to produce the enzymes required to make this compound for itself. This condition is described in more detail under Bacterial Genetics (see p. 73).

Handling Bacteria in the Laboratory

GROWTH MEDIA

It can be seen from the preceding sections that much is known about the growth requirements of bacteria. This information is used in the microbiology laboratory to isolate and identify bacteria by growing them on different media. A wide variety of media are used, differing in composition according to the purpose of the experiment. Most media consist of a solution of salts and nutrients in water, adjusted to the correct pH. The solution is prepared and sterilised in order to kill any unwanted bacteria. If a solid medium is required, a solidifying agent is added; this is usually **agar,** a complex polysaccharide extracted from seaweed.

Chemically defined media

A **chemically defined medium** is one whose exact chemical composition is known. It is prepared by weighing out exact amounts of pure chemicals, and dissolving them in distilled water. This type of medium is used in research when, for example, the effect of growth factors is being studied, or a fastidious organism is being isolated.

Complex media

For routine work, a **complex medium** is used. In this type of medium, most of the organic nutrients are supplied by protein hydrolysates. These are small peptide or peptone fragments produced by partial digestion of large protein molecules. Vitamins and growth factors are supplied by extracts of yeast or meat. A commonly used medium is called nutrient broth. Its composition is listed in Table 4.2. When it is required in solid form, agar is added and it is called nutrient agar. Agar itself is not metabolised by bacteria and thus does not provide a source of nutrition. Agar is a useful gelling agent as it has the unusual property of melting at a much higher temperature (90°C) than it sets (45°C).

Blood agar

In routine clinical laboratories, **blood agar** is used for the initial isolation of a clinical specimen. It consists of nutrient agar to which defibrinated horse blood has been added. It is especially useful in identifying organisms that damage red blood cells, such as the haemolytic streptococci.

Selective media

A **selective medium** contains substances that suppress the growth of unwanted bacteria while permitting the growth of the desired organisms. For example, MacConkey medium contains crystal violet and bile salts which inhibit the growth of Gram-positive organisms, but allow the growth of most Gram-negatives.

Differential media

A **differential medium** is used to distinguish between organisms growing on the same plate. An indicator, usually a dye, is added to the medium and it undergoes a colour

TABLE 4.2
COMPOSITION OF COMPLEX MEDIA

NUTRIENT BROTH	
Water	1L
Peptone	5g
Beef extract	3g
Sodium chloride	8g
NUTRIENT AGAR	
Add agar 15g/L to nutrient broth	

change if certain organisms are present and able to metabolise the nutrients supplied.

Some media are both selective and differential. For example, **mannitol salt (MS) agar** contains the sugar alcohol, mannitol, as the carbon source, together with a high concentration of salt. When a clinical specimen is grown on MS agar, the salt-tolerant staphylococci will survive and grow, but other organisms will be inhibited. The strains of staphylococci present can be further differentiated because *Staphylococcus aureus* metabolises mannitol, producing an acid that turns the indicator dye from pink to yellow. *Staphylococcus epidermidis* does not produce acid so there is no colour change (see Figure 2.19).

A huge range of prepared culture media is available commercially.

LABORATORY TECHNIQUES

Clinical samples

In order to isolate and identify a particular bacterial species, it is necessary to obtain pure cultures, that is, a culture containing only one type of bacterium. Microorganisms that occur in clinical samples are almost invariably a mixture of normal flora and the invading pathogen. To isolate individual bacterial types, clinical specimens are usually grown on an agar plate and 'streaked out' to obtain single colonies (see Chapter 15). The thick suspension of bacteria is spread out on the plate until single bacteria are isolated, each of which will give rise to a single separate colony. These are considered 'pure', having arisen from a single cell and therefore consisting of only one cell type.

Growth of bacterial cultures

Most of the known kinds of bacteria are maintained as pure cultures in culture collections. They can easily be grown in the laboratory under controlled conditions. This is one reason why bacteria have been used extensively for research—it is possible to produce a uniform homogeneous population of cells that will all behave in an identical manner. Much of our knowledge of cell structure and metabolism, as well as our understanding of DNA replication and protein synthesis, has come from experiments with bacteria. Bacterial cultures are also used to prepare various food products as well as other important metabolites (see Chapter 2).

It is important to use sterilised equipment and media so that only the desired bacteria will be grown. The cells may be grown in liquid culture or on solid media, depending on the type of work being done. To grow bacteria in liquid medium, a solution of nutrients, salts and other growth requirements is prepared in a test tube or flask. The container is loosely stoppered and then sterilised in an autoclave. A small sample of the bacteria is introduced into the flask in a sterile manner, the flask is covered tightly, and the culture incubated at a constant temperature, with shaking if aeration is required. A solid medium is prepared from a similar solution of nutrients, to which agar has been added to solidify it. The medium is sterilised and then poured aseptically into sterile petri dishes or 'plates', covered and allowed to set. Samples of bacteria are inoculated onto the surface of the plate, spread and incubated at constant temperature.

Storage of bacteria

It is sometimes necessary to preserve cultures of bacteria, either for later laboratory use or for reference. In the laboratory, organisms can be grown on nutrient agar slopes in tubes or bottles and stored in the refrigerator for 2–3 months. For longer-term storage, a thick suspension of cells is deep frozen at –70°C in a protective suspending medium. Freeze-drying is another method whereby a suspension of cells is frozen and then dehydrated under vacuum. The dehydrated culture is stable for years and the bacteria can be revived by the addition of water. Throughout the world there are national culture collections of pure cultures of bacteria which have been preserved in this way for reference and are available to microbiologists.

PATTERN OF BACTERIAL GROWTH

Phases of growth

When bacteria are grown in the laboratory in liquid medium, the medium becomes cloudy or turbid. It is possible to measure the increase in numbers of bacteria at various time intervals and plot the values on a graph representing a growth curve. When cells are first inoculated into fresh medium containing all the nutrients they require, they take a short time to adapt before they start to divide. This is termed the **lag phase**. The cells then begin to duplicate their contents and undergo binary fission, doubling the cell numbers with each generation time. Thus, for each cell present initially, there are two cells after one generation, four, (or 2^2) cells after two generations, eight cells (2^3) after three generations, and so on. In other words, the number of cells increases by a power of 2 each generation time. Mathematically, this is described as a **logarithmic** or **exponential** increase. It can be seen from the graph in Figure 4.12 that a huge number of bacterial cells can be produced in a short time. This phase of growth is termed the **logarithmic** or **log phase** and the cells are generally reproducing at a maximum rate. This type of growth rate is very sensitive to environmental conditions.

The logarithmic rate of bacterial growth continues only while conditions are optimal. As the number of bacteria increases, nutrients are used up and there is an accumulation of waste products. These may inhibit essential enzyme reactions in the cell, or cause a change in the pH of the medium, both of which will slow growth. As the density of cells in the culture increases, the availability of oxygen may decrease. The rate of cell division therefore slows down and eventually cell division ceases, or some cells

FIGURE 4.12
RATE OF GROWTH OF BACTERIAL CULTURE

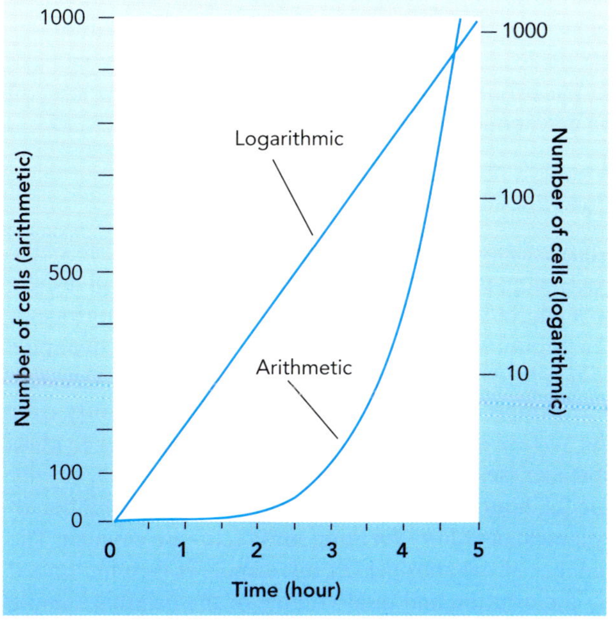

FIGURE 4.13
TYPICAL GROWTH OF CURVE FOR A BACTERIAL CULTURE

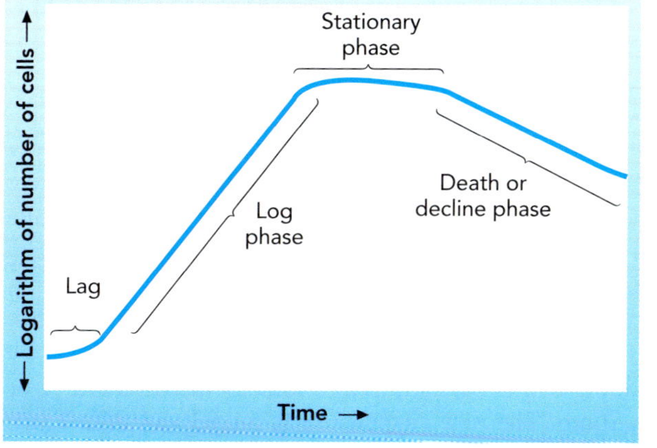

may die instead of dividing. When the rate of cell division equals the rate at which cells are dying, the culture is said to be in the **stationary phase** of growth. Many important secondary metabolites are produced under the limited nutritional conditions encountered in the stationary phase (see Chapter 2, p. 39).

Gradually the rate of cell division stops completely, some of the cells die, so the number of viable cells is reduced and the culture enters the **decline** or **death phase**. Figure 4.13 illustrates the four phases of growth that are usually observed in batch cultures grown in the laboratory in liquid medium.

When cells are grown on solid medium, the dynamics of growth are similar. Single cells rapidly divide until a colony becomes visible to the naked eye. (A colony about 0.1 mm in diameter usually contains 10^4 to 10^5 cells.) Cells at the edge of the colony have a source of nutrients, so continue to divide, but cells in the centre of the colony pile up on top of each other and, without space or access to nutrients, gradually die off.

Continuous culture

Our description of bacterial growth has been confined to cultures in closed or limited environments, such as a tube or flask of liquid medium. Under these conditions, growth is limited by the volume of culture medium contained in the tube or flask. The composition of this medium is continually being altered by the depletion of nutrients and accumulation of wastes. The rate of growth therefore slows down.

In the laboratory it is possible to devise a vessel called a **chemostat** which allows continuous additions of fresh medium and removal of spent medium (Figure 4.14). Cells can also be harvested so that bacterial growth can be maintained in the logarithmic phase. Large quantities of bacteria can be produced by this method. A chemostat can be used for experiments to determine the effect of limiting the amount of various nutrients on the growth of a culture, to prepare large quantities of bacterial cells when required for research or commercial use, or to encourage the formation of secondary metabolites.

Measurement of Bacterial Growth

It is often necessary to determine the number of bacteria present in a sample or to measure the rate at which the bacteria are multiplying. Several methods have been developed in order to measure the number of viable (living) cells present at any given time. Bacterial populations are often very large and it is then necessary to dilute the sample before attempting to measure the number of bacteria present. On the other hand, when estimating the level of faecal contamination in sea water, for example, the

FIGURE 4.14
DIAGRAM OF A CONTINUOUS CULTURE APPARATUS (CHEMOSTAT)

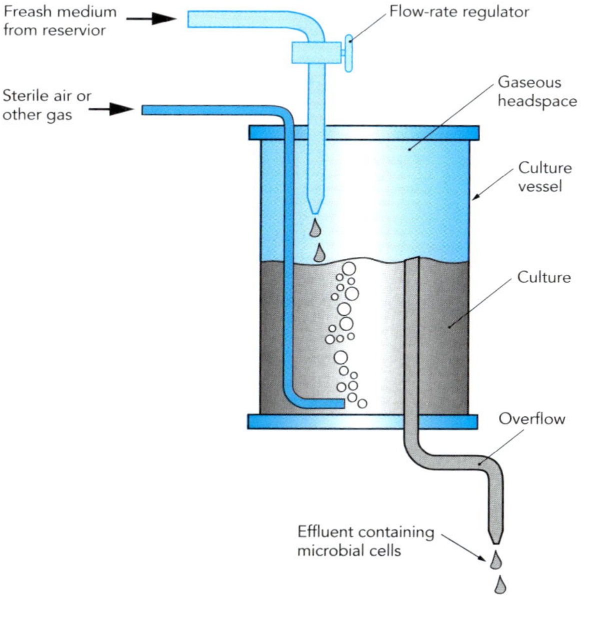

number of bacteria per millilitre may be very small, so it becomes necessary to concentrate the sample to be able to detect accurately the number of bacteria present.

Several methods of measurement are described below.

SERIAL DILUTIONS

In many samples, the number of bacteria present is very large. To ensure that the bacterial count will be as accurate as possible, the inoculum is diluted so that fewer cells are spread on the plate. This makes counting easier and it is more likely that the observed colony has arisen from a single cell. The technique is known as **serial dilution**.

The original suspension of bacteria is diluted 1:10 by adding 1 mL of sample to 9 mL of distilled water or medium. The new suspension is mixed and then 1 mL is taken and further diluted in 9 mL of fresh medium or water in another tube (Figure 4.16). The procedure is continued until a suspension is obtained that appears to be clear and therefore has a measurable number of cells. Then 0.1 mL of this suspension is plated and counted as described below. Each dilution reduces the number of bacteria in the original suspension by a factor of 10. If the original suspension contained 1 million (10^6) cells per millilitre, after three dilutions it would contain 1000 (10^3) cells per millilitre. A 0.1 mL sample would give rise to 100 colonies, which can be accurately counted.

This method is used to determine bacterial populations when a heavy growth is present. It is used in food microbiology and public health laboratories. A weighed sample of food, suspected of being contaminated, is suspended in a known volume of liquid. Serial dilutions are made and a plate count carried out. Multiplying back to the original sample, the level of contamination can be determined.

PLATE COUNT

This technique is based on the assumption that each single bacterium, when inoculated onto an agar plate, gives rise to a single visible colony under specified conditions of temperature, time and culture medium. One advantage of this method is that only viable (live) cells are counted. The sample (usually 0.1 mL) is spread uniformly over the surface of a prepared agar plate, using a sterile glass spreader (see Figure 4.15). The plate is incubated, usually for 24 hours. It is then examined and the number of colonies, or **colony forming units** (cfu) are counted. The number of colonies per 0.1 mL sample is then multiplied by the dilution and total volume of the original sample to determine the number of bacteria present. Disadvantages of this method include the time taken to obtain a result and the fact that sometimes bacteria are clumped together so that more than one bacterium may have given rise to the observed colony. This is why the results are usually expressed as colony forming units.

FIGURE 4.15
SERIAL DILUTIONS AND PLATE COUNTS
The number of bacteria present in a suspension is determined by carrying out serial dilutions. The bacterial suspension is diluted tenfold in a series of test tubes until a dilution is reached which enables an accurate colony count to be made when a sample from the tube is grown on a plate.

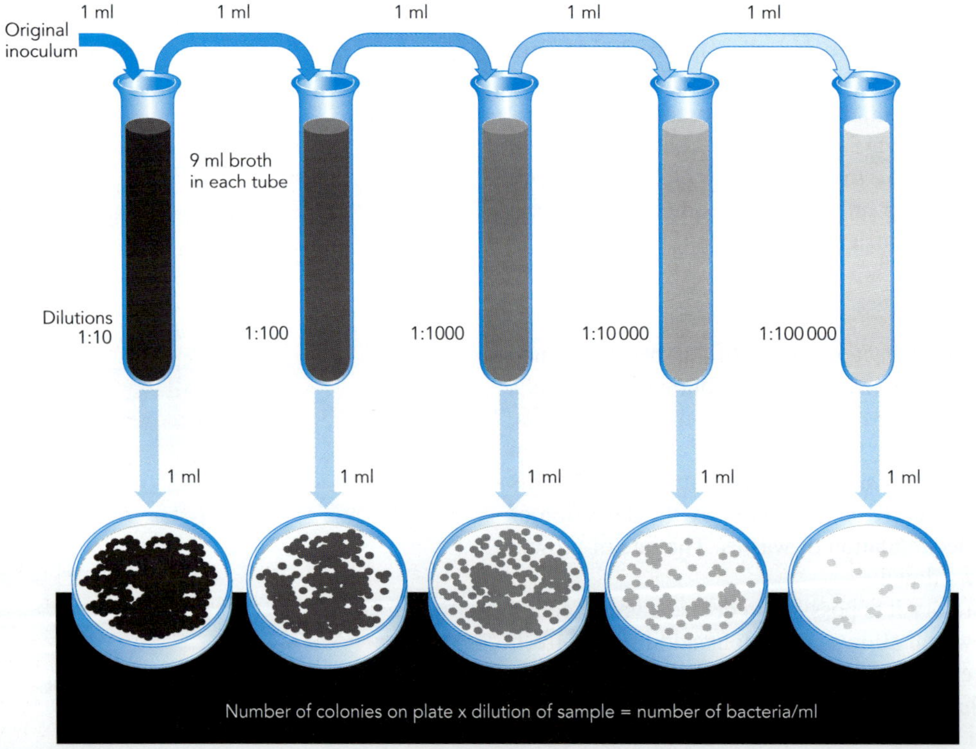

Another method is to place the sample on a layer of agar in a plate and then pour a thin layer of agar on top, mixing them together before the agar sets. Disadvantages are that this method is more time-consuming, and occasionally the hot liquid agar may destroy heat-sensitive organisms.

FILTRATION

When the concentration of bacteria is very small, as in water samples for example, it is necessary to concentrate the sample to obtain an accurate measurement. A known volume, say 100 mL, is passed through a sterile filter equipped with a filter paper which retains bacteria. The paper is then transferred to an agar plate and incubated. The number of colony forming units can be counted and the level of contamination in the original sample determined. Growth on different selective media can be used to help identify the bacteria.

DIRECT MICROSCOPIC COUNT

This method is useful when a quick estimate of the number of bacteria is required. It is used in routine diagnostic laboratories, especially for urine samples. A measured volume is placed on a special microscope slide with a calibrated chamber. The organisms present in each square of the grid are counted, an average number determined and the concentration of the bacterial cells in the original sample calculated. This method requires a bacterial concentration of at least 10^7 cells per millilitre and does not distinguish between living and dead cells. It is useful because it is possible at the same time to report on the presence of red blood cells, epithelial cells and pus cells, all of which are an aid in clinical diagnosis (see Chapter 15).

TURBIDITY

As bacteria multiply in liquid medium, the culture becomes cloudy or turbid. One simple way to measure growth is by measuring the level of turbidity using a spectrophotometer or colorimeter. This machine measures the amount of light passing through a solution. As the bacterial suspension becomes thicker, the amount of light transmitted through the bacterial culture decreases and can be measured by placing the culture tube in the path of a beam of light. A calibration curve is established relating the number of bacteria present to the amount of light transmitted (**absorbance**). This method is useful within certain limits of cell concentration (10^6 to 10^{12} cells per mL). If the suspension is too thin it does not absorb light and if too thick the direct proportionality no longer applies.

In research laboratories, turbidity is a useful method of monitoring the growth of a culture so that the bacteria can be harvested at a certain phase of their growth. Some culture flasks have a special photometer tube attached to the flask so that the turbidity of the culture can be continuously monitored. However, no distinction is made between live and dead cells.

METABOLIC ACTIVITY

Metabolic activity can be used as an indicator of the presence of bacteria. Rather than estimating the number of viable bacterial cells directly, the level of a specific metabolic product or an enzyme is measured. It is then assumed that the amount of this product is proportional to the number of bacteria present. For example, the rate at which a gas such as CO_2 is produced can be measured. These tests are useful to show the presence of a particular bacterial species but are not very accurate.

Classification of Bacteria

The previous sections have described the appearance and structure (morphology) of bacteria and their growth requirements. There are many thousands of different strains of bacteria and it is essential to have some method of grouping or classifying them.

NOMENCLATURE AND PROPERTIES

As we explained in Chapter 1, bacteria belong to the **Monera** or **Procaryotic** kingdom in the five-kingdom classification. Within this classification all bacteria are given two names: the **genus**, usually signified by a capital letter, followed by the **species**. For example, *Staphylococcus aureus* and *Staphylococcus epidermidis* are the names of two different species within the same genus. A species may consist of a collection of similar strains that differ slightly from each other. The strain is usually designated by a letter or number after the species, for example, *Escherichia* (genus) *coli* (species) K12 (strain).

The formidable task of classifying bacteria has been undertaken by a team of microbiologists and published under the title of *Bergey's Manual of Systematic Bacteriology*. The basis for the classification includes properties such as cell wall structure, Gram stain, shape, motility, oxygen requirements and biochemical properties. It is beyond the scope of this text to discuss the classification scheme, but it is important for students to be aware of the enormous diversity of microorganisms and the complexity of isolation and identification procedures. Some of this diversity is shown in the photographs in Figure 4.16. A brief description of the bacteria in some sections of Bergey's manual is included below.

PHAGE-TYPING OF BACTERIAL STRAINS

Another useful method of classification should be mentioned here. Some bacteria are attacked by viruses that are specific for a particular strain of bacteria within a species. A bacterial virus is called a **bacteriophage** or **phage**. Bacteria isolated from different sources can be tested for their susceptibility to a particular phage. This helps to identify the strain of bacteria and can assist in epidemiological studies when clinicians are trying to

FIGURE 4.16

DIVERSITY OF BACTERIAL MORPHOLOGY

The differences in size, shape and arrangement of cells can be seen in Gram-stained preparations (a) Staphylococcus aureus; (b) Bacillus subtilis; (c) Kelbsiella pneumoniae; (d) Colstridium tetani.

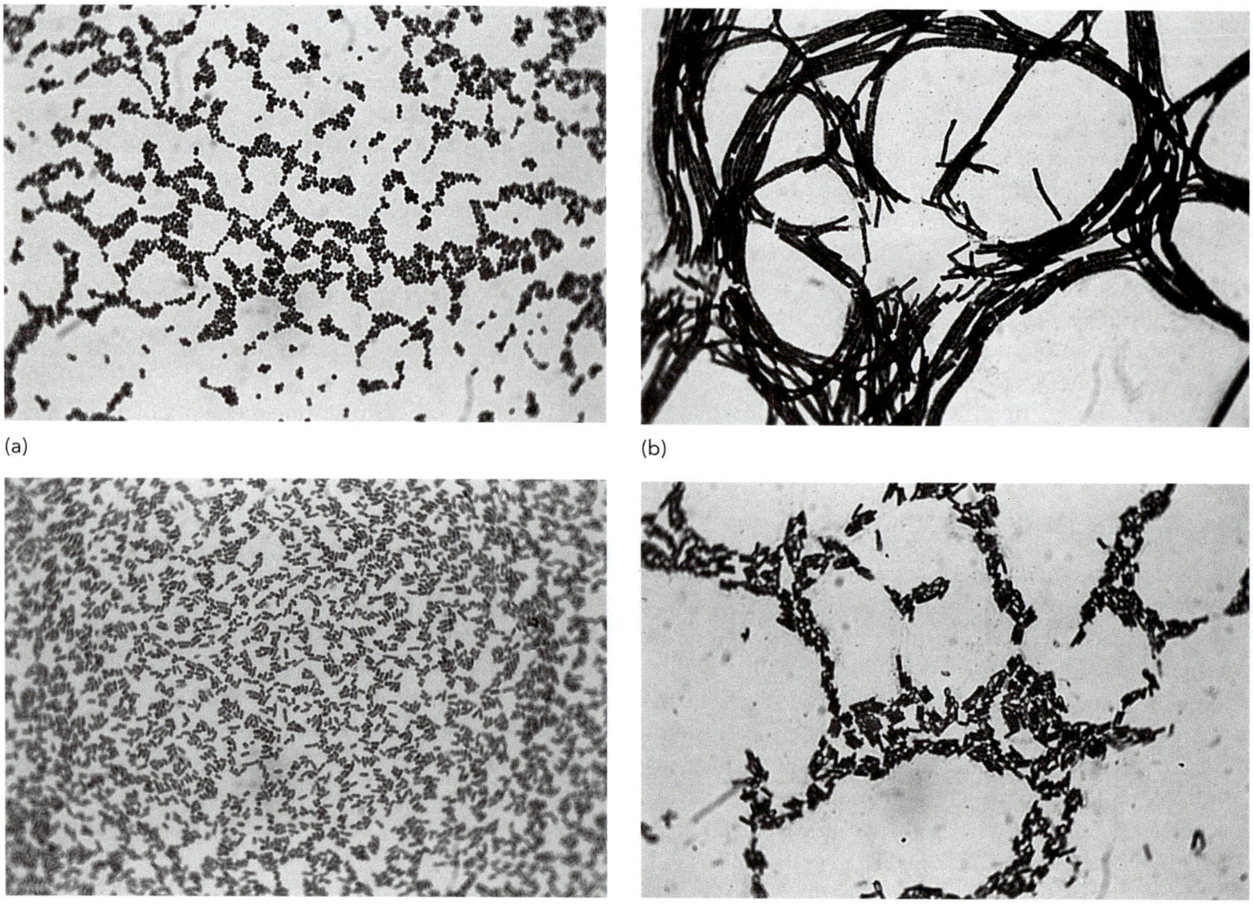

(a) (b) (c) (d)

identify the source of an outbreak of infection. For example *Staphylococcus aureus* is frequently isolated from the noses of health personnel. Phage typing of the strain of *Staphylococcus* and comparison with the phage type of the outbreak can help identify the source or carrier of the infection. (See Figure 4.17.)

FIGURE 4.17

PHAGE TYPING OF *STAPHYLOCOCCUS AUREUS*

A culture of the strain to be tested is spread over the whole plate and different phages inoculated in rows on the plate. The development of areas of lysis or 'plaques' indicates that the strain of *Staphylococcus* is sensitive to infection by some of the phages and allows identification of the strain.

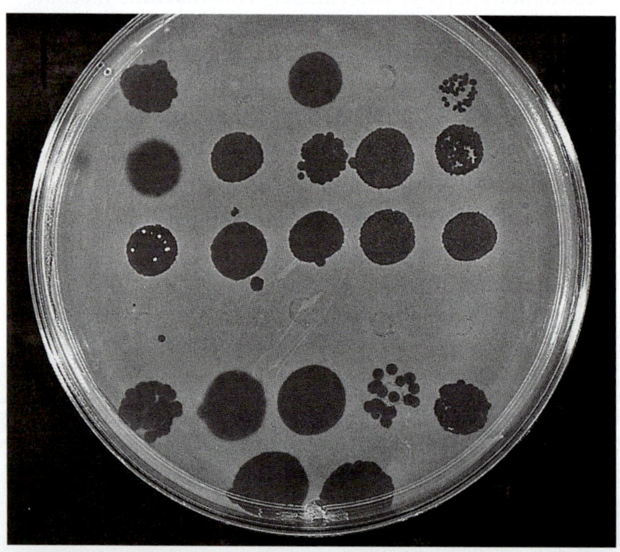

A POSSIBLE NEW APPROACH TO CLASSIFICATION

Bergey's manual relies on established methods of identification and classification—that is, morphology (appearance), and chemical and physical properties such as staining. New methods in molecular biology and DNA analysis mean that it is now possible to compare the composition of the genetic material of different bacteria. This new approach has already resulted in some revision of the accepted classifications and there may be more in the future.

Bacteria of Medical Importance

Bergey's system of classification consists of four divisions and 33 sections and covers hundreds of genera and thousands of species. We deal briefly here with some of the sections which contain organisms of medical importance. (Note that each of the following headings refers to one of Bergey's sections.)

SPIROCHAETES

The **spirochaetes** are long (10 μm) Gram-negative helical bacteria containing two or more axial filaments for motility, giving them a distinctive corkscrew-like appearance. Some are free-living, occurring in sewage, mud and decaying organic matter. Others inhabit humans and animals as part of the normal flora. Among the spirochaetes are the causative organism of the sexually transmitted disease, syphilis—*Treponema pallidum* (see Chapter 21). Members of the genus *Borrelia*, which are usually transmitted by ticks, are responsible for relapsing fever and Lyme disease (see Chapter 19). *Leptospira* species are often acquired from water contaminated with animal faeces or urine and cause a disease characterised by kidney and liver damage.

AEROBIC/MICROAEROPHILIC, MOTILE, HELICAL/VIBRIOID, GRAM-NEGATIVE BACTERIA

These spiral bacteria do not have an axial filament but use flagella for motility. *Campylobacter jejuni* is an important pathogen responsible for food-borne gastrointestinal infections. *Helicobacter pylori* has been shown to be associated with gastric ulcers in humans.

GRAM-NEGATIVE AEROBIC RODS AND COCCI

This is a very large group of organisms, many of which are important human pathogens. The **pseudomonads** are aerobic rods with flagella. Many of these synthesise distinctive pigments ranging in colour from blue through greenish-yellow to brown. They exist mainly in water and soil.

Pseudomonas aeruginosa is an important opportunistic pathogen. It is often responsible for serious infections in immunocompromised patients, especially in burns units. Its ability to grow in water with only minimal nutrients and its resistance to many disinfectants, antiseptics and antibiotics means that it poses a particular threat in the hospital environment.

Legionella is a genus that was only recently discovered after an outbreak of atypical pneumonia in the United States. It is the cause of Legionnaires' disease and is spread mainly in water as aerosol droplets dispersed by wind from reservoirs such as the water cooling towers of air conditioning plants, where the bacteria are growing.

The genus *Neisseria* comprises non-endospore-forming diplococci which only grow well at body temperatures. It includes two important pathogens: *Neisseria gonorrhea*, the causative agent of gonorrhea and *Neisseria meningitidis* (meningitis) (see Chapter 21).

Other important pathogenic organisms in this section include: *Moraxella*, aerobic coccobacilli that cause conjunctivitis; *Brucella* (brucellosis); and *Bordetella pertussis*, the causative organism of whooping cough. *Francisella tularensis* is a fastidious organism that requires media enriched with blood or tissue extracts for growth, and causes tularemia. The *Acetobacter* are aerobic organisms which convert alcohol to vinegar and are used industrially.

FACULTATIVELY ANAEROBIC GRAM-NEGATIVE RODS

These form an important group of bacteria. Some of them are found on the human body as part of the normal flora and many of them are responsible for causing diseases of the gastrointestinal tract and other organs.

The **Enterobacteriaceae (enterics)** form a large group of organisms, many of which inhabit the human intestine. Because they are so important, a series of diagnostic tests for biochemical properties and serology of surface antigens has been developed for their identification (see Chapter 15). The most important genera are *Escherichia, Salmonella, Shigella, Klebsiella, Serratia, Proteus, Yersinia* and *Enterobacter*.

Escherichia coli (*E. coli*) is one of the most common inhabitants of the human intestine. Its presence is often used as an indication of faecal contamination ('coliform' count). It is generally considered to be part of the normal flora and relatively non-pathogenic, unless it is transferred to body sites other than the colon. It is one of the most common causes of urinary tract infections and some strains produce enterotoxins that can cause diarrhoea. Almost all the members of the genus *Salmonella* are pathogenic. *Salmonella typhi* is responsible for typhoid fever. Other *Salmonella* are responsible for various gastrointestinal diseases associated with food poisoning. The different strains are identified on the basis of their surface antigens which are referred to as 'serovars' or 'serotypes'. Species of *Shigella* are responsible for a severe type of diarrhoea called bacillary dysentery or shigellosis, caused by the ingestion of contaminated food.

Among other enterics, *Klebsiella pneumoniae* is a major cause of pneumonia, especially in children and susceptible patients, *Proteus* is an inhabitant of the large intestine and a common cause of urinary tract and wound infections. It has a distinctive 'swarming' appearance when grown on plates in the laboratory and an unpleasant odour. *Enterobacter cloacae* and *E. aerogenes* are opportunistic pathogens which may cause urinary tract or nosocomial infections. *Serratia marcescens* grows at room temperature with the production of a distinctive red pigment. In recent years it has been recognised as a significant cause of opportunistic hospital-acquired infections. The most pathogenic of all the enterics is *Yersinia pestis*, the cause of bubonic and pneumonic plague (see Chapter 19).

The **Vibrionaceae** are a family of curved Gram-negative rods. The most important members are *Vibrio cholera*, which causes cholera, and *Vibrio parahaemolyticus*, which is often found in shellfish and causes a form of gastroenteritis.

Pasteurellaceae are very small Gram-negative bacilli and coccobacilli. They are non-motile and are very fastidious in their nutritional requirements. *Pasteurella* species infect mainly animals but can be transmitted to humans.

Haemophilus influenzae is an important human pathogen. Although it is often present as part of the normal flora in the upper respiratory tract, it is a common cause of middle ear infections and is responsible for potentially fatal meningitis and epiglottitis in young children. A vaccine for *Haemophilus influenzae* type b (Hib) is now available in Australia.

ANAEROBIC, GRAM-NEGATIVE, STRAIGHT, CURVED AND HELICAL RODS

The most important of this group are members of the genus *Bacteroides*, which live in the human gastrointestinal tract. They are non-motile, do not form endospores and are often responsible for infections due to puncture wounds or surgery, and for peritonitis.

RICKETTSIAS AND CHLAMYDIAS

These are very small, obligate, intracellular parasites and were not at first classified as bacteria, because they can only reproduce inside a living cell. **Rickettsias** are rod-shaped bacteria or coccobacilli that are **pleomorphic** (have many forms). They are Gram-negative and non-motile and most of them are transmitted to humans by insects and ticks. Some of the diseases caused by rickettsias include epidemic and endemic typhus, Rocky Mountains spotted fever in the United States, and scrub typhus in Australia. Q fever, caused by *Coxiella burnetii*, is harboured by ticks but can also be transmitted in aerosols and milk.

Chlamydias are also Gram-negative, non-motile, intracellular parasites and are transmitted by close person-to-person contact. They have a complex developmental cycle. In the host cell they develop inside membrane-bound cytoplasmic vacuoles, forming large metabolically active reticulate bodies. These divide many times by binary fission, rupture and release the smaller infectious particle, or elementary body, which can attack other cells. *Chlamydia trachomatis* is the agent responsible for trachoma. The organism can also be sexually transmitted and is a primary cause of non-gonococcal urethritis and pelvic inflammatory disease. *C. pneumoniae*, a cause of pneumonia, has recently been identified. *C. psittaci* is the agent responsible for psittacosis in birds and can also infect humans.

MYCOPLASMAS

Mycoplasmas are very small bacteria that do not form cell walls. They are mainly aerobic or facultatively anaerobic. Since they are not bound by a rigid cell wall, they are capable of assuming many shapes (**pleomorphic**), often producing fungus-like filaments. *Mycoplasma pneumoniae* is the cause of atypical pneumonia. The mycoplasmas and the **ureaplasmas** are often inhabitants of the vagina and are thought to be involved in intrauterine infections in pregnancy which may result in abortion.

GRAM-POSITIVE COCCI

Many of the medically important bacteria are Gram-positive cocci. The staphylococci and streptococci which are responsible for many skin and wound infections, belong to this group. **Staphylococci** appear as grape-like clusters when viewed under the microscope. They are very tolerant in their growth requirements, surviving in conditions of relatively low moisture and high osmotic pressure (e.g. high salt concentration).

Staphylococcus aureus and *Staphylococcus epidermidis* are two common inhabitants of the human body, being found in areas of low moisture such as the nose or skin. Because of their tolerance for salt and dry conditions, staphylococci are often present in salted or preserved meats, such as bacon. *Staphylococcus aureus* produces various toxins which contribute to its pathogenicity. It is a common cause of food poisoning, producing an enterotoxin that causes diarrhoea and vomiting. It has also been identified as the agent responsible for toxic shock syndrome and is a major cause of wound infections in hospitals. Here it poses a serious threat because of its ability to quickly develop a resistance to antibiotics. *Staphylococcus aureus* can be distinguished from *Staphylococcus epidermidis* (also a major cause of wound infections) by its ability to produce the enzyme, coagulase, and also by growth on the differential medium, mannitol salt, in which it produces a yellow colour due to a pH change in the medium. (See Figure 2.19.)

Streptococci are Gram-positive cocci that usually occur in chains of varying length (although *Streptococcus pneumoniae* typically occurs in pairs). They are responsible for a wide variety of diseases: wound and throat infections, scarlet fever, glomerulonephritis, pneumonia etc. (described in Unit IV). They are often classified by their growth on blood agar. Beta (ß)-haemolytic streptococci produce an enzyme that lyses red blood cells, creating clear areas of haemolysis on blood agar plates. Alpha (α)-haemolytic species reduce haemoglobin (red) to methaemoglobin (green), causing a colour change on blood plates. Gamma (γ) or non-haemolytic streptococci have no effect on red blood cells.

ENDOSPORE-FORMING, GRAM-POSITIVE RODS AND COCCI

Some organisms form endospores as a means of survival under adverse environmental conditions. Some of these organisms are important pathogens. The two most important genera are *Bacillus* and *Clostridium*. *Bacillus anthracis* is the agent responsible for anthrax, a serious disease of cattle which can also affect humans. *Bacillus thuringiensis* is an insect pathogen.

Members of the genus *Clostridium* produce endospores that are highly resistant to heat. They are obligate anaerobes and produce toxins that are responsible for some serious human diseases. These include tetanus (*Clostridium tetani*), botulism (*Cl. botulinum*), and gangrene and food poisoning (*Cl. perfringens*).

REGULAR NON-SPORING GRAM-POSITIVE RODS

This group includes the genus *Lactobacillus*, whose members are able to produce lactic acid during carbohydrate fermentation. In humans they are found in the vagina, where they maintain a protective, slightly acid environment; they also occur in the intestinal tract and oral cavity. They are used extensively in the food industry in the production of cheese, soured milk products and pickles, the lactic acid acting as a food preservative.

Listeria monocytogenes is a Gram-positive rod which sometimes contaminates dairy products. It poses a serious threat to pregnant women, causing damage to the foetus or even stillbirth.

IRREGULAR NON-SPORING GRAM-POSITIVE RODS

This group includes some organisms that tend to be pleomorphic (i.e. their shape varies, often with the age of the cells). Best known are the **corynebacteria**, which tend to be club-shaped. *Corynebacterium diphtheriae* is the causative agent of diphtheria. *Propionibacterium acnes* is found on the skin and is thought to be implicated in the skin infection, acne. Members of the genus *Actinomyces* are commonly found in the mouth and throat of humans and animals. They often form branched filaments. *A. viscocus* is involved in the colonisation of tooth surfaces, as a prelude to plaque formation by *Streptococcus mutans* and subsequent tooth decay.

MYCOBACTERIA

Mycobacteria are aerobic rod-shaped organisms that occasionally form filaments. They do not stain well with the Gram stain as they are surrounded by a waxy outer layer. The acid-fast stain is used instead (see Chapter 3). Among the pathogenic species (acid-fast bacilli), *Mycobacterium tuberculosis* causes tuberculosis and *Mycobacterium leprae* is the causative organism of leprosy.

NOCARDIOFORMS

Nocardia are filamentous aerobic organisms. Their cell wall is similar to the mycobacteria; and are acid fast. *Nocardia asteroides* is the major pathogen in this group, causing skin abscesses and lung infections.

OTHER SECTIONS OF *BERGEY'S MANUAL*

The other major groups of bacteria—**gliding bacteria**, **appendaged bacteria**, **chemoautotrophs**, **archaeobacteria**, the **photosynthetic bacteria** and the **actinomycetes**—will not be described here as they are not significant pathogens. Members of the genus *Streptomyces* are important as a source of antibiotics (see Chapter 11).

Bacterial Genetics

The study of bacterial genetics has become an increasingly important area of research in recent years. A full description is beyond the scope of this book, but some aspects of this topic have special significance for the health professional. This section examines the structure of the genetic material (genes), its method of replication, the way in which cells synthesise nucleic acids, their involvement in protein synthesis, and the way genes direct and control cellular function. The effect on the cell when the composition of the DNA is altered by mutation or manipulation by scientists is discussed. The material presented here is an overview of the topic to help 'demystify' some of the jargon that is used, and show how an understanding of genetic processes can assist in the control and treatment of disease. The references at the end of the chapter offer a more detailed description.

All the characteristics of bacterial cells described in this chapter are determined by the genetic material, or genes, of the cell.

What are genes and how do they control cellular activity?

Genes are linear sequences of nucleotides of DNA (deoxyribonucleic acid). Each gene consists of a specific sequence of nucleotides and is responsible for determining a particular characteristic of the cell. **Nucleotides** consist of nitrogen-containing compounds, called 'bases', joined to the sugar, deoxyribose, and to phosphate. The nucleotide bases are the purines, **adenine** and **guanine**, and the pyrimidines, **thymine** and **cytosine** (see Figure 4.18(a)).

A number of genes are joined together to form a structure called a **chromosome**. In bacteria, all the genetic material is contained in a single circular chromosome containing many thousands of genes. Some bacteria contain one or more additional pieces of DNA called **plasmids**. Eucaryotic cells usually have more than one chromosome and the DNA exists in association with proteins called **histones**.

STRUCTURE OF DNA

The name 'nucleic acid' is derived from early studies which showed that the substance carrying hereditary traits was located in the nucleus of the cell. When DNA was first isolated and chemically analysed in the 1940s, it was found that the amount of thymine present was approximately the same as the amount of adenine and the amount of cytosine was approximately equal to guanine. However, the significance of this finding was not readily apparent and it was necessary to further elucidate the unique structure of DNA in order to understand that the pairing of these bases provided a mechanism for genetic information to be preserved and transferred accurately during cell division.

Careful research by the English scientists, Max Wilkins and Rosalind Franklin, using X-ray crystallography of DNA, led James Watson and Francis Crick in 1952 to propose a structure for DNA that has laid the basis for our understanding of genetic inheritance.

The double helix

DNA consists of two strands of nucleotides twisted around each other into a double helical structure. The nucleotide bases are arranged in a specific sequence in each strand. The strand has a backbone of sugar and phosphate from which the bases protrude (see Figure 4.18(a)).

FIGURE 4.18
STRUCTURE OF DNA
(a) pairing of nitrogenous bases in sugar-phosphate backbone; (b) helical structure of DNA.

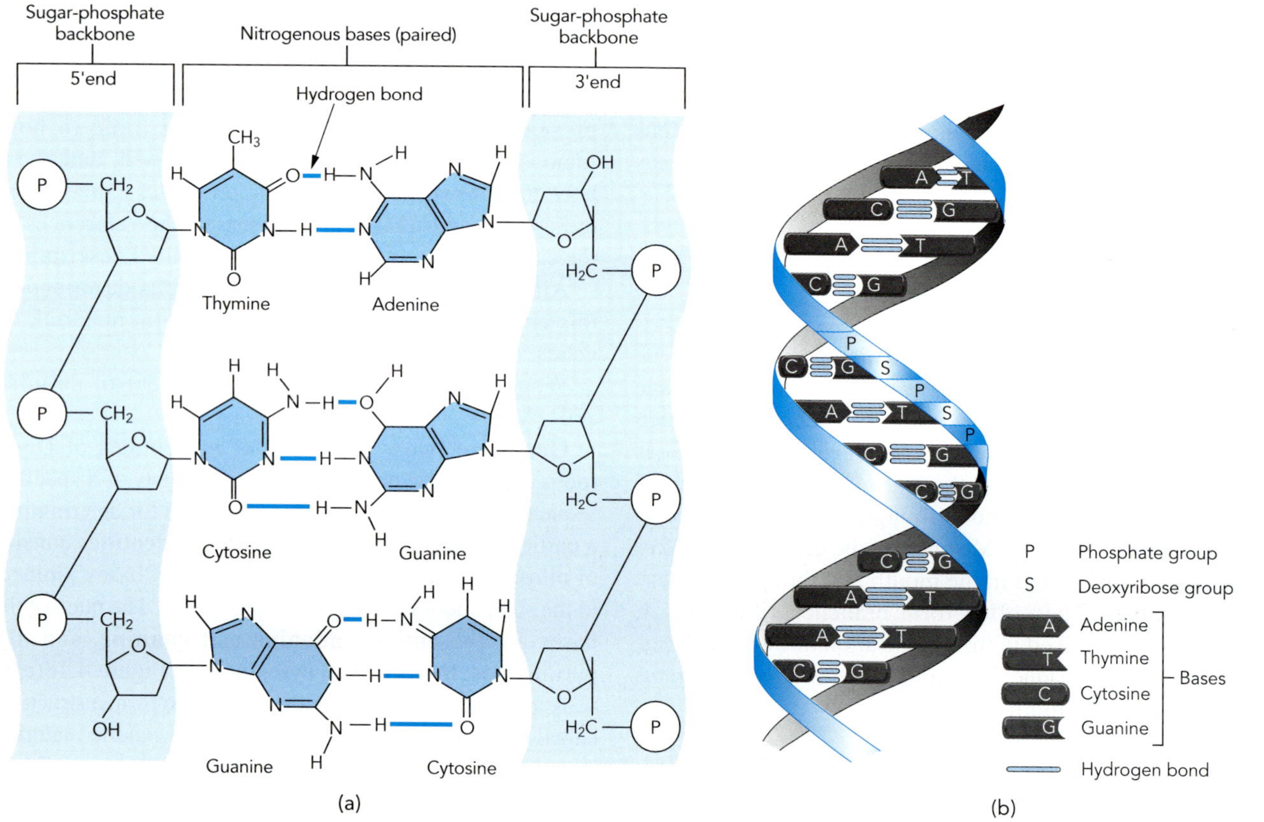

To enable the two strands to fit together into a double helix, the bases have to be held together by hydrogen bonds between the opposing strands, with adenine opposite thymine and guanine opposite cytosine. This explains the equal ratios of adenine to thymine and guanine to cytosine.

Figure 4.19(b) shows the simple, elegant structure proposed for DNA. It explains the unique properties of the genetic material and, in particular, allows for the exact replication of the nucleotide sequence. The sequence of nucleotides in one strand exactly complements the sequence in the other strand, but runs in the opposite direction. A gene consists of a number of nucleotides, and one DNA molecule may contain thousands of genes.

Nucleic acid synthesis

The elucidation of the structure of DNA showed how genetic properties could be preserved from cell to cell. The sequence of nucleotides in each strand acts as a pattern, or **template**, for the synthesis of the new strand. DNA replication involves the separation of the two strands of DNA, and the building up of a new strand of DNA on each of the original strands. Base pairing ensures two new identical double helices are formed (see Figure 4.19).

PROTEIN SYNTHESIS

Most activities of the cell are carried out by proteins. Enzymes are proteins, as are many of the structural components of the cell. The information needed for the synthesis of these proteins is contained in the DNA, so the cell needs a way of using this information to direct the synthesis of the correct proteins. This is done by involving another type of nucleic acid called **RNA** (**ribonucleic acid**). Ribonucleic acid differs from DNA in that the sugar molecule is ribose and one of the bases, thymine, is replaced by the closely related purine molecule, uracil. In addition, RNA does not occur as a double helix, but usually in single strands.

There are three distinct types of RNA, varying in molecular size and function.

1. **Ribosomal RNA (rRNA)** is a large molecule that combines with protein to form particles called ribosomes, which are the site of protein synthesis in all cells.
2. **Messenger RNA (mRNA)**, which carries the information or 'message' from the chromosome to the site of protein synthesis, is a single strand of RNA that is synthesised on the DNA template.
3. **Transfer RNA (tRNA)** is a small molecule, the function of which is to transfer amino acids to the mRNA strand on the ribosomes in the cytoplasm, and ensure that the correct amino acid is added to the growing peptide chain.

Mechanism of protein synthesis

The synthesis of a functional protein with the correct amino acid sequence is dependent on the information in the genes of the DNA being correctly transferred. Special terms are used to describe this process.

FIGURE 4.19
REPLICATION OF DNA

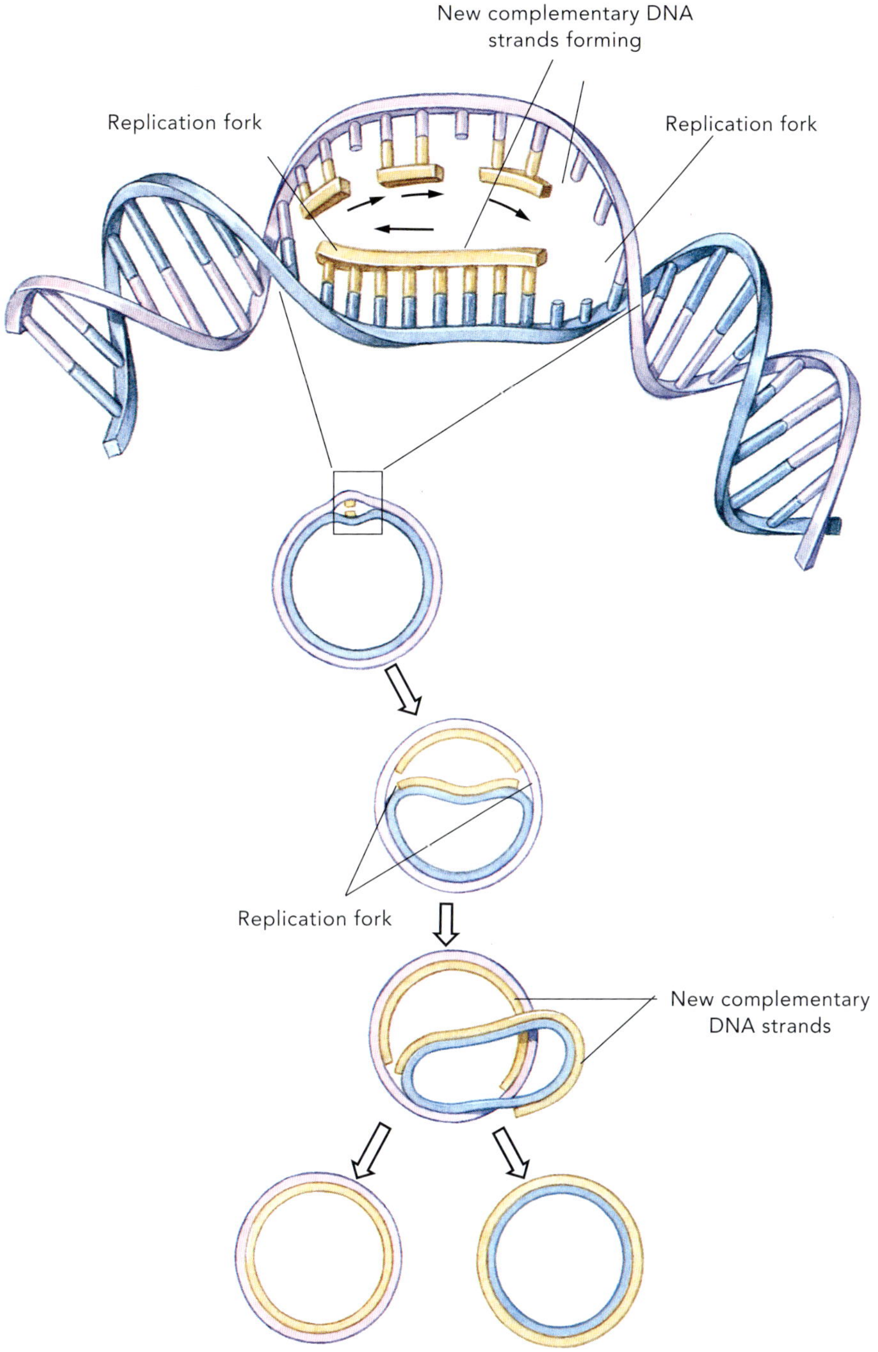

- **Transcription** is the term applied to the synthesis of mRNA on the DNA template, i.e. the formation of a single strand of ribonucleic acid with a base sequence complementary to the base sequence of the DNA. The DNA is *transcribed* into a different form. The process could be likened to changing handwritten information into a typewritten form, but keeping the same language.
- **Translation** refers to the formation of a protein or polypeptide composed of a chain of amino acids, using the mRNA as a template or pattern to ensure that the correct amino acid is inserted into the correct place. The product here is a compound composed of amino acids instead of the nucleotides of the RNA and DNA. This process, therefore, can be likened to translating a message from one language to another (English to French, for example). In this case the information in the nucleic acid is *translated* into protein.

The process can be summarised as follows:

$$\text{DNA} \xrightarrow{\text{transcription}} \text{mRNA} \xrightarrow{\text{translation}} \text{protein.}$$

During **transcription**, the double strands of DNA are pulled apart and an enzyme called RNA polymerase binds to one of the strands of DNA at a site called the promoter.

RNA nucleotides are then paired with the complementary DNA bases—adenine with thymine, uracil with adenine, and guanine with cytosine. As the messenger RNA is synthesised, the section of DNA that has been transcribed rejoins. When a terminator gene is reached, the RNA polymerase and the new mRNA are released. The mRNA that is produced may be a sequence containing the information for only one gene or for several closely related genes. The newly formed mRNA moves from the DNA to the ribosomes, where it is attached and acts as a template or pattern for the formation of protein molecules.

Proteins consist of long chains of amino acids, in a specific sequence. During **translation**, the mRNA has to be able to direct the incorporation of amino acids into polypeptide chains in the correct sequence. How is this achieved?

In the 1960s several scientists working in the United States realised that the sequence of the four nucleotide bases in the nucleic acid molecules could determine which amino acid was incorporated into the protein. They were able to show that a specific sequence of three nucleotide bases, called a **codon**, was responsible for the binding of each particular amino acid.

There are four different nucleotides. It can be calculated that they can be arranged in $4 \times 4 \times 4 = 64$ different codons, more than enough for the 20 amino acids found in proteins. We now know that some amino acids have more than one codon and some codons contain other messages, such as 'stop' and 'start'. Table 4.3 shows the nucleotide codon for each amino acid.

One further discovery was necessary to complete the picture. It was already known that small molecules of RNA, called **transfer RNA** (tRNA), could bind to amino acids. It was found that there was a specific tRNA for each amino acid and that this tRNA had a corresponding sequence of three nucleotides that could recognise the correct codon on the messenger RNA (see Figure 4.20). It was now possible to visualise a scheme whereby the genetic information in the DNA could be translated into functional proteins (see Figure 4.21).

The accurate transfer of the genetic information contained in the DNA of the cell into functional proteins is of primary importance in all living cells. It is sometimes said that a gene is **expressed** or **not expressed.** This refers to whether or not the cell is actually producing a particular protein for which it has the gene. Most cells carry information for characteristics (proteins) which they do

FIGURE 4.20
TRANSCRIPTION FROM DNA TO RNA
The two-dimensional structure of a molecule of transfer RNA. The anticodon end will pair up with a codon on a strand of messenger RNA and deliver the desired amino acid, which is bonded to its other end. The molecule is maintained in its cloverleaf pattern by hydrogen bonding between strands that form the arms (dotted lines).

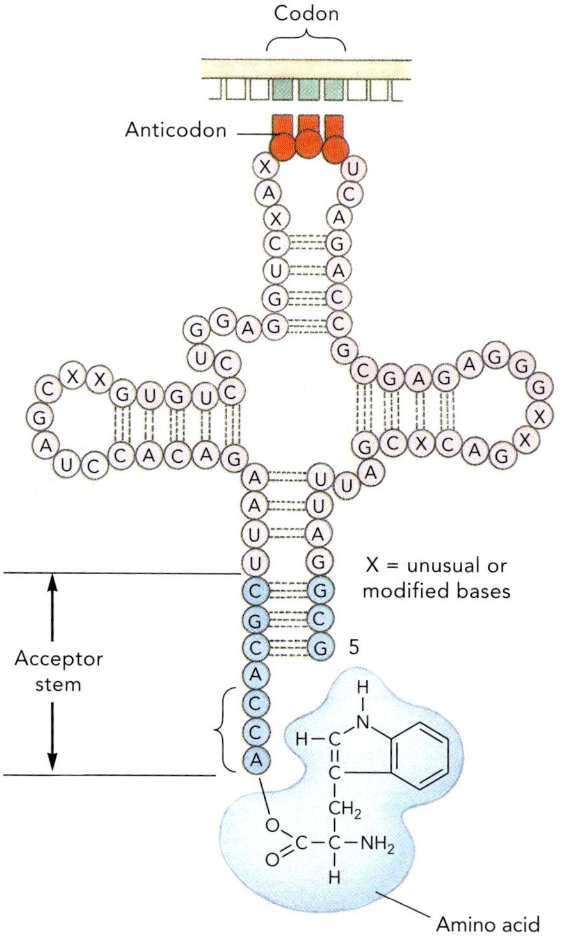

TABLE 4.3
THE GENETIC CODE

Codons are written with the 5'-terminal nucleotide on the left. Note that most amino acids are represented by more than one codon and that variation at the third nucleotide in a codon is common.

Amino acids are written as follows:

Ala	Arg	Asp	Asn	Cys	Glu	Gln	Gly	His	Ileu	Leu	Lys	Met	Phe	Pro	Ser	Thr	Trp	Tyr	Val	Stop
GCU	CGU	GAU	AAU	UGU	GAG	CAG	GGU	CAU	AUU	CUU	AAG	AUG	UUU	CCU	UCU	ACU	UGG	UAU	GUU	UGA
GCG	CGG	GAC	AAC	UGC	GAA	CAA	GGG	CAC	AUC	CUG	AAA		UCC	CCG	UCG	ACG		UAC	GUG	UAG
GCC	CGC						GGC		AUA	CUC				CCC	UCC	ACC			GUC	UAA
GCA	CGA						GGA			CUA				CCA	UCA	ACA			GUA	
	AGG									UUG					AGU					
	AGA									UUA					AGC					

FIGURE 4.21
MAIN STEPS IN PROTEIN SYNTHESIS
Diagrammatic representation of the events in protein synthesis. Genetic information encoded in DNA is transcribed into messenger RNA. The mRNA attaches to ribosomes in the cytoplasm and acts as a template for the insertion of the correct sequence of amino acids into the growing peptide chain by matching the codons on the transfer RNA.

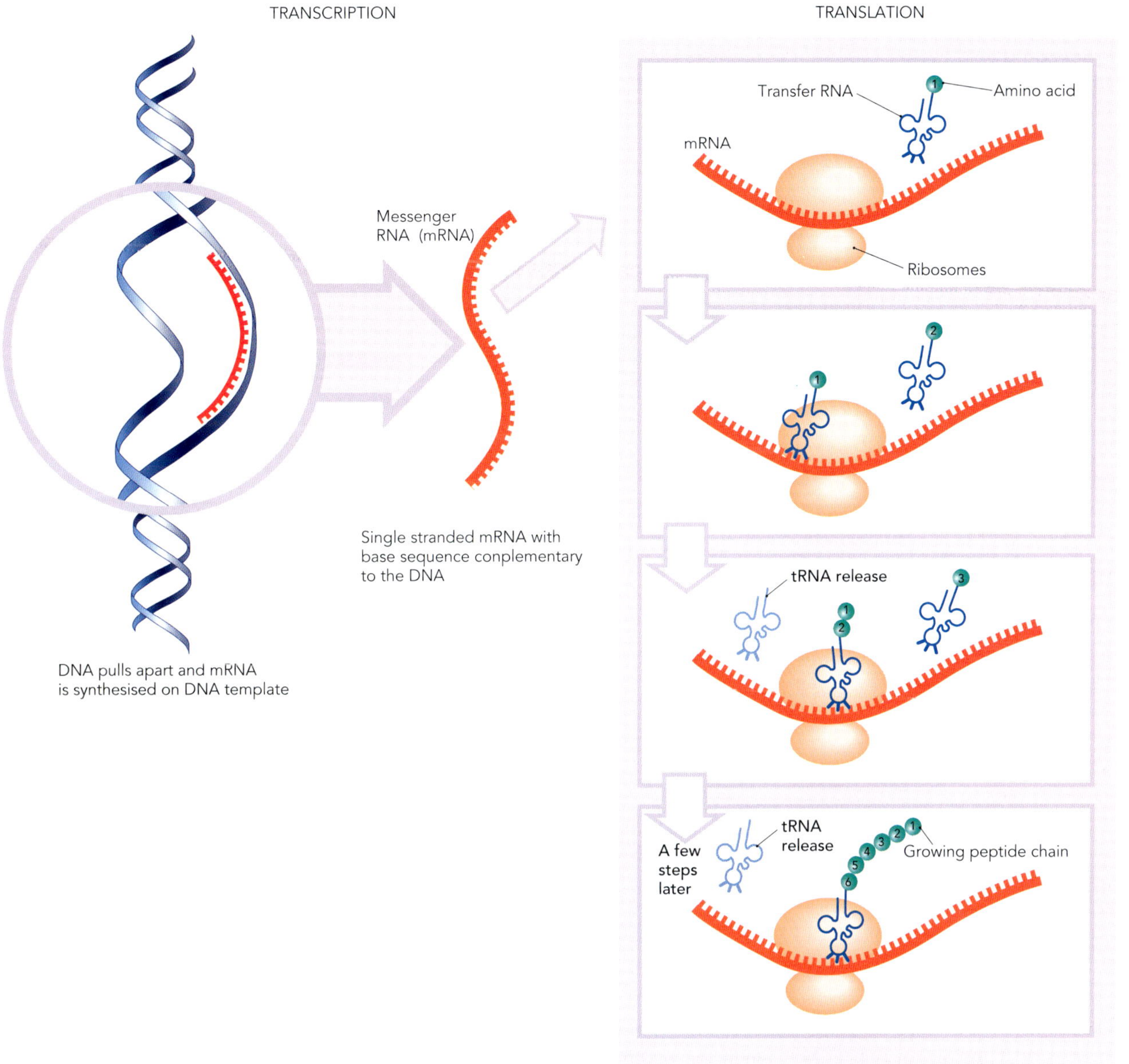

not need to use all the time. Bacteria, especially, are very small and there is no space in the cell for proteins that are not actually carrying out a function. Thus, although the bacteria may carry the gene, it may not necessarily be expressed. It is rather like having a book full of recipes (the DNA) which are only used when required. This characteristic enables bacteria to make best use of their nutritional environment. This property of bacteria was discovered when it was found that *E. coli* only synthesised the enzymes necessary for the metabolism of lactose when it was grown in a medium containing lactose.

The mechanism that hinders the expression of a gene is called **repression**, and is usually mediated by special proteins called **repressors**, which interfere with the transcription of the gene to mRNA. On the other hand, substances such as lactose act as **inducers** to induce the transcription of the genes responsible for coding of enzymes necessary for lactose metabolism. Such enzymes are termed **inducible enzymes** because they are not part of the normal cellular makeup and are synthesised only when required.

Mutation

A **mutation** is defined as a permanent change in the sequence of the nucleotide bases in the DNA. From the foregoing discussion it can be seen that a change of even one base is likely to result in the formation of a protein with an altered amino acid sequence. Some mutations involve the change of only one base, a **point mutation**.

FIGURE 4.22

POSSIBLE EFFECT OF BASE SUBSTITUTION IN A GENE CODING FOR A PROTEIN

The substitution of one base in the DNA sequence of the gene for haemoglobin gives rise to a different mRNA codon and leads to the insertion of the non polar amino acid valine instead of the charged amino acid glutamic acid. The 'sickle cell' haemoglobin molecules that are produced stick together causing the red blood cells to change shape or 'sickle' and get stuck in the blood capillaries.

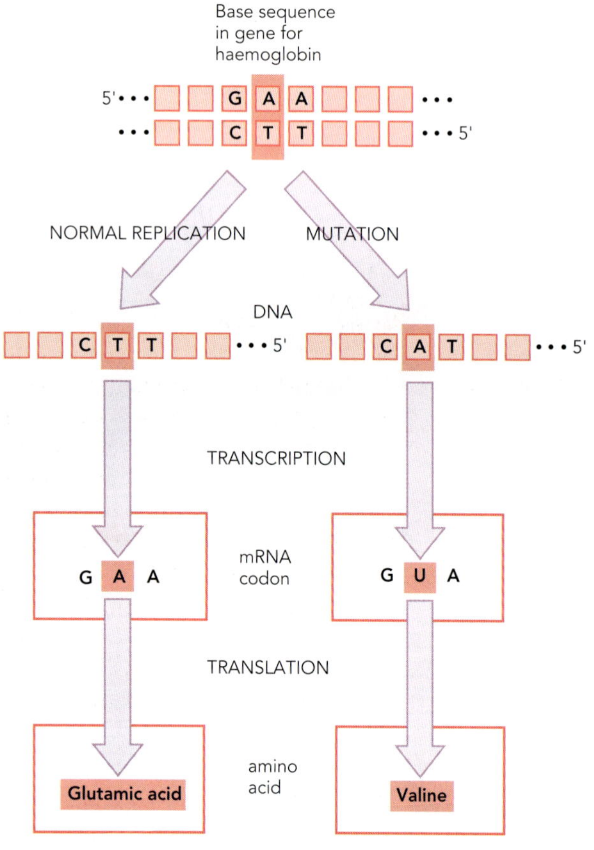

FIGURE 4.23

GENETIC RECOMBINATION BETWEEN TWO ADJACENT CHROMOSOMES

The two homologous chromosomes R and r carry a copy of the genes A to E and a to e respectively. When the DNA strands break, cross over and rejoin, two recombinant chromosomes are formed carrying information from each parent.

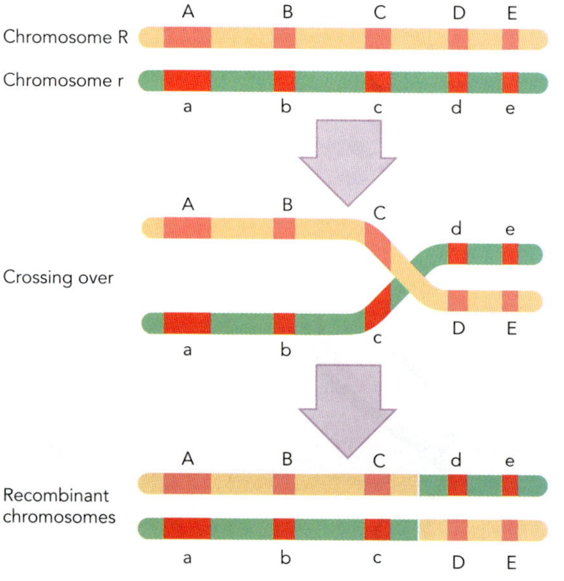

SPOTLIGHT

SICKLE CELL ANAEMIA

The inherited genetic disorder known as sickle cell anaemia is due to a single base substitution in the DNA which gives rise to a haemoglobin molecule with one altered amino acid. The change in the amino acid composition gives the molecule a different charge and so the haemoglobin molecules stick together and cause the red blood cell to sickle and become stuck in the capillaries.

Others involve a more dramatic change; for example, a **frame-shift mutation** that occurs when the reading of the code misses a base or bases and gets out of phase. The protein formed as a result of a mutation may be non-functional or, on the other hand, it may have useful properties. Another outcome of mutation could be the formation of a **'nonsense' codon** which would give a 'stop' signal, resulting in the synthesis of an incomplete peptide chain. In fact, many mutations do not have any observable effect, as there is no significant alteration to the cellular proteins, but some are lethal (see Spotlight box on this page). The possible effects of base substitution is illustrated in Figure 4.23.

HOW DO MUTATIONS OCCUR?

Many mutations occur spontaneously. The cell may make a mistake during the replication of the DNA during cell division. In bacteria the rate of spontaneous mutation is considered to be 1 in every 10^9 cell divisions. This may not seem very great but, considering the enormous rate at which bacterial cells divide, mutation is a very common event. Many of these mutations are not noticed because the change produces a cell that is not viable. Sometimes, the mutation may result in the appearance of a cell with a characteristic which allows it to survive better, and so these cells flourish and multiply. A particularly important example is the development of resistance to antimicrobial drugs or antibiotics. Mutants that have resistance to a particular drug will survive and multiply in the presence of the antibiotic. Therapeutic or prophylactic use of the antibiotic, therefore, has the potential to select for antibiotic-resistant mutants. Continued exposure to antibiotics, especially in the hospital environment, has led to the emergence of a population of resistant microorganisms (see Chapter 12).

Chemical mutagens

Some chemicals damage DNA and cause an alteration to the nucleotide sequence. These chemicals are called **mutagens**. The chemical may act by altering the structure of the base so that it is incapable of pairing with its correct partner. This results in an abnormal DNA being formed with different properties to the DNA of the parent cell. Chemicals that cause damage to human cells so that they mutate and become cancerous are called **carcinogens.**

Radiation

Ionising radiation, such as X-rays and gamma rays, causes damage to the DNA by producing errors in replication. These rays penetrate tissue easily, and can break the DNA chain, destroying chromosomes and leading to the death of the cell. Non-ionising radiation such as UV light, also causes significant damage to cellular DNA by the production of **thymine dimers**. These distorted molecules are incapable of correct replication, and this may lead to the death of the cell or an alteration in its properties. UV light is used to destroy bacteria in clinical areas. The UV rays do not have great penetrating power but are useful for disinfecting air spaces and surface areas (see Chapter 11). Bacteria and some other organisms have enzymes that can repair radiation damage. Sometimes, an error occurs during the process of repair and gives rise to a mutant cell. The enzymes that are involved in DNA synthesis and repair have been isolated and are used by scientists in the process of genetic engineering (see below).

Damage or alteration to DNA has a profound effect in all types of cells. UV radiation damage to the DNA in skin cells may produce mutations that cause the cell to become cancerous, leading to the development of skin cancer or melanoma. Much of our current knowledge about mutation has come from research with bacteria. A useful test for determining the potential carcinogenic properties of a chemical substance is the **Ames test**. A specific test strain of bacteria is exposed to the chemical. If it causes an observable change to the properties of the bacterial strain, then it is considered to have potentially mutagenic or carcinogenic properties and requires further testing.

Transfer of Genetic Material

The simplest kind of transfer of genetic information occurs during asexual cell division. In this process, the DNA molecule replicates itself exactly and each new DNA molecule moves into one of the two new daughter cells. However, in nature there are many variations on this simple process, and these are described below. DNA replication may involve any of the following processes: genetic recombination, 'crossing over', transformation, transduction and conjunction.

Genetic recombination is the term used to describe the transfer of genes from one DNA molecule to another, thus forming a new combination of genes on a chromosome. In eucaryotic cells, recombination usually takes place during **meiosis** when chromosomes containing DNA molecules from each parent are lined up beside each other. If these chromosomes break and the chromosomes then rejoin, DNA from one chromosome can be transferred to the other in a process called '**crossing over**'. This is an ordered process that occurs regularly during sexual reproduction in eucaryotes and gives rise to the necessary genetic diversity observed in higher organisms. (See Figure 4.23.)

In bacteria, genetic recombination occurs relatively infrequently, and requires special conditions. However, research into the mechanisms of DNA replication and transfer in bacteria has contributed greatly to our knowledge of the whole genetic process. DNA transfer between bacteria always requires a donor cell and a recipient cell, and the new DNA formed in the recipient cell is referred to as **recombinant DNA**.

TRANSFORMATION IN BACTERIA

In the 1940s, experiments with pathogenic bacteria were responsible for identifying DNA as the carrier of genetic information. In brief, heat-killed bacteria from a pathogenic encapsulated strain of *Streptococcus pneumoniae* were mixed with live bacteria from a non-pathogenic strain that did not form a capsule. Growth was allowed to take place and it was found that a live, encapsulated pathogenic strain was produced. This showed that a heat-resistant 'factor' carrying the genes for capsule formation and pathogenicity had somehow entered the non-pathogenic cells and 'transformed' them into a pathogenic strain. This 'factor' was identified as DNA, which is not destroyed by heat, and the phenomenon that had occurred was termed **transformation** (see Figure 4.24).

Considerable research has been carried out since these early experiments and it is now known that, under certain conditions, live bacteria are able to take up fragments of DNA from their environment and incorporate them into their cellular DNA, thus 'transforming' their genetic properties. These fragments usually come from the lysis of dead cells. Not all bacteria are capable of undergoing transformation and it usually occurs only between cells of the same genera. *Bacillus, Haemophilus, Streptococcus* and *Staphylococcus* are some of the genera that have been shown to readily undergo transformation. Other cells have walls that do not easily allow the entry of large DNA molecules. The transformed cell, containing the recombinant DNA, continues to replicate and so the transferred genes are passed on to subsequent generations.

TRANSDUCTION

Bacteriophage, or **phage**, is the name given to viruses that attack bacteria. Viruses are very simple, consisting of genetic material, RNA or DNA, enclosed in a protein coat. As discussed in Chapter 5, viruses are quite specific for the cell they infect and this specificity can be used to target a particular strain of bacteria.

FIGURE 4.24
TRANSFORMATION
Griffith's experiment with pathogenic and non pathogenic strains of *Streptococcus pneumoniae*. Mixing of heat killed encapsulated pathogenic bacteria with live non pathogenic bacteria resulted in the production of live capsulated pathogenic bacteria. The genetic information in the DNA of the heat killed cells was transferred to the live cells and transformed their properties.

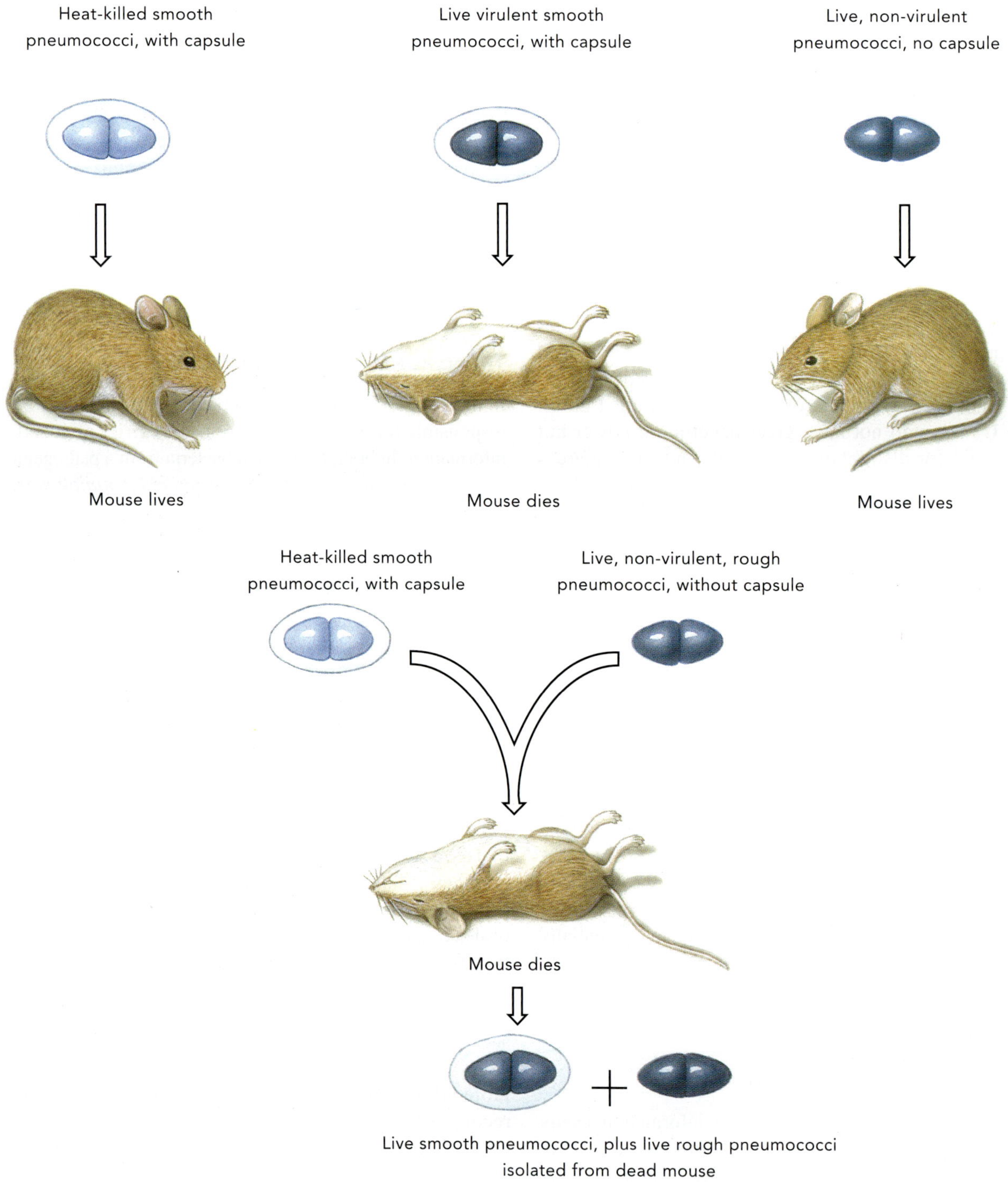

Lytic cycle and generalised transduction

When a bacterium is infected by a phage, the phage first attaches to a specific receptor site on the outside of the cell. It then injects its DNA into the cell, leaving its protein coat outside. The nature of viral replication is such that the virus uses the host cell's metabolic machinery in order to replicate. Once inside the cell, the phage DNA directs the synthesis of phage nucleic acid and proteins and assembles them into new phage particles. Eventually, the infected cell ruptures (lyses), releasing the new phage particles, and the cell is destroyed. This is termed a **lytic** cycle. During this process, phage enzymes break the bacterial chromosomal DNA into small fragments.

When the newly synthesised phage particles are being assembled, some of the bacterial DNA fragments may be included at the expense of some of the phage DNA. Thus, when the phage particle is released and infects another cell, it may take with it some of the bacterial DNA which has been accidentally included. This phenomenon is referred to as **generalised transduction**. It involves the transfer of genetic material from one bacterial cell to another by a lytic phage and allows the transfer of bacterial characteristics from a donor to a recipient cell. Because the phage is carrying slightly altered DNA, some phage genes are lacking and it may not kill the cell it attacks. The phage DNA becomes incorporated into the recipient bacterial cell which acquires new characteristics from the donor cell. (See Figure 4.25.)

Specialised tranduction

A different type of transduction, **specialised transduction,** occurs under some circumstances. **Temperate phages** are phages which, instead of lysing the host cell, insert their DNA into the bacterial chromosome. The inserted phage DNA is called a **prophage** and replicates along with the bacterial DNA, a state called **lysogeny**. The phage DNA may confer additional characteristics on the infected cell. For example, pathogenic strains of *Corynebacterium diphtheriae* contain a temperate phage that carries the gene for toxin production. The toxin is largely responsible for the symptoms of diphtheria. Strains that do not carry the phage are not pathogenic.

A bacterial cell infected with a temperate phage may revert spontaneously to a lytic cycle, in response to an external stimulus. The phage DNA replicates, producing phage DNA and proteins and assembling them into new phage particles. These particles may contain fragments of bacterial DNA that will be transferred to the next bacterial cell the phage infects. The difference between generalised and specialised transduction is that the bacterial DNA carried to the new cell will usually be the DNA that was adjacent to the phage DNA when it was in the lysogenic state. This phenomenon can be used to provide information about the location of specific genes on the bacterial chromosome, and can also be used to select particular genes to be transferred.

Transduction has been used by scientists to manipulate the DNA composition of bacterial cells. Bacteria that have a desired characteristic are infected with phage and the phage allowed to reproduce. Then the newly synthesised phages are transferred to another bacterial cell which can be tested to see whether the desired characteristic has been transferred—that is, whether transduction has occurred.

CONJUGATION

Conjugation is another important method whereby genetic information is transferred from one bacterial cell to another. It differs from transformation and transduction in that it requires the two bacterial cells, the donor and the recipient, to actually come into contact with each other. This is achieved by the formation of a **sex pilus**, a tubular structure that forms a bridge or channel between two cells to allow the passage of pieces of DNA from one cell to the other.

Very often, the DNA that is transferred is in the form of a plasmid. As mentioned earlier, **plasmids** are small, circular, extra-chromosomal pieces of DNA that occur in some bacteria and replicate independently of the bacterial chromosome. They are not essential for growth of the cell, but have been shown to code for a number of other important characteristics. The first plasmid to be described was the **F⁺ plasmid** of *E. coli*. F stands for fertility factor and refers to its ability to direct the formation of a sex pilus. Cells containing a plasmid that codes for a sex pilus are called

FIGURE 4.25
GENERALISED TRANDUCTION
Bacteriophage infection of a host bacterium breaks the bacterial chromosome into fragments which are carried (transduced) to the next bacterium the phage infects.

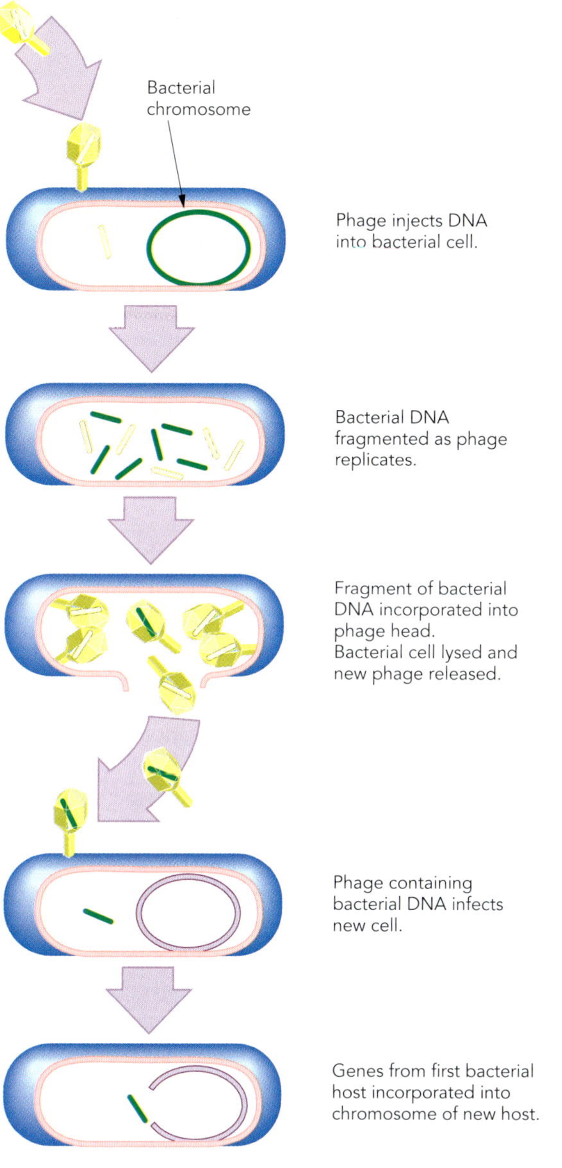

FIGURE 4.26
DIAGRAMMATIC REPRESENTATION OF CONJUGATION
(a) When an F^+ plasmid is transferred to a recipient F^- cell, the F^- cell is converted to F^+; (b) If the plasmid is integrated into the recipient chromosomal DNA, the cell becomes Hfr.

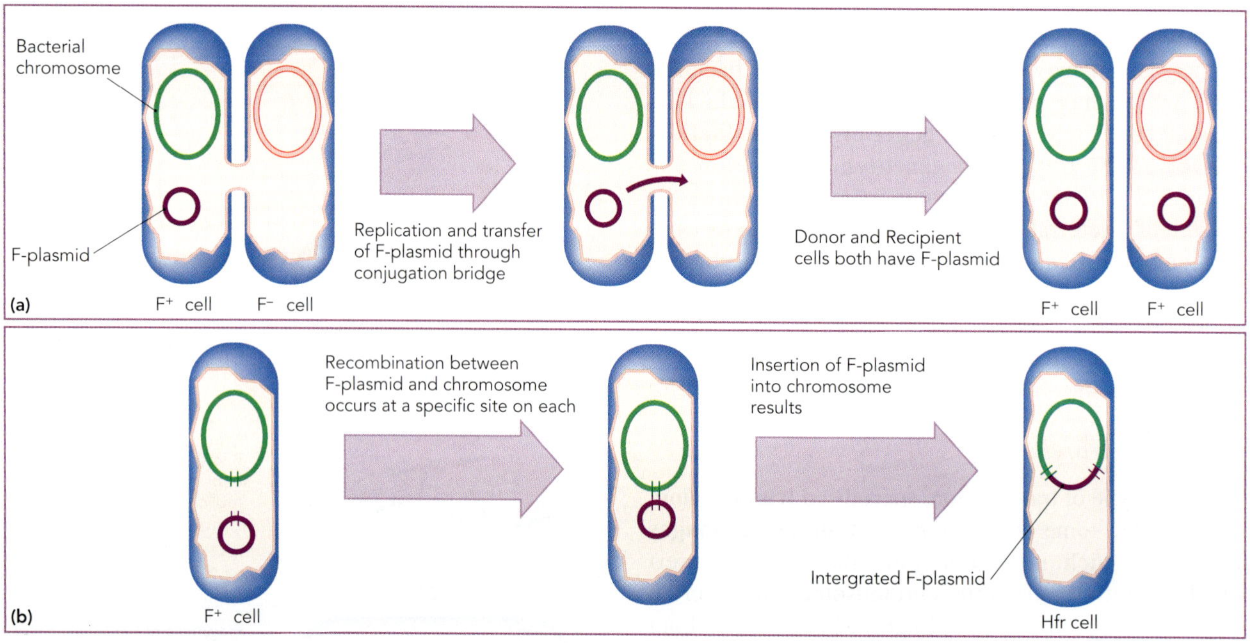

F^+ and those that cannot form a pilus are F^-. Figure 4.26 illustrates the mechanism whereby the F^+ plasmid transfers its genes to another cell during conjugation. In the recipient cell, the plasmid either continues to replicate independently of the chromosomal DNA or it may fuse (recombine) with the chromosome. If this occurs, the recombinant DNA will then carry the genes for conjugation. These cells are called **Hfr strains** (**H**igh **f**requency of **r**ecombination) because they exhibit a very high frequency of bacterial chromosomal transfer. Hfr cells are capable of acting as donor cells in conjugation processes with new recipient cells. During this process, a copy of part of the chromosomal DNA from the donor cell is usually transferred and incorporated into the recipient cell DNA.

Transfer of plasmids during conjugation is an important method of transfer of genes from one bacterial cell to another. Plasmids containing the genes for a number of important properties have been described. Some carry genes for the production of toxins or virulence factors (see Chapter 10). A plasmid-containing strain of *E. coli* is responsible for the toxin production associated with 'traveller's diarrhoea'.

For clinical microbiologists, the most important plasmids are those carrying **resistance factors (R)**. These are genes that enable the cell to display resistance to various antibiotics, either by interfering with the entry or action of the antibiotic or by destruction of the antibiotic molecule. For example, most strains of *Staphylococcus aureus* currently isolated in hospitals carry an R plasmid with a gene which codes for the formation of the enzyme beta-lactamase, which destroys penicillin.

Resistance plasmids may carry genes for resistance to more than one antibiotic and, as described above, can be rapidly passed from cell to cell. Transfer can also occur between closely related genera, which gives rise to populations of organisms that are highly resistant to a range of antibiotics. Whereas mutation usually gives rise to resistance to one antibiotic at a time, plasmid transfer allows for the development of resistance to several antibiotics in one step. This is of increasing importance in the hospital environment.

Genetic Engineering

The brief description of the ways in which genetic information can be transferred between bacterial cells was given as an introduction to the subject of genetic engineering. Scientists have developed laboratory techniques that enable them to transfer genes from one cell to another and to manipulate the activities of the bacterial cell in order to obtain desired products. These techniques are based on the types of transfers described above and use many of the enzymes from bacterial cells. Of particular use is a group of enzymes found only in bacteria called **restriction endonucleases**. These enzymes recognise a particular sequence of nucleotides in the DNA molecule and hydrolyse (break) each strand at a specific point in the sequence. Because the DNA is a double strand, the break is always jagged, exposing a 'sticky' end. The enzymes are usually named after the bacteria from which they were isolated. For example, Eco I comes from *Escherichia coli* (**E.co** *li*) and hydrolyses the sequence GAATTC between guanine and adenine, giving rise to two fragments each with the sequence AATT on the end of a single strand (the 'sticky' end). New pieces of DNA (genes) can be inserted into these breaks. (See Figure 4.27.)

FIGURE 4.27
THE ROLE OF RESTRICTION ENZYMES IN MAKING RECOMBINANT DNA

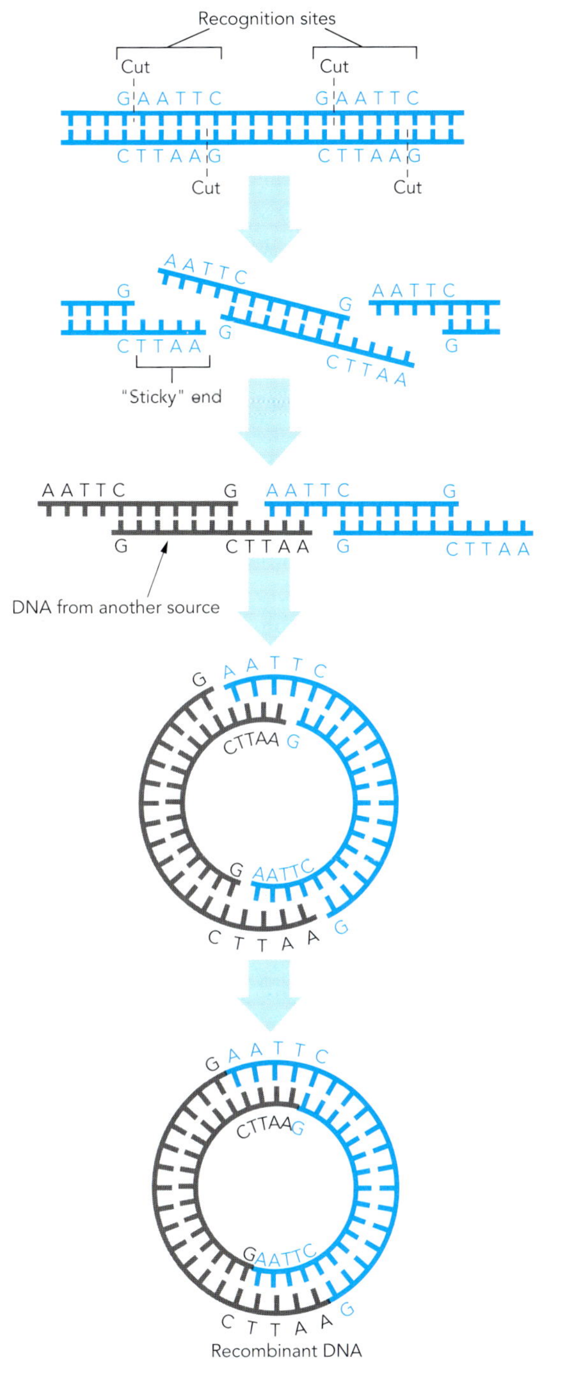

(a) Recognition sites of this particular restriction enzyme in double-stranded DNA are shown in red. Arrow indicate where the cuts occur.

(b) Cuts by this restriction enzyme produce a fragment with two sticky ends.

(c) When two fragments of DNA cut by the same restriction enzyme come together, they can join by base pairing.

(d) A circle can be formed—as for a plasmid

(e) The enzyme DNA liagse is used to unite the backbones of the two DNA fragments, producing a molecule of recombinant DNA. (It may be linear or circular.)

Plasmids are used as vectors, or carriers, to introduce a foreign piece of DNA carrying the desired gene into a cell. A restriction enzyme is used to cut both the plasmid and the foreign DNA. This gives rise to fragments of DNA from both sources which have corresponding sticky ends, with the sequence coding for the particular gene somewhere in between. When these are mixed, some of the foreign DNA can be inserted into the plasmid. An enzyme called DNA ligase is added to join the nucleotides together and the result is a plasmid vector carrying the desired gene. In the laboratory the plasmid is usually introduced into the recipient cell by transformation. If the host cell does not normally take up DNA, the cell wall can be modified by chemical treatments. (See Figure 4.28.)

RECOMBINANT DNA TECHNOLOGY

The procedures used in genetic engineeering result in the formation of DNA molecules that have been modified in some way; that is, they have become 'recombinant DNA'. Recombinant DNA is a term widely used to refer to DNA that has been produced using DNA from two different sources. It can mean:

- the DNA produced by spontaneous crossing over during cell division; or
- the DNA produced in the laboratory by genetic engineering.

Scientists have developed ways of using genetic engineering to benefit humans. For example, a gene from a eucaryotic cell can be inserted into a bacterial cell. The recipient bacterial cell containing the recombinant DNA can then be induced to express this gene. Because of the rapid rate of growth of bacterial cells, large amounts of the substance coded for in the eucaryotic gene can be produced quickly and in a relatively pure form. One of the first examples of the use of this technique was the production of human insulin by cells of *E. coli.*

Vaccines such as the one for hepatitis B, hep B surface antigen (HBsAg), have also been genetically engineered. The gene responsible for the synthesis of one particular sequence of the hepatitis B viral protein coat is introduced into a yeast cell. The yeast produces multiple copies of this fragment of the protein coat, which is then isolated, purified and used as a vaccine in humans to stimulate production of protective anti-hepatitis B antibodies.

There are several advantages to the use of recombinant DNA in the production of compounds such as hormones or vaccines for human use. Previously, many of these compounds had to be derived from human or animal tissue. The presence of animal proteins often gave rise to an adverse immune reaction (see Chapter 9). The need to use blood or tissue from human sources limited the amount of the substance that could be produced and increased the cost. There is also a slight risk of transferring another human pathogen that may be present in the extracts. There is some evidence that this has occurred with the use of preparations of human growth hormone from pituitary extracts of cadavers. Some patients treated with these hormone preparations have developed Creutzfeldt-Jakob syndrome, a disease of the nervous system (see Spotlight box, p. 94). The use of purified genetically engineered products, synthesised by microbial cells, removes the risk of adverse effects from preparations contaminated with human pathogens or other substances that may cause hypersensitivity reactions.

Biotechnology is the term used for all the many and varied techniques involving manipulation of genes or genetic information. Table 4.4 lists some of the products of biotechnology.

DNA ANALYSIS

Techniques are now available which allow the determination of the sequence of nucleotides in a piece of DNA. Very often, a genetic characteristic can be ascribed to a particular nucleotide sequence. In other words, it is now possible to detect the presence or absence of a particular gene. This method is being used to study the genetic composition of higher organisms. The human genome project is a worldwide cooperative study by scientists and aims to map the complete sequence of the 100 000 genes that make up the human chromosomes. This will require the determination of the sequence of about 3 billion nucleotide pairs.

DNA analysis is also used for identification of human tissue. No two humans (except identical twins) look exactly alike. This is because we all have a different complement of DNA in our genes. Methods have been developed to compare DNA from different sources. The DNA fragments

TABLE 4.4
MICROBIAL PRODUCTS OF GENETIC ENGINEERING

PRODUCT	ORGANISM	COMMENT
Medical		
Insulin	*E. coli*	Treatment for diabetes
Interleukin 2 (IL-2)	*E. coli*	Stimulates immune system
Interferon α and γ	*E. coli* *S. cerevisiae*	Possible therapy for viral diseases
Tumour necrosis factor	*E. coli*	Attacks cancer cells
Human growth hormone	*E. coli*	Corrects growth deficiencies
Colony stimulating factor (CSF)	*E. coli* *S. cerevisiae*	Stimulation of immune system and treatment of infections
Vaccines		
Hepatitis B	*S. cerevisiae*	HBsAg for vaccine
Modified organisms		
Pseudomonas syringae		Prevents frost damage to plants
Pseudomonas fluorescens		Insecticide properties derived from *Bacillus thuringiensis*

FIGURE 4.28

INSERTION OF FOREIGN GENES INTO A BACTERIUM USING A PLASMID AS THE VECTOR

Foreign DNA and plasmid DNA are cut with a restriction enzyme. The foreign DNA is inserted into the plasmid. The recombinant plasmid is introduced into a new bacterial cell which acquires the characteristics coded of the foreign DNA and can be cloned.

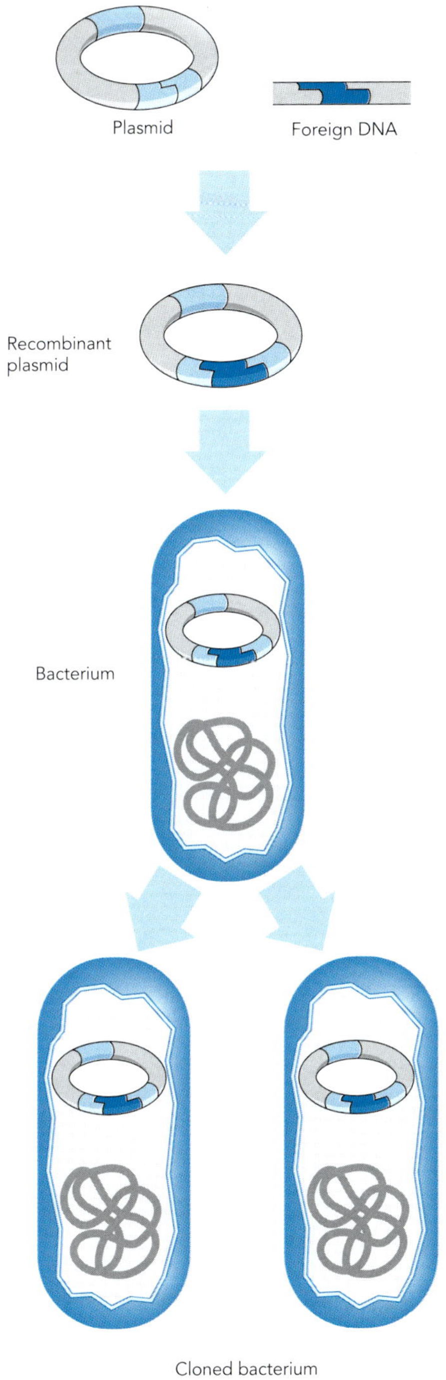

by hydrolysis are separated by electrophoresis on a gel and a pattern, or fingerprint, of the DNA content is obtained. DNA fingerprinting is used in forensic science to compare, for example, the DNA in a sample of semen with the DNA in a blood sample to help establish the identity of a criminal, or determine paternity. It can also be used to identify different strains of bacteria.

DNA analysis also allows scientists to identify defective genes that may be responsible for a particular disease. Some attempts are being made to introduce DNA into embryonic cells in order to correct defects, but these experiments are in the early stages and are the subject of much discussion regarding the ethics of such procedures.

AMPLIFICATION OF DNA

Another technique with widespread use involves the amplification of DNA molecules in order to produce multiple copies of the DNA, or genes. If the sequence of nucleotides is to be determined, large amounts of DNA are required. In this technique, fragments of the DNA of interest are copied until enough molecules are obtained to carry out an analysis (such as the fingerprinting described above). The method is called the **polymerase chain reaction** or **PCR**. PCR can make billions of copies of a particular nucleotide sequence in just a few hours. A small piece of the DNA to be copied is heated so that the strands are pulled apart. The solution is then cooled and the four DNA nucleotides and synthesising enzymes are added. The nucleotides are incorporated, pairing with their corresponding base on the exposed single strand. The DNA strand is then 'zipped up' by the action of a polymerase enzyme, effectively doubling the amount of DNA each time. (See Figure 4.29.)

PCR must be carried out under very strictly controlled laboratory conditions, as it is an extremely sensitive technique. The researcher must ensure that the equipment and solutions are not contaminated with any extraneous DNA from the wrong source.

THE FUTURE OF BIOTECHNOLOGY

One use for PCR in the future will be to test for the presence of bacteria in a sample when the concentration of cells is too low to be detected by any other means (see Chapter 15). PCR amplification followed by reaction of the DNA with a radioactively labelled nucleotide probe may aid in the detection of slow-growing organisms such as *Legionella*.

The last 15 years have seen an explosion in our knowledge of genes and our ability to manipulate genetic characteristics. However, this has been accompanied by many legal and ethical questions. Should scientists be allowed to release genetically modified organisms into the environment? Should doctors manipulate the genes in unborn babies?

The use of bacteria to produce vaccines and other substances of benefit to humans is expanding at an incredible rate. One of the strategies currently being investigated to produce an AIDS vaccine involves the modification of the *Vaccinia* virus to carry HIV antigen, by the use of recombinant DNA technology.

FIGURE 4.29
POLYMERASE CHAIN REACTION

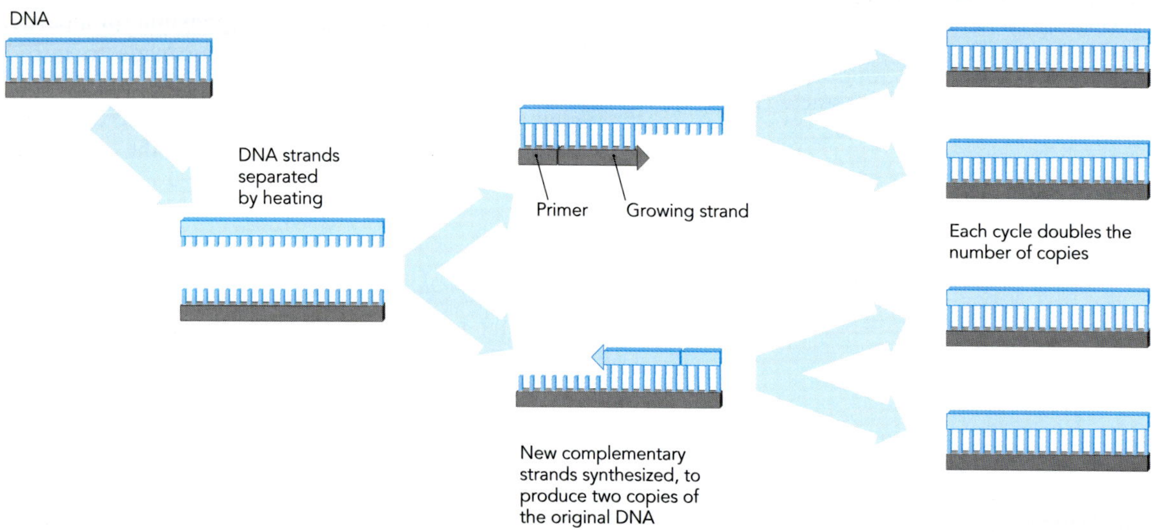

Summary

SIZE, SHAPE AND APPEARANCE OF BACTERIAL CELLS

- Bacteria occur in three main shapes—spherical (cocci), rod-shaped (bacilli) and spiral (spirilla, spirochaete or vibrio).

STUDY OF BACTERIA

- Bacterial cell walls are complex, semi-rigid structures.
- Depending on the structure of the wall, bacteria are classified as Gram-positive or Gram-negative. Gram-positive walls consist of a thick layer of peptidoglycan with a thin layer of teichoic acid. Gram-negative walls consist of a thin layer of peptidoglycan and an outer layer of lipopolysaccharides, lipoproteins and phospholipids.
- Mycobacteria have a waxy outer layer that necessitates their identification by the acid-fast stain.
- The cell wall can be damaged by certain chemicals or enzymes such as lysozyme. The synthesis of peptidoglycan is inhibited by penicillin.
- Bacterial cells are enclosed in a plasma membrane, consisting of a phospholipid bilayer with proteins embedded in it.
- The membrane is a semi-permeable barrier, controlling the passage of substances into and out of the cell.
- Bacterial cell membranes are the site of metabolic reactions which occur in the organelles of eucaryotic cells.
- The cytoplasm contains water, enzymes, ribosomes, inclusion granules and a single, circular chromosome of DNA.
- In some bacteria, additional genetic information is carried on a plasmid.
- Ribosomes are the site of protein synthesis.
- Some bacteria are surrounded by a polysaccharide-containing capsule, the glycocalyx, which allows the bacteria to bind to surfaces and evade phagocytosis.
- Flagella are thin, rigid filaments which enable the bacteria to swim.
- Pili are short, hair-like appendages which aid in the attachment of bacteria to mucosal cells. Some are involved in bacterial conjugation.
- Some Gram-positive bacilli form resistant endospores when environmental conditions are unfavourable.

BACTERIAL GROWTH

- Bacteria reproduce by binary fission.
- The time taken for a cell to reproduce itself is called the generation time.
- Special techniques are used to grow and store pure cultures of bacteria.
- When grown in the laboratory under controlled conditions, bacteria have four phases of growth: lag, logarithmic, stationary and death.

REQUIREMENTS FOR GROWTH

- Bacteria require various physical factors for growth, including correct temperature, correct pH, correct osmotic pressure and the correct amount of oxygen.
- Nutritional requirements include water and the elements carbon, nitrogen, sulphur, phosphorous and various trace elements. Autotrophic bacteria use carbon dioxide from the atmosphere. Some bacteria require specific organic compounds.

HANDLING BACTERIA IN THE LABORATORY

- Bacteria can be grown, isolated and identified in the laboratory by growing them on defined media.

MEASUREMENT OF BACTERIAL GROWTH

- The number of bacteria in a sample can be measured by growth on agar plates and counting the number of colonies present.

CLASSIFICATION OF BACTERIA

- *Bergey's Manual of Systematic Bacteriology* classifies bacteria on the basis of their cell wall structure, Gram stain, shape, motility, oxygen requirements, biochemical properties and some genetic data.
- Phage typing of bacterial strains is important for epidemiological studies.
- New techniques in DNA analysis are contributing to classification.
- Bergey' classification system includes many different types of bacteria that are of medical importance.

BACTERIAL GENETICS

- The characteristics of bacterial cells are determined by their genetic material or genes, which are linear sequences of nucleotides of DNA.
- DNA consists of two strands of nucleotides twisted around each other to form a double helix.
- In protein synthesis, the genetic information contained in the DNA is first transcribed to messenger RNA, which then acts as a template for the synthesis of proteins.

MUTATION

- Mutation (which can occur as a result of exposure to chemicals or radiation) is a change in the nucleotide bases in the DNA which gives rise to different properties in the cell.
- Favourable mutations, such as the development of drug resistance, allow some bacteria to survive instead of others.

TRANSFER OF GENETIC MATERIAL

- Genetic recombination refers to the exchange of DNA between two molecules.
- Transformation, transduction and conjugation are different ways in which one bacterial strain acquires the characteristics of another strain.

GENETIC ENGINEERING

- The processes of transformation, transduction and conjugation, which occur in bacterial cells, have been used by scientists to manipulate the genetic information in some cells.
- Recombinant DNA technology is being used in a number of ways to develop products which are of benefit to humans (e.g. vaccines, hormones).

Study Questions

1. Describe the major shapes of bacterial cells.
2. What is meant by morphology?
3. How does the structure of Gram-positive cell walls differ from Gram-negative cell walls?
4. What is meant by an acid-fast bacillus?
5. Where is the genetic information in bacterial cells located?
6. What is the function of these extracellular bacterial structures—glycocalyx, flagella and pili?
7. What are the main requirements for bacterial growth?
8. Describe the four phases of bacterial growth.
9. At what temperature would you incubate bacterial cultures of clinical specimens? Why?
10. What are the properties used to classify bacteria by Bergey's method of classification?
11. How are proteins synthesised in bacterial cells?
12. What is meant by the term 'gene expression'?
13. What happens when a mutation takes place in a bacterial cell?
14. What is meant by 'recombinant DNA'?
15. Describe the ways in which recombinant DNA technology is being used to benefit humans.

Test Your Understanding

1. How does the structure of the plasma membrane control the passage of substances into and out of the cell?
2. Why is correct osmotic pressure important for bacterial cell growth?
3. Why is it important to use methods of sterilisation that destroy endospores?
4. How would you measure the level of bacterial contamination in a food sample?
5. Why are tetanus and/or gangrene sometimes treated by placing the patient in a hyperbaric oxygen chamber?
6. How can phage typing help to identify the source of an infection?
7. How is the information for antibiotic resistance transferred from one bacterial cell to another? What are the implications for the control of infectious diseases?
8. How can the polymerase chain reaction (PRC) contribute to the classification of bacteria?

FURTHER READING

Holt, J.G., ed. *Bergey's Manual of Systematic Bacteriology*, 1st edn., 4 volumes. Baltimore: Williams & Wilkins, 1984–1989. (This is a standard reference for identification and classification of bacteria.)

Mulligan, R.C., 1993, 'The Basic Science of Gene Therapy', *Science 260*, pp. 926–935.

Sleigh, J.D. & M.C.Timbury, *Notes on Medical Bacteriology*, 4th edn., London: Churchill Livingstone, 1994.

Watson, J.D., *Recombinant DNA*, 2nd edn., New York: Scientific American Books, W.H. Freeman, 1992.

chapter 5

viruses and viral diseases

Chapter focus

- *What are the special characteristics of viruses?*
- *How do viruses replicate in cells?*
- *What are the different ways in which viruses can produce disease in humans?*
- *What are the major routes of transmission of viral diseases?*
- *How are viral diseases diagnosed, treated and prevented?*

There are over 600 different viruses known to infect humans and most of these have been identified only in the last 50 years. Before then, many unexplained illnesses were attributed to the presence of toxins or poisons, or to exposure to 'bad air'. The word **virus** means venom, or poison, and the original name given to the infective agents that caused these diseases was 'filterable viruses.' This was because infectivity, present in samples obtained from diseased animals or plants, was not lost when passed through a filter that was known to retain bacteria. Viruses are too small to be seen under the light microscope and cannot be cultured in the laboratory on the media normally used for growth of bacteria.

We now know that viruses can reproduce only inside a living (host) cell. They lack most of the enzymes necessary for the metabolism and synthesis of complex molecules and so must replicate inside a cell using the host cell's machinery to do so. As a result, they have been called *obligate intracellular parasites*. In most instances, viruses cause damage or changes to the cells in which they replicate. There are many different kinds of viruses and they attack not only humans but also other animals, plants and even bacteria. We shall look at some of their properties in this chapter.

Structure of Viruses

Viruses are among the smallest infectious agents known. They range in size from the tiny polio virus (0.02 µm diameter) to the large vaccinia (smallpox) virus which is 0.4 µm in diameter. This is still smaller than even the smallest bacteria which are 1–2 µm in diameter. For comparison, human erythrocytes are 7–8 µm in diameter. Viruses cannot be seen under the light microscope, requiring the higher resolution of electron microscopy in order for their structure to be visible. They have a simple structure consisting of only one type of nucleic acid enclosed in a protein coat called a **capsid**. Some of the more complex viruses have in addition a protein core, which encloses the nucleic acid. Viruses are not cells and they do not contain any of the subcellular organelles that are important for the function of eucaryotic organisms; they do not even contain a plasma membrane. They are unable to carry out any metabolic processes without the involvement of some type of living cell. Each type of virus has a distinctive shape and structure which is used as a basis for classification (see Figure 5.1).

NUCLEIC ACID

A virus possesses only one type of nucleic acid, which carries its genetic information. This is either single-stranded RNA (ss-RNA), double-stranded RNA (ds-RNA), single-stranded DNA (ss-DNA) or double-stranded DNA (ds-DNA). The size of the viral genome is limited and does not carry all the information necessary for the synthesis of a complete virus. Instead, the viral genes code mainly for structural viral proteins and a limited number of viral enzymes, as well as regulatory genes which direct the host cell pathways required.

THE VIRAL CAPSID

The protein coat covering the nucleic acid is called a **capsid** and is made up of repeating protein units called **capsomeres.** These are often arranged in symmetrical patterns which enable the purified virus particles to be crystallised. Capsids occur in distinctive shapes. (See Figure 5.1.) Many consist of a regular polyhedron such as the icosahedral (20-sided) structure found in, for example, the adenovirus. Others are helical, forming hollow cylinders which may be either rigid or flexible. Although viral capsids contain only a minimum number of protein molecules, the capsid proteins have a number of important functions. They may have antigenic properties and they participate in the attachment and entry of the virus particle to the host cell during infection (see below). They also protect the nucleic acid against inactivation by nuclease enzymes.

ENVELOPE

Some viruses are surrounded by an envelope. This is usually a lipid bilayer derived from the membrane of the host cell, into which some viral proteins and glycoproteins have been inserted. The viral glycoproteins often appear as 'spikes' protruding from the envelope (see Figure 5.2). The structure of the envelope usually assists the virus to attach to the host cell. This can be demonstrated in the laboratory by incubating red blood cells with influenza virus, which causes agglutination of the cells. This is due to the attachment of the spikes on the influenza virus to the red blood cells, which have similar surface receptors to the cells of the respiratory epithelium that the virus attacks naturally. Viruses that lack envelopes are called **naked viruses**. They are generally more resistant to environmental conditions

FIGURE 5.1
RELATIVE SIZES AND SHAPES OF DIFFERENT VIRUSES

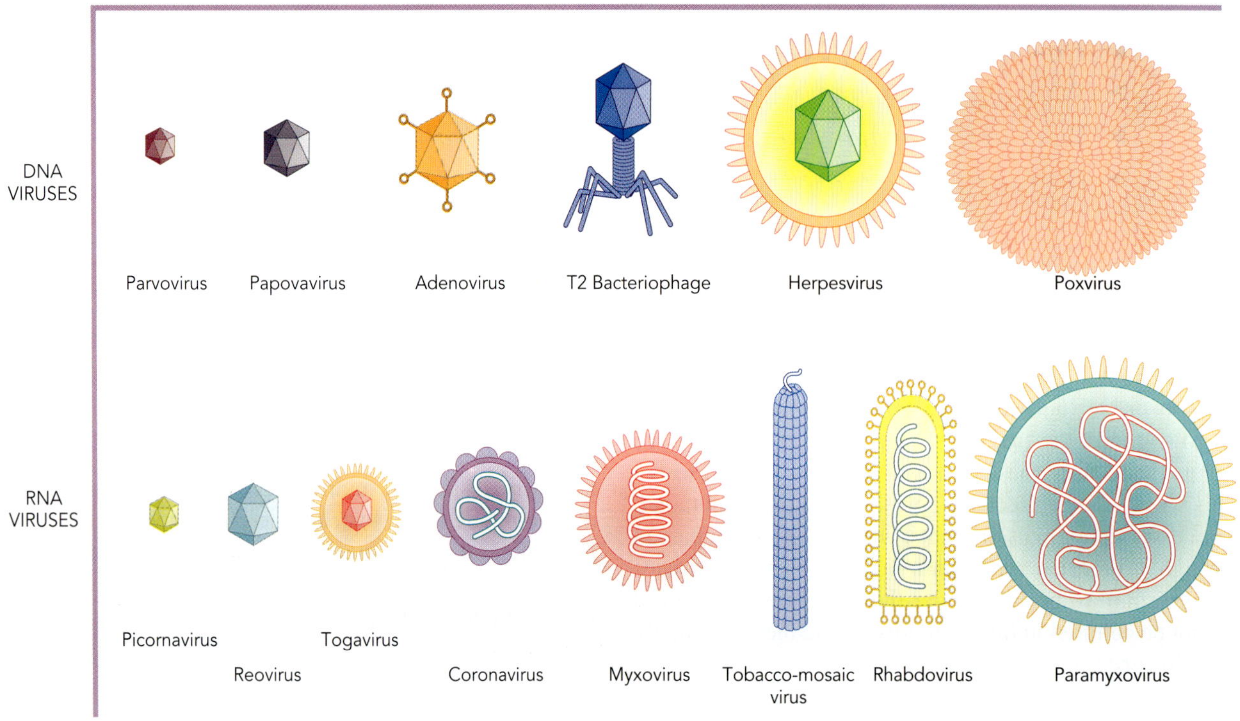

FIGURE 5.2
INFLUENZA VIRUS
A drawing of the influenza virus, showing haemagglutinin and neuraminidase spikes on its outer surface and RNA in the core.

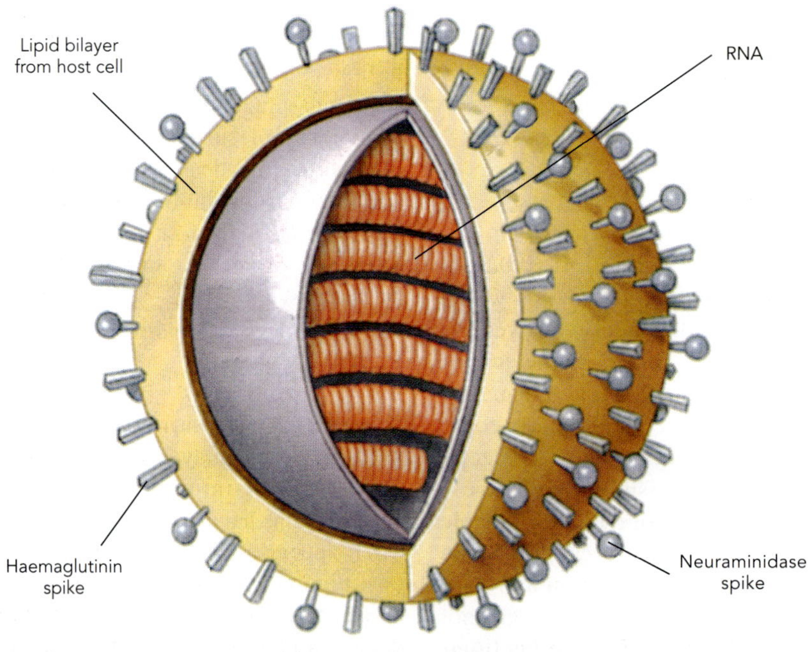

than enveloped viruses. This is because the envelope is easily damaged by chemicals or extremes of pH or temperature.

The surface protein components of both enveloped and naked viral particles participate in the attachment of the viral particle to the specific receptor site on the susceptible cell. They also determine the antigenic characteristics of the virus. The immune system of the host produces antibodies directed against the proteins and glycoproteins present on the viral surface (see Chapter 9).

FIGURE 5.3
HERPES VIRUS
An example of an enveloped virus containing double stranded DNA surrounded by an icosahedral capsid.

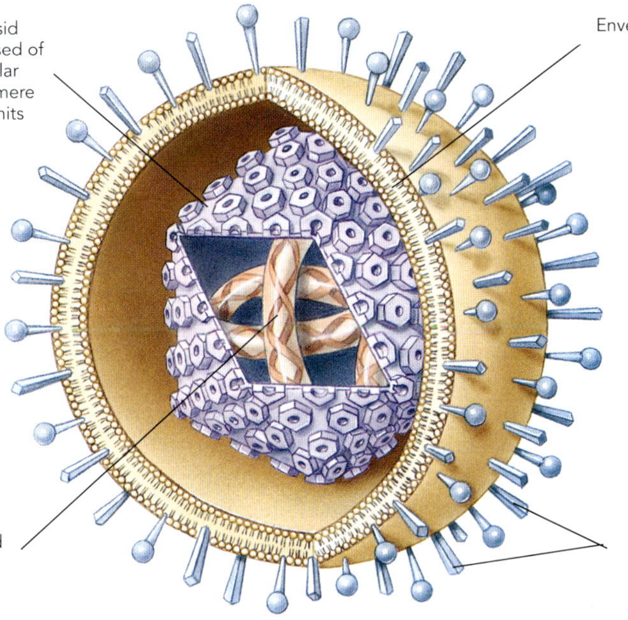

Figure 5.3 is a schematic diagram of the herpes simplex virus, an example of a virus containing double-stranded DNA, surrounded by an icosahedral capsid and an envelope.

VIRAL ENZYMES

Viruses do not carry out any metabolic processes outside the host cell. However some viruses contain enzymes that are important for the infective process. Most of these are involved with nucleic acid transcription—for example, RNA polymerase, which is necessary for the transcription of the viral nucleic acid into messenger RNA. Reverse transcriptase carries out the initial step in the replication of the retroviruses, the synthesis of DNA from viral RNA. Neuraminidase, an enzyme located in the spike of the influenza virus, appears to be important for virus assembly and release. These enzymes are not generally found in the host cell so they are good targets for antiviral therapy (see Chapter 12).

TERMINOLOGY

Sometimes, only parts of viruses are isolated from the infected host. Studies have shown that some of these are infective and some can stimulate an immune response. As a result, a number of different terms are used in relation to viruses.

- **Virion** is used to describe an entire mature virus particle consisting either of nucleic acid and capsid (naked virus) or nucleic acid, capsid and envelope (enveloped virus). Virions are found outside the host cell and are capable of transmission from one host to another.
- **Virus**, or **viral particle**, refers to the intracellular infectious particle consisting of nucleic acid and a protein coat.
- The **viral genome** is the genetic information of the virus, either RNA or DNA.
- **Viroids** are infectious agents which lack a capsid and consist only of a closed circular RNA molecule. They are usually plant pathogens and will not be discussed further in this text.
- A **prion** is a novel kind of infective particle that appears to consist only of protein, without any nucleic acid component. Prions have been implicated in some unusual transmissible neurodegenerative disorders, known as **spongiform encephalopathies.** These include kuru and Creutzfeldt-Jakob syndrome in humans, scrapie in sheep and BSE, bovine spongiform encephalopathy or 'mad cow disease' (see Spotlight box on CJD, p. 94). Prions are particularly resistant to procedures that normally modify nucleic acids, such as treatment with disinfectants and autoclaving.

Host Range and Specificity

Viruses are selective for the range of hosts and the type of cells they infect. In general, plant viruses infect only plants, bacterial viruses infect only bacteria and animal viruses infect only animals. Within these broad categories, most viruses will attack only one type of animal or plant (its host range) and may even be specific for only one kind of cell or tissue within that organism (**tissue tropism**).

The ability of a virus to infect a particular kind of cell is dependent on the presence of an attachment site

SPOTLIGHT
CREUTZFELDT-JACOB DISEASE

In October 1990 an article was published in the *Australian & New Zealand Journal of Medicine* describing the death in 1988 of a 41-year-old Adelaide woman, from the rare Creutzfeldt-Jakob disease (CJD). Another Australian woman who had been on the in-vitro fertilisation (IVF) program died soon after. They had both received injections of a fertility hormone preparation, human pituitary gonadotrophin (HPG). These cases caused great concern in the medical community and among the estimated 1400 women and 62 men who had received injections of the extract. To date, a total of four Australian women have died from CJD acquired through hormone injections. The tragic deaths of these women occurred because they were treated with a hormone preparation that had been extracted from pituitary glands obtained from human cadavers. Since the preparation involved pooling of the gland material, contamination of the whole batch could occur even if only one gland was infected.

Creutzfeldt-Jakob syndrome belongs to a group of diseases called spongiform encephalopathies* because of the distinctive lesions found in the brain on autopsy. They include diseases such as kuru, a neurologic disease which used to occur in New Guinea natives who practised ritual cannibalism, scrapie, a disease of sheep, and 'mad cow' disease in cattle. These diseases are thought to be caused by infectious particles called prions, which consist of protein without any nucleic acid. They are highly resistant to conventional methods of sterilisation and disinfection. The method of preparation of HPG apparently did not destroy the infectious agent of CJD and so the patients were accidentally injected with the CJD prions.

Creutzfeldt-Jakob disease is a neurologic disorder first described in 1920. Cases occur sporadically with an incidence of about one case per million population. Its origin is largely unknown, although recent research has shown that, while the disease is transmissible under some circumstances, unlike other transmissible diseases, it can also be caused by a mutation in the chromosomal gene PrP.

Early symptoms include lack of balance, followed by lack of muscular coordination, loss of speech and/or vision, development of jerking movements and dementia. The disease may take many years to develop but, once the symptoms appear, the neurological changes progress rapidly and the disease is usually fatal in less than one year.

The development of CJD in patients treated with HPG followed the discovery that some children who had been treated with human growth hormone (HGH) had developed CJD up to 20 years after treatment. Prior to 1985, human pituitary glands were used to prepare human growth hormone, which was administered to over 40 000 'abnormally short' children worldwide. Athletes and body builders also received injections of the hormone.

About 80 people worldwide are thought to have died from CJD acquired as a result of iatrogenic (medical) procedures, such as corneal grafts, dura mater transplants and administration of hormone preparations. The long incubation time for the development of the disease makes it difficult to predict how many of the recipients of hormone preparations will develop CJD. The infection does not provoke an immune (antibody) response so it is impossible to detect exposure to the disease before symptoms appear. Although it is not known whether the disease can be transmitted in ways other than by exposure to brain tissue, most of the hormone recipients in Australia have been contacted and advised against donating blood or any other body tissue. The advances in molecular biology techniques mean that HPG and HGH are now prepared by methods involving genetic engineering, so there is no risk of disease from preparations currently in use.

Of major concern to health workers are the possible risks of occupational exposure to blood or tissue of an infected patient who may not be showing symptoms of the disease. The routes of transmission are not certain. Kuru is transmitted by ingestion of infected brain tissue (cannibalism) and mad cow disease has been linked to the ingestion of scrapie-infected offal in feed supplements. Recent cases of CJD in Great Britain have been linked to the ingestion of meat from infected cows. Iatrogenic infections in humans have occurred from corneal grafts, dura mater transplants and the hormone treatments described above. There is one report of transmission to a laboratory technician who handled formalin-fixed brain tissue from a CJD patient.

Infection control procedures should include scrupulous adherence to Standard Precautions especially when handling cerebrospinal fluid (CSF), or brain biopsies, and at post mortems. Recommendations for handling tissues, fluids and other contaminated materials from patients with CJD, or suspected cases with rapidly progressing dementia, include steam autoclaving at 132°C for one hour or 121°C for 2 hours, or soaking in IN NaOH for one hour at room temperature. Disposable equipment should be incinerated.

* See Chapter 20 for a discussion of spongiform encephalopathies.

for the virus on the surface of the host cell. **Ligands** (chemical groups) in specific proteins (**viral attachment proteins**) on the surface of the virion bind to receptor molecules on the surface of the plasma membrane of the target cell. For some viruses the chemical structure of the ligands and corresponding receptor molecules have been determined. For example, the orthomyxoviruses bind to a terminal sialic acid molecule located on a side chain of a membrane glycolipid or glycoprotein. The gp120 attachment protein of the human immunodeficiency virus, HIV, binds to the CD4 receptor molecule on the membrane of T4 lymphocytes.

The recognition of specific receptors by particular viruses is not absolute. Sometimes unrelated viruses may use the same receptor which means that a cell with that receptor may be vulnerable to attack by a number of different viruses. On the other hand, similar viruses may use quite different receptors. In addition, certain viruses are able to recognise more than one kind of receptor. If the receptor is on a different type of cell this will extend the **tissue tropism** (i.e. the range of cells the virus can attack), or even the host range of the virus. For example, the rabies virus can attach to the acetyl choline (ACh) receptor as well as sialyted gangliosides, and this greatly extends its range of susceptible cells. The more common the receptor molecule, the wider the range of cells the virus can attack.

In general, it appears that viruses have evolved in such a way as to make maximum use of the available glycoprotein molecules on the host cell membrane as their receptors. It should be noted, however, that these molecules are an integral part of the host cell membrane and have functions other than merely serving as an attachment site for viruses. The presence or absence of these receptor molecules is a fundamental determinant of the susceptibility of the host cell to viral attack. The polio virus, for example, binds to specific receptors that are present in primate cells but not in other animals. Hence the polio virus can attack humans and monkeys, but not mice. However, replication of the polio virus occurs only in neurone and muscle cells so it appears that the existence of the appropriate receptors on the primate cells is not the only determinant of successful infection. The other kinds of primate cells may be non-permissive for other reasons.

It is thought that, after penetration of the host cell by the virus, viral replication depends on the activity of a number of regulatory factors, variously called promoters, enhancers and transcriptional activators. These regulatory factors may be restricted to certain types of cells and tissues where they exert an important role as an additional determinant of successful viral infection.

Because viruses are host-specific, few viruses cause disease in both humans and other animals. Those that do so usually occur under conditions that allow transmission from the animal reservoir to humans. One of these is the rabies virus, which is widespread throughout the animal kingdom and can be transmitted to humans by the bite of an infected animal. Other viruses which persist in nature in an animal reservoir (usually rodent) can be transmitted to humans by close contact with the animal or infected droppings. Among these, the hanta virus, which was responsible for a serious outbreak of an influenza-like disease in New Mexico in 1993, was linked to a plague of deer mice. The equine morbillivirus, recently identified in Australia as responsible for the death of a horse trainer and 14 racehorses (see Spotlight box, p. 172), is another example of a virus that can apparently cross the species barrier. Some viruses persist in animal or bird reservoirs and are transmitted to other animals or humans by the bite of insects such as mosquitoes. The virus causes a subclinical infection in the animal reservoir and multiplies in both the vertebrate host and invertebrate vector. These are called arboviral infections and are described later in this chapter.

Classification of Viruses

The clinical classification of viruses, based on the disease they produce or the part of the body they affect, is useful but not completely satisfactory for the scientist who is interested in other properties. Viruses with very different structures may cause diseases that are superficially similar; for example, hepatitis A,B,C,D and E all affect the liver but are really quite different. Some of the viruses responsible for known diseases have not yet been isolated or seen under a microscope (e.g. hepatitis C virus) and others have not been cultured in the laboratory (e.g. human papilloma virus). New techniques in immunology and molecular biology are now providing information about the structure of viruses. This knowledge may give rise to different grounds for classification. At present, viruses are separated into major groups or families, based on the type of nucleic acid they contain, their shape and structure and their method of replication.

Table 5.1 lists the major families of viruses responsible for human infections.

Viral Replication

As was mentioned earlier, viruses always need to use a host cell in order to replicate. Viruses do not contain the genetic information required to produce all the enzymes necessary for the synthesis of new viral particles. Instead, they use the host cell DNA and some host cell enzymes to produce viral components. The assembly of the new components into viral particles is under the direction of the viral genes.

REPLICATION OF BACTERIAL VIRUSES

Although we are not primarily concerned in this text with the infection of bacteria by viruses, we include a brief description here because the phenomenon has provided much information about many of the important processes that occur in the infection of animal cells. Viruses that infect bacteria are called **bacteriophage** or **phage**. They have been extensively studied, as they provide a simple model for investigating the mechanisms of viral infection. A bacterial culture contains many millions of identical cells. It is easy to infect a culture of bacteria with phage and observe the results in a uniform population.

Phage exert the same specificity for their host cell as do viruses which infect higher organisms. This property is often used to differentiate strains of bacteria. For example, different strains of the bacterium *Staphylococcus aureus* are susceptible to different bacteriophage. **Phage typing** is used to determine which particular strain of the bacterium is responsible for an outbreak of infection. Bacterial specimens obtained from infected patients are cultured in the laboratory and then exposed to different phage preparations. Susceptible strains are killed by the

TABLE 5.1
CLASSIFICATION OF VIRUSES INTO FAMILIES BY CHEMICAL AND PHYSICAL PROPERTIES

VIRAL FAMILY	CAPSID SYMMETRY	VIRION NAKED OR ENVELOPED	SIZE (NM)	NUCLEIC ACID
Parvoviridae	Icosahedral	Naked	18–26	ss DNA
Papovaviridae		Naked	45–55	ds DNA (circular)
Adenoviridae		Naked	70–90	ds DNA
Herpes viridae	Icosahedral	Enveloped	90–130	ds DNA
Poxviridae	Complex		230 x 400	ds DNA
Hepadna viridae			42	ds DNA (circular)
Picornaviridae	Icosahedral	Naked	20–30	ss RNA
Calciviridae		Naked	35–39	ss RNA
Reoviridae		Naked	60–80	ds RNA (segmented)
Togaviridae	Icosahedral	Enveloped	50–70	ss RNA
Flaviviridae	Unknown	Enveloped	45–50	ss RNA
Arenaviridae	or	Enveloped	50–300	ss RNA (segmented)
Coronaviridae	complex	Enveloped	80–160	ss RNA
Retroviridae		Enveloped	~ 100	ss RNA (diploid)
Bunyaviridae	Helical	Enveloped	90–100	ss RNA (segmented)
Orthomyxoviridae	Helical		80–120	ss RNA (segmented)
Paramyxoviridae	Helical		150–300	ss RNA
Rhabdoviridae	Helical		75 x 80	ss RNA

Source: Adapted from Brooks, G.F., Butel, J.S. and Ornston, L.N. (1991) *Jawetz, Melnick & Adelberg's, Medical Microbiology*, 19th ed., Appleton & Lange, Table 32.1, p. 368

FIGURE 5.4
BACTERIOPHAGE
(a) Electron micrograph and diagram of T even bacteriophage; (b) diagrammatic representation of lytic and lysogenic cycles of bacteriophage infection.

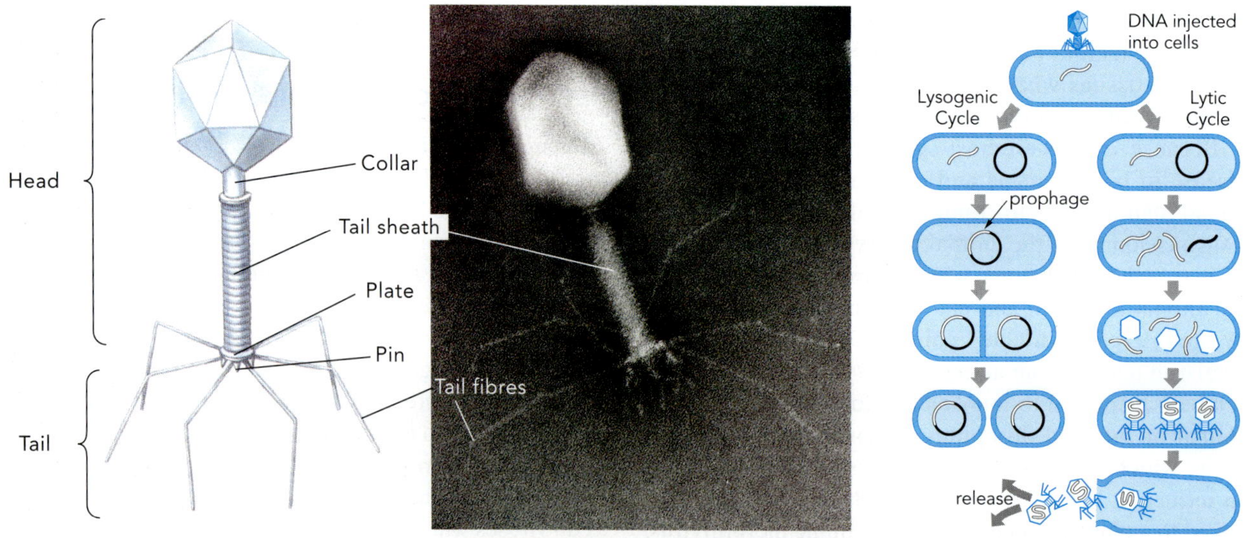

(a) Electron micrograph of bacteriophage

(b)

phage and this allows identification of the particular strain present. This technique is useful for epidemiological studies to determine the source of the infection and the method of transmission. (See Figure 4.17.)

Infection of a bacterium by the phage involves first, the attachment of the phage to a specific receptor site on the target cell wall. Since the bacterial cell is relatively small, only the viral nucleic acid is injected into the bacterium during infection. This is illustrated in Figure 5.4. Once the phage DNA has entered the cell, a number of different events may occur. The most usual outcome is that the phage takes over the cell machinery, produces many new phage particles and then causes lysis of the cell as the new phage are released into the surrounding medium. This is called the **lytic cycle**.

Sometimes, the phage enters the cell but, instead of reproducing itself, the phage DNA is incorporated into the host cell DNA. In this state, called **lysogeny**, the phage is **latent** and does not produce new phage or cause lysis. The phage DNA that has been inserted into the bacterial chromosome is called a **prophage.** When the bacterium divides, the phage DNA is also copied, with the result that all the bacterial daughter cells contain the phage genes. One possible outcome of lysogeny is that the host cell may exhibit new properties. For example, *Corynebacterium diphtheriae*, the bacterium that causes diphtheria, is only pathogenic when it is carrying the prophage that has the gene for the production of the diphtheria toxin. Scarlet fever, a possible complication of a streptococcal infection, occurs only when the particular strain of streptococci is carrying the gene for the erythrogenic scarlet fever toxin on its prophage DNA.

Lysogeny can also give rise to **specialised transduction**, in which bacterial genes are transferred with the phage DNA to another bacterial cell (see Chapter 4). A similar process to lysogeny can occur in animal cells, and may involve the transformation of the animal cell by the incorporation of viral DNA into the host cell genome. This usually results in the production of abnormal or cancerous cells. This is discussed further on page 103.

Viral Infection in Animal Cells

Of more interest to health professionals is the sequence of events that takes place when an animal (human) cell is infected by a virus. This process can be broken down into six steps.

1. **Adsorption**. The first step in viral infection is the attachment of the virion to the specific receptor site on the outside of the host cell. The part of the viral capsid or envelope that binds to the host has a specific chemical structure and often forms part of the viral antigen.
2. **Penetration**. After the virion has attached to the host cell, the whole virion penetrates the cell by a process in which the host cell membrane engulfs the viral particle. Animal cells are so much larger than viruses that there is plenty of room for the whole virion to enter.
3. **Uncoating**. The virus is then dismantled, the envelope and capsid removed and broken down into their component amino acids, and the nucleic acid is released into the cytoplasm.

   Adsorption, penetration and uncoating occur very rapidly, usually taking only a few minutes.
4. **Synthesis**. The nucleic acid is then copied many times, the viral genes directing the synthesis of viral messenger RNA and new viral capsid proteins and enzymes.
5. **Assembly**. The viral nucleic acid and the newly synthesised capsomeres are assembled in either the nucleus or the cytoplasm of the cell.
6. **Release**. Naked viruses are released from the host cell, usually resulting in cell lysis and death. Enveloped viruses 'bud' out through the cell membrane, acquiring their envelope from the host cell membrane which has been modified by the insertion of viral glycoproteins. (See Figure 5.5.)

The complete cycle occupies several hours.

When many viral particles are synthesised and released at once, lysis and death of the host cell inevitably occurs. Sometimes, virus formation is slower and the new virions are released continuously. This does not necessarily cause the immediate death of the cell.

REPLICATION OF ANIMAL VIRUSES

Synthesis of new viral components takes place in the nucleus and cytoplasm of the host cell. The actual method of viral replication varies, depending on whether the viral nucleic acid is RNA or DNA, and whether it is single- or double-stranded. The replication of double-stranded DNA (dsDNA) viruses essentially follows the usual pathways for nucleic acid and protein synthesis, except that the host cell provides most of the necessary enzymes. The viral DNA directs the synthesis of viral messenger RNA and proteins and the assembly of the viral components into new viral particles.

This process is illustrated in Figure 5.6 for a DNA-containing virus.

Most RNA viruses contain single strands of RNA (ssRNA) which are described as either positive or negative sense strands. Positive (+) sense strands can function directly as messenger RNA (i.e. as a template for protein synthesis). The details of the method of replication of the different ssRNA-containing viruses are beyond the scope of this text. A brief overview is given here. In general, the single RNA strands need to synthesise new viral RNA and viral protein via a series of steps involving positive and negative sense RNA strands. The viruses containing double-stranded RNA have a slightly different method of replication. This family includes the human rotavirus, an important cause of infantile gastroenteritis. A completely

FIGURE 5.5
HERPES BUDDING OUT OF CELL

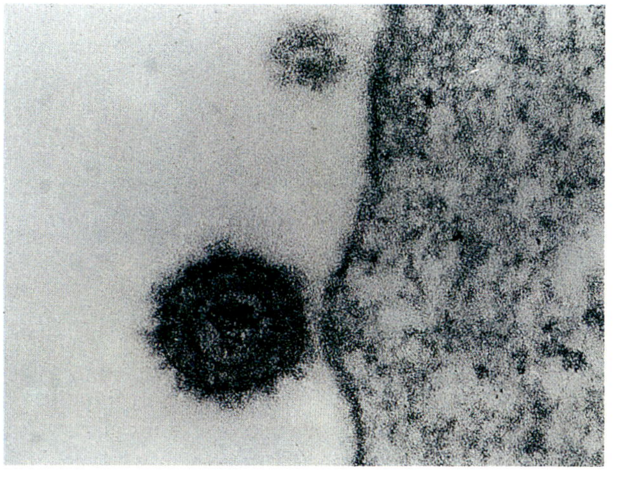

FIGURE 5.6
INFECTION OF ANIMAL CELL BY DNA VIRUS

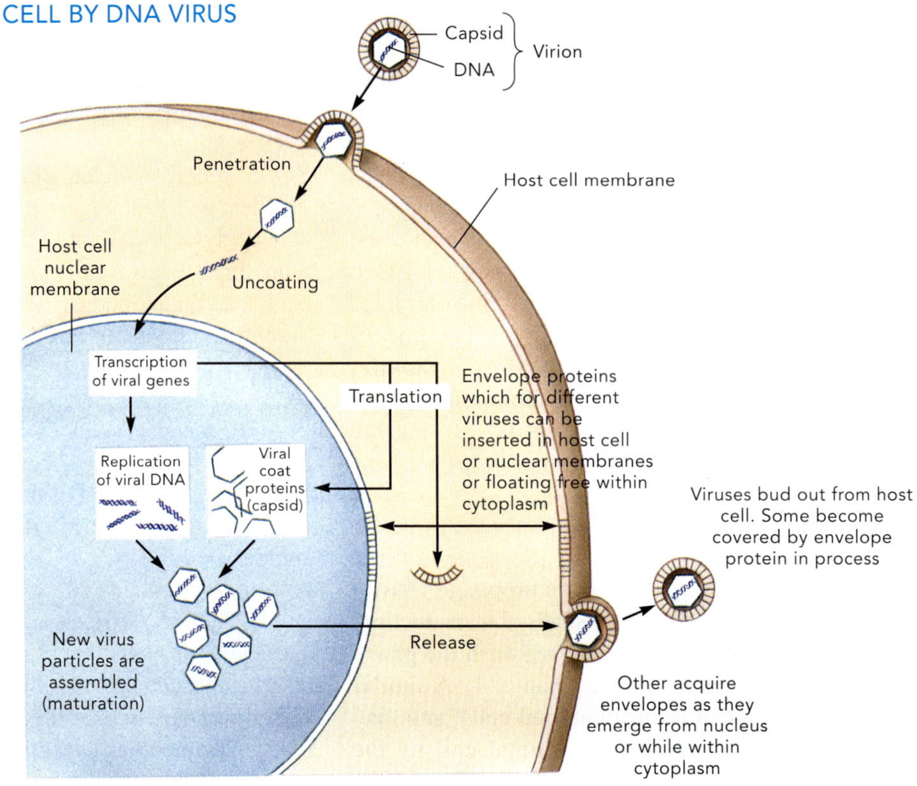

different pathway of synthesis occurs in an important family of RNA viruses known as the **retroviruses**. Replication in these viruses initially involves a reverse process whereby viral DNA is synthesised from the single-stranded viral RNA, using a viral enzyme called reverse transcriptase. The viral DNA is then transcribed into viral messenger RNA, protein and new viral RNA. A number of very important pathogens belong to this group, including the human immunodeficiency virus, HIV.

Figure 5.7 is a diagrammatic comparison of the steps involved in the synthesis of a positive sense ssRNA virus and a retrovirus.

An understanding of the different pathways of viral synthesis allows scientists to identify critical steps that could be the target for antiviral drugs. For example, the enzyme reverse transcriptase is unique to retroviral synthesis. The drug zidovudine (AZT), an analogue of thymine that is used to treat HIV-positive patients, is readily incorporated by this enzyme into the viral DNA, resulting in an inactive DNA and preventing further viral replication.

Antiviral drugs are discussed more fully in Chapter 12.

Types of Viral Infections in Humans

In this book we are concerned with viral infections of humans, the outcome for the host and the implications for transmission, treatment and prevention. A knowledge of the method of replication and the course of the disease can aid in the development of suitable treatments or preventative measures. We now look at the different ways in which viruses infect human cells and examine the implications for transmission and prevention of viral infections.

Table 5.2 is a list of common viral infections of humans. New viruses are constantly being described so a table such as this requires continual updating. The diseases listed are described in detail in other chapters of this book under the appropriate body system (see references in table).

Viral infection of human cells can follow any one of a number of different pathways. The outcome of any infection is determined by the genetic makeup of the virus and the susceptibility of the host. Some viruses produce a range of disease symptoms and the same disease can be produced by a variety of different viruses (e.g. the common cold is caused by adenoviruses, rhinoviruses, parainfluenza viruses, enteroviruses etc.). Viral infections can be described as acute, subclinical, latent, chronic (carrier), persistent, slow or oncogenic. The familiar, acute, highly contagious viral illness, that follows a defined course, characterised by recognisable signs and symptoms and leading to complete recovery, is only one of the outcomes of viral infection. Many viral infections do not produce recognisable symptoms of disease at all and are said to be **subclinical**.

Much of our current knowledge is gained from studies aimed at detecting viral antigens and the antibodies to those antigens in different tissues. These studies have shown that some viruses tend to persist in the host and cause recurrent bouts of disease. Another important feature of viral diseases is the ability of some infective virions to be transmitted from an asymptomatic carrier to a

FIGURE 5.7
INFECTION AND REPLICATION BY VARIOUS RNA VIRUSES

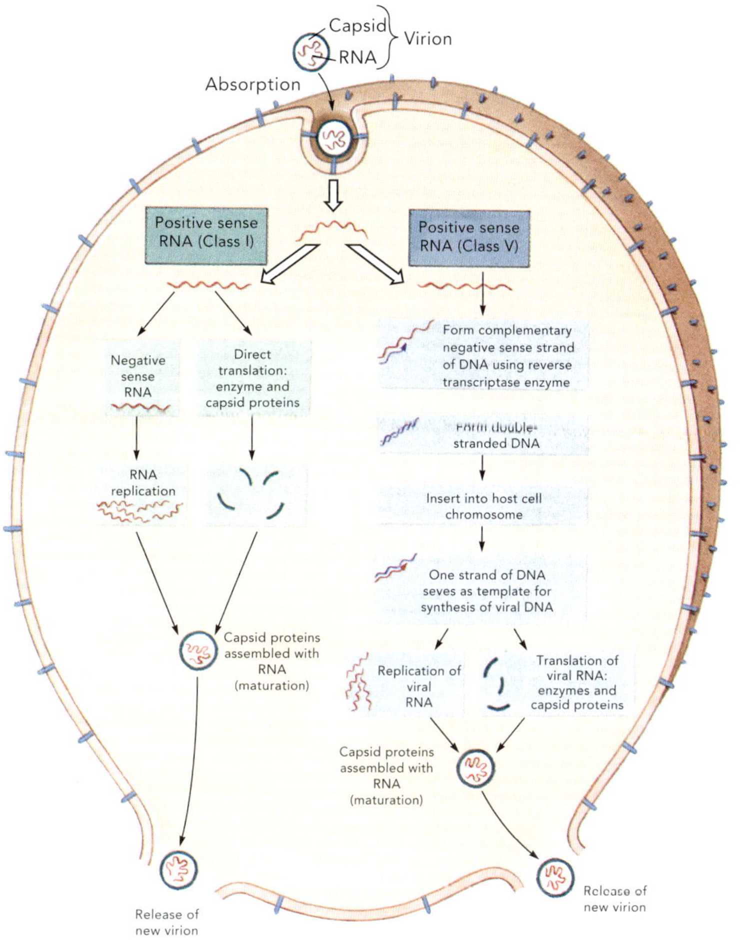

Two of the mechanisms used for the replication of RNA animal viruses. The one shown at the left is found in Class I RNA viruses, which have positive sense, single-stranded RNA genomes. The viral RNA serves as mRNA—it is translated immediately to produce proteins needed for reproduction of the virus. A negative sense copy is then made, which serves as a template for production of more positive sense viral RNA. The one at the right is found in Class V RNA viruses. The positive sense RNA is copied with the help of reverse transcriptase to make a negative sense strand of DNA, which serves as a template for the synthesis of a complementary positive sense strand. The double-stranded DNA is then inserted into the host chromosome, where it can remain for some time. When replication occurs, one strand of the DNA becomes the template for the synthesis of viral RNA.

susceptible host. We now look at each of these phenomena in some detail.

ACUTE LYTIC INFECTION

Acute lytic infection is typified by an acute, well-defined, recognisable infection, such as mumps, influenza or the common cold. The virion gains entry to the host, attaches to its specific target cell, enters and takes over the host cell machinery, making many copies of the virus. The release of the new virions causes cell lysis and death. The new viral particles then infect neighbouring cells. Eventually, the host produces an immune response that is successful in eliminating the invading virus, and immunological memory is established to protect against further infections by the same virus.

For many diseases (e.g. mumps), this acute infection will give rise to long-lasting immunity. However, some viruses, such as those responsible for influenza, have the ability to mutate and alter the structure of their outer envelope or capsid. This means that the antibodies produced against one particular strain of influenza virus will not recognise and be effective against another strain (see Chapter 9 for discussion of antigen-antibody reactions). Exposure to this new or altered strain of influenza virus will *apparently* give rise to the same disease again.

SUB-CLINICAL INFECTIONS

Very often a host is infected by a virus but does not exhibit any recognisable clinical signs or symptoms. A general feeling of malaise, slight fever or **lymphadenopathy**, 'swollen glands', may be the only signs that the patient is unwell. In this type of infection, the patient recovers, often unaware of having had any disease. Frequently, the only evidence of infection is that an immune response has been provoked resulting in the production of antibodies to the virus. These can be detected in the bloodstream of the patient who, depending on the level of antibodies present, is usually then considered to be protected from future attacks by the same virus. Rubella (German measles) can be a very mild disease and is often subclinical. However, when this disease occurs during the first trimester of pregnancy, it can cause serious congenital abnormalities in the foetus, even though the mother may experience few, if any, symptoms. Similarly, cytomegalovirus infection produces only very mild cold-like symptoms, but can cause serious congenital defects in a developing foetus.

Polio is another disease that can occur subclinically as well as in the more acute paralytic form. When the polio virus was first isolated and tests were developed for the detection of antibodies, it was found that a large percentage of the population was carrying antibodies to the virus

TABLE 5.2
SOME COMMON VIRAL INFECTIONS OF HUMANS

DISEASE	VIRUS	MAJOR ORGANS AFFECTED	REFERENCE	
Chickenpox	Varicella zoster	Generalised symptoms/skin rash	Chapter 16	p. 353
Common cold	Various	Respiratory tract	Chapter 17	p. 374
CMV	Cytomegalovirus	Generalised/salivary glands	Chapter 19	p. 457
Dengue fever	Dengue virus	Generalised	Chapter 19	p. 455
Encephalitis	Various/some arthropod-borne	Nervous system/brain	Chapter 20	p. 480
Gastroenteritis	Rotavirus Norwalk Enterovirus	Gastrointestinal system	Chapter 18	p. 404 ff.
Glandular fever (infectious mononucleosis)	Epstein-Barr	Immune system	Chapter 19	p. 456
Hepatitis	Hepatitis A,B,C,D,E	Liver	Chapter 18	p. 419 ff.
Herpes	Herpes simplex type 1, type 2	Skin	Chapter 16 Chapter 21	p. 354; p. 506
HIV/AIDS	Human immunodeficiency virus	T4 cells of immune system	Chapter 19	p. 446
Influenza	Various orthomyxoviruses	Generalised/respiratory system	Chapter 17	p. 381
Lassa fever	Lassa virus	Generalised/haemorrhagic	Chapter 19	p. 457
Measles	Rubeola	Generalised/skin rash	Chapter 16	p. 352
Meningitis	Various	Nervous system/meninges	Chapter 20	p. 478 ff.
Mumps	Paramyxovirus	Salivary glands		
Polio	Polio	Nervous system	Chapter 20	p. 486
Bronchiolitis	Respiratory syncytial virus	Respiratory tract	Chapter 17	p. 381
Rubella (German measles)	Rubella	Generalised/skin rash	Chapter 16	p. 351
Shingles	Herpes zoster (latent form of varicella zoster)	Skin/nervous system	Chapter 16	p. 353
Warts	Papilloma	Skin/mucous membranes	Chapter 16	p. 254
Yellow fever	Yellow fever	Generalised/liver	Chapter 19	p. 457

without any previous history of the disease. It has been suggested that this was most probably the result of a subclinical infection in an earlier childhood exposure.

Other viral diseases that are known to occur subclinically include glandular fever (Epstein-Barr virus) and hepatitis B. Both can also have other serious outcomes.

Persistence of Viral Infections

Viral infections are usually self-limiting—that is, the host immune system overcomes the virus and it is completely eliminated from the system. However, sometimes the virus persists in the human host for long periods. This persistence may have a number of different outcomes, which are variously described as latent, chronic or slow infections.

LATENT VIRAL INFECTIONS

In some cases the virus remains dormant in some host cells and can be reactivated at a later stage, causing a recurrence of the disease. Many of the latent viral infections are caused by viruses belonging to the herpes family.

The viruses generally produce an initial recognisable disease, followed by apparent recovery. However, instead of the virus being completely cleared from the host by the immune system, some viral particles remain. They often 'hide' in cells that are not the usual target of attack. Reactivation of the virus may occur when the physiological state of the host is altered. This may be due to conditions of physical or psychological stress or other illnesses.

The most familiar example of latent infection are the blisters produced by herpes simplex virus (HSV), types 1 and 2. Many patients only ever report one initial attack of herpes. However, others suffer repeated attacks associated with colds ('cold sores', 'fever blisters'), exposure to UV light (sunburn) or other stress factors. The virus has been shown to be dormant in the nerve cells of the sensory ganglia. Other herpes viruses also produce latent infections. These include the varicella zoster virus which is responsible for **varicella** (chickenpox) and **zoster** (shingles). After an attack of chickenpox, the virus may remain dormant in the sensory nerve ganglia and give rise to shingles many years later.

Epstein-Barr virus (EBV), which is responsible for glandular fever, and cytomegalovirus (CMV) can also establish latent infections.

An important characteristic of latent infections is that they tend to be reactivated when the immune system is compromised. This may be a serious complication for elderly patients, for those receiving immunosuppressive therapy or for immunodeficient patients.

In some types of latent infection, the virus responsible for the disease persists in the host for many years after the initial infection. New disease symptoms occur, usually slowly and over a long period. These symptoms are not the same as the original disease. **Subacute sclerosing panencephalitis** (SSPE) is a rare late complication of measles infection, and usually occurs in teenagers and young adults. It has been attributed to the persistence of the measles virus which lodges in the brain cells. The disease is characterised by slow (1–2 years) progressive mental deterioration and degeneration of the nervous system, and is invariably fatal. Other persistent viral infections may play an important role in human disease. Some have been shown to be associated with the development of leukaemia and sarcomas in animals.

The recently described 'post-polio syndrome' may be an example of a persistent viral infection. Patients who suffered from polio up to 40 years ago, but who had apparently completely recovered, have recently reported symptoms of muscle weakness, fatigue and other neurological problems, similar to the original polio disease.

CHRONIC VIRAL INFECTIONS (CARRIER STATE)

An important outcome of viral disease occurs when the virus remains in the host and gives rise to a continuous low level of viral production and shedding. This may occur after an acute illness or a subclinical infection. Patients do not have any disease symptoms and are often unaware that they are chronic carriers of the virus and are therefore, infectious to others. Hepatitis B is one important viral infection that may have a number of outcomes. Exposure to the virus can cause an acute infection, leading either to death or complete recovery. However, it may also result in a milder or subclinical disease. This type of exposure often gives rise to the chronic carrier state.

Hepatitis B can also be acquired by vertical transmission from a carrier mother to her baby. The baby may not exhibit any symptoms of hepatitis, but may be a chronic carrier. Serological testing for the presence of the various hepatitis B antigens and antibodies is used to establish the infectious status of the patient. (See Chapter 18 for a discussion of hepatitis and the significance of the presence of the various viral antigens.) Chronic active hepatitis B infection may cause liver damage, **cirrhosis** and in some cases **hepatocellular carcinoma**.

Hepatitis C is another virus considered to be a chronic infection. A test for hepatitis C has only been available since 1990 and there is still much to be learnt about this virus. Human immunodeficiency virus (HIV) is the primary cause of AIDS (**A**cquired **I**mmune **D**eficiency **S**ydnrome). It is described as a chronic infection because the virus is considered to be transmissible throughout the illness.

ONCOGENIC VIRUSES

Viruses thought to be implicated in the formation of cancers are called **oncogenic**. The role that viruses play in the development of cancer has not been fully established. However, various types of cancers have been shown to be associated with a previous or current viral infection. These are listed in Table 5.3. A number of viruses have been shown to cause tumours in animals and to be able to transform human cells in tissue culture. All known tumour viruses either have DNA as their nucleic acid (genome) or generate proviral DNA after infection of the cell (e.g. the retroviruses, Figure 5.7). There are two ways in which it is thought that a virus can alter normal cells.

1. The oncogenic virus introduces a new 'transforming' gene into the cell, or,
2. The virus induces or alters the expression of a pre-existing cellular gene (a 'proto' oncogene).

The result in either case is that the cell loses control of normal regulation of growth processes. One of the most important of these regulatory mechanisms is contact inhibition. Transformed cells replicate in an uncontrolled way, piling up on top of each other into a tumour-like mass.

There is a large amount of evidence linking certain types of papilloma virus to the occurrence of cervical cancer. Early changes in cervical cells can be detected by a Pap smear. (See Spotlight Box, p. 102.)

EFFECT OF HOST AGE AND IMMUNE STATUS

The age of patients and the status of their immune systems are important determinants of their susceptibility to viral infection. It is well known that the immune system matures in the first year of life and that it is less effective in the

TABLE 5.3
HUMAN CANCERS RELATED TO VIRAL INFECTIONS

CANCER	VIRUS	FAMILY	GENOME
Adult T cell leukaemia	HTLV-I	Retrovirus	ssRNA
Skin carcinomas; genital carcinomas	Papilloma, HPV5, 8 HPV 16,18	Papovavirus	DNA
Hepatocellular carcinoma	Hepatitis B ? Hepatitis C	Hepadnavirus Flavivirus	DNA RNA
Nasopharyngeal carcinoma	Epstein-Barr	Herpes	DNA
Burkitt's lymphoma	Epstein-Barr	Herpes	DNA

SPOTLIGHT
CERVICAL CANCER

Mrs Y, a 32-year-old mother of two children was admitted to hospital with advanced cervical carcinoma. Although she had been sexually active since she was 20, she had never had a Pap smear. A hysterectomy was performed to remove the diseased uterus, followed by radiation treatment and chemotherapy. However, the cancer had already spread through her body and she died 18 months later.

Comment

In Australia there is an average of 1000 new cases of cervical cancer and 350 deaths each year. More than 80% of cases are associated with a previous infection by the human papilloma virus (HPV), the cause of genital warts. All women who have ever been sexually active are at risk of developing cervical cancer, even if they have never suffered from genital warts. The risk is highest in women with multiple partners who do not use protection such as condoms.

There are more than 70 different types of human papilloma viruses that attack skin and mucosal cells. About 30 types have been identified with genital infections. Of these, types 16 and 18 are most frequently associated with abnormal Pap smears, and type 18 has been shown to have the highest risk of recurrence.

HPV induces characteristic changes in the epithelial cells of the cervix. These can be detected by microscopic examination of a smear of cells obtained from the cervix (the Papanicolaou test—Pap test) and appear even before the first evidence of malignancy.

The changes to the epithelial cells progress through stages described as cervical intraepithelial neoplasias (CIN) to carcinoma in situ (CIS), which is a precancerous condition and can lead to invasive squamous cell carcinoma. The stages are described as:

CIN I	minor dysplasia
CIN II	moderate dysplasia
CIN III	severe dysplasia—carcinoma in situ

If abnormal cells are detected by a Pap smear, the patient is referred for colposcopy. This involves examination of the cervix after a painless application of 3% acetic acid (vinegar). The lesion appears as a flat white plaque and can be removed by laser treatment. If detected early, the treatment is successful, but the woman is advised to have regular follow-up Pap smears. If the disease has progressed further, a cone biopsy can be performed. Early treatment of cervical cancer is very successful and in all countries where routine Pap smears are available the mortality from the disease has been reduced.

Unfortunately, there are limits to the accuracy of the Pap test. Incorrect results may occur because of poor sampling or from laboratory error. Approximately 20% of tests may return false negative results. Recently, some laboratories have introduced computerised scanning of microscope slides to improve the accuracy of diagnosis. Women are advised to have a Pap test at least every two years, or more frequently if there are any abnormal symptoms.

There are moves in some States to establish a central register to encourage women to return for regular checkups.

aged. On the other hand, there also seems to be an age-related susceptibility to different viral infections. The so-called childhood diseases, such as mumps and chickenpox are usually much more severe in adults. During pregnancy, the mother's immune system is also somewhat compromised to accommodate the foetus. This may explain the ability of viruses such as rubella and cytomegalovirus to cross the placenta and cause congenital defects. A very high level of maternal mortality is associated with hepatitis E infection in pregnancy.

Transmission of Viral Diseases

Effective prevention and treatment of viral diseases depends partly on an understanding of the mechanisms of transmission of these infectious agents. Infections are transmitted from one host to another when complete viral particles (virions), shed by the infected host, reach a susceptible host. Most viruses do not survive for long periods outside living cells, so transmission usually involves their direct transfer in body fluids or tissues, close contact between hosts, or transmission via an insect vector.

The rate and number of virus particles being shed varies during the course of the infection. Very often virus production and shedding is high just before recognisable clinical symptoms develop (the **prodromal phase**). This helps to explain the occurrence of epidemics, as transmission can take place before patients are aware they have a disease (e.g. chickenpox outbreaks in schools).

AIRBORNE TRANSMISSION

Viruses are shed mainly from the area of the body where the infection is localised. Thus, infection of the mucosal cells of the upper respiratory tract by the cold virus results in virions being shed in aerosol droplets when the patient coughs or sneezes. These viruses travel only short distances and do not survive for long. Other viruses which enter via the respiratory route are mainly shed in the same way.

Viral infections that produce pustules or vesicles, such as chickenpox and herpes, also shed virions from these lesions. Transmission of herpes is considered to occur mainly when visible vesicles are present, although there is some evidence that, in genital herpes, virus shedding can occur when there are no apparent symptoms.

FAECAL-ORAL TRANSMISSION

Many viruses are transmitted by the faecal contamination of food or water. For example, hepatitis A and rotavirus, which cause gastrointestinal infections, are usually shed in the faeces. Special care must be taken to prevent transmission of rotavirus among babies and small children in hospitals and child-care centres, as it can cause rapid and severe dehydration in infants. The polio virus is also shed in faeces. Although polio has been almost eradicated from some parts of the world, all viruses transmitted by the faecal-oral route are still a cause for concern in developing countries or in areas where sanitation is poor. A vaccine is available for polio but as yet there is no preventative treatment available for any of the gastrointestinal viral infections.

TRANSMISSION IN BODY FLUIDS

In recent years considerable attention has focused on viruses that can be transmitted in blood or other body substances. These include the hepatitis B (HBV) and hepatitis C (HCV) viruses, and the human immunodeficiency virus (HIV). The discovery of a previously unknown and potentially fatal virus (HIV) has drawn attention to the possibility of there being other unidentified viruses present in body substances. This has led to the adoption of a system of infection control procedures in hospitals and health care facilities that is designed to minimise the risks of transmission of viral infections (see Chapter 13).

TRANSMISSION BY INSECTS

Arboviruses are viruses that are transmitted by **arthropod vectors**, that is, by insects which carry the virus from an infected host to a susceptible human. Transmission by arthropods requires the ingestion of the virus from an infected human or animal reservoir while the insect is feeding. The virus replicates in the gut of the insect vector, spreads to the salivary glands and is injected into a susceptible host during the next blood meal. The replicative phase may take several days and the rate is affected by the ambient temperature.

About 80 arboviruses are known which are capable of infecting humans, although only a limited number occurs in Australia. Most arboviruses are maintained in nature in animal hosts, which usually sustain a subclinical infection and develop immunity. One of the most common arthropod vectors is the mosquito, and specific breeds of mosquito act as vectors for different viruses. An outbreak of a viral disease can occur if there is a pool of infected hosts present in the community, together with favourable conditions for breeding of the particular type of mosquito. Control is best achieved by mosquito eradication programs.

Some important viral diseases that are endemic to Australia and transmitted by mosquitoes include Ross River fever, Murray Valley encephalitis, and dengue fever. Of these, Ross River fever is the most widespread; the mosquito vector (*Aedes* species) is found throughout the Eastern states. Other serious arboviral diseases found outside Australia are yellow fever, Lassa fever and Japanese encephalitis.

Table 5.4 lists the major arboviral infections occurring in Australia.

FOETAL AND NEONATAL TRANSMISSION

Viral infections in the mother can have serious repercussions for the foetus or neonate. These include teratogenic (congenital) effects, the tranmission of infection to the neonate, and the acquisition of viral diseases during birth.

Teratogenic effects

Several viruses have been proven to cause serious damage to the unborn foetus. One of the earliest of these to be recognised was the effect of the rubella (German measles) virus on the foetus during the first trimester of pregnancy. The connection was first observed in Sydney in 1941, when a severe epidemic of German measles was followed by a very high incidence of congenital abnormalities.

TABLE 5.4
MAJOR ARBOVIRAL INFECTIONS IN AUSTRALIA

FAMILY	VIRUS	MOSQUITO VECTOR	REFERENCE	
Flaviviridae	Murray Valley encephalitis (MVE)	*Culex annulirostris*	Chapter 20	p. 480
	Kunjin (KUN)	*Culex annulirostris*	Chapter 20	p. 480
	Dengue	*Aedes aegypti*	Chapter 19	p. 455
Togaviridae (Alphavirus)	Ross River (RR)	25 species including *Aedes vigilax* and *Aedes camptorynchus*	Chapter 19	p. 454
	Barmah Forest (BAR)	*Culex annulirostris*	Chapter 19	p. 454
	Sindbis (SIN)	*Culex annulirostis* *Aedes normanensis*		

These included congenital heart defects, total or partial blindness, and growth or mental retardation. Work carried out by Sir Norman Gregg at the Royal Alexandra Hospital for Children in Camperdown, Sydney, correctly identified the rubella virus as the causative agent. A vaccine to prevent rubella is now available and is given routinely to all infants (male and female) at 15 months of age and again at 12–16 years.

Another virus that has been shown to cross the placenta and cause congenital abnormalities is the cytomegalovirus CMV. The extent of damage caused by CMV depends on the state of gestation at which infection occurs. *In utero*, infections may result in death or premature birth. Growth retardation and developmental malformations such as congenital heart defects, cataracts, deafness and central nervous system defects may result. There is no vaccine available for CMV, but fortunately there is a high level of immunity in the community from previous, mainly subclinical, exposure.

Recent studies have shown that there is also a slightly increased risk of congenital defects if the mother acquires chickenpox during pregnancy. Viral infection during pregnancy is suspected of being associated with the occurrence of other birth defects, and of causing severe foetal damage leading to abortion. However, not enough data are available at present to link specific viruses with specific outcomes.

Transmission of infection to the neonate

If the mother is infected with HIV or HBV, there is a significant risk of the infection being passed on to the baby. It is not certain whether the virus crosses the placenta during the last few weeks of pregnancy, or whether the virus is acquired by the neonate when blood from the mother and baby mix at the time of delivery. Probably both situations occur. Babies born to mothers who are known hepatitis B carriers are given anti-hepatitis B immunoglobulin antibodies at birth. The hepatitis B antibodies neutralise any live virus particles transmitted at, or just prior to, birth. The baby is then started on a course of hepatitis B vaccination to prevent development of the disease by future exposure to the maternal carrier. Usually breast feeding is not recommended in this situation. Babies treated this way have a very good chance of not acquiring hepatitis B, and of not suffering any ill effects.

Babies born to HIV-positive mothers will usually be carrying antibodies to the virus (IgG) which have been derived from the mother across the placenta. It will usually be 6–12 months before the maternal antibodies disappear from the neonate and it is therefore not possible, during this period, to test specifically for neonatal antibodies to find out whether the baby is infected with the virus. Tests for the HIV virus itself are often not conclusive as the virus may be 'hiding' inside a white blood cell or lymph mode, rather than being free in the blood stream. Breast feeding by HIV-infected mothers is usually not recommended. Present data indicate the risk of vertical mother to baby transmission at less than 20% for HIV and about 70% for hepatitis B. Reliable data for hepatitis C are not yet available.

Viral diseases acquired at birth

Viruses acquired during birth may also pose a serious risk to the neonate. The most serious of these is herpes simplex. If the mother has an active genital herpes infection at the time of birth, the baby may acquire the virus during passage through the birth canal. Usually the eyes are infected first, but in severe cases **herpes encephalopathy, viral infection of the brain,** may result. The latter can be fatal. If the mother has had a long-established genital herpes infection, the baby will already have maternal IgG antibodies that will provide some protection. The greatest risk to the neonate is from a recently acquired active maternal infection. In such cases, caesarean section is often performed to avoid exposure of the baby to the virus during passage through the birth canal.

Inactivation of Viruses

There is great variability in the length of time that a virus particle (virion) can survive outside the host cell, as well as the range of physical and chemical conditions it can withstand.

- Most viruses are destroyed by heating at 60°C for 30 minutes although some, such as the hepatitis B and papova viruses, can withstand much higher temperatures. The surface proteins are inactivated in a few minutes at 60°C, with the result that the virus is no longer capable of surface attachment or uncoating. The rate of inactivation is slower at room temperature, some viruses being able to survive for several hours. Many viruses can survive for several days in the cold (4°C).
- Some viruses are stable in the presence of salt solutions and buffers. This property is useful for the preparation and storage of viral vaccines, but also means that the virus can persist in food or body substances for significant periods of time.
- Viruses are usually stable at neutral pH (pH 5–9) but most are destroyed by alkaline conditions. Some viruses, like the enteroviruses, are resistant to acid pH, which allows them to survive the acidity of the stomach.
- The effect of detergents varies, depending on the presence or absence of lipid or a lipid-containing envelope in the structure of the virus. Disruption of the outer capsid or envelope structure by detergent prevents the virus from attaching and gaining entry to the host cell, even though the nucleic acid may be intact.
- Disinfectants such as the quaternary ammonium salts, organic iodine compounds and alcohols are not very effective against viruses. Higher concentrations of chlorine are needed to kill viruses than are required to kill bacteria, especially in the presence of organic matter such as faeces. For example, the polio virus can be inactivated by 1 ppm of chlorine, but much higher concentrations are required when the virus is present in faecal specimens in sewage. The polio virus is also protected when in the presence of milk products such as ice-cream. Nevertheless, chlorine compounds (sodium hypochlorite) are useful disinfectants for the inactivation of viruses.

  Standard Precautions (Chapter 13) specify a concentration of 0.1% chlorine for the disinfection of spills of blood and body substances that may contain blood-borne pathogens including viruses.
- Treatment of viruses with the chemical, formaldehyde, destroys infectivity by reacting with the viral nucleic acid, but has little effect on the capsid proteins. It has been used in the preparation of some viral vaccines, such as the Salk polio vaccine, as the antigenic properties of the capsid proteins are retained but the virus is no longer infective.
- Antibacterial antibiotics and the sulphonamide drugs are not effective against viruses. A limited number of antiviral drugs has been developed. These are described in Chapter 12.

Diagnosis of Viral Infections

Most viral infections are diagnosed by signs and symptoms. Very often, a general feeling of malaise and slight fever is suddenly explained when a distinctive rash appears (e.g. chickenpox). Usually, by the time these symptoms appear in an acute infection, the body's immune system has already responded. Treatment of the patient is therefore largely symptomatic. Sometimes, however, it is important to have an accurate diagnosis as early as possible. It may be necessary to determine the level of infectivity of the patient and the consequent risk of transmission to other patients. Specimens are collected from the affected tissues of the patient and one of the following methods is used to detect the presence of the virus.

IMMUNOFLUORESCENCE

If large numbers of viral particles are present in the specimen, they can often be detected by reaction with a fluorescently labelled antibody, followed by observation with a fluorescence microscope (see Figure 5.8). This method can give a quick definitive answer in 2–3 hours, but is limited to situations where there is a large viral population and to diseases for which appropriate labelled antibodies are commercially available.

CELL CULTURE

Culture of viruses in the laboratory is more difficult, expensive and time-consuming than the culture of bacteria, because viruses must be grown inside a living cell. When there are not sufficient virus particles present in the specimen to detect by immunofluorescence, a sample is usually inoculated into a cell culture and grown for 2–5 days. The cells are then observed for **cytopathic effects (CPE)** (see Figure 5.9 on p. 106). The cell culture can also be tested for the presence of a specific virus by immunological methods (see Chapter 15). These include the direct enzyme-linked immunoabsorbent assay (**ELISA**), which produces colour reactions linked to antibody-antigen reactions, and the immunofluorescent antibody method described above.

SEROLOGY

An alternative, and often easier, method is to test for the patient's immune response by serology. A blood sample is taken from the patient and tested for the presence of antibodies to the suspected virus. The presence of specific IgM antibodies generally indicates a recent infection. IgG antibodies indicate that the infection occurred some time before. As described in Chapter 15, this method is limited by the time required after infection for the body to mount an immune response and produce detectable antibodies. On the whole, this method is reliable for acute infections. For some important persistent infections, the methods currently used detect only the presence of antibodies and not the virus itself. This imposes some limitations on

FIGURE 5.8
DETECTION OF VIRUS PARTICLES BY IMMUNOFLUORESCENCE

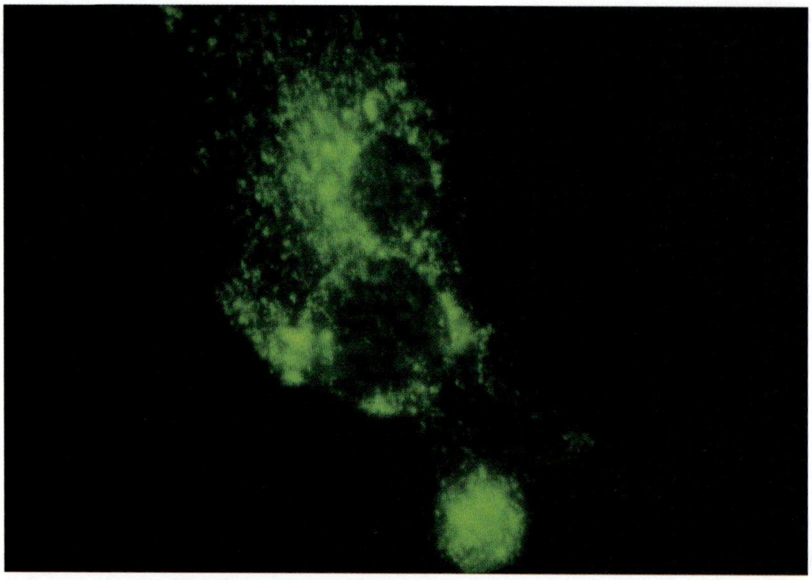

FIGURE 5.9
CYTOPATHIC EFFECTS OF VIRAL INFECTIONS IN CELL CULTURE
(a) Normal and (b) infected cells. Such transformation is a cytopathic effect (CPE) caused by infection with certain viruses, in this case polio virus.

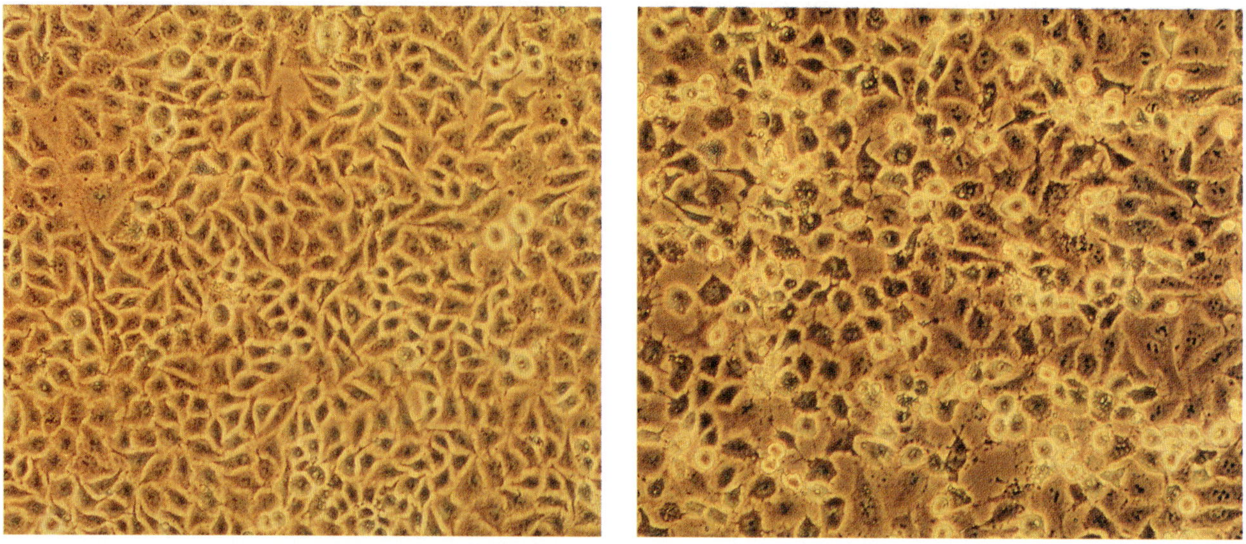

(a) (b)

the interpretation of the results in terms of the infectivity of the patient's serum.

Tests for the presence of live viruses in serum may require the use of PCR and DNA typing and are still limited by cost and sensitivity (see below).

The serology methods are discussed in more detail in Chapter 15.

NUCLEIC ACID PROBES

The use of DNA probes is a new technique with the potential to detect viral nucleic acid (i.e. live viruses) in clinical specimens. It utilises the reaction of nucleic acid 'probes'—that is, specific nucleotide sequences which have been identified and which match corresponding sequences in the viral genome. For example, a probe for the detection of the human papilloma virus in cervical cells is available commercially. This technique will no doubt become more widely used as more specific viral probes become available and the sensitivity of the tests is improved.

Growth of Viruses in the Laboratory

As we know, viruses can replicate only inside a living cell. This characteristic places strict limitations on the methods that can be used to cultivate viruses. In general, viruses are grown in the laboratory for one of the following reasons:

- diagnosis of infection;
- research;
- preparation of a vaccine.

The actual method employed depends on the number of viral particles which are required and the availability of suitable cell cultures. Early attempts to grow viruses relied on the use of animals or embryonated eggs. The inoculation of viral specimens into live animals is costly and in many cases inconclusive. It is used mainly for the primary isolation of 'new' viruses or for studies of *in vivo* pathogenesis or oncogenesis. This method has been largely replaced by growth of viruses in cell culture.

Growth of viruses in embryonated eggs is a convenient and cheap alternative to whole-animal experiments. Several different membranes in the egg are able to support the growth of viruses. The effects of viral infection are measured by death of the embryo or production of typical lesions or other damage. Early vaccine preparations were made from viruses harvested from egg cultures. There were some problems associated with this method as the vaccine sometimes contained residual egg proteins which provoked an allergic response in some individuals. Most viral cultures are now carried out using the techniques of cell culture (tissue culture). Some vaccines (e.g. hepatitis B) are produced by genetic engineering.

Cell cultures are preparations of animal (usually human) cells which are grown in a special cell culture medium under strictly controlled aseptic conditions. The cells adhere to the walls of the flask and spread out to form a confluent monolayer. Cell lines for culture can be obtained in several different ways. **Primary cell lines** are cultures of cells extracted from fresh tissue and induced to grow as monolayers in cell culture flasks. They are useful, but tend to die out after a few generations. **Diploid cell lines** consist of cells that have been developed from human embryonic tissue. Among the most widely used are **fibroblasts** (immature cells that give rise to collagen, connective tissue and skin). They are capable of rapid growth and tend to be able to continue to reproduce for 50–100 generations. They are essentially normal cells so their response to viral infection can often be an indicator of true *in vivo* effects.

Continuous cell lines are cultures derived from malignant tissue and are therefore capable of prolonged or indefinite growth. They are usually 'transformed' cells, that is, cells that are no longer normal, do not exhibit contact inhibition and have unusual chromosome patterns. Although these cells are useful as a medium for virus culture, they do not really provide information about the effect of virus infection on normal cells.

The selection of which cell culture to use depends on the specificity of the particular virus and the kind of information required. Viral specimens are inoculated into the culture and the effect of the virus on the host cell can be observed microscopically. The changes that occur in infected cells are called **cytopathic effects** and are usually typical of the infecting virus. These effects include:

- production of 'inclusion bodies'—granules in the cytoplasm of the infected cell;
- fusion of several cells, forming giant, multinucleated or 'syncytial' cells;
- transformation of the cell into a spindle-shaped cell that does not exhibit contact inhibition;
- cell death.

Cell culture is the main method used in specialist viral laboratories. The cells are grown in special culture flasks and may also be grown in small volumes in the wells of microtitre plates. Different dilutions of the virus preparation are inoculated into the wells to observe the cytopathic effects produced by the virus infection and to quantify the amount of virus present (see Figure 5.9) and Chapter 15). After the virus has been allowed to multiply in the cells, it may also be further identified by the ELISA test or by reaction with specific fluorescent antibodies, as described above.

Treatment and Prevention of Viral Infections

Viral infection produces several kinds of response by the host's immune system in order to eliminate the virus and prevent reinfection. A rapid immune response often results in a mild or subclinical infection. The response includes activation of T cells, production of lymphokines and other cytokines, as well as the activation of B-lymphocytes and production of antibodies and memory cells (see Chapter 9). As well, interferon is released from infected cells and binds to uninfected cells to prevent further viral replication. The activation of the immune system and the production of interferon and cytokines is responsible for many of the symptoms associated with viral infections—swollen glands (lymphadenopathy), malaise, headache and myalgia, for example.

Treatment of most viral infections is aimed mainly at relieving the symptoms, which are to a large extent an indication of the body's immune system fighting the infection. Bed rest and administration of analgesics and antipyretics to alleviate symptoms are the main methods available. Recovery from the disease will depend largely on the ability of the host's immune response to recognise the foreign invader and produce antibodies and T cells to combat it.

ANTIVIRAL DRUGS

An understanding of the methods of viral replication is important in order to appreciate the difficulties associated with finding suitable antiviral drugs. One of the basic requirements for a safe, effective drug is **selective toxicity**; that is, the ability to kill the pathogen without harming the host cell. Since viruses use the host cell machinery to replicate, any drug that inhibits or interferes with viral multiplication is also likely to affect the host cell adversely. Most drugs that interfere with viral replication are too toxic to be used therapeutically. It is therefore necessary to identify steps in the replicative process that are unique to the virus, or to identify and target one of the few virus-specific enzyme reactions.

At present, the most successful antiviral drugs are those that are analogues of the various nucleotide bases found in viral DNA—that is, they have a structure that is similar to, but not identical with, the naturally occurring base. They are able to be incorporated by the viral enzymes into viral DNA, but the DNA is inactive and not able to be replicated. Zidovudine (AZT), an analogue of thymine, is one such compound; it is incorporated into the DNA of the AIDS virus by an enzyme unique to retroviruses, called **reverse transcriptase**. This enzyme is used by the virus to synthesise DNA from RNA. Incorporation of the analogue into the viral DNA gives rise to an inactive DNA which is not able to be replicated and so prevents further viral replication. However, although zidovudine is readily incorporated into viral DNA by reverse transcriptase, it is also incorporated to some extent by DNA polymerase into normal cell DNA causing severe side effects in the host, such as bone marrow depression.

Another useful drug is **acyclovir**, an analogue of guanosine. This compound is phosphorylated by the enzyme thymidine kinase, present only in herpes viruses, to produce an inactive nucleotide triphosphate which, when incorporated into viral DNA, interferes with DNA replication. Acyclovir has been used successfully for the treatment of a number of infections due to the herpes family, including shingles and genital herpes.

Interferons are naturally occurring antiviral proteins that are produced by animal (host) cells in response to viral infection. There are several different interferons, commonly grouped into three classes: alpha interferon (α-IFN), beta interferon (ß-IFN) and gamma interferon (γ-IFN). The exact mechanism of the action of the interferons is not clear. They appear to act by interfering with the translation of viral messenger RNA into viral protein, thus preventing the further production and spread of virus after the initial infection has occurred. Interferons are host cell specific, not virus specific. There are, however, serious limitations in their therapeutic use since they have a very short half-life in the human body, and a number of toxic side effects. They have been used with some success in the treatment of chronic viral infections such as hairy cell leukaemia, and hepatitis B and C, but the symptoms of viral infection recur when treatment is halted.

Antiviral drugs are discussed in more detail in Chapter 12.

VACCINATION

The observation by Edward Jenner in the 18th century that milkmaids who had recovered from cowpox did not usually contract smallpox laid the basis for our modern vaccination programs. Vaccination (or immunisation) is the major weapon available against viral disease, and is the means whereby smallpox has been eradicated.

Vaccination involves the exposure of a person to only a part of the virus, or to an inactive or weakened form of the virus in order to elicit an immune response. The aim is to produce specific antibodies and specific B- and T-lymphocyte memory cells, without producing any clinical symptoms of disease. These antibodies and memory cells protect the patient against subsequent exposure to the virulent form of the disease-causing agent. The mechanism of the immune response is discussed in Chapter 9.

It has been possible to derive attenuated (weakened) forms of many viruses for use in vaccines. Other vaccines consist of killed or inactivated viral preparations which retain their antigenic properties; that is, they are still able to stimulate an immune response. Recent developments in genetic engineering have seen the production of vaccines consisting of fragments of the virus produced by cloning a part of the viral DNA in a yeast or bacterial cell. Hepatitis B vaccine is one example of this type of vaccine. One of the major advantages (apart from the ease of production) is that there is no risk of causing the actual disease since the vaccine consists of only part of the viral coat.

Prevention of viral disease by mass immunisation campaigns is an important aspect of primary health care. Table 5.5 lists the viral diseases for which vaccines are currently available. Figure 5.10 illustrates the dramatic fall in the incidence of many diseases since the introduction of vaccines. It is possible that viral diseases for which humans are the only reservoir, and which are caused by viruses that do not survive for long periods outside the human body, can be eradicated by effective vaccination campaigns. Smallpox has officially been eradicated worldwide. Polio has almost been eradicated from the Americas and there have been no cases in Australia since 1986.

Future Directions in Virus Research

It has become apparent in recent years that there are many viruses yet to be discovered. Some of these may be responsible for presently unexplained illnesses. People in Africa were dying from 'wasting disease' long before HIV was identified as its cause, and 'post-transfusion hepatitis' was described long before it was shown to be caused by the hepatitis C virus. New techniques in molecular biology make it possible to identify a viral genome without isolating or culturing the virus itself, as has been the case for hepatitis C. This virus has still not been observed microscopically or cultured in the laboratory, despite the fact that there are sophisticated tests available to detect the presence of both viral antibodies and antigens in blood.

The ability to amplify fragments of viral RNA or DNA (e.g. for hepatitis C in blood) by the polymerase chain reaction (PCR) has far-reaching consequences for diagnostic virology. The sensitivity of PCR (see p. 85) means that it is easier to probe for the viral nucleic acid, rather than try to isolate the virus itself. The identification of another hepatitis virus that appears to be transmitted in blood (hepatitis G or GB) opens up the possibility of many other still unidentified viruses.

However, despite our detailed understanding of viral replication, we still have a lot to learn about how viruses cause disease. Cytopathic effects, leading to the destruction of infected cells, are obvious consequences, but there

TABLE 5.5
VIRAL DISEASES FOR WHICH VACCINES ARE AVAILABLE

DISEASE	RECOMMENDED SCHEDULE IN AUSTRALIA
Chickenpox	Not yet licensed for use in Australia.
Hepatitis A	Three doses: two 1 month apart, and a booster at any age.
Hepatitis B	Three doses: 1, 2, 6 months apart, can be given at any age.
Influenza	Different vaccine produced each year for prevalent strain. Recommended for elderly and 'at risk' patients.
Measles	MMR: two doses, 12–15 months, 10–16 years.
Mumps	MMR: two doses, 12–15 months, 10–16 years.
Rubella	MMR: two doses, 12–15 months, 10–16 years. Booster may be required before becoming pregnant. Antibody titre should be checked.
Polio	Sabin oral vaccine (OPV): 2, 4, 6 months; boosters at 18 months, 5 years, 15 years.
Rabies	Usually only after exposure to rabies virus.
Yellow fever	Recommended when travelling to endemic countries.

FIGURE 5.10
EFFECT OF INTRODUCTION OF VACCINES ON INCIDENCE OF VIRAL DISEASES
The fall in incidence of poliomyelitis, measles, rubella and mumps in the USA following the introduction of vaccination against diseases (arrows). Inactivated poliovirus vaccine was introduced in 1954, live vaccines in 1963. The other three, for measles (introduced in 1963), mumps (1967) and rubella (1969) are live vaccines. (Compiled from data kindly supplied by the US Centers for Disease Control.) (From White, D. O. and Fenner, F. (1994) *Medical Virology*, 4th ed., Academic Press.)

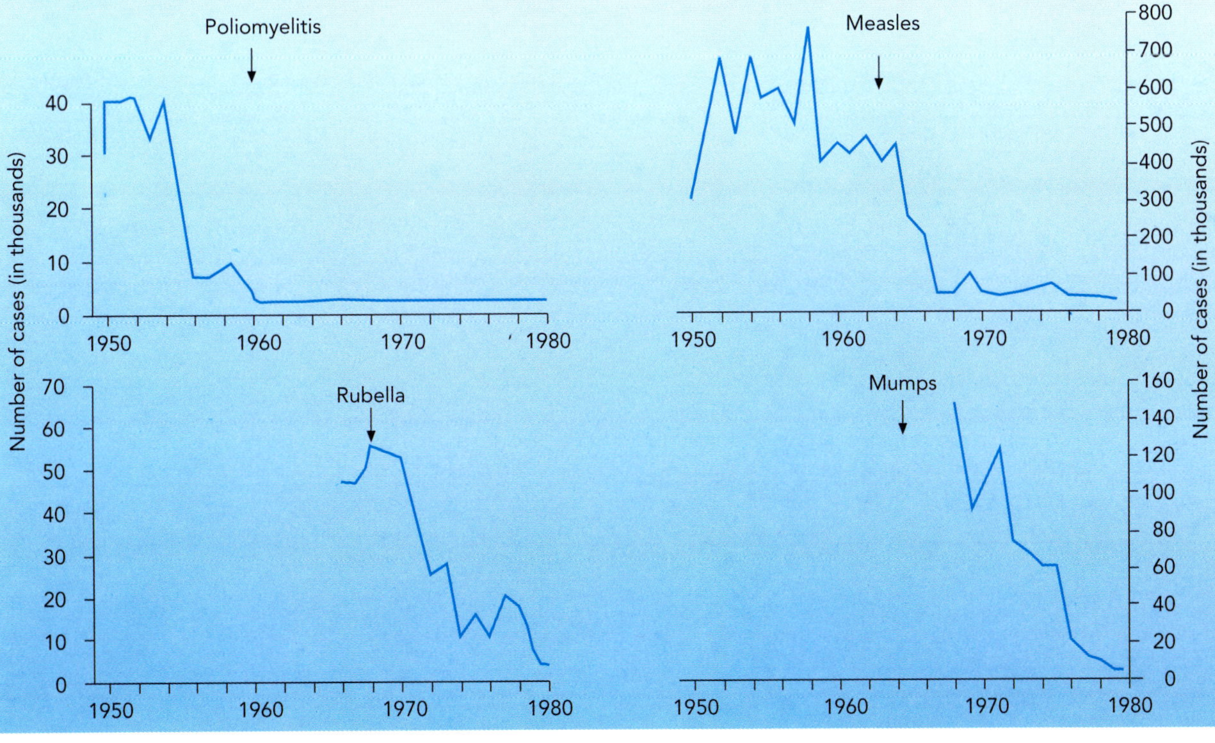

are more subtle physiological changes that appear to be due to non-cytocidal viruses. The ability of some viruses to evade host defences, to undergo specific mutations, or to lie dormant and be reactivated under certain conditions has far-reaching implications for human health in general. Persistent viral infections, such as measles and possibly polio, which produce symptoms many years after the patient has apparently fully recovered from the disease, pose a particular challenge. The World Health Organization is mounting a worldwide campaign aimed at eradicating both these diseases. This requires education and the cooperation of both individuals and governments.

The significance of the role that viruses play in multifactorial diseases such as hepatocellular carcinoma has yet to be fully elucidated. One of the most interesting aspects of viral infection that needs further study is the involvement of viruses in autoimmune reactions and the possible viral suppression of the immune system with consequent reactivation of, or superinfection by, other microbial species.

Summary

STRUCTURE OF VIRUSES

- Viruses are the smallest type of infectious particle.
- Each viruses possesses only one type of nucleic acid—RNA or DNA—enclosed in a protein coat or capsid made up of capsomeres.
- Capsids occur in distinctive shapes (e.g. icosahedral, helical).
- Some viruses are enclosed by an envelope which helps the virus attach to the host cell.
- Viruses use the host cell enzymes for synthesis, but some viruses direct the synthesis of additional enzymes specific for their replication.

HOST RANGE AND SPECIFICITY

- Viruses are specific for the type of organism and the type of cell which they infect.
- This specificity depends on the presence of a suitable target site for viral attachment to the susceptible cell.

CLASSIFICATION OF VIRUSES

- Viruses are classified into groups or families based on the type of nucleic acid they contain, their shape, structure and method of replication.

VIRAL REPLICATION

- Viruses always replicate inside another living cell.
- Bacteriophage infect bacteria, resulting in lysis, lysogeny or specialised transduction.

VIRAL INFECTION IN ANIMAL CELLS

- Viral infection of animal (human) cells involves six steps: adsorption, penetration, uncoating, synthesis, assembly and release.
- The method of replication inside the host cell depends on the type of nucleic acid the virus contains.

TYPES OF VIRAL INFECTIONS IN HUMANS

- Many common human diseases are caused by viruses.
- Viral infections may be acute, subclinical, chronic, latent, slow or oncogenic.
- Viral infections usually stimulate the immune system to produce antibodies which protect the host against subsequent infection.
- The susceptibility of a person to viral infection is influenced by age and immune status.

TRANSMISSION OF VIRAL DISEASES

- Viruses are shed mainly from the area where the infection is localised.
- Control of the spread of virus disease is helped by an understanding of the method of transmission of the virus.
- Transmission may be via air-borne route as aerosol droplets, from vesicles or pustules, via the faecal-oral route, or in blood and other body fluids.
- A system of infection control procedures for the handling of blood and body substances has been introduced to prevent the transmission of blood-borne pathogens.
- Arboviruses are transmitted by insects, the most common of which is the mosquito.
- Some viruses are transferred vertically from mother to baby, transmission occurring *in utero*, during birth or through breast milk.
- Some viruses are teratogenic, causing congenital defects in the foetus when the mother contracts the infection during pregnancy.

INACTIVATION OF VIRUSES

- Most viruses are destroyed by heat, detergents and chlorine.
- Many viruses are stable in the presence of salt solutions and buffers, and between pH 5 and pH 9
- Treatment of viruses with formaldehyde destroys their infectivity but leaves their antigenicity intact.

DIAGNOSIS OF VIRAL INFECTIONS

- Viral diseases are diagnosed mainly by signs and symptoms.
- The presence of virus particles in tissues can often be detected in the early stages of infection by reaction with fluorescent antibodies.
- To diagnose viral infections, specimens are grown in cell culture which is observed for cytopathic changes.
- The presence of antibodies to the virus in the patient's blood indicates infection.
- Some viruses are identified by DNA typing, using nucleic acid probes.

GROWTH OF VIRUSES IN THE LABORATORY

- Viruses may be grown in the laboratory in animals, embryonated eggs or cell culture.

TREATMENT AND PREVENTION OF VIRAL INFECTIONS

ANTIVIRAL DRUGS

- It is difficult to find antiviral drugs that do not also harm the host cell.
- The most successful antiviral drugs are analogues of DNA bases which react with specific viral enzymes.
- Interferons are naturally occurring antiviral compounds.

VACCINATION

- Vaccines are available for many serious viral diseases and are the most effective means of prevention.
- Effective mass vaccination campaigns can lead to the eradication of some viral diseases (e.g. smallpox).

Study Questions

1. Describe the structure of a virus.
2. What type of nucleic acid occurs in viruses?
3. Where do viruses replicate?
4. What is meant by virus specificity?
5. What is (a) a capsomere, (b) a capsid?
6. Describe the major shapes of viral particles.
7. How does the newly synthesised virus acquire its envelope?
8. What is meant by a complex virus?
9. What is (a) a viroid, (b) a prion?
10. How are viruses classified?
11. What are bacterial viruses called?
12. Differentiate between lysis and lysogeny when applied to viral infection of bacterial cells.
13. List the six steps involved in the replication of a virus in an animal cell.
14. What is meant by a subclinical infection?
15. List the viruses that can cause latent infections.
16. List the major routes of virus transmission.
17. What is meant by viral shedding? When and where does it occur?
18. How can you control the transmission of blood-borne viruses?
19. What is meant by an arbovirus? Give examples.
20. Which viruses have teratogenic effects?
21. What are the most effective ways of inactivating viruses?
22. How are viral diseases diagnosed?
23. What are interferons?
24. What is meant by an attenuated virus?
25. What is the most effective way of preventing viral diseases?

Test Your Understanding

1. How does the replication of the retroviruses differ from other RNA-containing viruses?
2. Differentiate between the processes that occur in the host during an acute and a chronic viral infection.
3. What types of viral infections elicit an immune response?
4. What are the major advantages of being vaccinated against measles, rather than acquiring the disease naturally?
5. How are viruses able to transform normal cells?
6. Why is it difficult to design antiviral drugs?

FURTHER READING

Frontiers in Medicine: Vaccines, 1994 *Science 265*, pp. 1371–1401. (A collection of news reports, policies etc. relating to the prevention of viral infections.)

Timbury, M.C. *Notes on Medical Virology*, 10th edn., London: Churchill Livingstone, 1994.

White, D.O. & F. Fenner, *Medical Virology*, 4th edn., San Diego: Academic Press, 1994.

chapter 6

eucaryotic microorganisms

fungi, protozea and multicellular organisms

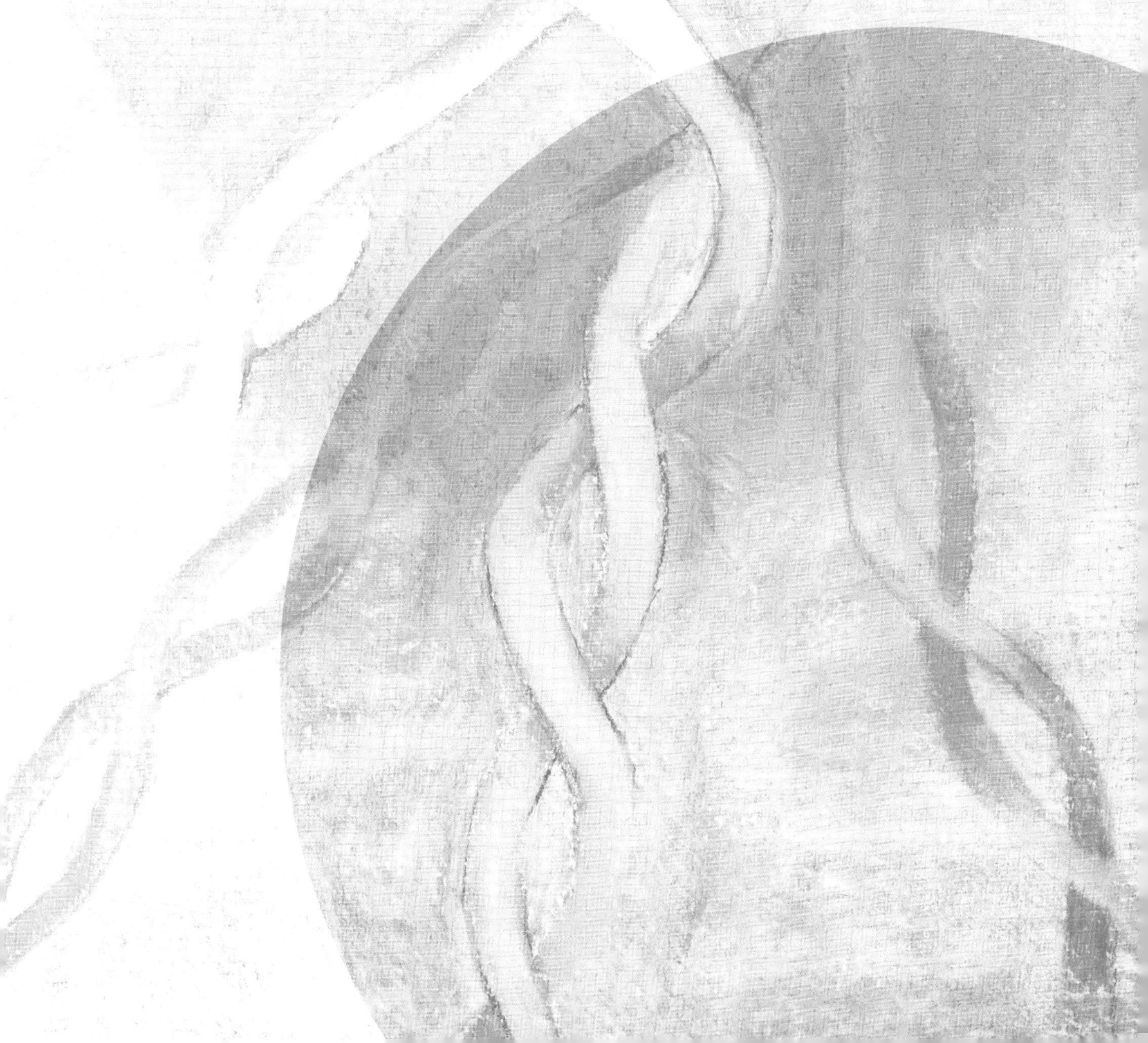

Chapter focus

- *What are the major groups of eucaryotic microorganisms that cause disease?*
- *What are the main characteristics of fungal infections?*
- *Which are the most important protozoal diseases?*
- *How do parasitic diseases caused by protozoa and helminths differ from other infectious diseases?*
- *What factors affect a patient's susceptibility to fungal and protozoal diseases?*
- *What is the role of insects in the transmission and cause of infections?*

Chapters 4 and 5 deal in with the properties of bacteria and viruses. These microorganisms are responsible for a large proportion of infectious diseases. A smaller, but significant number of diseases are caused by eucaryotic organisms that are either microscopic (e.g. protozoa and yeasts) or have a microscopic stage in their life cycle (e.g. some fungi, worms, and other parasites).

Some of these eucaryotes cause only minor diseases in healthy individuals, but can have serious effects on a person whose immune system is compromised in some way. They are then referred to as opportunistic pathogens. **Opportunistic infections** are defined as infections caused by microorganisms that would not normally cause disease in individuals whose immune system is intact, but may do so in people with altered defence mechanisms. Opportunistic infections caused by protozoa or fungi are a major cause of mortality in AIDS patients.

Eucaryotic microorganisms have very similar properties to their host cells, which means that it is often difficult to find drugs that can destroy them without having significant side effects on the host. This is of special importance in the treatment of systemic infections, where the infection is spread throughout the body and various body organs. When this occurs, the antimicrobial drug has to be administered in such a way as to reach the pathogen, and the method of administration may mean that susceptible host cells are exposed to the drug.

In this chapter we look at the properties of these organisms and discuss briefly the diseases they cause and the implications for health care.

Fungi

Fungi comprise two major groups—yeasts and moulds. There are literally thousands of different types of fungi, ranging from microscopic single-celled yeasts to multicellular, filamentous moulds and large fleshy moulds, or mushrooms. Only about 50 of these fungi cause disease in humans although many more of them are known to attack plants. Very few fungi are truly pathogenic. Most serious fungal infections are opportunistic, occurring in patients with a deficient immune system.

Fungi exhibit a wide range of morphology (appearance). All fungal cells are surrounded by a cell wall. They are distinguished from plants and algae in that they do not contain chlorophyll and cannot carry out photosynthesis. Fungi are widely distributed in nature and play an important role in the decomposition of organic material. They are described as heterotrophic; that is, they require an organic source of carbon for growth. Many of them are saprophytes, feeding off dead, woody plant materials, which are not readily decomposed by bacteria. Most fungi can grow under conditions where bacteria are not able to thrive. For example, many moulds grow on substances with a very low moisture content (e.g. bread and cereals) and are resistant to extremes of osmotic pressure (e.g. they are able to grow in high sugar or salt concentrations). Many prefer an acid pH and can tolerate cold conditions (e.g. the household refrigerator).

TYPES OF FUNGI

Yeasts

The yeasts are unicellular organisms, usually spherical to oval in shape and bounded by a cell wall. They are slightly larger than bacteria and contain various subcellular organelles. A number of pathogenic strains exhibit **dimorphism**, that is, the ability to grow in two different forms. Dimorphic fungi are usually filamentous at room temperature and grow as yeast cells in the body or when incubated in the laboratory at 35°C on enriched medium such as blood agar. *Candida albicans*, the organism responsible for thrush, exhibits several forms of growth, both at 28°C and in the host tissues. At 28°C it may exhibit a single-celled budding yeast form or produce rudimentary filaments called pseudohyphae, or even produce true **hyphae**. The production of pseudohyphae appears to aid in the invasion of the mucocutaneous host tissues and indicates a pathogenic rather than commensal role for the organism (see Figure 6.1).

Reproduction in yeasts is mainly asexual, by a process called 'budding'. A small outgrowth, or bud, appears on the parent cell; it gradually enlarges and then separates, forming a new daughter cell, which then rapidly increases in size (Figure 6.2). Some non-pathogenic yeasts exhibit sexual reproduction, in which two haploid cells fuse to form a zygote, followed by the production of spores.

Yeasts occur widely in the environment and are found on the surfaces of plants and fruit. They are able to ferment sugars with the production of alcohol. Strains of the yeast *Saccharomyces cerevisiae* are used in bread making and in wine and beer production. *S. cerevisiae* has also been

FIGURE 6.1
CANDIDA ALBICANS: GROWTH ON AGAR, YEAST AND FILAMENTOUS FORM

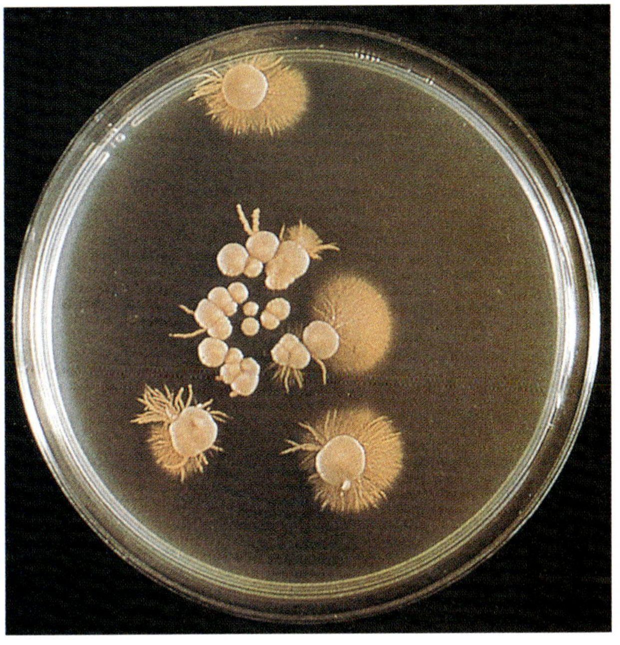

FIGURE 6.2
YEAST REPRODUCING BY BUDDING
Circular scars can be seen on the surface of the cell on the left, representing sites of previous budding.

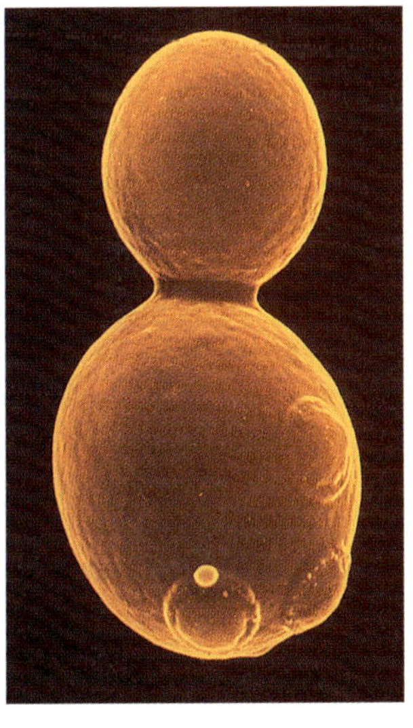

used by molecular biologists for the production of genetically engineered products, such as the vaccine for hepatitis B (see Chapter 4).

Moulds

The moulds are filamentous fungi that are capable of growth in many different habitats. They are commonly found growing on stale bread, cheese and vegetables. They consist of filaments or **hyphae** (singular: hypha) which grow by extending the terminal cell at the tip of the filament. As they grow, the hyphae branch and form a dense mat of filaments called a **mycelium**, which is usually visible to the naked eye. The cells of this vegetative structure often contain more than one nucleus. After the dense mycelial mat has formed, **aerial hyphae** are produced and extend up into the air above the mycelial mat.

The most common method of reproduction in moulds is by the production of asexual spores in specialised structures on the ends or off the sides of these aerial hyphae. Asexual spores are produced by mitotic division of the parent cell. There are two main types.

1. **Sporangiospores** are produced inside a sac, or **sporangium**, on the tip of a stalk, or **sporangiophore.** These spores are released when the sporangium ruptures.
2. **Conidia** (**conidiospores**) are not enclosed in a sac. They develop by being pinched off from the tip of an aerial hypha. Conidiospores are the most common type of asexual spores. They are usually pigmented, ranging in colour from blue or green to black or red, so the growing fungus changes in appearance from a white mat to its own particular colour with a dusty surface.

The structure of the spore-bearing hyphae is distinctive for each mould and is useful for identification. The spores are dispersed on air currents and carried to a new site where they germinate and grow into new hyphae. Some typical moulds are illustrated in Figures 6.3 and 6.4.

Some filamentous fungi produce chemicals with

FIGURE 6.3
STRUCTURE OF MOULDS
(a) Distinctive appearance on agar plates of dermatophyte; (b) microscopic appearance of spores of Trichophyton mentagrophytes.

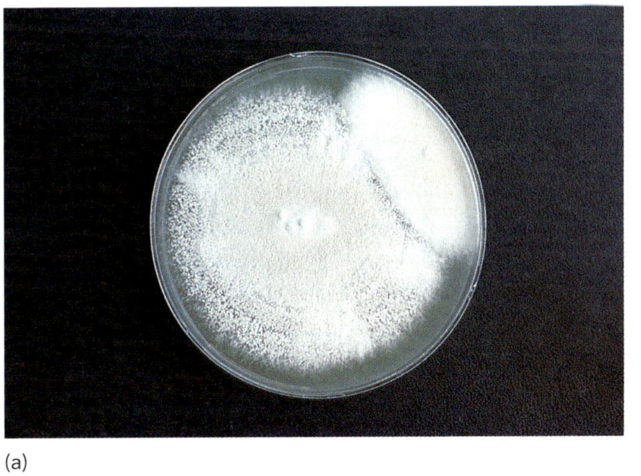

(a)

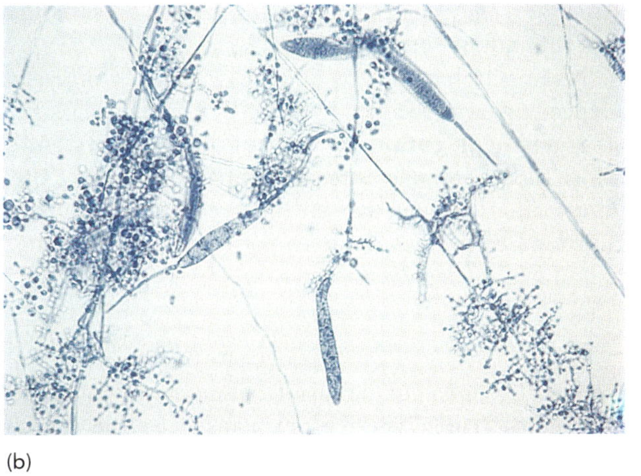

(b)

FIGURE 6.4
STRUCTURE OF MOULDS
(a) Growth of Microsporum cookei on Agar; (b) microscopic appearance of spores of M. cookie.

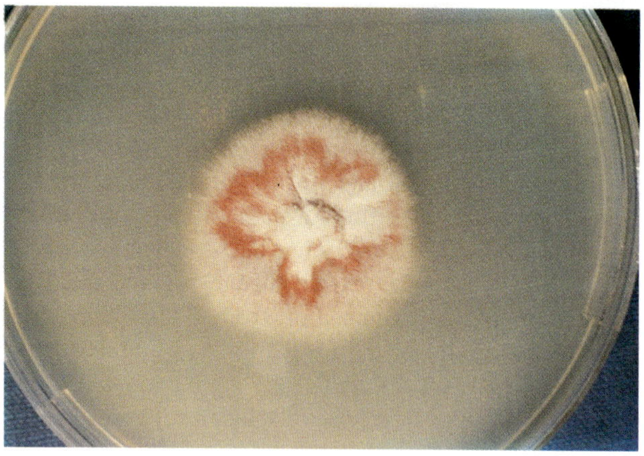

(a)

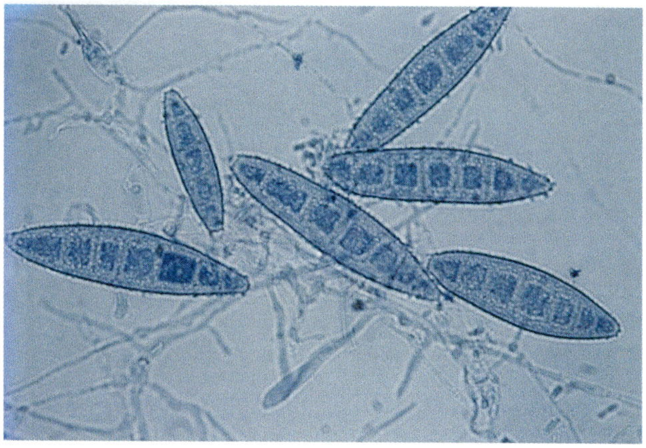

(b)

antibacterial properties. The most important of these is penicillin, which is produced by several species of *Penicillium* (see Chapter 2).

Mushrooms are filamentous fungi in which the aerial hyphae form a fleshy structure called a 'fruiting body'. During most of its life, the mushroom exists as a mycelium of hyphae in the soil and when conditions are favourable a fruiting body or 'mushroom' is formed. Spores are produced on the coloured gills underneath the cap, and are dispersed when the mushroom matures and dries. The various members of the mushroom family are an important food source.

FUNGAL INFECTIONS

For many years, infections caused by fungi were regarded as a nuisance rather than life-threatening. More recently, however, fungal infections have become increasingly important in patients whose immune system is compromised in some way. Such people are not necessarily confined to hospitals. Many of them are living in the community. They include transplant patients who are being treated with immunosuppressive drugs, patients with leukaemia, other cancer patients, and diabetics, as well as people suffering from immune disorders such as AIDS. All these individuals are likely to suffer severe morbidity (illness) if they contract a fungal infection even though it would not be serious in a healthy person.

An infection caused by a fungus is called a **mycosis.** Depending on its location in the body, it may be classified as **superficial**, **cutaneous**, **subcutaneous** or **systemic.** Most superficial and cutaneous infections are not life-threatening, although they are often resistant to treatment and tend to persist for long periods with associated inflammation and discomfort.

Superficial mycoses

The most common of the superficial mycoses is pityriasis versicolor (**tinea versicolor**), caused by the fungus *Malassezia furfur* (Figure 6.5). It is a mild infection of the skin and produces lesions that range from white, or non-pigmented (usually seen in darker-skinned people—e.g., in New Guinea it is colloquially called 'white spot') through to brown, which is more common in fair-skinned people. The lesions are purely cosmetic. No inflammatory response is involved and the infection responds to topical antifungal treatment, such as selenium.

Cutaneous mycoses

Cutaneous mycoses comprise the familiar skin infections commonly referred to as **tinea** or **ringworm**. They are caused by fungi called **dermatophytes** which invade keratinised tissue (skin, hair and nails). Most important of these are organisms belonging to the genera *Microsporum, Trichophyton* and *Epidermophyton*. Dermatophyte infections may be identified by microscopic examination of skin scrapings. When grown in the laboratory the

FIGURE 6.5
PITYRIASIS VERSICOLOR
Distinctive rash caused by the dermatophyte *Mallassezia furfur.*

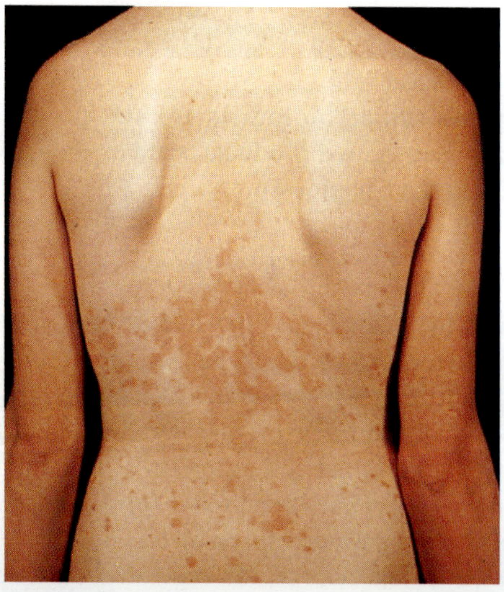

arrangement of their hyphae and the structure of their conidiospores are distinctive for each species. They can be identified by culture on Sabouraud's agar.

Cutaneous fungal infections are transmitted by person to person contact or by the shedding of infected skin scales or hair clippings. Tinea infections can occur on any part of the body and are named accordingly.

- **Tinea pedis** (athlete's foot) is the most common dermatophyte infection. Usually, the skin between the toes becomes infected, followed by the development of small vesicles that burst and cause peeling and cracking of the skin (Figure 6.6). *Tinea pedis* is frequently contracted from fungal cells present in communal showers and change rooms.
- **Tinea corporis** may occur anywhere on the body. The lesion usually consists of a central scaly patch surrounded by a circular border of vesicles that are red and inflamed, giving the appearance of a ring—hence the name 'ringworm'.
- **Tinea cruris** (jock itch) occurs in the groin.
- **Tinea capitis** is the name given to infections on the scalp. These may also involve the roots of the hair.

Subcutaneous mycoses

Subcutaneous infections occur when a fungus penetrates beneath the skin and establishes an infection. They are usually caused by soil or plant microorganisms that are introduced when the skin is broken or damaged, such as when a thorn or splinter penetrates the skin while gardening. Many of the fungi associated with plants cause this type of infection—for example, *Sporothrix schenckii*, which lives on wood or plants and produces a chronic granulomatous infection that can spread along the lymphatic system. **Paronychia** is an infection which occurs under the fingernail. It is caused by any of the soil or plant fungi but can also be caused by the yeast, *Candida albicans* (Figure 6.7). Subcutaneous mycoses are difficult to treat and can persist for long periods.

Systemic mycoses

Systemic (deep) fungal infections are caused by pathogenic fungi or by opportunistic fungi that have invaded an immunosuppressed patient. Very few fungi are truly pathogenic; that is, very few will cause an infection in an individual with normal immune defences. Table 6.1 is a list of pathogenic fungi which may give rise to systemic infections. They are predominantly dimorphic, free-living, soil organisms and tend to be restricted to defined geographical habitats. These fungi are a common source of infection in the United States (see Table 6.1). They do not occur in Australia, with the exception of *Histoplasma*, a few cases of which have been reported.

In endemic areas these pathogenic fungi are usually introduced into the body by inhalation of spores. In the majority of cases the result is a mild lung infection. In

FIGURE 6.7
PARONYCHIA DUE TO *CANDIDA ALBICANS*
Candida infections of the nails are very difficult to eradicate.

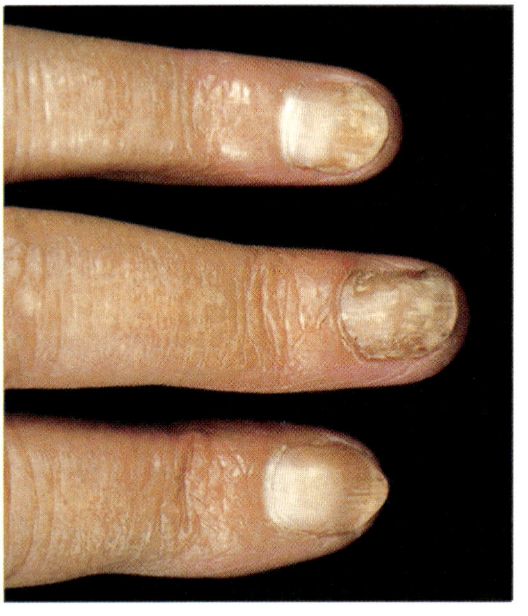

FIGURE 6.6
TINEA PEDIS—ATHLETE'S FOOT
Ringworm of the foot, or athlete's foot (*tinea pedis*). Moisture between the toes favours fungal infections.

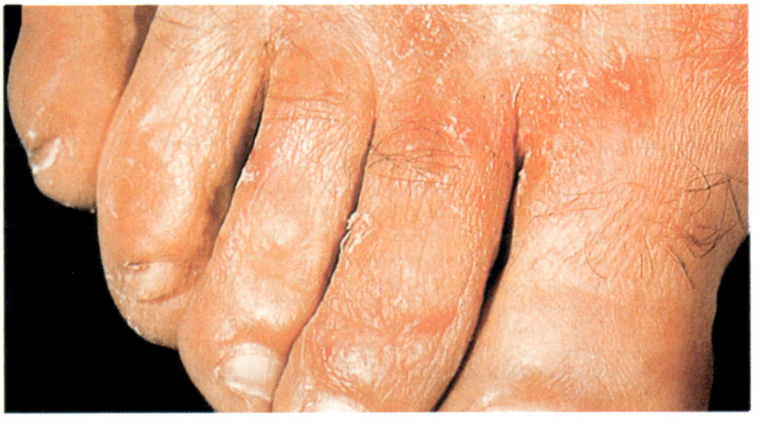

a small percentage of cases, the fungus may be disseminated (spread) through the body, affecting other body organs and progressing to a full-blown, sometimes fatal, disease. Patients' ability to withstand invasion by these fungi depends on the integrity of their cell-mediated immune response (see Chapter 9). Although these fungi may infect any individual exposed to them, they have much more serious consequences in immunosuppressed patients and are commonly found as opportunistic infections in AIDS patients in the United States.

Apart from the pathogens described, the major cause of systemic mycoses are opportunistic fungi, which occur mainly in immunosuppressed patients.

Opportunistic fungal infections

A number of fungi are opportunistic pathogens; that is, they cause disease only when the host defences are weakened (see Table 6.1). Among these, the yeast *Candida albicans* and related *Candida* species are the most common. *Candida* is a commensal of human mucosal surfaces, especially the mouth, vagina and intestinal tract, but may become a pathogen when the body's defence mechanisms are impaired or when the balance of microbial flora is disrupted.

Candida infections may be either **mucocutaneous** or **systemic**. **Thrush** is the name commonly given to mucocutaneous infections of the mouth or vagina. Outbreaks of thrush are usually indicative of a local or systemic weakness in the immune system. A number of factors can contribute to the proliferation of *Candida* and production of disease (candidiasis). For example, oral thrush is frequently seen in neonates (especially low birth weight infants) where the immune system is immature and the population of protective normal flora has not yet been established. It is commonly associated with the use of corticosteroid puffers for asthma. Thrush often occurs after long-term treatment with broad spectrum antibiotics, which alters the composition of the normal bacterial flora. **Chronic mucocutaneous candidiasis** (CMC), which presents first in childhood but is also seen in adults, is usually an indication of an underlying deficiency in cellular immunity.

Vaginal candidiasis in adult females is often associated with diabetes, pregnancy or the use of the contraceptive pill. Alterations in the body's physiological state, such as hormonal imbalance or stress, appear to favour the growth of the yeast cells. Prolonged antibiotic therapy can also destroy the normal flora in the vagina. Species of *Lactobacillus*, a normal inhabitant of the vagina, help to maintain an acid environment, limiting the growth of *Candida* which prefers a neutral pH (pH 7). Destruction of the lactobacilli by prolonged broad spectrum antibiotic therapy allows the pH to rise and an overgrowth or **superinfection** of *Candida* may result.

Candida can also cause skin infections in obese or diabetic patients. The yeast flourishes in the warm moist parts of the body (axillae, skin folds, under the breasts in females), causing inflammation and red weeping vesicles. It can also be a cause of skin infections in elderly patients, who may have problems with hygiene and adequate care. Nappy rash in babies due to the constant moisture on the skin can also be caused by *Candida*. Mucocutaneous candidiasis can be treated with topical antifungal preparations.

Systemic candidiasis (candidaemia) generally occurs in association with another severe underlying disease such as leukaemia or other cancers. The incidence of systemic

TABLE 6.1
SYSTEMIC FUNGAL INFECTIONS

ORGANISM	DISEASE	DISTRIBUTION/HABITAT
Pathogenic fungi		
Blastomyces dermatitidis	Blastomycosis	North America
Coccidioides immitis	Coccidioidomycosis	Soil; south-west United States, Mexico
Histoplasma capsulatum	Histoplasmosis	Central and eastern United States, South America, Africa
Paracoccidioides brasiliensis	Paracoccidioidomycosis	Soil; Latin America
Opportunistic fungi		
Candida spp.	Candidiasis	Normal human flora
Aspergillus spp.	Aspergillosis	Ubiquitous; soil, grains
Cryptococcus neoformans	Cryptococcal pneumonia Cryptococcal meningitis	Birds
Rhizopus, *Mucor*	Zygomycosis	Soil, plants

infections is also high in patients subjected to traumatic medical procedures, such as organ transplantatin with consequent immunosuppressive therapy. Invasive procedures such as intravenous therapy with **total parenteral nutrition (TPN)**, or **endotracheal intubation** increase the risk of systemic infections. *Candida* infections are frequently associated with central lines and Hickman catheters. Severely compromised babies in intensive care may develop systemic *Candida* infections, often with a significant mortality rate.

The ability of *Candida* to develop into a systemic infection appears to be related to the immune status of the patient. *Candida* typically grows in the extracellular speaces and is subject to phagocytosis by neutrophils and macrophages. **Neutropenia** (a deficiency of neutrophils) appears to render a patient more susceptible to systemic *Candida* invasion. However, *Candida* infections also occur in association with a reduction in T cells and teh cell-mediated immune response (see Chapter 9). Mucocutaneous candidiasis is commonly seen in patients with the human immunodeficiency virus (HIV positive) but it does not appear to be readily disseminated in patients who have progressed to AIDS.

Cryptococcal infections are caused by *Cryptococcus neoformans* var. *neoformans*, an encapsulated yeast found in the excreta of pigeons and othe birds in most parts of the world. The organism enters the body via the respiratory tract and is responsible for causing a mild, largely asymptomatic pneumonitis in humans. However, in immunosuppresse patients, the organism can become invasive and cause severe cryptococcal pneumonia. It may also spread to the brain, causing cryptococal meningitis. This occurs in about 80% of AIDS patients. Cryptococcal infections are frequently seen in patients receiving steroids or in transplant patients on immunosuppressive drugs.

The varietyy, *C. neoformans* var. *gattii*, is found mainly in areas where the Australian Red River gum (*Eucalyptus camaldulensis*) is growing; that is, in certain parts of Australia and in other countries to which the tree has been exported. Infections seem to occur mainly during the flowering season. Aborigines who live in dry river beds in Northern and Central Australia are often infected with this variety. It is rarely seen in immunocompromised patients in urban areas.

Aspergillus infections are opportunistic infections caused predominantly by *Aspergillus fumigatus*. Members of the *Aspergillus* genus are widely distributed in nature and release spores that are inhaled into the lungs. If the fungus invades the lung tissue it is able to enter the bloodstream and be disseminated throughout the body, causing potentially fatal abscesses in various body organs. Aspergillosis is a major problem for immunosuppressed patients and transplant patients, especially bone marrow recipients.

TRANSMISSION OF FUNGAL INFECTIONS

Most fungi live in the soil or on plants, and are transmitted to humans by contact with the fungus or its spores. They are frequently inhaled (e.g. *Aspergillus* spores and *Cryptococcus*), but they can also enter through broken skin. Some of the cutaneous mycoses are transmitted by contact with infected skin scales, or by direct contact with a lesion on the skin of an infected human or animal (e.g. ringworm on cats).

A notable exception is Candida. Since Candida species are normal human commensals, they tend to cause infection when there is a lowering of the host resistance, as described above.

FACTORS CONTRIBUTING TO FUNGAL INFECTIONS

It should be apparent that most fungal infections are of only minor importance in healthy individuals. The overall integrity of the host immune system is of utmost importance in avoiding fungal infections.

A number of factors contribute to patient susceptibility. Neutropenia is a predisposing factor for many infections. Certain medical procedures also affect susceptibility, including:

- Transplant surgery with administration of immunosuppressive drugs.
- Prolonged broad specrum antibiotic therapy which destroys the normal flora.
- Other invasive therapies such as intravenous total parenteral nutrition (TPN). This involves the use of solutions containing high concentrations of glucose which inhibit bacterial growth but favour the growth of fungi such as *Candida albicans*. The use of fat emulsion in TPN also encourages the growth of *Malassezia furfur*, an otherwise harmless superficial fungus.
- **CAPD** (**C**ontinuous **A**mbulatory **P**eritoneal **D**ialysis). This therapy is used as an alternative to hemodialysis for patients with renal failure. The main problem is the risk of fungal infections as well as bacterial infections through the indwelling cannulae.
- Fungal infections may also occur in prosthetic devices. The organisms originate from contaminated equipment or materials.

DIAGNOSIS OF SYSTEMIC INFECTIONS

Diagnosis of fungal infections is very difficult because the symptoms are often not definitive and laboratory growth of funci is very slow. Fungal infections are usually suspected if the patient is immunocompromisedd and does not respond to empirical antibacterial therapy. Careful collection and processing of specimens is very important.

TREATMENT OF FUNGAL INFECTIONS

Cutaneous fungal infections are treated with topical antifungal preparations. Systemic infections are more difficult to treat as there are few antifungal drugs that do not have serious side effects on the host. Amphotericin is the most effective drug for neutropenic patients. Candidiasis and cryptococcosis in AIDS patients (who are usually not neutropenic) are treated with fluconazole. No vaccines are available for any of the fungal infections.

HARMFUL EFFECTS OF FUNGI

Apart from causing infections, fungi can have other harmful effects. These include the induction of allergic responses to fungal spores and the harmful effects associated with the ingestion of fungal toxins.

Allergic reactions

Allergic bronchopulmonary reactions may result from the repeated inhalation of mould spores. Workers in farm industries are particularly at risk of occupational exposure due to inhalation of spores of fungi such as *Aspergillus* species, which are commonly formed in grain storage bins, haystacks, silos and sugar cane piles (bagasse). The introduction of spores into sensitised lungs causes a hypersensitivity reaction, usually associated with severe breathing difficulties (farmer's lung).

Fungal toxins

Some fungi produce chemicals that are toxic to humans. The poisonous effects of eating some species of mushroom (commonly called toadstools) are well known. Symptoms such as nausea, severe diarrhoea, damage to body systems, muscle spasms, and death may occur. Other fungi infect food and produce toxins that are ingested with the food. Among these is aflatoxin produced by the mould *Aspergillus flavus* when it grows on peanuts and other grains. It has been linked to the occurrence of liver cancer.

Another interesting toxin is ergotamine, produced by *Claviceps purpurea*, a mould that infects rye grain. It is a chemical similar to LSD (lysergic acid diethylamide) and also produces hallucinogenic effects. It has been suggested that some of the witchcraft incidents of the Middle Ages were due to the ingestion of this mind-altering toxin in contaminated rye bread. It is important to have strict health controls to prevent the contamination of food with fungal toxins. The presence and possible harmful effects of fungal toxins in animal feed is also of concern to farmers.

Parasites

A **parasite** is defined as an organism that derives its nutrients from another living organism, the host. Thus, most pathogens are considered to be parasites. However, parasitic diseases usually refer to those caused by protozoa, helminths and arthropods, which live at the expense of their host. As discussed in Chapter 7, parasitism encompasses a wide range of relationships, from those in which the host is only slightly harmed to those in which it is killed. The most successful parasites are those that maintain their own life processes without killing their host.

Parasitic infections are often given very little coverage in microbiology courses. However, each year they cause disease in more than one billion people throughout the world and lead to several million deaths, mostly in developing countries. Major diseases such as malaria, sleeping sickness, schistosomiasis and leishmaniasis are still widespread in many areas, causing severe debilitation and death among the populations they affect. Other parasitic infections that were once considered minor are becoming more important because of their occurrence in immunocompromised individuals. These include the infections caused by the protozoa, *Pneumocystis*, *Toxoplasma* and *Cryptosporidium*.

In Australia, serious parasitic diseases are still relatively uncommon. However, an increasing number of individuals in our community are immunodeficient and therefore potentially susceptible. These include AIDS patients, cancer patients, and transplant patients on immunosuppressive therapy. There is also a significant number of people who are susceptible because of their lifestyle and other contributing factors. Many Aborigines in remote communities have an increased susceptibility to parasitic infections because of pre-existing conditions such as malnutrition, alcoholism and diabetes. Their lifestyle (e.g. the custom of going barefoot) places them at risk of contracting the parasitic worms, hookworm and strongyloides, which gain entry to the body by burrowing through the skin.

There are several ways in which parasitic infections differ from those caused by bacteria or viruses.

- Parasites frequently have a complex life cycle involving the formation of resistant cyst forms of the organism. These cysts can survive for long periods outside the host.
- The life cycle may involve an insect vector (carrier) that is essential for the transmission of the disease. Elimination of the vector should effectively control the spread of the disease, but this has proved impossible in most cases.
- Some parasites are capable of infecting both humans and other animals. In this case both the animal and humans can act as reservoirs for the infection. This is especially true for many of the protozoal infections carried by insects.
- Many of the helminths (worms) have two or more hosts in their life cycle. The **definitive host** harbours the mature adult form of the parasite, and the **intermediate host** has the immature or larval form. Frequently, humans are an 'accidental' host, and obtain the parasite by eating infected meat (e.g. the beef tapeworm).
- Many parasites have life cycles that need sufficient time to allow for the various stages to mature, either in soil or in an insect or host.

We will now go on to describe the properties of the protozoa and helminths and discuss the problems associated with the prevention and control of the infections they cause.

Protozoa

CHARACTERISTICS

Protozoa are the smallest organisms in the animal kingdom. They are single-celled eucaryotic organisms about 20–50 μm in size, containing various subcellular organelles and are surrounded by an outer membrane rather than

FIGURE 6.8
PROTOZOA
Diagrammatic representation of three different protozoa. (a) Flagellate; (b) ciliate; (c) amoeba; (d) scanning electron micrograph of a flagellate protozoan *Giardia lamblia.*

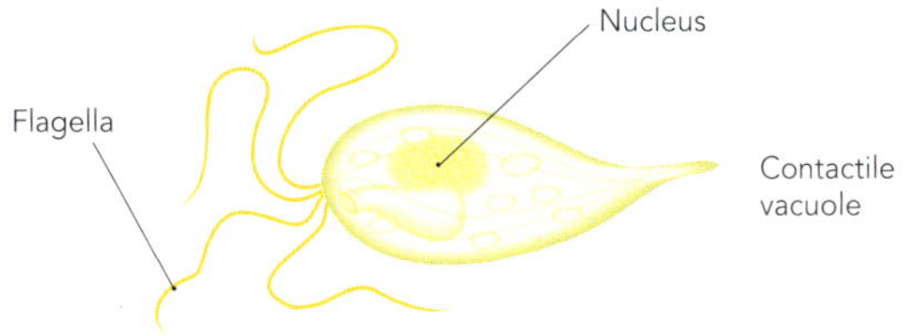

(a)

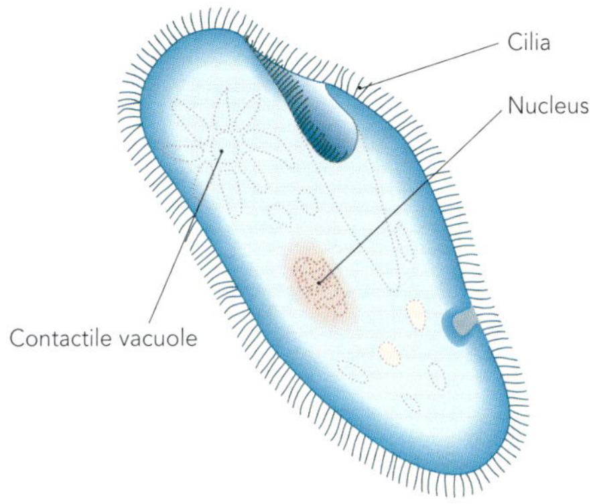

(b)

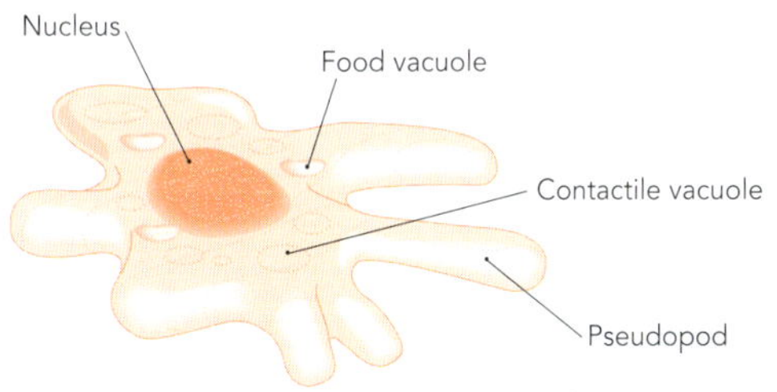

(c)

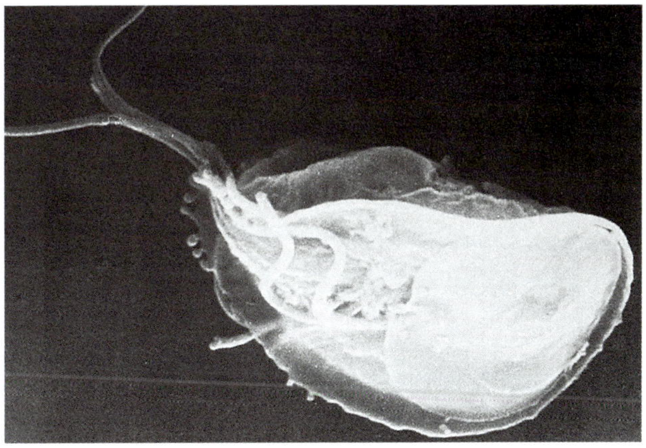
(d)

a cell wall. In the environment they are generally found in water habitats, but a number exist as parasites in animals (including humans) and insects. Protozoa obtain their nutrients by absorption of small molecules, or ingestion of food particles or even microorganisms from their environment. Some protozoa have a clearly defined gullet and anal pore (e.g. the paramecia) (Figure 6.8(b)). Others obtain food by phagocytosis. The cell surrounds the food particle and engulfs it, drawing the food inside the cell where it is contained in a vacuole, or sac, and then digested (e.g. amoeba, see Figure 6.8(c)). Intracellular parasites obtain their food by absorption of nutrients from the host cytoplasm through their outer layer.

REPRODUCTION

Many of the protozoa have a complex life cycle involving a number of different forms or stages—for example, the malaria parasite, *Plasmodium*. The simplest form of reproduction is asexual by a process of binary fission or multiple fission (**schizogony**) of the infective stage (**trophozoite**). Sexual reproduction occurs mainly in protozoa that have an insect vector stage, although *Cryptosporidium*, which is a cause of diarrhoea in humans, can undergo sexual reproduction. Most protozoa are capable of encystment—that is, the production of a resistant cyst form of the cell. **Cysts** are surrounded by a protective layer that is resistant to drying and enables them to survive for long periods (even years) in the soil. Some cysts are also resistant to the chlorine compounds used in water purification, and to stomach acid.

PROTOZOAL INFECTIONS

Protozoa are responsible for causing some important human diseases. They may be found as intracellular or extracellular parasites in blood, intestines and other organs. Like opportunistic fungi, protozoal infections have a more serious outcome in the immunocompromised (e.g. *Cryptosporidium* in AIDS patients).

Most protozoal infections are acquired by one of two main routes.

1. The first route of transmission is by the ingestion of the infective stage of the parasite in contaminated food or water; or, as is the case for *Toxoplasma*, by the inhalation of dried oocysts.
2. The other route of transmission is via the bite of a blood-sucking insect. In some cases the insect acts purely as a vector, in others the parasite multiplies and undergoes a developmental stage in the insect (e.g. malaria).

The incidence of a disease and ease of transmission depends on a number of factors, including climatic conditions and the distribution of the appropriate insect vector.

A knowledge of the stages in the life cycles of the pathogenic protozoa is important for the prevention of transmission of the organisms and for the development of vaccines.

TABLE 6.2
PROTOZOAL INFECTIONS IN HUMANS

PHYLUM	ORGANISM	DISEASE	HABITAT SOURCE/VECTOR	REFERENCE
Sarcodina (amoebae)	*Entamoeba histolytica*	Amoebic dysentery	Contaminated water	Chapter 18, p. 411
Mastigophora (flagellates)	*Giardia lamblia*	Giardiasis	Contaminated water	Chapter 18, p. 410
	Trichomonas vaginalis	Vaginosis	Vagina	Chapter 21, p. 508
	Trypanosoma brunei gambiense	Sleeping sickness	Tsetse fly	Chapter 6, p. 123
	Trypanosoma cruzi	Chagas disease	Kissing bug	Chapter 6, p. 123
	Leishmania spp.	Cutaneous: visceral (kala-azar)	Sandflies	Chapter 6, p. 123
Ciliata	*Balantidium coli*	Balantidial dysentery	Contaminated water	Chapter 6, p. 123
Sporozoa	*Plasmodium* spp.	Malaria	Anopheles mosquito	Chapter 19, p. 458
	Toxoplasma gondii	Toxoplasmosis	Cat faeces	Chapter 19, p. 461
	Cryptosporidium	Diarrhoea	Humans/animals	Chapter 18, p. 411
	Microsporidium	Diarrhoea	Humans/animals	Chapter 18, p. 403

For example, patients suffering from diseases that require an insect vector for transmission are not considered infectious to other patients or health workers, unless a suitable vector is present. The development of a vaccine for malaria has proved particularly difficult because of the existence of multiple stages in the life cycle of the parasite (see p. 124).

The protozoa that cause infections in humans are listed in Table 6.2. Not all these protozoa are found in Australia. Several of the more serious infections are transmitted by insect vectors, and so their incidence is limited to the geographical regions where these insects are found. A successful life cycle also depends on climatic conditions of temperature and humidity that favour the survival and replication of the insect vectors and the different stages of the parasitic life cycle. The references in the table are to the pages of this text where the diseases are discussed in more detail.

CLASSIFICATION

Protozoa are usually classified into four main groups depending on the way they move—sarcodina, mastigophora, ciliata and sporozoa.

Sarcodina

This group consists of the **amoebae**, large cells surrounded by a membrane and lacking a definitive shape. They move by extending the cell membrane and allowing the cytoplasm to flow into this extension, called a **pseudopod** (false foot). Amoebae absorb nutrients from their environment through their membrane, or engulf food particles by phagocytosis.

There are several different species of amoeba that may inhabit the human intestine. Many of these are non-pathogenic (e.g. *Entamoeba coli*). They form cysts in the host that are excreted in the faeces and can then be ingested by another host (human) in contaminated food or water. The pathogenic amoeba, *Entamoeba histolytica*, is the major cause of amoebic dysentery worldwide, with most infections occurring in tropical and subtropical regions. The disease may range from mild diarrhoea to severe dysentery or ulcerative colitis, characterised by blood, pus and mucus in the faeces. It is only rarely seen in Australia, but travellers to endemic tropical areas may contract it there. Despite treatment, some individuals become asymptomatic carriers and continue to shed cysts of *E. histolytica* in the faeces, thus contributing to the spread of the disease (see Chapter 18).

Su pseudomonas.

Mastigophora (flagellates)

These protozoa move by the action of flagella, whip-like tails that propel the organism through water environments. They are usually oval in shape and reproduce asexually by longitudinal binary fission. Most of them are able to form cysts for survival. Several of the flagellates are important human pathogens.

Giardia lamblia (*Giardia intestinalis*) is a common intestinal parasite found throughout the world, including Australia. It exists in two forms: the infective trophozoite stage, which has four pairs of flagella and a 'sucker' that allows it to attach to the wall of the intestine; and the resistant cyst stage which is shed in the faeces and is able to survive for weeks in a moist environment (see Figure 6.8(a)).

Contaminated drinking water is the main source of infection. Symptoms may take several weeks to appear so it is often difficult to establish when and where the infection was contracted. *Giardia* is notoriously difficult to diagnose. Symptoms may range from abdominal pain and prolonged bouts of diarrhoea to weight loss and general lack of energy. Examination of faeces is often inconclusive as the cysts and trophozoites tend to be shed intermittently. Physicians who are aware of the high incidence of giardia infections often treat patients who have prolonged gastrointestinal symptoms empirically with drugs like metronidazole or tinidazole.

Drinking water should be filtered and chlorinated to remove *Giardia* cysts, as outbreaks frequently occur when drinking water supplies become contaminated with sewage. In urban areas, broken water pipes or an overflow of sewage during storms can cause problems. In rural areas, water supplies are often derived from natural creeks which may have become contaminated with sewage. There is some evidence that other animals (dogs and beavers) can harbour the same species that infects humans. Bushwalkers should avoid drinking unboiled water from creeks and water courses.

Trichomonas is a flagellated protozoan that occurs as a commensal in a large percentage of the population. *Trichomonas hominis* is found in the large intestine and *Trichomonas vaginalis* is a frequent inhabitant of the female genital tract. A condition called **trichomoniasis**, characterised by a smelly greenish vaginal discharge, may occur when the pH of the vagina becomes less acid and *T. vaginalis* is able to multiply (see Chapter 21). The organism is sexually transmitted, so treatment should include both partners.

The **haemoflagellates** are a group of flagellated protozoans responsible for a number of serious diseases with a high morbidity and mortality rate. They are mentioned briefly here, even though they do not occur in Australia, because they are the cause of millions of deaths in other parts of the world. Also, they illustrate some principles of epidemiology—that is, the requirement for a reservoise. Neither of these diseases occurs in Australia as the appropriate insect vector is not found in this part of the world. *Trypanosoma brunei gambiense*, found in West Africa, and *Trypanosoma brunei rhodesiense* in East Africa, are both carried by the tsetse fly and are the cause of African sleeping sickness. The protozoa affect the nervous system leading to coma and death.

Trypanosoma cruzi, the cause of Chagas disease, is also carried by an insect vector, the reduviid or kissing bug. This flightless insect is found in South America, usually in areas of poor quality housing. The disease has a slow progression with increasing debilitation and eventual death, often due to myocarditis.

The *Leishmania* are another closely related group of haemoflagellates, responsible for the serious illness **leishmaniasis**. There are several different species, distributed over South and Central America, India, the Middle East and Africa. Sandflies are the vector for all the species of *Leishmania*. The disease takes two forms. Some species attack the skin, causing cutaneous leishmaniasis; others that affect certain organs, mainly the liver and spleen, cause visceral leishmaniasis (also called kala-azar). Untreated kala-azar is invariably fatal. Several different drugs are used, but in many Third World countries access to treatment is difficult and the cost of drugs prohibitive. Prevention of these diseases depends on an effective campaign to control the specific sandfly vectors. Animals other than humans can serve as a reservoir for *Leishmania*, so it is very difficult to limit the incidence of the disease.

Ciliates

The third group of protozoa are the ciliates. These organisms have cells with a large number of small hair-like appendages that move in a synchronised wave to propel the cell along. There are many ciliates found in the environment (e.g. paramecia), but the only human pathogen is *Balantidium coli*, a large protozoan that causes diarrhoea. Although it is widely distributed throughout the world, infections are rare.

Sporozoa

Sporozoans are non-motile protozoa; that is, the adult forms do not have any mechanism or appendages to enable them to move. This group contains several important human pathogens.

Sporozoa belonging to the genus *Plasmodium* are responsible for causing **malaria**. They are non-motile protozoa and require an insect vector, in this case the Anopheles mosquito for transmission. It is estimated that worldwide there are 200 million cases of malaria annually and between 1 and 2 million deaths. The disease is widespread in tropical areas, but is not endemic in Australia at present. However, the north of Australia (above latitude 19°S) is a receptive area where Anopheles mosquitoes are found.

Malaria parasites produce disease symptoms when they replicate inside the red blood cells of the human host. However, the parasite has three distinct stages in its life cycle. The first involves the injection of the **sporozoite** into the human host via the bite of an infected female Anopheles mosquito. The sporozoite migrates to the liver where, over a period of several days or weeks, it replicates asexually, producing hundreds of **merozoites**. The second asexual stage occurs in the red blood cells of the human host. The merozoites that were released from the liver into the bloodstream invade the red cells and multiply, causing haemolysis and releasing hundreds more merozoites into the bloodstream. It is this stage that produces the typical symptoms of malaria—headache, nausea, fever and chills. These symptoms occur at regular intervals, coinciding with the synchronised release of the merozoites from the red cells.

As the life cycle continues, some merozoites produce **trophozoites** which develop into male and female gametes. The gametes are ingested by the feeding Anopheles mosquito and undergo the third and sexual stage in the mosquito. Gametes fuse to form a zygote which matures into a sporozoite that is released through the salivary glands of the mosquito when it bites a new host, thus completing the cycle.

The sexual stage in the mosquito takes from 7–10 days,

There is an interesting relationship between the occurrence of red blood cell disorders and susceptibility to malaria. Individuals who carry the genetic trait (i.e. are heterozygous) for sickle cell anaemia appear to have an increased level of immunity to malaria (see Spotlight box, p. 78). The red blood cells of these carriers are not as susceptible to *Plasmodium* as are normal blood cells. This also seems to apply to other genetically inherited blood disorders—thalassaemia and glucose-6-phosphate dehydrogenase deficiency.

Programs for the prevention of malaria have been aimed at control or eradication of mosquitoes. These have not been very successful, partly because of bureaucratic inefficiency, but also because the mosquitoes have become resistant to pesticides such as DDT. Another serious problem confronting the medical profession at present is the widespread appearance of strains of *Plasmodium* that are resistant to the anti-malarial drugs currently in use. Research into producing a vaccine for malaria has so far been unsuccessful, although a number of field trials of candidate vaccines are at present in progress. It is made very difficult because the complex nature of the life cycle means that each stage of the parasite has a different antigenic structure. To be effective, a vaccine would have to be active against more than one stage in order to eliminate the parasite. The sexual stage of the life cycle also allows for genetic variation to occur, so that there is a continual change in the antigenic structure of the parasite.

Pneumocystis carinii is an organism that causes an atypical pneumonia, **Pneumocystis pneumonia** (PCP), especially in immunosuppressed patients. There is still considerable discussion about whether this organism should be classified as a protozoan or a fungus, as it resembles a fungus in many of its properties. It is very difficult to isolate and grow in the laboratory. The usual diagnosis is by observation of other clinical symptoms, X-ray of the lungs, or examination of an induced sputum specimen. (See Figure 6.9.)

Pneumocystis is probably present in the respiratory tract of many healthy individuals, but only becomes invasive in immunosuppressed patients. It is a primary cause of pneumonia in AIDS patients and responsible for a large number of AIDS deaths.

Toxoplasma gondii is a sporozoan responsible for a mild flu-like illness in humans, **toxoplasmosis.** The life cycle of the parasite and characteristics of the disease are described in detail in Chapter 19. Humans can be infected by the accidental ingestion of oocysts that have been shed in cat faeces, or by the consumption of undercooked meat containing cysts. Like many of the parasites discussed in this chapter, *Toxoplasma* has much more serious effects in patients whose immune system is deficient. These include the foetus during pregnancy, and immunocompromised patients such as those with AIDS.

The organism produces congenital defects when a non-immune mother is infected during pregnancy. The type of congenital abnormality depends on whether infection occurred during the first, second or third trimester of pregnancy. The outcome of infections during the first trimester are the most serious and include still birth and

FIGURE 6.9
PNEUMOCYSTIS CARINII
(a) Conventional stain, structures are difficult to identify; (b) Fluorescent antibody stain clearly showing the cysts which block the alveoli.

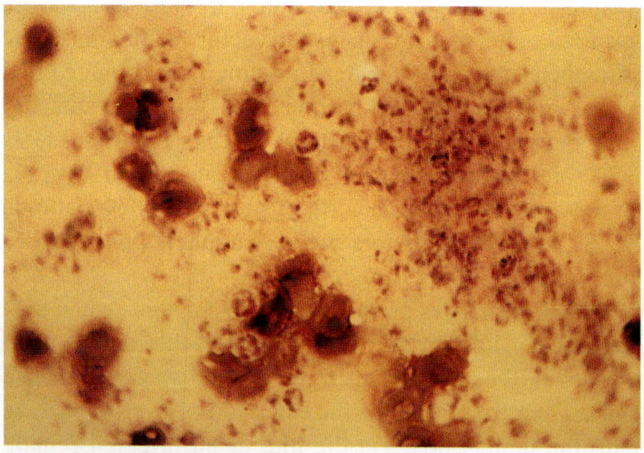

(a)

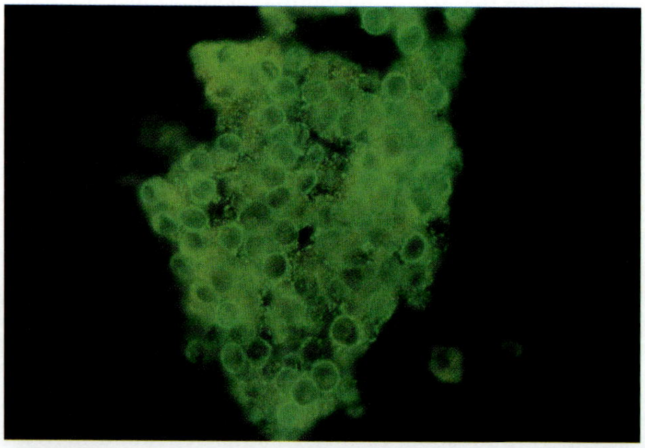

(b)

neurological defects such as blindness. If infection occurs later in pregnancy, the effects are not so severe and may not be clinically apparent until later in life. Neurological problems and learning difficulties are sometimes an outcome of late prenatal toxoplasmosis. *Toxoplasma* is widely distributed and many Australians carry antibodies in the protozoan. Women considering becoming pregnant can be tested to determine their level of immunity and, if necessary, avoid contact with cat faeces and undercooked meat (see Chapter 19). *Toxoplasma* can be treated successfully if detected but, at present, routine screening of pregnant women is not considered cost-effective in Australia, due to the low infection rate in pregnancy and the difficulty of establishing whether the infection is a recent one.

In patients who are immunodeficient (AIDS) or immunosuppressed (transplant), latent *Toxoplasma* can be reactivated to a fulminating fatal infection. Other serious consequences of reactivation include retinitis, encephalitis and pneumonia.

Cryptosporidium and *Microsporidium* are non-motile protozoa that commonly inhabit the intestines of various animals and birds. They are a probable cause of transient mild diarrhoea in humans, which can be quite serious in children. There have been recent reports of outbreaks of diarrhoea due to *Cryptosporidium* in day-care centres, and one report that was traced to a public wading pool. Children are particularly susceptible to the organism, which is transmitted via the faecal-oral route. In individuals who are HIV positive, *Cryptosporidium* and, more recently, *Microsporidium* have been found to be responsible for chronic diarrhoea with loose watery stools. *Cryptosporidium* can be identified in faecal specimens using a special staining technique. (See Figure 18.6.)

Helminths

Helminths, or worms, are a common cause of parasitic infection throughout the world. In general, their occurrence in humans is linked to low socioeconomic conditions and poor sanitation. Although infections are widespread, especially in developing countries, they are rarely fatal on their own. Many individuals carry a significant worm 'load' without apparent ill effect, but in some cases the parasites contribute to significant morbidity.

Many helminths have a complex life cycle, often involving more than one host. Some require an insect vector for transmission. An understanding of the life cycle of each parasite is essential in order to develop appropriate strategies for prevention and treatment of infection. The **definitive host** harbours the sexually mature adult form of the parasite whereas the cyst or larval stages are found in the **intermediate host**. The human host is not necessarily an essential part of the life cycle of the parasite. Very often humans are an 'accidental' host—that is, they acquire the parasite by ingestion of contaminated food or water. With rare exceptions, helminths do not replicate within their human hosts. However, the production of eggs in the human intestine, with subsequent shedding in the faeces, contributes to the continuation of the life cycle.

Classification

The parasitic helminths that occur in humans belong to two phyla—the **Platyhelminthes**, or flatworms, which include the **trematodes** (flukes) and **cestodes** (tapeworms); and the **Aschelminthes**, which contain the **nematodes** (roundworms). Helminths are usually large organisms with a complex body structure. However, the larval stages may be quite small, only 100–200 μm in size, and the eggs are microscopic.

Distribution

Table 6.3 lists the common species of worms that cause human infections in Australia. Other serious parasitic helminth infections—such as filariasis, onchocerciasis and schistosomiasis—occur in many parts of the world but are not usually seen in Australia. This is mainly due to the lack of the appropriate insect vector, the lack of a suitable intermediate host for the parasite, or to the absence of a reservoir of infection. Many of these infections are associated with tropical climates and poor sanitary practices. In this section we concentrate mainly on helminth infections that are prevalent in Australia.

FLATWORMS

The **cestodes**, or **tapeworms**, live as intestinal parasites in their definitive host. They consist of a head, or **scolex**, and a long body made up of segments, or **proglottids** (Figure 6.10). The scolex has hooks or suckers, enabling the worm to attach to the mucosal cells lining the intestine. The worm obtains its food by absorption of predigested nutrients directly from the intestine of the host, through pores on the surface of the proglottids. Each segment contains both male and female sexual organs and is thus capable of egg production. Mature proglottids containing thousands of eggs are shed in the faeces. Other animals ingest vegetation or water contaminated with the eggs. In the new host, the eggs hatch into larvae which bore through the intestinal wall and establish cysts in the tissues of the infected animal (intermediate host). Ingestion of cysts in meat by the definitive host completes the cycle.

Humans act as the definitive host for the beef tapeworm, *Taenia saginata*, and the pork tapeworm, *Taenia solium*. Of these, only the beef tapeworm occurs in Australia, mainly in cattle-raising areas. Strict meat inspection procedures at abattoirs prevent contaminated meat from reaching the markets and, up to now, quarantine regulations have prevented the pork tapeworm from reaching Australia. Humans can often unknowingly harbour large tapeworms without any apparent symptoms.

The dwarf tapeworm *Hymenolepsis nana* is sometimes found in Northern Australia. It is unusual in that it does not require an intermediate host. Ingested eggs can develop into mature worms in the human intestine.

Humans are the intermediate host for the dog tapeworm *Echinococcus granulosis*, giving rise to a condition known as **hydatid cysts**. Dogs and cats are the definitive host for this tiny tapeworm, which is 2–8 mm in length. Eggs

TABLE 6.3
ENDEMIC HELMINTH INFECTIONS IN AUSTRALIA

ORGANISM	DEFINITIVE HOST	INTERMEDIATE HOST	TRANSMISSION TO HUMANS	MEDICATION
Taenia saginata (beef tapeworm)	Humans	Cattle	Ingestion of undercooked beef	Praziquantel Niclosamide
Echinococcus granulosis (dog tapeworm)	Dogs	Humans/Tissues (hydatid cysts)	Ingestion of eggs	Albendazole
Hymenolepsis nana (dwarf tapeworm)	Humans Intestine		Ingestion of eggs	Praziquantel
Ascaris lumbricoides (roundworm)	Humans Intestine		Ingestion of eggs	Mebendazole
Enterobius vermicularis (pinworm)	Humans Intestine		Ingestion of eggs	Albendazole
Ancylostoma duodenale *Necator americanus* (hookworm)	Humans Intestine		Penetration of skin by larvae	Albendazole
Strongyloides stercoralis	Humans Intestine/other tissues		Penetration of skin by larvae	Thiabendazole
Trichuris trichiura (whipworm)	Humans		Ingestion of eggs	Mebendazole

are shed in the faeces and may be transmitted to humans from faeces on the fur or tongue of the animal. The eggs hatch in the human intestine and migrate to various parts of the body, where they form large fluid-filled sacs of larvae, called hydatid cysts. Cysts may form in any tissue but those which form in the liver, lungs and brain are the most common and have the most serious consequences. Hydatids can be avoided by worming domestic animals regularly and not feeding them raw meat.

The **trematodes**, or **flukes**, have a flat, leaf-shaped body and a rudimentary digestive system consisting of a mouth and intestine but no anus. Most of the body is taken up by a complex reproductive system. On the outside surface of the fluke are muscular suckers that enable it to attach to host tissue. (See Figure 6.11.) Two main groups of flukes cause disease in humans.

1. The tissue flukes attach to the lungs (e.g. *Paragonimus westermani*) or liver (e.g. *Clonorchis sinensis*, *Opisthorchis felineus*, *Opisthorchis viverrini* and *Fasciola hepatica*).
2. The blood flukes (e.g. *Schistosoma*) reside in the vascular system of their human hosts.

The life cycle of all the flukes is very complex, often involving more than one intermediate host. They all require a species of freshwater snail which is usually specific for each of the fluke species and occurs only in certain habitats. Tissue flukes usually have a second intermediate host, a crustacean or fish, which acts as a source of infection for the definitive human host. The schistosomes (blood flukes) are released from the snail as the free-swimming fork-tailed infective form, **cercariae**, which invade humans by direct penetration through the skin. **Schistosomiasis** is a major world health problem and is discussed further in Chapter 19.

With the exception of *Fasciola hepatica*, infections by flukes do not occur in Australia. Good sanitation, combined with the absence of the specific snail hosts, keep the parasite out of this country. However, cases of schistosomiasis, acquired from contaminated water or fish, have been seen recently in Australia in travellers returning from endemic tropical areas.

ROUNDWORMS

Nematodes, or roundworms, are widely distributed throughout the world. They are long, cylindrical worms, with a complete digestive system comprising a mouth, intestine and anus. Male and female sex organs are located on different organisms, the female worm often being significantly larger than the male. In general, nematodes have a less complex life cycle than flatworms. Several roundworms are able to parasitise humans and other

FIGURE 6.10
BEEF TAPEWORM, *TAENIA SAGINATA*
The adult tapeworm has suckers and hooks to attach to the mucosa of the host intestine. Eggs are excreted in faeces and eaten by the cow which is the intermediate host. Humans are infected by eating contaminated meat.

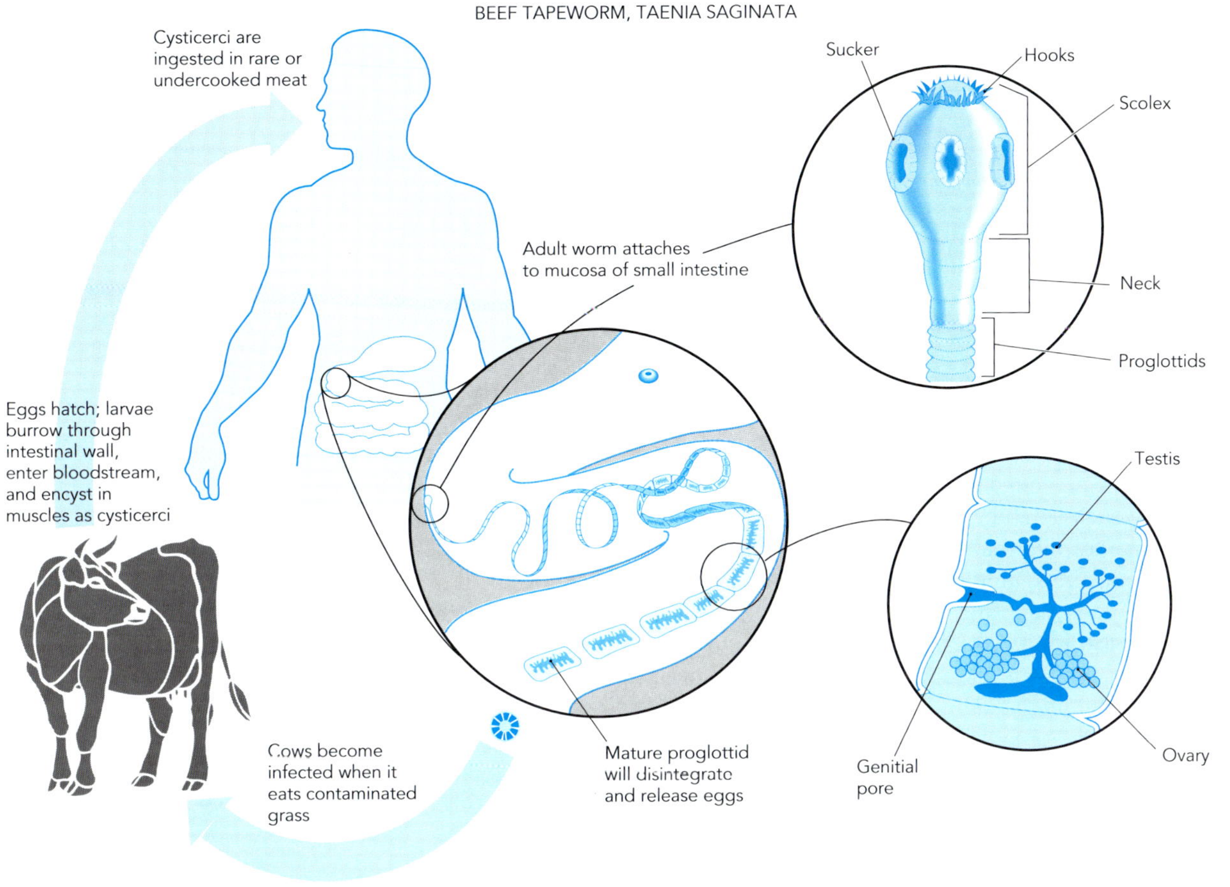

FIGURE 6.11
FLUKES
This generalised diagram of the anatomy of an adult fluke shows the oral and ventral suckers. The suckers attach the fluke to the host. The mouth is located at the centre of the oral sucker. Flukes are hermaphroditic; each animal contains both testes and ovaries.

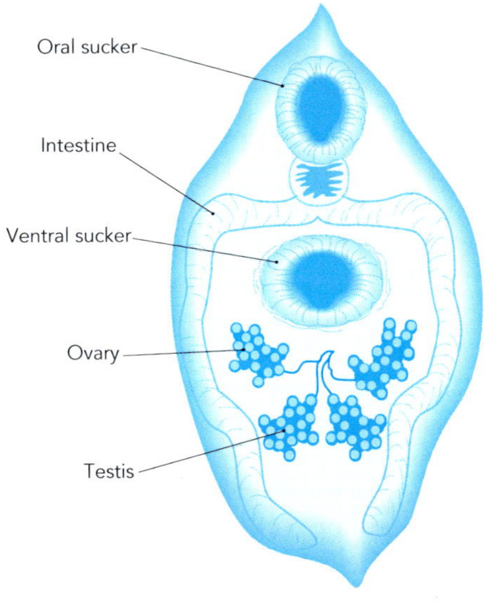

animals, as well as insects and plants. For humans, the important parasites include the common roundworms, hookworms and threadworms. Many of these occur in Australia (Table 6.3).

The common **pinworm** or **threadworm** *Enterobius vermicularis* is universally distributed. The tiny (0.5 cm) worm lives in the large intestine, the female emerging at night to lay eggs around the anus. The main symptom is anal pruritis (itching) due to irritation of the skin. Transmission of the worm occurs when the eggs are picked up on the fingers and ingested by the same host (reinfection) or another host. Eggs are frequently shed into clothing and bedding, which can also serve as a source of infection. Threadworm infections do not really have any major adverse effects on the host, and are usually easily treated.

Strongyloides stercoralis is another threadworm infection, commonly seen in tropical and subtropical regions, especially in Aboriginal people. It is acquired by larval penetration of the skin. The adult worms, which are only 2–3 mm long, are found lodged in grooves in the intestinal mucosa, but the larvae circulate constantly through the body. The worm is unusual in that it can replicate within the human host, so the infection may

FIGURE 6.12
STRONGYLOIDES INFECTION
A patient with disseminated *Strongyloides* infection. Trails under the skin indicate the migrations of the worms.

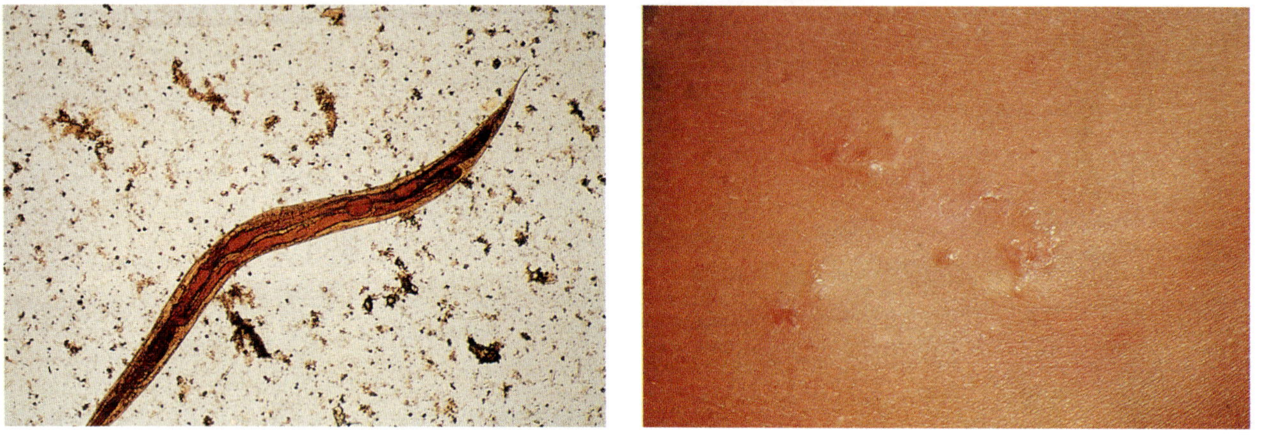

(a) Worm (b) Infection

persist for long periods. If only a few worms are present, patients may be asymptomatic but, with heavy infestations, symptoms such as abdominal pain, rashes and pruritis occur. Immunocompromised or debilitated patients often have more severe symptoms and treatment may need to be repeated at regular intervals (Figure 6.12).

The roundworm *Ascaris lumbricoides* is a large worm that may reach 30 cm in length. It usually lives in the small intestine, producing mild symptoms of abdominal discomfort. Occasionally, a bolus of worms may cause intestinal obstruction in children. The female worm produces thousands of eggs that are passed in the faeces. They can survive for long periods in the soil. When ingested by another host, the eggs hatch in the intestine, mature in the lungs and then migrate back to the intestine. Occasionally, adult worms are excreted in the faeces.

Hookworm infections are caused by *Ancylostoma duodenale* and *Necator americanus*. Hookworms are about 1 cm in length and have a mouth with hooks or suckers which enable them to attach to the wall of the intestine and suck blood. Depending on the level of infection (worm load), symptoms may range from slight discomfort to anaemia and abdominal pain. Eggs are shed in the faeces and develop into larvae in the soil. Infection takes place when the larvae burrow through the skin, enter the blood vessels of the host and are carried to the lungs. The larvae are coughed up in sputum, swallowed and finally arrive in the intestine where they attach to the mucosal cells and establish an infection. Hookworm occurs mainly in remote areas of Australia, when sanitation is poor. The Aboriginal population is particularly susceptible because of chronic malnutrition and the practice of walking barefoot.

Trichinosis is a serious infection caused by the roundworm *Trichinella spiralis*. It is acquired by eating raw or undercooked pork that is contaminated with cysts of the worm. Although widespread in America, trichinosis is not a problem in Australia; the pork sold in Australia is currently free of this parasite.

Several other roundworms that do not occur in Australia are responsible for severe infections in other parts of the world. Among these are the **microfilariae**, tiny worms that are carried by insects. **Filariasis**, or **elephantiasis**, is caused by *Wuchereria bancrofti*, and transmitted by mosquitoes. (see Chapter 19). The worm blocks the lymphatics, preventing drainage of fluid from the tissues and causing gross distortion of parts of the body—for example, legs, arms, breasts, vulva and scrotum. Filariasis is common in the Pacific Islands.

Onchocerca volvulus is a tiny worm carried by the black fly and is responsible for river blindness, a debilitating blindness that affects many thousands of people in developing countries. Guinea worm (*Dracunculus medinensis*) is another nematode acquired from contaminated drinking water; it produces large painful abscesses when the worm emerges from the body.

The cat and dog roundworms, *Toxocara cati* and *Toxocara canis*, are transmitted to humans, mainly children, by the ingestion of eggs in dog or cat faeces. After ingestion, the eggs hatch and the larvae migrate to various body organs, including the eye, when blindness may result. The worm occurs in Australia although it is more widespread in other parts of the world. Regular worming of pets is an effective control.

TREATMENT AND PREVENTION OF HELMINTH INFECTIONS

In recent years the attitude of the medical profession to the treatment of helminth infections has altered significantly. This is due to a number of factors.

1. We know now that most helminths do not replicate inside their definitive human host.
2. It is now recognised that worms only really cause significant damage to their host when the infestation is very heavy and that, in general, most infected individuals do not carry a sufficient population of worms to cause disease.
3. More importantly, in recent years a number of effective antihelminthic drugs have become available. These are listed in Table 6.3.

For Australia, this means that there are safe, effective drugs available to treat any worm infestations that may occur. These drugs, combined with education about proper sanitation and improved awareness of the importance of nutrition, should improve the health of people in remote areas.

In developing countries, there has been a shift in the strategies employed for the control of helminth diseases. It should be apparent from this discussion that the life cycles of the various helminths are very complex. Attempts to prevent worm infections by destruction of intermediate hosts, elimination of vectors, or alteration of environmental conditions to destroy larvae are all very costly and have not proved effective. The availability of effective drugs means that public health measures aimed at prevention and treatment now concentrate on the administration of these drugs at regular intervals. A worldwide policy for the treatment of worm infestations in children in developing countries has been proposed. This involves the regular administration of antihelminthic drugs at yearly intervals. Since 1993 this has been implemented for 100 000 children in five developing countries, along with the administration of nutritional supplements. It is hoped that these programs will reduce morbidity and improve growth and development in children in these countries.

Ectoparasites

A number of arthropods (insects) are capable of existing in a parasitic relationship on the outside surface of the human body. These are called **ectoparasites**. The most common are fleas, ticks, lice, and mites such as scabies. (See Figure 6.13.)

SCABIES

Scabies is an itchy skin infection caused by a tiny mite about 0.4 mm in diameter, called *Sarcoptes scabei*. The female mite burrows under the surface of the skin, forming a tunnel in which she lays two or three eggs each day. The infection is visible as a red, inflamed line, caused by an allergic reaction to the faeces left in the tunnel by the mite. Infection may occur anywhere on the body but is most common on the hands and forearms, or in warm, moist areas such as the armpits or groin. The mites are transmitted directly from person to person, but they

FIGURE 6.13
ECTOPARASITES
Representative examples of arthropods that are parasitic or can serve as disease vectors. (a) False-colour SEM of the pubic louse, *Phthirus pubis*, also known as a crab louse, clinging to a human pubic hair. The lice suck blood, feeding about 5 times a day. (b) The *Aedes* mosquito. (c) A flea, *Ctentocephalides*.

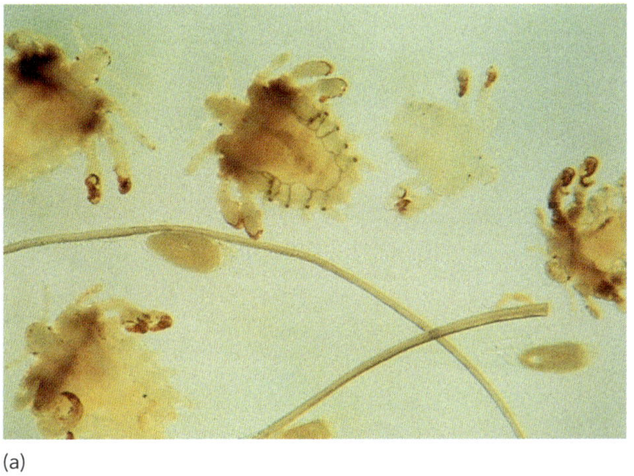

(a)

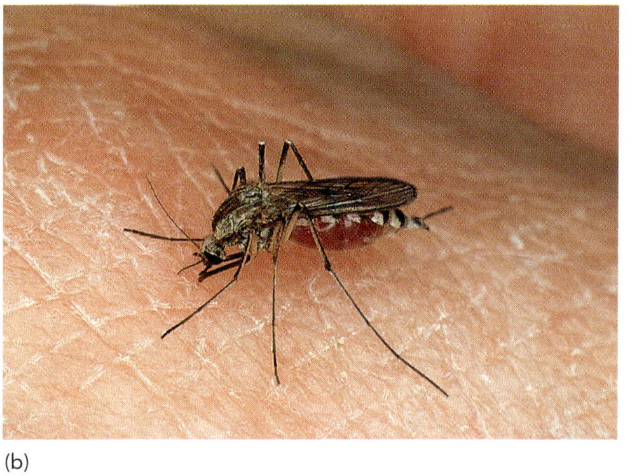

(b)

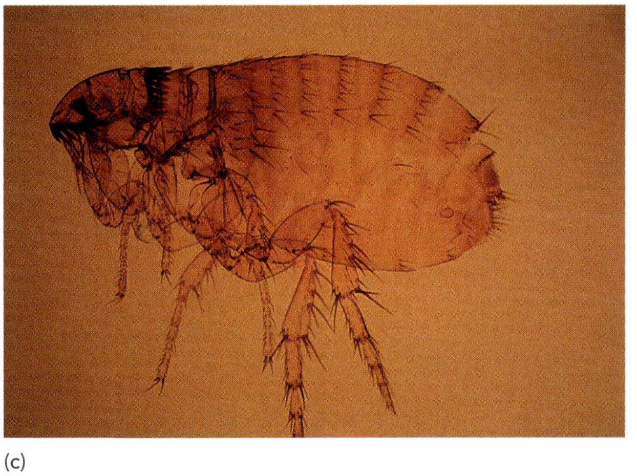

(c)

are also found on bedding and clothing and can survive for 2–3 days away from a human host. Treatment with benzyl benzoate or a cream containing 5% permethrin is effective, but eradication requires that all clothing and bed linen is washed and household contacts are also treated.

Scabies is endemic within Aboriginal communities in Northern Australia, and also occurs in urban areas where there is close human contact. Prevalence rates in Northern Territory Aboriginal schoolchildren are 30-65%. One of the major problems associated with scabies infection is that the itching and subsequent scratching allow secondary bacterial infections to occur.

Group A streptococcal infections are commonly associated with scabies. They can be readily treated with penicillin, but if the scabies infection is not eliminated the bacterial infection may recur and antibiotic-resistant strains of bacteria may invade. If untreated Group A streptococci can give rise to bacteraemia and kidney diseases such as acute post-streptococcal glomerulonephritis (see Chapter 14).

FLEAS

Fleas are blood-sucking insects which live parasitically on any warm-blooded animal. Occasionally, they will move from their usual animal host (cats, dogs, rats, wild animals) to humans. Usually, they do not create a problem, other than a brief irritation, and can easily be removed by improved hygiene or, if necessary, treating houses with insecticides. Fleas are the carrier (vector) of the bacterium that causes bubonic plague, *Yersinia pestis*. Usually, the infection occurs in rodents (rats, squirrels), but when the animal dies the infected fleas may move to a human host. Plague is not endemic in Australia although there have been outbreaks in the past (see Chapter 19).

LICE

The louse, *Pediculus humanus*, is a small insect that lives on the outside of the body, particularly on the scalp and in the hair. The parasite causes redness and itching where it bites, with some lymph exudate which can provide a medium for secondary infections. Lice infestation is easily diagnosed by the presence of small white eggs (nits) which are attached to the hair shaft. The lice are transmitted directly by person to person contact. Outbreaks of lice are common in school children and can be treated with preparations obtained from the chemist. Bedding and clothing should also be disinfected. The crab louse, *Phthirus pubis*, is found mainly in the pubic region and is transmitted by sexual contact.

ARTHROPOD VECTORS

A number of ectoparasites—ticks, mites and lice—can harbour rickettsia-like organisms in the cells of the alimentary canal. The insect acquires the organism by biting an infected animal or human and transmits the infection by biting, or by faecal excretion onto the skin of another human. Scratching the bite allows the organism to penetrate the skin and enter the new host. Of these infectionsthe most serious is epidemic typhus, which is carried by the human body louse. The disease is limited to developing countries or conditions of poor hygiene. Mites are responsible for carrying scrub typhus, which occurs in Northern Queensland and the Northern Territory. Other diseases carried by insect vectors are described in Chapter 8.

Summary

- A number of infectious diseases are caused by eucaryotic microorganisms.
- Patients who are immunocompromised are very susceptible to opportunistic infections caused by protozoa and fungi.

FUNGI

- Fungi comprise two groups: yeasts and moulds. Fungal cells are surrounded by a cell wall; they lack chlorophyll and cannot carry out photosynthesis.
- Fungi can grow at extremes of pH, temperature and osmotic pressure and are important for the decomposition of organic material.
- Yeasts are unicellular organisms that reproduce by budding. Some pathogenic yeasts (e.g. *Candida*) exhibit dimorphism.
- Moulds are filamentous fungi; they grow by producing a mat of hyphae called a mycelium as well as aerial hyphae that extend up above the mycelium.
- Asexual reproduction takes place by the formation of spores on the tips of the aerial hyphae.

FUNGAL INFECTIONS

- A fungal infection (mycosis) may be superficial, cutaneous, subcutaneous or systemic.
- Cutaneous infections (tinea) are caused by fungi called dermatophytes.
- Subcutaneous infections occur when the fungus is inoculated beneath the skin surface due to a wound or penetration of an object such as a splinter or thorn.
- Systemic mycoses are caused by pathogenic fungi, or fungi that have invaded an immunocompromised patient.
- Most serious fungal infections are opportunistic.

TRANSMISSION OF FUNGAL INFECTIONS

- Some fungi are transmitted by direct contact with an infected lesion or skin scales.
- Fungal spores are spread throughout the atmosphere on wind currents.
- Patient susceptibility to fungal infection is affected by use of immunosuppressive drugs, invasive procedures, IV therapy, and prolonged antibiotic therapy.

TREATMENT OF FUNGAL INFECTION

- Topical antifungal preparations are useful for cutaneous infections.
- Systemic infections are difficult to treat as most drugs have side effects.

HARMFUL EFFECTS OF FUNGI

- Allergic bronchopulmonary reactions occur from repeated inhalation of fungal spores.
- Some fungi produce toxins that are poisonous to humans.

PARASITES

- Parasites are organisms that derive their nutrients from another living organism.
- Parasites often have a complex life cycle, involving two or more hosts. The definitive host harbours the mature adult form of the parasite. The intermediate host has the immature or larval form.
- Serious parasitic diseases are relatively uncommon in Australia.
- Lifestyle factors and deficiencies in the immune defences increase susceptibility to parasitic infections.

PROTOZOA

- Protozoa are single-celled animals surrounded by a cell membrane. They are found mainly in water habitats.
- Reproduction is mainly asexual by binary or multiple fission.
- Protozoa form cysts that are able to survive for long periods under adverse conditions.
- Protozoa can exist as intracellular or extracellular parasites in humans and animals.
- Protozoal infections can be acquired by ingestion of the parasite or via the bite of a blood-sucking insect.
- Protozoa are classified by the way they move.
- Sarcodina (amoebae) move by extending the cell membrane to form a pseudopod and allowing the cytoplasm to flow into it.
- Protozoa that move by means of flagella include *Giardia*, which is responsible for gastrointestinal infections, and *Trichomonas vaginalis*, a sexually transmitted pathogen.
- Ciliates move by hair-like appendages called cilia.
- Sporozoa are non-motile protozoa.
- The genus *Plasmodium* is the cause of malaria and requires the Anopheles mosquito for transmission.
- *Pneumocystis carinii* is a non-motile protozoan that causes opportunistic lung infections in immunocompromised patients.
- *Toxoplasma gondii* is a non-motile sporozoan carried by cats. It produces only a mild illness in healthy people, but has serious effects on immunosuppressed patients and can cause congenital defects.
- *Cryptosporidium* and *Microsporidium* cause chronic diarrhoea in immunodeficient patients.

HELMINTHS

- Helminths (worms) include the phylum *Platyhelminthes* (flatworms, i.e. flukes and tapeworms) and the phylum *Aschelminthes* (roundworms).
- Many helminths have a complex life cycle involving an intermediate and a definitive host.
- Cestodes (tapeworms) consist of a head (scolex) and a body made of proglottids (segments) with both male and female organs on each segment. Eggs are produced and excreted in the faeces.
- Trematodes (flukes) have a flat body with muscular suckers for attachment.

- Nematodes (roundworms) are cylindrical worms with male and female organs located on different worms.

TREATMENT AND PREVENTION OF HELMINTH INFECTIONS

- Several antihelminthic drugs are available.
- Adequate nutrition and good sanitation are effective control measures.

ECTOPARASITES

- Arthropods such as scabies mites, fleas and lice can exist on the surface of the human body, causing skin irritation and carrying infection.

Study Questions

1. What are opportunistic infections?
2. Name the two main groups of fungi.
3. Describe the structure and method of replication of yeasts.
4. Describe the structure of moulds and their method of asexual reproduction.
5. What is a mycosis?
6. Differentiate between superficial, cutaneous and subcutaneous mycoses.
7. What is tinea?
8. Under what conditions is *Candida albicans* likely to cause infections?
9. How are fungal infections transmitted?
10. List two harmful effects of fungi other than mycoses.
11. What is a parasite?
12. What are some of the predisposing factors that allow parasitic infections to occur?
13. How do diseases caused by protozoa and helminths differ from those caused by bacteria or viruses?
14. What is the difference between an intermediate host and a definitive host?
15. What are protozoa?
16. How do protozoa reproduce?
17. What is the importance of the cyst form of protozoa?
18. How are protozoa classified?
19. Describe the causative organism, transmission and symptoms of amoebic dysentery.
20. Describe two important flagellate diseases present in Australia.
21. What is the most important sporozoal infection worldwide?
22. What role does the domestic cat play in the transmission of *Toxoplasma*?
23. What is a common cause of diarrhoea in AIDS patients?
24. How are worms classified?
25. How do tapeworms reproduce?
26. What are the main differences between human infections due to the beef tapeworm and those caused by the dog tapeworm?
27. Why are infections due to flukes not commonly seen in Australia?
28. What is the most common roundworm infection of children?
29. Why are worm infestations more common in people of lower socioeconomic status?
30. Which helminth infections are carried by insects?
31. How are helminth infections (a) prevented, (b) treated and (c) controlled?
32. What is scabies? Describe the major problems associated with scabies infections.
33. What is an ectoparasite? Give three examples.
34. Which diseases can be carried by ectoparasites?

Test Your Understanding

1. What is the difference between a cutaneous and a systemic mycosis?
2. Why are many hospitalised patients at risk of acquiring systemic fungal infections?
3. Why is it difficult to find an effective vaccine for malaria?
4. What other health problems would you suspect in a patient who is diagnosed with atypical pneumonia due to *Pneumocystis carinii*? Why?
5. Why should pregnant women avoid soiled kitty litter, sand pits and undercooked meat?
6. How do climate and environmental conditions influence the occurrence of parasitic infections? Explain your answer.
7. Discuss why effective drug therapy for diseases caused by eucaryotic organisms is difficult to achieve.

FURTHER READING

Ashman, R.B. & J.R. Warmington, 1991, 'New Perspectives on Candida and Candidiasis', *Today's Life Science*, 3, No. 12, pp. 22–26.

Doolan, D.L & M.F. Good, 1993, 'Developing a Malaria Sporozoite Vaccine', *Today's Life Science*, 5, No. 6, pp.18–27.

Grove, D.I., 1993, 'Worms in Australia', *Medical Journal of Australia*, 159, pp. 464–466.

Parasitology, 1994, *Science*, 264, pp. 1857–1884. (A collection of articles and reports on various parasitic diseases.)

Pritchard, R., 1989, 'The Immunocompromised Patient: New Opportunities for Fungi', *Today's Life Science*, 1, No. 3, pp. 36–45.

Warren, K.S., 1993, 'For the new millenium: control of helminth diseases throughout the world', *Medical Journal of Australia*, 159, pp. 461–463.

unit II

host-microbe interactions

chapter 7

host-microbe interactions

and principles of disease

Chapter focus

- *What kinds of relationships exist between living organisms?*
- *What are the properties of the microorganisms that inhabit the human body?*
- *What is an infectious disease?*
- *What factors determine whether a microorganism will cause an infection?*
- *What are the signs, symptoms and pattern of infectious diseases?*

Chapters 4–6 describe in some detail the properties of the major types of microorganisms. Some of these organisms are responsible for causing specific diseases and these are described more fully in Unit IV, which deals with infections of various body systems.

- But how do we know that microorganisms cause disease?
- Why do some organisms cause disease and others don't?
- What is the definition of disease?
- Why do some people get sick and others don't?
- How does disease spread from one person to another?

The chapters in this unit describe the interactions that occur between humans and microorganisms that can give rise to states of health, disease, epidemics and/or death. We describe the immune system—the complex system of defences that the human body uses to protect itself from invasion by microorganisms—and discuss the consequences for the human host when this system fails. The ways in which microorganisms are equipped to overcome human host defences and produce damage and disease are also described.

In this chapter we focus on what is meant by infection and infectious disease, pathogens, pathogenicity and virulence, and discuss the ways in which the delicate balance between microorganisms and humans can be altered, thus giving rise to a state of disease.

Symbiosis

All living organisms exist in some kind of relationship with each other. Sometimes the organisms do not interact unless they are physically brought together, for example, humans and animals. Sometimes the relationship is very close, as with members of a family. The biological term used to describe two organisms living together is **symbiosis**. The study of how organisms interact in an environment is called **ecology** and each particular defined environment is termed an **ecosystem**.

The human body can be regarded as a special type of ecosystem. At any moment in time, the human host may be interacting with numerous microorganisms and is subjected to physical, nutritional and traumatic alterations in environmental conditions that may have a marked influence on this interaction. Within this ecosystem, microorganisms live either permanently or transiently and, depending on various other factors, they may or may not cause an infection.

Not all symbiotic relationships are equally beneficial to both organisms. There are three broad categories of symbiotic association, based on the degree of benefit each organism receives—mutualism, commensalism and parasitism. In practice, the categories overlap to some extent, especially when applied to the human body, as the type of interaction may vary depending on physiological circumstances.

Mutualism

Mutualism usually refers to a situation where two independent organisms live together to their mutual benefit. The most commonly cited example is that of bacteria living in the stomach of ruminant cattle, where they aid in the digestion of cellulose in the animal's diet and in return receive a constant supply of nutrients. In humans, the bacteria living in the large intestine (colon) are of benefit to the host by producing vitamin K and some B vitamins; these are absorbed from the large intestine into the bloodstream and contribute to the host's requirements for those vitamins. The bacteria also help in the breakdown of waste material and the formation of faeces. In return, the bacteria benefit because they have a sheltered environment and an assured food supply.

Commensalism

Commensalism is an association between two organisms where one benefits while not causing any harm to the other. This is the term normally used to describe the relationship between the human host and the many and varied microorganisms that reside in or on the human body (see 'normal flora' below). For the most part, these organisms are harmless, living on the body surfaces and making use of the waste products (oils and fatty acids) that are excreted through pores on the skin surfaces (see Figure 7.1). Indeed, by preventing colonisation by harmful bacteria, they may also be regarded as being of indirect benefit to the host. However, when environmental conditions alter, these commensals may sometimes gain entry to other parts of the host and set up an infection. This situation is called 'opportunism' and is discussed later in this chapter. The definition of commensalism is therefore not clear-cut, as the relationship between host and resident microbes may vary with conditions.

FIGURE 7.1

BACTERIA ON HUMAN SKIN

Most of these organisms are commensals, which indirectly benefit us by competing with harmful organisms for nutrients and preventing them from finding a site to attach and invade tissues.

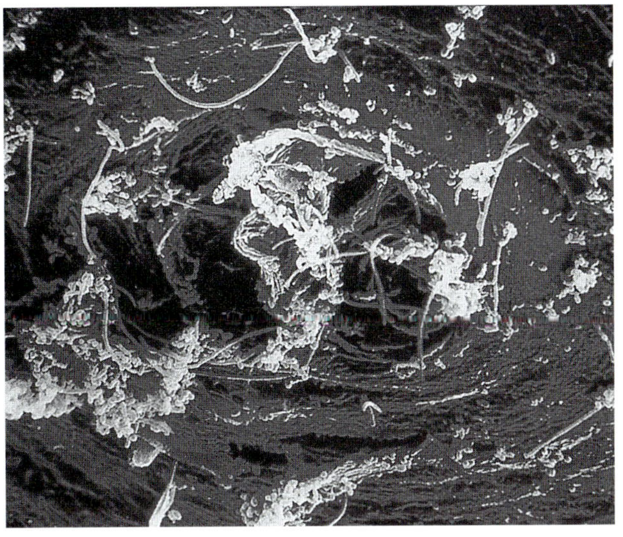

Parasitism

Parasitism is defined as a situation where one organism benefits at the expense of the other, usually larger, organism—the host. This usually means that the host is damaged or disadvantaged in some way. Most infections caused by microorganisms result in some degree of damage to the host cells. Parasitism, therefore, encompasses a wide range of relationships, from those in which the host is only slightly harmed, to those in which it is killed. The most 'successful' parasites are those that maintain their own life processes without killing their host, which is their source of nourishment. Many bacteria are commensals and are usually only considered to be in a parasitic relationship when they cause an infection. However, other microorganisms, such as the viruses and some protozoa and helminths, are true parasites in that they are unable to live outside their host and so always cause an infection and produce some degree of damage (see Chapter 6).

As will become apparent in the following sections, the relationship between the human host and the microorganisms that may be present on it is complex and continually changing, due to alterations in the physiological and nutritional states of both. This relationship determines whether a clinically identifiable infection or disease will occur.

Microorganisms of the Human Body: Normal Flora

Before discussing the process of infection and disease, we should examine the human body as a habitat for microorganisms. Microorganisms are ubiquitous in the environment and a very rich population of microbes, especially bacteria, resides on the human body. These are called the **normal flora** or **microflora** of the body.

The human foetus develops in a sterile environment in the uterus and at birth the neonate is free of microorganisms. However, within days, even hours of birth, a population of microorganisms, mainly bacteria, take up residence on the various body surfaces. They are derived from the baby's immediate environment, usually the birth canal of the mother, the hands of the people who care for the infant, the surfaces in the hospital nursery and other parts of the hospital environment. Because of the different organisms to which they are exposed, babies who are bottle fed tend to have different bacteria in the large intestine to those who are breast fed.

For the rest of their lives, humans are constantly exposed to a changing population of microorganisms. Some of these take up permanent residence on the skin and on the mucosal surfaces of the upper respiratory tract, mouth, gastrointestinal system and genital tract. These are called normal or **resident flora**. Others (some of which may be pathogens) establish themselves briefly in suitable areas (e.g. nose and throat), and are said to **colonise** these surfaces. They are **transient flora** and, after some time, are excluded from the site by competition with the normal flora or by the host's immune defence mechanisms. Other microorganisms are carried for a brief time on hands or other skin surfaces; they are usually considered to be contaminants and can be removed by physical means such as handwashing.

The human body provides an excellent shelter and source of nourishment for microbes. The various areas of the body have different conditions of temperature, moisture, pH, nutrients and oxygen so that different species can select the most suitable environment in which to reside. Most body surfaces (internal and external) that are exposed to the environment can, and do, harbour microorganisms. The bloodstream and the internal organs, however, are usually maintained in a sterile state by the various body defence mechanisms. When microorganisms enter these sites and persist, a state of disease exists.

The normal flora have a number of useful and protective effects. Once established in a suitable area, they can modify their environment—they may alter the pH (e.g. lactobacilli in the vagina), excrete chemicals with antibacterial activity (e.g. bacteriocins and organic acids in the large intestine) or occupy sites in the body so that other organisms cannot invade. The microbes that make up the normal flora are relatively stable but can be influenced by factors such as age, nutritional status, exposure to antibiotic therapy, or a change in environment, such as a prolonged stay in hospital. Studies have shown that the composition of the microbial population alters very rapidly after a patient enters hospital, the normal flora being replaced with hospital strains that are generally resistant to antibiotics. Infection with these hospital strains has serious implications for the patient as they are usually more difficult to treat. Normal body flora can also be the cause of infections if the delicate balance between host and microbe is upset (see 'Opportunism', p. 143).

NORMAL FLORA: TYPES OF ORGANISMS

By far the most predominant kinds of organism found on the human body are bacteria (see Figure 7.2). They can be easily identified by standard laboratory techniques and their role in maintaining the human ecosystem has been accepted for some time. The yeast, *Candida*, is the major fungal inhabitant and there are a few protozoa that appear to live in harmony with the human host (e.g. *Trichomonas intestinalis, Entamoeba coli*).

Because viruses are always thought of as disease-producing, they are not generally considered part of the normal flora. However, it may be that some viruses are able to reside in the human body without producing disease symptoms unless there is a change in the immune status of the host. An example of these would be latent viruses, such as members of the herpes family—herpes simplex, Epstein-Barr and cytomegalovirus (CMV)—but there may be others that have not yet been identified (see Chapter 5).

NORMAL FLORA OF THE SKIN

The skin harbours a diverse population of microorganisms. Bacteria reside in or on the dead layers of skin, obtaining nutrients from the secretions of the sebaceous glands and hair follicles. There are two distinct cutaneous populations: contaminants and resident flora. The **contaminants**, or exposed organisms, cling to the skin surfaces but do not usually replicate there. They include any organisms that the body (especially the hands) may have come into contact with during normal daily activities. Contaminants are greatly influenced by the personal hygiene of the individual. For health workers, the organisms carried on the hands are important as a mechanism in the transmission of disease.

The **resident flora** of the skin usually live in deep crevices in the skin layers, in hair follicles and in sweat glands. There are relatively few organisms present on the exposed, dry areas of the skin surfaces, the population of bacteria being much greater in warm, moist areas of the body such as the axillae (armpits) and groin. The organisms usually present include species of *Staphylococcus, Corynebacterium, Propionibacterium* and some fungi. *Staphylococcus epidermidis* is found mainly on dry areas of the skin, whereas *Staphylococcus aureus* prefers a moister environment such as the nasal passages. The organisms that populate the axillae metabolise the chemicals in sweat, producing breakdown products with a distinctive odour (body odour). Most commercial deodorants act by inhibiting the metabolic action of the bacteria or by drying the skin surface so that the bacteria cannot multiply.

NORMAL FLORA OF THE RESPIRATORY TRACT

The upper respiratory tract has a rich population of resident flora, including streptococci, staphylococci, dipththeroids and Gram-negative cocci. *Staphylococcus aureus* is found mainly in the nasal passages. Alpha- and beta-haemolytic

FIGURE 7.2 LOCATION OF NORMAL FLORA ON THE HUMAN BODY

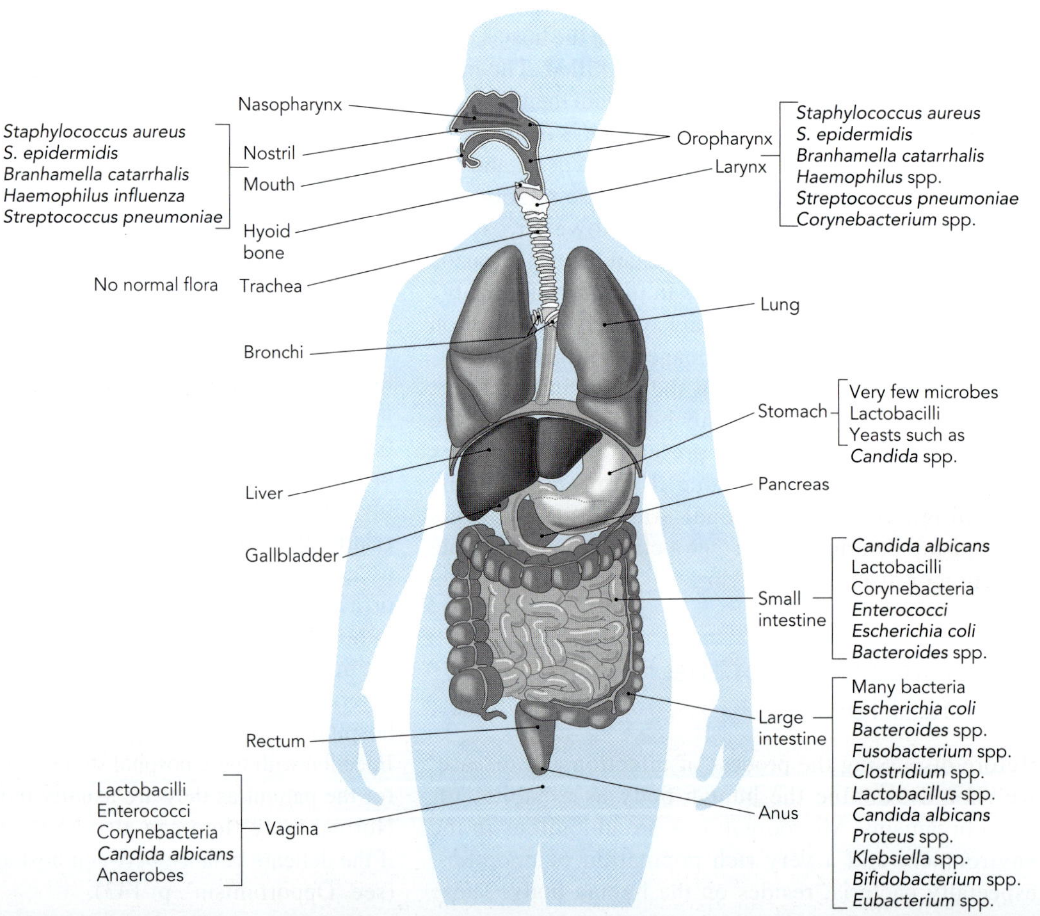

streptococci and *Haemophilus influenzae* are frequently found in the throat. *Streptococcus pneumoniae* may be present and is often responsible for middle ear infections (otitis media). Other organisms that may be present include *Neisseria meningitidis* and *Candida albicans*. Some people carry *Pneumocystis carinii* without any apparent ill effect. The bronchial tubes and lungs are relatively free of organisms in healthy individuals.

NORMAL FLORA OF THE GASTROINTESTINAL SYSTEM

The gastrointestinal system consists essentially of a long tube extending from the mouth to the anus. Varying conditions of oxygen tension, availability of nutrients and pH occur along this system and this is reflected in the different microbial populations that exist in each region.

The mouth contains a distinctive population of oral bacteria, the mucous membranes of the mouth supporting as many as 10^{11} bacteria per gram wet weight of tissue. These bacteria are usually present as commensals but can also be responsible for diseases in the mouth. The viridans group of streptococci are common members of the flora of the upper respiratory tract. They include the aerobes *Streptococcus mutans* and *Streptococcus sanguis* which can contribute to dental decay (**caries**) by secreting glucan, a sticky polysaccharide that attaches to the enamel of the tooth surface. **Plaque** consists of a film of bacterial cells anchored in a matrix of glycoproteins and polysaccharide that the organisms have secreted. This matrix provides a stable environment in which other oral bacteria thrive and metabolise sugars, producing acid that contributes to dental decay. Other bacteria, including *Lactobacillus, Fusobacterium* and *Actinomyces*, which prefer an anaerobic environment, thrive on the gums or in crevices between the teeth. Sometimes these organisms are responsible for an infection of the gums known as **gingivitis**.

The pH of the stomach is acid due to the secretion of hydrochloric acid, and inhibits the growth of most microorganisms. A few acid-tolerant lactobacilli may be present in the gastric mucosa. *Helicobacter pylori*, a bacterium that is thought to be intimately involved in the occurrence of gastric ulcers, can also tolerate this environment, but is not considered to be part of the normal flora. The upper part of the ileum (duodenum) is slightly alkaline and is also relatively free of bacteria. The lower intestine, the caecum and colon, harbours a large population of bacteria (approximately 10^{12} bacteria per gram of intestinal contents) and they can comprise up to 30% of the faecal volume.

The predominant flora are anaerobes or facultative anaerobes (Table 7.1), but strict anaerobes such as *Bacteroides* are also present in large numbers, *Escherichia coli, Klebsiella* and *Enterobacter* are among the bacteria that are usually present. The presence of *E. coli* in water samples is often used as a test for faecal contamination. Bacteria in the colon are of benefit to the host by digesting waste material and converting it to faeces. They are also largely responsible for the formation of gas (flatus) and various breakdown products with a strong, distinctive odour, as well as the production of short chain fatty acids

TABLE 7.1
REPRESENTATIVE EXAMPLES OF NORMAL HUMAN BODY FLORA[a]

Skin	*Propionibacterium acnes, Staphylococcus aureus, Staphylococcus epidermidis, Corynebacterium xerosis, Candida* spp. (yeast)
Eyes	*Staphylococcus aureus, Staphylococcus epidermidis*, diphtheroids
Upper respiratory tract	*Staphylococcus aureus, Staphylococcus epidermidis*, diphtheroids (mainly in nose).
Nose/throat	*Streptococcus pneumoniae, Haemophilus influenzae, Neisseria* in throat *Brahnamella* spp., *Micrococcus* spp.
Gastrointestinal system	
Mouth	*Streptococcus* spp., *Lactobacillus, Fusobacterium, Actinomyces, Bacteroides, Veillonella, Candida* (yeast)
Stomach	*Lactobacillus*
Large intestine	More than 300 species including *Bacteroides, Enterococcus, Enterobacter, Escherichia coli, Proteus, Klebsiella, Bifidobacterium, Candida* (yeast), *Clostridium perfringens*
Genital tract	*Lactobacillus, Streptococcus*, Corynebacterium, diphtheroids, *Staphylococcus, Candida* (yeast), *Trichomonas vaginalis* (protozoan)
Urinary tract[b]	*Staphylococcus, Streptococcus, Proteus, Enterococcus, Lactobacillus, Klebsiella*

a. Unless otherwise indicated, these organisms are bacteria.
b. In females, flora exist in the lower portion of the urethra. The population is similar to that found in the large intestine. In males, the urethra has a much smaller population of organisms.

(SCFA) which are important in maintaining the health of the colon. A number of non-pathogenic protozoa exist in the intestine.

NORMAL FLORA OF THE GENITOURINARY TRACT

The major components of the urinary system—the kidneys, bladder and upper part of the urethra—are usually sterile. The lower portion of the urethra, especially in females, may harbour microorganisms that are representative of those present on the skin, vagina or colon. They are usually flushed out regularly by the flow of urine.

The composition of the normal flora of the vagina illustrates how the flora change depending on age and physiological conditions. Before puberty, the pH of the vagina is about 7 and the predominant inhabitants are staphylococci, streptococci, dipththeroids and some coliforms. After puberty, the hormone oestrogen stimulates the secretion of glycogen by the vagina. Fermentation of glycogen is carried out by lactobacilli with the production of acid, which lowers the pH to about 5. This acidic pH is protective, inhibiting the growth of many other organisms (e.g. *Candida albicans*) and establishing conditions suitable for fertilisation. When the lactobacilli of the vagina are destroyed by prolonged antibiotic therapy, or the pH is altered by hormonal or physiological disturbances, an overgrowth of other organisms frequently ensues (e.g. *Candida*, causing thrush). Other principal residents include beta-haemolytic Group B streptococci (*Streptococcus agalactiae*).

The presence of normal flora in the body is of significant benefit to the human host as they prevent other organisms from becoming established and possibly causing an infection. The products of their metabolism contribute to the establishment of an environment unfavourable for harmful organisms (e.g. acid pH) and produce substances of benefit to the host (e.g. vitamins). The value of the normal flora to the human host is apparent when their numbers are reduced by long-term broad spectrum antibiotic therapy. A frequent side effect of such therapy is an overgrowth of undesirable organisms; for example, *Clostridium difficile* may flourish in the large intestine causing diarrhoea and pseudomembraneous colitis. As described above, vaginitis or thrush is another common occurrence. Cessation of antibiotic therapy usually allows the normal flora to become re-established.

Infection and Disease

Up to now we have been considering the microorganisms that live on the human body as a normal part of our environment. However, a delicate balance exists between health and disease. Under certain conditions many of the normal flora, as well as organisms from the external environment have the potential to cause disease.

The first step is for microorganisms to become established or colonise the human body. They then have an opportunity to penetrate the host defences, invade the tissues, multiply and set up an **infection**. When the results of the infection produce clinical symptoms, a disease results. **Disease** is defined as any harmful alteration to the physiological or metabolic state of the host. An **infectious disease** occurs when this alteration is caused by a microorganism, or its products, such as **toxins** (see Chapter 10). Any organism capable of causing disease is called a **pathogen**. The microorganisms responsible for the infection may come from anywhere in the environment or from the human body itself.

Pathogenicity is defined as the capacity to produce disease. This capacity depends on certain characteristics of the organism, such as the ability to:

- gain entry to the host;
- attach to the host tissues and multiply;
- evade the host defences;
- damage tissue and produce disease symptoms.

Some diseases are not as serious as others, and this depends on the type of pathogen involved. The degree of pathogenicity of different types of microorganisms ranges from mild to serious or even fatal. For example, the cold virus is a pathogen, but the disease it causes is usually only mild, whereas infection with the influenza A virus is much more serious, and an infection with the rabies virus is nearly always fatal. Differences in pathogenicity are also related to the **virulence** of the organism or strain of that organism. Virulence refers to the intensity of the disease symptoms produced by a particular organism. It depends on a number of factors, such as the ability of the organism to invade the host cell and produce damage. Some organisms are able to carry this out more effectively than others and so are described as being very virulent. For example, encapsulated strains of *Streptococcus pneumoniae* are more virulent than unencapsulated strains. The presence of the capsule allows the bacterium to attach to and invade the host tissues, and also contributes to its ability to evade phagocytosis by the host's white blood cells.

Other virulence factors include the ability to produce enzymes and toxins that damage the host cell. Different strains of the same organism may show a variation in virulence. For example, some strains of *Streptococcus pyogenes* are very invasive and cause rapid, severe, sometimes fatal infections (e.g. puerperal fever). Other strains are not as virulent and produce milder symptoms (e.g. 'strep throat'). The difference in virulence between strains is related to the virulence factors they produce. Some strains of influenza are more virulent than others, causing serious epidemics throughout the world. The mechanisms used by pathogens to produce disease are discussed in detail in Chapter 10.

The virulence of a particular organism may be increased by its passage through a series of susceptible animal hosts. Sometimes this change occurs spontaneously, when a disease such as influenza spreads through the human population. The strain of the virus isolated at the end of an epidemic is frequently more virulent than the original pathogen. The mutational changes that cause this alteration in virulence are not well understood. In the laboratory, the virulence of a particular organism can often be decreased or *attenuated* by repeated passage through cell culture, or prolonged growth in artificial media. This technique has been used successfully to produce weakened strains of organisms which can then be used as vaccines (e.g. the MMR vaccine contains attenuated strains of measles, mumps and rubella viruses).

Another important factor in determining whether a disease will occur is the **infective dose**, or the number of cells of the organism that are able to penetrate the human body and become established. If only a few cells are present, then the host defences may be able to destroy them. However, if the numbers are large they may overwhelm the defences. For example, the stomach acid may be sufficient to neutralise the few bacteria normally contained in food, but is not able to inactivate all the microbes in a heavily contaminated food sample. In general, the more virulent the organism, the fewer the number of cells that will be needed to establish an infection and produce disease symptoms. For example, a gastrointestinal infection due to *Shigella* may require as few as 100 organisms to be present in contaminated food or on the hands, whereas one million *Salmonella* cells might be needed under similar circumstances.

OPPORTUNISTIC INFECTIONS

Up to now we have been describing the characteristics of true pathogens—that is, microorganisms that are always able to overcome the natural host defences and cause disease in an otherwise healthy host. However, a significant number of diseases are caused by microorganisms that set up an infection because they have been moved from their normal habitat, or because the host defences are compromised in some way. For this reason, we will define another type of relationship that may occur.

Opportunism refers to a situation where microorganisms that would not normally cause an infection do so because of an alteration in physiological conditions in the host, or a change in the environment where the organism is located. These organisms are called **opportunistic pathogens**. They are able to gain entry and set up an infection in a host when the host defences are lowered or compromised in some way. Often such infections are caused by normal flora of the host that have been displaced from their usual habitat. For example, many of the infections in surgical wounds are due to *Staphylococcus epidermidis*, derived from the patient's own skin.

This is also true of infections associated with intravenous catheters or central lines. Many urinary tract infections are caused by bacteria that are normally resident in the large intestine but which have been transported from the anus to the opening of the urethra, from where they can gain entry to the bladder. The seriousness of the infection and the ease of treatment depends on the properties of the particular organism causing the infection and the site of infection.

Frequently, an alteration in the physiological or hormonal state of a patient encourages the overgrowth of one of the normal flora. For example, as described above, the yeast *Candida albicans*, a normal inhabitant of the vagina, is often the cause of vaginitis, or thrush.

Opportunistic infections occur when the normal defences of the host are lowered. This fact is becoming of increasing importance in hospitals where many of the patients have a real or induced deficiency of their immune system, placing them at great risk of acquiring infection.

HOST RESISTANCE OR SUSCEPTIBILITY

One of the most important factors to consider when discussing infectious disease is the ability of the host to resist invasion by the pathogen. The human body has a complex system of specific and non-specific mechanisms to deal with foreign particles and microorganisms. These are discussed fully in Chapter 9. One of the most important of these is the mechanical barrier provided by an intact skin. Once this barrier is broken (e.g. in wounds, surgery or burns), microorganisms are able to gain easy access to the tissues.

The general health of the host is also very important in determining the outcome of exposure to a pathogen. A healthy person is often able to ward off an infection, whereas someone with an additional, often unrelated, illness may succumb. One of the most difficult problems for health workers is when a patient presents with an infection or infectious disease which is really an expression of a number of underlying diseases. This is especially true of patients in some remote areas of Australia, and among Aborigines or people in lower socioeconomic groups. Underlying illnesses such as diabetes or leukaemia may contribute to patient susceptibility. Those with a lowered white blood cell count (**neutropenia**) are at greater risk of infection. Many patients receive treatment that affects the functioning of their immune system (e.g. cancer patients receiving chemotherapy and radiotherapy). Transplant patients receive immunosuppressive drugs to prevent rejection of the transplanted organ. Most of these drugs also interfere with the body's ability to fight foreign microorganisms, rendering these patients at risk from infectious diseases.

Patients with immune disorders are obviously more susceptible to infection. Most people who acquire the human immunodeficiency virus (HIV) develop AIDS, and the cause of death is usually an opportunistic infection (see Chapter 19).

General lifestyle and nutritional status affect the susceptibility of the host. Malnutrition and alcoholism both contribute to lowered body defence mechanisms. Intravenous drug users are at risk of acquiring blood-borne pathogens such as hepatitis B, hepatitis C and HIV. Cigarette smokers tend to be at greater risk of lung infections and bronchitis. Many people who die from Legionnaires' disease have a previous history of lung problems associated with smoking.

Age is an important factor, as it often reflects the status of the immune system. Neonates and infants up to about one year of age have a poorly developed immune system and so are particularly susceptible to infection, even though they have some protection from maternal antibodies. As their immune system matures they are able to deal with invading pathogens and develop their own immunity. The system appears to decline in old age, so the elderly are at a greater risk of infection. Males and females show a different pattern of susceptibility. For example, females suffer more urinary tract infections because of the comparative shortness of the female urethra and the proximity of the anus to the urethra. During pregnancy, the immune system is slightly compromised and so pregnant women tend to be more susceptible to some infections. Hepatitis E and malaria are two diseases with an increased risk of a fatal outcome during pregnancy.

There is considerable evidence that the genetic makeup of an individual plays a part in susceptibility to infection. The reason for this is not well understood at present, but there are documented cases of differences in the ability of various individuals to resist disease that can only be explained on the basis of genetic differences in their immune system. (See Table 7.2.)

PREDISPOSING FACTORS

As well as individual susceptibility, a number of external factors contribute to the likelihood of someone acquiring an infectious disease. High on the list are the environment in which they live and the general hygiene of their surroundings. The climate often has an effect, as it may favour the persistence of a pathogen or its vector. The weather, winds, temperature or natural disasters such as floods will facilitate the spread of microorganisms. Air pollution affects the lungs and lowers resistance to respiratory pathogens. Many infectious diseases have a seasonal occurrence; for example, influenza occurs more often in the winter months, chickenpox usually in spring. Patients who are hospitalised are often at greater risk of acquiring an infection than they would be outside the hospital environment. This is largely due to their lowered resistance because of illness, but is also related to the invasive procedures they may have undergone. In the hospital environment, they are likely to be exposed to large numbers of microorganisms, many of which are resistant to antibiotics. Hospital-acquired (nosocomial) infections are discussed in Chapter 13.

Koch's Postulates

How do we know that microorganisms cause disease? Today, we take for granted that microorganisms are responsible for the clinical signs and symptoms of an infection. This was not always the case—in 1876, when the German microbiologist Robert Koch proposed his **germ theory of disease**, he had to overcome significant opposition to his ideas. Koch investigated the cause of a disease, anthrax, that was killing the cattle in Europe and discovered that a bacterium he named *Bacillus anthracis*, was responsible. He subsequently went on to isolate other bacteria that were responsible for tuberculosis and cholera. Based on his research he put forward a set of criteria that should be met when deciding whether an organism is responsible for causing a particular disease.

TABLE 7.2
FACTORS THAT INCREASE SUSCEPTIBILITY TO INFECTION

FACTORS	SUSCEPTIBILITY
Age	Neonates have immature immune system. Elderly have decreased immune system. Some pathogens have increased virulence in different age groups.
Pregnancy	More susceptible to some diseases, e.g. hepatitis E, malaria.
Nutrition	Malnutrition and alcoholism lower immune response.
Illness	Underlying illnesses, e.g. diabetes, cancer, liver disease contribute to susceptibility.
Immunosuppressive drugs	Transplant patients have lowered immune response.
Chemotherapy	Cancer patients susceptible, due to effects of drugs.
Atmospheric pollution	Lung damage increases susceptibility to respiratory infections.
Surgery/Trauma	Provides portal of entry for pathogens.
Physical defects	Provides site for infection.
Stress	Lowers immune response.
Immune diseases, acquired or genetic	Lowers immune response.
Gender/Genetic predispositon	Variable effect on susceptibility to different diseases.

They are called **Koch's Postulates** and can be summarised as follows:

- The organism must always be present in every case of the disease.
- It must be possible to isolate the organism from the diseased host and grow it in pure culture.
- The pure culture of the organism, when inoculated into a new susceptible host, must produce the same symptoms of disease.
- It must be possible to recover the organism from the experimental host.

Koch's work was important in developing the concept of 'one germ, one disease'—that is, that a single type of organism is responsible for causing a disease with a characteristic group of symptoms. These postulates provided a sound scientific approach to the problem of identification of the causative agents of infection and, during the following 30 years, scientists around the world adopted his methods and were successful in isolating and identifying the bacteria responsible for many of the major diseases then known (see Table 1.2, p. 8).

These methods were very useful for bacterial diseases but, during the 20th century, diseases caused by viruses were identified. Although the basic principles of Koch's postulates still stand, they need some modification in the light of current technology, the type of pathogens that have been described in recent times and our understanding of the nature of infectious diseases. For example, some organisms are difficult to grow in pure culture away from the host. *Mycobacterium leprae*, the causative organism of leprosy, has never been grown on artificial media. Viruses and rickettsiae can be grown only in cell culture. Recently, a previously unknown organism, *Legionella pneumophila*, was identified as the bacterium responsible for Legionnaires' disease. Although it is now possible to grow it in the laboratory on special medium, the bacterium was originally isolated from infected patients by injecting samples of lung tissue into guinea pigs. Instead of testing this culture and producing the same disease in a susceptible human host, as would be required to fulfil Koch's postulates, modern immunological methods were used. Patients who had had Legionnaires' disease were tested and found to have antibodies to the same bacteria that had produced the disease symptoms in the guinea pigs.

TABLE 7.3
SOME MICROBIAL CAUSES OF PNEUMONIA

Bacteria	*Streptococcus pneumoniae* *Staphylococcus aureus* *Haemophilus influenzae* *Escherichia coli* *Klebsiella pneumoniae* *Pseudomonas aeruginosa* *Legionella pneumophila* *Mycobacterium tuberculosis* *Mycoplasma pneumoniae*
Chlamydia	*Chlamydia* spp.
Rickettsia	*Coxiella burnetii*
Viruses	Influenza virus Respiratory syncytial virus
Protozoan (? fungus)	*Pneumocystis carinii**
Fungus	*Histoplasma capsulatum**

* in immunosuppressed patients

Some diseases can be caused by more than one type of pathogen. For example, pneumonia, which is really an infection of the lungs, can be caused by any one of a number of organisms, some of which are listed in Table 7.3.

We also know that some organisms apparently cause more than one disease. For example, streptococci, which are responsible for 'strep sore throat', may also release bacterial antigens into the bloodstream and elicit a post-streptococcal hypersensitivity response involving the heart, known as rheumatic fever.

Sometimes pathogens may be present in the body, giving rise to a **subclinical infection** where there are no clinically identifiable disease symptoms (see p. 151). This is often the case with diseases such as rubella (German measles) and glandular fever. Other pathogens, especially the viruses belonging to the herpes family, can remain in the body in a *latent* form, and be reactivated when the physiological state of the host changes. Neither of these situations fulfils the criteria used by Koch. It is now thought that some diseases may occur because of an interaction between more than one infectious agent; for example, post-viral syndrome may be related to previous unresolved viral diseases. We also need to take into account the differences in host susceptibility (discussed above).

Even with these modifications, however, Koch provided a set of scientific principles that formed the basis for a sound experimental approach to the investigation of the **aetiology** (cause) of infectious diseases.

Signs and Symptoms of Disease

In the previous sections, we have distinguished between situations where microorganisms are normally present in or on the human body and those cases in which an infection or disease occurs. In order to decide whether a state of infection or disease exists, it is usual to observe the individual for indications of the presence of microorganisms and, in the case of disease, for the presence of tell-tale signs or symptoms. These represent pathological changes or damage to the host cells and tissues; they are often characteristic of the type of infection and so are useful for diagnosis.

Signs are measurable changes in the patient that can be observed by examination of the patient or their body fluids. They include occurrences such as fever, swelling (oedema), rashes, vomiting and diarrhoea, as well as data derived from laboratory tests.

Symptoms are changes that are felt and reported by the patient, such as pain, headache, nausea, or a general feeling of illness (**malaise**). Sometimes these categories overlap. The combination of signs and symptoms that characterise a particular disease state is called a **syndrome** (e.g. AIDS stands for acquired immune deficiency **syndrome**).

FEVER

Fever (**pyrexia**) almost invariably accompanies infection and is one of the most useful early warning signs. Constant monitoring of a patient's temperature will often indicate that an infection is present, long before other symptoms appear.

The body temperature is maintained within narrow limits by the temperature-regulating centre in the hypothalamus in the brain. A fever is produced when chemicals called **pyrogens** that are circulating in the bloodstream act on the hypothalamus and reset the thermostat to a higher temperature. **Endogenous pyrogens** are derived from within the human body. The main ones are **interleukin-1** (IL-1) and **tumour necrosis factor** (TNF), which are released by the phagocytic white blood cells, monocytes and macrophages. **Exogenous pyrogens** are products of infectious organisms. One of the most important is an endotoxin that is part of the lipopolysaccharide found in the cell wall of Gram-negative bacteria (see Chapter 4). Exogenous pyrogens act by stimulating the release of endogenous pyrogens such as IL-1, which in turn act on the hypothalamus as described above. Fluids to be administered to patients (such as IV solutions) are frequently labelled 'pyrogen-free'. This means they do not contain any fever-producing substances such as fragments of dead microorganisms. Endotoxins can also cause other serious effects in the human host (see Chapter 10).

INFLAMMATION

Inflammation is a common non-specific response that often occurs at the site of injury or infection. The syndrome, which consists of heat, pain, redness, vasodilation and swelling, is described in Chapter 9. When the host tissue is damaged, one of the first reactions is the activation of the inflammatory response, which is mediated by a number of chemicals released by the damaged cells and other cells of the immune system.

Important among these chemicals is **histamine**, which causes vasodilation and an increase in permeability of the capillaries. Fluids and white blood cells (phagocytes) move into the tissues, resulting in redness, swelling and pain. A localised increase in temperature at the site of inflammation is due to this vasodilation. Other chemicals released by the damaged cells attract phagocytic white blood cells (monocytes and macrophages) to the site. They may release pyrogens such as interleukin-1 (IL-1) which act on the hypothalamus (as described above) and produce a rise in temperature throughout the body (fever). The pus that forms at the site of an infection is a mixture of dead microbial cells, dead or damaged host cells and white blood cells. Many of the signs and symptoms observed are actually a result of the host's own defence system attempting to counter the infection.

IMMUNE REACTIONS

The reaction of the body to infection involves an immune response that is discussed in detail in Chapter 9. Some of the signs of this immune response can be detected and serve as an indication of the presence of infection. Stimulation of the immune system results in increased activity in the lymph nodes or glands, causing **lymphadenopathy** (swollen glands). Changes in the white blood cell population are typical of the body's response to infection and are indicative of certain kinds of disease. **Leukocytosis** is an increase in the white cell count, while **leukopenia** is a decrease in the number of white cells circulating in the bloodstream. The specific immune response also results in the formation of **antibodies** to the organism responsible for the infection. These can be detected in the blood and their number and type are indicative of the progress of the disease in the patient.

SKIN SIGNS

Skin rashes are often non-specific, but some are quite distinctive and play a major role in diagnosis. For example, the pustular lesions of chickenpox are easy to identify. The reaction of the skin during infection can be described in various ways.

- **Lesion**—any area of damaged tissue.
- **Erythema**—reddening of the skin, due to dilation of the surface capillaries.
- **Macule**—a small, flat, reddish patch.
- **Papule**—a slightly raised red spot, such as a pimple.
- **Vesicles**—small blisters, often filled with clear, yellowish fluid (serum).
- **Pustule**—a lesion containing creamish opaque material (pus).
- **Ulcer** or **erosion**—a skin lesion that is deep and reaches subcutaneous tissue.
- **Abscess**—a localised collection of pus.

The signs and symptoms of disease are usually indicative of the body system affected. Infections of the gastrointestinal system typically cause nausea, stomach cramps, vomiting and diarrhoea. Headache, stiff neck and confusion indicate infection of the nervous system. Some symptoms are common to a number of diseases. For example, headache, nausea and fever may be caused by any of a number of organisms. Frequently, the presence of a high fever will induce vomiting that may be unrelated to the true cause of the illness. For this reason, the laboratory examination of swabs or specimens plays an essential role in diagnosis of the causative agents of an infection (see Chapter 15).

Laboratory tests

Tests are carried out on specimens of blood, urine, cerebrospinal fluid (CSF) and other tissue samples in order to detect or confirm other signs of infection. The presence of microorganisms in a specimen or swab from a normally sterile body site may indicate infection. Cultures derived from sites that carry normal flora usually contain more than one type of organism and are more difficult to interpret. Blood specimens are useful in the detection of some infections that are not visible on the body surface. Microorganisms can enter the bloodstream through breaks in the capillary walls. The presence in the blood of bacteria (**bacteraemia**) or viruses (**viraemia**) is not necessarily significant unless symptoms are produced. **Sepsis** occurs when the organisms multiply in the bloodstream and result in a systemic inflammatory response (SIR).

Development of Disease

The course of infection and disease in the human body generally follows a defined pattern or sequence of events (see Figure 7.3). These are the incubation period, the prodromal phase, the invasive or acute phase of disease (which sometimes involves a peak or crisis) and the convalescence. The outcome of the disease may be either complete recovery, death, or the establishment of a latent or chronic infection (see below).

INCUBATION PERIOD

After successfully gaining entry to the body, the pathogen has to overcome the host defences in order to establish itself, multiply and cause disease. The **incubation period** is the time interval that occurs between the exposure of the host to the pathogen and the appearance of any signs or symptoms of disease. The incubation time is affected by a number of factors, including the properties of the pathogen, its virulence, the infective dose, the place of entry of the pathogen into the host relative to its target organ, and the resistance of the host. In gastrointestinal infections, the length of time before the onset of symptoms depends on whether the disease is due to bacterial contamination of food or to the presence of preformed toxins.

Table 7.4 shows typical incubation times for some infectious diseases. During the incubation period, patients are often unaware that they have been exposed to the pathogen. However, during this period as well as the following prodromal period, they may be infectious and thus able to spread the disease to others.

PRODROMAL PERIOD

As the pathogen continues to multiply, non-specific disease symptoms are produced such as headache, nausea and general malaise. This is termed the prodromal period and signals the beginning of disease. Sometimes the host defences overcome the pathogen at this stage and the symptoms disappear before a recognisable disease syndrome develops. The host may or may not be left with an acquired resistance (antibodies and memory cells) to the pathogen but, if so, is said to have experienced a subclinical infection (see p. 151). Not all diseases have a prodromal phase. Many start suddenly with acute symptoms of pain and fever, reflecting the nature of the infection.

FIGURE 7.3
STAGES IN THE PROGRESSION OF DISEASE

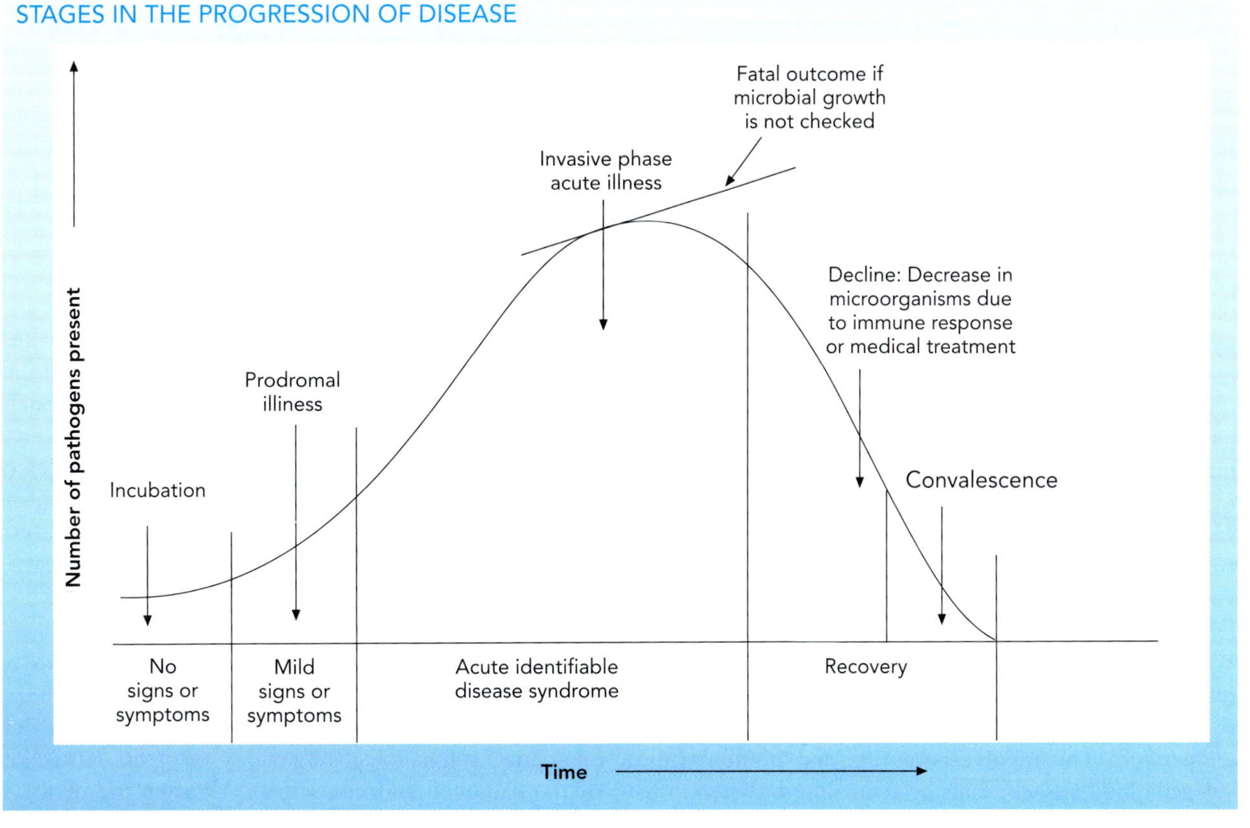

TABLE 7.4
INCUBATION TIMES FOR SOME COMMON INFECTIOUS DISEASES

DISEASE	TIME
Chickenpox	2–3 weeks
Measles	8–14 days
Mumps	12–25 days
Diphtheria	2–6 days
Tuberculosis	4–12 weeks
Rubella (German measles)	14–21 days
Influenza	2–3 days
Food poisoning	12–36 hours
Gangrene	24–48 hours
Tetanus	24–48 hours after injury
Whooping cough	7–10 days
Glandular fever	4–6 weeks
Hepatitis A	3–5 weeks
Hepatitis B	2–6 months
Hepatitis C	6–8 weeks
HIV	Minimum 3 weeks; may be months or years
Gonorrhoea	2–5 days
Syphilis	2–3 weeks

ACUTE OR INVASIVE PHASE

If the early host defences do not overcome the pathogen, the prodromal stage is followed by a period of acute disease, the **invasive phase**, during which the pathogen invades and damages the host tissue. Fever and chills, caused by the presence of pyrogens, are typical symptoms of the invasive phase of the disease. As mentioned earlier, pyrogens are chemicals that act on the hypothalamus and reset the normal body temperature control to a higher temperature. They are breakdown products of some pathogens or are produced by phagocytes during the inflammatory reaction. The body's immediate response to an increase in the temperature set point is to try to raise the body temperature by involuntary muscle contraction (shivering) and the narrowing of surface blood vessels to prevent heat loss (**vasoconstriction**). The effect is that the patient becomes pale and feels cold or chilled. When further fluctuations occur in the set point control, returning it to the normal lower temperature, the body responds by trying to increase heat loss to lower the body temperature. This involves sweating, and dilation of the surface blood vessels, causing reddening of the skin or flushing. The patient feels hot and has a fever.

Some diseases, such as malaria, have repeated episodes of fever and chills, mediated by the synchronised release of the merozoites from the red blood cells (Chapter 6). Others have a longer period of sustained elevated temperature before a sudden drop or a slow decline. There is some evidence that a moderate increase in temperature (up to 40°C) is protective. The multiplication of some microorganisms (e.g. rhinoviruses, gonococci) is inhibited or slowed by higher temperatures. In addition, the higher body temperature may stimulate the rate of the inflammatory immune response. Nearly all fever is caused by infection. **Pyrexia of unknown origin (PUO)** is a term used to describe a situation where the patient has an unexplained fever. In more than 50% of such cases, an infection is present. There are a few non-infective causes of fever, including some malignancies and some vascular diseases.

Some invasive phases reach a crisis or peak over a period of time, after which symptoms (especially fever) quickly subside. Other diseases are characterised by a longer invasive phase during which additional symptoms occur, such as cough, diarrhoea, jaundice, loss of muscle control, swelling, pain and discharge. These additional symptoms may be due to the action of toxins produced by the pathogen (see Chapter 10). For example, the cough associated with whooping cough develops as the disease progresses and is due to inflammation and damage to the trachea caused by the toxins produced by the invading pathogen (*Bordetella pertussis*). The cough persists long after the invasive phase has ended and the patient is no longer infectious.

The ability of the host to overcome the invasive phase determines the outcome of the disease—that is, recovery or death (terminal outcome). A **fulminating disease** is an acute infection that progresses very rapidly, often with a fatal outcome. The symptoms appear suddenly and develop quickly into a serious infection (e.g. pneumonic plague or meningococcal meningitis). In this situation, the pathogen overcomes the host before protective immunity can develop.

DECLINE PHASE

If the immune system responds to the infection and overcomes the effects of the pathogen, the symptoms subside, the disease enters the decline phase and the patient begins to recover. In some cases, however, the host defences are unable to eliminate the pathogen completely from the body and the disease progresses to a latent or chronic state (see section below, on types of infection).

EFFECTS OF DRUG THERAPY

This description of the progress of a disease needs to be modified when drug therapy (antimicrobials, antipyretics, analgesics) is used. Often, the use of an appropriate antimicrobial drug will speed up the destruction of the pathogen and dramatically shorten the invasive phase, sometimes averting a fatal outcome. However, one of the undesirable outcomes of antibiotic use is that endotoxins may be released from the breakdown of certain types of dead Gram-negative bacteria. These endotoxins can produce serious, sometimes fatal, effects such as fever and septic shock, leading to haemorrhage, collapse of the circulatory system and sequential failure of essential body organs—as can occur in meningococcal meningitis (see Chapter 10).

There is also considerable discussion about the merits of using antipyretics, especially aspirin, to reduce fever in the early stages of infection. As mentioned above, fever may sometimes be beneficial, provided body temperature does not exceed 40°C, when organ damage may occur. There is some evidence that the use of aspirin in children during episodes of some viral diseases (influenza and chickenpox) is associated with the development of **Reye's syndrome**. This is a sometimes fatal disease characterised by brain damage and degeneration of some internal organs.

CONVALESCENCE

Convalescence is the time when the body repairs itself and regains strength. The energy that has been used to activate and support the immune response is directed back to the normal processes of cell regeneration and tissue repair. In today's busy society, many people fail to allow sufficient time for convalescence and so are frequently exposed to another pathogen before regaining their full strength. The result is a series of illnesses because the immune system is too weak to protect the body effectively.

Types of Infection

When microorganisms invade host tissue an infection occurs. The type of infection depends on the nature of the invading organism, the site of entry and the susceptibility of the host. The definitions of many of the terms commonly used to describe infection and disease are listed in Table 7.5.

LOCALISED INFECTIONS

Infections that are confined to the site where the pathogen enters the body are said to be **localised**. Some examples are an infected wound (usually due to bacteria), cutaneous fungal infections, and warts (papilloma virus). In the case of cutaneous infections (warts and fungi), the infection remains localised because the pathogen preferentially attacks epidermal tissue. Other organisms remain on body surfaces because they prefer the lower temperature on the skin (33°C). *Mycobacterium leprae*, the causative organism of leprosy, is one such example, usually occurring only on the nasal mucosa, skin and superficial nerve cells.

Wound infections, ulcers and abscesses remain localised because they are contained by the inflammatory reactions described above. Inflammation involves fibrin deposition and causes swelling; this effectively walls off the site of the infection and prevents the escape of the infectious agent (usually bacteria) into the surrounding tissue and blood vessels. Large numbers of phagocytic cells are attracted to the infected site by chemotaxis and attack the pathogen.

Superficial localised infections can be treated with topical antimicrobial drugs. A combination of antimicrobial treatment and the non-specific immune response often limits the pathogen to the original site of infection. More serious infections require **debridement** (removal of necrotic tissue and debris) and/or wound cleansing, which may be accompanied by the administration of oral or intravenous antibiotics.

DISSEMINATED INFECTIONS

A **disseminated infection** occurs when the pathogen escapes from its primary site of infection into the bloodstream or lymphatic system and spreads to other parts of the body where it establishes another infection. Disseminated infections include situations such as the spread of *Streptococcus pyogenes* from the throat (pharyngitis) to the ears (otitis media), or when opportunistic infections spread in immunocompromised patients (e.g. *Histoplasma* or tuberculosis in AIDS patients).

Minor skin infections due to streptococci can also be disseminated throughout the body (see Case History 7.1). Usually, the bacteria gain entry to the lymphatic system via a break in the skin and are carried to the lymph nodes. The inflammation that occurs in the lymph capillary appears as a red line running from the site of the infection towards the lymph node. The stimulation of the lymphocytes of the specific defence system in the lymph nodes causes swelling, producing 'swollen glands', which are an indication of the immune system being activated to fight the invading pathogen.

The presence of bacteria or viruses in the lymphatic system or bloodstream does not always lead to an infection or disease. Sometimes, microorganisms gain entry and circulate, producing transient viraemia or bacteraemia without any disturbance to body functions. Occasionally, the bacteria lodge in susceptible locations such as the ends of growing bones, causing osteomyelitis, or on defective heart valves, causing endocarditis. Sometimes, infections from the ear or the lungs can spread to the brain and cause meningitis. In some cases, Group A streptococci (GAS) can spread from a localised infection on the skin to the kidneys and establish a serious condition known as acute post-streptococcal glomerulonephritis (APSGN), or to the heart and initiate a hypersensitivity reaction known as rheumatic fever. This type of spread is a major health problem among the Aboriginal population in the Northern Territory (see Chapter 14).

SYSTEMIC DISEASES

A **systemic disease** occurs when the pathogen affects several different organs or tissues in the body during the normal course of the infection (e.g. typhoid, measles, chickenpox). The pathogens gain entry to the body via mucosal or skin surfaces and are then spread to other body organs via the

TABLE 7.5
DEFINITIONS OF INFECTION AND DISEASE

TERM	DEFINITION
■ Infection	Situation where microorganisms invade the host tissue and multiply
■ Disease	Harmful alteration to the physiological or metabolic state of the host
■ Infectious disease	A disease caused by a microorganism
■ Pathogen	A microorganism capable of causing disease
■ Infective dose	The number of cells of a pathogen that are required to produce disease symptoms
■ Virulence	The severity or intensity of the disease symptoms produced by a pathogen
■ Signs	Measurable changes in the patient as the result of an infection
■ Symptoms	Changes felt by the patient as a result of an infection
■ Syndrome	The combination of signs and symptoms
■ Bacteraemia	Presence of bacteria in the blood
■ Viraemia	Presence of viruses in the blood
■ Septicaemia	Multiplication of bacteria in the blood
■ Toxaemia	Presence of toxins in the blood
Disease	
■ Acute	Characteristic symptoms appear and the disease runs its course quickly.
■ Fulminating	The symptoms appear suddenly and the disease proceeds rapidly, often to a fatal outcome.
■ Chronic	The disease progresses slowly and persists for long periods with continuous shedding of the pathogen.
■ Latent	The pathogen remains dormant in the host and may be reactivated under certain conditions.
■ Subclinical	The infection produces an immune response without recognisable symptoms.
Infections	
■ Localised	Confined to one area of the body.
■ Systemic	The pathogen progressively affects more than one organ.
■ Primary	The first sign of infection in a healthy host.
■ Secondary	Develops when the defences are lowered by the primary infection.
■ Superinfection	Results from overgrowth of opportunistic organisms, following destruction of normal flora.

blood or lymph. They often undergo a stepwise invasion of various tissues before reaching the final site of replication, disease production and shedding of the pathogen. For example, typhoid enters via the gastrointestinal system, then spreads via the blood and lymphatic system to the liver, spleen and bone marrow, causing fever, septicaemia, haemorrhage and diarrhoea. The measles virus enters via the upper respiratory system and spreads slowly via the lymphatic system to the lymph glands and then to the bloodstream. It finally invades various epithelial cells, causing cold-like symptoms in the upper respiratory tract, distinctive white patches (Koplik's spots) in the oral mucosa and a maculopapular skin rash.

Some infections remain localised, but the organisms produce toxins that have a systemic effect. For example, *Clostridium tetani*, the cause of tetanus, sets up an anaerobic infection at the site of entry, or in the wound itself, and produces a powerful neurotoxin that circulates through the bloodstream and causes muscular spasms.

MIXED INFECTIONS

Some diseases are due to the effects of more than one pathogen; that is, they are mixed infections. In such cases the pathogens act *synergistically* (they help each other)

CASE HISTORY 7.1
SIGNS AND SYMPTOMS ARE NOT ALWAYS WHAT THEY SEEM

Nine-year-old Jenny complained of feeling unwell and of severe pain in the lower right abdomen. The child was not hungry and was flushed and lethargic. Her mother took her temperature, which was 39.5°C, and, suspecting appendicitis, called the doctor.

On examination, the doctor could find no evidence of rigor or inflammation in the region of the appendix. The child's bowel movements were normal. The doctor noticed a scab that had almost healed on Jenny's right knee and asked when it had happened. Jenny had fallen over in the school playground about a week before and suffered the usual grazed knee. The wound was not cleaned or treated with antiseptic until the evening. The wound site had not become infected and was almost healed by the time it was seen by the doctor.

The doctor diagnosed a disseminated bacterial infection that must have entered Jenny's body at the time of the injury. After about a week, the bacteria had spread to the lymph glands in the groin and caused a serious infection. After checking that Jenny was not allergic to penicillin, the doctor gave her an injection and prescribed a course of oral medication. Jenny recovered completely after 2–3 days.

Comment

The bacteria that entered the wound at the time of the injury did not remain localised, but spread into the lymphatic system. The immune system was not able to overcome the pathogen, which lodged in the lymph glands and multiplied. If not diagnosed and treated, the infection could have had a serious outcome. It was essential to give prompt treatment, so a broad spectrum antibiotic (amoxycillin) was used since the most likely organism was a Gram-positive *Staphylococcus* or *Streptococcus*, from the skin or environment.

by breaking down tissue or providing a favourable environment for another microorganism to multiply. For example, gas gangrene is often associated with the presence of more than one organism. The initial wound infection may involve a mixture of organisms but, once the tissue is infected and damaged, **necrosis** (death of tissue) occurs. This produces an anaerobic environment that favours the growth of *Clostridium perfringens*, the cause of gangrene.

PRIMARY AND SECONDARY INFECTIONS

Sometimes, the disease symptoms change or develop over a period of time. The first or **primary infection** may lower the host's resistance, allowing another or **secondary infection** to occur. Often, an upper respiratory tract infection (URTI), caused by one of the cold viruses, weakens the host immune system so that a secondary bacterial infection develops, such as bronchitis or a middle ear infection (otitis media). Diseases that involve itchy skin lesions (e.g. chickenpox, scabies) encourage scratching which allows easy access for secondary streptococcal or staphylococcal infections.

A **superinfection** is a type of secondary infection that occurs as a result of the destruction of the normal flora, usually by the prolonged use of broad spectrum antibiotics in the treatment of a primary infection. It involves the overgrowth of an opportunistic pathogen, which occurs when the normal flora are suppressed (e.g. *Candida albicans* in vaginal thrush, or *Clostridium difficile* in pseudomembranous colitis).

SUBCLINICAL INFECTIONS

Although many infections are obvious and produce identifiable symptoms, it is sometimes possible for a pathogen to cause a subclinical infection. When this occurs, the patient/host does not exhibit any symptoms of the disease, but the pathogen multiplies in the host and elicits an immune response that can be detected by the presence of antibodies in the bloodstream. For example, people often have antibodies in their blood to diseases such as polio, rubella or glandular fever, without any previous history of disease symptoms.

PERSISTENT INFECTIONS

A number of infectious agents are able to persist in the human body for long periods after the original disease symptoms have disappeared. These are classified as **latent** or **chronic**, depending on the activity of the pathogen over time. Two unusual persistent, or 'slow', infections—subacute sclerosing panencephalitis (SSPE) and Creutzfeldt-Jakob disease (CJD)—are discussed in Chapter 5.

Latent infections

Latent infections refer to the situation where the pathogen (usually a virus) remains in the body after disease symptoms have subsided (see Chapter 5). The viral DNA replicates inside the cell with the host cell DNA but mature viral particles are not formed or shed; in other words, the host is not infectious. Reactivation of the infection may occur when the host defences are lowered. During reactivation, the host again becomes capable of transmitting the disease. Many of the viruses belonging to the herpes family are capable of latency, the most common ones being herpes simplex, herpes zoster (the cause of chickenpox, which reactivates as shingles) and Epstein-Barr (glandular fever).

Chronic infections

Chronic infections occur when multiplication and shedding of the pathogen continues at a low level after disease symptoms have disappeared. The host is still capable of transmitting infection and in this situation is said to be a **carrier**. Typical examples are pathogens that lodge in the liver, such as typhoid and hepatitis B (HBV) and hepatitis C (HCV). In chronic hepatitis, the viruses HBV and HCV persist and after many years can cause permanent liver damage (**cirrhosis**), which may develop into liver cancer.

The Spread of Infectious Diseases

Infectious diseases are diseases caused by microorganisms. In this chapter we have examined the characteristics of the different types of infection and the factors that lead to the development of a state of disease. The ability of a microorganism to cause disease depends on its ability to gain entry to and damage the host. Another way of classifying infectious diseases is according to the source or reservoir of the causative organisms and their method of transmission. This is discussed fully in Chapter 8.

COMMUNICABLE AND NON-COMMUNICABLE DISEASES

Infectious diseases that can spread from one host to another are said to be **communicable diseases**. Some are spread more easily than others and are described as very infectious or **contagious.** The term 'contagious' is used to describe the *ease* of spread, not whether the disease can be spread or not. Communicable diseases include colds, influenza, measles, chickenpox, rubella, diphtheria and polio, as well as gastrointestinal diseases and sexually transmitted diseases. These diseases are transmitted in various ways:

- by contact with aerosols from an infected host;
- via body fluids such as blood, urine, sputum and faeces;
- by infected skin cells that have been shed;
- from open lesions or wounds.

Non-communicable diseases are those that would not normally be spread from an infected host to a healthy person during the course of usual contact and normal daily activities. They include diseases that are acquired by the mechanical transfer of a pathogen from the environment into the host tissue, such as occurs with tetanus. Tetanus spores are usually carried on an implement into a puncture wound where they germinate, multiply and produce the toxin responsible for disease symptoms. Diseases such as cystitis (urinary tract infections), which are caused by displacement of normal body flora from one site to another, are not usually considered to be communicable.

Diseases transmitted by insects are unlikely to be communicable unless all the conditions for spread are ideal; that is, there is a large reservoir of infected hosts and an unlimited number of vectors. Parasitic diseases that require an intermediate host are not directly communicable from one definitive host to another.

Some non-communicable diseases are caused by the ingestion of a preformed toxin produced by a microorganism. Strictly speaking, this should be defined as **intoxication** rather than infection. For example, the symptoms of botulism are caused by the ingestion of a preformed neurotoxin produced by the bacterium, *Clostridium botulinum*, which grows anaerobically in inadequately sterilised canned or bottled food. The bacterium does not multiply in the human body and is shed in the faeces. For transmission to occur, the spores would have to find their way into unsterilised canned or bottled food.

In practice, there is some overlap between the strict definitions of communicable and non-communicable but it is a useful grouping that enables health workers to assess the risk of transmission of infection from a person with a disease to another individual—non-communicable diseases have essentially a low or minimum risk of transmission, communicable diseases have a high risk of transmission.

ENDOGENOUS AND EXOGENOUS INFECTIONS

Most of this chapter has examined what happens when pathogens enter the human host. We now briefly examine the major sources of these pathogens. Depending on the source, infectious diseases can be classified as endogenous or exogenous.

Endogenous infections occur when the source of the pathogen is the human host itself. Thus, diseases caused by normal flora are endogenous. The flora usually cause the infection when they are displaced from their normal habitat to a susceptible body site. For example, skin bacteria such as *Staphylococcus epidermidis* are a major cause of infection in surgical wounds and intravenous lines. Nasal carriers of *Staphylococcus aureus* can transfer bacteria from the nose to an open wound or sore. Cells of *E. coli* may be carried from the colon to the bladder and cause a urinary tract infection. Latent viral infections may be reactivated when the host immune defences are reduced.

Congenital infections are a type of endogenous disease that occur when the source of the pathogen is the mother. Sometimes the pathogen crosses the placenta during pregnancy and causes congenital defects such as occur with rubella, syphilis, cytomegalovirus and toxoplasmosis. If the mother is a carrier of a disease, the baby may become infected, usually late in pregnancy or at the time of birth, as occurs with hepatitis B and HIV. Sometimes, the foetus is infected *in utero* by normal flora from the vagina (e.g. Group B streptococci or *Mycoplasma*). These infections have been implicated as a cause of premature labour.

Exogenous infections are caused by organisms from the external environment. They may be acquired by cross-infection from patients in the hospital environment, or from people in the wider community. Most infectious diseases are acquired in the community and are transferred from person to person by various routes (see Chapter 8). If the infectious disease is treated at home, the pathogen remains in the community. Sometimes the disease requires hospitalisation and so the pathogen is introduced into the hospital environment, where it may spread.

Exogeneous infections acquired during a patient's stay in hospital are called **hospital-acquired infections (HAI)** or **nosocomial infections** (see Chapter 13). It is not always possible to distinguish between a hospital-acquired infection and one that is acquired in the community. It is usually considered to be nosocomial if the patient has no signs or symptoms on admittance and does not develop them until after about 48 hours. Similarly, if the patient develops the symptoms within 48 hours of discharge, they are usually regarded as having been acquired in hospital. Wound infections post-surgery are the most common nosocomial infection, followed by urinary tract infections. They usually develop during the hospital stay. Infections due to pathogens acquired in hospital are often very serious as the hospital environment harbours a large population of antibiotic-resistant organisms, and hospitalised patients are frequently very susceptible. The major risks to patients are from contact with health workers' hands or clothing, or from invasive procedures they may undergo. When such infections can be largely attributed to invasive medical procedures they are called **iatrogenic.**

Summary

- The interaction between host and microorganisms determines whether an infectious disease will occur.
- The biological term used to describe two organisms living together is symbiosis.
- Mutualism occurs when two organisms live together to their mutual benefit.
- Commensalism is an association where one organism benefits without harm to the other.
- Parasitism is when one organism benefits at the expense of the other (host) organism.

MICROORGANISMS OF THE HUMAN BODY: NORMAL FLORA

- Normal flora are the microorganisms found on the human body. They may be present on the skin, or in the gastrointestinal, respiratory or genitourinary tract.
- Normal flora may protect the host from invasion by pathogens.
- Bacteria are the most common kind of organism found on the human body. Other organisms are the yeast *Candida*, some protozoa and latent viruses.
- Some microorganisms reside permanently. Others are transient. Some are contaminants.
- Contaminant microorganisms cling to skin surfaces, but do not replicate there. Resident flora live in skin crevices, and comprise species of staphylococci, streptococci, corynebacteria and some fungi.
- In the gastrointestinal system, oral bacteria (e.g. *Streptococcus* spp.) are found in mucous membranes and in plaque attached to the teeth. The stomach, which has an acid pH, inhibits the growth of most bacteria; the lower intestine harbours a large population of bacteria.
- The upper respiratory tract has a large population of resident microorganisms, but the bronchial tubes and lungs are free of microorganisms in healthy individuals.
- The major components of the urinary system are sterile, but the lower region of the urethra may harbour organisms representative of those found in the genital tract and colon.
- The normal flora of the vagina may vary depending on factors such as hormonal influences, stress, puberty or antibiotic therapy.
- When normal flora are destroyed by long-term antibiotic therapy, opportunistic pathogens often flourish.

INFECTION AND DISEASE

- It is important to be able to define the terms: infection, disease, infectious disease, pathogen, pathogenicity, virulence, infective dose.
- Opportunistic pathogens are able to gain entry to the host and set up an infection when the normal host defences are lowered or compromised.
- The ability of the host to resist invasion by a pathogen determines whether a disease will occur.
- Factors that contribute to patient susceptibility include: underlying diseases such as diabetes or leukaemia; immunosuppression; chemotherapy and diseases of the immune system; poor nutritional status; alcoholism and IV drug use; age; genetic make-up.
- Other factors that influence the occurrence of an infection include: general environment and hygiene; climatic conditions; air pollution; seasonal variations.

KOCH'S POSTULATES

- In the germ theory of disease, German microbiologist Robert Koch proposed a set of criteria to determine whether an organism was responsible for a particular disease. They are known as Koch's postulates.

SIGNS AND SYMPTOMS OF DISEASE

- Signs are measurable changes in the patient.
- Symptoms are changes that are felt and reported by the patient.
- The combination of signs and symptoms is called a syndrome.
- Signs of infection include: fever; inflammation; lymphadenopathy; changes in white blood cell count; formation of antibodies; skin rashes.
- Signs and symptoms of a disease are usually related to the body system affected.

DEVELOPMENT OF DISEASE

- The pattern of disease consists of the incubation period, the prodromal phase, the invasive or acute phase, and convalescence.
- A fulminating disease develops very rapidly, often with a fatal outcome.
- Drug therapy modifies the progress of disease.

TYPES OF INFECTION

- Infections may be localised, disseminated or systemic.
- Some pathogens produce toxins that have systemic effects.
- Some diseases are due to the presence of more than one pathogen.
- Primary infections may lower the host's resistance, allowing a different or secondary infection to develop.
- Superinfections result from an overgrowth of opportunistic pathogens.
- Infections that do not have symptoms may be subclinical, latent or chronic.

THE SPREAD OF INFECTIOUS DISEASES

- Communicable diseases are easily spread from one host to another.
- Non-communicable diseases are not usually spread during the normal course of activities. They may be opportunistic or require a vector, or caused by a toxin.

- Endogenous infections occur when the source of the pathogen is the human host (e.g. normal flora, congenital infections).
- Exogenous infections are those where the pathogen is derived from the external environment.
- Hospital-acquired infections (nosocomial) develop more than 48 hours after admittance or within 48 hours of discharge.
- Iatrogenic infections are due to medical procedures.

Study Questions

1. What is meant by the terms: symbiosis, commensalism, mutualism, parasitism?
2. Define normal flora.
3. How does the presence of the normal flora benefit the human host?
4. List two bacterial species that may be found as normal flora of (a) the skin, (b) the gastrointestinal system, (c) the upper respiratory tract, and (d) the vagina.
5. What is a pathogen?
6. What characteristics are required for pathogenicity?
7. What is meant by virulence?
8. What is meant by the infective dose of a pathogen?
9. Define opportunism.
10. Give two examples of opportunistic infections.
11. Who was the microbiologist responsible for the germ theory of disease?
12. What criteria are used to determine whether an organism is the cause of a disease?
13. What is the difference between signs and symptoms of disease?
14. List four of the common signs of an infection or infectious disease.
15. Why is fever sometimes considered to be beneficial?
16. What is inflammation?
17. Describe each of these skin signs: erythema, vesicle, lesion, pustule, ulcer.
18. Describe the stages in the development of an infectious disease.
19. What is pyrexia of unknown origin (PUO)?
20. What is a fulminating disease?
21. List two diseases that are often the result of a disseminated infection.
22. What is meant by a systemic disease?
23. What is the difference between primary and secondary infections?
24. What is meant by the terms: superinfection, subclinical infection, latent infection, chronic infection?
25. What is the difference between a communicable and a non-communicable disease?
26. What is the difference between endogenous and exogenous infections? Give examples of each.
27. How is a nosocomial infection defined?
28. What are the most common types of nosocomial infections?

Test Your Understanding

1. What external factors affect the composition of the normal flora?
2. A patient, Mrs B, is diagnosed with a urinary tract infection. The causative organism is *E. coli.* Explain the significance of this finding and how the infection may have occurred.
3. Why are some organisms more virulent than others?
4. How do opportunistic infections differ from those caused by other pathogens?
5. Describe the factors that contribute to a host's susceptibility to infection.
6. Discuss how the criteria in Koch's postulates need to be modified in the light of current knowledge of infectious diseases.
7. How is fever produced in the course of an infectious disease?
8. What factors determine whether an infection remains localised?
9. Why are hospital-acquired infections often more difficult to treat than those acquired in the community?

chapter 8

epidemiology: how diseases are spread

Chapter focus

- *What are the major reservoirs of infection?*
- *How do organisms gain entry to the human body?*
- *What are the major portals of exit from the human body?*
- *How are diseases transmitted from one person to another?*
- *How does the science of epidemiology help to control the spread of infectious diseases?*

In Chapter 7 we examined the relationships between microorganisms and the human host and described situations that can give rise to a state of infection or disease. You will recall that some infectious diseases are communicable, that is, easily spread from one person to another (e.g. chickenpox and influenza), while others are considered to be non-communicable, or not readily transmitted from person to person (e.g. tetanus).

In this chapter we describe the ways in which microorganisms gain access to the human body, how they are transmitted from one host to another and how outbreaks of disease occur. An understanding of the methods of transmission of infection is essential if the spread of disease is to be prevented or controlled.

Reservoirs of Infection

We described earlier the occurrence and properties of the various kinds of microorganisms. By now it should be apparent that there are thousands of different types of microbes living in our environment and that humans are in constant contact with these organisms during the course of their normal daily activities. Some of these organisms are able to cause disease in healthy individuals (natural pathogens), while others cause disease only in compromised people (opportunistic pathogens). Some are easily spread from one person to another, while others are only introduced into the human body by mechanical means. In order to acquire an infectious disease, an individual must be exposed to a reservoir or source of the potential pathogen and a situation must exist whereby the pathogen can be transmitted to the human body and gain entry in sufficient numbers to cause an infection.

Many of the organisms that cause disease in humans survive for only a limited period outside the human body unless they are provided with a suitable alternative environment. For a disease to persist in a community, there has to be a permanent reservoir of the infectious agent. This **reservoir** is a habitat where the microorganisms can persist for long periods. It may be a favourable environment where they are able to survive or even increase in numbers, or it may be an unfavourable environment where the organism survives in a resistant form—for example, protozoal cysts or bacterial endospores. It may be a human or other animal host or a non-living environment such as soil or water. For some infectious diseases, humans are the only reservoir (e.g. syphilis, gonorrhoea, the hepatitis viruses, smallpox and measles). Other pathogens (e.g. many kinds of bacteria) can survive in the external environment, in soil and water. Some microorganisms infect animals as well as humans, in which case the animal acts as the reservoir of the pathogen.

We can distinguish between a reservoir of infection and a source of infection. The **source** is the individual or object from which the infectious agent is actually acquired. The reservoir may also be a source if an opportunity exists for the microorganisms to pass directly from the reservoir to a susceptible host. For example, infected humans are both the reservoir and source for diseases such as measles and syphilis. However, sometimes the reservoir and source are different. For example, if the nose is colonised by staphylococci, it can be considered a reservoir of staphylococcal infection, but when the staphylococci from the nose are present as a contaminant in food, the food is the source of the infection.

A source may also be contaminated water, or a fomite. A **fomite** is an inanimate object that can carry microorganisms (usually bacteria) on its surface. In the hospital environment, fomites are important sources of infection. They include such items as medical equipment and instruments, soiled linen and dressings, keys and other utensils. Diseases such as polio or hepatitis A have human reservoirs, but the source of the infectious agent (virus) is usually food or water contaminated by infected human faeces. This applies to most diseases transmitted by the faecal/oral route (see p. 167).

HUMAN RESERVOIRS

By far the most important reservoir of pathogenic microorganisms is the human body itself. Patients who are suffering from an infectious disease are constantly producing and shedding the pathogens responsible for the disease and these can be readily spread to others. This may occur during the incubation period or the early (prodromal) phase of the disease before symptoms appear, as well as later when the disease is fully established.

Individuals with an obvious symptomatic infection are usually regarded as a reservoir for the pathogen and a potential source of infection. However, as we saw in Chapter 7, not all infections are clinically obvious. There is a number of situations where a person is infected without showing any apparent signs of illness. These include patients who have subclinical infections—they have been infected by the pathogen but do not exhibit recognisable symptoms. They still produce and shed pathogens and are able to spread the disease to others. Other reservoirs are those people who are chronic asymptomatic carriers of a disease. They may have had the disease and recovered, but instead of the pathogen being completely eliminated from their system it remains in one of their body organs, such as the liver or gall bladder. These people have a constant low level of infection with consequent shedding of the pathogen. This can occur in diseases such as typhoid or hepatitis B and C. Humans with latent viral infections are also important reservoirs for viral pathogens. The virus persists in the human body in a latent or dormant form and is able to multiply and spread when conditions in the host change (e.g. herpes infections).

In Chapter 7 we described the normal flora of the human body. This is a rich and diverse population of microorganisms that represents a significant reservoir of potential pathogens if they are displaced from their normal habitat or if their host is compromised in some way. For example, most urinary tract infections are caused by normal flora of the colon such as *E. coli.* A large number of the infections that occur in surgical or other wounds are caused by normal skin flora such as *Staphylococcus epidermidis*. *E. coli*. may also be the cause of diarrhoea when toxin-producing strains of the bacteria are ingested in contaminated food or water (see Spotlight Box on Haemolytic Uraemic Syndrome, p. 407).

ANIMAL RESERVOIRS

Many animals, both wild and domestic, harbour microorganisms that can cause disease in humans. About 150 of these diseases—termed **zoonoses** (singular: **zoonosis**)—are known. In some cases (e.g. rabies), both animals and humans suffer from a similar disease. In others (e.g. typhus or viral encephalitis), the animal does not appear to suffer from the disease at all but the organism is pathogenic for humans. Transmission of many of these diseases from an animal reservoir to humans requires a vector in the form of a blood-sucking insect. For other diseases, transmission requires direct contact with the animal, its fur, feathers or body secretions. Some types of ringworm (tinea) are acquired from exposure to infected domestic animals or pets. Some of the protozoal and helminthic parasites have complex life cycles involving both animals and humans.

Humans may be either an accidental or a definitive host, while the animal may be an intermediate or definitive host for the parasite (see Chapter 6). For example, the beef tapeworm exists in the larval or cyst form in the muscle tissue (meat) of cattle, from where it is ingested by humans who are the definitive host. *Toxoplasma gondii* is harboured in the intestine of domestic cats and other animals and excreted as oocysts in their faeces. From there it may be ingested by animals, lodging in the muscle tissue which is then eaten by humans. An alternative route is the direct inhalation or ingestion of oocysts from soil or kitty litter. Most of the zoonoses are impossible to eradicate as to do so would require the destruction of all animal reservoirs. Table 8.1 lists some of the common zoonoses.

NON-LIVING RESERVOIRS: SOIL AND WATER

Many microorganisms thrive in the external environment, especially in soil and water.

Soil

Bacteria may be present as vegetative cells or, in some cases, as resistant endospores. Some of the spore-forming bacteria are important pathogens, especially species of the genus *Clostridium*, which are commonly found in the soil. For example, spores of the bacillus responsible for tetanus (*Clostridium tetani*) are excreted in faeces and remain viable for long periods in the soil. They are transferred to humans when a person sustains an injury from an object contaminated with the tetanus spores. Gas gangrene (*Clostridium perfringens*) spores are also very resistant and widely distributed in the environment. If they gain entry to the body at the site of tissue injury or via surgical wounds they can cause gangrene but, if the spores are ingested in food, gastroenteritis may result.

Botulism is caused by the ingestion of poorly preserved food in which spores of *Clostridium botulinum,* commonly found in the soil, have germinated and grown under anaerobic conditions, producing the neurotoxin responsible for botulism. Anthrax spores are able to survive for many years in soil and infect animals or humans who come in contact with the contaminated soil. Species of Gram-negative pseudomonads are commonly found in soil and on plants and can be introduced into the hospital environment on flowers and plants. They are important opportunistic pathogens and a common cause of hospital infections, especially in burns patients. Many protozoa form cysts as a stage in their life cycle and these survive for long periods in the soil before entering the human or animal hosts (e.g. *Toxoplasma*). Helminth eggs or larvae (e.g. hookworm and tapeworm) may be found in soil. Many different kinds of fungi are found in soil.

Water

Water is a reservoir for a number of pathogens that live and multiply best in an aqueous environment. These include protozoa such as *Giardia* and *Entamoeba* which are frequently present in natural water environments, especially where sewage pollution occurs. Many different kinds of bacteria can be found in water. *Legionella* is found in natural streams and has been isolated from water in the cooling towers of air-conditioning plants. *Pseudomonas,* which has minimal nutritional requirements, is often present in the water in cooling towers, drinking water coolers and bubblers. Water contaminated with faeces can be the source of a large number of pathogens responsible for infectious diseases, including typhoid, cholera, polio and hepatitis A. *Leptospira* may be found in water contaminated with animal urine. The blood fluke *Schistosoma* has a

TABLE 8.1
SELECTED ZOONOSES OCCURRING IN AUSTRALIA

ORGANISM	DISEASE	ANIMAL RESERVOIR	TRANSMISSION
Bacteria			
Brucella spp.	Brucellosis	Cattle	Direct contact
Borrelia spp.	Lyme disease	? Native animals	Tick bites
Chlamydia psittaci	Psittacosis (ornithosis)	Birds/parrots	Direct contact
Coxiella burnetii	Q fever	Cattle	Direct contact
Leptospira	Leptospirosis	Wild mammals, cats/dogs	Contact with urine/water
Listeria monocytogenes	Listeriosis	Domestic animals	Unpasteurised milk
Salmonella spp.	Salmonellosis	Poultry	Ingestion of contaminated
Campylobacter	Gastroenteritis	Domestic livestock	food, water
Viruses			
Influenza virus	Influenza (some types)	Pigs, ducks	Direct contact
Flavivirus	Murray Valley encephalitis	Fowl/birds	Mosquitoes
Orf virus (parapoxvirus)	Orf	Sheep, goats	Direct contact
Alphavirus	Ross River fever	Native animals	Mosquitoes
Protozoa			
Toxoplasma gondii	Toxoplasmosis	Cats/other mammals	Ingestion of contaminated meat, contact with faeces
Fungi			
Trichophyton	Ringworm (tinea)	Domestic animals	Direct contact
Microsporum			
Epidermophyton			
Helminths			
Echinococcus granulosis	Hydatid cysts	Dogs	Contact with faeces
Taenia saginata	Tapeworm	Cattle	Ingestion of contaminated meat

free-living larval stage in water—the cercariae—and people swimming where these occur are at risk of acquiring the infection. Outbreaks of diarrhoea caused by *Cryptosporidium parvum* have been associated with children's wading pools.

Portals of Entry

To cause disease, the infectious agent must first gain entry to the human body. The microorganisms may come from any of the reservoirs described above. Some infections are caused by the microorganisms already present on the human body, which acts as the reservoir (**endogenous infections**). They include diseases such as:

- **cystitis,** an infection of the bladder usually caused by normal flora from the colon;
- **thrush**, an opportunistic infection caused by *Candida albicans*;
- recurrent **herpes**, due to the reactivation of a latent infection; and
- disseminated infections such as those due to *Streptococcus* species, which spread from the throat and set up infections in the ears, lungs or kidneys.

Infections acquired by the foetus *in utero* across the placenta are also considered to be endogenous.

Other infections are caused by **exogenous** pathogens, that is, microorganisms derived from the external environment. An intact layer of skin provides a protective barrier for the body and anything that damages or penetrates this barrier allows the entry of microorganisms. Other major portals of entry are via the mucous membranes lining the walls of the respiratory, gastrointestinal and genitourinary tracts. Most pathogens have a **preferred portal of entry**, one that gives ready access to an immediate environment suitable for the establishment of growth, or one that allows the pathogens to reach their target tissues or organs. See Table 8.2.

Sometimes the portal of entry is quite specific for the disease. For example, bacteria such as *Salmonella*, which cause gastrointestinal infections, enter via the mouth. If *Salmonella* comes into contact with intact skin, a gastrointestinal infection will not occur. In other cases, pathogenic organisms are able to gain entry to the body via more than one portal. *Mycobacterium tuberculosis* can enter via both the gastrointestinal and respiratory tracts.

Some diseases take different forms depending on the portal of entry. *Yersinia pestis*, the bacterium responsible for plague, produces buboes in the lymph glands (bubonic plague) when it is introduced via the bite of an infected

TABLE 8.2
PREFERRED PORTAL OF ENTRY FOR SOME COMMON PATHOGENS

PORTAL OF ENTRY	DISEASE	PATHOGEN
Skin		
Infections of skin and mucosal surfaces	Herpes	*Herpes simplex*
	Thrush	*Candida albicans*
	Skin infections	Staphylococci
		Streptococci
		Pseudomonads
Conjunctiva	Trachoma	*Chlamydia trachomatis*
	Gonorrhoea	*Neisseria gonorrhoeae*
Puncture wounds	Tetanus	*Clostridium tetani*
	Gangrene	*Clostridium perfringens*
IV drug users Needlesticks	Hepatitis B	Hepatitis B virus
	Hepatitis C	Hepatitis C virus
	AIDS	Human immunodeficiency virus
Burrowing parasites	Hookworm	Hookworms
	Schistosomiasis	*Schistosoma*
Insect-borne infections	Plague	*Yersinia pestis*
	Malaria	*Plasmodium*
	Arboviral infections	Various viruses (see Table 5.4)
Respiratory tract		
Localised infections of the respiratory tract and lungs	Diphtheria	*Corynebacterium diphtheriae*
	Common colds	Various adeno, rhino viruses
	Tuberculosis	*Mycobacterium tuberculosis*
	Pneumonia	Various organisms, see Table 7.3 e.g. *Streptococcus pneumoniae*
	Whooping cough	*Bordetella pertussis*
Systemic infections	Chickenpox	*Varicella zoster* virus
	Measles	Morbillivirus
	German measles	Rubivirus
	Glandular fever	Epstein-Barr virus
	Influenza	Influenza virus
	Meningococcal meningitis	*Neisseria meningitidis*
Gastrointestinal tract		
Gastroentestinal infections	Gastroenteritis	Various organisms, e.g. *Shigella, Salmonella, Staphylococcus aureus, Campylobacter, E. coli, Cl. perfringens*, enteroviruses
	Cholera	*Vibrio cholera*
	Hepatitis	Hepatitis A, hepatitis E viruses
Parasitic infections	Tapeworm	*Taenia saginata*
	Hydatids	*Echinococcus granulosis*
	Amoebic dysentery	*Entamoeba histolytica*
	Giardiasis	*Giardia instestinalis*
Systemic infections	Toxoplasmosis	*Toxoplasma gondii*
	Polio	Enterovirus
	Mumps	Paramyxovirus
	Typhoid	*Salmonella typhi*
Urogential tract		
Sexually transmitted diseases (STDs)	Gonorrhoea	*Neisseria gonorrhoeae*
	Syphilis	*Treponema pallidum*
	Trichomoniasis	*Trichomonas vaginalis*
	Chlamydia	*Chlamydia trachomatis*
	Genital warts	Human papilloma virus
	Herpes	*Herpes simplex*
	Thrush	*Candida albicans*
Systemic infections	Hepatitis B and C	Hepatitis B, hepatitis C viruses
	AIDS	Human immunodeficiency virus

flea. However, it can also be inhaled directly into the lungs, causing pneumonia and giving rise to a much more severe form of the disease (pneumonic plague).

SKIN AS A PORTAL OF ENTRY

Infections of the skin are described in Chapter 16. Intact skin is a major barrier to the entry of microorganisms (see Chapter 9). Cracks or splits in the skin, due to swelling or drying, allow microorganisms to enter and set up infections (described in detail in Chapter 16) in the cutaneous or subcutaneous layers. Fungal dermatophytes are responsible for cutaneous mycoses such as tinea and the herpes virus also enters through the skin and infects epithelial cells. Bacteria such as *Staphylococcus aureus* and *Streptococcus pyogenes* can infect hair follicles or sebaceous glands, causing pimples and boils. Damage to the skin caused by scratching itchy insect bites or scabies infections also allows these organisms to enter and become established, causing infections such as impetigo.

The conjunctiva of the eye provides protection against infection, and so damage to the conjunctiva by dust or foreign bodies can allow entry of microorganisms. As well, pathogens such as *Neisseria gonorrhoeae* and *Chlamydia trachomatis* can infect the intact conjunctiva because they have attachment devices to avoid the flushing action of tears. Other important pathogens (e.g. hepatitis B) can gain entry via the conjunctiva as a result of splashes of blood or body fluids into the eyes.

The larvae of helminths such as hookworm enter the body by burrowing through the skin, as do the cercariae of *Schistosoma*. The bite of an insect vector that breaches the skin barrier and carries pathogens directly into the bloodstream is an important method of entry for many infectious agents. Mosquitoes can carry a variety of diseases—malaria, encephalitis, yellow fever, dengue fever, and Ross River fever. Fleas and ticks can carry other diseases, including plague and typhus (see Chapter 6).

The use of hypodermic syringes by intravenous drug users breaks the skin and provides ready access for microorganisms. Sharing of needles and syringes allows the spread of blood-borne pathogens such as hepatitis B, hepatitis C and HIV, as well as bacterial infections.

Other microorganisms are able to gain entry to the body through puncture wounds in the skin; they then multiply and cause infections in the deeper tissues. For example, spores of the agents that cause tetanus and gangrene are usually carried into the body through breaks in the skin caused by puncture wounds, or they may lodge in wounds where there has been extensive tissue damage. They are then able to reproduce under the favourable anaerobic conditions that exist in deep or necrotic tissue, causing disease by the production of harmful toxins.

The importance of intact skin is especially apparent in the hospital environment, where many patients are particularly susceptible to infection due to the nature of their illness or the procedures they undergo. Breaks in the skin caused by wounds due to surgical procedures provide a easy portal of entry, especially if the wound has a drainage device attached postoperatively. Even though surgical aseptic techniques are followed, approximately 10% of all surgical wounds become infected while the patient is in hospital.

Microorganisms can also gain access via invasive procedures such as the insertion of intravenous (IV) lines (in particular, central venous lines) and catheters. Manipulation of the IV lines and care of the catheters by nursing staff provide further opportunities for microorganisms to enter via breaks in the skin. Aseptic procedures must be carefully followed. Central venous lines pose an additional hazard when used for total parenteral nutrition, as the nutritious solutions used are ideal growth media for bacteria and fungi. Infections acquired as a result of medical procedures are termed **iatrogenic infections**.

Another group of patients susceptible to infection via the skin are those suffering from burns. These patients may have large areas of damaged skin and are particularly vulnerable to infections by many bacteria, of which *Staphylococcus aureus* and *Pseudomonas aeruginosa* are the most serious.

RESPIRATORY TRACT AS A PORTAL OF ENTRY

Infections of the respiratory tract are described in Chapter 17. The mucous membranes of the respiratory tract are a major portal of entry for many pathogens, which may be inhaled as aerosols, spores, or on dust particles. If they are not washed away by the mucous secretions, they adhere to the cells lining the upper respiratory tract, and may cause infections in the nasopharynx, tonsils, throat and larynx. If they are not eliminated by other defence mechanisms, they may travel further—to the bronchial tubes, causing bronchitis, or to the lungs, causing pneumonia.

Common bacterial diseases that are acquired via the upper respiratory tract (URT) include whooping cough (*Bordetella pertussis*), diphtheria (*Corynebacterium diphtheriae*), meningitis (*Neisseria meningitidis*), streptococcal infections and tuberculosis (*Mycobacterium tuberculosis*). Tuberculosis enters via the URT and infects the lungs.

The viruses of influenza, measles, chickenpox, rubella, mumps and the common cold also enter via the mucous membranes of the upper respiratory tract. From there, some of these organisms spread to other parts of the body and produce systemic symptoms, such as a skin rash or enlarged lymph nodes. Some fungi are able to infect the lungs (see Chapter 6). Certain infections that enter initially via the respiratory tract may be disseminated to other organs of the body, especially in immunocompromised patients (e.g. histoplasmosis).

Pneumonia is an inflammation of the lungs that can be caused by a number of different viruses and bacteria that enter via the respiratory tract and penetrate to the lung tissue (see Table 7.3, p. 145). The occurrence of pneumonia in hospitalised patients is potentially very serious because of the type of organisms usually responsible and the susceptibility of the patients.

The respiratory tract is an important portal of entry for nosocomial pathogens. Patients may inhale any of the pathogens carried on air currents around the hospital. Viral infections such as those caused by the respiratory syncytial virus and influenza virus may be serious and even fatal to infants or elderly hospitalised patients. The use of respiratory equipment such as ventilators can create conditions that allow microorganisms to be introduced directly into the respiratory tract. Water from the humidification of the inspired air and the condensation of expired air collects in the ventilator tubing and may support the growth of bacteria, especially Gram-negative rods such as *Pseudomonas aeruginosa*. Tubes should be changed regularly to minimise this risk. Adequate cleaning and disinfection of all respiratory equipment is of the utmost importance.

Another hazard exists in the use of nebulisers for humidification as the equipment has the potential to spray the patient with contaminated water. Endotracheal intubation for mechanical ventilation bypasses the defence mechanisms normally present in the mouth and throat and allows entry of microorganisms directly to the lungs. The wound associated with the tracheostomy provides another portal of entry for infection as it may become colonised with organisms such as *Staphylococcus aureus* during handling of the tracheal tube. The maintenance of good oral hygiene is important in preventing the spread of bacteria from the mouth to the respiratory tract and lungs.

GASTROINTESTINAL TRACT AS A PORTAL OF ENTRY

Infections of the digestive tract are described in Chapter 18.

The ingestion of contaminated food or drink via the gastrointestinal tract (GIT) is a major way for pathogens to enter the body. To gain access by this route, the pathogen must be able to resist the acid conditions in the stomach (pH 1–2), as well as the other defences of the GIT. Resistant microbes may be ingested as eggs (e.g. helminths), cysts (e.g. *Giardia*) or endospores (e.g. *Clostridium perfringens*). In order for other kinds of organisms to enter by this route, they must be resistant to acid (e.g. cholera, some *E. coli*, enteroviruses), need only a low infective dose (e.g. *Shigella*) or be ingested in such large numbers that enough organisms survive to penetrate into the intestine. In some cases, the pathogens may be protected by the food in which they are carried. Most of the microorganisms responsible for gastrointestinal infections have specialised structures for attachment to the mucosal cells lining the intestine (see Chapter 10).

As well as being the entry route for the microorganisms that cause gastroenteritis, such as *Campylobacter, Salmonella* and *Shigella*, the GIT also acts as a portal of entry for various bacterial toxins that are produced in food before it is ingested. These include the neurotoxin of botulism and the enterotoxin of *Staphylococcus aureus*. These toxins are resistant to stomach acid and are absorbed in the small intestine, producing symptoms within hours of ingestion. Other diseases which enter via the GIT, but are disseminated to other parts of the body, include hepatitis A which affects the liver, and polio which is absorbed in the intestine and affects other parts of the body including nerve cells.

THE UROGENITAL TRACT AS A PORTAL OF ENTRY

Infections of the urinary and genital systems are discussed in Chapter 21.

The lower section of the urinary tract, the urethra, is frequently contaminated with normal flora, similar to those found in the colon. In females these organisms are likely to ascend the relatively short urethra to the bladder, causing cystitis; and if not treated they may reach the kidneys and cause pyelonephritis. A high percentage of all hospital-acquired infections are of the urinary tract and are associated with the use of urinary catheters. The use of indwelling catheters, especially in elderly or incontinent patients, gives bacteria ready access to the bladder, usually on the outside of the catheter. The infecting organisms are generally derived from the patient's own flora, but in hospitalised patients, or patients undergoing long-term antibiotic treatment, there is the likelihood that these infections will be caused by antibiotic-resistant strains of bacteria. The most serious complication of urinary tract infections occurs when damage to the cells lining the mucosa of the urinary tract allows the organisms to gain access to the bloodstream, causing sepsis.

The genital tract is the main portal of entry for a number of diseases, usually transmitted by intimate contact during sexual intercourse. Organisms responsible for diseases that enter this way include *Neisseria gonorrhoeae*, *Treponema pallidum* (syphilis), chlamydia, human papilloma virus (genital warts), herpes and *Trichomonas vaginalis*. Some of these microorganisms have special structures such as pili, which enable them to attach to and infect the mucosal cells lining the genital tract and prevent their being washed away by urine or mucosal secretions (e.g. *Neisseria gonorrhoeae)*. Blood-borne viruses present in semen and vaginal secretions (e.g. hepatitis B, C and HIV) can enter the bloodstream through breaks in the skin or mucosal lining of the genital tract, although this is not considered their major portal of entry.

The prevalence of sexual practices other than vaginal intercourse means that sexually transmitted organisms can enter and infect other areas of the body such as the anus or mouth and throat, provided that specific attachment sites exist in these areas. *Neisseria gonorrhoeae* is one such organism that can infect any of these sites as well as the genital tract.

CONGENITAL INFECTIONS

Microorganisms that infect the foetus, *in utero*, gain access by crossing the placenta. The placenta is usually an efficient barrier, allowing nutrients and waste to pass through, while excluding larger, possibly harmful, cells and molecules. However, some microorganisms are able to cross the placental barrier and infect the foetus. In the process, they can cause abortion or various degrees of foetal damage, depending on the type of organism involved and the stage of pregnancy when the infection occurs. Organisms that can cause congenital defects include:

- rubella virus (congenital rubella syndrome);
- *Toxoplasma gondii* (toxoplasmosis);
- cytomegalovirus (congenital CMV);
- *Treponema pallidum* (syphilis); and
- *Listeria monocytogenes* (congenital listeriosis).

Hepatitis B and HIV may also infect the foetus, but this usually occurs at the end of pregnancy or during birth and gives rise to a chronic infection in the neonate without cogenital defects.

Perinatal infections (infections acquired at birth) are caused by microorganisms present in the mother's birth canal; they infect the baby by entering via any of the portals described above. Most serious for the neonate are herpes infections of the eyes (which can spread to the brain and cause herpes encephalitis), chlamydial and gonorrhoeal infections of the eyes, and pneumonia due to Group B streptococci or chlamydia. *Candida* (thrush), derived from the mother's genital tract, is a common infection of the mucosal lining of the mouth of the neonate.

Portals of Exit

In earlier sections of this chapter, we described the human body as an important reservoir for infectious microorganisms, and the body's secretions and excretions as a potential source of pathogens. Microorganisms are continually being shed from the human body during such normal activities as coughing, sneezing, defecating and changing clothing. A healthy person sheds mainly normal flora which do not generally pose any special risk to other healthy members of the population. When a person is suffering from an infectious disease, the pathogens responsible for that disease are also shed in large numbers and may infect other susceptible people. Very often, the pathogen is shed from the same area (portal) by which it entered (see Table 8.3). In the hospital environment, it is important for the nurse to be aware of the way in which pathogens exit the human body in order to ensure the safe and effective disposal of contaminated material and to prevent cross-infection. Health workers also need to be aware of the potential risks to themselves of occupational exposure to pathogenic organisms (see Chapter 13).

UPPER RESPIRATORY TRACT: NOSE AND MOUTH

Organisms that infect the nasopharynx, throat and lungs are usually present in large numbers in the watery mucosal secretions and in sputum. They are expelled as aerosols by talking, coughing and sneezing. The fine aerosol droplets allow rapid dispersal of such pathogens as the cold and flu viruses, which do not survive long outside the body. These aerosol droplets are able to infect other people, directly through inhalation, or indirectly by contamination of a fomite. Pathogens, such as those responsible for measles, chickenpox and tuberculosis, are also carried in respiratory secretions for short distances to their next host. Some bacteria, such as *Mycobacterium tuberculosis* (TB) persist in a dried form on dust particles and are carried by air currents for greater distances. Viruses such as the mumps virus (which infects the salivary glands), herpes simplex virus, Epstein-Barr virus (glandular fever) and cytomegalovirus (CMV) are secreted and shed in saliva. CMV is also present in urine and other body fluids.

GASTROINTESTINAL SYSTEM

A major portal of exit of potential pathogens from the human body is via the bowel. It has been estimated that faeces contain up to 10^{12} bacterial cells per gram of faeces. In a healthy person, these consist mainly of the organisms that make up the normal flora. However, as well as normal flora from the colon, faeces may contain pathogenic organisms. Some of the pathogens responsible for gastrointestinal infections affect the gut, causing irritation

TABLE 8.3
MAJOR DISEASES TRANSMITTED IN BODY SECRETIONS

SECRETION	DISEASE
Sputum, mucosal secretions	Tuberculosis Diphtheria Whooping cough Influenza Measles Rubella
Saliva	Mumps Glandular fever Hepatitis B, (C?) Cytomegalovirus
Semen/vaginal secretions	Sexually transmitted diseases Hepatitis B, AIDS
Urine	Cytomegalovirus Leptospirosis
Faeces	Polio Typhoid Cholera Hepatitis A, hepatitis E Gastroenteritis—bacterial and viral
Blood	Hepatitis B Hepatitis C AIDS

of the lining of the large intestine and interfering with water absorption, giving rise to watery stools or diarrhoea. When this occurs, large numbers of the pathogens are shed in the faeces. Organisms responsible for other diseases such as cholera, typhoid, hepatitis A and polio, as well as protozoal cysts and helminth eggs and larvae are also excreted in faeces. If any of these pathogens contaminates the water supply, the pathogen can spread easily and the disease can become an epidemic (e.g. cholera outbreaks often occur after natural disasters).

Faeces are therefore a major source of microorganisms and there is a continual risk of transmission of organisms from faecal material to wounds or other susceptible sites in hospitalised patients. Health workers need to be aware of the importance of handwashing, the correct method of disposal of faeces and the correct cleaning and disinfection of contaminated equipment in order to prevent transmission.

In the community, faecal contamination of water is an important public health issue. Pathogens derived from faeces are frequently found in the sea water on Australian beaches and in stormwater run-off. In some countries, untreated sewage is used as a fertilizer for vegetable crops, which creates a serious health risk when unpeeled or unwashed fruit or vegetables are eaten. Faecal contamination of food and water is a major cause of gastrointestinal infections in developing countries.

SKIN

The dead outer layers of the skin (dermis) are constantly being shed, and these may carry the bacteria that are resident or transient on the skin. These skin scales are widely dispersed like dust particles on air currents. Bacteria contained in dried particles from crusts or scabs of wounds may also be carried this way. In the hospital environment, pathogenic organisms shed from the skin of infectious patients adhere to dust particles and skin scales. They can be disturbed by activities such as bedmaking, dry dusting, or excessive movement of equipment, and dispersed around the hospital on air currents. Exudates from skin lesions, boils and pustular rashes (e.g. chickenpox), usually contain large numbers of pathogens and are thus a potential source of infection. Other skin diseases in which microbes are shed into the environment include herpes, warts and syphilis. Some of these organisms survive for a long time in the environment (e.g. chickenpox) while others (e.g. syphilis) are quite fragile and do not survive for long outside the human body.

UROGENITAL TRACT

The organisms responsible for most sexually transmitted diseases are present in semen and vaginal secretions and so are discharged from the body in this way. Others such as herpes or warts, which infect the skin, are shed from lesions on the genital organs. Organisms that infect the bladder or kidneys are usually present in urine, but do not pose a significant health risk to others. Cytomegalovirus is a major pathogen shed in urine, but there is no evidence that HIV or hepatitis B or C viruses are present in urine in significant amounts. However, urine from animals infected with *Leptospira* contains the bacterium and can be a source of infection when it contaminates water supplies.

BLOOD

Blood is not usually considered a portal of entry for pathogens unless contaminated blood is given in a transfusion. In Australia, the careful screening of blood donors and blood products has essentially eliminated the risk of transmission of these organisms by blood transfusion. However, blood is a significant portal of exit for several important blood-borne pathogens that are released when bleeding occurs, or when blood is removed from the body for some other purpose. Viruses such as HIV, hepatitis B and hepatitis C are transmitted in blood, blood-tinged body fluids, and blood products. They may be transmitted by the sharing of needles for intravenous (IV) drug use, or through breaks in the skin or mucous membranes that allow blood containing the virus to enter the body. These pathogens can also be transmitted from an infected patient to another individual (patient or staff) during dental or medical procedures where bleeding occurs, if there is a breakdown in aseptic technique or if contaminated instruments are not adequately cleaned and sterilised. Another risk for health workers is transmission occurring as a result of needlestick injuries (see Chapter 13).

Some diseases are transmitted in blood by the bite of a bloodsucking insect such as a mosquito. One of the most important of these is *Plasmodium*, the protozoan responsible for malaria, which is present in the blood of infected humans (see also pp. 170–71). In rare cases, malaria can be transmitted by a blood transfusion. The Ebola virus, responsible for the recent outbreak of haemorrhagic fever in Zaire, causes massive bleeding from body organs and is shed and transmitted in blood.

Transmission of Microorganisms

So far in this chapter we have looked at the reservoirs of infection, where microorganisms can persist, and the ways in which microorganisms enter and exit the human body. For a disease to spread, the causative organism or pathogen has to move or be transmitted from a reservoir or source to a susceptible host. A knowledge and understanding of the possible means of transmission is very important for health professionals, especially when working in a hospital, where there is a huge reservoir of pathogens and a population of susceptible patients. To prevent the spread of infection, it is important to be able to break the chain of transmission. This is discussed more fully in Chapter 13. In this section we outline the major routes of transmission.

Transmission of microorganisms within the community usually occurs horizontally—that is, from person to person. Vertical transmission—that is, from mother to foetus, occurs across the placenta. Organisms can be spread horizontally by **direct contact,** by **indirect contact** with the reservoir or source, by means of a **common vehicle**, or by a **mechanical vector** or **biological vector**. (See Figure 8.1.)

CONTACT TRANSMISSION

Many pathogens are too fragile to exist for any length of time outside their host. For these organisms to spread, there has to be some kind of direct or very close contact between the infected host and a suitable portal of entry in the next host. Organisms may be passed from one person to another by actually touching the skin or body secretions of the infected person, or by touching an object that has recently been contaminated with the pathogen.

Direct contact

Direct contact refers to close or intimate contact between the infected person and a susceptible individual, resulting in the spread of pathogenic organisms. Exposure to skin and body secretions, such as occurs during kissing and sexual activity, is a major route of transmission of many infectious diseases. The transmission of pathogens present in the genital area, or in semen or vaginal secretions, can be prevented by adopting 'safe sex' practices, particularly the wearing of a condom. Skin infections such as herpes, cutaneous fungal infections, and bacteria from infected wounds can also be transmitted by contact.

Infections may also be transmitted from one part of the body to another by direct contact. For example, if the hands touch the genital region and then the eyes, infections such as gonorrhoea or herpes can be transferred from the genitals to the eyes. Similarly, normal flora from different parts of the body can be transmitted to an open wound. Once the hands are contaminated, organisms can be transmitted to other parts of the body or to another susceptible individual. For this reason, health workers should be aware of the need to wash their hands regularly and to wear gloves whenever caring for patients with a communicable infection, in order to protect both themselves and other patients.

A number of diseases of animals (**zoonoses**) can be transmitted to humans by direct contact with the infected animal. People working in the livestock industry may acquire the zoonoses Q fever and brucellosis, both of which are diseases of cattle and can be transmitted by direct contact with the animals as well as eating or handling contaminated meat. Although not found in Australia, rabies and anthrax are two serious diseases transmitted by direct contact. Rabies is transmitted by contact with the saliva of an infected animal, usually via a bite. Direct contact with the exudate from the lesions of anthrax allows transmission from an infected animal to a human or other animal. Other zoonoses transmitted by direct contact include tinea (ringworm), which is common in domestic

FIGURE 8.1
METHODS OF TRANSMISSION

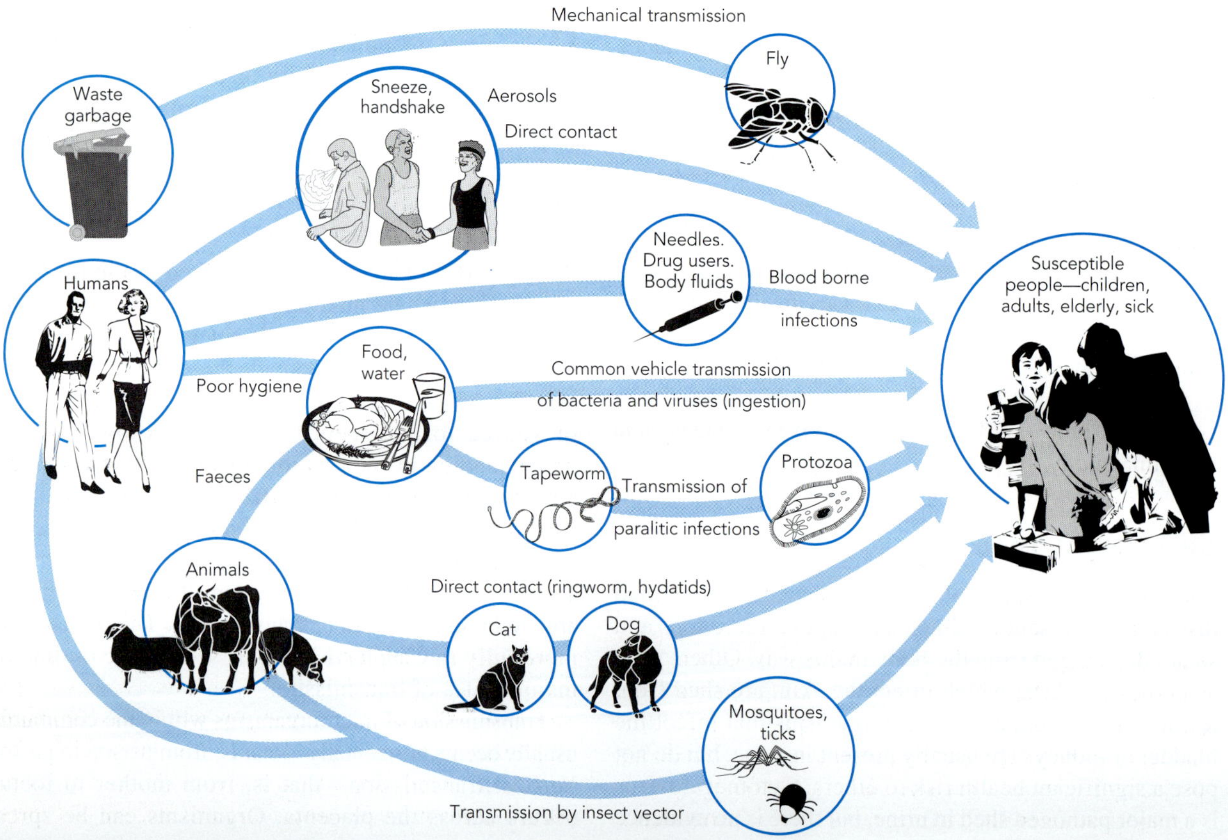

cats and dogs. A number of viruses (e.g. hantaviruses) that are endemic in the rodent population can find their way from wild rodents to domestic animals and then to humans. They are generally transmitted in saliva and urine by direct contact, or by indirect contact with dried urine or droppings.

Indirect contact

Indirect contact occurs when microorganisms from an infected host or other reservoir are deposited on an inanimate object, or **fomite**, and then transmitted to a susceptible host. This type of transmission can easily occur in the hospital environment unless health personnel take special precautions. Fomites that can become sources of infection include medical equipment and instruments, eating utensils, bedpans, clothing, bedding, dressings, soap, taps, cupboard handles, refrigerators, sinks, telephones, toilet bowls, keys, money and handkerchiefs. The pathogen leaves the human body by any of the portals described above and is deposited on a fomite. From there it can be spread directly to a new host. The pathogen may also be picked up on the hands of a health worker after handling the contaminated fomite and transferred to a susceptible patient. Adequate cleansing and disinfecting procedures, careful handwashing and wearing of gloves are the main ways of preventing transmission by this route.

Droplet transmission

Droplet transmission is also considered a form of contact transmission. Microorganisms contained in body secretions, usually from the upper respiratory tract, are expelled from the body by coughing, sneezing or talking and may immediately come into contact with a susceptible person. The major pathogens transmitted in this way are the viruses responsible for colds and influenza as well as whooping cough, measles and tuberculosis. The organisms are carried in droplets over a distance of less than 1 metre and inhaled directly into the respiratory tract of the new host. Simple actions like covering the nose and throat when coughing or sneezing help to prevent the spread of these organisms.

COMMON VEHICLE TRANSMISSION

Microorganisms can be transmitted over a wide area by means of a vehicle such as air, water or food. When a number of people are infected with the same organism by one of these routes, it is called **common vehicle transmission**.

Air-borne transmission

Air-borne transmission occurs when disease-causing microorganisms are carried on air currents over distances greater than 1 metre. The pathogens may be present in fine water aerosol sprays that are too light to settle. The spray may be a watery secretion from the respiratory tract, containing pathogenic bacteria or viruses. The bacterium *Legionella pneumophila,* which is responsible for causing Legionnaires' disease (see Spotlight box, p. 168), is transmitted in aerosol sprays derived from the exposed reservoirs of water-cooled air-conditioning plants. The bacteria are present in the water and are dispersed in a fine aerosol spray that can be blown by wind currents over a wide area before entering a susceptible person via the respiratory tract.

Bacteria and viruses often adhere to dust particles or skin scales and can be dispersed on air currents. To be transmitted in this way, the pathogen must be able to survive outside the host and tolerate dry conditions. These pathogens include fungal spores, bacterial endospores and cysts or ova of various parasites. Certain bacteria, such as some staphylococci and the tubercle bacilli, are also resistant to dry conditions and can remain viable (alive) for long periods. The oocysts of *Toxoplasma gondii* can be transmitted by inhalation of the dust from cat faeces in kitty litter.

Although pathogens are easily spread by the air-borne route, they will only cause disease if they are able to gain access in sufficient numbers to a susceptible host through a suitable portal of entry. Organisms transmitted by the air-borne route do not multiply in air, but their spread is facilitated in modern air-conditioned buildings, such as hospitals, which have controlled temperatures and moist, recirculating air.

In the hospital environment there is a large reservoir of disease-causing microorganisms, constantly being shed in the form of aerosols, infected skin scales, and dried bacteria in crusts from infected wounds and herpes lesions. These organisms fall to the floor, some adhering to dust particles, or to equipment and clothing. Activities such as cleaning, bedmaking or movement of equipment disturb them and they can then be carried on air currents throughout the hospital (see Figure 8.3).

The use of wet mops and dusters when cleaning can reduce the spread of pathogens by this route. Bed linen should be folded carefully and not shaken. The use of masks and special protective clothing helps to prevent air-borne transmission in operating theatres, burns wards and intensive care units, where patients are particularly susceptible (see Chapter 13).

Water-borne transmission

Water is a major vehicle for the transmission of microorganisms. Many diseases are transmitted by the faecal-oral route; that is, the pathogen enters via the mouth and is excreted in the faeces. Faecal contamination of the water supply used for drinking or bathing is a major source of infectious agents. These include most of the bacterial and viral pathogens responsible for diarrhoeal infections, as well as the causative organisms of hepatitis A, hepatitis E, typhoid and polio. Protozoa such as *Giardia* and *Entamoeba* live and multiply in fresh water habitats and can be acquired by drinking or swimming in the water. As mentioned above, the bacterium *Legionella pneumophila* multiplies in water reservoirs, and is dispersed

SPOTLIGHT
LEGIONNAIRES' DISEASE: AN EPIDEMIOLOGICAL INVESTIGATION

From time to time there is an outbreak of a disease that has not been previously documented. This occurred in 1976 in the United States when 29 people from various parts of the country died from an unusual type of pneumonia. Perhaps it would have gone unnoticed even then, if it were not for the fact that all the victims were members of the American Legion and had recently attended their annual convention in Pittsburgh, Pennsylvania. When reports of the sudden deaths of a number of their members simultaneously reached headquarters of the Legion, they decided to investigate the cause.

Epidemiologists from the Centers for Disease Control (CDC) in Atlanta, Georgia, were called in to determine the cause of death. In all, 182 people reported being ill and 29 died. The link between the affected people was that they had all been in or around the hotel where the convention was held.

All the routine microbiological tests failed to isolate any known microorganisms or to detect antibodies to them in the blood of the infected people. The investigation took on the character of a murder mystery. The hotel, its surroundings, the food that had been served, the water supply, and all the equipment and utensils that had been used were tested for microorganisms, food toxins and poisonous chemicals. At one stage, newspapers published reports of a 'communist plot to kill American war veterans'. A senate investigation was held and the scientists at CDC were accused of being incompetent.

Finally, one of the scientists at CDC re-examined some tissue from the spleen of a guinea pig that had been infected with lung tissue from one of the victims. Using a special staining technique, he found an unusual rod-shaped organism. After much experimentation, they were eventually able to grow this organism in the laboratory. DNA testing showed that it was a previously unidentified bacterium, a completely new genus. It was named *Legionella* (after the Legionnaires) *pneumophila* (lung-loving).

Outbreaks in other parts of the country helped to confirm the reservoir of the infectious agent and the method of transmission. The bacterium was found growing on top of the hotel in the open water tanks that were part of the air-conditioning system. Wind blowing across the tanks produced a fine aerosol spray carrying the bacteria which were then blown around the street and into the foyer of the hotel. Anyone who happened to be present when the air currents were circulating in a certain way was at risk of inhaling the bacteria and contracting the infection.

Once the bacteria had been identified, methods were developed to grow it in the laboratory and to test for the presence of antibodies. It was found to be a very fastidious organism requiring iron and sulphur for growth, and taking about five days to produce a visible colony on an agar plate.

Further investigations revealed that the bacterium is found throughout the world, living in water environments. Tests on the stored blood and tissue samples of patients who had died from atypical pneumonia over a number of years revealed the presence of *Legionella* in several instances. Since 1976 there have been other outbreaks of pneumonia that have been attributed to *Legionella*.

It has been shown that *Legionella* is:

- transmitted by inhalation of the bacteria in fine aerosol sprays;
- not transmitted person to person within a household;
- sensitive to erythromycin.

Note: Outbreaks of Legionnaires' disease occur from time to time in Australia. Usually, there are one or two deaths, mainly in older people who have associated illness or lung impairment. The disease can be successfully treated if diagnosed early. Health authorities require that all water tanks of water-cooled airconditioners be regularly cleaned and chlorinated. Deaths from *Legionnella* each year represent only a small percentage of the deaths from pneumonia caused by other organisms.

FIGURE 8.2
Water cooled air conditioning plants can be a reservoir for *Legionella*.

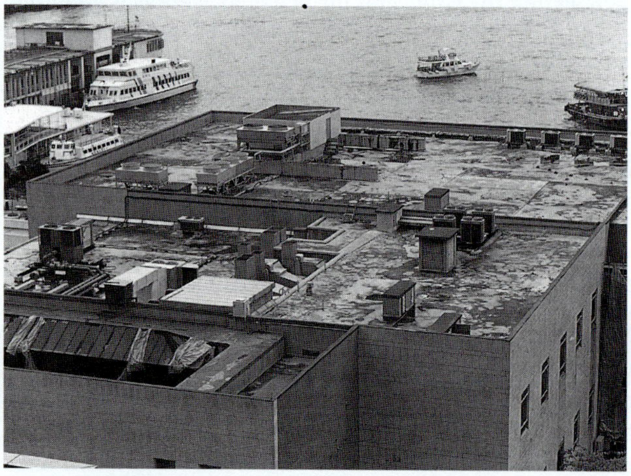

in water aerosols. Water also acts as a vehicle for transmission of some parasitic diseases such as the cercariae of *Schistosoma* (blood flukes). The bacterium *Leptospira* is generally transmitted in water contaminated with animal urine.

We should all be aware of the importance of a clean, uncontaminated water supply. In developed urban areas, government authorities are responsible for ensuring the quality of the water. However, in remote areas or in developing countries the condition of the water supply is often uncertain. If there is any question about the quality of the water, drinking water should be boiled and people should not swim in areas where pathogens are known to be found.

FIGURE 8.3
AIR CURRENTS IN A HOSPITAL
Some common modes of transmission of nosocomial infections in a hospital setting.

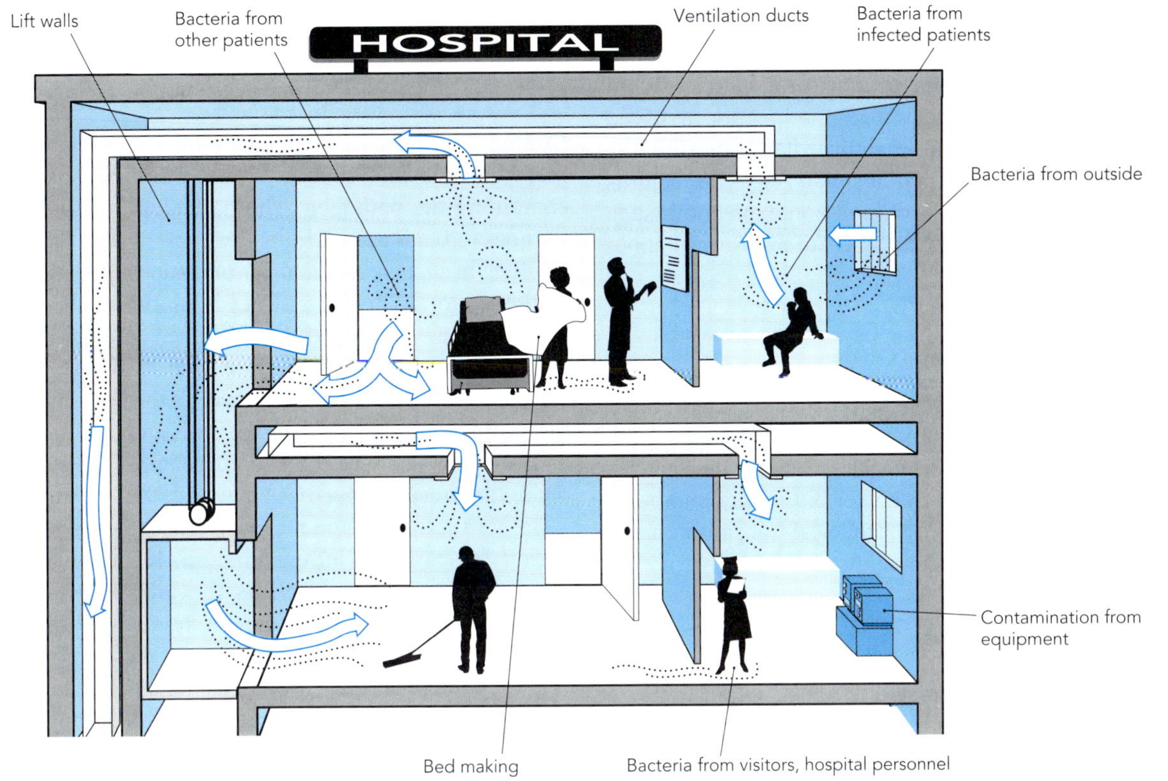

Food-borne transmission

Food is an ideal medium for the growth of microorganisms. Food spoilage due to microbial growth is a well-recognised problem in the home as well as in the food industry. In general, humans do not consume food that is obviously contaminated with microorganisms. We tend to discard mouldy bread, rotten fruit and food that smells 'off'. However, food can be contaminated with microorganisms and still be palatable. The handling, storage and preparation of food provide many opportunities for microorganisms to be deposited in or on the food, and for the organisms then to multiply. In this way, food can serve as an efficient vehicle for the transmission of disease.

Disease-producing microorganisms may be present in food at its source: for example, meat from animals infected with parasites such as tapeworms or *Toxoplasma*. Careful inspection of meat at abattoirs can usually detect helminth infections. Bacteria that cause diseases such as anthrax, brucellosis and listeriosis, as well as the rickettsia, *Coxiella burnetii* (responsible for Q fever), are also sometimes found in or on meat for human consumption. Thorough cooking destroys most pathogens, but the ingestion of raw or inadequately cooked products can cause disease.

Salmonella is commonly found on raw chicken and can be transmitted to humans if the chicken is not thoroughly cooked. It can also be transmitted by poor food-handling procedures from raw chicken to other foods, which are then eaten raw. Health department regulations do not allow the handling of raw meats with the same utensils that are used for processed food that is eaten without further cooking. Pathogenic *Escherichia coli*, derived from humans or animals, may be present on raw meat or badly processed food (see Spotlight box, p. 407).

In South-East Asia, raw fish is often contaminated with the larval stages of parasites such as the flukes. Shellfish that are eaten raw (e.g. oysters) can transmit a variety of gastrointestinal infections.

Milk can be a major means of disease transmission. It may be contaminated with pathogenic organisms from the cow, such as *Listeria monocytogenesis*, *Mycobacterium* species, *Brucella*, etc. Adequate pasteurisation destroys most pathogens in milk.

The transmission of infectious diseases in contaminated food occurs most frequently when the organisms, mainly bacteria, are introduced into the food by poor hygiene and sanitation, or inadequate handling procedures. The source of the contamination is frequently the food handlers, who may be shedding pathogens from their person or in their faeces and transferring them to food because of poor personal hygiene. Once they are present in the food, bacteria may multiply, especially in food stored at room temperature or left in a warming oven, reaching the numbers needed for an infective dose (see Chapter 7). A common contaminant is *Staphylococcus aureus* (which usually comes from the nose or skin of a carrier). When allowed to multiply at room temperature before the food is eaten, some strains produce an enterotoxin that is heat-stable and resistant to stomach acid. The toxin does not alter the taste of the food but causes rapid, severe symptoms after ingestion.

It is clear that many pathogens are excreted in large numbers in the faeces; they can be transferred on to food and then ingested if proper hygiene procedures are not followed. It is therefore essential that people involved in food preparation should wash their hands thoroughly. In institutions such as mental hospitals, day-care centres or nursing homes, outbreaks of food-borne infections such as hepatitis A can occur if the staff are not careful about hygiene.

TRANSMISSION BY VECTORS

Vectors are living agents, usually insects, that are responsible for the transmission of an infectious agent from one host to another. The major vectors are mosquitoes, fleas, ticks, lice, sandflies and other biting flies and bugs. We can distinguish between mechanical transmission and biological transmission.

Mechanical transmission

Mechanical transmission is the passive transport of microorganisms on the outside of the insect's body from a source of infection to a susceptible host, either directly or indirectly. The source may be rotten food, faeces, or a contaminated wound or dressing; the vector may be a household fly. **Direct mechanical transmission** might involve a fly alighting on the source and then going to a portal of entry such as an open sore, a wound, or even eyes. **Indirect mechanical transmission** might involve an insect carrying the pathogen from the source and depositing it on food that was later consumed, or on a dressing or equipment which then came into contact with a susceptible patient.

Biological transmission

Biological transmission occurs when an insect bites an infected host and ingests some blood or body fluid containing the pathogen. The pathogen then multiplies (or goes through a stage in its life cycle) inside the vector, resulting in an increased number of organisms being present in the vector. When the insect bites the next host, the pathogen may be present in regurgitated blood or in faeces deposited at the site of the bite, and is introduced into the body when the bite is scratched. In the case of malaria, the protozoa are present in the saliva of the mosquito, and are injected into the bloodstream of the new host when the mosquito feeds.

Insect vectors are the means of transmission for many serious diseases including malaria, leishmaniasis and sleeping sickness, as well as the arboviral diseases, encephalitis, yellow fever, dengue fever and Ross River fever (described in Chapter 5). Many of these are zoonoses (i.e. they infect animals as well as humans) and can only be transmitted from the animal reservoir to humans by a vector. Mosquitoes are the most important insect vectors. Vector-borne diseases are listed in Table 8.4.

The best method of control of vector-borne diseases is to interrupt the transmission by destroying the vectors or their habitats. Sometimes, the development of an area for farming or settlement interferes with the natural

TABLE 8.4
SOME DISEASES TRANSMITTED BY INSECT VECTORS

ORGANISM	DISEASE	VECTOR
Bacteria		
Yersinia pestis	*Plague	Flea
Borrelia spp.	Lyme disease	Tick
Rickettsia		
Rickettsia prowazekii	*Typhus	Louse
Rickettsia australis	Queensland tick typhus	Tick
Protozoa		
Plasmodium spp.	*Malaria	Mosquito
Leishmania donovani	*Leishmaniasis (kala-azar)	Sandfly
Viruses		
Alphavirus	Ross River fever	Mosquito
Flavivirus	Murray Valley encephalitis	Mosquito
Alphavirus	Barmah forest fever	Mosquito
Flavivirus	Dengue fever	Mosquito
Flavivirus	*Yellow fever	Mosquito

*Not endemic in Australia

ecosystem and creates areas where the vector can breed, and so the disease may be introduced. Drainage of swamps and emptying of containers of stagnant water help to reduce mosquito breeding grounds. In Australia, the major arboviruses are Ross River fever, Murray Valley encephalitis, Barmah forest fever and dengue fever. Control of the mosquito population and avoidance of mosquito bites are the most effective means of preventing outbreaks of these diseases, for which there are no vaccines or antibiotics available.

Epidemiology

Epidemiology is the study of the occurrence, spread and control of disease. The word applies to all kinds of disease, including cancer, heart disease, drug addiction and mental illness, as well as infectious diseases. It involves the collection and processing of information about all aspects of the disease: its **aetiology** (cause), the method of transmission and various other factors that contribute to the spread of the disease or the susceptibility of the population. For infectious diseases, the causative agent is a microorganism.

The science of epidemiology is generally regarded as having been founded by John Snow, an English physician who worked in London in the 1850s. He was intrigued by the fact that some of his patients contracted cholera while others did not. Although the causative agent of cholera was not known at that time, he suspected that it was being transmitted in water. His investigations showed that the inhabitants of London who received their water supply from the River Thames *downstream* from London (i.e. after the river had passed through the city and been polluted with all the sewage and wastes from the city) were much more likely to contract cholera than those who received water drawn from the Thames *before* it reached London. He concluded that the agent responsible for cholera was being excreted by people suffering from the disease into the sewage which was dumped in the river, contaminating the water used by other inhabitants.

His work was confirmed by Robert Koch in Germany who was investigating an outbreak of cholera in Hamburg at about the same time. He noticed that, although there was a high incidence of cholera in Hamburg, the nearby town of Altona, which filtered the dirty river water through sand before use, was essentially free of disease. The work of these two scientists laid the basis for our modern ideas of 'common vehicle transmission' and water purification.

In this chapter we have examined the ways in which microorganisms enter and exit the human body, where they are found and how they are transmitted from the reservoir or source to a susceptible host. In today's society, people share many common sources of food and water and live or work in close proximity to each other. They also travel extensively and are exposed to a wide variety of microorganisms which they may pick up on their bodies and transport from one habitat to another, thus spreading disease.

When there is an outbreak of disease, or sometimes even an isolated case, the epidemiologist is called in to determine the facts surrounding the incident. An **outbreak of infection** is defined as the occurrence of a number of cases of the disease in excess of the number expected in a given time or place. During the investigation, information is collected about the patients, their lifestyle, people they have been in contact with, food they have eaten and places they have visited, to try to pinpoint the source and method of transmission of the disease-causing microorganism. Statistics may be collected giving the levels of **morbidity** (serious illness) and **mortality** (death) from a particular disease.

To contain an outbreak of disease, it is essential that the causative agent be identified and its source located, so that the chain of transmission can be broken. Sometimes, the source may be a single person who has entered the community and is infected with a particular disease which then spreads. This person is called the **index case.** The exact source can sometimes be determined by identifying the strain of the pathogen isolated from the index case and comparing it with the strains causing the disease in later cases. Modern techniques of DNA analysis have contributed to scientists' ability to differentiate between bacterial strains and viral types. In Sydney, where it was alleged that transmission of the AIDS virus from patient to patient had occurred in 1993 in a doctor's surgery, the claim was substantiated by showing that all four infected patients had the same type of virus as the original patient (i.e. the index case).

Occasionally, the epidemiologist is confronted with a totally new disease, one caused by a previously unknown microorganism. The outbreak of the atypical pneumonia, Legionnaires' disease, which occurred in the United States in 1976, was found to have been caused by *Legionella pneumophila*, a bacterium that had not been isolated before (see Spotlight box, p. 168). The virus responsible for acquired immune deficiency syndrome (AIDS) only appeared in Western society in about 1980. Several other viruses have been isolated for the first time in recent years but, unless they have a high morbidity or mortality rate, they do not attract a great deal of publicity. In 1994, a previously unknown morbillivirus was responsible for the death of a horse trainer in Brisbane (see Spotlight box, p. 172).

As well as determining the cause and source of an infectious disease, epidemiologists also study the pattern of its occurrence. The **incidence** of a disease is the number of *new* cases of the disease seen in a specific period of time. Incidence statistics are important in determining whether the number of new cases of the disease is increasing or decreasing; that is, whether the outbreak is being contained. **Prevalence** is the number of people who are infected with the disease at any one time. If a count is made of people suffering from the disease on a particular day, it would include both old and new cases. So, depending on the duration of the disease, a single case may be counted more than once. Thus, if prevalence studies are carried out once a week, but the disease lasts three weeks, then the same patient will contribute to the prevalence statistics each week (i.e. three times altogether).

SPOTLIGHT

A NEW ZOONOSIS

An outbreak of severe respiratory disease in humans and horses due to a previously unrecognised paramyxovirus.

In September 1994, a racehorse in Brisbane, Queensland died from a severe respiratory disease which, on autopsy, showed evidence of heavy, wet lungs and interstitial pneumonia.

A number of other horses in the same stable became sick and, over a period of two weeks, a total of 14 horses died. Within days of the first horse's death a stablehand and the trainer who had cared for the horse became ill with an influenza-like illness. The stablehand was ill for more than two weeks but gradually recovered fully. The trainer died about two weeks after becoming ill. At autopsy there was evidence of heavy, wet lungs and interstitial pneumonia.

Extensive investigations were carried out by the Queensland Health Department and the Queensland Department of Primary Industry (QDPI) to determine the cause of the illness. Samples were sent to Australian laboratories and to reference laboratories overseas. Tests were carried out to detect unusual microorganisms which were known to produce pneumonia-like symptoms, such as *Legionella* and hantavirus. The horse samples were tested for the presence of various exotic viral diseases.

A previously unidentified virus with characteristics of the Paramyxoviridae family was isolated from the lungs of six of the dead horses and from the kidneys of the trainer. It was identified at the CSIRO Australian Animal Health Laboratory (AAHL) by electron microscopy. It was shown to belong to a group known as morbilliviruses, but is only distantly related to other members of the group, such as the measles virus. It is a new addition to the list of viruses that can affect both humans and animals.

The affected horses and stables were placed in quarantine. Fluorescent antibody tests were developed by the scientists at CSIRO and the QDPI and a further 2500 horse samples and 150 human samples were tested, but no new cases were found. Because of the rapid identification of the virus a possible disaster for the racing industry was averted.

The virus appears to be transmitted by close contact with blood or secretions from the nose or mouth. The severity of the symptoms and the final outcome is probably dependent on the level of exposure to the virus and the susceptibility of the patient. The virus is able to infect humans and horses and also some other animals, such as cats.

In October 1995, the death was reported of a man from Mackay in Queensland who had assisted at the autopsy of a horse in August 1994, before the Brisbane outbreak. He died from encephalitis, but blood tests showed the presence of antibodies to the equine morbillivirus, so there is evidence that the virus is not only confined to the Brisbane area.

FIGURE 8.4
(a) Electron micrograph of equine morbillivirus. (b) Scientists working with morbillivirus use special protective clothing.

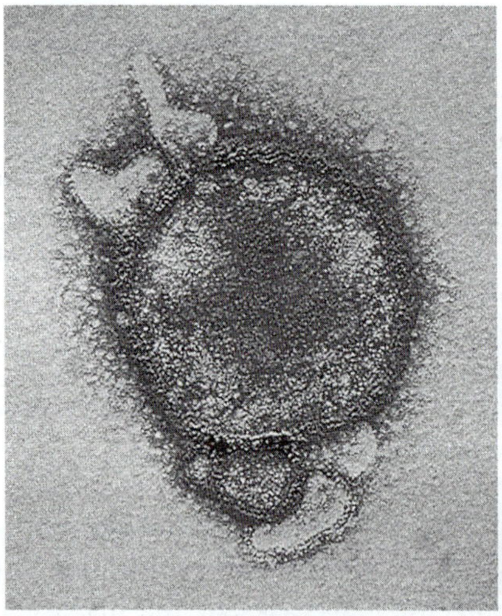
(a)

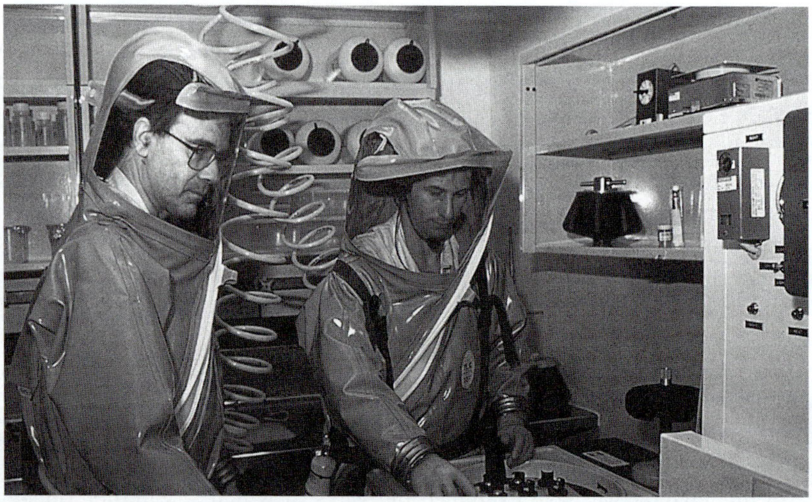
(b)

Source: Adapted from the CDI report Vol.18, October 1994, p. 499 and *Today's Life Science*, Vol. 7, April 1995.

If only incidence statistics are collected, the patient will only be counted once. Incidence statistics more accurately reflect the occurrence, and therefore rate of transmission, of the disease.

Seroprevalence is the number of people who are carrying antibodies to a particular disease at any time. The presence of antibodies in the blood gives information about a person's immune status or a present or past infection. The person is not necessarily infected or symptomatic. For example, in a disease such as AIDS, detection of antibodies to the human immunodeficiency virus (HIV) in the blood gives an indication of the prevalence of the infection in the community. People who are HIV-positive are infected, even though they may be largely asymptomatic. However, the incidence—that is, the number of new people testing positive—will indicate whether the spread of the disease is being contained.

Epidemiologists classify diseases according to their incidence in our society. The incidence can be affected by seasonal variation or climatic changes. A disease is said to be **endemic** in a particular geographical region if a reservoir of the causative organisms is always present in that area and able to give rise to an outbreak of disease at any time. For example, the childhood diseases of measles, mumps and chickenpox are endemic in most parts of the world, but may have seasonal variation. Most outbreaks of chickenpox occur in the spring. Rotavirus, which causes severe diarrhoea in infants, is usually seen in winter. Outbreaks of endemic diseases may be **sporadic**; that is, they may occur as unrelated isolated cases, anywhere in the country.

Epidemics occur when there is a sudden rapid rise in the incidence of a disease in a particular locality. This may be due to a number of factors. For example, an epidemic may occur when a new organism or strain of an organism is introduced into a population that is not immune, such as occurs with the regular outbreaks of influenza due to mutations in the virus. Travellers may carry organisms to areas where they were not previously found. The early settlers in Australia brought with them European diseases, such as smallpox, which killed many of the Australian Aborigines who had not previously been exposed to them. During 1993 and 1994, there were several serious outbreaks of measles in Australia that were classed as epidemics. They occurred mainly because, despite the availability of a vaccine, many people were not immune to measles, because of poor compliance with the recommended vaccination schedules (see Chapter 14). Endemic diseases can become epidemics given the right conditions—for example, lack of immunity in a large proportion of the population of the community. Sometimes epidemics are due to the emergence of a particularly virulent strain of the pathogen, such as occurs in influenza epidemics.

A **pandemic** is a series of epidemics that occur when the disease spreads worldwide. Examples include the devastating influenza epidemic of 1918, which killed 21 million people worldwide, and the new threat of AIDS, which has spread from Africa throughout the rest of the world.

SURVEILLANCE

An important aspect of epidemiology that is necessary for effective control of disease is ongoing **surveillance**—that is, the collection and analysis of data on all aspects of the occurrence and spread of a disease. Included in surveillance data are the laboratory results on the isolation and identification of causative organisms, morbidity and mortality statistics, results of field investigations, and reports of adverse reactions to immunisation or exposure to chemical or biological hazards. Epidemiologists are also concerned with all the factors that determine a person's susceptibility to a particular disease. They collect information about age, sex, lifestyle, occupation and history of immunisation together with data about exposure to common vehicles (food, water) or sources of the infectious agent. These data can be analysed and used to predict the likelihood of future outbreaks of the disease.

Epidemiological surveillance may be carried out within a particular hospital environment by members of the infection control team. Its purpose may be to investigate an outbreak or to measure or reduce the incidence of nosocomial infections (see Chapter 13).

Epidemiology is the scientific discipline underlying much infection control work and the science on which public health guidelines are based. Infectious diseases are one type of disease where intervention strategies of proven efficacy are available to treat and prevent the spread of those diseases. Among these strategies are immunisation programs, antibiotic therapy and prophylaxis, infection control programs in hospitals, and public health programs for infection control. The surveillance data from the community at large are used to develop health department policies and provide guidelines for the prevention of the spread of infectious diseases.

Public health authorities are responsible for collecting and recording data on outbreaks of infectious diseases. In Australia a number of diseases are classified as notifiable (see Chapter 14). When a patient is diagnosed with a notifiable disease, the doctor or hospital involved is obliged to inform the appropriate health authority.

In this way, it is possible to keep statistics on the incidence of disease and for the health authorities to formulate policies to try to control the spread of infectious diseases. This is discussed further in Chapter 14. Information about the incidence of notifiable diseases and outbreaks of infection in Australia is contained in a fortnightly publication, *Communicable Diseases Intelligence (CDI)*, by the Commonwealth Department of Human Services and Health. In New Zealand, a similar publication is obtainable from the Public Health Commission.

The Centers for Disease Control (CDC) in the United States publishes the *Morbidity and Mortality Weekly Report (MMWR)*, which covers the United States and important epidemics throughout the world. In the United Kingdom, the PHLS Communicable Diseases Surveillance Centre publishes the *Communicable Diseases Report (CDR)* weekly.

Summary

RESERVOIRS OF INFECTION

- For a disease to persist in a community, there has to be a permanent reservoir of the infectious agent. It may be human, animal or non-living.
- The source of an infection is the individual or object from which the infection is acquired.
- Human reservoirs include patients who have an acute, latent or chronic infectious disease.
- Normal flora of the body also act as a reservoir of infection.
- Diseases that occur in both animals and humans are called zoonoses.
- Transmission of the infectious agent from animal to human may be by direct contact with fur, feathers or body secretions, by the ingestion of cysts, or via the bite of an insect vector.
- Soil and water are major reservoirs of infectious agents.

PORTAL OF ENTRY

- Endogenous infections are caused by flora which are already present on the human body.
- Exogenous pathogens are microorganisms derived from a source outside the human body; they enter via a characteristic portal of entry.
- Many pathogens have a preferred portal of entry. It may be via the skin, respiratory tract, GI tract or genitourinary system.
- Intact skin is a major barrier to the entry of pathogenic microorganisms.
- Puncture wounds, injuries, insect bites and the use of hypodermic syringes break the skin and facilitate the entry of microorganisms.
- Nosocomial infections may occur in surgical patients or patients subjected to procedures such as the use of central lines, IV lines and catheters.
- Microorganisms gain entry by adhering to the mucosal cells lining the upper respiratory tract.
- The use of respiratory equipment creates conditions where microorganisms can be introduced directly into the respiratory tract.
- A major portal of entry for pathogens is the ingestion of contaminated food or drink.
- Urinary tract infections are very common in catheterised patients in hospital.
- The genital tract is the portal of entry of sexually transmitted diseases.
- Some microorganisms cross the placenta and infect the foetus *in utero*.
- The neonate is susceptible to infections acquired during passage through the birth canal.

PORTALS OF EXIT

- Microorganisms are continuously shed from the body.
- Health workers need to be aware of the ways in which pathogens are shed.
- Organisms such as viruses are expelled as fine aerosols by coughing and sneezing.
- Faeces contain normal flora as well as pathogens that may contaminate food and water.
- Microorganisms are shed on dead skin scales, as particles from dried crusts on wounds, and from skin lesions.
- Organisms responsible for sexually transmitted diseases are present in semen and vaginal secretions.
- Urine contains bacteria from urinary tract infections, as well as pathogens such as cytomegalovirus and *Leptospira*.
- Blood-borne pathogens such as HIV, and hepatitis B and C, are present in blood and body fluids.

TRANSMISSION OF MICROORGANISMS

- Transmission of microorganisms occurs horizontally from person to person or vertically from mother to baby.
- Transmission may be by direct or indirect contact, via a common vehicle such as air, water or food, or by insect vectors.

EPIDEMIOLOGY

- Epidemiology is the study of the occurrence, spread and control of disease.
- There is an outbreak of infection when the number of cases that occur is in excess of that expected in a given time or place.
- The index case is the person who is the primary source of the infection.
- The incidence of a disease is the number of new cases of the disease seen in a specific period of time. Prevalence is the number of people infected at any one time. Seroprevalence is the number of people carrying antibodies to a particular disease at any time.
- A disease is endemic if there is a constant reservoir of causative organisms in the area.
- Epidemics occur when there is a sudden rapid rise in the incidence of disease in a particular locality.
- A pandemic is a worldwide epidemic.
- Surveillance data are used to develop public health guidelines and infection control policies.

Study Questions

1. What is meant by a reservoir of infection?
2. Give examples of some of the major reservoirs of infection for human pathogens.
3. What is the difference between the source of an infection and the reservoir of infection?
4. Give some examples of fomites found in the hospital environment.
5. What is a zoonosis? Give examples.
6. Describe three diseases caused by members of the genus *Clostridium*.
7. What are the major non-living reservoirs for microorganisms?
8. What is the difference between endogenous and exogenous infections.
9. What is meant by a cutaneous infection? Give two examples.
10. Which diseases flourish in deep puncture wounds?
11. Which hospital procedures are likely to allow pathogens to enter the body via breaks in the skin?
12. Describe how microorganisms gain entry to the body via the respiratory tract.
13. What is pneumonia?
14. What are the risks to patients associated with the use of mechanical ventilation?
15. What is cystitis?
16. What are the major organisms that can cross the placenta?
17. How are pathogens shed from the human body?
18. Which diseases are likely to be transmitted in blood or blood products?
19. What is meant by vertical transmission?
20. What is the difference between direct contact and indirect contact?
21. What is meant by common vehicle transmission?
22. How can the spread of air-borne microorganisms be controlled in the hospital?
23. Why is it important to use different utensils for handling raw and cooked food?
24. Why should we drink only pasteurised milk?
25. Which insects can act as vectors for infectious disease?
26. What is the best method to control vector-borne diseases such as malaria?
27. What is the difference between the rates of morbidity and mortality?
28. What is meant by the index case?
29. What is meant by seroprevalence?
30. What is the difference between an epidemic and a pandemic?

Test Your Understanding

1. Why can a person who is suffering from a subclinical infection, or who is a chronic carrier, transmit the disease to another person?
2. Under what circumstances can the normal flora of the body cause an infection?
3. What is meant by the 'preferred portal of entry'?
4. Why is an intact skin so important?
5. How do microorganisms evade the hostile pH in the stomach in order to gain entry via the gastrointestinal route?
6. Why do patients with urinary catheters suffer from urinary tract infections?
7. What is meant by faecal-oral transmission?
8. How does epidemiology benefit the community?
9. What is the difference between incidence and prevalence statistics?
10. What is the value of carrying out surveillance programs?

FURTHER READING

Ashbolt, N., 1995, 'Public Health Water Microbiology for the 21st Century', *Recent Advances in Microbiology*, 3, pp. 173–214.

Grohmann, G.S., G.J. Logan, P.T. Cox & C.P. Gerba, 1994, 'Viruses: the Hidden Hazard', *Today's Life Science*, 6, No. 8, pp. 32–35.

Leggett, P.A., 1989, 'Legionnaires' Diseases on the March', *Australian Microbiologist*, 10, pp. 29–31.

Mackenzie, J.S., D.W. Smith, T.M. Ellis, M.D. Lindsay, A.K. Brown, R.J. Coelen & R.A. Hall, 1993, 'Human and Animal Arboviral Diseases in Australia', *Recent Advances in Microbiology*, 2, pp. 1–91.

Murray, K. & N. Byrne, 1995, 'Solving the Horse Virus Mystery', *Today's Life Science*, 7, No. 4, pp. 56–61.

chapter 9

the body's defence systems

Chapter focus

- *What are the non-specific defences of the body?*
- *How do the skin and mucous membranes protect the body against infection?*
- *What cells act non-specifically to protect the body against foreign particles and microorganisms?*
- *What is inflammation and what is its role in defence?*
- *What are the characteristics of the acquired immune system?*
- *What cells and tissues comprise the acquired immune system?*
- *What is humoral immunity and what are the functions of antibodies?*
- *What is cell-mediated immunity?*
- *What are the principles of immunisation?*
- *What disorders are associated with the failure or improper function of the immune system?*

In Chapters 7 and 8 we looked at the relationship between microorganisms and the human host. Whether or not a person becomes infected by a certain microorganism depends on the balance between the powers of the microbe to cause disease and the powers of the body to resist it. In this chapter we examine the ways in which the human body wards off infection. In Chapter 10 we look at some of the mechanisms that microorganisms possess that enable them to overcome or evade the body' s defences and cause disease. The ability of the body to prevent infection occurring is called **resistance**, whereas a lack of resistance, or vulnerability to an infection, is called **susceptibility**.

Given the multitude of microorganisms present in our environment and on our bodies, it is rather miraculous that we are not continually suffering from some kind of infection. We owe this to a highly complex and efficient system of defences. The body's resistance to infection depends on two major types of defences:

1. **Non-specific defences** act as the body's first line of defence and offer general protection against all potentially harmful agents, including pathogens (infectious agents) and foreign substances. These defences do not discriminate one agent from another, and act in a similar way each time the same agent enters (or attempts to enter) the body.
2. **Specific defences** are the body's second line of defence. They protect it against the pathogens that succeed in circumventing the non-specific defences and also protect the host against future attack by the same pathogen.

As you will see, the specific and non-specific defences overlap and interact with each other to protect the body. Many of the specific defence mechanisms have the function of directing or enhancing the action of non-specific defences, especially the activity of the body's phagocytic cells (see pp. 178–80). The specific defences, and some of the non-specific defences, comprise the body's **immune system**, the system the body has to eliminate foreign microorganisms and substances, and to provide long-term immunity to them.

Non-specific Defences

The function of the non-specific defences (also called **non-specific immunity**, **innate immunity**, **natural immunity**) is to prevent the entry of pathogens into the body, or to destroy them immediately if they do manage to enter. These defences include the skin and mucous membranes (and their secretions), cellular defences, inflammation, certain antimicrobial proteins and fever.

SKIN AND MUCOUS MEMBRANE BARRIERS

The body's first line of defence against invasion by microorganisms is the skin and the mucous membranes. These are very resilient physical barriers which protect against the entry of potentially pathogenic microorganisms and other foreign particles. The skin consists of two distinct layers, the epidermis and the dermis (see Figure 9.1). The epidermis is the outer layer and consists of multiple layers of tightly packed epithelial cells. The outermost of these cells contain the strong protein, **keratin**. Keratin is not affected by weak acids and bases and is resistant to bacterial enzymes and toxins. As long as the epidermis is unbroken, this thick, tough layer represents a formidable barrier to most microorganisms.

In the dermis there are sebaceous glands that secrete sebum, an oily substance containing fatty acids, which lowers the pH of the skin and inhibits the growth of certain bacteria and fungi. There are also sweat glands. The high salt concentration in sweat inhibits many microorganisms, although the normal flora that live on the skin's secretions are tolerant to salt and low pH (e.g. some staphylococci).

Intact mucous membranes provide similar physical barriers within the body. Mucosal membranes line all the body cavities that are open to the environment; that is, the digestive, respiratory, urinary and reproductive tracts. Although these surfaces suffer considerable wear and tear, the damaged cells are rapidly replaced and their integrity restored. Also, a film of sticky mucous secretion traps foreign particles and microorganisms that attempt to enter the body via these routes. The mucous helps to prevent microbes from attaching to the epithelial surface and entering the tissues. Inside the nose there is a meshwork of tiny hairs that, together with mucous, traps inhaled particles. There are mechanisms (described below) which then move the mucous and entrapped particles out of the body.

The mucosal membranes are the sites of secretion or formation of a large variety of other substances that contribute to defence. For example:

- **Lysozyme**. This enzyme breaks down the cell wall of many bacteria. It is found in saliva, sweat, tears, and nasal and vaginal secretions.
- Acids. The hydrochloric acid secreted in the stomach (pH 2) kills most microorganisms, and is a highly effective protection against the enormous numbers of microbes that enter the body in food and beverages. The pH of the vagina in adult females is acidic (pH 4) due to the conversion of glycogen to lactic acid by lactobacilli.
- **Digestive enzymes** and **bile salts**. These substances, which are secreted into the gastro-intestinal tract for digestion, also kill microorganisms and inactivate viruses.
- **Lactoferrin**. This substance inhibits the growth of some microorganisms by binding free iron, a necessary growth factor for them. It is found in a number of secretions, including saliva, milk and seminal fluid.
- **Spermine**. This is an antibacterial substance found in semen.

The movement of foreign particles over mucosal surfaces is a highly effective mechanism that eliminates many potential pathogens from the body. A vital non-specific defence mechanism is the ciliated epithelium of the upper respiratory tract (see Figure 9.2). The cilia move mucous and anything trapped in it upwards toward the throat, either to be expelled or swallowed, thus preventing it from entering the lower respiratory passages. This **mucociliary escalator** is enhanced by two other forms of movement: coughing and sneezing.

The movement of fluids over mucosal surfaces creates a washing effect, which helps to eliminate microbes from the body. Thus, tears wash foreign particles from eyes and the flow of urine in the urinary tract flushes the urethra. In fact, normal urine flow is one of the most important defences in the urinary tract, and people with urinary obstruction often suffer urinary tract infection.

The skin and mucous membranes are highly effective barriers. However, sometimes microorganisms are able to break through these barriers, either because their integrity is disrupted by cuts, wounds or abrasions, or because the particular microbes possess special properties that enable them to bypass these barriers. When this happens, and microorganisms are able to gain entry to the tissues, there are other non-specific mechanisms that come into play, as will be described in the following sections. However, the vital contribution that these barriers play should not be underestimated. This is clearly demonstrated in situations where some of these defences are disrupted or lost. For example, burns patients are highly susceptible to infection, and infection is one of the more common causes of death in badly burned patients.

NON-SPECIFIC CELLULAR DEFENCES

When microorganisms or foreign substances penetrate the skin or mucous membranes and enter the tissues, the body has certain cellular defences for protection. The most important of these are phagocytes and natural killer cells. The vital role played by phagocytes in particular is reflected in the serious infections suffered by people with a deficiency in these cells.

Phagocytes

Phagocytes are body cells that actively ingest and digest foreign particles (see Figure 9.3). They also break down dead tissue cells and remove cellular debris from the tissues. The two major types of phagocytes in the body are the macrophages and the neutrophils.

Macrophages are large phagocytic cells derived from blood monocytes. They are located in most tissues and organs of the body, where they search for cellular debris, or foreign cells or particles. Some of the macrophages in certain parts of the body are given different names—Kupffer cells in the liver, microglia in nerve tissue, Langerhans cells in skin, and histiocytes in connective tissue (see Table 9.1). At sites of infection, extra monocytes can migrate from the circulation into the tissue where they mature into macrophages.

Neutrophils, the most abundant type of white blood cell, are highly phagocytic and actively motile cells. Neutrophils are also referred to as **polymorphonuclear leukocytes (PMNs)**, **polymorphs** or **pus cells**. Neutrophils phagocytose foreign material in the bloodstream, but also migrate from the bloodstream into the tissue in the early stages of infection and inflammation.

The process of phagocytosis involves four major phases (see Figure 9.4):

TABLE 9.1
THE MONOCYTE/MACROPHAGE SYSTEM OF THE HUMAN BODY

ANATOMICAL SITE	CELLS
alveoli	macrophages
spleen	macrophages
blood	monocytes
lymph nodes	macrophages
brain	microglia
liver	Kupffer cells
connective tissue	histiocytes
bones	osteoclasts

FIGURE 9.1

A SECTION THROUGH SKIN

The top layers of the cells contain the tough protein called keratin.

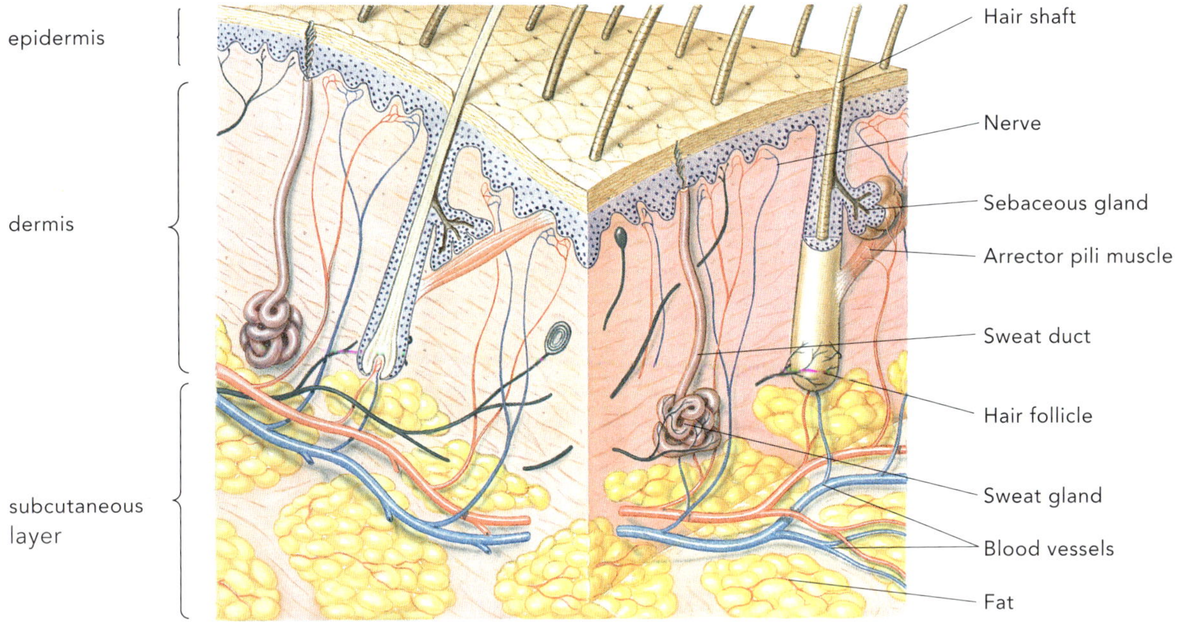

FIGURE 9.2

THE MUCOCILIARY ESCALATOR

The cilia of the upper respiratory tract, sweep mucus and any foreign material caught in it upwards away from the lungs.

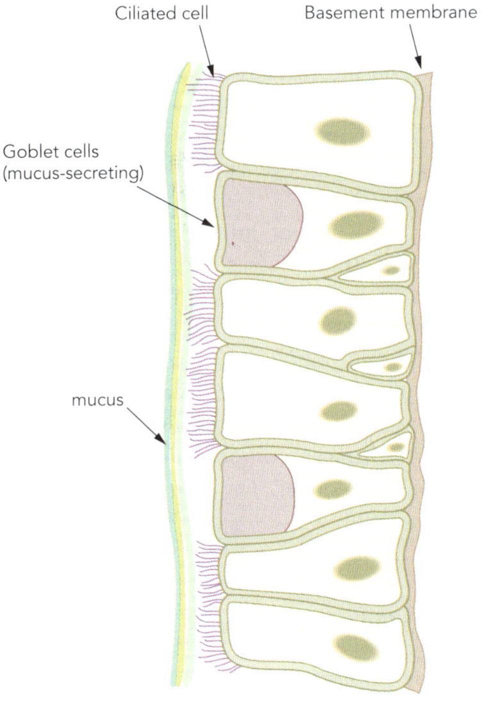

FIGURE 9.3

A SCANNING ELECTRON MICROGRAPH SHOWING A MACROPHAGE ENGULFING BACTERIA

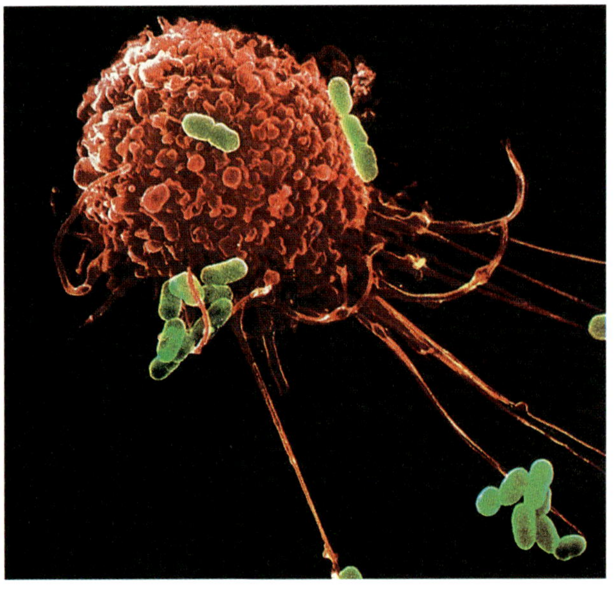

1. Chemotaxis;
2. Attachment;
3. Ingestion;
4. Digestion.

Phagocytes are attracted to sites of damaged tissue or microbial invasion by chemicals released at the site. This attraction is called **chemotaxis**. A variety of chemical substances act as attractants, including substances released from damaged tissues and some components of microorganisms. These chemical attractants cause the phagocytes to move along an increasing concentration gradient of the attractant towards its source—the site of infection or tissue damage.

FIGURE 9.4
THE MECHANISMS OF PHAGOCYTOSIS
Phagocytosis of a bacterial cell, showing the major steps of attachment, ingestion and killing/destruction of the microbe.

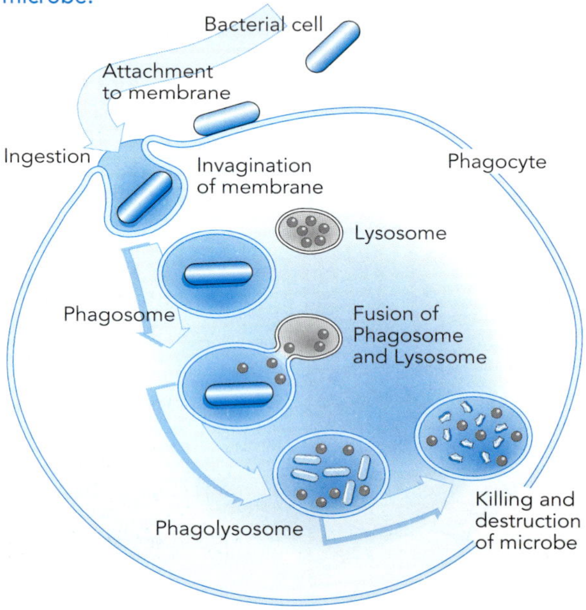

The phagocyte must first be able to attach to the foreign particle or microorganism in order to ingest it. Attachment appears to occur via non-specific receptor sites on the surface of the phagocyte. Some microorganisms have structures, such as polysaccharide capsules, which enable them to avoid being bound to the phagocyte surface (see Chapter 10). Host factors, particularly complement and antibodies, enhance the adherence of microorganisms to phagocytes, a process called opsonisation.

Phagocytes ingest foreign material by a process called **endocytosis**. The cytoplasm invaginates at the point where the particle is attached and then encloses around it. Having been taken up, the particle is contained within a membrane-bound vacuole. A **phagosome** or phagocytic vacuole is thus formed within the cytoplasm of the phagocyte.

Digestion of the foreign material is brought about by fusion of the phagosome with lysosomes, to form a **phagolysosome**. Inside the phagolysosome, the lysosomal digestive enzymes break down the foreign material. Toxic oxygen-containing substances, such as hydrogen peroxide and hypochlorite, are also produced by lysosomal enzymes to assist in the killing process. Some microbes, such as the bacteria that cause tuberculosis and Legionnaires' disease—which appear to be resistant to intracellular digestion—are thought to prevent, somehow, the fusion of lysosomes with the phagosome. Other organisms, like the *Rickettsiae,* appear to avoid destruction by escaping from the phagosome before it merges with the lysosome. Since lysosomal enzymes are not released into the cytoplasm, the bacteria are not digested.

The importance of phagocytosis as a defence mechanism is clearly reflected by the number of microorganisms that have developed means of escaping the process. This is discussed more fully in Chapter 10.

Natural killer cells

Natural killer (NK) cells are a unique group of cells that are capable of destroying cancer cells and virus-infected cells. They are part of a distinct group of lymphoid cells called 'large granular lymphocytes'. As we see later in this chapter, lymphocytes can recognise and respond in specific fashion to virus-infected or tumour cells, releasing substances or activating other cells that ultimately destroy them. NK cells act directly against these targets, apparently by recognising changes on the surface of the cells. The name 'natural killer' reflects the fact that they do not recognise specific cells, but are able to attack a variety of such targets. NK cells appear to bring about killing of the target cell by insertion of protein molecules, called **perforins**, into the cell membrane, creating a pore through which the cell contents leak out. NK cells can be stimulated by factors (called **cytokines**) released in specific immunity, and they then show greater killing activity (see cell-mediated immunity, p. 196).

INFLAMMATION

The **acute inflammatory response** is a non-specific defence that is the body's response to tissue injury. It occurs in response to any injury, including physical harm (e.g. cuts and abrasions), burns, radiation (e.g. sunburn) and chemical injury (e.g. acids), as well as to infection by microorganisms. Although acute inflammation can be initiated by a wide variety of injurious agents, the physiologic events are similar each time. However, the inflammatory response produced is usually appropriate to the cause and the extent of the injury. Inflammatory conditions are named by adding the suffix *-itis* to the affected organ or tissue (e.g. conjunctivitis for inflammation of the conjunctiva of the eye, appendicitis for inflammation of the appendix).

The major function of inflammation is to clear the injured site of cellular debris and any foreign material or pathogens (if present), thereby preparing the area for repair processes. In the case of infection, it can also serve to localise the microorganisms, preventing their spread to adjacent areas. When effective, the inflammatory response eliminates any pathogen or foreign material, removes injured tissue components and enables tissue repair processes to occur. The four main signs of acute inflammation are:

- redness;
- heat;
- swelling; and
- pain.

The major events of the inflammatory process are described below and summarised in Figure 9.5.

Vasodilation and increased vascular permeability

Once an injury has occurred, several events take place, leading to the activation or release of a variety of chemicals. These chemicals are responsible for the physiological events that occur in inflammation and are called the

FIGURE 9.5
A SUMMARY OF THE EVENTS IN ACUTE INFLAMMATION

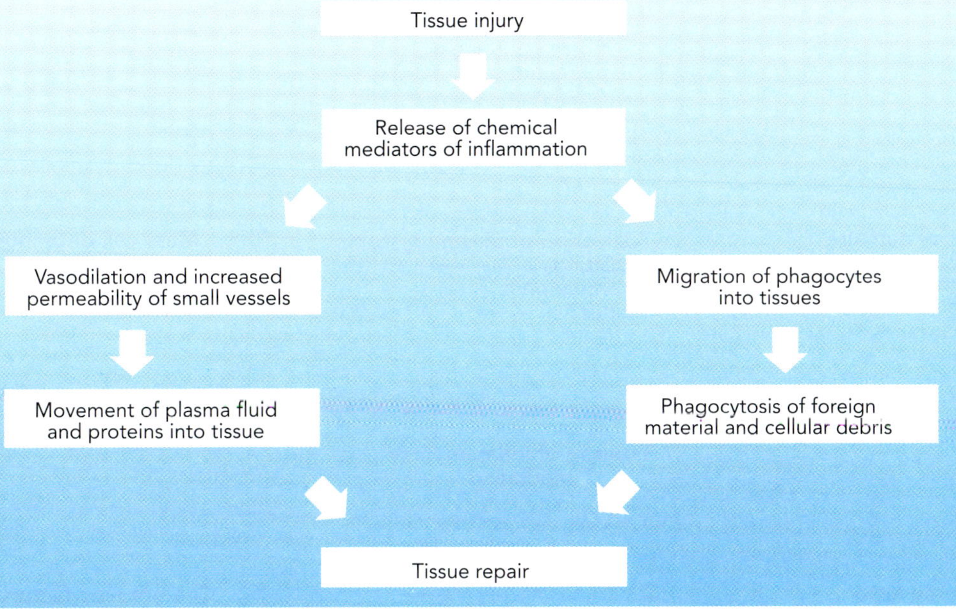

chemical mediators of inflammation. Derived from a variety of sources, the most important are histamine, kinins, prostaglandins, leukotrienes, tumour necrosis factor, and complement. The sources and activities of inflammatory mediators are summarised in Figure 9.6. Many of these mediators cause dilation of the arterioles in the area of damage. This causes more blood to flow into the area, accounting for the redness and warmth of inflamed tissue.

Some mediators also increase the permeability of local capillaries and post-capillary venules by causing retraction of the endothelial cells of these vessels. As a result, plasma fluid and proteins, such as clotting factors, complement and antibodies, are able to move from the bloodstream into the tissue spaces. This fluid is called an **exudate**, and its accumulation in the tissue is the cause of the **oedema**, or swelling. The pain that is usually associated with inflammation is due to compression of adjacent nerve endings by this swelling, as well as to the direct effects of prostaglandins and kinins on pain receptors. Depending on the site of injury, swelling and pain may cause temporary loss of function of a body part (e.g. in a joint), and this is sometimes regarded as the fifth sign of acute inflammation.

The different chemical mediators of inflammation come from a variety of different sources. **Histamine** is present in many different body cell types, especially in mast cells in connective tissue, and in basophils and platelets in the bloodstream. It is released when these cells are injured or stimulated, and it has a potent action on blood vessels, causing them to dilate and allow the leakage of plasma fluid and proteins. **Antihistamines** are used to alleviate the redness and swelling prominent in some clinical conditions such as hay fever and hives.

Kinins (bradykinin is the best known one) are small peptides present in blood and other body fluids in an inactive form (kallikrein). The kinin system is activated by tissue injury. Kinins cause vasodilation and increased vascular permeability as well as inducing pain.

Prostaglandins and **leukotrienes** are vasoactive mediators synthesised from a long chain fatty acid called arachidonic acid, which is released from mast cell membranes. They cause dilation of post-capillary venules, increased vascular permeability and neutrophil chemotaxis. Prostaglandins also induce pain. Several of the leukotrienes cause sustained constriction of bronchioles, as occurs in bronchial asthma.

The importance of prostaglandins and leukotrienes as inflammatory agents is reflected in the action of some commonly used anti-inflammatory drugs. Aspirin, indomethacin and certain other non-steroidal anti-inflammatory agents act by blocking the synthesis of prostaglandins, as shown in Figure 9.7. Steroidal anti-inflammatories are very potent because they block both prostaglandin and leukotriene synthesis. Some of these drugs (e.g. aspirin) also have an analgesic (pain-reducing) effect because of their inhibition of prostaglandin synthesis.

The complement system amplifies many of the processes in acute inflammation. The activation and actions of this system of proteins are discussed on page 185.

The purpose of local vasodilation and increased vascular permeability is to provide the injured site with a variety of blood-borne substances that assist in tissue repair. The plasma fluid that enters injured tissue contains oxygen and nutrients necessary for the repair process, as well as important proteins like antibodies, complement and clotting proteins. In some infections, the clotting proteins form a fibrin barrier around the site, to isolate the injured area and prevent the spread of bacteria or other harmful agents into surrounding tissues. As we describe later in this chapter, antibodies and complement are substances that help to eliminate foreign organisms.

FIGURE 9.6
THE SOURCES AND ACTIVITIES OF THE CHEMICAL MEDIATORS OF INFLAMMATION

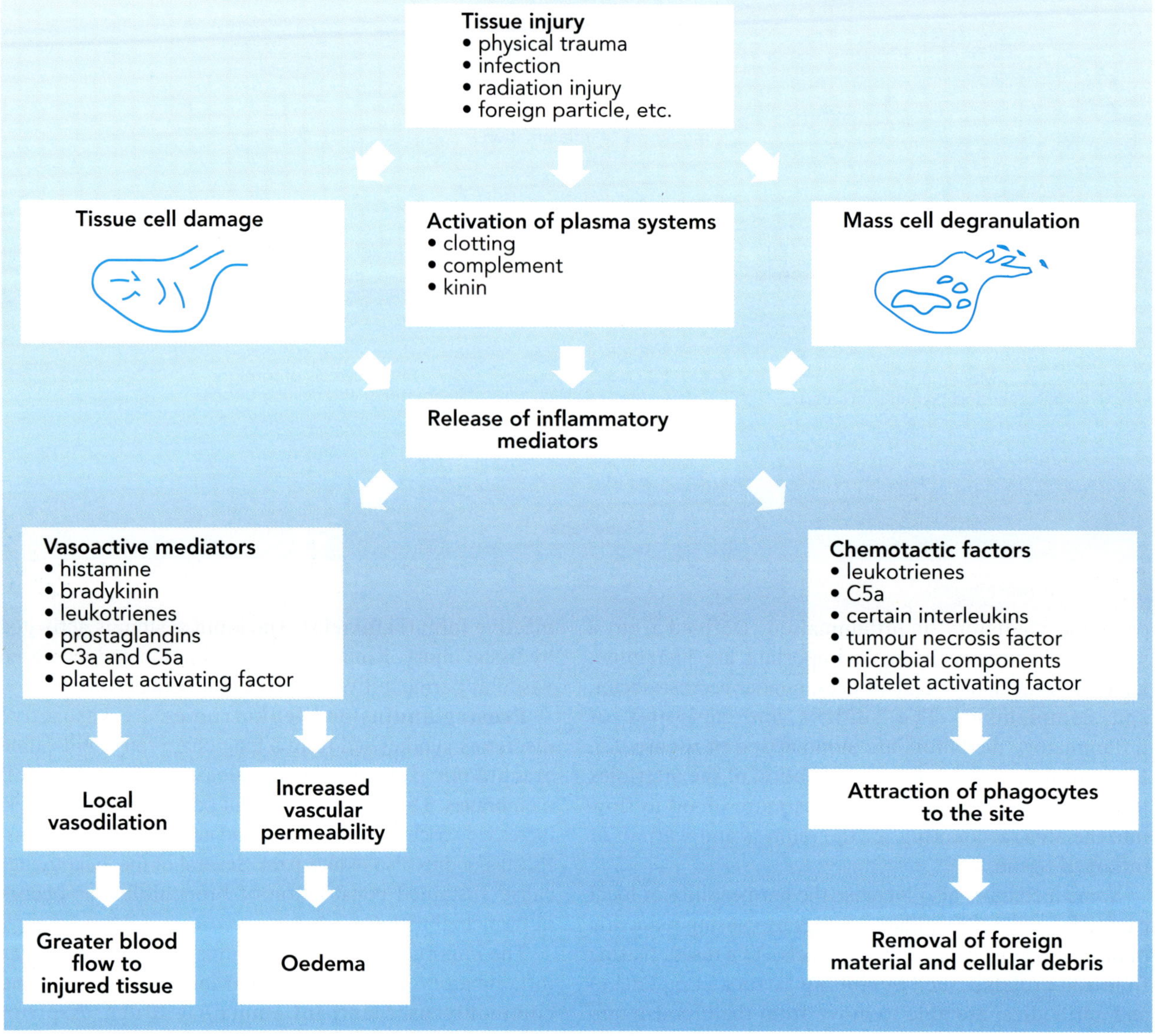

FIGURE 9.7
THE SYNTHESIS OF PROSTAGLANDINS AND LEUKOTRIENES AND THE ACTIONS OF SOME ANTI-INFLAMMATORY DRUGS

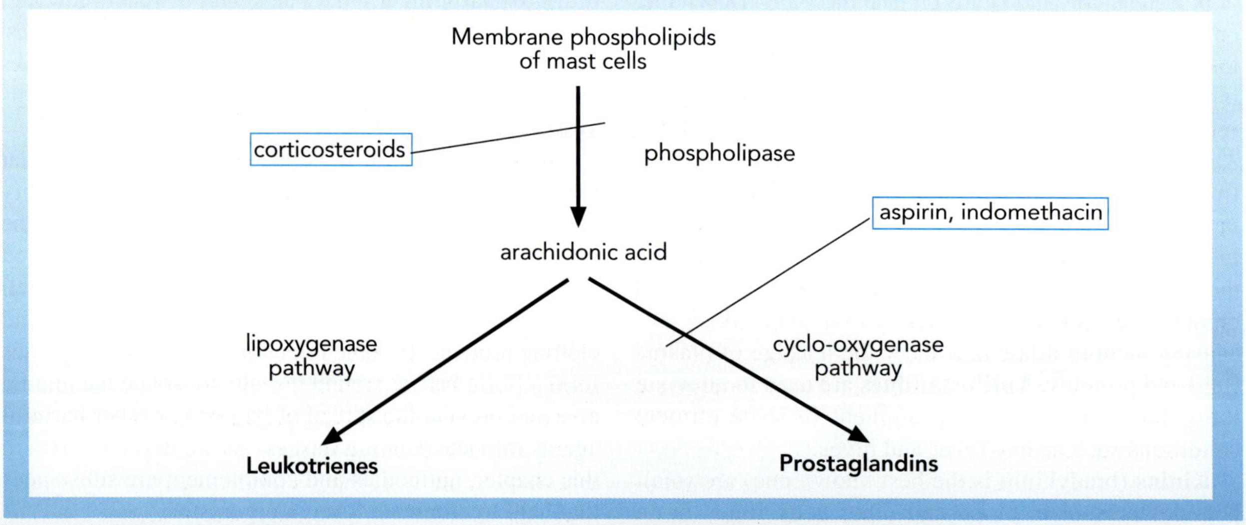

Although inflammation is an important defence mechanism, there are situations where it can actually harm the body. For example, the swelling and pain associated with a disorder such as rheumatoid arthritis are hardly beneficial; in fact, in this disorder an unnecessary degree of inflammation occurs. The role of inflammation in the production of disease is discussed below.

Phagocyte migration

During inflammation there is an influx of phagocytic cells into the injured tissue. First, the neutrophils arrive, and later the macrophages. Activated mediators from plasma and injured cells stimulate the release of extra neutrophils from the bone marrow into the blood. In severe infections, the number of neutrophils in the blood may increase four to five times within several hours . A significant increase in the number of white cells in blood is called a **leukocytosis** and, when neutrophils predominate (called a **neutrophilia**). Neutrophilia is a characteristic sign of severe bacterial infection. Some of the inflammatory mediators, such as complement factors, prostaglandins and kinins, act as chemotactic agents for phagocytes, attracting them to the site of the injury. During inflammation, the blood flow in the region of the injury slows and neutrophils begin to stick to the inner walls of the capillaries. This phenomenon is known as **margination** (see Figure 9.8). The neutrophils then begin to squeeze between the endothelial cells of the capillary walls (a process called **diapedesis)** and move into the tissue spaces, where they immediately begin to devour dead or damaged tissue cells and any foreign particles that are present.

Late in the inflammatory response, monocytes from the bloodstream begin to enter the area, replacing the neutrophils, which leave or die *in situ*. Monocytes are only weakly phagocytic, but after entering the tissues they swell and develop large numbers of lysosomes to become mature, highly active macrophages. Macrophages are responsible for the final clearing of cell debris and foreign matter from the injured area so that the tissue can be repaired.

In sites of bacterial infection, pus may accumulate in the wound. **Pus** is a thick, creamy-coloured fluid comprising a mixture of dead or dying neutrophils, tissue debris and remaining pathogens. Neutrophils are the major component of pus because many die *in situ*, having expended themselves in voracious phagocytic activity. Pus formation is typically induced by bacteria, but not by viruses. This can sometimes be helpful in distinguishing between bacterial and viral infections. Certain bacteria (e.g. staphylococci, gonococci) are particularly strong attracters of neutrophils and are termed **pyogenic**, or pus-forming, bacteria. When the sac of pus is walled off by a layer of fibrin, an **abscess** is formed. This represents the body's attempt to localise the infection and the potentially damaging neutrophil enzymes, which are released from these cells as they die. The pus remains locked up in the abscess. Thus, physical drainage of abscesses is often necessary before healing can occur.

FIGURE 9.8
MARGINATION AND DIAPEDESIS OF PHAGOCYTES
During inflammation phagocytes stick to the insides of capillaries (margination) at the site of injury and then enter the tissue spaces by passing between the endothelial cells (diapedesis).

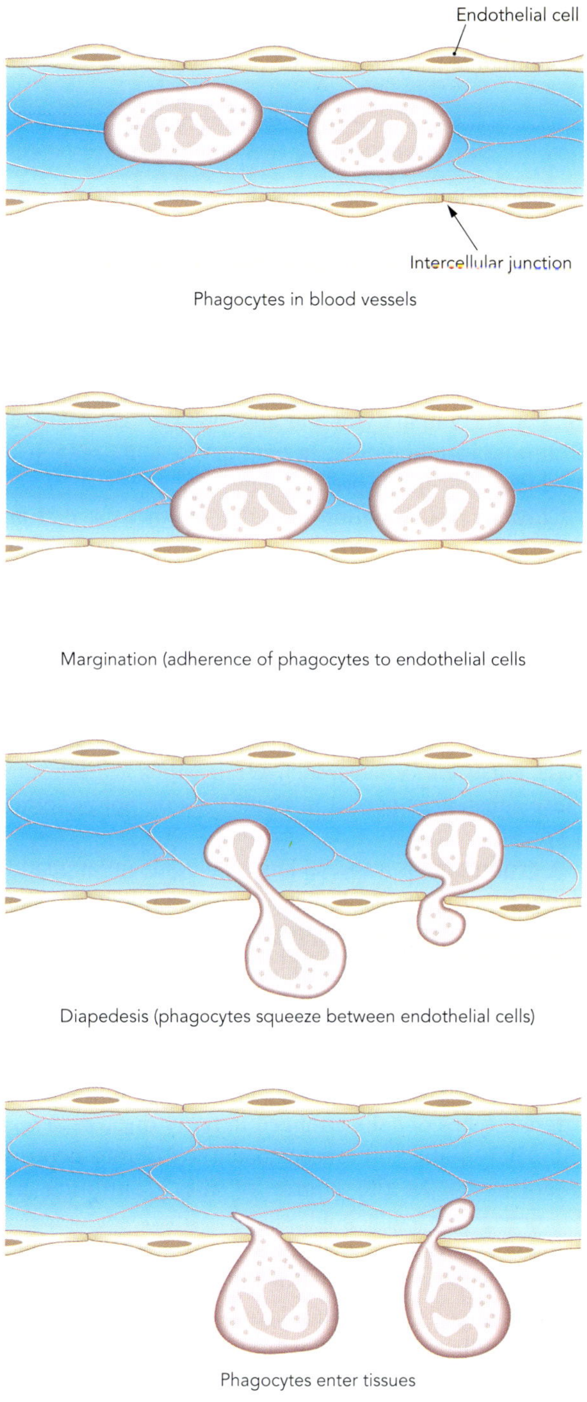

Repair

During the final stages of inflammation, tissue repair begins, but can only be completed if all microbes, other foreign material and damaged tissue cells have been effectively removed from the area. The most favourable outcome is the restoration of the tissue's original structure and physiologic function by **regeneration**, the proliferation of remaining cells by mitosis. This occurs if the destroyed tissue is capable of regeneration, if the damage is minor, or if there are no other complications. If the tissue is incapable of regeneration (e.g. nerve tissue), or is extensively damaged, or if the clean-up is incomplete (e.g. in abscess formation), the tissue is repaired by **scar tissue replacement**. Scar tissue is comprised mainly of collagen. It fills in the lesion but it does not have the physiological functions of the destroyed tissue.

Chronic inflammation

Chronic inflammation occurs if the acute inflammatory response is unsuccessful in eliminating the organisms or foreign material from the tissues. For example, if foreign objects (e.g. glass, dirt) and/or bacteria persist in a wound, the inflammatory response may continue beyond two weeks. In chronic inflammation, pus may be formed continuously, sometimes for months or even years. Large number, of lymphocytes and macrophages are involved in chronic inflammation, in contrast to acute responses in which neutrophils predominate.

Chronic inflammation can also occur as a distinct process from the outset, in the absence of acute inflammation. Certain microbes, such as the bacteria that cause tuberculosis, leprosy, and brucellosis, induce chronic inflammation because of their resistance to intracellular digestion by phagocytes. The persistence of these organisms continues to stimulate an inflammatory response. Other agents that typically evoke chronic inflammation are low-grade, persistent irritants, such as talc, silica and asbestos. These substances persist in tissues but do not penetrate or spread.

A **granuloma** is a special kind of chronic inflammation produced in response to certain microorganisms, such as the bacteria that cause leprosy, tuberculosis and syphilis, the fungus that causes histoplasmosis and the protozoan of toxoplasmosis. Granulomas are formed in these infections because the macrophages are unable to eliminate the organisms, so the body responds by walling off the infected site. Granulomas typically consist of a mass of different types of cells arranged in fairly discrete layers, completely walled off (encapsulated) by fibrous deposits of collagen. At the centre of the granuloma are macrophages or 'epithelioid cells' (modified macrophages) clumped in a mass, or coalesced together to form a multi-nucleated cell. Around these giant cells is a layer of epithelioid cells and then a layer of lymphocytes. This mass of cells represents the body's attempt to surround and isolate the foreign agent. Granulomas are sometimes given special names such as 'gummas' in syphilis and 'tubercles' in tuberculosis.

In the past, surgical gloves were dusted with talc powder so that they would slip on easily, but it was found that particles of talc often entered the surgical field and caused granulomas to develop there after surgery. Gloves are now dusted with an absorbant starch to eliminate this problem.

Fever

Inflammation is the local response to tissue damage. **Fever**, higher than normal body temperature, is a possible systemic response to microorganisms and often accompanies severe or systemic inflammation. Body temperature is regulated by a cluster of neurons in the hypothalamus, considered to be the body's thermostat. Normally, the thermostat is set at approximately 37°C. Fever occurs when the set-point of the thermostat is raised to a higher temperature.

Pyrogens are chemical substances which produce fever. They are referred to as **exogenous pyrogens** if they come from outside the body and **endogenous pyrogens** if they are formed inside the body. Exogenous pyrogens are, in the main, components of microorganisms, the best characterised being the lipopolysaccharide (endotoxin—see Chapter 10) of the cell wall of Gram-negative bacteria. Endogenous pyrogens are released from macrophages and neutrophils during inflammation or in response to the presence of exogenous pyrogens. The best known endogenous pyrogens are interleukin-1 (IL-1) and tumour necrosis factor (TNF). These are the substances that actually alter the set-point in the hypothalamus, whereas exogenous pyrogens act indirectly by causing their release. This is summarised in Figure 9.9.

The clinical approach to the treatment of fever has changed in recent years. In the past, **antipyretic** (fever-reducing) drugs and physical measures (e.g. tepid baths) were routinely used to reduce fever. Now, there are many who advocate allowing a slight to moderate fever to run its course. Although high fevers (above 40°C) are dangerous because of the possibility of thermal damage to nerve cells, and convulsions, mild or moderate fever may have some benefit for the body. The rate of cell division of

FIGURE 9.9
THE PRODUCTION OF FEVER

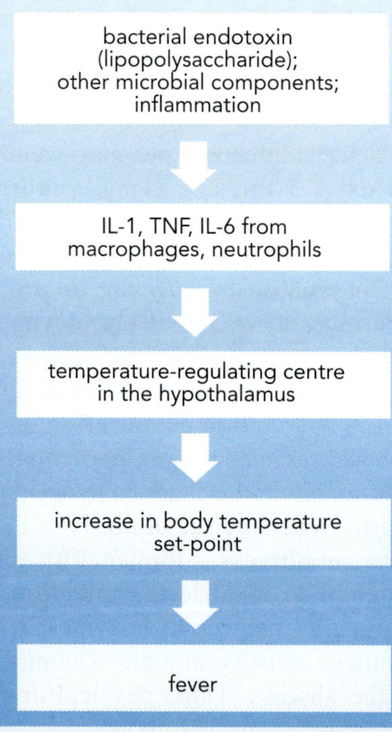

bacteria is slowed at temperatures above 37°C. Also, bacteria require iron and zinc for growth, but during fever the liver and spleen sequester these nutrients, making them less available. A small increase in body temperature may also increase the metabolic rate and activity of defence cells, such as T-lymphocytes and phagocytes, and is also thought to speed up repair processes.

It is accepted, however, that high fever, or fever in patients with cardiovascular disease, seizures or respiratory disorders, should be treated immediately. Antipyretic drugs such as aspirin appear to reduce fever by restoring the temperature set-point in the hypothalamus to normal.

ANTIMICROBIAL PROTEINS

Apart from the various protective chemicals mentioned earlier in this chapter, the body also has certain antimicrobial proteins that act non-specifically. The most important of these are the complement proteins and interferon.

Complement

The complement system, or simply **complement,** comprises a complex system of plasma proteins that are present in the blood in an inactive state. The major components of the system are designated as factors C1 through to C9 (C stands for complement), and factors B, D and properdin. It is an enzymatic cascade system, similar to the blood coagulation system. When it is activated, the complement system enhances the inflammatory response and is largely responsible for the destruction of foreign cells in the body. Its major functions are to:

- enhance phagocytosis;
- produce inflammation;
- directly lyse foreign cells.

Although complement acts non-specifically, it 'complements' or enhances the action of many non-specific and specific defences, and is in turn enhanced by specific defences.

Complement can be activated by either of two pathways or cascades (outlined in Figure 9.10): the classical pathway or the alternate pathway. The **classical pathway** is initiated by the binding of antibodies to antigen (see p. 193). Complement proteins are activated and fixed to a receptor on antibody molecules in a step called **complement fixation**. The **alternate (alternative) pathway** is initiated by an interaction between properdin, factors B and D, and the polysaccharides that are present in the walls of many microorganisms.

In both pathways the complement proteins are activated in a particular sequence, with each protein activating the next one in the sequence. Both pathways lead to the cleavage of large amounts of C3 into two fragments (C3a and C3b). These fragments are responsible for the induction of three different processes which result in the destruction of foreign cells and substances. They are cytolysis (cell breakage), opsonisation (enhancement of phagocytosis) and inflammation.

FIGURE 9.10
THE PATHWAYS OF COMPLEMENT ACTIVATION AND ITS BIOLOGICAL ACTIVITIES

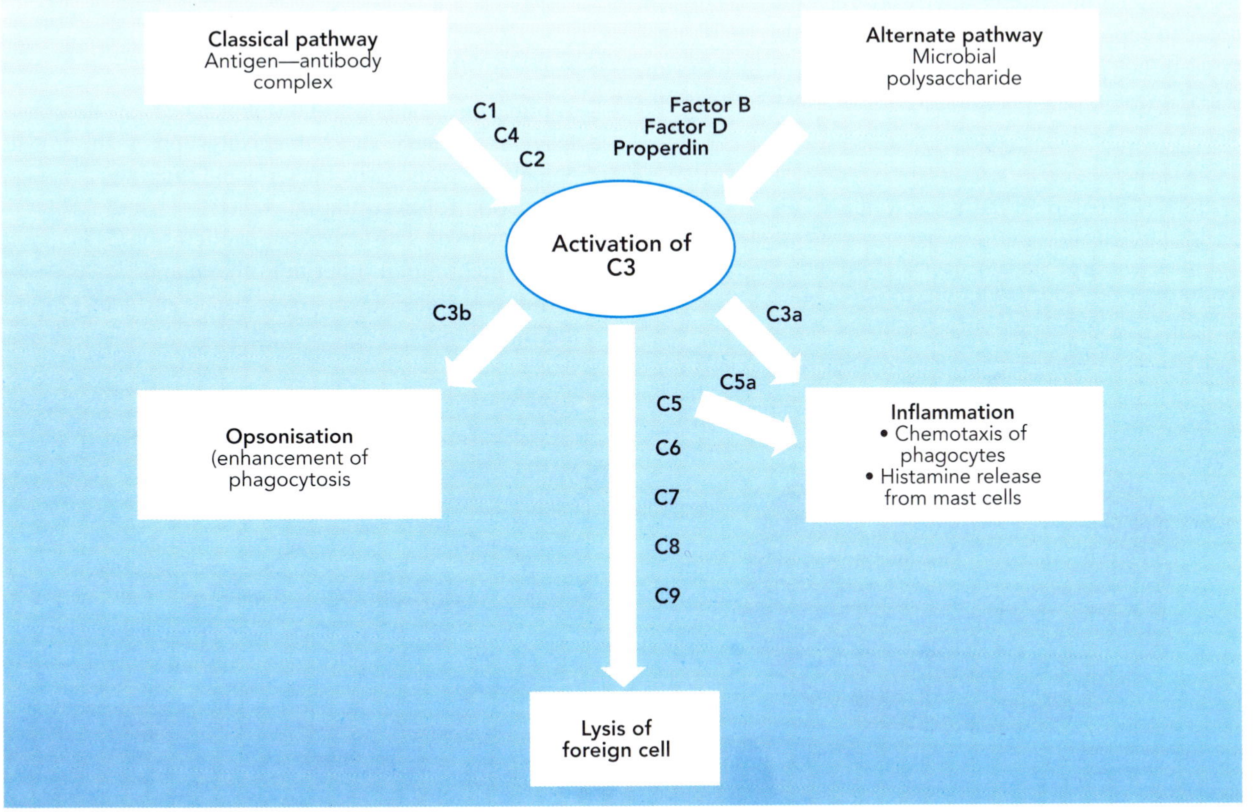

The complement proteins are able to destroy foreign cells by damaging their cell membranes. This **cytolysis** is initiated by the C3b fragment and other components which activate the C5 to C9 sequence of reactions. The activated proteins produced from these reactions form a complex which is inserted into the foreign cell membrane (see Figure 9.11). This **membrane attack complex** acts as a trans-membrane channel which allows the leakage of water and electrolytes out of the cell and, ultimately, cytolysis. Complement-mediated cytolysis is important in protection against microorganisms, and is also the basis for other reactions, such as transfusion reaction following transfusion of incompatible blood, transplant rejection and some autoimmune diseases.

The C3b fragment can also bind covalently to the surface of microorganisms and then bind with specific C3b receptors on phagocytes. By binding to both the microbe and the phagocyte, the C3b effectively holds the microorganism against the surface of the phagocyte (see Figure 9.12), thereby promoting the phagocyte's ability to ingest the organism. This enhancement of phagocyte activity is termed **opsonisation** and the C3b is called an **opsonin**.

C3a (the other cleavage product of C3) and C5a (the cleavage product of C5) are **anaphylatoxins**; that is, they bind to mast cells, basophils and platelets, triggering the release of histamine and other substances (see Figure 9.10). As mentioned earlier in this chapter, histamine and leukotrienes are major inducers of inflammation. C5a also contributes to inflammation by acting as a potent chemotactic factor, attracting phagocytes to the site of injury.

Interferon

As explained in Chapter 5, viruses must invade cells in order to reproduce. It was discovered in the 1950s that virus-infected cells secrete a protein called **interferon (IFN)**, which helps neighbouring cells resist infection.

FIGURE 9.11
THE MEMBRANE ATTACK COMPLEX OF COMPLEMENT
Complement proteins are inserted into the membrane of the foreign cell, forming a pore through which the cell contents can leak out.

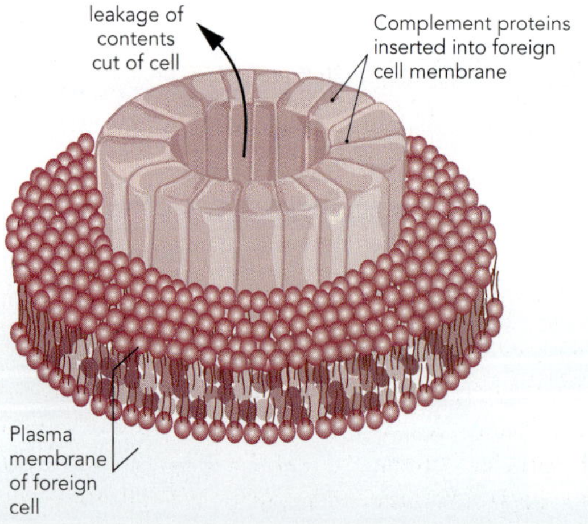

It is thought that the IFN molecules bind to specific receptors on nearby cells, where they stimulate the synthesis of enzymes that interfere with viral replication in those cells. The IFN, however, does not kill viruses and has no effect on cells already infected. One of the important features of the 'antiviral state' induced by IFN is that it is *not virus-specific*; that is, IFN produced against a particular virus protects against a variety of other viruses. However, interferons are host-specific. That is, only human IFN is effective in humans.

When attempts were made to purify interferon it was discovered that it is actually a group of related proteins produced by different body cells. Leukocytes produce alpha interferon (IFN-α), whereas fibroblasts, epithelial cells, macrophages and possibly all body cells secrete beta interferon (IFN-β). The third type, gamma interferon (IFN-γ), is secreted by lymphocytes. In addition to their antiviral activity, the interferons play important roles in enhancing the actions of macrophages, natural killer cells and other defence cells.

When interferons were discovered, it was hoped they would be useful in the treatment of viral diseases. Interferons are made only in very small amounts in the body, so it was not until the 1980s, when genetic engineering techniques were successfully used to produce these proteins synthetically, that clinical trials were commenced. Unfortunately, interferon has been only partially successful in a few situations (e.g. in chronic hepatitis B and C, and herpes zoster infections). One of the major problems with the therapeutic use of interferons is the possible side effects of long-term use (e.g. fatigue, muscle pains, toxicity to the kidneys and bone marrow). However, because of the theoretical potential of interferon, the search for therapeutic applications continues.

THE NORMAL MICROBIAL FLORA

The normal microbial flora of the human body are described in detail in Chapter 8. These organisms suppress the growth of potentially pathogenic bacteria and fungi by:

- competing for essential nutrients;
- secreting toxic substances (e.g. colicins of *Escherichia coli*, which inhibit other microbes); and
- forming bacterial layers over tissue surfaces (e.g. in the intestine).

FIGURE 9.12
OPSONISATION OF A BACTERIAL CELL BY COMPLEMENT

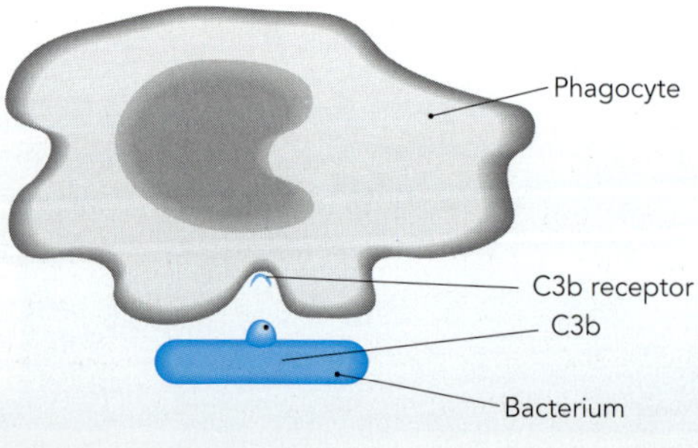

The importance of the normal flora in preventing infection is clearly demonstrated when broad spectrum antibiotics are administered to a patient. In some cases, such drugs can reduce the normal flora and allow infection to occur. Thrush, caused by the yeast *Candida albicans*, is an infection of the oral cavity, or gastrointestinal or genital tracts, that often follows broad spectrum antibiotic therapy.

Specific Body Defences: The Acquired Immune System

The specific body defences, or **acquired immune system** (also called the **specific immune system**, **adaptive immune system**), is a functional system consisting of a variety of cells, especially lymphocytes and macrophages, and various organs such as the thymus gland and lymph nodes. It is the body's second line of defence and protects it from infection and from damage by other foreign cells and substances that enter the body; it is also active against cancer cells. If it fails or is disabled, serious diseases such as cancer or life-threatening infections may result. **Immunity** is the capacity of the immune system (the acquired immune system plus some components of the non-specific immune system) to successfully defend the body against a potentially infectious agent. **Immunology** is the study of the immune system and immunity.

CHARACTERISTICS OF THE ACQUIRED IMMUNE SYSTEM

The non-specific immune system is highly effective in quickly eliminating microorganisms from the body, but many microbes find ways around these defences. When a microbe is able to persist in the tissues, the body reacts by producing a response specifically directed against the invading organism. This is the **immune response**. It is responsible for:

- identifying the antigens (foreign molecules) of the microbes;
- producing a specific defence reaction to destroy the microbes;
- providing memory, which enables the body to react more vigorously on subsequent exposures to the same microbes.

The immune response also amplifies the inflammatory response and enhances the activation of complement.

It has been known for centuries that, once someone has an infectious disease, they are unlikely to have the same disease again. The basis of this immunity was revealed in 1890, when Emil von Behring and Shibasaburo Kitasato demonstrated that animals that survive an infection have protective factors (now called antibodies) in their blood that protect them against future attacks by the same pathogen. It was further shown that serum from surviving animals, when injected into other animals, protected them from the same infection. These and subsequent studies revealed some important characteristics of the acquired immune system.

- It is able to distinguish between host substances (self) and foreign substances (non-self)—that is, it *recognises* foreign substances.
- It is directed only against the particular pathogen or foreign substance that stimulated it—that is, it is *specific*.
- It recognises and mounts a more rapid and stronger response to a previously encountered pathogen—that is, it has *memory*.

THE DUAL NATURE OF THE ACQUIRED IMMUNE SYSTEM

In the 1960s it was found that, for some diseases, injection of antibody-containing serum did not protect recipients from the disease the donor had survived, but that injection of the donor's lymphocytes did provide immunity. Jacques Miller in London, and Warner and Szenberg (of the Walter and Eliza Hall Institute in Melbourne) determined that there are two different populations of lymphocytes, termed **B lymphocytes** (or **B cells**) and **T lymphocytes** (or **T cells**). Each type is responsible for a different form of immunity.

Humoral immunity is immunity provided by **antibodies**, which are present in the body's 'humors' or fluids. The antibodies are produced and secreted by plasma cells (derived from B lymphocytes) and they then circulate in the blood and other body fluids. Antibodies are most effective against bacteria, their toxins and viruses *before* they enter host cells. They act by binding to microbes or their products, leading to their inactivation and destruction or elimination by various means (see p. 195).

Because antibodies are unable to enter cells, another type of defence is needed to deal with intracellular pathogens. This is called **cellular immunity** or **cell-mediated immunity**, because of the direct involvement of cells in the immune processes. In cell-mediated immunity, T lymphocytes act against target cells by directly lysing the cells, or by releasing chemicals that enhance the inflammatory response and/or activate other defence cells to bring about destruction of the target cells. Cell-mediated immunity provides the major form of defence against viruses and bacteria that have invaded host cells, and also against fungi, other eucaryotic parasites and cancer cells.

Before describing the humoral and cell-mediated responses separately, we will consider the cells involved in these two components of the immune response and the foreign substances that trigger their activity.

CELLS AND TISSUES OF THE ACQUIRED IMMUNE SYSTEM

Cellular components

The cells that are primarily responsible for a specific immune response are the lymphocytes and macrophages. As stated above, the **B lymphocytes** are mainly responsible for humoral immunity and the **T lymphocytes** provide the cell-mediated immunity. These two types of lymphocytes interact with macrophages to produce a specific immune response to a large variety of pathogenic microorganisms and other foreign substances and cells.

Lymphocytes are the second most numerous type of white cell in blood, and their total number in the body is among the highest of all body cells. Like all blood cells, lymphocytes originate in the bone marrow. Immature lymphocytes are released from the marrow and mature into B cells or T cells depending on the site in the body where they undergo final maturation and become immunocompetent. T cells are lymphocytes that migrate from the bone marrow to the thymus, where they undergo a maturation process under the direction of thymic hormones (hence the term T cell). After puberty the thymus regresses in size and becomes replaced by fatty tissue; other sites, such as the skin and mucosal lymphoid tissue, are then thought to become responsible for T cell maturation.

B cells are believed to mature in the bone marrow itself (or in the liver in the foetus). B cells are so called because they were first identified in the 'bursa of Fabricius', a pouch of lymphatic tissue associated with the digestive tract in birds. Since the thymus and the bone marrow are the sites of lymphocyte maturation, they are referred to as the **primary lymphoid organs** (see Figure 9.13). The collection of lymphoid organs and tissues described in the next section are the sites in the body where immune reactions occur, and are referred to as the **secondary lymphoid organs**.

On the surface of mature lymphocytes there are numerous receptors of a single, unique type that enable the cells to recognise and bind to a single, specific antigen (foreign substance). This means that each lymphocyte reacts with one particular antigen, and no others, because all the antigen receptors on its surface are the same and specific for that antigen. For example, receptors of one lymphocyte can recognise only the toxin of the tetanus-causing bacterium, whereas those of another lymphocyte might bind to the cold virus. Generally, there will be populations of both T lymphocytes and B lymphocytes that recognise each type of antigen.

The exact processes involved in lymphocyte processing and maturation are still not clear, but it is known that lymphocytes become immunocompetent and specific for a particular antigen before actually coming into contact with that antigen. That is, the specific foreign substances that the immune system is able to recognise and respond to are predetermined. Importantly, they are predetermined by genes, not by the antigens that are contacted. This means that, to be effective, the immune system must consist of precommitted lymphocytes for all the possible antigens that people are likely to contact over the whole of their lifetime. Obviously, only some of the possible antigens our lymphocytes are programmed to recognise will ever be encountered and, therefore, only some of the immunocompetent cells present in the body will ever be utilised.

Immunocompetent T cells and B cells migrate to lymph nodes, the spleen, and other lymphoid organs, where encounters with foreign antigens occur. In the next section we describe how these lymphoid organs are strategically placed throughout the body to contact foreign substances when they enter. Many lymphocytes move about freely between lymphoid organs and the tissues, transported in the bloodstream and lymphatic system.

We have already examined the role of macrophages in non-specific immunity, particularly in relation to inflammation and the phagocytosis of foreign material, but these cells also play an important role in specific immunity. They are widely distributed throughout the lymphoid organs, as well as connective tissues, and interact significantly with lymphocytes. In fact, macrophage-lymphocyte interactions form the basis of many of the processes of the immune system.

The lymphatic system

The lymphatic system is a network of vessels, cells and specialised organs. Lymph is the fluid that is formed in tissues from certain blood components that enter the extracellular spaces. The lymph is drained from the tissues and carried in lymph capillaries that converge into larger vessels, ultimately returning the lymph back to the circulatory system. On its way, the lymph is filtered through numerous lymph nodes. The **lymph nodes** are small, bean-shaped organs that tend to occur in clusters along lymphatic channels. Because lymph capillaries carry substances and pathogens absorbed from nearly all body tissues, immune

FIGURE 9.13
THE MATURATION OF LYMPHOCYTES
The maturation of immature lymphocytes occurs in the thymus and bone marrow, where they become antigen-specific T cells and B cells respectively. After puberty, the thymus gland begins to decrease in size and T cell maturation occurs in other sites.

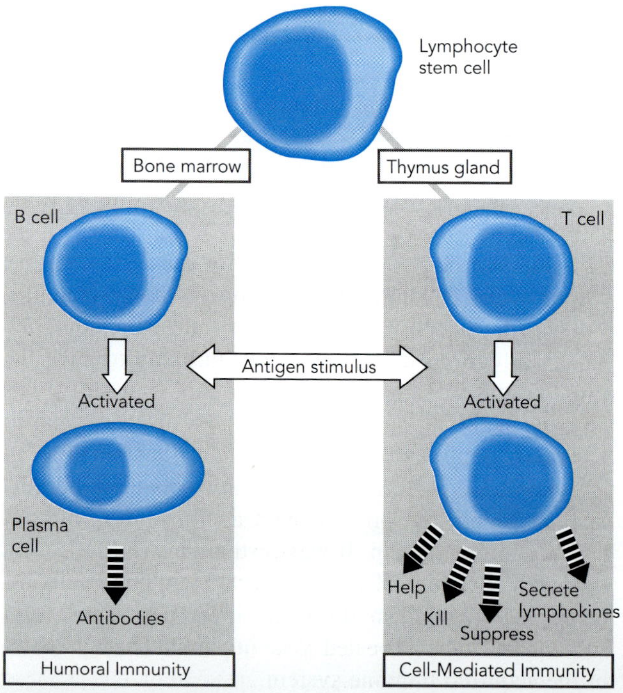

cells in lymph nodes are in a strategic position to encounter antigens that have entered tissues.

The secondary lymphoid organs comprise the lymph nodes as well as the spleen, tonsils and clusters of lymphoid cells in the gastrointestinal tract, respiratory tract and other mucosal surfaces. The clusters of lymphoid cells lining the mucosal surfaces are called gut-associated lymphoid tissue (GALT), bronchi-associated lymphoid tissue (BALT) and so on, or are collectively referred to as the mucosa-associated lymphoid tissue (MALT).

The lymphoid organs have a common structure that is a loose framework housing numerous lymphocytes and macrophages. Moreover, they are strategically placed throughout the body to provide defence where it is likely to be needed (see Figure 9.14). For example, lymphocytes and macrophages in the tonsils act primarily against microorganisms that invade the oral and nasal cavities, whereas the spleen acts as a filter to trap blood-borne antigens. Collections of lymphocytes underlying mucosal surfaces provide local defence at those sites.

The **thymus** is found in the upper thoracic region beneath the sternum (breastbone). Its size, proportional to the rest of the body, is greatest at birth. It continues to grow until puberty, after which it progressively shrinks to become largely replaced by fatty tissue in later adulthood. As mentioned earlier, immature lymphocytes develop into mature T cells under the influence of thymic hormones. By adulthood enough mature T cells have been produced so that thymus size and function can be reduced. The importance of the thymus gland is clearly demonstrated in babies born without a functional thymus (DiGeorge syndrome). These children are highly susceptible to infection—even common childhood infections like chickenpox can be very serious, and even fatal.

Macrophages in lymphoid organs tend to remain there, whereas lymphocytes, especially the T cells, circulate continuously between the bloodstream and lymphoid organs. This enables the lymphocytes to come into contact with antigens present in different parts of the body, as well as with other lymphocytes and antigen-presenting cells.

To summarise: the acquired immune system's ability to identify and destroy foreign substances is based on the ability of its cells, the lymphocytes, to recognise and respond to foreign substances (antigens) in the body. Different lymphocytes interact with one another and with other cells to mount a concerted response specific to each antigen.

ANTIGENS

Antigens are foreign substances (i.e. different to substances in the body) that activate the acquired immune system of the body and induce an immune response. The word 'antigen' is in fact a contraction of the term '*anti*body *gen*erating'. Most antigens are large, complex molecules (macromolecules) of the following types: proteins (and polypeptides), lipoproteins, glycoproteins, nucleoproteins and polysaccharides. Antigens are present on the surfaces of viruses, bacteria and other microorganisms, and human and animal cells.

Complete antigens and haptens

Complete antigens are foreign substances that stimulate specific T and B lymphocytes, inducing them to produce an immune response. Complete antigens are thus said to be **immunogenic** (or **antigenic**), that is, capable of inducing an immune response. A large variety of substances can be complete antigens, including proteins, nucleic acids, some lipids and large polysaccharides. In general, proteins tend to be the strongest antigens. Microorganisms are highly immunogenic because they possess many different foreign molecules (antigenic determinants), many of which are proteins exposed on the cell surface.

In contrast, smaller molecules, such as peptides, nucleotides and saccharides, are generally not immunogenic, even though they are foreign. However, some of them become immunogenic if they become attached to the body's own proteins, and the immune system recognises the combination as foreign. A small molecule such as this is called a **hapten**. Although haptens

FIGURE 9.14
THE COMPONENTS OF THE LYMPHATIC SYSTEM
The lymph vessels, lymph nodes, thymus, spleen, tonsils and aggregates of lymphocytes lining the small intestine (gut-associated lymphoid tissue, GALT), bronchi (BALT) and other mucosal surfaces.

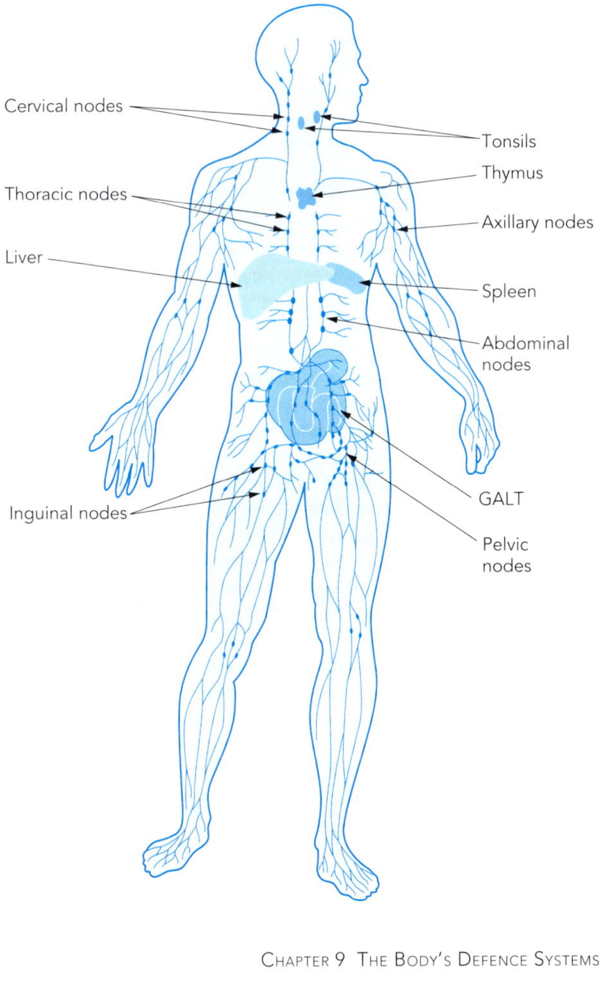

cannot initiate an immune response on their own, they can react with antibodies or activated T cells produced against them. A good example of a hapten is penicillin, which can bind with a serum protein in some people and induce an immune response. In this case the immune response is manifested as an allergic reaction (see p. 202), which can be life-threatening.

Epitopes

Although antigens are foreign molecules of a certain size, only a small part of the whole antigen molecule is immunogenic. This important part of the molecule is called the **epitope** (or **antigenic determinant**), and is the part to which free antibodies or activated B or T lymphocytes can bind.

Most naturally occurring antigens are very complex molecules and consist of a number of different epitopes (see Figure 9.15). Different epitopes are recognised by different lymphocytes; thus, a single, complex antigen may activate many different lymphocytes, stimulating the formation of many different kinds of antibodies. Large proteins often comprise hundreds of different epitopes, which is why these substances are so strongly immunogenic. In contrast, substances made of large molecules, formed from many identical repeating units, such as plastics, are often non-immunogenic. Such substances are ideal for making artificial body implants (e.g. bone replacements) because they are not recognised as foreign by the immune system, and therefore not rejected.

HUMORAL IMMUNITY

Antigen processing

If foreign cells or particulate antigens enter the body and evade the non-specific defences, they then encounter the cells and tissues of the lymphatic system. Macrophages

FIGURE 9.15
DIFFERENT EPITOPES (ANTIGENIC DETERMINANTS) ON A BACTERIAL CELL
Bacteria generally have multiple epitopes on their surface, each one capable of stimulating a different antibody response.

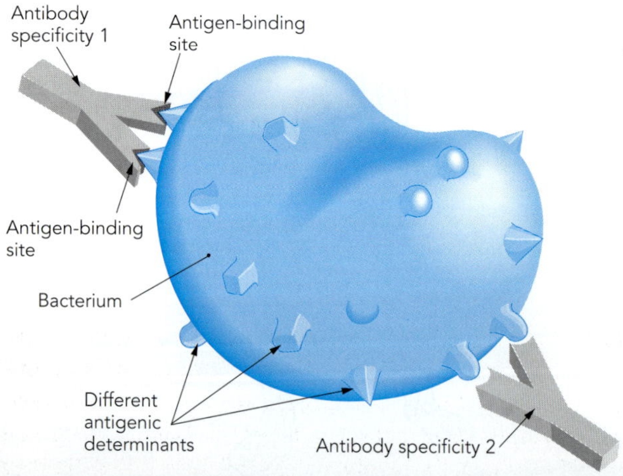

or dendritic cells (highly branched cells in lymphoid tissues) are usually the first cells to recognise the antigens. They are called antigen-presenting cells because they engulf and process antigen for presentation to lymphocytes. This processing, which involves partial degradation of antigen and its attachment to special recognition molecules on the surface of presenting cells, enables lymphocytes to recognise and respond to the antigen. Antigen processing and presentation by these specialised cells is the trigger necessary for lymphocyte activation to occur (see Figure 9.16). The first encounter between an immunocompetent lymphocyte and an invading antigen often takes place in the spleen or a lymph node, but may happen in any lymphoid tissue. If the lymphocyte is a B cell, the challenging antigen provokes a **humoral immune response**, in which antibodies are produced against the foreign antigen.

Activation of B cells and formation of antibodies

Each mature B lymphocyte carries molecules of specific antibody (the antigen receptor) on its membrane. It is activated when an antigen binds to this specific receptor. As described on p. 197, T cells usually collaborate in this process as well. Following the activation of B cells, there are two distinct phases:

1. Proliferation—to expand the number of cells capable of reacting to the particular antigen; and
2. Differentiation—to obtain functional cells from the newly formed population.

The activating event first stimulates the B cell to transform into a 'blast cell', which is an enlarged, highly active cell prepared for mitotic division. The blast multiplies through successive mitotic divisions to produce a large population of cells all bearing the same antigen receptors (Figure 9.17). This population of cells, all with the same specificity, is called a **clone**. Thus, it is the antigen that does the selecting in clonal selection by 'choosing' a lymphocyte with complementary receptors. This is the basis of the **clonal selection theory**, first proposed by the Australian immunologist Sir Frank Macfarlane Burnet in the 1950s.

After multiplication, the clone cells differentiate into functional cells. Some of them become **plasma cells**, which are the cells responsible for synthesis and secretion of antibodies in humoral immunity. Plasma cells are able to synthesise enormous amounts of antibody (as many as 10 million antibody molecules per hour!) for several days and they then die. Each antibody has the same antigen specificity as the receptor molecules on the surface of the parent B cell. The antibodies are secreted by the plasma cells into the blood and other body fluids, where they can bind to specific antigens and prepare them for destruction by other specific or non-specific mechanisms.

The clone cells that do not become plasma cells become long-lived **memory cells**, which persist in the body for months to years, and can react with the same antigen if it enters the body again at a later time. Memory cells

FIGURE 9.16

ANTIGEN PROCESSING

Specialised antigen-presenting cells, such as macrophages, ingest antigens, process them, and join them to a recognition molecule (called an MHC protein) so that lymphocytes can respond to the antigen

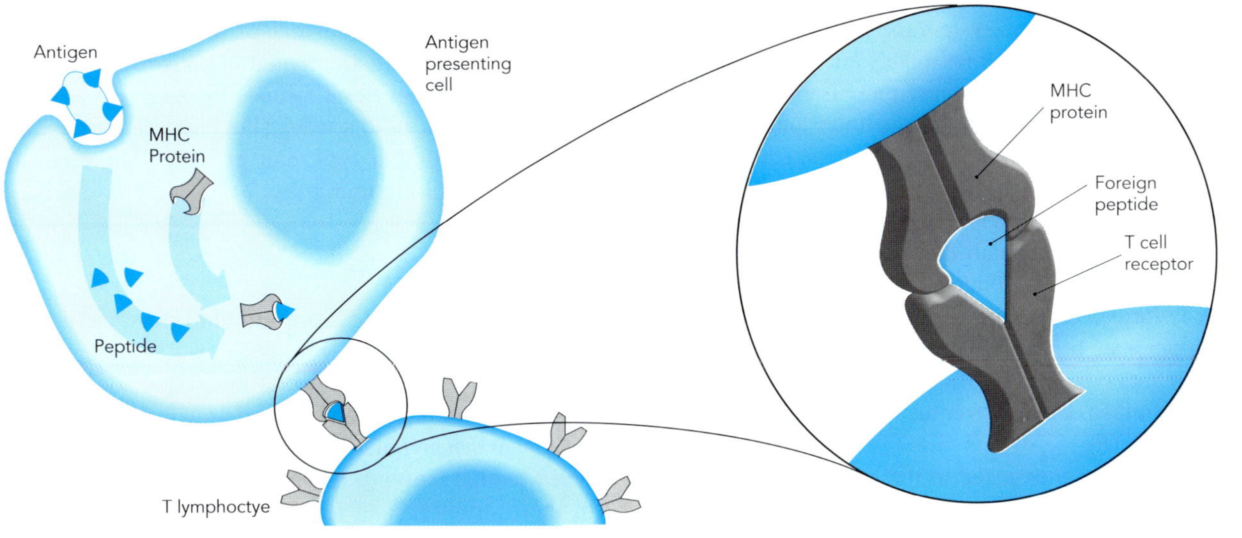

FIGURE 9.17

CLONAL SELECTION

There is a multitude of different lymphocyte populations in the body, each population being able to recognise a single antigen. When an antigen enters the body it virtually selects the clone that is specific to it. When activated by antigen, that small clone proliferates and then differentiates to produce a much larger clone, comprising antibody-secreting plasma cells and long-lived memory cells. All cells in this large clone are specific for the same antigen.

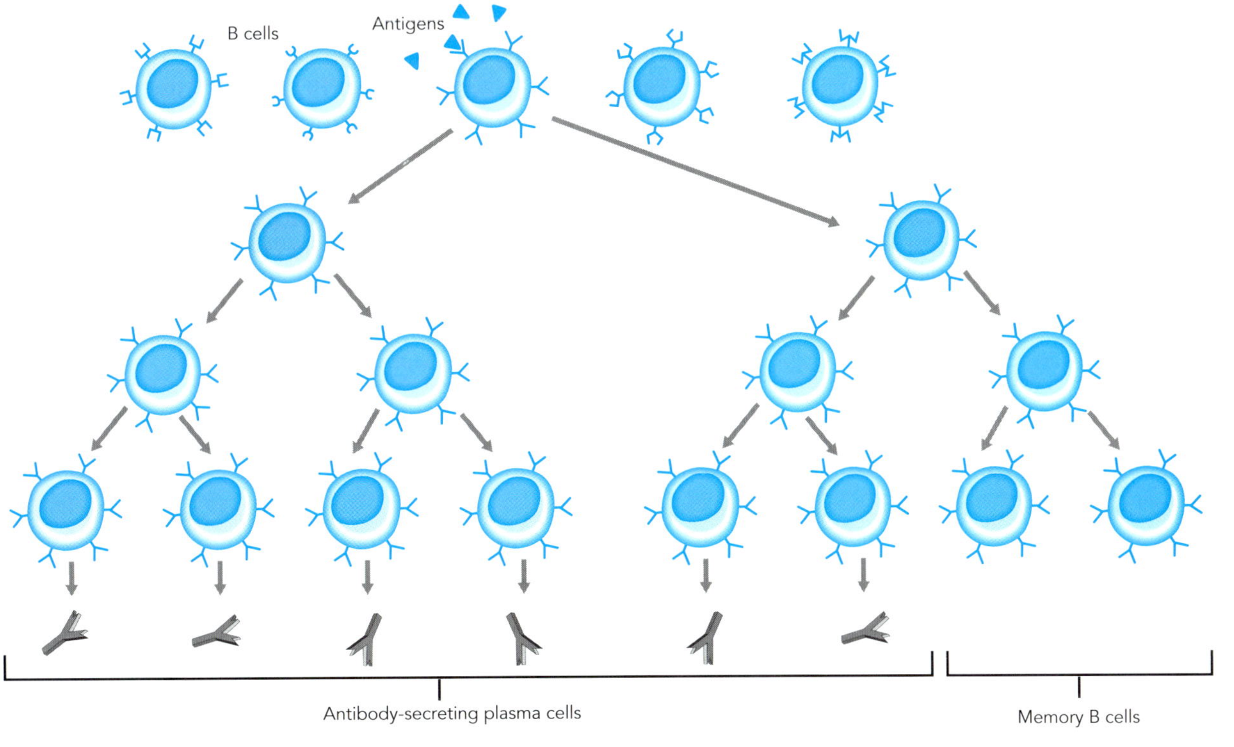

respond to antigenic stimulation in the same way that the original parent B cell responded to antigen, again increasing the clone size, producing even more cells with the same specificity. The larger population of memory cells is able to respond more rapidly and more strongly than the group of cells in the original B cell population.

In the activation of the B lymphocyte, an antigen-presenting cell (e.g. a macrophage) and a certain type of T lymphocyte (called a T helper lymphocyte, see p. 197) are usually involved. The cells act on each other by releasing soluble factors, called **cytokines** (see p. 202), which bind to surface receptors on the target cell and regulate their activity.

The events described so far in this section constitute the **primary immune response**; that is, the response of the acquired immune system the first time it is exposed to a particular antigen. Immediately after antigen challenge in a primary immune response there is characteristically a lag period of several days (sometimes longer), in which there is no observable increase in the specific antibody levels in blood (or serum). During this time there is much activity; the lag period is the time required for processing of antigen, for the small number of B cells specific for the antigen to be activated and proliferate, and for the newly formed cells to differentiate into plasma cells. Once antibodies are being produced in large amounts, the specific serum antibody level begins to rise, peaking within several weeks; it then declines over the next few weeks to months (Figure 9.18).

If a person is exposed to the same antigen a second time, a **secondary immune response** occurs that is:

- faster,
- stronger and
- longer-lasting (Figure 9.18).

The secondary response is very different because the immune system has been primed to the antigen in the primary response, which produced large numbers of memory B lymphocytes. The increased numbers of lymphocytes in the memory pool specific for the antigen give rise to this powerful secondary response. The advantage of this response is that it provides a quick and potent reaction on re-exposure. These memory cells provide what is commonly called **immunological memory**. This memory effect is the basis for giving boosters when using some vaccines. When a booster is given, even more memory cells are produced and the antibody levels in the blood can remain high for many years.

It should be stressed that the primary antibody response described above relates to the injection of non-living (and therefore non-replicating) antigen. In the case of infection or vaccination with a living organism, the antibody reponse is more like that of a combination of primary and secondary responses. The reason for this is that living organisms stimulate the immune system repeatedly as they are replicating in the body. Effectively, it is the equivalent of having multiple boosters of a non-living antigen. Vaccines containing attenuated organisms (see p. 199), which replicate but don't cause disease, stimulate the immune system in this way. Thus, infection or a single vaccination of this type can provide long-term and sometimes lifelong immunity.

Basic antibody structure

Antibodies, also called **immunoglobulins**, are proteins found in blood and other body fluids, including lymph, urine, CSF and mucosal secretions. They constitute the **gammaglobulin** fraction of blood proteins. All antibodies in humans can be grouped into one of five immunoglobulin types (called isotypes or classes), based on differences in their structure and function. We look at how these immunoglobulin classes differ on pages 196–98.

All antibody molecules have a basic structure consisting of four polypeptide chains linked together by disulphide bonds (Figure 9.19). Two of these chains are long and identical to each other, and are called **heavy (H) chains.** The other two chains, the **light (L) chains**, are also identical to each other, but much shorter. The molecule has a Y-shaped structure, which can change to a T shape because of a flexible hinge region, which allows the arms of the molecule to change position. This is the basic, single antibody molecule or *monomer*.

As shown in Figure 9.19, the two 'arms' of the antibody molecule are called **antigen-binding fragments (Fab)**, and at the ends of the arms are grooves called the **antigen-binding sites**, which is where the molecule binds to its antigen. The remainder, or tail part, of the molecule is called the **crystallisable fragment (Fc)**. There are two antigen-binding sites per monomer. The high specificity of the antigen-binding sites for their antigens is similar to that

FIGURE 9.18
THE PRIMARY AND SECONDARY ANTIBODY RESPONSES TO INJECTION OF A NON-REPLICATING ANTIGEN
The secondary response is faster, larger and longer-lasting.

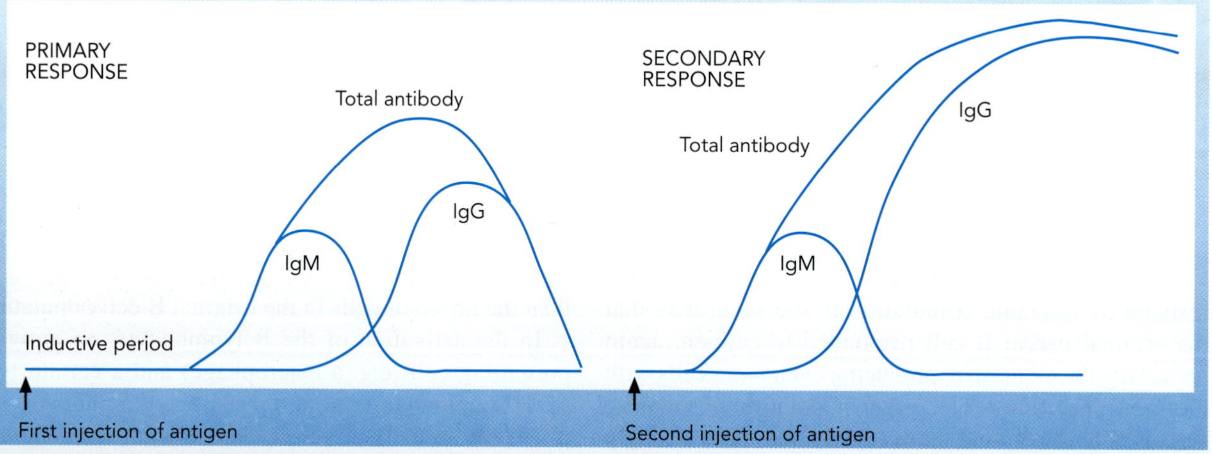

FIGURE 9.19

THE BASIC STRUCTURE OF AN ANTIBODY MOLECULE

The four polypeptide chains (two heavy and two light) are joined together by disulphide bonds. In each chain there is a variable region (V) and a constant region (C). Antigen binding occurs in the variable region of the antigen-binding fragment (Fab). The molecule binds the complement proteins and binds to a phagocyte via parts of the Fc region.

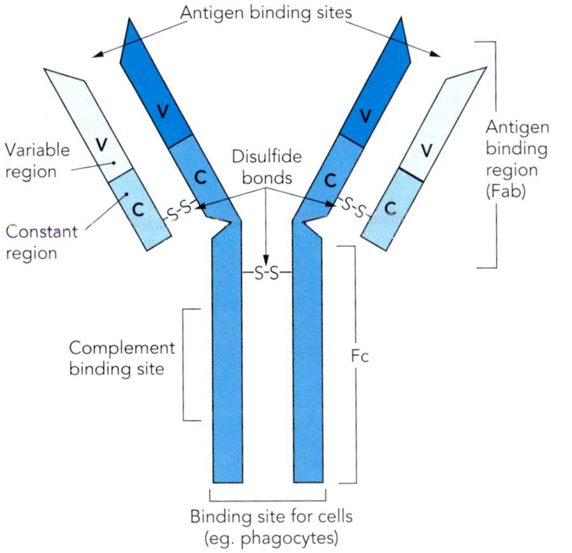

of the active site of enzymes for their substrates. The binding sites are complementary to the antigen. These binding sites have to be different for different antigens, and are part of what is called the *variable (V) region* of the molecule. The specific sequence of the amino acids in the variable region determines the antigen specificity of the antibody. The other end of the molecule is the *constant (C) region*, where the amino acid sequence is the same (or very similar) in all antibodies of the same class. The Fc fragment, which is part of the C region, is involved in binding to other molecules and cells of the immune system.

Antibody classes

Five major immunoglobulin classes have been identified in humans and are designated IgD, IgM, IgG, IgA and IgE, on the basis of differences in the C regions of their heavy chains. 'Ig' stands for immunoglobulin, followed by a letter designating the different types of heavy chains. As illustrated in Figure 9.20, IgG, IgD and IgE have the single, basic Y-shaped structure and therefore exist as monomers. IgA exists as either a monomer or dimer (two linked monomers). Also different to other antibody classes, IgM is made from five linked monomers.

Each class of antibody has a different biological function. For example, IgM is the first type of antibody that is produced after primary antigenic stimulation, and lasts for only a short time (weeks to months) in body fluids. IgG is the most abundant antibody in blood and is the type that persists for months to years after antigenic stimulation (see Figure 9.18), thus providing long-term protection. It is the only antibody class that is able to cross the placental barrier from mother to foetus.

IgA is found primarily in the mucous that covers the body's mucosal surfaces. In these secretions it exists as a dimer and has an extra component, called a secretory piece, which makes it resistant to proteolytic digestion by enzymes in these fluids. IgA plays a major role in preventing pathogens from gaining entry into the body by stopping them from crossing the epithelium. IgA aggregates antigens and keeps them in the secretions, and when the secretions are expelled so, too, are the antigens.

The monomeric forms of IgM and IgD are membrane proteins present on the surface of B lymphocytes where they act as antigen receptors. IgE antibodies are thought to be involved in immunity to worm infections of the intestinal tract, and also in some allergic reactions. These and other characteristics unique to each of the immunoglobulin classes are summarised in Table 9.2.

The basis of antibody diversity

It is thought that the acquired immune system of a person can make antibodies to millions of different antigens. Given the number of possible antigens in the world that the body might contact, this would seem to be necessary if the immune system is to protect us against most microorganisms. Since antibodies, like all proteins, are coded for by genes, it might be expected that an individual has millions of genes just for antibodies. However, this cannot be the case, since humans are thought to have only about 100 000 genes for all the proteins that the body's cells must make. There are believed to be only about 600 genes for antibodies.

The critical question that vexed immunologists for many years was how so few genes could produce so many different antibody proteins. The answer began to unfold in the 1970s when it was shown that the genes that code for antibodies are not present as such in embryonic cells. Instead of containing a complete set of antibody genes, embryonic cells contain sets of mini-genes that act as an 'erector set' for antibody genes. Antibody diversity

FIGURE 9.20

THE STRUCTURES OF THE FIVE CLASSES OF HUMAN IMMUNOGLOBULINS

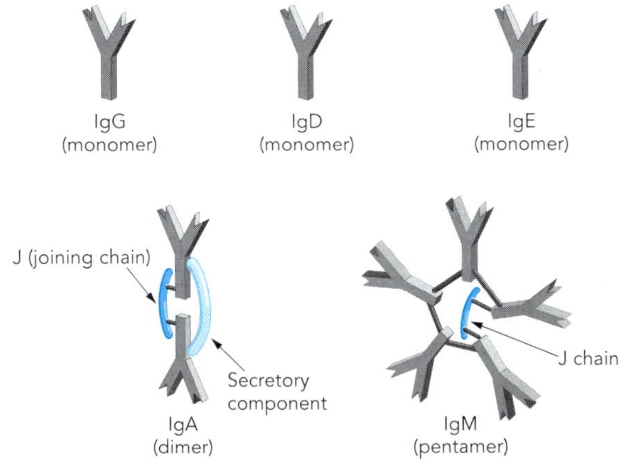

TABLE 9.2
THE BIOLOGICAL PROPERTIES OF HUMAN IMMUNOGLOBULINS

	IgG	IgM	IgA	IgE	IgD
Bind to antigen	yes	yes	yes	yes	yes
Cross the placenta (protects foetus)	yes	no	no	no	no
Trigger complement system	yes	yes	no	no	no
Fix to mast cells and basophils (involved in allergic reactions)	no	no	no	yes	no
Bind to phagocytic cells (enhances phagocyte activity)	yes	no	sometimes	no	no

comes from the shuffling and combining of these gene segments in different ways by each B cell as it becomes immunocompetent. The information of these reassembled genes is then expressed as the surface receptors of B cells, and in the antibodies later released by their clone members. The light and heavy chains are manufactured separately and then joined to form the antibody molecule.

This has been likened to using a child's building block set—the set contains a small number of different blocks, but they can be used to build numerous different objects. It is estimated that the diversity in the light and heavy chains allows for almost two million different antibody genes.

However, the random mixing of gene segments to make antibody genes, plus the diversity that results from different combinations of H and L chains, account for only part of the huge number of antibody specificities. The joining process adds even more diversity. The enzymes that combine the gene segments add random DNA bases to the segments as they are being joined.

As a result of gene shuffling and mutation on a large scale, the lymphoid system is thought to be capable of producing millions of different clones of lymphocytes. And according to the clonal selection theory:

- each mature lymphocyte is preprogrammed;
- each mature lymphocyte can respond to one antigen only; and
- each clone of specific lymphocytes is selected and expanded only when the appropriate antigen enters the body.

Because the total lymphocyte population must express such a large number of different specificities, it follows that there can only be a relatively small number of lymphocytes that have the same specificity before first contact with the antigen. A considerable part of the lag period in the antibody response is spent increasing this small number of cells to a larger population, capable of producing large amounts of antibody.

Activities and functions of antibodies

The basic function of antibody molecules is to bind specifically with their antigens and form **antigen-antibody** (or **immune**) **complexes**. Once they have bound to antigen, antibodies help to bring about removal of the antigen from the body in a number of different ways:

- opsonisation;
- complement fixation;
- neutralisation; and
- agglutination or precipitation.

Different actions of antibodies are necessary for different types of antigens. These functions are summarised in Figure 9.21.

Antibodies can **opsonise** antigens in a similar way to complement (Figure 9.22). Microorganisms or other particles, when coated with opsonising antibody, become more readily recognised and ingested by phagocytes. Opsonising antibodies are particularly important defences against microbes that have capsules or other structures that enable them to avoid being ingested by phagocytes (see Chapter 10).

Antibody attachment followed by **complement fixation** (or activation) is an important defence against foreign cells, such as bacteria and cancer cells. When antibodies bind to cellular targets, complement-binding sites are exposed on the Fc fragments of the antibody molecules. This triggers complement fixation which leads to the insertion of complement proteins into the plasma membrane of the foreign cell, creating holes in the membrane and resulting in cell lysis.

Neutralisation is a process in which antibodies bind to and block specific attachment sites on viruses or bacterial exotoxins (toxic substances secreted by bacteria, see Chapter 10). As a result of being coated by antibody, the virus or toxin is prevented from binding to receptor sites on tissue cells, thus preventing invasion or injury. The antigen-antibody complexes are eventually destroyed by phagocytes. **Antitoxin** is the name given to antibodies that neutralise bacterial toxins.

Because antibodies have two or more antigen-binding sites, they can bind to the same epitope on different antigen molecules. In this way, antibodies can cross-link antigens to form large lattices (see Figure 9.21). When cell-bound antigens are cross-linked, clumping of the foreign cells occurs, and this is called **agglutination**. IgM, with

FIGURE 9.21
THE FUNCTIONS OF ANTIBODIES
Antibodies have different functions depending on the class of the antibody and the nature of the antigen. Once bound to antigen, antibodies can enhance the phagocytosis of particulate antigens (called opsonisation), aggregate particulate antigens (called agglutination), coat toxins and viruses (called neutralisation) or, in conjunction with the complement system, cause lysis and death of foreign cells.

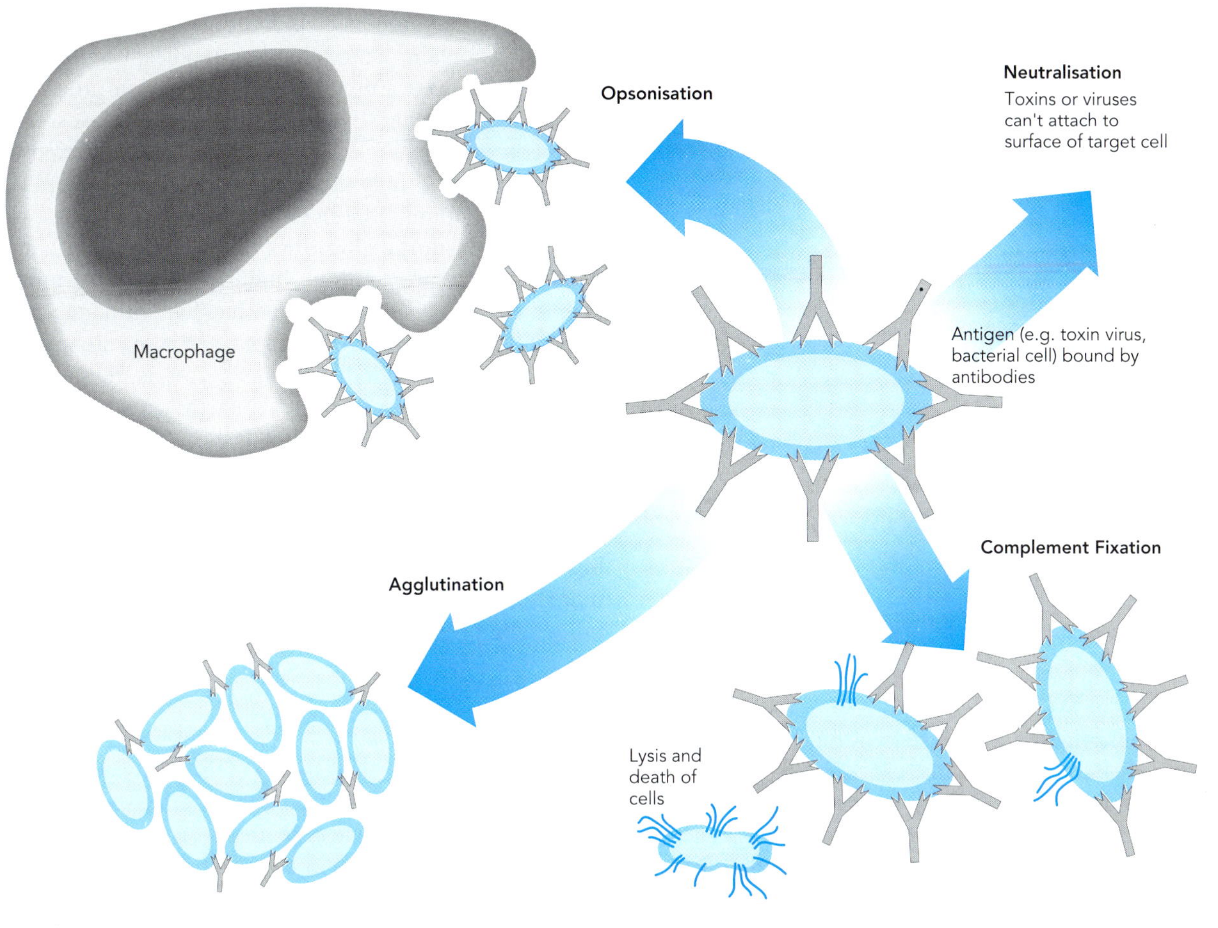

(theoretically) ten antigen-binding sites (see Figure 9.20), is a very potent agglutinating antibody. Examples of this type of reaction occur with bacterial cells and with foreign red cells when mismatched blood is transfused. In **precipitation**, soluble molecules (instead of cells) are cross-linked into large complexes which then precipitate out of solution. The benefits of these reactions are that agglutinated bacteria and precipitated foreign molecules are much more easily identified and captured by phagocytes.

The Fc part of the antibody molecule also has functions. Once antigen is bound, areas of the Fc fragment become activated and can bind to receptors on some host defence cells, including macrophages, neutrophils and mast cells. In opsonisation, the antibody binds to the foreign cell or particle via its binding sites, and then the Fc part of the antibody binds to the surface of neutrophils or macrophages, effectively binding the antigen to these phagocytes. Some antibodies have receptors for the fixing (activating) or complement. IgE antibodies bind specifically to mast cells and basophils and, when antigen is bound, they cause the release of allergic mediators such as histamine (see pp. 202–3).

Active versus passive immunity

Specific immunity can be acquired either actively or passively (see Figure 9.23). **Active immunity** is the immunity developed when the acquired immune system responds to microorganisms or other foreign substances that enter or are introduced into the body. Active immunity is *naturally acquired* during microbial infections, and *artificially acquired* as a result of vaccination (see pp. 199–200). Generally, active immunity is long-lasting, often for a lifetime, especially when naturally acquired.

Passive immunity is the immunity resulting from the transfer of pre-made antibodies (or immune cells) from an immune person (or animal) to a non-immune person. The recipient becomes immune, but only for a short time (up to several months) until the transferred antibodies are naturally degraded in the body. The immunity is short-

FIGURE 9.22
OPSONISATION OF MICROORGANISMS
Adherence of microbes to phagocytes can be facilitated by (a) antibodies, or (b) antibodies together with complement. The mechanisms are similar to opsonisation with complement alone (illustrated in Figure 9.12).

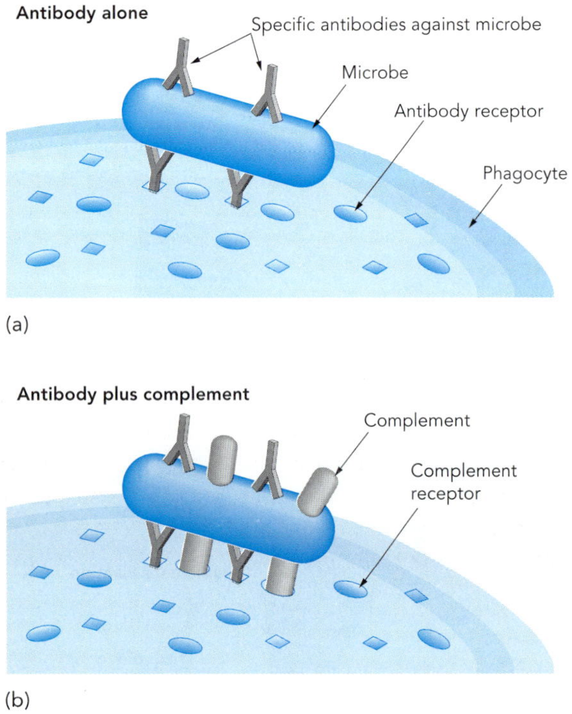

lived because the immune system of the recipient is not stimulated. Passive immunity can also be naturally or artificially acquired. Passive immunity is conferred naturally on a foetus as the mother's antibodies pass across the placenta into the foetal circulation. Antibodies are also transferred to an infant in colostrum and breast milk. These antibodies protect the foetus and then the young infant for several months after birth against the wide variety of microbes to which the mother is immune. In the meantime, the baby's own immune system is maturing.

Passive immunity is artificially conferred when a person is injected with antibodies from an immune human or animal. In the early 1990s, horse serum containing antitoxins was used to prevent tetanus and diphtheria, but now antisera produced in animals are not often used because of the chance of developing a hypersensitivity (see p. 202) to the foreign animal proteins. Products of human origin are now more often used. **Gammaglobulin** is an immunoglobulin preparation extracted from the pooled serum of large numbers of blood donors. Each batch of this serum contains a mixture of antibodies, which offers protection against a broad range of common infectious diseases. It is generally used to prevent diseases such as rubella and hepatitis A in people who have been exposed to these viruses. It is also sometimes used to replace antibodies in immunodeficient patients.

Specific immune globulin (SIG), on the other hand, is an antibody preparation obtained from the serum of people who are convalescing and in a hyperimmune state after an infection. Specific immune globulins are usually prepared against such diseases as pertussis, tetanus and hepatitis B. For example, a health worker who is accidentally exposed to hepatitis B virus by a neddlestick injury is given hepatitis B immune globulin in an attempt to prevent establishment of infection. These preparations are preferable to gammaglobulin because they contain higher titres of specific antibodies against these potentially more serious diseases. The injected antibodies provide immediate protection, but their effect is short-lived.

CELL-MEDIATED IMMUNITY

Usually, at the same time that B cells are responding to an antigen, a clone of specific T cells is similarly activated. The cell-mediated immune response involves the activation, differentiation and actions of chemical mediators by some of them.

T cells and their functions

There are several different types of T cells involved in the process of cellular immunity. Their classification and functions are much more complex than that of B cells.

FIGURE 9.23
THE DIFFERENT TYPES OF ACQUIRED (SPECIFIC) IMMUNITY

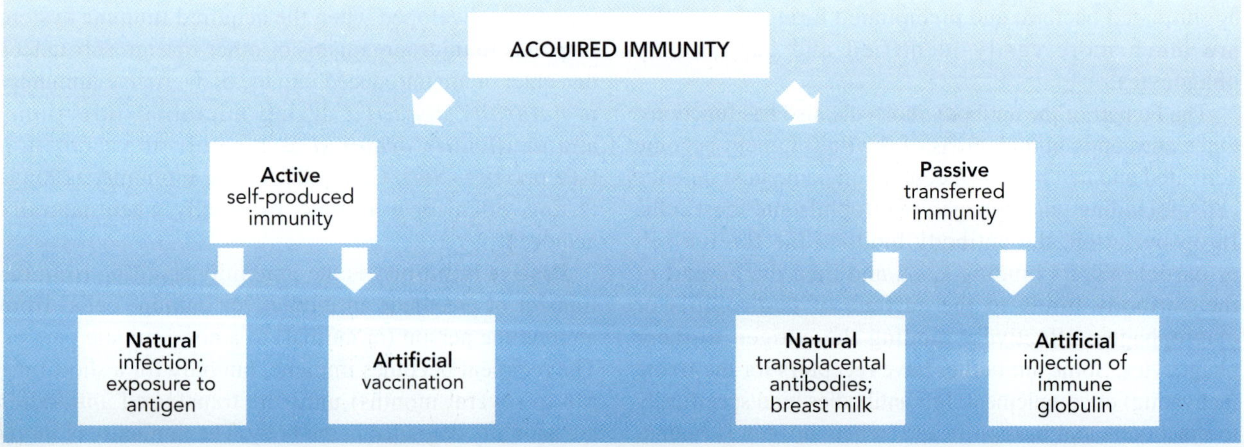

Based on their general functions and distinct cell surface markers, the two major populations of T cells are effector cells, called **cytotoxic T cells**, and regulatory cells, called **helper T cells**. T cells possess a number of different glycoproteins on their surface. Like B cells, T cells also have antigen receptors, although the nature of T cell receptors is different to that of B cell receptors. Two T cell surface glycoproteins that are important in distinguishing between different functional types are the CD4 and CD 8 markers. T cells that possess the CD4 marker, called **CD4 cells** or **T4 cells**, are primarily the helper T cells, whereas T cells with the CD8 marker, the **CD8 cells** (or **T8 cells**), are cytotoxic T cells.

Helper T cells are regulatory cells that play a central role in the immune response. Once activated by antigen, their major function is to help B cells and other T cells to respond to antigen (Figure 9.24). Helper T cells are so important in the activation of other lymphocytes that, without them, the immune response to most antigens is severely diminished. This is starkly demonstrated in infections caused by the human immunodeficiency virus (HIV). The HIV attacks the helper T cell population, rendering the patient incapable of mounting immune responses, and thus highly susceptible to infection and cancer.

When helper T cells are activated by exposure to specific antigen, they secrete a variety of different molecules called **lymphokines**. Some of these lymphokines act on other B and T lymphocytes to induce them to divide and differentiate (Figure 9.24), while others promote inflammation. The lymphokines are described more fully on page 199. Most antigens require the involvement of T cells in order for activation of B cells to occur. These are called **T-dependent antigens**.

Cytotoxic T cells directly attack and kill target cells. Activated cytotoxic T cells circulate in the bloodstream and lymphatic system in search of cells displaying the antigens they specifically recognise. They mainly attack virus-infected cells, but they are also involved in defence against intracellular bacteria and cancer cells. The cytotoxic T cell recognises viral antigens on the surfaced of an infected cell and binds tightly to the cell; it then releases protein molecules call **perforin**, which are inserted into the plasma membrane of the target cell. The proteins form a pore in the cell membrane, causing death of the cell in a way that is similar to the complement mechanism. By killin virus-infected cells they interrupt virus replication and expose the viruses to extracellular defences, thus reducing the spread of infection. However, the infected host cell is also destroyed. Cytoxic T cells secrete potent cytokines, including gamma interferon and **tumour necrosis factor (TNF)**, which limit viral replication inside an infected cell and also attract phagocytes to the cell to destroy it.

Some T lymphocytes appear to have suppressor activity, that is, they down-regulate immune responses. Lymphocytes with suppressor activity often bear the CD8 marker, like the cytotoxic T cells. T lymphocytes with suppressor activity may be involved in the winding down of the immune response after an antigen has been successfully eliminated. This would help to prevent uncontrolled or unnecessary immune system activity. Such cells may also be important in preventing autoimmune reactions and maintaining tolerance to self-antigens (see p. 204).

The cell-mediated immune response

In cell-mediated immunity, the stimulus for clonal selection and T lymphocyte activation, proliferation and differentiation is the binding of antigen. The T cell receptor is not an antibody, but consists of two amino acid chains (α and β), each with constant and variable regions. However, T cells are unable to recognise free antigens carried in blood or lymph; they recognise and respond only to processed fragments of antigens displayed on surfaces of the body's own cells. This means that T cell activation requires a simultaneous recognition of non-self (the antigen) and self (a glycoprotein of the body cell).

FIGURE 9.24
THE CENTRAL ROLE OF HELPTER T CELLS IN HUMORAL AND CELL-MEDIATED IMMUNITY
Helper T cells are activated by antigen presented by an antigen-presenting cell; the activated helper T cells then release various lymphokines (cytokines) which help to activate other helper T cells, cytotoxic T cells and B cells.

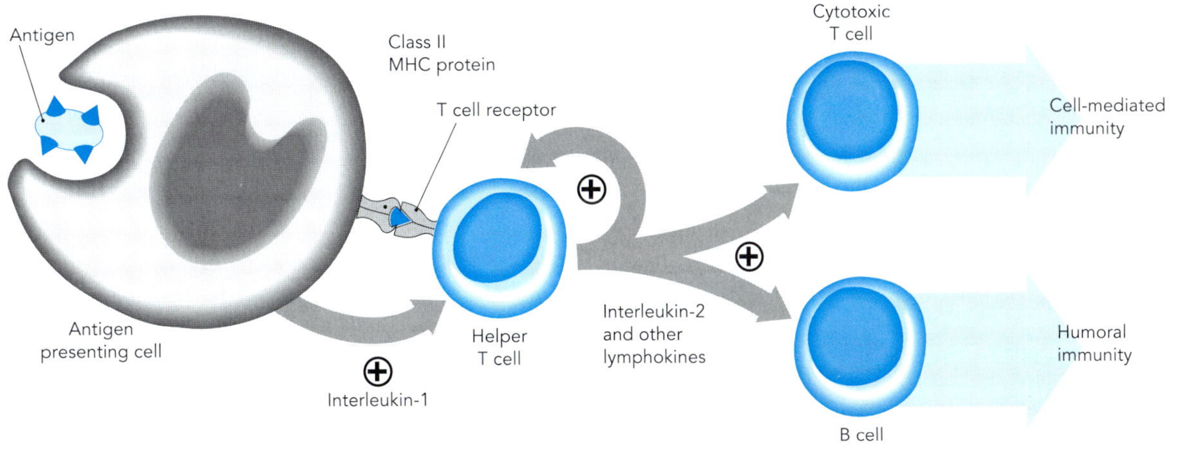

A protein, coded for by a gene of the **major histocompatibility complex (MHC)**, brings the antigen fragment to the surface of the antigen-containing cell, where the T cell can bind to it. Infected cells display microbial antigens in conjunction with one type of MHC protein (called class I MHC) which are recognised primarily by cytotoxic T cells (see Figure 9.25), whereas antigen-presenting cells (see p. 190) display foreign antigens in conjunction with a different type of MHC protein (class II MHC), which are recognised by helper T cells, as well as B cells (see humoral immune response, p. 190).

Once a T cell is activated it enlarges and proliferates to form a clone of cells that differentiate and perform functions according to their T cell class (see Figure 9.26). Helper T cells recognise antigen fragments on the surface of macrophages and other antigen-presenting cells. They then become activated and produce large amounts of lymphokines. Cytotoxic T cells are activated by antigen fragments on infected cells or tumour cells, which they ultimately lyse by punching holes in the cell membranes. In every case, some clone members become memory T cells; they persist, perhaps for life, providing a reservoir of T cells that can mediate secondary responses to the same antigen.

FIGURE 9.25

ACTIVATION OF CYTOTOXIC T LYMPHOCYTES

Cytotoxic T lymphocytes are activated by binding to an MHC class I molecule together with an antigen fragment on the surface of an infected cell.

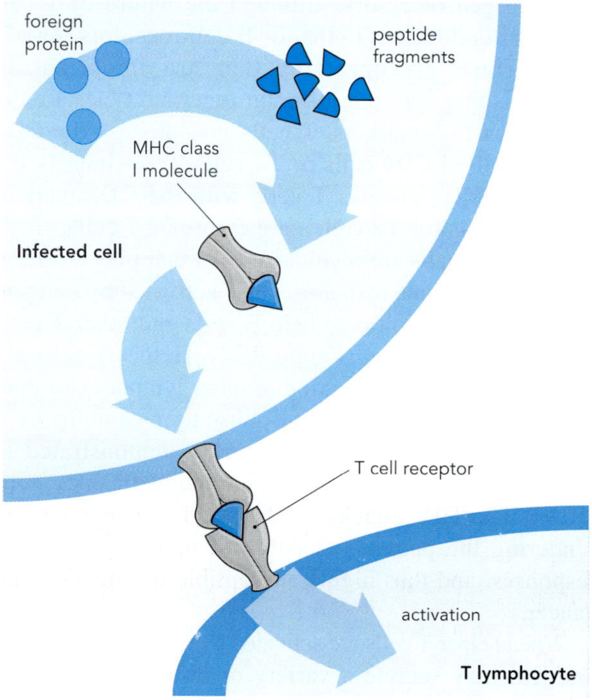

FIGURE 9.26

CELL-MEDIATED IMMUNITY

T cells are activated by antigen-presenting cells and/or infected cells and can perform a variety of functions, depending on their type.

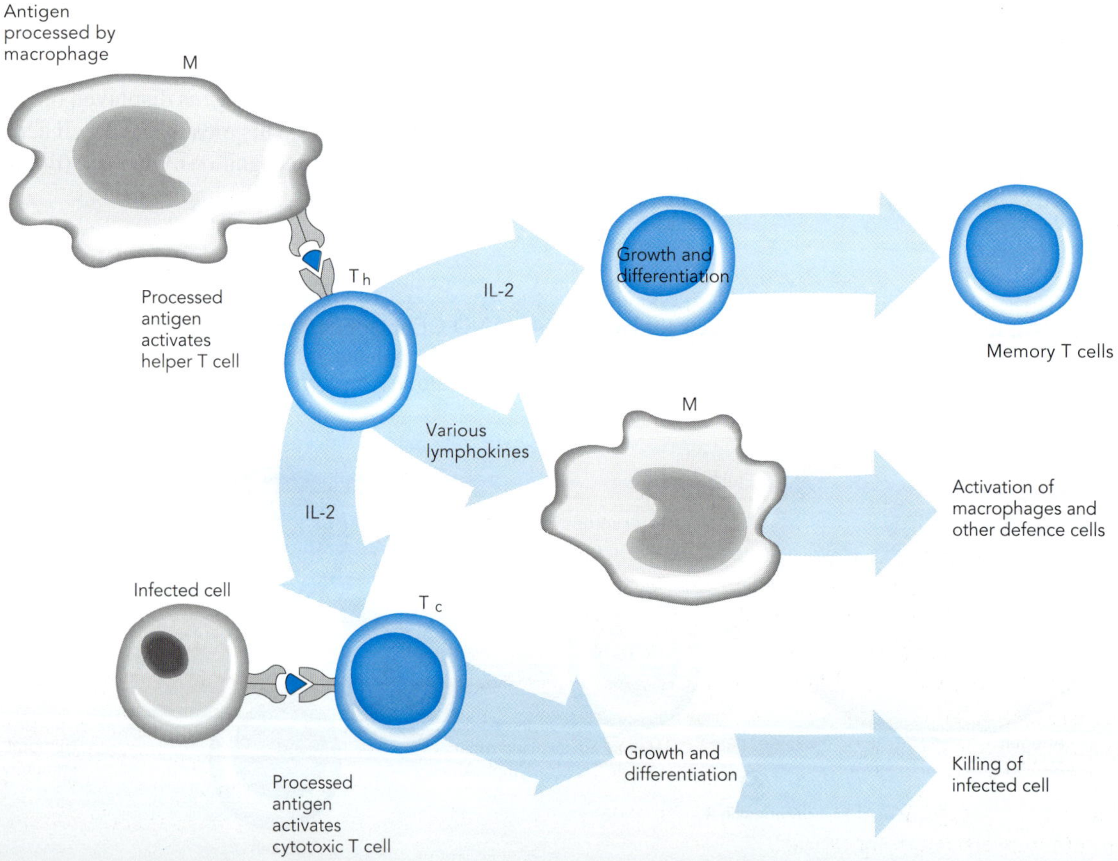

Cytokines and lymphokines

As for the inflammatory response, chemical mediators also drive the immune response. The chemical mediators involved in cellular immunity are collectively called **cytokines**, and include the mediators released by activated T cells themselves, which are called **lymphokines**. Many lymphokines mobilise other lymphocytes; others act primarily on macrophages and other white cells. The terminology for these substances is still in a state of flux, and some cytokines that act specifically between leukocytes are called **interleukins**. Furthermore, the **interferons**, mentioned earlier in this chapter, are also cytokines. However, all these substances provide communication between cells and have a central role in regulating the immune response. In general, cytokines have multiple activities and sources and usually have different effects on different cell types.

Two important cytokines are interleukin-1 and interleukin-2. **Interleukin-1 (IL-1)** is released by macrophages and other cells, and stimulates antigen-activated T cells to liberate **interleukin-2 (IL-2)** and to synthesise more IL-2 receptors. Interleukin-2 encourages activated T cells to proliferate and differentiate. IL-1 also enhances the inflammatory response, as do IL-6 and IL-8. Gamma interferon (IFN-γ) is produced by activated T cells and is an important activator of macrophages and NK cells. **Tumour necrosis factor (TNF)** has been shown to kill virus-infected cells as well as being important in inflammation and lymphocyte proliferation. The cytokines obviously comprise a very complex regulatory system, which we know relatively little about.

IMMUNISATION

Active immunity may be conferred artificially by **immunisation (vaccination)**, which involves exposing a person to material that is antigenic but not pathogenic. The discovery of vaccination was one of the farthest reaching and most important developments in medical science. It profoundly reduced the prevalence and impact of a number of infectious diseases that were once common and often deadly. Vaccines for viral diseases are particularly important because of the lack of effective treatment for so many of these diseases. In this section, we examine the nature of vaccines and aspects of their usage.

Types of vaccines

In natural, acquired immunity, an infectious agent stimulates specific B and T lymphocytes and creates clones of memory cells which often give lifelong immunity. In immunisation, the objective is to obtain this same response with a modified version of the microbe or its components. A safe and effective vaccine should mimic the natural protective response but not cause the infection, have long-lasting effects in a few doses, and be easy to administer. Most vaccine preparations comprise one of the following:

- killed, whole bacterial cells or inactivated viruses;
- live, attenuated bacteria or viruses;
- inactivated bacterial toxins;
- parts of bacterial cells or viruses.

The types of common vaccines in use are listed in Table 9.3.

Killed vaccines are prepared by cultivating the required bacterium or virus and treating it with formalin, radiation, or some other agent that kills it but does not destroy its immunogenicity. The vaccine contains whole, killed organisms. The vaccines for pertussis, typhoid fever and influenza are of this type, as is the Salk polio vaccine. Because the microbe does not multiply in the host, and therefore strongly stimulate the immune system, killed vaccines often require several boosters to be effective.

A number of vaccines are prepared from live, attenuated microbes. **Attenuation** is any process that substantially reduces or (preferably) eliminates the virulence of microorganisms, while still keeping them alive. It can be achieved by growing the organism in unusual conditions or by manipulating its genes in a way that eliminates virulence factors. Long-term cultivation *in vitro* or passage of the microbe through unnatural hosts have proved to be successful methods of attenuation for some organisms. For example, the vaccine for tuberculosis (the BCG—Bacille Calmette et Guerin) was obtained by Calmette and Guerin after more than 10 years of subculturing the agent of bovine tuberculosis on an artificial culture medium. Vaccines for measles, mumps, polio (Sabin) and rubella contain live, non-virulent viruses.

The advantages of attenuated vaccines are that viable microorganisms can multiply and produce mild or subclinical infection, which will confer long-lasting protection. Many attenuated vaccines provide lifelong

TABLE 9.3
TYPES OF VACCINES IN COMMON USE

TYPE OF VACCINE	DISEASE
Killed bacteria	cholera whooping cough typhoid
Inactivated viruses	influenza rabies
Live, attenuated bacteria	tuberculosis
Toxoids (inactivated toxins)	tetanus diphtheria
Attenuated virus	measles polio (Sabin) mumps rubella smallpox
Microbial subunit	*Haemophilus* infections (polysaccharide) hepatitis B (viral surface antigen)

immunity without the need for boosters. The major disadvantage of using live vaccines is the inherent risk that the organism might mutate back to a virulent strain (see polio, Chapter 20). Live vaccines, however, are generally preferred to killed types, where available, because of their greater efficacy.

For protection against diseases that are due primarily to the actions of a bacterial exotoxin (see Chapter 10), immunity to the toxin is often more appropriate than immunity to the whole bacterium. A special type of vaccine is the **toxoid,** which consists of a bacterial exotoxin that has been inactivated (usually with formaldehyde), but is still antigenic. Toxoids elicit the production of **antitoxins**—antibodies that neutralise the toxin and prevent it from causing disease. Examples of toxoids are the highly effective vaccines for diphtheria and tetanus, which are two of the components of the triple antigen vaccine for children.

If the exact antigenic determinants that stimulate good immunity are known, it may be possible to produce a vaccine based on that particular part of a microorganism. These are called **subunit vaccines.** Examples of subunit antigens are the capsular of polysaccharides *Haemophilus influenzae* (Hib vaccine), pneumococcus and meningococcus, and the surface antigen of hepatitis B virus.

The immunogenic components of some subunit vaccines are prepared by genetic engineering techniques. In this process, the gene for the synthesis of the protective antigenic determinant (epitope) is introduced into a bacterium or yeast cell. These microbes are grown in large amounts and the antigen is harvested for use in the vaccine. The hepatitis B vaccine is a subunit vaccine prepared in this way. A list of the major vaccines in use in Australia is provided in Chapter 14.

Subunit and toxoid vaccines are non-living, and thus need to be administered several times in order to produce strong, effective immunity.

Side effects of vaccines

Before vaccines are licensed they must undergo stringent trials in experimental animals and humans. However, even after such rigorous testing, they can cause problems. The most common of these are local hypersensitivity reactions at the injection site, other allergic reactions or fever. For certain vaccines there are rare complications, for example:

- encephalitis following measles vaccine (although the incidence of this is much lower than following infection);
- back mutation of attenuated organisms to the virulent strain (e.g. polio vaccine); and
- allergic reactions to the vaccine medium (eggs or tissue culture).

Health professionals involved in giving vaccinations should be aware of the possible risks, but also aware that the risk of contracting the disease could be far more serious (see Chapter 14). Extreme caution must be exercised in giving live vaccines (a) to the immunocompromised, because even low-virulence organisms can produce disease in such people, and (b) to pregnant women, because of the possible risk to the foetus.

Another major advantage of immunisation is the establishment of **herd immunity** in the population. This is based on the principle that individuals who are immune to an infectious disease will not be carriers of the organism, reducing the occurrence of that microbe and, therefore, the number of susceptible people who will encounter it. In other words, mass immunisation confers indirect protection on the whole population, including the non-immune. Herd immunity helps to avert epidemics. This is discussed more fully in Chapter 14.

Disorders of the Immune System

There are certain situations where the immune system fails or functions inappropriately. When it fails, the individual becomes more susceptible to infectious diseases and sometimes cancer, and when it functions inappropriately it can cause disease and sometimes damage to the body. These disorders of the immune system can be classified as an immunodeficiency, hypersensitivity, or an autoimmune disease, although some disorders are a combination of them.

IMMUNODEFICIENCY

Immunodeficiency includes both inborn and acquired conditions in which the production or function of lymphocytes, phagocytes or complement is abnormal. These are the key components of the immune system, and a person with a defect in one or more of them is said to be **immunocompromised**. **Primary immunodeficiency** is generally due to the improper foetal development of one or more of these components. **Secondary immunodeficiency** results from damage to otherwise normal components and may be due to infection, cancer, malnutrition, or the use of drugs and other therapies that suppress the immune system. With respect to infectious diseases, immunodeficiency is the most important disorder of the immune system.

Primary immunodeficiency

Selected primary immunodeficiencies are listed in Table 9.4. Phagocytes, lymphocytes and complement are the key components of the immune system, so a defect in any one of them will lead to impaired ability to resist infection and/or cancer. The most serious primary immunodeficiency diseases are congenital thymic hypoplasia or aplasia, caused by a failure of the thymus to develop fully, and severe combined immunodeficiency disease (SCID), in which lymphocyte precursors in the bone marrow fail to develop properly, resulting in a marked deficiency in both B and T cells. Since T cells are required for the proper functioning of both humoral and cell-mediated immunity, individuals afflicted with either condition have little or no protection against infection. Even normally minor infections can be fatal.

TABLE 9.4
SELECTED PRIMARY IMMUNODEFICIENCY DISEASES

DISEASE	NATURE OF DEFECT
Defects in B lymphocytes	
■ X-linked infantile agammaglobulinaemia (Bruton's disease)	Pre-B cells do not mature—no circulating B cells
■ acquired hypogammaglobulinaemia	B cells respond to antigen but do not secrete antibody
■ selective IgA deficiency	IgA is synthesised but not released
Defects in T lymphocytes	
■ congenital thymic aplasia (DiGeorge syndrome)	Improper development of the thymus gland—few T cells
Defects in both T and B lymphocytes	
■ severe combined immunodeficiency	Stem cell defect resulting in T and B cell deficiency
■ Nezelof's syndrome	Thymic hypoplasia and T and B cell deficiency
Defects in phagocytes	
■ chronic granulomatous disease	Phagocyte enzyme deficiency
Defects in complement	
■ Complement defect	Deficiency in any component of complement

X-linked (Bruton's) agammaglobulinaemia is a primary immunodeficiency caused by incomplete maturation of B lymphocytes. Children with this disorder suffer repeatedly from infections such as pneumonia, otitis media, meningitis and septicaemia caused by staphylococci, streptococci and other bacteria.

Different types of immunodeficiency will result in increased susceptibility to different types of pathogenic microorganisms. In general, a T cell deficiency will mainly increase susceptibility to viruses, intracellular bacteria and other intracellular parasites like the malaria protozoan and fungi, since it is the T cell which attacks infected host cells. A selective deficiency in B cells or antibodies, on the other hand, will greatly increase susceptibility to most bacterial infections and, to a lesser extent, viruses. A deficiency in both cell types, as occurs in SCID, will make the individual highly susceptible to all pathogenic microbes and even to organisms with low virulence. Complement mainly attacks foreign cells in extracellular fluids, so a deficiency in any one of the cascade proteins will increase the risk of bacterial infections. A defect in macrophage activity will greatly impair defences against bacteria, and defence against viruses will also be affected, but to a lesser extent.

Secondary immunodeficiency

There are numerous potential causes of secondary immunodeficiency. Any agent that causes a suppression or malfunction of the bone marrow or lymphoid organs may cause a secondary immunodeficiency. For example, in leukaemia, a massive number of cancer cells are produced in the bone marrow, preventing the normal production of white cells. In Hodgkin's disease, the immune system is suppressed because of the growth of tumour cells in the lymph nodes.

The treatments for certain diseases can also cause immunodeficiency. For example, the cytotoxic drugs and radiation therapy used for treatment of cancer suppress white cell production in the bone marrow. Corticosteroids, used to reduce inflammation in certain diseases, can reduce the number of leukocytes in the blood. Immunosuppressive drugs are used to prevent rejection of organ transplants, but they also make the patient more susceptible to infection.

The most obvious and devastating of the secondary immunodeficiencies is the **acquired immunodeficiency syndrome (AIDS)**, caused by the human immunodeficiency virus (HIV). The HIV severely damages the immune system by infecting and destroying helper T cells (this is described more fully in Chapter 19). A large variety of other microbes cause less severe suppression of the immune system, including the measles virus, mumps virus, *Mycobacterium leprae* (leprosy) and the protozoa that cause malaria.

The common predisposing factors that can lead to secondary immunodeficiency are summarised in Table 9.5.

In addition to these secondary immunodeficiency diseases, non-specific defences can be impaired in certain situations. They are not regarded as immunodeficiency disorders because the defences affected are not part of the immune system, but nevertheless they increase the risk of infection. For example, broad spectrum antibiotics can temporarily lower the body's non-specific defences by reducing the normal flora of the body. When the skin barrier is disrupted by burns, surgical wounds or other trauma, infection becomes more likely. A urinary catheter

TABLE 9.5
EXAMPLES OF FACTORS THAT CAUSE SECONDARY IMMUNODEFICIENCY

FACTOR	EFFECT ON BODY DEFENCES
Some tumours	
■ leukaemia	Production of dysfunctional bone marrow cells
■ Hodgkin's disease	Disease of lymph nodes
Tumour therapy	
■ cytotoxic drugs	Suppression of white cell production
■ radiotherapy	Suppression of white cell production
Malnutrition	
■ protein deficiency	Poor lymphoid organ development, low antibody and complement concentrations, low lymphocyte numbers
Immunosuppressive therapy	
■ in transplant patients	Suppression of lymphocyte function
Anti-inflammatory therapy	
■ corticosteroids	Reduction of white cell production, impairment of lymphocyte function and antibody and cytokine production
Infection	
■ human immunodeficiency virus	Destruction of helper T lymphocytes

predisposes a person to urinary tract infection because of the loss of the flushing action of urine over the urethral surface, and impairment of mucociliary activity in the airways as a result of cigarette smoking is an important factor in some types of lower respiratory infection.

HYPERSENSITIVITY

Hypersensitivity is an overreaction of the immune system to an antigen it has previously encountered. There are different types of hypersensitivity reactions, which may be classified according to whether antibodies or T cells are the principal elements involved. The British immunologists Phillip Gell and Robin Coombs categorised them into four types. The first three types in their scheme are due primarily to the action of antibodies, and the fourth type is due to the action of T cells. Some disorders are actually a combination of more than one type.

Type I: Immediate hypersensitivity

An **immediate hypersensitivity**, also called **allergy**, occurs within minutes to several hours after a sensitised, susceptible person comes into contact with a foreign antigen. The term **allergen** is used to distinguish this type of antigen, which has the potential to elicit this type of adverse immune reaction. Typical allergens include pollens, dust mites, fungal spores, certain foods, and some antibiotics and other drugs. The predisposition for allergies is an inherited trait, and is associated with the production of IgE antibodies to some antigens.

The basis of immediate (Type I) hypersensitivity is the production of the IgE class of antibodies after initial exposure to the allergen. If this class of antibody is produced, the person becomes sensitised to the allergen, whereas the production of any other class of antibody to the allergen does not sensitise the person. The IgE molecules have a special affinity for mast cells and basophils and attach to these cells via their Fc fragments. The sensitised cells may remain in the tissues for years. On subsequent exposure to the allergen, the allergen molecules cross-link the IgE antibodies attached to mast cells or basophils, stimulating the cells to degranulate, releasing histamine and other inflammatory chemicals that rapidly induce an inflammatory response (Figure 9.27). Activation of these cells also induces them to synthesise other powerful inflammatory mediators, particularly the prostaglandins and leukotrienes.

Most allergic reactions are local, occurring typically where the allergen enters the body. Thus, most involve the skin, the respiratory passages or the gastrointestinal tract, because of local binding of allergen to mast cells. Because the mediators cause dilation and increased permeability of blood vessels, local reactions are usually characterised by redness and swelling. Other familiar signs and symptoms, such as a runny nose, watery eyes, and itching reddened skin (hives) are related to the specific tissues affected. When the allergen is air-borne and inhaled, symptoms of asthma may appear as a result of bronchiolar smooth muscle contraction, which constricts the bronchioles, restricting air flow. Excessive mucous production further constricts the airways. When the allergen

FIGURE 9.27

THE MECHANISMS OF ALLERGY

Following first contact with an allergen, B lymphocytes are stimulated to produce IgE antibodies. These antibodies bind to mast cells and basophils, via their Fc region, thereby sensitising those cells. On subsequent contact with the allergen, it is bound to the sensitised cells, causing release of various inflammatory mediators which cause allergic reactions.

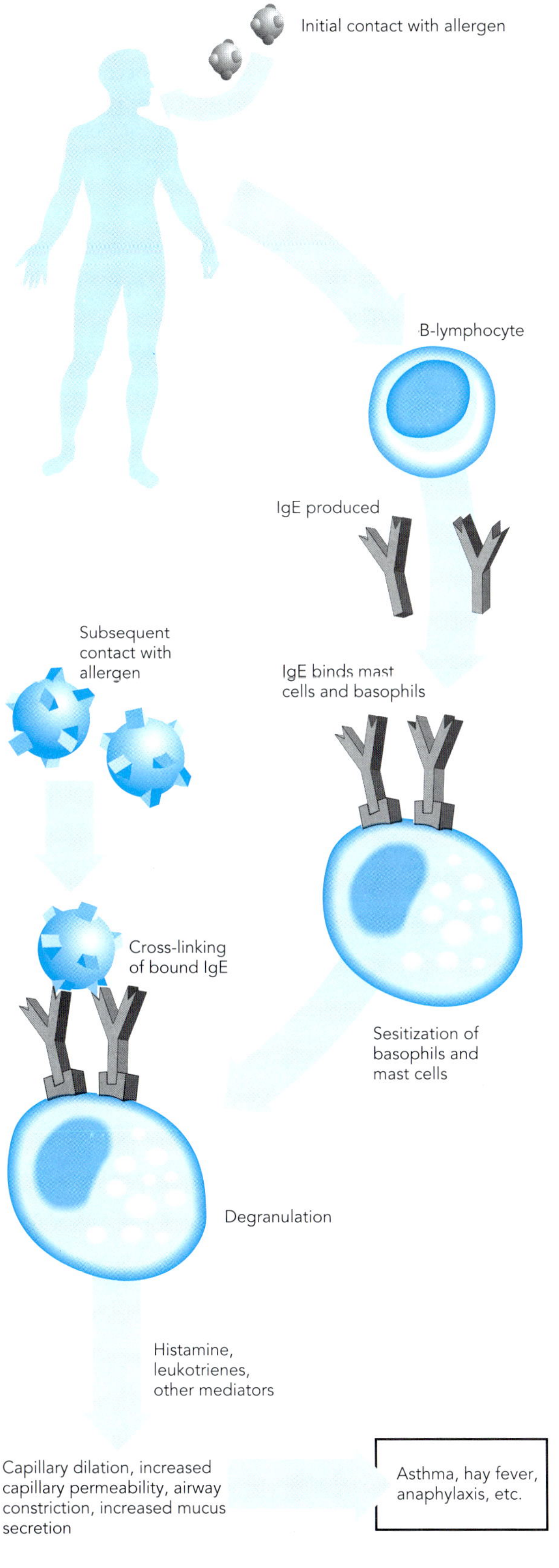

is ingested (e.g. in food), gastrointestinal hypersensitivity occurs (cramping, vomiting or diarrhoea), and sometimes a skin rash.

Fortunately, systemic reactions, referred to as **anaphylaxis**, are far less common than local allergy. Anaphylaxis typically occurs when the allergen enters the blood and circulates through the body, as may happen with bee stings. It may also follow injection or ingestion of a foreign substance, such as penicillin, or other drugs, in a susceptible individual. Anyone who has had any adverse reaction to penicillin, such as hives or throat or chest constriction, should not be given the drug again. The mechanism of anaphylaxis is essentially the same as that of local responses but, when mast cells and basophils are degranulated throughout the body, the generalised inflammatory response can be life-threatening. The sudden vasodilation may cause lowered blood pressure, circulatory collapse and physiological shock and, together with constriction of bronchiolar smooth muscle, can cause death within minutes. This serious form is called **anaphylactic shock**.

Type II: Cytotoxic hypersensitivity

Cytotoxic (Type II) hypersensitivity results from the binding of antibodies to antigens on the surface of a cell, followed by complement activation and lysis of the target cell. The cell may be a foreign cell or a cell of the person's own body that is recognised as foreign. Examples of this type of hypersensitivity include reactions following transfusion of the wrong blood type, and a disease referred to as haemolytic disease of the newborn (or erythroblastosis foetalis). In both these cases, red cells are recognised as foreign, and antibodies in conjunction with complement cause lysis of the cells. In the case of transfusion reaction, red cells with foreign ABO or Rh antigens are present in the donor blood. In haemolytic disease of the newborn, the baby's Rh positive (D antigen) red cells are destroyed by maternal anti-D antibodies of the IgG class, which are able to cross the placenta. Cytotoxic (Type II) reaction is the major cause of damage in many autoimmune diseases (see p. 204).

Type III:Immune complex hypersensitivity

Immune complex hypersensitivity results when antigen-antibody complexes are formed and are not cleared quickly from the body. Normally, immune complexes are engulfed and destroyed by phagocytes, but if the complexes persist or are being formed continuously, this type of hypersensitivity occurs. If the number of circulating complexes is large, they may be deposited in the basement membranes in certain sites, such as the kidneys, lungs, joints, and blood vessels of the skin. The complexes activate complement and an inflammatory reaction occurs that can damage local tissues (Figure 9.28).

Acute glomerulonephritis is an example of an immune complex disease in which the complexes are deposited on the basement membrane of kidney glomeruli. Certain skin rashes result from the deposition of immune complexes in the basement membrane of surface blood vessels. Rheumatoid arthritis is due to a combination of immune complex hypersensitivity and autoimmune disease.

Type IV: Delayed type hypersensitivity

Delayed type hypersensitivity reactions (also called **cell-mediated hypersensitivity**) are mediated by T cells and take a day or more to appear after the introduction of antigen, compared to the few minutes or hours in antibody-mediated hypersensitivity reactions. The mechanism involved is basically that of a cell-mediated immune response. A subgroup of sensitised T cells, sometimes called **delayed type hypersensitivity T cells**, when stimulated by antigen, secrete lymphokines which activate macrophages and cause inflammatory reactions, such as eczema, oedema and granuloma formation. A massive infiltration of mononuclear white cells (macrophages and lymphocytes) often occurs. This reaction represents a normal cell-mediated response in which host tissue cells are unfortunately damaged.

The Mantoux test for assessing immunity to tuberculosis depends on a delayed hypersensitivity reaction. When protein antigens of the tuberculosis bacterium are inoculated intradermally (just under the skin), a small, hard inflammatory reaction occurs two to three days later if the person has been previously sensitised to the antigen. Contact dermatitis to haptens in cosmetics, metals, soaps and dyes are other examples of delayed type hypersensitivity.

AUTOIMMUNE DISEASES

Occasionally, the immune system loses its ability to distinguish self; from non-self, that is, it loses its **tolerance** to one or more self-antigens. When this happens, the body produces antibodies (**autoantibodies**) and sensitised T lymphocytes against its own tissues, causing damage to them. If the damage is significant and disease results, it is called an **autoimmune disease** (Table 9.6).

In most cases, it is not known what precipitates autoimmunity, but genetic factors, sex and age are known to influence its incidence. In some disorders, the body's own cells are thought to appear 'foreign' because they are distorted or altered in some way. Autoimmune haemolytic anaemia is a condition in which red cells are destroyed by autoantibodies in conjunction with complement. In this disease, an alteration to the surface composition of red cells (often for unknown reasons) causes the immune system to recognise them as foreign and produce antibodies to these antigens.

In rheumatoid arthritis, an altered antibody molecule (an IgG) is thought to be the basis of the disease. First, the IgG to some unknown antigen is formed within a joint. Then, also for some unknown reason, this IgG becomes altered, and eventually appears sufficiently foreign to stimulate an immune response in the form of antibodies (usually IgM). These anti-IgG antibodies can also be found in serum, and are called the **rheumatoid factor**. The immune complexes formed by the binding of IgM to the altered IgG antibodies activate complement, leading to chronic inflammation and joint damage. This disorder is thus a combination of autoimmune disease and immune complex hypersensitivity.

Antibodies made against a foreign antigen sometimes cross-react with a self-antigen that has a similar structure and composition. For instance, antibodies produced during a streptococcal throat infection have been found to cross-react with components of heart muscle, causing inflammation and damage to the heart muscle and valves. This rare autoimmune sequela of streptococcal sore throat is called rheumatic fever (see Chapter 19). It affects only a small percentage of people, those with the genetic makeup to produce the cross-reacting antibodies.

FIGURE 9.28
THE MECHANISM OF IMMUNE COMPLEX HYPERSENSITIVITY
Immune complexes that are not rapidly removed by phagocytes are deposited in tissues where complement activation causes inflammation and tissue damage.

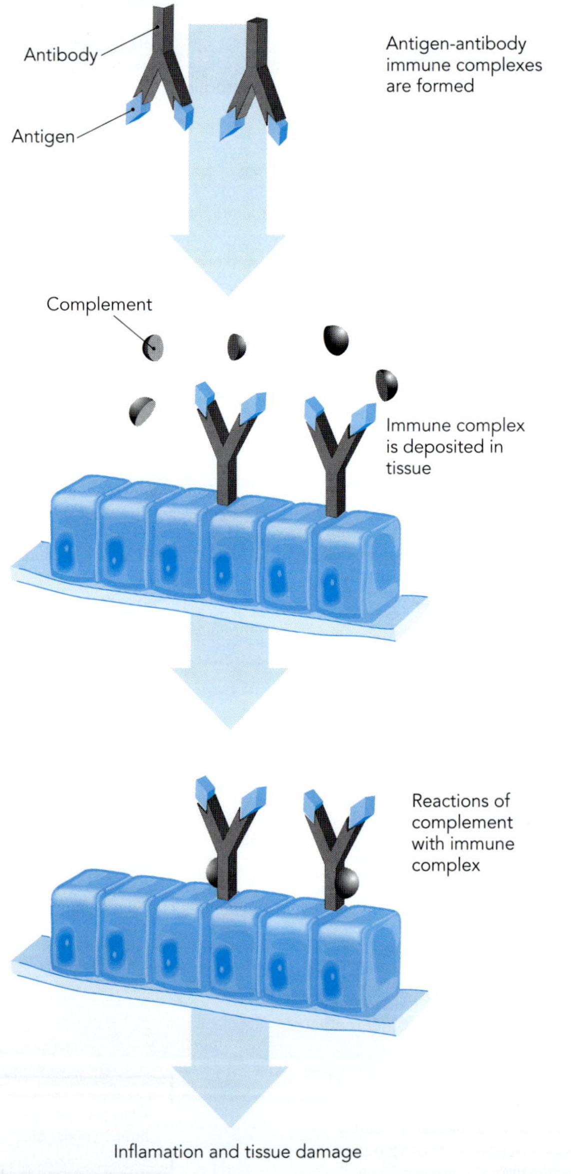

TABLE 9.6
EXAMPLES OF AUTOIMMUNE DISEASES

DISEASE	TARGET OF THE AUTOANTIBODY
Autoimmune haemolytic anaemia	Red blood cells
Idiopathic thrombocytopaenic purpura	Platelets
Grave's disease	TSH receptor on thyroid cells
Rheumatic fever	Cardiac muscle
Myasthenia gravis	Acetylcholine receptor at the neuromuscular junction
Goodpasture's syndrome	Basement membrane in kidney and lungs
Systemic lupus erythematosis	Nucleic acid, red blood cells, platelets, etc.
Insulin-dependent diabetes mellitus	Pancreatic beta cells
Rheumatoid arthritis	Antibodies, connective tissue

Summary

- The ability of the body to prevent infection is called resistance.
- The lack of resistance, or vulnerability to an infection, is called susceptibility.
- The body's resistance to infection depends on non-specific defences (the body's first line of defence) and specific defences (the body's second line of defence).
- The specific and non-specific defences overlap and interact with each other to protect the body.
- The specific defences and some of the non-specific defences comprise the body's immune system.

NON-SPECIFIC DEFENCES

- The function of the non-specific defences is to prevent the entry of pathogens into the body, or to destroy them immediately if they do manage to enter.

SKIN AND MUCOUS MEMBRANE BARRIERS

- The body's first line of defence against invasion by micro-organisms is the skin and the mucous membranes.
- The epidermis is the outer layer of the skin and consists of multiple layers of tightly packed epithelial cells which contain the strong protein, keratin.
- In the inner layer, the dermis, there are sebaceous glands that secrete sebum, which lowers the pH of the skin and inhibits the growth of certain micro-organisms.
- Mucosal membranes line all the body cavities that are open to the environment. They are coated with a film of sticky mucus that helps to prevent microbes from attaching to the epithelial surface and entering the tissues.
- The mucosal membranes are the sites of secretion or formation of a large variety of other substances that contribute to defence.
- A vital non-specific defence mechanism is the ciliated epithelium of the upper respiratory tract. This mucociliary escalator moves mucus and anything trapped in it upwards toward the throat, either to be expelled or swallowed.
- The movement of fluids, such as tears and urine, over mucosal surfaces creates a washing effect, which helps to eliminate microbes from the body.

NON-SPECIFIC CELLULAR DEFENCES

- When microorganisms or foreign substances penetrate the skin or mucous membranes and enter the tissues, the body has certain cellular defences for protection.

Phagocytes

- Phagocytes are body cells that actively ingest and digest foreign particles and remove cellular debris from the tissues. The two main types of phagocytes are the macrophages and the neutrophils.
- Macrophages are derived from blood monocytes, and are located in most tissues and organs of the body.
- Neutrophils are the most abundant type of white blood cell.
- The process of phagocytosis involves four main phases: chemotaxis, attachment, ingestion and digestion.
- Phagocytes are attracted to sites of damaged tissue or microbial invasion by chemicals released at the site—a process called chemotaxis.
- A variety of chemical substances act as attractants for phagocytes, including substances released from damaged tissues and some components of microorganisms.
- The phagocyte must be able to attach to the foreign particle or microorganism in order to ingest it.
- Phagocytes ingest foreign material by a process called endocytosis in which the cytoplasm invaginates at the point where the particle is attached and then encloses it.
- Inside the phagocyte, the foreign particle is contained within a membrane-bound vacuole called a phagosome.
- Digestion of the foreign material is brought about by fusion of the phagosome with lysosomes containing digestive enzymes.
- Toxic oxygen-containing substances, such as hydrogen peroxide and hypochlorite, are also produced by lysosomal enzymes to assist in the killing process.
- Some microbes are able to avoid intracellular digestion.

Natural killer cells

- Natural killer (NK) cells are a unique group of cells that are capable of destroying cancer cells and virus-infected cells.
- NK cells appear to bring about killing of the target cell by insertion of protein molecules, called perforins, into the cell membrane, creating a pore through which the cell contents leak out.

INFLAMMATION

- The acute inflammatory response is a non-specific defence that is the body's response to tissue injury.
- Inflammatory conditions are named by adding the suffix *-itis* to the affected organ or tissue.
- The major function of inflammation is to clear the injured site of cellular debris and any foreign material or pathogens, thereby preparing the area for repair processes.
- In the case of infection, inflammation also serves to localise the microorganisms, preventing their spread to adjacent areas.
- The four main signs of acute inflammation are redness, heat, swelling and pain.

Vasodilation and increased vascular permeability

- The chemicals responsible for the physiological events that occur in inflammation are called the chemical mediators of inflammation.
- The most important mediators of inflammation are histamine, kinins, prostaglandins, leukotrienes, tumour necrosis factor and complement.
- Some inflammatory mediators cause dilation of the arterioles which causes more blood flow to the area, resulting in redness and warmth.

- Some mediators increase the permeability of local capillaries and post-capillary venules; as a result, plasma fluid and proteins are able to move from the bloodstream into the tissue spaces. The fluid is called an exudate, and its accumulation in the tissue is the cause of the oedema, or swelling.
- The pain that is usually associated with inflammation is due to compression of adjacent nerve endings by oedema, as well as to the direct effects of mediators on pain receptors.
- Histamine is present in many different body cell types, especially in mast cells in connective tissue, and basophils and platelets in the bloodstream.
- Histamine has a potent action on blood vessels, causing them to dilate and allow the leakage of plasma fluid and proteins.
- The kinin system is activated by tissue injury and causes vasodilation and increased vascular permeability, as well as inducing pain.
- Prostaglandins and leukotrienes are synthesised from arachidonic acid, which is released from mast cell membranes. They cause dilation of post-capillary venules, increased vascular permeability and neutrophil chemotaxis. Prostaglandins also induce pain.
- Several of the leukotrienes cause sustained constriction of bronchioles, as occurs in bronchial asthma.
- Aspirin, indomethacin and certain other non-steroidal anti-inflammatory agents act by blocking the synthesis of prostaglandins.
- Steroidal anti-inflammatory drugs are very potent because they block both prostaglandin and leukotriene synthesis.

Phagocyte migration

- During inflammation there is an influx, first of neutrophils, and then of macrophages, into the injured tissue.
- Late in the inflammatory response, monocytes from the bloodstream begin to enter the area, replacing the neutrophils, which leave or die *in situ*. After entering the tissues, monocytes become mature, highly active macrophages.
- Pus is a thick, creamy-coloured fluid comprising a mixture of dead or dying neutrophils, tissue debris and remaining pathogens.
- Pus formation is typically induced by bacteria, but not by viruses.
- When a sac of pus is walled off by a layer of fibrin, an abscess is formed.
- Physical drainage of abscesses is often necessary before healing can occur.

Repair

- During the final stages of inflammation, tissue repair begins. The most favourable outcome is the restoration of the tissue's original structure and physiologic function by regeneration.
- If the tissue is incapable of regeneration or is extensively damaged, it is repaired by scar tissue replacement.

Chronic inflammation

- Chronic inflammation occurs if the acute inflammatory response is unsuccessful in eliminating the organisms or foreign material from the tissues.
- Large numbers of lymphocytes and macrophages are involved in chronic inflammation.
- Chronic inflammation can occur as a distinct process from the outset due to infection by microbes that are resistant to intracellular digestion by phagocytes.
- Other agents that typically evoke chronic inflammation are low-grade, persistent irritants, such as talc, silica and asbestos.
- A granuloma is a special kind of chronic inflammation produced in response to certain microorganisms.

Fever

- Fever represents a systemic response to invading microorganisms and often accompanies severe or systemic inflammation. It occurs when the set-point of the body's thermostat is raised to a higher temperature.
- Pyrogens are chemical substances which produce fever.
- Exogenous pyrogens are mainly components of microorganisms, especially the lipopolysaccharide of the cell wall of Gram-negative bacteria.
- Endogenous pyrogens are released from macrophages and neutrophils during inflammation or in response to the presence of exogenous pyrogens.
- The best known endogenous pyrogens are interleukin-1 (IL-1) and tumour necrosis factor (TNF).
- High fevers (above 40°C) are dangerous because of the possibility of thermal damage to nerve cells, and convulsions, but mild or moderate fever may have some benefit for the body.

ANTIMICROBIAL PROTEINS

Complement

- The complement system is a complex system of plasma proteins that normally circulate in an inactive state.
- It is an enzymatic cascade system which, when activated, can enhance phagocytosis, produce inflammation and directly lyse foreign cells.
- Complement can be activated by either the classical pathway or the alternate pathway.
- The classical pathway is initiated by the binding of antibodies to antigen.
- The alternate pathway is initiated by an interaction between certain complement factors and polysaccharides present on the surface of some microorganisms.
- Complement-mediated cytolysis is important in protection against some microorganisms.
- The C3b complement fragment can bind to the surface of microorganisms and then with specific receptors on phagocytes. This enhances phagocyte activity and is termed opsonisation.
- The C3a and C5a complement fragments bind to mast cells, basophils and platelets, triggering the release of histamine and other inducers of inflammation.

Interferon

- Virus-infected cells secrete protein molecules called interferon (IFN) which help neighbouring cells resist infection.
- One of the important features of the antiviral state induced by IFN is that it is not virus-specific.
- In addition to their antiviral activity, the interferons play important roles in enhancing the actions of a number of other defence cells.

THE NORMAL MICROBIAL FLORA

- The normal microbial flora of the body suppress the growth of potential pathogens by competing for essential nutrients, secreting toxic substances and forming bacterial layers over tissue surfaces.

SPECIFIC BODY DEFENCES: THE ACQUIRED IMMUNE SYSTEM

- The specific body defences, or acquired immune system, is a functional system consisting of a variety of cells, especially lymphocytes and macrophages, and various organs.
- The acquired immune system is the body's second line of defence and protects it from infection, damage by other foreign cells and substances, and cancer.
- Immunity is the capacity of the immune system to defend the body successfully against a potentially infectious agent.
- Immunology is the study of the immune system and immunity.

CHARACTERISTICS OF THE ACQUIRED IMMUNE SYSTEM

- When a microbe is able to persist in the tissues, the body reacts by producing an immune response.
- The immune response is able to recognise foreign substances, is specific and has memory.

THE DUAL NATURE OF THE ACQUIRED IMMUNE SYSTEM

- There are two different populations of lymphocytes: the B lymphocytes (B cells) and T lymphocytes (T cells).
- Humoral immunity is provided by antibodies present in the body's fluids.
- Antibodies are produced and secreted by plasma cells (derived from B lymphocytes); they then circulate in the blood and other body fluids.
- In cell-mediated immunity, T lymphocytes act against target cells.

CELLS AND TISSUES OF THE ACQUIRED IMMUNE SYSTEM

Cellular components

- Lymphocytes and macrophages are the cells primarily responsible for a specific immune response.
- B cells are mainly responsible for humoral immunity and T cells provide cell-mediated immunity.
- T cells undergo a maturation process under the direction of thymic hormones.
- B cells are believed to mature in the bone marrow.
- The thymus and the bone marrow are the primary lymphoid organs.
- On the surface of mature lymphocytes there are receptors of a single, unique type, which enable the cells to recognise and bind to a single, specific antigen.
- Macrophage-lymphocyte interactions form the basis of many of the immune system's processes.

The lymphatic system

- The lymphatic system is a network of lymph vessels, cells and specialised organs.
- The lymph is drained from the tissues and carried in lymph capillaries that converge into larger vessels, ultimately returning the lymph back to the circulatory system.
- Lymph is filtered through numerous lymph nodes.
- Immune cells in lymph nodes are in a strategic position to encounter antigens that have entered tissues.
- The secondary lymphoid organs comprise the lymph nodes, spleen, tonsils and clusters of lymphoid cells in mucosal surfaces.

ANTIGENS

- Antigens are foreign substances that activate the body's acquired immune system and induce an immune response.
- Most antigens are large, complex molecules of proteins, lipoproteins, glycoproteins, nucleoproteins or polysaccharides.
- Antigens are present on the surfaces of microorganisms and human and animal cells.

Complete antigens and haptens

- Complete antigens are foreign substances that stimulate specific T and B lymphocytes, inducing them to produce an immune response.
- Some small foreign molecules, such as peptides, nucleotides and saccharides, are not usually immunogenic, but become so if attached to the body's own proteins. These are called haptens.

Epitopes

- Only a small part of the antigen molecule is immunogenic (the epitope or antigenic determinant); it is the part to which free antibodies or activated B or T lymphocytes can bind.
- Most naturally occurring antigens consist of a number of different epitopes.

HUMORAL IMMUNITY

Antigen processing

- Macrophages or dendritic cells are usually the first cells to recognise antigen. They are called antigen-presenting cells because they engulf and process antigen for presentation to lymphocytes.
- Antigen processing involves partial degradation of antigen and its attachment to special recognition molecules on the surface of presenting cells.

Activation of B cells and formation of antibodies

- Each mature B lymphocyte carries molecules of specific antibody (the antigen receptor) on its membrane and is activated when an antigen binds to this receptor.
- Following the activation of B cells there are two distinct phases: proliferation, to expand the number of cells capable of reacting to the particular antigen; and differentiation into plasma cells or long-lived memory B cells.
- A population of lymphocytes, all with the same specificity, is called a clone.
- Antibodies are secreted by the plasma cells into body fluids.
- In the activation of the B lymphocyte, an antigen-presenting cell and a T helper lymphocyte are usually involved.
- The primary immune response is the response of the acquired immune system the first time it is exposed to a particular antigen.
- If a person is exposed to the same antigen for a second time, a secondary immune response occurs that is faster, stronger and longer-lasting.
- The secondary response is different because the immune system has been primed to the antigen in the primary response, and produced large numbers of memory B cells (immunological memory).

Basic antibody structure

- Antibodies (or immunoglobulins) are proteins found in blood and other body fluids.
- All antibody molecules have a basic Y-shaped structure consisting of four polypeptide chains linked together by disulfide bonds. Two of these chains are long and identical, and are called heavy (H) chains.
- The two 'arms' of the antibody molecule are called antigen-binding fragments; at the ends of the arms are the antigen-binding sites.
- The high specificity of the antigen-binding sites for their antigens is similar to that of the active site of enzymes for their substrates.

Antibody classes

- Five major immunoglobulin classes have been identified in humans: IgD, IgM, IgG, IgA, and IgE.
- IgM is the first type of antibody produced after primary antigenic stimulation and lasts for only a short time (weeks to months) in body fluids.
- IgG is the most abundant antibody in blood and persists for months to years after antigenic stimulation; it is the only antibody class able to cross the placenta from mother to foetus.
- IgA is found primarily in the mucus that covers the body's mucosal surfaces and plays a major role in preventing pathogens from crossing the epithelium.
- The monomeric forms of IgM and IgD are membrane proteins present on the surface of B lymphocytes that act as antigen receptors.
- IgE antibodies are responsible for in allergic reactions and also thought to be involved in immunity to worm infections.

The basis of antibody diversity

- The acquired immune system can make antibodies to millions of different antigens.
- There are believed to be about 600 genes for antibodies.
- Antibody diversity comes from the shuffling and combining of gene segments in different ways by each B cell as it becomes immunocompetent.
- As a result of gene shuffling and mutation on a large scale, the lymphoid system is thought to be capable of producing millions of different clones of lymphocytes.

Activities and functions of antibodies

- The basic function of antibody molecules is to bind specifically with their antigens and form antigen-antibody (or immune) complexes.
- Microorganisms or other particles, when coated with opsonising antibody, become more readily recognised and ingested by phagocytes.
- Antibody attachment, followed by complement fixation (or activation), can lead to lysis of foreign cells, such as bacteria and cancer cells.
- Neutralisation is a process in which antibodies bind to and block specific attachment sites on viruses or bacterial toxins.
- Antitoxin is the name given to antibodies that neutralise bacterial toxins.
- When cell-bound antigens are cross-linked by antibodies, clumping of the foreign cells occurs; this is called agglutination.
- In precipitation, soluble antigen molecules are cross-linked into large complexes which then precipitate out of solution.
- Agglutinated bacteria and precipitated foreign molecules are much more easily identified and captured by phagocytes.

Active versus passive immunity

- Active immunity is developed when the acquired immune system responds to microorganisms or other foreign substances entering the body.
- Active immunity is naturally acquired during microbial infections, and artificially acquired as a result of vaccination. It is long-lasting, often for a lifetime, especially when naturally acquired.
- Passive immunity results from the transfer of premade antibodies (or immune cells) from an immune person (or animal) to a non-immune person. The recipient becomes immune, but only for a short time.
- Passive immunity is conferred naturally on a foetus as the mother's antibodies pass across the placenta into the foetal circulation; they are also transferred via colostrum and breast milk.
- Passive immunity is artificially conferred when a person is injected with antibodies from an immune human or animal.
- Gammaglobulin is an immunoglobulin preparation extracted from the pooled serum of large numbers of blood donors. Each batch of this serum contains a

mixture of antibodies, which offers protection against a broad range of common infectious diseases.
- Specific immune globulin is an antibody preparation containing a high titre of antibodies against a specific disease.

CELL-MEDIATED IMMUNITY

- The cell-mediated immune response involves the activation, differentiation and actions of different types of T cells.

T cells and their functions
- The two main populations of T cells involved in the process of cellular immunity are (a) effector cells (called cytotoxic T cells) and (b) regulatory cells (called helper T cells).
- T cells that possess the CD4 marker (CD4 cells or T4 cells) are primarily the helper T cells; T cells with the CD8 marker (CD8 cells or T8 cells) are cytotoxic T cells.
- Helper T cells are regulatory cells whose major function is to help B cells and other T cells to respond to antigen.
- When helper T cells are activated by exposure to specific antigen, they secrete a variety of different molecules called lymphokines.
- Cytotoxic T cells directly attack and kill target cells, especially virus-infected cells.
- Cytotoxic T cells secrete potent cytokines that limit viral replication inside an infected cell and also attract phagocytes to the cell to destroy it.
- Some T lymphocytes appear to have suppressor activity (i.e. they down-regulate immune responses).

The cell-mediated immune response
- In cell-mediated immunity, the stimulus for clonal selection and T lymphocyte activation, proliferation and differentiation is the binding of antigen.
- The T cell receptor consists of two amino acid chains (a and b).
- T cells recognise and respond only to processed fragments of antigens displayed on surfaces of the body's own cells.
- Once a T cell is activated, it enlarges and proliferates to form a clone of cells that differentiate and perform functions according to their T cell class.

Cytokines and lymphokines
- The chemical mediators involved in cellular immunity are called cytokines; they include the lymphokines released by activated T cells.
- Some cytokines that act specifically between leukocytes are called interleukins.
- Cytokines provide communication between cells and have a central role in regulating the immune response.

IMMUNISATION

- Active immunity may be conferred artificially by immunisation (vaccination).
- Vaccines for viral diseases are particularly important because so many viral diseases lack effective treatment.

Types of vaccines
- Most vaccine preparations comprise one of the following: killed, whole microorganisms; live, attenuated microorganisms; inactivated bacterial toxins; or parts of bacterial cells or viruses.
- Killed vaccines are prepared by cultivating the required bacterium or virus and treating it with formalin, radiation or other agent that kills it but does not destroy its immunogenicity.
- Several vaccines are prepared from live, attenuated microbes that have lost their virulence but are still alive.
- A toxoid is a type of vaccine consisting of a bacterial exotoxin that has been inactivated, but is still antigenic.

Side effects of vaccines
- The most common side effects of vaccination are local hypersensitivity reactions at the injection site, fever or other allergies.
- Health professionals involved in giving vaccinations should be aware of the possible risks, but also aware that the risk of contracting the disease could be far more serious.
- Extreme caution must be exercised in giving live vaccines to the immunocompromised and to pregnant women.
- Herd immunity is based on the principle that individuals who are immune to an infectious disease will not be carriers of the organism, thus reducing the occurrence of that microbe and the number of susceptible people who will encounter it.

DISORDERS OF THE IMMUNE SYSTEM

IMMUNODEFICIENCY

- Immunodeficiency includes both inborn and acquired conditions in which the production or function of lymphocytes, phagocytes or complement is abnormal.
- Primary immunodeficiency is generally due to the improper foetal development of one or more of these components.
- The most serious primary immunodeficiency diseases are (a) congenital thymic hypoplasia or aplasia, caused by a failure of the thymus to develop fully, and (b) severe combined immunodeficiency disease, in which lymphocyte precursors in the bone marrow fail to develop properly, resulting in a marked deficiency in both B and T cells.
- Any agent that causes a suppression or malfunction of the bone marrow or lymphoid organs may cause a secondary immunodeficiency.
- The treatments for certain diseases can cause immunodeficiency (e.g. cytotoxic drugs, radiation therapy, corticosteroids, and immunosuppressive drugs).
- The most serious infectious secondary immunodeficiency is the acquired immune deficiency syndrome (AIDS), caused by the human immunodeficiency virus (HIV).

HYPERSENSITIVITY

- Hypersensitivity is an overreaction of the immune system to an antigen it has previously encountered.

Type I: Immediate hypersensitivity

- An immediate hypersensitivity, or allergy, occurs within minutes to several hours after a sensitised, susceptible person comes into contact with a foreign antigen.
- The term 'allergen' is used to distinguish the type of antigen that has the potential to elicit a Type I reaction.
- The predisposition for allergies is an inherited trait, associated with the production of IgE antibodies to allergens.
- IgE molecules have a special affinity for mast cells and basophils and attach to these cells. On subsequent exposure to the allergen, the allergen molecules cross-link the IgE antibodies, stimulating the cells to degranulate, releasing histamine and other inflammatory chemicals that rapidly induce an inflammatory response.
- Most allergic reactions are local, occurring where the allergen enters the body.
- Systemic reactions, referred to as anaphylaxis, occur when the allergen enters the blood and circulates through the body.

Type II: Cytotoxic hypersensitivity

- Cytotoxic hypersensitivity results from the binding of antibodies to antigens on the surface of a cell, followed by complement activation and lysis of the target cell.
- Type II cytotoxic reaction is the major cause of damage in many autoimmune diseases and in haemolytic disease of the newborn.

Type III: Immune complex hypersensitivity

- Immune complex hypersensitivity results when antigen-antibody complexes are formed and are not cleared quickly from the body by phagocytes.
- If circulating complexes are deposited on the basement membranes of certain tissues, the complexes activate complement and an inflammatory reaction occurs that can damage the tissues.

Type IV: Delayed type hypersensitivity

- Delayed type hypersensitivity reactions (cell-mediated hypersensitivity) are mediated by T cells and take a day or more to appear after the introduction of antigen.
- A subgroup of previously sensitised CD4 cells, called delayed type hypersensitivity T cells, are responsible.
- The Mantoux test for assessing immunity to tuberculosis depends on a delayed hypersensitivity reaction.

AUTOIMMUNE DISEASES

- Occasionally, the immune system loses its ability to distinguish self from non-self; that is, it loses its tolerance to one or more self-antigens.
- When the body produces autoantibodies and sensitised T lymphocytes against its own tissues, disease can result, called an autoimmune disease .

Study Questions

1. What are the major differences between the non-specific and specific defences of the body?
2. What factors make intact skin such an effective barrier against infection?
3. Describe the functions of mucus in preventing infection.
4. What is the mucociliary escalator and what is its function?
5. What are the major phagocytic cells of the body and what are their functions?
6. Describe the process of phagocytosis.
7. What are the major events in acute inflammation, and what are their functions?
8. What are chemical mediators of inflammation?
9. What is pus and what is its significance?
10. Explain the physiological basis of fever.
11. What is complement and what are its functions?
12. Describe the types and activities of interferon.
13. Define the terms: immune system, acquired immune system, immune response.
14. What are the three important characteristics of the acquired immune system?
15. What are the major differences between humoral immunity and cell-mediated immunity?
16. List the primary and secondary lymphoid organs in humans.
17. Distinguish between an antigen, a hapten and an epitope.
18. Describe the functions of plasma cells.
19. Describe the functions of memory cells.
20. Draw a graph showing the major differences between a primary and secondary immune response.
21. Draw a basic antibody molecule showing its antigen-binding sites.
22. What is an antitoxin?
23. Distinguish between gammaglobulin and specific immune globulin.
24. List the major types of T lymphocytes and describe their functions.
25. What is meant by the term 'immunodeficiency'?
26. Give two examples of secondary immunodeficiency.
27. What is meant by the term 'hypersensitivity'?

Test Your Understanding

1. Why are regular booster doses needed for some vaccines, but not for others?
2. Explain the principle behind the clonal selection theory.
3. A 25-year-old nurse pricks herself with a needle after using it to collect blood from a patient with hepatitis B. She has not been vaccinated against hepatitis B. What prophylactic treatment should she receive, and why?
4. Describe four conditions that would directly reduce a person's non-specific immunity and the effects each of these conditions would have.
5. What is opsonisation? Why is opsonisation important in the defence against microorganisms like *Streptococcus pneumoniae*?

FURTHER READING

Janeway, C.A., 1993, 'How the immune system recognises invaders', *Scientific American* 269, p. 41. (A detailed explanation of the basis of antibody diversity.)

Janeway, C.A. & P. Travers, *Immunobiology. The Immune System in Health and Disease*, London: Current Biology Ltd/Garland Publishing Inc., 1994. (A comprehensive text of immunology, detailing the molecules, cells, organs and processes that comprise the immune system.)

Marrack, P. & J.W. Kappler, 1993, 'How the immune system recognises the body', *Scientific American* 269, p. 48. (A detailed explanation of how the body's immune system is able to distinguish between foreign substances and self substances.)

Nossal, G.J.V., 1993, 'Life, death and the immune system', *Scientific American* 269, p. 20. (A succinct overview of the immune system, summarising the important components and how they protect the human body.)

Paul, W.E., 1993, 'Infectious diseases and the immune system', *Scientific American* 269, p. 57. (A summary of the mechanisms of the immune system that protect the body against infection.)

Seymour, G.J., N.W. Savage & L.J. Walsh, *Immunology. An Introduction for the Health Sciences*, Sydney: McGraw-Hill, 1995. (A well-written text giving a concise and readable overview of the concepts of immunology.)

Weissman, I.L. & M.D. Cooper, 1993, 'How the immune system develops', *Scientific American* 269, p. 32. (A summary of the development of immunocompetent lymphocytes from stem cells produced in the bone marrow.)

chapter 10

pathogenic mechanisms

and evasion strategies of microorganisms

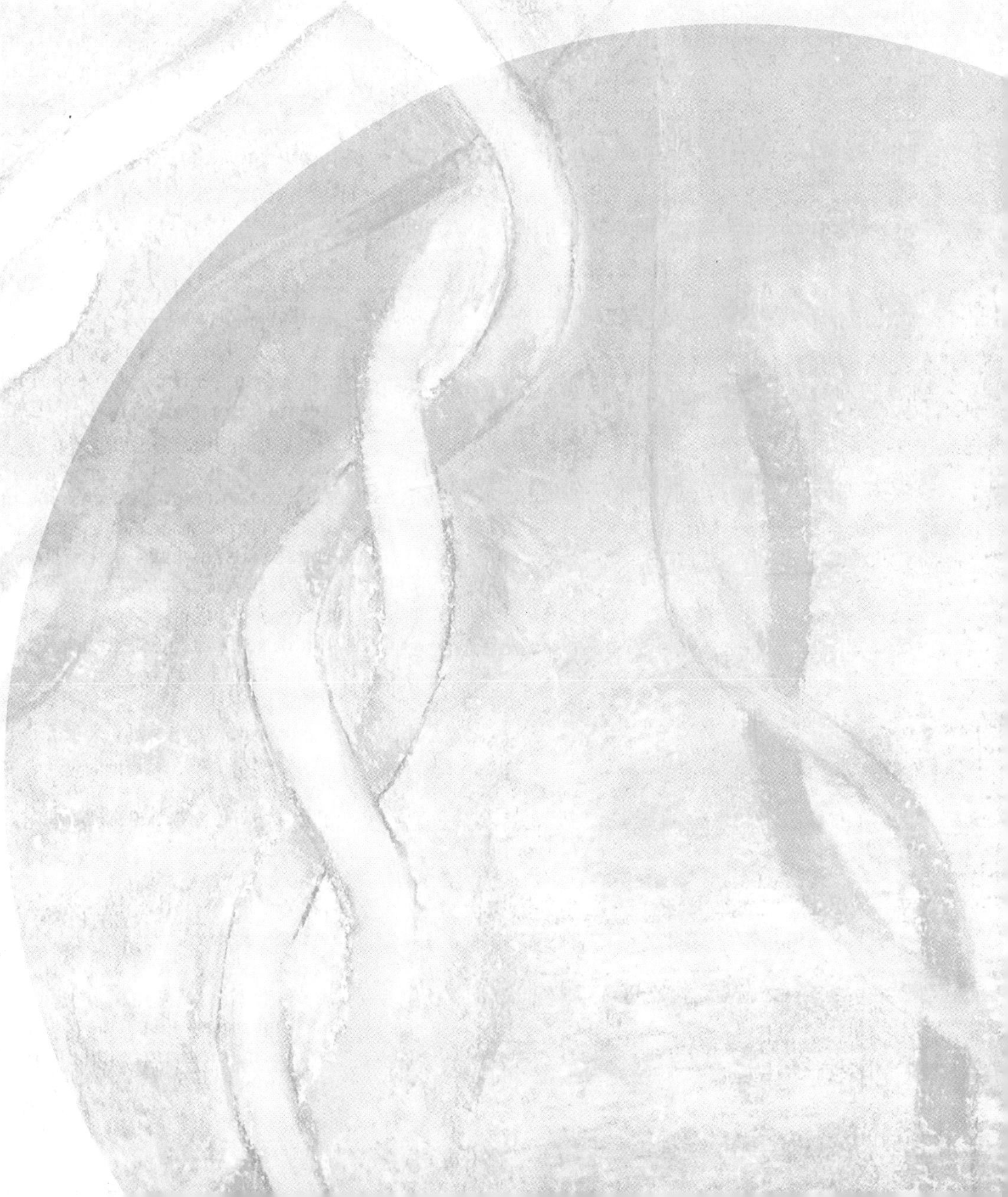

Chapter focus

- *How do microorganisms cause disease?*
- *What substances do microorganisms produce that enable them to cause disease?*
- *How do microorganisms damage human cells?*
- *How do pathogenic microorganisms evade the defence systems of the body?*

Chapter 9 described the ways in which the human body protects itself against infection and against certain other types of diseases. In this chapter we look at the other end of the balance between infection and health (see Figure 10.1). In order to cause disease, pathogenic microorganisms have to possess characteristics and/or properties that enable them to bypass or overcome the host's defences. As described in Chapter 7, the ability of an organism to cause disease is referred to as its **pathogenicity**. The factors that contribute to an organism's ability to cause disease are called **virulence factors**. For many organisms the factors involved are either unclear or not known. However, for some, we do know what characteristics or properties enable them to overcome the host's defences and cause disease. We will examine these factors in detail in this chapter.

FIGURE 10.1
THE BALANCE BETWEEN DISEASE AND HEALTH
When the resistance of the host is greater than the pathogenicity of the microbe, the host remains healthy; when the pathogenicity of the microbe is greater than the resistance of the host, disease occurs.

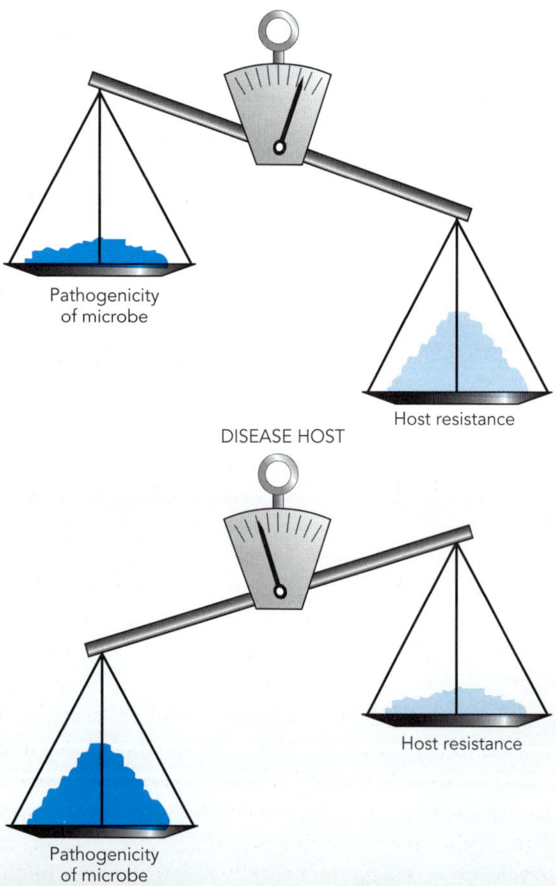

Most microorganisms enter the human body by way of a mucous membrane or a break in the skin. In order to establish themselves, most microbes must first adhere to specific tissues within the host. Once inside the body, pathogenic microorganisms may cause damage to the host, and hence disease, in a variety of ways. This usually involves the invasion of tissues and cells, and/or the release of substances that cause cell damage or cellular dysfunction. Some microbes have to enter cells to damage them, whereas others can cause damage from outside the cell. As described in Chapter 7, some pathogens enter the lymphatic or circulatory systems and spread to other parts of the body where further foci of infection may be established. In other diseases, the organisms remain localised at or near their site of entry, but cause damage at remote sites by secreting toxic substances which are transported in body fluids to other parts of the body.

Adherence

Adherence is the process by which microorganisms attach to host tissues. It is an important step in the pathogenicity of many organisms, particularly those that enter the body via mucous membranes. If, after entering the body, the microorganism is quickly expelled (e.g. as a result of coughing, sneezing or urination), then it will be unable to cause infection. Often adherence involves a specific interaction between surface components of a microorganism and surface receptors on host cells. For example, fibronectin, a protein found on the surface of many human cells, is the receptor to which *Streptococcus pyogenes* and other Gram-positive bacteria attach when colonising the upper respiratory tract. In some cases, this specific interaction helps to explain why a certain organism can only infect a particular host species and even a particular cell type in that species. It is this specificity that largely determines the potential sites of infection of a given microorganism. This is especially true for viruses.

The substances on the surfaces of microorganisms that enable them to attach to cell surfaces are called **adhesins**. The adhesins of some bacteria are found on specific attachment structures called pili or fimbriae (see Chapter 4). Strains of *Escherichia coli* that cause urinary tract infections usually have attachment pili that enable them to establish infection in the bladder and kidneys. The piliated strains are much more commonly associated with urinary tract infections than the non-piliated strains; that is, the piliated strains are more virulent. Other strains of *E. coli* that cause diarrhoea adhere specifically to cells of the small intestine by way of pili (different to those for the urinary tract). Similarly, pathogenic strains of *Neisseria gonorrhoeae*, the cause of gonorrhoea, have pili which allow them to attach to epithelial cells in the urogenital tract, whereas non-piliated strains rarely cause disease.

The adhesins of other organisms are surface substances such as sticky slime layers (glycocalyx), proteins or polysaccharides (Figure 10.2). For example, *Streptococcus mutans*, one of the organisms largely responsible for tooth decay, has a glycocalyx. The organism attaches to the tooth surface by this sticky layer and, by colonising this site and producing acids, contributes to plaque formation.

Adherence is also important in the pathogenesis of bacterial meningitis. In order to cause meningitis, the bacteria must enter the central nervous system from the bloodstream, and to do this they have to cross the highly specialised capillaries that comprise the blood-brain barrier. Although the exact way in which bacteria cross this barrier is not clear, it is thought that polysaccharide capsules may play a critical role in the attachment of the bacteria to the endothelial cells of the capillaries. Indeed, the three major causes of acute bacterial meningitis—*Neisseria meningitidis*, *Haemophilus influenzae* and *Streptococcus pneumoniae*—are all encapsulated.

Viruses attach to specific membrane receptors on the cells that they infect. Some have specialised attachment structures like tail fibres (as in bacteriophages) or envelope spikes (see Chapter 5). Generally, the presence of a particular receptor on the membrane of a cell is the key determinant of whether a particular virus can infect that cell or not. For example, the human immunodeficiency virus (HIV) preferentially infects cells that possess a glycoprotein called the CD4 receptor on their surfaces (see Chapter 19). This receptor is found mainly on helper T lymphocytes, which are therefore the major targets for this virus. Many parasitic helminths fasten to host tissues by way of suckers or hooks (see Chapter 6). Similarly, the protozoan *Giardia intestinalis* attaches to epithelial cells lining the intestine via an adhesive disc.

FIGURE 10.2
MECHANISMS OF ADHERENCE OF PATHOGENIC MICROORGANISMS
(a) attachment pili; (b) adherent slime, capsule or other sticky substance; (c) viral envelope spikes.

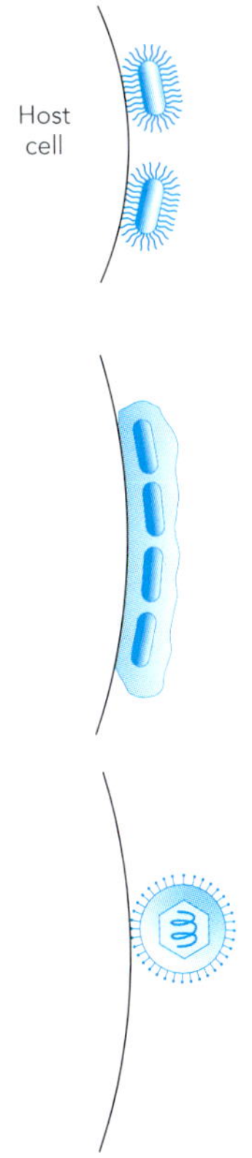

Toxins

Toxins are substances produced by some microorganisms that interfere with the normal functioning of host cells or tissues. They do this either by directly damaging cells or tissues or by altering normal cellular processes. Not all microorganisms produce toxins, but the production and release of toxins are, for some bacteria, the most important determinants of their ability to damage tissues and thus cause disease. A loss of their ability to produce toxins results in their loss of pathogenicity. We know most about bacterial toxins, but still only understand in detail the action of some of them. Some species of protozoa, fungi and helminths also produce toxins. Viruses, on the other hand, do not produce toxins, but cause cell damage by multiplying in cells, leading to cell destruction or alteration of function.

Bacterial toxins are classically divided into two broad groups:

- **Exotoxins** are toxins secreted into the surrounding environment in which the bacteria are growing (e.g. host tissues, food, soil, water).
- **Endotoxins** are toxins that form part of the outer membrane of Gram-negative bacteria; they are not actively secreted but are released when the bacterial cell is damaged or lysed.

EXOTOXINS

Exotoxins are heat-labile proteins that are usually released as the organism grows, although in some spore-forming bacteria, like the clostridia, toxin release occurs as a by-product of spore formation. While many different forms of toxins occur, there is a general structure to which a number conform. This is a two-subunit structure—one subunit is responsible for initial binding of the toxin to the target cell and its entry into the cell; and a separate subunit, which is the active component, is responsible for the inhibition or alteration of some cellular function.

Some bacteria produce a single exotoxin, and the major manifestations of the disease are due to the action of that toxin. Others produce many toxins, which have a number of different effects on the host. The more common exotoxin-producing bacteria are listed in Table 10.1. Some exotoxins are extremely potent and include some of the strongest poisons known. One gram of botulinum toxin, for example, is sufficient to kill 10 million people, and 300 grams would be enough to kill the entire population of the world! The tetanus and *Shigella* toxins are similarly potent.

Most bacteria secrete their toxins while growing in the host. But some, like *Clostridium botulinum* and *Staphylococcus aureus*, secrete their toxins into food and the preformed toxin is ingested when a person eats the contaminated food. To produce disease these organisms don't need to grow inside the host. In fact, they don't survive well in the body even when ingested. Since the toxin is responsible for disease, and not the growth of the organism itself, this type of disease is often referred to as an **intoxication**, rather than infection.

Bacterial exotoxins vary greatly in their degree of specificity. Some affect a wide range of cells and tissues. Others have specific targets and are sometimes grouped and named according to the tissues they primarily affect. The major groups are **neurotoxins**, which act pre-

TABLE 10.1
EXAMPLES OF DISEASES CAUSED BY EXOTOXINS

ORGANISM AND DISEASE	EXOTOXIN	ACTION OF TOXIN	SYMPTOMS PRODUCED
Bacillus anthracis (anthrax)	cytotoxin	Increases vascular permeability	Pulmonary oedema
Bordetella pertussis (whooping cough)	pertussis toxin	Damages respiratory mucosal cells	Paroxysmal cough
Clostridium botulinum (botulism)	neurotoxin	Blocks acetylcholine release at neuromuscular junctions	Flaccid paralysis
Clostridium perfringens (gas gangrene, food poisoning)	α-toxin enterotoxin	Lysis of various cell types Causes excessive loss of fluid and electrolytes from intestinal cells	Tissue destruction Diarrhoea
Clostridium tetani (tetanus)	tetanus toxin	Interferes with transmission in inhibitory interneurones	Severe muscle spasm
Corynebacterium diphtheriae (diphtheria)	diphtheria toxin	Damages many cell types by stopping protein synthesis	Damage to throat, heart, and nerve tissue
Entamoeba histolytica (amoebic dysentery)	enterotoxin	Lysis of epithelial cells lining the colon	Bloody, mucoid diarrhoea
Escherichia coli (gastroenteritis)	enterotoxin	Causes loss of fluid and electrolytes from intestinal cells	Diarrhoea
Listeria monocytogenes (listeriosis)	listeriolysin	Lysis of many cell types	Tissue damage, loss of red cells and white cells
Pseudomonas aeruginosa (various infections)	exotoxin A	Inhibits protein synthesis in cells	Tissue damage
Shigella dysenteriae (dysentery)	shiga toxin	Inhibits protein synthesis in many cell types	Uncertain
Staphylococcus aureus (various infections)	α-toxin leukocidin enterotoxin exfoliatin TSST-1	Lysis of red and white cells Kills white cells Stimulates intestinal cells Unclear Stimulates T cells to release certain cytokines	Infection and abscess Infection and abscess Vomiting, diarrhoea Scalded skin syndrome Toxic shock syndrome
Streptococcus pyogenes (scarlet fever and other infections)	pyrogenic exotoxin streptolysin O and S	Vasodilation of skin capillaries Lysis of red and white cells	Diffuse rash and fever Tissue damage
Vibrio cholerae (cholera)	cholera toxin	Causes severe loss of fluid and electrolytes from intestinal cells	Profuse diarrhoea

dominantly on nervous tissue, and **enterotoxins**, which act specifically on the small intestine. However, for a clear understanding of how exotoxins produce disease, it is most appropriate to examine them in terms of their mode of action; that is, what the toxins actually do to damage the host tissues or interfere with normal processes.

Toxins that break down cells

A large number of exotoxins act by damaging host cell membranes, resulting in lysis and death of the cells. Some of these toxins are phospholipases, like the α-toxin of *Clostridium perfringens*, a cause of gas gangrene. Phospholipase enzymes lyse cells by hydrolysing the phospholipid lecithin (phosphatidylcholine), a common component of mammalian cell membranes. Other lytic toxins damage host cell membranes by inserting themselves into the cell membrane, creating pores or channels. The membrane becomes more permeable to water and, because of the higher concentration of the cytoplasm compared to the environment, water rushes into the cell, causing it to swell and rupture. The α-toxin of *Staphylococcus aureus* and the streptolysin-O of *Streptococcus pyogenes* are examples of pore-forming toxins.

Many phospholipase and pore-forming types of toxins break down red cells, and are therefore referred to as **haemolysins**, although they usually break down other cells as well. When bacteria that secrete haemolysins are grown on culture media containing blood (e.g. sheep blood agar), distinct zones of red cell clearing can be seen around the bacterial colonies. The soluble exotoxins diffuse into the agar and cause destruction of red cells around the colony (see Figure 10.3). This property is useful in the identification of some bacteria.

FIGURE 10.3
BACTERIAL HAEMOLYSIS
Clearing or complete haemolysis of blood agar caused by colonies of *Streptococcus pyogenes*.

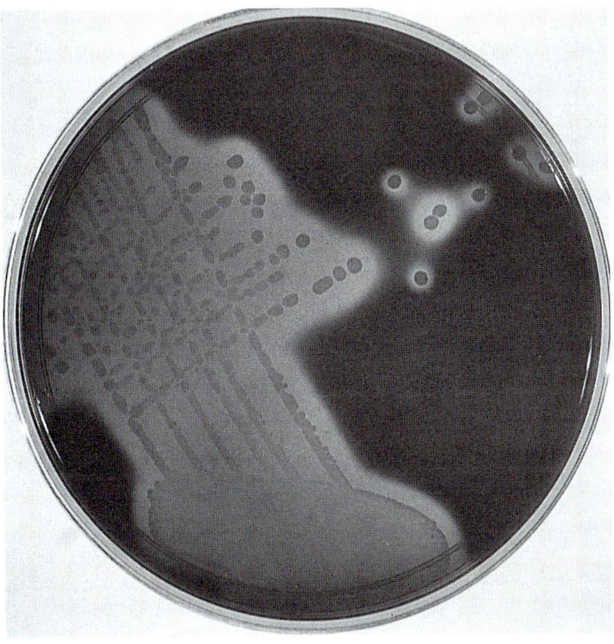

Some bacteria, such as *S. aureus* and *S. pyogenes*, secrete toxins called **leukocidins** that kill phagocytic leukocytes (neutrophils and macrophages). The leukocidins of these organisms induce the release of the lysosomal enzymes into the cytosol of the white cell itself. These highly destructive enzymes are normally packaged up safely within the lysosomal membrane but, once released, cause lethal damage to the cell by breaking down cellular components. Destruction of phagocytic white cells in this way presumably increases the ability of leukocidin-producing organisms to survive and persist longer in the body. In addition, release of the lysosomal enzymes from dead phagocytes can cause further damage to the surrounding tissue.

Toxins that enhance microbial spread or survival in tissues

Many bacteria secrete enzymes that help them to break down tissues. These enzymes increase the *invasiveness* of bacteria by breaking down substances that would otherwise impede their spread through tissues. **Hyaluronidases** are produced by many bacteria, including staphylococci, streptococci and clostridia. These enzymes break down hyaluronic acid, a component of the ground substance of virtually all connective tissue, making the tissue less viscous and easier to penetrate. **Collagenases** are enzymes that break down collagen, the tough fibres that give strength and a supporting network to connective tissues. *C. perfringens* and some helminths (worms) are examples of organisms that secrete collagenases.

Skin is a highly protective coating against microbial infection, due mainly to the presence of the relatively indigestible protein called keratin. However, the fungi that cause tinea (ringworm) are able to infect skin because they secrete a keratin-degrading enzyme, or **keratinase**. Some organisms (e.g. *Vibrio cholerae*) secrete a **mucinase** which digests a glycoprotein in mucus, thereby enhancing their ability to colonise mucous membranes.

The body's defence against local infection sometimes includes the deposition of a layer of fibrin around the infected site. This is designed to wall off the infection, preventing the spread of microorganisms into adjacent tissue. **Kinases** are a group of enzymes produced by certain bacteria that help them to dissolve fibrin clots and hence break through this barrier. **Streptokinase** is produced by some streptococci, including *S. pyogenes*, and **staphylokinase** is produced by *S. aureus*. Streptokinase is in fact used therapeutically as a thrombolytic agent in patients with thromboses (see Spotlight box, p. 221).

Coagulase is an enzyme produced by some staphylococci, which has almost the opposite effect to kinases. This enzyme coagulates fibrinogen to form a deposit of fibrin material around the bacterial cells which is thought to offer them some protection against host phagocytic cells. The pathogenicity of staphylococci depends largely on their ability to produce coagulase. Some coagulase-negative staphylococci are pathogenic, but generally they are much less frequently associated with disease than the coagulase-positive species.

> **SPOTLIGHT**
> **STREPTOKINASE**
>
> Streptokinase is an enzyme produced by some streptococci that breaks down fibrin clots by converting plasminogen into the proteolytic enzyme, plasmin. Streptokinase assists the bacteria to spread and produce disease, but a therapeutic use for the enzyme has been uncovered.
>
> Because of its action in breaking down thrombi (blood clots), streptokinase is used in patients with disorders where clots may develop and obstruct vital blood vessels. Its use is thus indicated in patients with acute myocardial infarction, pulmonary embolism or arterial thrombosis.
>
> Streptokinase, however, is a foreign protein and so a patient may develop some immunity to the substance. For this reason, it may not be effective in patients who have previously been administered with the substance or who have recently had a streptococcal infection. Its use is contraindicated in people with an existing or recent haemorrhagic (bleeding) disorder.

Toxins that interfere with cellular metabolism

There are several toxins that enter cells and alter their metabolism in some way. *Corynebacterium diphtheriae* secretes a toxin that is one of the best understood of all bacterial toxins. The toxin first binds to a receptor on the host cell membrane and then enters the cell by an endocytotic process. The toxin blocks protein synthesis by inactivating elongation factor 2, an enzyme necessary for the growth of the polypeptide chain in translation. The cell dies because it can no longer synthesise proteins. The exotoxin A of *Pseudomonas aeruginosa* appears to have a similar mode of action to that of diphtheria toxin.

Diphtheria toxin is highly potent; one molecule is thought to be sufficient to kill a cell. The pathogenicity of *C. diphtheriae* is entirely due to this toxin; strains that do not have the gene for toxin production are non-pathogenic. Although *C. diphtheriae* remains localised in the throat during the infection, the secreted toxin is absorbed and enters the bloodstream. The actions of the toxin in the throat cause considerable damage to mucosal cells, resulting in a membrane (called a pseudomembrane) over the mucosal surface, consisting of fibrin, bacteria and inflammatory cells. When the larynx is involved, a life-threatening obstruction of the airway can occur (see Chapter 17). The action of diphtheria toxin on other organs, especially the heart, can result in irregular heartbeat, coma and death.

The enterotoxin of *Vibrio cholerae*, the causative agent of cholera, is an exotoxin that alters the regulatory control in a cell, rather than directly damaging it. Cholera toxin binds specifically to intestinal epithelial cells. It then enters the cell and causes increased and uncontrolled production of cyclic AMP, the mediator of a number of regulatory systems in cells. The increased levels of cyclic AMP cause unregulated secretion of chloride and bicarbonate ions from the epithelial cells lining the intestine. This change in ionic balance results in a massive outflow of water from the cells into the lumen of the intestine, manifested as a profuse diarrhoea (see Figure 10.4). The loss of water can be so great that cholera victims may die from extreme dehydration if their fluids and electrolytes are not replaced. The toxins of enteropathogenic *Escherichia coli* and *Salmonella* are believed to have a similar action.

Toxins that affect nerve cell function

The neurotoxins of the anaerobic bacteria *Clostridium tetani* and *Clostridium botulinum* are two of the most potent toxins known. *Clostridium tetani* usually grows in deep, necrotic puncture wounds where anaerobic conditions exist. The bacterium itself does not spread far from the initial site of infection, but the exotoxin that it secretes travels to the central nervous system to cause severe neuromuscular dysfunction. *Cl. tetani* is a good example of an organism that produces only a single toxin. The toxin binds to the surface of nerve cells, is internalised, and is then transported to the spinal cord, where it becomes fixed to nerve synapses. It interferes specifically with synaptic transmission in inhibitory interneurones, creating an imbalance in the excitatory and inhibitory transmissions to motor neurones. This causes an excessive stimulation of muscles, resulting in an uncontrolled, rigid muscle contraction, or spastic paralysis. Different muscles may be affected, such as the powerful masseter muscles of the jaw, resulting in the classic condition of tetanus known as *lockjaw*. Often, back muscles are affected, causing arching of the back and sometimes even crushing of spinal processes in severe cases (see Figure 20.4, p. 482).

Botulism occurs when the preformed toxin of *Cl. botulinum* is ingested in contaminated food, often inadequately prepared home-canned foods. The organism itself normally causes no problem if ingested because it is unable to compete successfully with the normal gut

FIGURE 10.4
THE MODE OF ACTION OF CHOLERA TOXIN
The toxin increases cyclic AMP production in epithelial cells of the intestine. This results in an outflow of water and ions from these cells, producing diarrhoea.

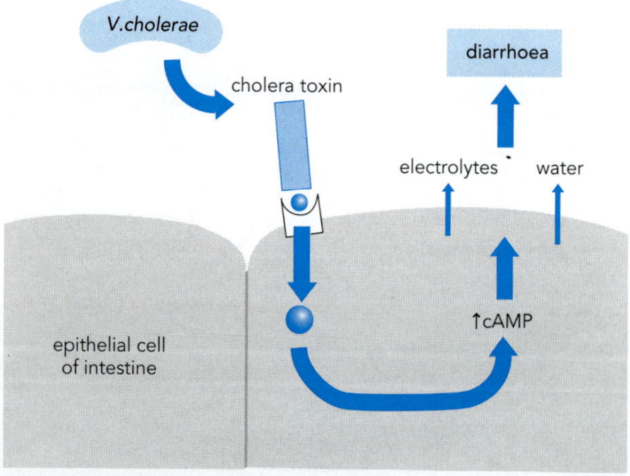

flora. As stated earlier, botulism is usually an intoxication, caused by toxins produced outside the body, rather than an infectious disease. The toxin is resistant to gastrointestinal digestion; after ingestion it crosses the gut wall and ultimately localises at the neuromuscular junctions. Infant botulism is different in that growth of the clostridia and production of toxin occur in the colon. In this disease the clostridia are able to grow and produce toxin because the infant colon has a poorly developed microbial flora which is unable to inhibit the pathogen.

In contrast to tetanus toxin, botulinum toxin acts on peripheral nerve endings. At neuromuscular junctions the toxin binds to presynaptic terminal membranes and blocks the release of acetylcholine, preventing transmission of impulses from the nerve cell to the muscle cell, and hence muscle contraction (see Figure 10.5). This flaccid paralysis in botulism can lead to the death of the patient due to dysfunction of the respiratory muscles and respiratory failure.

TOXOIDS AND ANTITOXINS

Exotoxins are proteins and, as such, are usually antigenic; that is, they are capable of stimulating the production of antitoxins (antibodies to the toxins) by the immune system (see Chapter 9). An antitoxin, once produced, is able to bind to the toxin and neutralise it; that is, prevent it from binding to its target cell or tissue. Exotoxins are thus effective immunogens, but of course cannot be used in their natural form in vaccines. Fortunately, many exotoxins can be chemically modified by heat, or chemical substances such as formaldehyde and phenol, in order to remove their toxicity but still retain their ability to elicit an immune response. Toxins modified in this way are called **toxoids**, and can be used in vaccines to stimulate immunity without causing disease. Toxoids are particularly useful in vaccines when the toxin is the major (or only) virulence factor of the organism. Toxoids for diphtheria and tetanus are used in the diphtheria-pertussis-tetanus (DPT) vaccine for young children.

It is interesting to note that in some diseases, such as tetanus, so little toxin is required to produce the symptoms of disease that the person's immune system may not be sufficiently stimulated by the toxin to produce antibodies. That is, the clinical disease does not confer immunity, and a person who survives clinical tetanus may not subsequently be immune to the disease, unless actively immunised.

The treatment of diseases caused by exotoxin-producing bacteria sometimes involves the use of **antitoxins** to neutralise the toxin already in the body. Antitoxins are antibody preparations derived from the serum of immune humans or animals. They are particularly important for diseases such as tetanus and botulism, which can have a rapidly fatal outcome. Injection of specific antitoxin (also called **specific immune globulin**) is aimed at immediate neutralisation of the toxin before it is able to bind to target cells. Without antitoxin, patients may die, because their immune systems do not have sufficient time to make the required antibodies. Thorough excision and cleansing of the wound and appropriate antibiotic therapy are important for elimination of tetanus organisms from the wound, but are of secondary importance to antitoxin therapy. Antibiotics are not necessary in botulism at all, since the organism does not survive inside the body.

ENDOTOXINS

Endotoxins consist of the lipopolysaccharides (LPS) of the cell walls of Gram-negative bacteria. As described in Chapter 4, the outer membrane of the Gram-negative cell wall consists of LPS, lipoproteins and phospholipids. The exact composition of LPS varies from genus to genus and species to species. The lipid A portion of LPS is the actively toxic component. Being a part of the bacterial cell wall, endotoxins only exert their effect once the cell wall breaks down. During infection, small amounts of LPS may be sloughed off as cells grow or may be released as older bacterial cells die. However, death of bacteria and release of endotoxin can be greatly accelerated once

FIGURE 10.5
THE MODE OF ACTION OF BOTULINUM TOXIN
The toxin blocks the release of acetylcholine at the neuromuscular junction causing a flaccid paralysis.

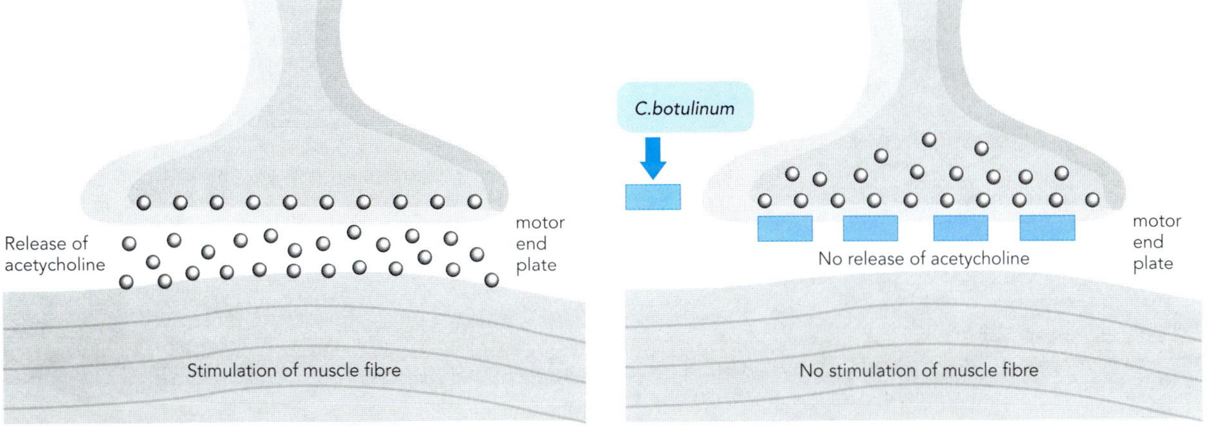

phagocytes begin to digest them or once antibiotics that kill the bacteria are administered. Thus, in some cases, antibiotics may initially cause a worsening of symptoms.

Other major differences between exotoxins and endotoxins are that the latter are generally less toxic, relatively heat-stable and cannot be toxoided. Although endotoxins can induce an immune response, they cannot be treated in a similar way to exotoxins to render them non-toxic while still preserving their ability to induce antibody formation.

Endotoxin, regardless of its source, produces similar signs and symptoms in the host. It can cause a variety of host responses, many of which involve some part of the immune system. Fever is one of the more common and important of the symptoms. Endotoxin produces fever by stimulating the release of endogenous pyrogens from mononuclear phagocytes. Currently, the best known of these pyrogens are the cytokines interleukin-1 (IL-1) and tumour necrosis factor (TNF) (see Chapter 9). These act on the temperature-regulating centre in the hypothalamus to reset the body temperature set-point (or thermostat) to a higher level, resulting in an increase in body temperature. Other possible responses of the host to endotoxin include muscle weakness, generalised aches, diarrhoea and malaise.

Large amounts of endotoxin may be released during a systemic infection caused by bacteria such as *E. coli, Neisseria meningitidis* or *Pseudomonas aeruginosa*. This can have severe effects on the body. **Endotoxic** (or **septic**) **shock**, the shock caused by large amounts of endotoxin, is frequently fatal. In this situation, endotoxin is believed to induce the release of TNF, IL-1 and other cytokines from a variety of cells, including monocytes, macrophages and lymphocytes. The systemic release of large amounts of these cytokines causes damage to blood capillaries and alters their permeability characteristics. Large amounts of fluid leak into the tissues, causing a severe drop in blood pressure, resulting in shock. Septic shock due to Gram-positive bacteria and other organisms is thought to be caused by a similar triggering of cytokine release from host cells.

Endotoxin may also cause a non-specific activation of blood coagulation mechanisms, resulting in the blockage of small vessels by thrombi in organs such as the kidney, brain and lungs. Tissue necrosis in the blood-deprived areas of these organs may then occur. This potentially fatal disorder is referred to as **disseminated intravascular coagulation**. In rare cases of *N. meningitidis* infection, infarction of adrenal glands can occur (called the Waterhouse-Friderichsen syndrome—see Chapter 20) leading to a rapid death.

Invasion of Cells

Viruses typically cause disease by invading and damaging host cells. As explained in Chapter 5, viruses are obligate intracellular parasites and are able to replicate only inside their specific target cells. Once inside the cell a virus can cause microscopically observable changes to the cell, called **cytopathic effects** (CPE). Different viruses cause different CPE in cells, and some of these can be observed by microscopic examination of the viruses grown in tissue culture (see Figure 10.6). Some viruses kill the cells they infect and are said to be cytocidal. They can do this by:

- diverting the cell's metabolic processes and stopping the synthesis of proteins or other macromolecules; or
- causing the release of lysosomal enzymes into the cytoplasm of the cell; or
- inserting viral proteins into the membrane of the cell during the release phase, resulting in rupture of the membrane and cell lysis.

Even if the virus does not directly kill the cell, it takes control of the regulatory mechanisms of the cell and produces viral proteins and nucleic acids, thus causing the cell to become dysfunctional. Some non-cytocidal viruses cause CPE characterised by the formation of inclusion bodies within the cell, such as the Negri bodies found in the brain cells of humans and animals infected with the rabies virus. These inclusion bodies are granules of unassembled viral components or deposits of viral remnants.

FIGURE 10.6
CYTOPATHIC EFFECTS CAUSED BY VIRUSES
(a) Uninfected fibroblasts; and (b) the same cells after being infected with herpes virus.

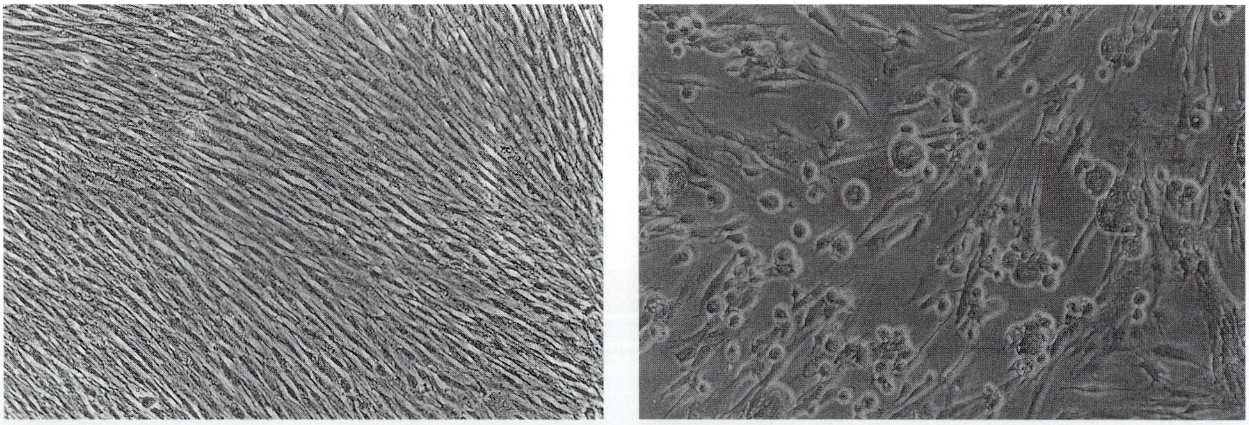

(a) (b)

Other viruses cause host cells to fuse with each other, producing multi-nucleated 'giant cells' (e.g. measles virus and respiratory syncytial virus). Eventually, the accumulated damage to the cell results in its death. However, some viruses, like the herpes simplex viruses, do not kill the cell; instead they remain dormant inside it for long periods, sometimes for life. These highly adapted parasites cause minimal damage to the nerve cells they infect, allowing them to remain there for years. Sometimes they may be reactivated many years later, and cause symptomatic disease (e.g. the herpes zoster virus and shingles).

Another important effect is the viral transformation of normal cells into cancer cells. This is discussed in the following section.

A few other organisms, apart from viruses, also invade cells and damage them. For example, chlamydia are bacteria which are obligate intracellular parasites. They enter epithelial cells and multiply quickly, lysing these cells within a couple of days. Rickettsia are also obligately intracellular bacteria which can invade many types of mammalian cells, especially vascular endothelium. They grow slowly in these cells, eventually breaking them open to release large numbers of organisms. *Plasmodium* spp., the causative agents of malaria, typically go through cycles of red blood cell invasion, multiplication, lysis of the red cells with release of large numbers of the merozoite form, and then infection of many more red cells.

Cellular Transformation into Tumour Cells

Some viruses cause disease by transforming host cells into tumour cells. Transformed cells differ markedly from normal cells in a number of ways. Typically, they have an altered morphology and do not have an ordered pattern of growth. Instead, they divide in an unregulated manner and form random aggregations of dysfunctional cells. These cells are not responsive to normal growth-regulating factors. Some human papillomaviruses (e.g. HPV 1, 2, 3 and 10) cause cutaneous warts, which are benign tumours. Other viruses are believed to be involved in malignant tumours, such as HPV types 16, 18, 31 and 33 in cervical cancer, and hepatitis B virus in hepatocellular carcinoma. Transformation of cells is brought about by the incorporation of viral nucleic acid into the host cell genome, which is then replicated along with the cell's DNA. The tumour-causing viruses and their relationship to oncogenes are described in Chapter 5.

Other Mechanisms of Pathogenesis

Microorganisms can cause disease in a variety of other ways. Sometimes, the clinical features of a disease arise from the physiological responses of the host to infection. For example, the major disease symptoms may be due to an abnormal response of the immune system. If the invading organism causes the host's immune response to be 'overreactive', then tissue damage may occur. This overreactivity of the immune system is referred to as **hypersensitivity**, and is the basis for many important diseases. For example, many pathogenic helminths release waste products during infection that induce allergic reactions. The bases of hypersensitivity reactions are described in Chapter 9. Each of the four classic types of hypersensitivity can be of a microbial or non-microbial origin. Examples of hypersensitivity reactions induced by microorganisms are listed in Table 10.2.

Microorganisms may also cause tissue damage by physical means. For example, a mass of *Ascaris* worms in the intestinal tract may cause obstruction. The larvae of a number of pathogenic helminths cause damage by blocking the flow of blood in small vessels, thus reducing the amount of oxygen and other nutrients to the adjacent tissues. In some diseases, other narrow, tubular structures, such as lymph vessels, may also be obstructed, such as occurs in elephantiasis, caused by the nematode *Wuchereira*. *Clostridium perfringens,* the major cause of gas gangrene, produces gas in the tissues where it is growing. The gas causes compression of the tissue and blood vessels in the area. The resultant lack of oxygen in the site allows further bacterial growth, causing more tissue necrosis. These physical effects may then be aggravated by the body's response to infection, in particular the exudation of fluid from the blood into the injured tissue. This fluid may compress the tissue further, causing more damage.

Evasion Strategies

When a microorganism invades the body it usually faces a hostile response from the host. The human body has developed numerous mechanisms by which it defends itself against microbial invasion and these are mobilised when organisms gain entry. However, many microbes are known to possess special structures or have attributes that protect them from the host's defences. Although these microbial countermeasures do not directly cause tissue damage, some are nevertheless largely responsible for the organism's pathogenicity, or capacity to cause disease.

ESCAPE FROM PHAGOCYTES

Phagocytes are vital components of the body's defence system. They are responsible for scouring the body's tissues, searching for foreign substances and microbes, which they then engulf and destroy. Their critical role in defence is described in Chapter 9. Many microorganisms have developed ways of escaping phagocytosis by blocking or avoiding some part of the phagocytic process. Indeed, the large variety of ways that microbes have developed to avoid being phagocytosed reflects the importance of phagocytosis in defending the body. You will recall from Chapter 9 that, once phagocytes have been attracted to a site of infection, phagocytosis involves:

1. binding to the microbe, followed by ingestion and containment of it within a membrane-bound vesicle called a phagosome;

TABLE 10.2
HYPERSENSITIVITY REACTIONS INDUCED BY MICROORGANISMS

TYPE OF HYPERSENSITIVITY INDUCED	EXAMPLES
Allergy/anaphylaxis	Some helminths, e.g. *Ascaris*
Autoimmunity	Rheumatic fever (*Streptococcus pyogenes*) *Mycoplasma* infections
Cytotoxic hypersensitivity	Hepatitis B
Immune complex disease	Malaria Acute glomerulonephritis (*Streptococcus pyogenes*) Syphilis Allergic alveolitis
Cell-mediated reactions	Tuberculosis Leprosy Tertiary syphilis Viral rashes

2. fusion of lysosomes with the phagosome to form a phagolysosome; and
3. the degradation of the microbe by the highly destructive lysosomal enzymes.

Avoidance of, or interference with, one of these steps can allow a microbe to escape destruction by these white cells.

Some organisms possess capsules or a surface slime layer (see Chapter 4) which prevents the phagocytes from ingesting them. The exact mechanism involved is not known, but it appears that the chemical composition of these structures is such that they prevent binding of the phagocyte. *Streptococcus pneumoniae* appears to lack any major virulence factor other than its capsule, but this enables it to avoid being ingested by alveolar macrophages, and thus to survive and multiply in the lungs. Mutant strains of the organism that do not have a capsule are unable to cause disease. Other organisms that rely on a capsule for pathogenicity include *Haemophilus influenzae, Neisseria meningitidis*, *Yersinia pestis* and *Cryptococcus neoformans*, the yeast that causes meningitis.

Host immunity to these organisms is based on the production of specific anti-capsular antibodies, which opsonise the bacteria and permit the phagocytes to engulf them (see Chapter 9). Instead of a capsule, *Streptococcus pyogenes* has a cell wall component, termed an M-protein, which helps it to avoid ingestion by phagocytes by interfering with complement-mediated opsonisation (see Chapter 9).

Some microorganisms allow themselves to be ingested by phagocytes but have developed ways of surviving inside them. Not only does this allow them to avoid destruction, but the phagocytes provide them with a place to hide and multiply, and may even help them to spread through the body. Some organisms, like the *Rickettsia*, appear to avoid being digested by exiting the phagosome and entering the cytoplasm of the phagocyte. This is a privileged site since lysosomes do not normally release their degradative enzymes into the cytoplasm.

Other organisms, like *Mycobacterium tuberculosis* and *Legionella pneumophila*, avoid intracellular digestion by somehow inhibiting the fusion of lysosomes with the phagosome. How they actually do this is not clear at the present time, but it probably relies on some modification of the phagosomal membrane by the bacteria. *Staphylococcus aureus* resists intracellular killing by producing the enzyme **catalase**, which breaks down hydrogen peroxide, one of the substances phagocytes produce to kill microbes.

Still other organisms, like the protozoa *Leishmania*, are innately resistant to lysosomal enzymes and can survive in the phagolysosome. Such organisms probably have resistant cell surface structures and/or secrete substances that inhibit the lysosomal enzymes.

The most aggressive strategy is to kill the phagocyte. As stated earlier in this chapter, certain bacteria, such as staphylococci and streptococci, secrete toxins called leukocidins, that kill phagocytes as well as other cells.

CONCEALMENT

Some microorganisms evade the host defences by hiding, usually inside cells or in other so-called 'privileged sites', where defence cells do not normally circulate. If a microorganism can remain inside a cell, without any sign of its antigens on the surface of the cell, then it will be unseen by defence cells. Even if specific immune responses are induced before the organism invades the cells, once inside, the antibodies or activated immune cells would be ineffective against these hidden enemies. Fortunately, in most cases, the microbe leaves some of its components or antigens on the cell surface when it enters the cell. This allows components of the immune system (especially cytotoxic T cells and natural killer cells—see Chapter 9) to recognise the infected cells and destroy them, thereby exposing the microbes to other immune factors.

In latent viral infections, however, the viruses don't display their antigens. The herpes simplex and varicella zoster viruses can remain in this way in sensory neurones for years, sometimes for a lifetime, despite the presence of specific immunity. Retroviruses, like the human immunodeficiency virus (HIV), are also thought to remain hidden in lymphoid cells or macrophages by first having their RNA transcribed into DNA and then having this integrated into the cell's DNA. Again, as long as there is no display of viral antigens on the surface of the cell, the virus remains undetected.

Other privileged sites include those areas of the body where complement, antibodies and lymphocyte activity are low. A good example is the central nervous system (CNS). Complement and antibody levels are very low in cerebrospinal fluid (CSF), and there are few white cells. Even though white cells may enter the CNS during infection, their activity appears to be limited by the lack of opsonic antibodies and complement proteins. Other such privileged sites include the joints and testes.

Some microorganisms are able to create their own privileged sites. Hydatid disease is caused by *Echinococcus granulosus*, a tiny tapeworm that can infect the liver, lung or brain. This parasite evades host defences by forming and residing within thin-walled capsules that resemble small bladders (see Figure 10.7). The worms can survive inside these fluid-filled cysts, even if there are protective antibodies in the blood of the patient. A connective tissue coating of host origin around the cyst prevents it from being attacked by host defences. The blood fluke, *Schistosoma*, conceals itself by becoming coated with various plasma glycoproteins and glycolipids. These host substances are not recognised as foreign and the worm escapes detection.

ANTIGENIC VARIATION

Antigenic variation is a phenomenon in which certain bacteria, viruses and protozoa repeatedly or progressively change their cell surface components, or antigens, enabling them to evade the immune system. If the microbe changes the antigens to which immune responses have been developed, it will be unaffected by any immunity directed at those original antigens. Microorganisms contain numerous antigens, but immunity to only some of these is protective. That is, the strategy of changing antigens to escape host defences depends on changes being made to critical antigens against which protective immune responses are directed. Antigenic variation can occur during the course of infection, enabling the organism to persist longer, or it may occur as the organism spreads through the community, allowing it to reinfect a given individual (see Figure 10.8). The ways by which microbial antigens can be changed are antigenic drift, antigenic shift and gene switching.

Antigenic drift is the term used for repeated minor mutations in the genes that code for antigens of microorganisms. The antigens are sufficiently critical, and the mutations change them sufficiently, to reduce the effectiveness of prior immunological memory, allowing the organism to cause infection again, despite immunity in the host to a prior infection. Influenza virus constitutes the classic example of this. The tendency for influenza to occur repeatedly in a population and in an individual is due partly to the ability of influenza viruses to undergo antigenic drift. The influenza viruses have two surface glycoprotein antigens (the haemagglutinin and neuraminidase 'spikes') to which neutralising antibodies are formed. Antigenic drift can occur when minor mutations in DNA result in small changes in the amino acid sequence of these antigens. If the changes occur in areas where antibodies bind to the antigen, the virus is not susceptible to antibodies produced in previous infections. The cold viruses (rhinoviruses) have a similar ability. We can thus have the flu or a cold year after year, partly because of antigenic changes to the viruses that cause them.

The HIV is also apparently capable of antigenic drift, while it is infecting a person. This is thought to occur partly because the infection persists for so long, and partly because the viral reverse transcriptase is prone to making mistakes in transcribing RNA into DNA. This antigenic drift may be part of the reason why the immune system is so ineffective in controlling this infection.

Antigenic shift is displayed by the influenza A virus. When two different strains of this virus infect the same cell, a recombination of the genes that code for the surface glycoproteins can occur. This results in a new strain that is different to previous strains, which can spread through a population because of the lack of protective antibodies in the population. Major pandemics of influenza in 1957, 1968 and 1977 are thought to have been due to the sudden appearance of a new strain of influenza A, as a result of antigenic shift.

Another form of antigenic variation results from the ability of some microorganisms to switch the genes (gene switching) that code for certain surface antigens. The best known example of this occurs in the protozoa that cause African sleeping sickness, the *Trypanosoma*. These organisms are covered with a thick coat made of proteins called 'variable surface glycoproteins'. These protozoa carry genes for several hundred or more distinct surface glycoproteins, but only one is expressed at any given time. Periodic switching of these genes (e.g. at weekly intervals) during the course of infection results in new antigenic forms being produced during infection. By the time antibodies are made to a given antigenic type, the gene has often been switched and a new antigenic type has appeared. There can be many successive variants of the parasite in a given host, and the immune system is constantly trying to catch up. Some bacteria are also thought to be capable of switching their surface antigens, such as *Neisseria gonorrhoeae* and species of *Brucella*.

IMMUNOSUPPRESSION

A number of microorganisms cause a depletion or reduction in the defences of the host. As a consequence, the immune response to the antigens of the microbe (and sometimes other unrelated antigens) may be depressed, resulting in little or no antibody production or cellular immunity (see Chapter 9) to these antigens. The human immunodeficiency

FIGURE 10.7

HYDATID CYSTS

Hydatid cysts are thin, fluid-filled sacs produced by the tapeworm *Echinococcus granulosus*. The worms hide from the body's defences by residing inside cysts.

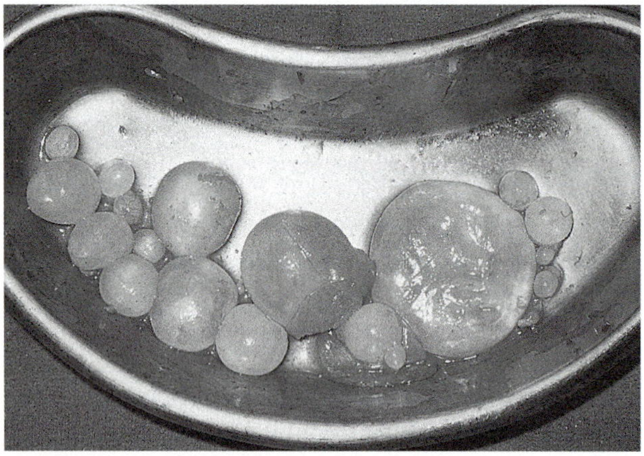

virus (HIV) is the most dramatic of microbial immunosuppressors, deriving its name in fact from this activity. The HIV suppresses the immune system in a number of ways. Much of it is believed to be due to infection, killing and depletion of T4 lymphocytes, which play a central role in immune responses. This greatly reduces the host's ability to produce adequate amounts of antibody or lymphokines (see Chapter 9). However, the virus is also believed to cause damage to the immune system in other ways, including:

- prevention of T4 cells responding to antigens by blocking the cell receptor sites;
- infection of lymph nodes leading to their damage or destruction;
- infection of other protective cells bearing the CD4 receptor, particularly macrophages and glial cells in the brain; and
- the initiation of autoimmune responses to T4 cells and other cells bearing the CD4 receptor.

The end result of this immunosuppression is that patients in the terminal stages of HIV infection are incapable of mounting an immune response to many infections and cancers that are normally readily dealt with by the immune system. Most AIDS patients die from one of these diseases.

Other microbes do not have such a dramatic and devastating effect on the immune system, but can cause immunosuppression nevertheless. For example, *Staphylococcus aureus* seems to interfere with immune defences by secreting toxins that are potent T cell mitogens (stimulators). These cause an uncontrolled and excessive activation of T lymphocytes, thus diverting the immune system to unproductive activity. Other microbes, such as the Epstein-Barr virus, may cause a similar diversion of the immune system by polyclonal activation of B lymphocytes, with the production of large amounts of irrelevant antibodies.

Some organisms release molecules that interfere with immunologically important molecules. For instance, many pathogenic strains of *Neisseria gonorrhoeae*, *Streptococcus pneumoniae* and *Haemophilus influenzae* secrete a protease that cleaves the IgA molecule, the major antibody type in mucosal secretions. This presumably facilitates the persistence of these bacteria on mucous membranes even if specific antibodies of this class are present. Strains of *Pseudomonas* secrete enzymes that inactivate components of the complement system. This is thought to inhibit the critical role that complement plays in opsonising (enhancing the phagocytosis of) foreign particles (see Chapter 9).

It appears that many microorganisms have mechanisms that inhibit the defence systems of the host in some way. Even a temporary suppression of host factors can give the microbe enough advantage to enable its establishment and growth in the body.

FIGURE 10.8

ANTIGENIC VARIATION

By repeatedly changing its critical antigens, an organism is not affected by prior immune responses to it, thereby evading the host's immune system.

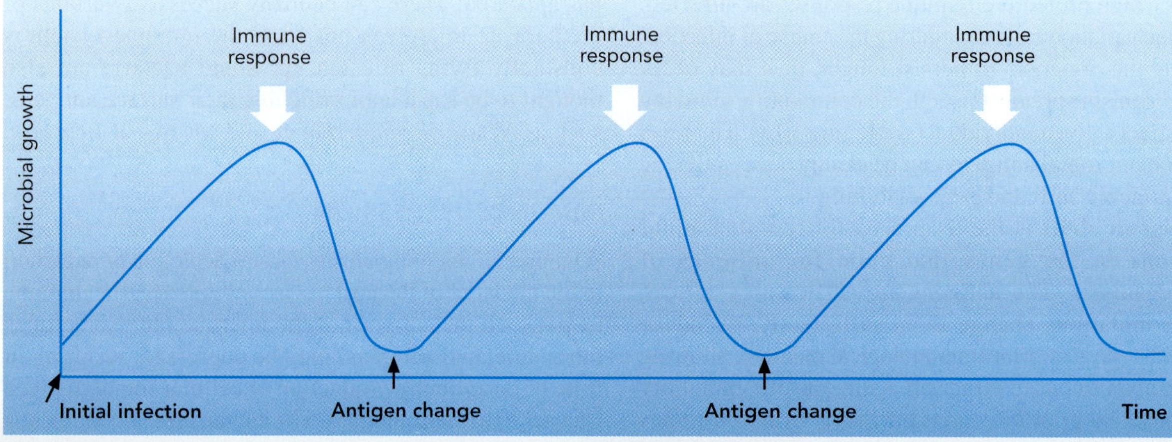

Summary

- The ability of an organism to cause disease is referred to as its pathogenicity.
- The factors that contribute to an organism's ability to cause disease are called virulence factors.
- Most microorganisms enter the human body by way of a mucous membrane or a break in the skin.

ADHERENCE

- Adherence is an important step in the pathogenicity of many organisms. It usually involves a specific interaction between surface components of a microorganism and surface receptors on host cells.
- The substances on the surfaces of microorganisms that enable them to attach to cell surfaces are called adhesins.
- The adhesins of some organisms are found on specific attachment structures called pili or fimbriae.
- The adhesins of other organisms are surface substances, such as sticky slime layers (glycocalyx), proteins or polysaccharides.
- Viruses attach to specific membrane receptors on the cells they infect.
- Many parasitic helminths fasten to host tissues by means of suckers or hooks.

TOXINS

- Toxins are substances produced by some micro-organisms that interfere with the normal functioning of host cells or tissues.
- The production and release of toxins are, for some bacteria, the most important determinants of their ability to damage tissues and thus cause disease.

EXOTOXINS

- Exotoxins are heat-labile proteins that are usually released as the organism grows.
- Some bacteria produce a single exotoxin, and the major manifestations of the disease are due to the action of that toxin, whereas others produce many toxins.
- Exotoxins include some of the strongest poisons known (e.g. the botulinum toxin).
- The main groups of bacterial exotoxins are neurotoxins, which act mainly on nervous tissue, and enterotoxins, which act specifically on the small intestine.
- A large number of exotoxins act by damaging host cell membranes, resulting in lysis and death of the cells.
- Some bacteria, such as *S. aureus* and *S. pyogenes*, secrete toxins called leukocidins that kill the phagocytic leukocytes, neutrophils and macrophages.
- Many bacteria secrete enzymes that increase their invasiveness by breaking down substances that would otherwise impede their spread through tissues.
- Hyaluronidases are enzymes produced by many bacteria; they break down hyaluronic acid, making tissues less viscous and easier to penetrate.
- Collagenases are enzymes produced by some bacteria and helminths; they break down collagen, the tough fibres that give strength and a supporting network to connective tissues.
- The fungi that cause tinea are able to infect skin because they secrete a keratin-degrading enzyme, keratinase.
- Kinases are a group of enzymes produced by certain bacteria that help them to dissolve fibrin clots.
- Coagulase is an enzyme produced by virulent staphylococci; it coagulates fibrinogen to form a deposit of fibrin material around the bacterial cells.
- Several bacterial exotoxins can enter cells and alter their metabolism.
- *Corynebacterium diphtheriae* secretes a toxin that blocks protein synthesis in cells, causing them to die.
- The enterotoxin of *Vibrio cholerae* is an exotoxin that alters the regulatory control in intestinal epithelial cells, causing a massive outflow of water from the cells, manifested as profuse diarrhoea.
- *Clostridium tetani* secretes a toxin that interferes with synaptic transmission specifically in inhibitory interneurones, resulting in an uncontrolled, rigid muscle contraction or spastic paralysis.
- *Clostridium botulinum* toxin acts on peripheral nerve endings, blocking the release of acetycholine and preventing muscle contraction.

TOXOIDS AND ANTITOXINS

- An antitoxin is an antibody that is able to bind to a toxin and neutralise it, thereby preventing it from binding to its target cell or tissue.
- Many exotoxins can be chemically modified to remove their toxicity, while still retaining their ability to elicit an immune response. Toxins modified in this way are called toxoids, and can be used in vaccines to stimulate immunity without causing disease.
- The treatment of diseases caused by exotoxin-producing bacteria sometimes involves the use of antitoxins to neutralise the toxin already in the body.

ENDOTOXINS

- Endotoxins consist of the lipopolysaccharides (LPS) of the cell walls of Gram-negative bacteria.
- The lipid A portion of LPS is the actively toxic component.
- Endotoxins only exert their effect once the cell wall breaks down.
- Release of endotoxin can be greatly accelerated once phagocytes begin to digest them or once antibiotics that kill the bacteria are administered.
- Endotoxin, regardless of its source, produces similar signs and symptoms in the host.
- Fever is one of the more common and important of the symptoms induced by endotoxin.
- Endotoxic (or septic) shock, the shock caused by large amounts of endotoxin, is frequently fatal.
- Endotoxin may also cause a non-specific activation of blood coagulation mechanisms, resulting in the

blockage of small vessels by thrombi. This disorder is referred to as disseminated intravascular coagulation.

INVASION OF CELLS

- Viruses typically cause disease by invading and damaging host cells.
- Once inside the cell, a virus causes changes to the cell that are called cytopathic effects (CPE).
- Cytocidal viruses kill the cells they infect.
- Even if the virus does not kill the cell directly, it takes control of the regulatory mechanisms of the cell and produces viral proteins and nucleic acids, causing the cell to become dysfunctional.
- A few organisms, other than viruses, also invade cells and damage them (e.g. the chlamydia and rickettsia).
- *Plasmodium* spp., the causative agents of malaria, typically go through cycles of red blood cell invasion, multiplication and lysis.

CELLULAR TRANSFORMATION INTO TUMOUR CELLS

- Some viruses cause disease by transforming host cells into tumour cells.
- Transformed cells differ markedly from normal cells in that they have an altered morphology and do not have an ordered pattern of growth.
- Some human papillomaviruses cause cutaneous warts, which are benign tumours.
- Some viruses are believed to be involved in malignant tumours, such as HPV types 16, 18, 31 and 33 in cervical cancer, and hepatitis B virus in hepatocellular carcinoma.

OTHER MECHANISMS OF PATHOGENESIS

- Some microorganisms cause the host's immune response to be 'overreactive', which results in tissue damage; this is referred to as hypersensitivity.
- Some microorganisms cause tissue damage by physical means (e.g. a mass of worms in the intestinal tract may cause obstruction).

EVASION STRATEGIES

ESCAPE FROM PHAGOCYTES

- Some organisms possess capsules or a surface slime layer which prevents phagocytes from ingesting them.
- Some microorganisms allow themselves to be ingested by phagocytes but have developed ways of surviving inside them.

CONCEALMENT

- Some microorganisms evade the host defences by hiding inside cells, or in 'privileged sites' where defence cells do not normally circulate.
- Some microorganisms create their own privileged sites, such as the tapeworm *Echinococcus granulosus*, which forms thin-walled cysts.

ANTIGENIC VARIATION

- Antigenic variation is a phenomenon in which microorganisms repeatedly or progressively change their cell surface antigens, enabling them to evade the immune system.
- Antigenic drift refers to repeated minor mutations in the genes that code for antigens of microorganisms.
- Antigenic shift occurs when two different strains infect the same cell, and a recombination of the genes that code for the surface glycoproteins occurs. This results in a new strain.
- Another form of antigenic variation results from the ability of some microorganisms to switch the genes that code for certain surface antigens.

IMMUNOSUPPRESSION

- Several microorganisms cause a depletion or reduction in the host's defences, resulting in little or no immunity to their antigens.
- The HIV suppresses the immune system in a number of ways, but much of it is believed to be due to infection, killing and depletion of T4 lymphocytes.

Study Questions

1. What are virulence factors?
2. By what routes do most microorganisms enter the body?
3. What are adhesins? Give two examples.
4. How do viruses attach to the cells they infect?
5. Define the terms 'endotoxin', 'enterotoxin' and 'neurotoxin'.
6. How do microorganisms break down the cell membranes of humans?
7. What are leukocidins and how do they operate?
8. What is coagulase and how does it increase the pathogenicity of staphylococci?
9. Describe how the tetanus and botulinum toxins cause disease.
10. Define the terms 'toxoid' and 'antitoxin'.
11. What is an endotoxin?
12. What is septic shock?
13. What are cytopathic effects?
14. How do viruses kill host cells?
15. Describe the ways by which microorganisms avoid being ingested by phagocytes.
16. How can microorganisms hide from the immune system?
17. What is meant by the terms 'antigenic variation' and 'antigenic drift'?
18. What is thought to be the main way in which the human immunodeficiency virus causes immunosuppression in the host?
19. How could an IgA protease assist microorganisms to cause disease?

Test Your Understanding

1. Describe the differences between exotoxins and endotoxins.
2. Why must many pathogenic microbes have specific mechanisms for adherence to tissues?
3. In a patient with tetanus, why is the administration of specific immune globulin more important than antibiotics?
4. Explain why the administration of antibiotics to a patient with an infection caused by Gram-negative bacteria can initially cause a worsening of symptoms.

FURTHER READING

Ewald, P.W., 1993, 'The evolution of virulence', *Scientific American* 268(4), pp. 56–62. (A discussion of microbial pathogenicity from an evolutionary viewpoint. It contends that the pathogenicity of microorganisms could be controlled if evolutionary pressures were controlled.)

Olsnes, S., J.V. Kozlov, B. van Deurs & K. Sandvig, 1991, 'Bacterial protein toxins acting on intracellular targets', *Seminars in Cell Biology* 2(1), pp. 7–14. (This review article describes the ways by which bacterial toxins enter target cells and modify cellular functions.)

Salyers, A. A. & D.D.Whitt, *Bacterial Pathogenesis*, Washington, DC: American Society for Microbiology, 1994. (Examines in depth the mechanisms by which bacteria cause disease and summarises recent research advances.)

Schaechter, M., G. Medoff & B.L. Eisenstein, *Mechanisms of Microbial Disease*, 2nd edn, Baltimore: Williams & Wilkins, 1993. (This comprehensive text focuses on the mechanisms of infectious diseases and how the host responds to them.)

unit III

control of microorganisms

chapter 11

principles of sterilisation

and disinfection

Chapter focus

- *What are the basic principles underlying the effective control of microbial growth?*
- *What are the main methods used to destroy or inactivate microorganisms?*
- *Why are thorough cleaning procedures an important part of disinfection and sterilisation procedures?*
- *What determines the method of sterilisation to be used?*
- *How are chemical disinfectants used?*

Microorganisms are an integral part of our environment. They play an essential role as part of the normal body flora, in the recycling of nutrients by the decomposition of organic material, in agriculture, in food production and in industry. However, they are also responsible for food spoilage and contamination of water supplies, and are the causative agents of disease in plants and animals. To avoid the harm that microorganisms can cause, it is essential to have methods of controlling their growth and spread.

In this chapter, we examine the physical and chemical methods used to control microbial growth and to prevent the spread of disease-causing microorganisms ('germs'). The most appropriate method to use in a given situation depends not only on the type of microorganisms that are present, but also on their location—for example, in the home, in a hospital ward, in the operating theatre, in a laboratory, on surgical instruments or pharmaceutical products.

Different methods of control or destruction of microorganisms are required for different situations. It is important for health professionals, especially nurses, to understand how the methods work, their limitations, and how to use them safely. It is also important to be familiar with the properties of the different types of microorganisms and to know how these properties can affect the ease, or difficulty, of destruction. For example, some bacteria are easily killed by relatively mild heat treatment: *Mycobacterium tuberculosis* is killed by the temperatures used in pasteurisation (63°C for 30 minutes). On the other hand, bacterial endospores have been shown to survive for several hours at 100°C, requiring the higher temperature of 121°C for 15 minutes to kill them.

Historical Background

PRESERVATION OF FOOD

The first attempts to control microbial growth were aimed at the prevention of food spoilage and the preservation of food for the winter months. Methods such as drying or curing (smoking) of meat and fish have been used for centuries. Vegetable seeds, such as beans and lentils, were dried. In areas where salt was available, meat and fish were salted in large barrels; other foods were pickled in vinegar. We now know that these methods create conditions of low water content, high osmotic pressure or low pH, all of which are unfavourable for the growth of bacteria.

The use of heat to destroy bacteria and preserve food arose from the work of Louis Pasteur in the 19th century (see Chapter 1). Pasteur was responsible for showing that microbes exist everywhere in the environment, in the air, on surfaces, and on food. He showed that food spoilage was due to microorganisms already present in the food and that these could be destroyed by the application of heat. Provided the food was in a container that prevented the re-entry of microbes, the food would remain unspoiled. The technique he developed, which now bears his name (**pasteurisation**), does not kill *all* microbes, but it does kill most of those that produce organic acids (mainly the lactic acid bacteria) which cause souring of wine and milk. Pasteur's work was of enormous economic importance to the wine industry in France in the 19th century.

When applied to milk, the method was found not only to prevent spoilage by lactic acid bacteria, but also to destroy certain pathogens, such as those responsible for tuberculosis. *Mycobacterium tuberculosis* can infect dairy cattle and can easily be transmitted to humans in unpasteurised milk. The early explorers, sailing for months or years around the world, took food that had been heated and stored in sealed containers. They knew it preserved the food, even though they did not understand the mechanism responsible for spoilage. The use of heat to destroy microorganisms is still one of the most efficient and reliable methods available today.

PREVENTION OF DISEASE

For centuries people have been aware of the seriousness of infections and infectious diseases (see Chapter 1) and have tried various methods to cure them or prevent their spread. During the plague in Europe in the Middle Ages, people burnt the bodies and clothes of those who had died and burnt sulphur and aromatic plants in their houses to try to 'purify the air'.

The middle of the 19th century saw the the first attempts at disinfection, or the use of chemicals to destroy microorganisms. Joseph Lister, a Scottish surgeon, was one of the first to use chemicals to prevent the death of patients from infection, especially following surgery (see Chapters 1 and 13). At about the same time, Ignaz

SEMMELWEIS, a Hungarian physician working in Vienna, introduced a procedure of handwashing in a solution of chlorinated lime for all nurses and physicians (see Chapters 1 and 13). The methods used by Lister and Semmelweis involved very crude, corrosive chemicals. Modern antiseptics and disinfectants are more effective. In addition, physical methods such as radiation have been developed for use on objects that might be damaged by heat or chemicals.

In this chapter, we describe the physical and chemical methods used to destroy microorganisms or to control their growth, and discuss the principles behind their use. The control of microbial growth can be achieved in a number of ways:

- by preventing the organisms from gaining access to a susceptible site;
- by killing all the organisms;
- by reducing the number of microbes to an 'acceptable level';
- by exposing them to conditions that inhibit their growth.

The terms commonly used to describe the destruction or control of microorganisms are listed in Table 11.1.

Pattern of Microbial Death

Any method used to kill microorganisms must interfere with their ability to reproduce. A number of different cellular components are essential for the structural and functional integrity of the cell and damage to any of these will kill or inactivate the cell. The nucleic acids, which contain the genetic information, are essential for reproduction and so agents that damage or destroy nucleic acid will prevent cell replication. A major component of all cells are the proteins, which are important for cellular structure and for enzymic activity. If the proteins are altered or denatured, cell function is impaired. Damage to the wall or membrane, which play an integral role in maintaining the structure and internal environment of the cell, will allow the cell contents to leak out, resulting in the death of the cell.

RATE OF DEATH

When a microbial population is exposed to a killing agent, the pattern of death obeys certain laws. In general, each microbial cell has actually to come into contact with the antimicrobial agent; in other words, heat or radiation must have time to penetrate throughout the whole population of cells. Chemical molecules must come into contact with each microbial cell so that they can interact chemically and produce lethal changes to the cell. This means that, under specified conditions, a certain number of microbes will be killed in a certain period of time; for example, 90% may be killed in one minute. After these cells are killed, it will take another minute for the killing agent to come into contact with 90% of the remaining live cells. So 90% will be killed in the next minute, and so on. This is called an exponential killing curve (see Figure 11.1). If the rate of death is plotted logarithmically it is a straight line.

Obviously, the more microorganisms that are present initially, the longer it will take to destroy them all. It is therefore essential that any process is continued for a sufficient period of time to ensure the death of all organisms. Most procedures are standardised and recommend that articles are treated for a specified period of time to ensure that all organisms present are destroyed. Failure to allow the article to be in contact with the antimicrobial agent for the correct period of time may jeopardise the efficiency of the killing procedure.

TABLE 11.1
TERMS USED IN THE DESTRUCTION OR CONTROL OF MICROORGANISMS

TERM	DEFINITION
Antiseptic	A type of chemical disinfectant, suitable for use on skin or living tissue, to kill or remove harmful microorganisms without damaging the tissue.
Decontamination	The removal of possible harmful microorganisms from an object by cleaning or disinfecting.
Disinfectant	A chemical substance normally used for the disinfection of inanimate objects.
Disinfection	The destruction, removal or reduction in numbers of harmful microorganisms to an acceptable level. Usually kills vegetative bacteria, not endospores or viruses.
Germicide	Any agent capable of killing microorganisms (germs).
Pasteurisation	A method developed to preserve milk and other liquids without altering their taste or quality. Destroys bacteria responsible for spoilage and some pathogens, but not all microorganisms.
Sanitisation	Thorough cleaning of an object or utensil to remove most microorganisms. Does not imply use of disinfectant.
Sterilisation	The complete destruction or removal of all microorganisms, including endospores.

FIGURE 11.1
KILLING CURVE

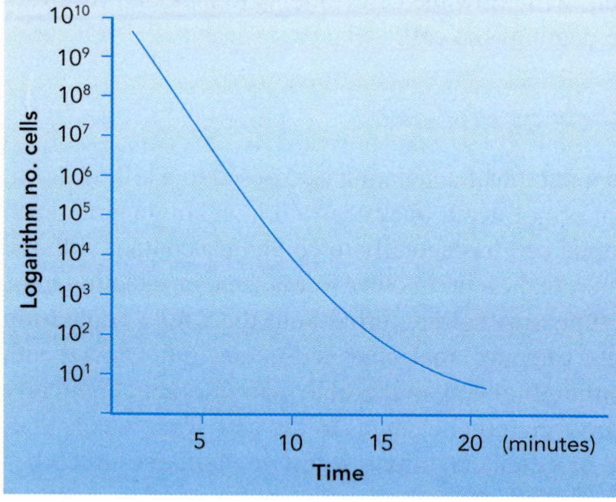

Several other factors can affect the rate of killing of microbes by heat or chemicals. A major factor is the type of microorganisms that may be present. Some chemicals have a different action depending on whether the bacterium is Gram-negative or Gram-positive. Some bacteria such as the pseudomonads and the mycobacteria, are particularly resistant to disinfectants. Bacterial endospores are highly resistant to heat and many disinfectants. Cysts of the protozoan *Giardia* are resistant to chlorine, which is used for water purification.

The phase of growth of the microorganisms also has a direct effect on the efficiency of the disinfection process. In general, when cells are dividing rapidly they are very susceptible to chemical damage, whereas cells in stationary phase are more resistant and many of them form highly resistant cysts or endospores.

For chemical inactivation of microorganisms to take place, there has to be a sufficient number of molecules of the chemical present to be able to interact with each of the cells present. Therefore, any disinfectant or antiseptic solution must be used at an adequate concentration to ensure that all the microbes will be killed. Usually, the concentrations recommended by the manufacturer specify the optimum concentration to be used to ensure that the chemical will be effective. The use of weaker or stronger solutions may compromise the effectiveness of the treatment.

In summary, it can be seen that the efficiency of an antimicrobial treatment will depend on both the concentration of the killing agent and the length of time it is in contact with the microorganisms.

Procedures for Cleaning, Disinfection and Sterilisation

RISK FACTORS

In the health care setting, the processes of cleaning, disinfection and sterilisation are of the utmost importance for the prevention of transmission of infection. Before we examine specific methods of sterilisation and disinfection, we will consider the need for each method to be applied according to the setting. It is essential to be able to recognise situations that have a high risk of transmission of infection, and to identify those patients who are particularly susceptible. Appropriate methods can then be selected and applied to remove or destroy microbes. Table 11.2 summarises the level of cleaning, disinfection and sterilisation required for different procedures.

The highest risk is associated with equipment that penetrates the skin or mucous membranes during surgery or during the insertion of devices such as catheters or intravenous lines. These procedures allow direct access for microbes to susceptible sites. An added risk factor is that these procedures are often performed on seriously ill patients (e.g. in intensive care) who usually have other contributing conditions that make them particularly susceptible to infection. Therefore, the equipment must be sterile and the highest level of aseptic technique must be followed.

Equipment that comes into contact with the patient's skin or mucosal surfaces, but does not necessarily breach it, should also be sterile whenever possible. Endoscopes and respiratory equipment are easily damaged and require special methods of decontamination. X-ray equipment, trolleys, beds and other furniture carry a low risk of cross-infection and adequate cleaning is usually sufficient.

TABLE 11.2
REQUIREMENTS FOR STERILISATION AND DISINFECTION OF EQUIPMENT

Sterilisation	■ All equipment that penetrates the skin or mucous membranes: surgical instruments, needles (syringes), IV and urinary catheters, endoscopes ■ All invasive devices, implants ■ All solutions that are administered parenterally ■ All objects that contact a break in the skin or mucosal surfaces: dressings, swabs ■ Surgical gowns, drapes and gloves
Disinfection (after cleaning)	■ Equipment that comes into contact with patients' skin but does not penetrate: X-ray machines, bedpans, thermometers
Cleaning	■ Equipment that does not pose significant risk to the patient from contact: beds, sinks, eating utensils

Some pieces of equipment are very large or have parts that are damaged by heat, so are difficult to sterilise. It is necessary to assess the risk category carefully in order to decide the best method of cleaning and disinfection to be used.

REUSE OF DISPOSABLE EQUIPMENT

Some equipment is designed to be discarded after use while other articles can be reused after cleaning and sterilisation. Often nurses are asked to 'reprocess' the equipment (that is, clean and disinfect, or sterilise). They must be confident of the safety and reliability of any method they are asked to use. The reuse of equipment that is not properly cleaned or sterilised may also have legal implications.

Any item of equipment that falls into the high-risk category must be sterile. Many items are labelled 'single use only' and these *must not be reprocessed*. Some articles of equipment are difficult to sterilise between patients and too expensive to be discarded as single use only. Each situation must be assessed by an appropriately qualified person to determine the best possible procedure for disinfection and/or sterilisation in order to prevent cross-infection and transmission of potential pathogens.

Cleaning

One of the most important aspects of the control of microbial growth is good hygiene. Bacteria thrive in moist organic matter such as tissue, blood, body fluids, soiled linen and dressings, food and garbage. Therefore, the removal of these materials by effective cleaning methods is of the utmost importance. Before any disinfecting or sterilising procedures are carried out on equipment or utensils, they must be freed of material such as blood, tissue, pus, mucus, grease and dirt which provide a protective barrier for the microorganisms and prevent the penetration of the killing agent. It is also important to remove organic matter as it may react with the chemical agent, rendering it less effective.

The washing of equipment with hot water and soap or detergent does not kill all bacteria, but it reduces their numbers to a level where disinfection and sterilisation procedures are usually effective. Ultrasonic cleaning equipment is useful for complicated instruments with parts that are difficult to reach. In this procedure, the equipment is placed in a solution of detergent and subjected to high-frequency sound waves which dislodge the dirt, blood and tissue from inaccessible areas of the instruments.

In hospitals, the cleaning of wards, bathrooms, floors and equipment is an important part of infection control (see Chapter 13). The equipment used for cleaning should be kept dry when not in use to prevent the growth of bacteria. Very often, a damp, contaminated mop head can be responsible for spreading pathogens around the hospital. Cleaning also helps to maintain medical equipment in good condition. In general, the use of disinfectants for routine cleaning tasks is not necessary. A description of the correct cleaning procedures to be followed for the various fixtures and equipment in the hospital is usually contained in each hospital's infection control manual.

Terminal cleaning of a room that has contained an infectious patient usually requires the use of a disinfectant. Guidelines for the decontamination and/or sterilisation of the equipment, bedding and other objects from an infectious area are provided in each hospital manual.

Sterilisation

Sterilisation involves the complete destruction or removal of all living organisms from an object. There are no degrees of sterility. An object is either sterile or non-sterile. Several methods can be used to sterilise an object, that is, render it completely free of all living microorganisms (Table 11.3). They include physical methods that utilise heat or radiation, mechanical methods such as filtration (used for air and fluids) and chemical methods that use ethylene oxide or glutaraldehyde or more recently hydrogen peroxide. The method employed depends on the nature of the object to be sterilised, the type of facility where it will be used and the subsequent use to which the object will be put.

HEAT

Heat is the most widely used of all methods of sterilisation. It is cheap, efficient and easily controlled. Dry heat kills microorganisms by inactivation of cell components by oxidation, whereas moist heat mainly destroys microorganisms by denaturation of essential cellular proteins. The presence of water and heat causes disruption of the hydrogen bonds holding the proteins in their specific 3-dimensional configuration. Microorganisms vary in their susceptibility to heat. To establish suitable protocols to be followed in order to render an object sterile, it is useful to determine the type of organisms that are likely to be present so as to ensure that the methods employed are sufficient to kill all the organisms. It is also essential to monitor the outcome regularly.

The **thermal death point (TDP)** is defined as the lowest temperature at which all the microorganisms in a liquid suspension will be killed in 10 minutes. As mentioned earlier, the time required to kill all the microorganisms will depend on the number of microorganisms present, or the level of contamination. We can therefore define another value, the **thermal death time (TDT)**, which is the minimum time it takes to kill all the organisms in a liquid culture at a given temperature. It is useful to determine these values for situations where the objects to be sterilised would be affected by prolonged exposure to excessive heat. They are especially relevant in the food industry, for example, in the preparation of canned food, in order to preserve the quality of the product. In the laboratory, these values are important in the preparation of culture media, or other sterile solutions where some of the essential ingredients might be broken down by extended exposure to high temperatures.

TABLE 11.3
METHOD OF STERILISATION

METHOD	ADVANTAGES/DISADVANTAGES
Autoclave Steam under pressure 121°C 15 mins	Requires special equipment; reliable, inexpensive to run; kills all microbes; *not* suitable for heat-sensitive objects or solutions.
Dry heat 160°C more than 1 hour	Inexpensive, slow; not suitable for heat-sensitive materials.
Incineration	Total destruction of contaminated articles.
Ionising radiation (gamma)	Requires access to commercial cobalt-60 source; good for prepacked materials.
Filtration	Used for sterilising heat-sensitive solutions; awkward to handle; difficult to monitor efficiency.
Ethylene oxide gas	Useful for heat-sensitive materials, disposable plastics; requires special facility in sterilising department; gas is toxic; flammable equipment; must be well aired before use; difficult to monitor efficiency.
Glutaraldehyde	Used for delicate instruments e.g. endoscopes; toxic, allergenic, expensive, unstable.
Hydrogen peroxide	Low temperature 'plasma' sterilisation; requires special unit. Suitable for delicate instruments; fast, non toxic; not suitable for cellulose, paper or fabric.

MOIST HEAT STERILISATION: USE OF THE AUTOCLAVE

In the hospital setting, patients must be protected from infection by the use of sterile equipment, instruments, dressings and IV solutions. To ensure these objects are sterile, they must be subjected to a reliable procedure that can be closely monitored. The most reliable method is moist heat sterilisation, which uses a machine called an autoclave. This process is able to kill endospores as well as vegetative bacterial cells and viruses.

Although boiling (in so-called 'sterilisers') is used to kill microorganisms, it is *not* an accepted method of sterilisation. Some organisms can withstand the temperature of boiling water (100°C at normal atmospheric pressure) for long periods. To achieve sterility, it is necessary to use higher temperatures. These can be reached by increasing the pressure in the sterilising chamber so that the temperature at which the water boils (i.e. the temperature of the steam) is raised. The higher the pressure, the higher the temperature that can be reached. For example, when steam from boiling water is placed under a pressure of 1 atmosphere (or 15 pounds per square inch, psi) in excess of normal atmospheric pressure (i.e. twice atmospheric pressure), the temperature of the steam is increased to 121°C. At three times atmospheric pressure, the temperature reaches 134°C. A temperature of 121°C is sufficient to kill all microorganisms, including endospores, in 15 minutes. At 134°C, the time required for sterilisation is reduced to 3.5 minutes. It is important to note that these times are measured from the time when steam penetrates to all parts of the object to be sterilised. This is especially important when thick or bulky items are being treated.

Domestic pressure cookers are able to reach high temperatures by placing steam under pressure. Commercial autoclaves work the same way, but need to be more sophisticated to ensure safety and reliability. They vary in size from small bench-top models, used in medical and dental surgeries, to large, fully automated commercial models used in hospitals and industry.

An autoclave consists of a double-walled or jacketed chamber made of thick steel. Steam is circulated through the outer jacket and then supplied under pressure to the closed inner chamber (see Figure 11.2). Both the inner chamber and the airtight doors are constructed to withstand the pressures and temperatures generated. For sterilisation to be effective, steam must be able to contact every part of the object to be sterilised (i.e. every microorganism that is present). To ensure the correct temperature is reached, all the air must be eliminated from the chamber and replaced with steam. There are five stages in the sterilising cycle:

1. The autoclave is loaded with the articles spaced sufficiently far apart to allow the steam to circulate and penetrate, and the door is closed securely.
2. The automatic cycle is started and the air is replaced by steam, usually by forcing steam into the chamber (although some autoclaves are evacuated before admitting the steam).
3. The chamber is heated until the correct temperature and pressure are reached and held there for the required period of time.
4. Drying of the load is carried out at the end of the cycle by removing the steam from the inner chamber, but allowing the steam to continue to circulate in the outer jacket so that the chamber remains hot and the moisture in the load evaporates.

FIGURE 11.2
DIAGRAM OF AUTOCLAVE
The entering steam forces the air out of the bottom (black arrows). The automatic ejector valve remains open as long as an air-steam mixture is passing out of the waste line. When all the air has been ejected, the higher temperature of the pure steam closes the valve, and the pressure in the chamber increases.

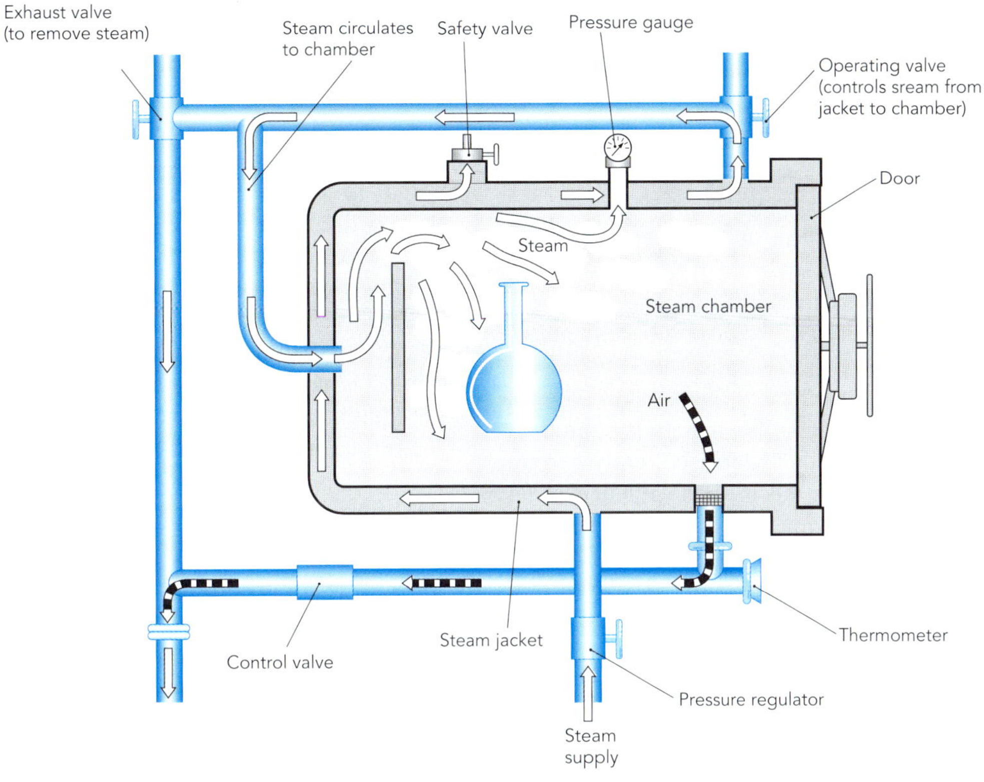

5. After the steam is removed, air is admitted to return the chamber to normal atmospheric pressure, and the load is then removed.

To maintain sterility after removal from the autoclave, dry equipment to be sterilised must be wrapped in a suitable material such as paper or fabric, which allows penetration of steam. Aluminium foil does not allow steam to penetrate and should not be used. The load should be allowed to dry inside the autoclave before being exposed to the outside air. This is to prevent bacteria from passing through the wet wrappings and contaminating the inside of the package. Liquids should be placed in loosely stoppered flasks and allowed to cool below 100°C before being removed from the chamber, to avoid explosions.

When properly used and maintained, an autoclave is a very efficient method of sterilisation. It should be regularly inspected by an engineer to ensure it is safe and is reaching the required temperatures and pressures. Its efficiency should also be monitored routinely to ensure that the articles are sterilised. This can be done by checking that the autoclave cycle has killed a sample of bacterial endospores. It is recommended that a specimen of endospores of *Bacillus stearothermophilus* is included with the load at least once a week. A spore strip and ampoule of medium are available in a vial which is placed in the centre of a loaded autoclave. After completion of the cycle the spores are incubated in the medium. If no growth is observed, the autoclave is considered to be functioning correctly. For daily checks, there are special tapes and indicators that change colour when the desired temperature is reached. The tape is placed in the middle of a wrapped package and should change colour evenly if the heat has penetrated uniformly. Care should be taken to ensure that wrapped articles remain sterile. Any water that comes into contact with the outside of a package allows the passage of microorganisms through the paper, and may cause contamination of the contents. Unless the wrapping of the package remains intact, the contents cannot be considered to be sterile.

DRY HEAT STERILISATION

To sterilise using dry heat, a temperature of 160°C for 60 minutes is required. Although relatively cheap and simple to use compared with an autoclave, hot air ovens are only suitable for sterilising equipment that is not harmed by long exposure to high temperatures. Glass and some metal objects can be sterilised in this way. Fabrics, and materials used for wrapping, usually cannot withstand these temperatures. Reusable equipment must be packaged in heat-proof containers (metal or glass). The time required to heat the oven, in addition to the sterilising time, makes this method less practical than an autoclave. The high temperature required is also a major limitation, although the dry atmosphere is preferable for some metal instruments, as it does not cause corrosion.

INCINERATION

Incineration of contaminated material is a certain method for the destruction of microorganisms present in biological materials, contaminated waste, soiled dressings, and disposable equipment. It is also used to sterilise the inoculating loops that are used to handle microorganisms in the laboratory. The platinum wire of the loop is heated to red hot, allowed to cool and then used to transfer organisms in a sterile manner.

RADIATION

Ionising radiation can damage or kill microorganisms by causing disruption to the structure of the DNA chains. Gamma rays from a radioactive cobalt-60 source are used industrially to sterilise much of the disposable equipment used in hospitals, such as prepackaged dressing packs, needles, syringes, suture material, catheters and prostheses. Because gamma rays can penetrate materials, a product can be packaged first and then sterilised. Only certain materials can be sterilised by this method without causing changes to their composition. Because of the highly dangerous nature of the radiation, this type of sterilisation treatment is carried out at a specially designed and centralised commercial facility.

FILTRATION

Filtration involves the passage of a liquid or air through a filter with pores small enough to prevent the passage of microorganisms. Filters are used to sterilise materials that cannot be sterilised by autoclaving. Many of the aqueous solutions used for intravenous therapy or total parenteral nutrition of hospitalised patients contain substances that are adversely affected by high temperatures. Some pharmaceutical preparations such as solutions of drugs and vitamins and various culture media used in microbiology laboratories are also sensitive to high temperatures. They can be sterilised by filtration through specially designed membrane filters (see Figure 11.3). These are made of nitrocellulose and are manufactured in a range of specific pore sizes capable of retaining different sized particles (Table 11.4).

To sterilise these solutions, a filter is selected with a pore size that will prevent the passage of *all* microorganisms (including viruses and mycoplasmas). Filters can also be used selectively to remove one type of microorganism—for example, to allow viruses to pass through but retain bacteria. It is more difficult to control sterility with filtration, as the equipment can be awkward to use and the efficiency of the filtration process is difficult to assess.

FIGURE 11.3
MEMBRANE FILTERS
Scanning electron micrograph showing red *Serratia marcescens* and yellow *Staphylococcus epidermis* cells trapped on the surface of a 0.22-μm Millipore membrane filter. Membrane pore size may be selected so as to allow viruses, but not bacteria, to pass through, or to prevent both from passing.

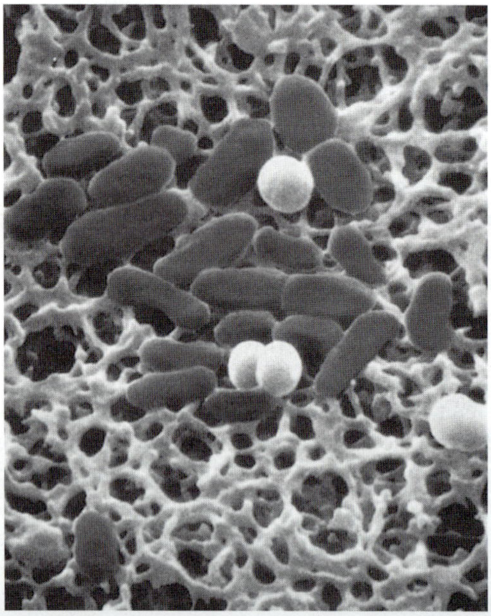

ETHYLENE OXIDE GAS STERILISATION

This method of sterilisation involves the use of ethylene oxide gas, which is odourless, highly toxic, flammable, and explosive when mixed with oxygen. For these reasons, the method is confined to industrial facilities or the central sterilising units of large hospitals. Careful control of the conditions is necessary, as time, temperature, humidity and gas pressure all affect the efficiency of the sterilisation. Because the gas is so toxic, items sterilised in this way must be aerated thoroughly before use to remove residual gas. This takes several hours or even longer if the article is porous or made of rubber, silicon or polyvinyl chloride (PVC).

The method is difficult to monitor, requiring the use of spore strips (specimens of endospores of *Bacillus subtilis*), which should be exposed during each sterilising cycle. The time required for aeration, and for assessing whether the spores have been killed, makes this a rather slow method of sterilisation; it is not suitable for reusable equipment that cannot be out of use for two days. It has

TABLE 11.4
PORE SIZES OF MEMBRANE FILTERS

PORE SIZE (μm)	FILTRATION USE
Less than 0.025 μm (ultrafilter)	Required to ensure removal of all bacteria, viruses and mycoplasmas.
0.22 μm	Allows passage of all viruses and molecules. Retains bacteria.
0.45 μm	Allows a few bacteria through. Retains yeasts, protozoa, blood cells.
1.2 μm	Allows viruses and most bacteria through. Retains yeasts.

good powers of penetration, however, and is most useful for sterilising prewrapped packages of disposable plastic equipment or delicate equipment that would be damaged by heat or liquids. The mechanism of action involves inactivation of proteins containing sulphydryl groups.

TREATMENT WITH GLUTARALDEHYDE

Many chemical solutions (e.g. strong acids) are able to kill the microorganisms present on the surface of an object. Unfortunately, many of them also cause irreversible corrosive damage to the surface. Glutaraldehyde is a non-corrosive chemical that acts as a sterilising agent when used at high concentrations and for sufficient exposure time. When used at a lower concentration and for shorter periods of time, it is regarded as a disinfectant. It appears to exert its effect by disrupting the structure of the microbial proteins. It is a broad spectrum antimicrobial chemical that can kill vegetative cells in a few minutes and endospores within a few hours.

Its advantages are that it is non-corrosive, and can be used on delicate heat-sensitive instruments such as endoscopes. It retains its potency even in the presence of organic material but, even so, equipment should be cleansed of grease and dirt before immersion in glutaraldehyde solutions. One disadvantage is that glutaraldehyde is somewhat unstable, especially at alkaline pH and high temperatures, so solutions may retain their activity for only a couple of weeks. It is preferable always to use fresh solutions, but the chemical is quite expensive and the expense cannot always be justified.

Glutaraldehyde is toxic and allergenic and equipment treated with it must be thoroughly rinsed in sterile water before use. There is increasing concern about its toxic properties, as contact with glutaraldehyde solutions, aerosols and vapours can cause irritation to the skin, eyes and the mucous membranes lining the nose, throat and lungs, as well as producing headaches and nausea. People working with glutaraldehyde can become sensitised to the chemical and develop allergic reactions. Worksafe Australia recommends a threshhold exposure limit of 0.2 ppm (0.7 mg/m^3) for short-term exposure. Gloves should always be worn when handling glutaraldehyde and it must be used only in an area with local exhaust ventilation. It is not recommended for routine cleaning or disinfection when a less toxic substance would be adequate; it should only be used when no other method is suitable, such as for the sterilisation of fibre-optic endoscopes.

LOW TEMPERATURE HYDROGEN PEROXIDE PLASMA STERILISATION

A recent development is the use of hydrogen peroxide vapour as a low temperature sterilant suitable for heat and moisture sensitive equipment (e.g. endoscopes). It is designed to replace both ethylene oxide and glutaraldehyde and is suitable for use in hospital central sterilising departments. The system uses hydrogen peroxide which is vapourised and exposed to radio waves giving rise to gaseous plasma (a mixture of high energy species of hydrogen peroxide, H_2O_2). This acts as an oxidising sterilant and is active against a wide variety of microorganisms including viruses, bacterial endospores and mycobacteria. The advantages of the process is that the products are non toxic (water and oxygen), low temperatures (around 45°C) are generated, the cycle is rapid (75 minutes) and no venting time is required. The process is suitable for sterilising medical devices made from stainless steel and most plastics, but should not be used for cellulosic materials which absorb liquids. Disadvantages are the cost of the unit and that items must be wrapped in special non cellulose wrap.

PERACETIC ACID STERILISATION

This system uses 35% peracetic acid at low temperatures (50–55°C) to sterilise surgical, diagnostic and dental instruments in about 30 minutes. The process involves an automatic cycle and the products are non toxic, but the instruments must be rinsed with sterile water. Peracetic acid is active against vegetative bacteria and endospores, fungi, viruses and mycobacteria.

Disinfection

Disinfection is a process that kills or inactivates large numbers of microorganisms, but does not sterilise. Disinfecting methods must be able to reduce the number of microbes present to an 'acceptable level'. The definition of what is an 'acceptable level' in the clinical environment depends on the purpose for which the article is to be used. An article that has been **disinfected** has usually been treated in one of the ways described below. Methods include the use of heat, radiation and various chemical agents that can destroy microorganisms.

Chemical disinfectants that are sufficiently mild to be used on skin, mucous membranes or exposed tissues are called **antiseptics**. Handwashing with antiseptic solutions is recommended as routine practice before carrying out medical and nursing procedures. As mentioned earlier, all articles to be disinfected should first be thoroughly cleaned. The presence of organic matter, grease or dirt interferes with the ability of the chemical to penetrate, contact and inactivate the microorganisms present.

Sanitisation is a poorly defined term. It usually means that an article has been cleaned, although it is used in some contexts to imply that the article is 'germ-free'. It does *not* usually mean that an object has been exposed to a disinfecting procedure, and health workers should not assume that an article that is 'sanitised' has been treated with a disinfectant.

PHYSICAL METHODS OF DISINFECTION

Heat

Heat is a very useful method of disinfection as it penetrates readily and is easier to control than most chemical disinfectants. Boiling water (100°C for 5 minutes) kills most microorganisms except for endospores and some viruses. As such, it is an inexpensive, easily controlled and reliable method for decontaminating many articles and utensils. It is *not* a method of sterilisation and should not be used for instruments that breach the body's defences (such as dental instruments, surgical equipment, vaginal speculae etc). As explained above, these should be sterilised in an autoclave.

Many organisms are killed by exposure to temperatures below 100°C. A temperature of 63°C for 30 minutes is the standard method for **pasteurisation** and destroys most pathogens likely to be present in food or milk, without causing deterioration to the quality of the food. Another method (flash pasteurisation) involves passing milk through a tube heated to 72°C, holding it there for 15 seconds and then cooling it quickly. Various heat treatments to preserve food have been developed. One involves the **ultra-high temperature process**, **UHT**, in which the milk is heated to 140°C for less than 5 seconds and then cooled rapidly back to 74°C.

Ultraviolet radiation

Many microorganisms are killed or damaged by exposure to short-wave ultraviolet (UV) light. UV light does not penetrate into liquids or through paper or even through a layer of dust. However, it is useful for killing bacteria on clean surfaces and for disinfecting limited air spaces such as microbiological safety cabinets and operating theatres. The amount of UV radiation received depends on the time of exposure and the distance the object is placed from the UV source (see Figure 11.4), the amount of radiation absorbed being inversely proportional to the square of the distance of the object from the source. Sunlight is a significant source of UV light, especially in Australia, and the exposure of articles to sunshine significantly reduces their microbial population.

TABLE 11.5
METHODS OF DISINFECTION

METHOD	USE
Heat	
100° boiling water	Instruments Food
63° pasteurisation	Food, milk products
Radiation	
Short wave UV	Surfaces, air spaces
Filtration	Air in safety cabinets, operating theatres, isolation units.
Chemicals	Surfaces, equipment. Decontamination of skin, blood spills, handwashing.

Ultraviolet light is absorbed by the DNA of the cell, causing the strands of nucleic acid to break which interferes with DNA and cell replication. Some bacterial cells are capable of repairing the DNA, thus restoring the original properties of the cell. In some cases a mutation occurs, producing DNA with a different base sequence.

Filtration

Microorganisms can also be removed from air with the use of special high-efficiency particulate air filters (HEPA). Some laboratory work involves the use of hazardous materials, such as infectious microorganisms or contaminated objects, and these can be safely handled in specially designed laminar flow cabinets that provide protection from dangerous aerosols (Figure 11.5). Air is drawn into the cabinet away from the worker and is filtered before leaving the cabinet. This method does not sterilise the air, but significantly reduces the number of organisms that are present in the exhaust and are released into the atmosphere. Filters are often used in ventilation systems to clean the air entering operating theatres, burns wards, isolation units and intensive care wards. They can also be used on exhaust systems in isolation units to trap pathogens that might be released from infectious patients. The filters should be changed regularly and decontaminated before disposal.

CHEMICAL DISINFECTANTS

A large number of chemicals are able to kill or inactivate microorganisms. However, not all of them can be safely used as disinfectants, usually because they are too toxic or corrosive. The widespread use of chemical disinfectants

FIGURE 11.4
EFFECT OF UV RADIATION ON THE GROWTH OF BACTERIA ON A PLATE
Effect on bacterial growth of different times of exposure to UV light (280 nm, d = 15 cm): (a) control, no exposure; (b) one minute; (c) five minutes.

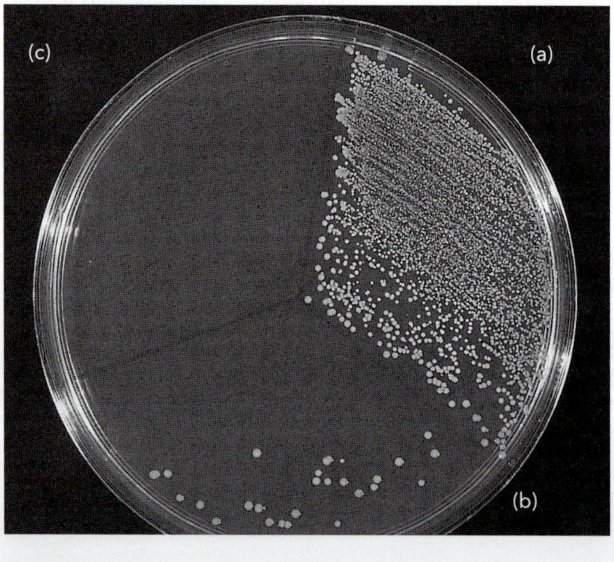

FIGURE 11.5
BIOLOGICAL SAFETY CABINET

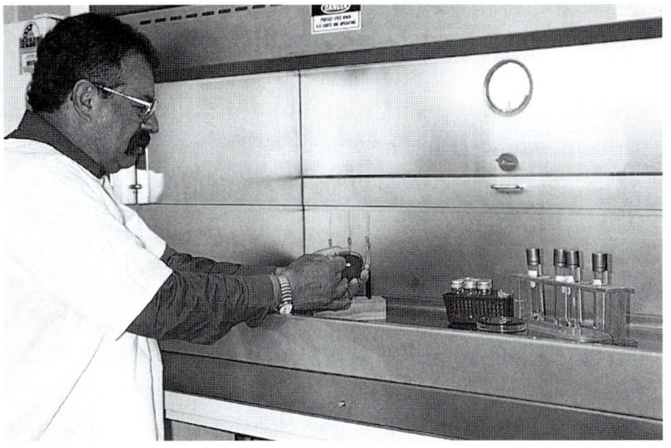

in hospitals for routine cleaning has been largely replaced by the use of neutral detergent. However, disinfectant chemicals are still used to clean contaminated articles or surfaces, to kill microorganisms present in accidental spills of potentially infected body fluids, and as antiseptics for disinfecting skin and tissue. The list of solutions that should be used for cleaning or disinfecting various areas under certain prescribed conditions is usually contained in the infection control manual for each hospital. It is important that health workers in the hospital environment understand the processes involved and are aware of the importance of using the correct concentration of chemicals and exposure times to achieve the desired result (see p. 233).

When using chemical disinfectants, care must be taken to ensure that every part of the article to be disinfected comes into contact with the disinfecting solution. The solution must be used at the correct concentration to ensure there are sufficient molecules of the disinfectant present to kill all the microorganisms. Some chemical disinfectants are unstable, especially in dilute solution, and so should always be used as freshly prepared solutions. It is also essential that the articles are immersed for a sufficient period of time, as the killing curve for chemical disinfection is similar to that for all sterilising and disinfecting methods (see Figure 11.1). Not all chemical disinfectants are equally useful. A major factor in their use is cost, as well as their stability, ability to penetrate, and residual activity on surfaces. The advantages and disadvantages of some disinfectants are listed in Table 11.6.

Some chemicals (e.g. alcohol) react very rapidly, but do not penetrate well into microbial cells in the absence of water. Others, like the hypochlorites, also act rapidly but are corrosive at high concentrations. Some chemicals are more active against one type of microorganism than another. Other factors that need to be taken into account when developing adequate procedures include the fact that some chemicals interact with (i.e. are neutralised by) the salts present in hard water, or with the plastics of which the containers or the articles to be disinfected are made.

TABLE 11.6
CHEMICAL DISINFECTANTS

DISINFECTANT	USE	ADVANTAGES/DISADVANTAGES
Phenolics	Environmental surfaces	Economical, not affected by organic material; unpleasant odour.
Iodine/Iodophores	Skin, preparation for surgery	Active against viruses, endospores; causes stains.
Chlorine (as sodium hypochlorite)	Environmental uses: ■ decontamination of blood spills; ■ terminal cleaning; ■ treatment of swimming pools; ■ purification of drinking water.	Inexpensive; active against viruses, spores, TB, bacteria; high concentrations are corrosive; unstable, inactivated by organic material.
Chlorhexidine	Skin, handwash, surgical scrub.	Non-toxic, antibacterial, good residual activity; not active against viruses, endospores.
Alcohol 70% ethyl or isopropyl alcohol	Skin decontamination before injections Alcohol wipes for equipment	Inexpensive; active against bacteria and fungi; flammable.
Quaternary ammonium compounds	Preservative in pharmaceutical preparations	Stable, non-toxic; effective against most microbes; easily contaminated with *Pseudomonas*.

Phenolic disinfectants

One of the earliest disinfectants used by Lister was the phenol, carbolic acid. Carbolic acid has a very powerful odour, is quite corrosive and has been replaced by derivatives of phenol with more acceptable properties. Phenols are active against a wide range of bacteria, including mycobacteria, but they do not kill endospores. They exert their effect by disruption of the cell membrane, denaturation of proteins and inactivation of enzymes, leading to cell death. Phenolic disinfectants are widely used as they remain active in the presence of organic material (e.g. pus, faeces, or other body substances) and they are inexpensive, stable and relatively non-toxic. However, they are slightly corrosive and should not be used on skin or tissue. Their strong odour makes them unsuitable for use on surfaces that come into contact with food.

The most commonly used phenolic disinfectant is **o-cresol**, which is the main ingredient in a number of commercial brands of disinfectants. A 1–2% solution of this 'clear' phenol is used for terminal cleaning of contaminated environments and high-risk areas and for decontamination of equipment.

Hexachlorophene is a phenol derivative that was once widely used as an antibacterial agent in soaps, lotions and surgical scrubs, and in various cosmetic and hygiene products. It has a bacteriostatic action and is effective against Gram-positive staphylococci and streptococci. Hexachlorophene emulsion was once used routinely to bathe babies in hospital nurseries in order to prevent staphylococcal infections. However, it has been shown to have toxic effects after excessive use, causing neurological damage, and so its use has been largely discontinued. Its main use in hospitals now is to contain outbreaks of nosocomial staphylococcal infections in neonatal wards.

Halogens

The halogens—iodine and chlorine—are very effective antimicrobial agents. **Tincture of iodine** is a solution of iodine in alcohol. It is not widely used now as it is irritating to the skin and causes brown staining of skin and clothing. More commonly, iodine is used in a preparation called an **iodophor**, which is a combination of the organic molecule, povidone, and iodine. The advantage of iodophors is that they are less irritating to the skin and the iodine is released slowly so that they have a good residual antiseptic activity on the skin. Povidone-iodine, when combined with detergent, is an effective antiseptic surgical scrub, and is used for disinfecting wounds. It has a broad spectrum of antimicrobial activity, including endospores, and is active against *Clostridium perfringens* (the causative agent of gangrene). For this reason it is widely used for skin disinfection preoperatively, before a surgical incision is made. The disadvantage is that it causes (temporary) discoloration of the skin and that *Pseudomonas* is able to grow in iodophor solutions.

Chlorine, in the form of **sodium hypochlorite (bleach)**, is an effective disinfectant that is active against a range of microorganisms. Chlorine kills bacteria and viruses and is active against the blood-borne viruses, HBV and HIV. It is relatively inexpensive and readily available for domestic use (swimming pools, bathroom cleaners, soaking baby's bottles and nappies). The chlorine released in aqueous solutions of sodium hypochlorite is a potent oxidising agent. However, because it is an oxidising agent it is inactivated by any organic material that may be present. It is therefore important to clean articles thoroughly before treating them with hypochlorite solutions.

The compound breaks down gradually, especially in sunlight, so fresh solutions should be used. A number of commercial preparations are available and the concentration of available chlorine varies from different manufacturers. It is therefore necessary to check the strength of the solution used (usually stated as percentage of available chlorine) and to ensure that the correct dilution is made. If the solution is too weak, the disinfecting action will not occur. However, chlorine is corrosive and care must be taken that the solution used is not too strong, especially if it comes into contact with skin or utensils used for babies.

Chlorine is used at a concentration of 10 000 ppm (parts per million) or 1% for decontamination of spillages of blood or body fluids. At this strength it is quite corrosive. It is sometimes replaced by sodium dichloroisocyanurate, a chlorine-releasing agent that is less corrosive. It comes in tablet or powder form and can be added as a solid to blood spills. Most commercial preparations for removal of mould contain 1–2% chlorine and are very corrosive. It is advisable to wear gloves when handling these solutions and to avoid inhaling the vapour.

For environmental decontamination, such as terminal cleaning of a room that has accommodated an infectious patient, or for the disinfection of contaminated equipment, chlorine is used at 1000 ppm or 0.1%. Chlorine is widely used to purify drinking water and in swimming pools, at a concentration of 1–5 ppm. **Chloramines** are organic chlorine-containing compounds that release chlorine slowly over a period of time. They are used to purify household water supplies as they do not have the unpleasant taste and odour sometimes associated with the chlorination of water.

Chlorhexidine

Chlorhexidine is a very effective antibacterial agent, widely used as an antiseptic for disinfection of skin and mucous membranes. A number of commercial preparations are available containing chlorhexidine in combination with various soaps or detergent, as alcohol rubs, or in skin lotions (various preparations of Hibitane®).

It is active against most bacteria, especially Gram-positive bacteria, where it acts by attacking the plasma membrane. It does not affect mycobacteria or endospores and *Pseudomonas* spp. are able to survive in aqueous solutions. It is effective against fungi, and some viruses including HIV. One of the main advantages of chlorhexidine is its low toxicity and its ability to persist on the skin for extended periods. This residual activity makes it useful for surgical scrubs. However, it is relatively expensive and is not used for routine cleaning or decontamination purposes.

Alcohol

Ethyl alcohol and **isopropyl alcohol** are effective antibacterial chemicals. Alcohols affect the cells by dissolving the lipids in the bacterial cell wall and membranes. They are most effective when mixed with water (usually 70% alcohol/water) as the water helps the alcohol to penetrate the cell. The alcohol/water preparation is also effective in the denaturation of proteins. Alcohols are used mainly to disinfect clean surfaces such as trolleys and thermometers, as alcohol wipes, and as a skin disinfectant before injections are given. The presence of organic material interferes with their action. They are often used in combination with other antiseptics such as chlorhexidine in alcohol rubs for the quick disinfection of the hands, the main advantage being the ease of evaporation which removes the need for rinsing or drying.

Quaternary ammonium compounds (QUATS)

These compounds are cationic detergents with a strong bacteriocidal action, due to the positive charge on the molecule. They are also effective against many fungi, some protozoa and enveloped viruses, but they do not affect endospores. They are thought to act by damaging the cell membrane. The main advantage of QUATS is that they are relatively stable, non-toxic, odourless and tasteless. However, some organisms—such as certain species of *Pseudomonas*—thrive in aqueous QUAT solutions. Because of the ease of contamination with *Pseudomonas*, which is a serious opportunistic pathogen, QUATS are no longer widely used in hospitals. Two of the most common substances in use are benzyl alkalonium chloride, which is used as a preservative in eye drops, and cetyl pyridinium chloride, which is used extensively in oral preparations such as antibacterial lozenges and mouthwashes.

Other Methods of Microbial Control

OXIDISING AGENTS

Some oxidising agents are also used to destroy bacteria; for example, **hydrogen peroxide** can act as an antiseptic and weak solutions are used for cleaning deep puncture wounds. Hydrogen peroxide (12%) is used in low temperature plasma sterilising units. **Benzoyl peroxide** is used to treat infections in anaerobic wounds and is also an ingredient in cosmetic preparations for the treatment of acne.

REFRIGERATION, FREEZING, DRYING

These methods are discussed here for completeness, but they are *not* methods of killing microorganisms. They are used mainly for control of microbial growth. Cold temperatures, such as are found in a domestic refrigerator (4°C), slow down the rate of cell division of most microorganisms but do not kill them. The rate of food spoilage can be slowed by refrigeration but, when the food is removed and warmed to room temperature, the microorganisms will continue to multiply.

Freezing is a more effective method of food preservation, but it does not kill microorganisms either. The rate of growth is negligible, so the food does not spoil. Some microbial cells may be destroyed by the formation of ice crystals, which disrupt the cell membranes, especially if repeated freezing and thawing occurs, but freezing does *not* cause significant death of microbes. In fact, a standard method for the preservation of bacterial cultures is rapid freezing in liquid nitrogen (–70°C).

Drying preserves food by reducing moisture but does not necessarily kill the organisms present; nor does the process of freeze-drying (**lyophilisation**) which involves the removal of water under vacuum from a frozen solution. Freeze-drying is also used to preserve microorganisms, which remain viable for long periods (months to years) at room temperature as a lyophilised powder.

CHEMICAL PRESERVATIVES

Chemicals are used as preservatives in food because they inhibit microbial metabolism or growth. Organic acids such as sorbic acid and benzoic acid inhibit the growth of mould at low pH. **Calcium propionate** is used as a fungal inhibitor in bread. The benzoic acid derivatives, methyl paraben and propylparaben, are used as preservatives in cosmetics and shampoos.

Summary

- Microorganisms are present everywhere in the environment but only some cause disease.
- Different methods of control are required for different situations and different types of organisms.

HISTORICAL BACKGROUND

- Food can be preserved by physical methods such as drying, heating, pickling and salting.
- Joseph Lister was the first to use chemical disinfection to prevent infections following surgery.
- Ignaz Semmelweis observed that pathogens could be transmitted on unwashed hands.

PATTERN OF MICROBIAL DEATH

- Damage to any of the structural or functional components of a cell will result in its death.
- The rate of death of a population of microorganisms follows an exponential curve.

PROCEDURES FOR CLEANING, DISINFECTION AND STERILISATION

- The highest risk of transmission of infection is associated with equipment that penetrates the skin or mucous membranes.
- The removal of organic matter, dirt and grease is essential before carrying out disinfection or sterilisation procedures.

STERILISATION

- Sterilisation involves the complete destruction or removal of all living organisms from an object.
- Physical methods of sterilisation use heat or radiation; mechanical methods use filtration; and chemical methods used glutaraldehyde, or ethylene oxide, or hydrogen peroxide.
- Dry heat kills by oxidation. Moist heat kills by denaturation.
- The cheapest and most effective method of sterilisation uses moist heat (steam under pressure in an autoclave). The efficiency of the autoclave should be monitored regularly.
- Heat-resistant metal and glass can be sterilised in a hot oven at 160°C for 60 minutes.
- Incineration is used for the complete destruction of contaminated articles.
- Ionising radiation kills microorganisms by disrupting the DNA chains.
- Filtration is used to sterilise heat-sensitive substances.
- Ethylene oxide gas is used to sterilise prepackaged disposable equipment.
- Glutaraldehyde is used to sterilise delicate heat-sensitive instruments.
- Low temperature plasma sterilisation uses hydrogen peroxide.

DISINFECTION

- Disinfection involves the removal or destruction of microorganisms to an 'acceptable level'.
- Antiseptics are chemical disinfectants that are mild enough to use on skin.
- Methods of disinfection include boiling at 100°C, pasteurisation, UV radiation, filtration and the use of chemicals.
- Some examples of chemical disinfectants are phenols, halogens (iodine and chlorine), chlorhexidine, alcohol and QUATS.
- Every part of the article to be disinfected must come into contact with the disinfecting solution.

OTHER METHODS OF MICROBIAL CONTROL

- Other methods of control include the use of oxidising agents, refrigeration, freezing, drying and the use of chemical preservatives.

Study Questions

1. What are some traditional methods of food preservation?
2. What is pasteurisation?
3. Who was the first doctor to use chemical disinfectants in surgery?
4. What contribution did Ignaz Semmelweis make to medicine?
5. What two factors determine the efficiency of the disinfecting process?
6. Why do instruments need to be cleaned before being treated with disinfectant?
7. What is the difference between sterilisation and disinfection?
8. What are the advantages of moist heat sterilisation?
9. How do you check whether an autoclave is functioning properly? Why is this important?
10. How do gamma rays have a sterilising effect?
11. When is filtration used to sterilise solutions?
12. What are the disadvantages of sterilisation with ethylene oxide?
13. Why is glutaraldehyde only recommended for use in special circumstances. What are they?
14. What is an antiseptic?
15. When is ultraviolet radiation used?
16. Why is hexachlorophene no longer used to bathe babies?
17. What are the advantages and disadvantages of phenolic disinfectants?
18. What antiseptics are the most effective for skin disinfection?
19. What disinfectant is used to decontaminate blood spills?
20. How is drinking water purified?
21. When is it appropriate to use alcohol as a disinfectant?
22. What is a major disadvantage of QUATS?
23. What happens to bacteria when they are stored in the refrigerator or freezer?
24. List two chemicals that are used as preservatives.

Test Your Understanding

1. Explain what you understand by the term 'killing curve' when applied to sterilising or disinfecting procedures.
2. How do you decide whether equipment needs to be sterilised or disinfected?
3. Why is boiling instruments at 100°C not considered to be a method of sterilisation?
4. How can hazardous substances or infectious microorganisms be safely handled in the laboratory?
5. Why is chlorine used extensively for disinfection?
6. Why is it important not to reuse disposable equipment?

FURTHER READING

Beneson, A.S. ed., *Control of Communicable Diseases Manual*, 16th edn, Washington: American Public Health Association, 1995.

Gardner, J.F. and Peel, M., *Introduction to Sterilization, Disinfection and Infection Control*, 2nd edn, London: Churchill Livingstone, 1991.

National Occupational Health and Safety Commission, *Workplace Control of Hazardous Substances: National Model Regulations and National Code of Practice*, Canberra: Australian Government Publishing Service, 1991.

Meers, P., W. Jacobsen & M. McPherson, *Hospital Infection Control For Nurses*, London: Chapman & Hall, 1992.

chapter 12

control of infection:

antimicrobial therapy

Chapter focus

- *Describe the discovery and development of antimicrobial drugs.*
- *What are the principles underlying the effective use of antimicrobial drugs?*
- *How do the major groups of antimicrobials kill or inhibit microbial cells?*
- *What guidelines are followed in prescribing antimicrobial drugs?*
- *What are the reasons for, and consequences of, the development of resistance to antimicrobial drugs?*
- *What are the responsibilities of the nurse in the administration of antimicrobial therapy?*

The end of the 19th century saw attempts being made to control the spread of infection by using physical or chemical methods that killed or inactivated microorganisms (see Chapter 11). The work of Robert Koch and other scientists who followed his principles (see Chapter 1) had resulted in the isolation and identification of the bacteria responsible for many of the known infectious diseases. However, the treatment of these diseases in humans still relied mainly on supportive methods that alleviated the symptoms. Chemical disinfectants that were used to kill bacteria on skin, wounds and some tissues were relatively non-specific in their action, and topical application sometimes caused local inflammation and interfered with healing.

For centuries, people have used extracts from plants and herbs to treat illness. We now know that some of these preparations contain valuable therapeutic drugs. For example: aspirin was first extracted from the bark of the willow tree; morphine is derived from the seeds of the opium poppy; quinine, used against malaria, comes from the bark of the chinchona tree; and digitalis, used in the treatment of heart disease, was first extracted from foxglove leaves. Ancient Chinese culture has traditionally used combinations of herbs to treat illness. The mouldy soybean preparation that was placed on infected wounds probably contained small amounts of an antibiotic such as penicillin. Plant extracts were used in a variety of ways—as medicinal teas, as inhalants, or as poultices placed on wounds or inflammation. Many of these treatments were successful but the mechanism by which they effected a 'cure' was unknown.

The idea of finding a chemical that could specifically kill the microbe responsible for the infection, without damaging the host cells (i.e. a 'magic bullet'), was proposed by the chemist Paul Ehrlich in 1908. It was known that the metal, antimony, was toxic to many bacteria, but it was also toxic to humans. Ehrlich set about trying to synthesise an organic compound containing antimony, that would retain the antimicrobial properties of the antimony but would be non-toxic to humans. He succeeded, and the compound, called 'salvarsan', was found to be effective against spirochaetes, in particular the agent responsible for syphilis, *Treponema pallidum*.

Ehrlich's work opened up a whole new approach to the treatment of disease. Chemists tried to repeat his success with salvarsan by synthesising various chemical compounds, but most of them were found to be too toxic to humans to be of use. However, the new science of chemotherapy had been created. **Chemotherapy** involves the introduction of a specific chemical compound, or drug, into the body in order to elicit a particular desired response, preferably without causing harm to the patient.

The Development of Antimicrobial Chemotherapy

SELECTIVE TOXICITY

The concept of **selective toxicity** is fundamental to the successful development, production and use of any chemotherapeutic agent, that is, the drug must be able to kill or inhibit the microorganism responsible for the disease without damaging the host cells in any way. It is relatively easy to find chemicals that will kill microorganisms. It is not so easy to find ones that will do so without harming the human host. To find such a compound, it is necessary to identify a reaction or structure that is unique to the target microorganism and that is altered or damaged by the drug in such a way as to prevent replication, or cause the death of the microbial cell. The principle of selective toxicity, therefore, exploits the differences in structure and metabolism between the microbial cell and the host cell. This is easier to achieve with procaryotic microorganisms (bacteria) than with eucaryotic microorganisms, which have more structural and functional similarities to human cells. It is difficult to achieve with viruses because their method of replication involves taking over the host cell, so that any compound that interferes with viral replication is also likely to damage the host cell. Sometimes, selective toxicity occurs as a result of the greater affinity of the drug for the microbial enzyme than for the host cell enzyme.

SULPHA DRUGS

Inspired by Ehrlich's synthesis of salvarsan, another chemist, Gerhard Domagk in Germany, tested a dye called 'prontosil' for its ability to kill streptococci. He found that it was active only in animal tissues, where it was converted to a compound called **sulphanilamide**, a potent inhibitor of bacterial replication. The discovery of sulphanilamide led to the synthesis of a large number of similar drugs, collectively named **sulphonamides** or **sulpha drugs**. These sulpha drugs exhibit activity against a variety of pathogens. However, many organisms are able to develop resistance to them and sulpha drugs also frequently cause allergies such as skin rashes. They are now used mainly in the treatment of urinary tract infections.

THE DISCOVERY OF ANTIBIOTICS

The real breakthrough in the treatment of infections came with the discovery of antibiotics. In 1928, at about the same time the sulpha drugs were being developed, ALEXANDER FLEMING noticed that the growth of a mould on an agar plate culture of *Staphylococcus aureus* had inhibited the growth of the bacteria. He correctly deduced that the mould had produced a chemical that diffused through the agar and killed the bacteria. He called the chemical **penicillin** from the name of the mould *Penicillium*. Attempts to isolate and purify significant amounts of it were largely unsuccessful and it was not until the beginning of World War II that interest in the compound was revived, as a treatment for infections of injuries sustained by soldiers.

Its isolation was largely due to an Australian physician, HOWARD FLOREY, who was working at Oxford and investigating the development of penicillin as a chemotherapeutic agent. He was invited to the United States and with the backing of the US Government and in collaboration with the chemist ERNST CHAIN, was largely responsible for the project that resulted in the production of large quantities of penicillin, which were then used successfully to treat infections in wounded soldiers.

The dramatic results obtained from the isolation, purification and therapeutic use of penicillin encouraged scientists to look for other naturally occurring substances, produced by microorganisms, that might also have antimicrobial activity.

The term **antibiotic** is used to describe a chemical produced by a microorganism, that in small amounts can kill or inhibit another microorganism. Antibiotics are natural products of various microorganisms, including fungi, actinomycetes and bacteria, many of which are found in soil. More than half the antibiotics in use are produced by different species of filamentous soil bacteria belonging to the genus *Streptomyces*. Although many antimicrobials are derived from natural sources, many of them are chemically modified in order to improve their antimicrobial properties and are, therefore, called 'semi-synthetic'.

ANTIMICROBIAL DRUGS

We have so far described the discovery of two different kinds of compounds that are active against microorganisms. Antibiotics such as penicillin are naturally occurring substances, whereas the sulpha drugs are completely synthetic. Attempts by scientists to find effective antimicrobial agents have resulted in the production of a range of naturally occurring, synthetic and semi-synthetic drugs, with varying activity against the different types of microorganisms. The term **antimicrobial** is used to describe a compound that is able to kill or inhibit the growth of a microorganism. Strictly speaking, antibiotics are a particular type of naturally occurring antimicrobial compounds, but in practice the terms 'antibiotic' and 'antimicrobial' are used interchangeably. Thus, an 'antibiotic sensitivity test', performed in a diagnostic microbiology laboratory, should correctly be called an 'antimicrobial sensitivity test' because it tests the sensitivity of a particular microorganism to a range of compounds, some of which are naturally occurring, but some of which may be chemically modified antibiotics, semi-synthetic (e.g. methicillin) or completely synthetic (e.g. sulpha drugs and quinolones).

We can further separate antimicrobials into groups depending on the type of organism they are active against. Thus, antibacterials are active against bacteria, antivirals against viruses, antifungals against fungi and antiprotozoals against protozoa. The reason that some drugs are active only against one type of organism (e.g. antibacterials do not kill viruses) is related to the compound's mechanism of action. To selectively kill or inhibit the microorganism, the compound must attack or interfere with a structure or a step in a metabolic or replicative process that is unique to that organism, and that is preferably not present in the host cell. Since different types of microorganisms have different cellular components and metabolic processes, the drugs that are most effective against one type of organism may not affect another type.

Compounds that are active against a number of different types of microorganisms are called **broad spectrum antimicrobial agents**, while those with a limited range of activity are called **narrow spectrum antimicrobial agents**. Some agents are able to kill microorganisms and are identified by the addition of the suffix *-cidal*—for example, penicillin is **bacteriocidal**. Others inhibit the replication of the organism without killing it and have the ending *-static*—for example, tetracycline is **bacteriostatic**. These properties are also related to the compound's mechanism of action. In general, compounds that are bacteriocidal result in the irreversible formation of an inactive compound (e.g. an unstable cell wall) so that the cell is no longer viable. In contrast, agents that are bacteriostatic interfere with metabolism or the synthesis of a compound such as an enzyme protein, but do not necessarily cause the death of the cell, and so their effect is reversed once they are removed from the cell. However, even though they do not cause the death of the cell, bacteriostatic agents are useful because, while they are present in the body, they prevent further replication of the microorganism and give the immune system time to mount its defences against the infection. In practice, the use of a bacteriocidal agent in preference to a bacteriostatic one is only important for immunocompromised patients whose own defences are not able to complete the task of eliminating the pathogens from the body.

One of the major problems associated with the use of antimicrobials today is the development of resistance by the organisms to the antimicrobial drug. This can take many forms and is discussed later in this chapter.

Antibacterial Drugs

There are four main target sites for antibacterial action:

1. synthesis of the bacterial cell wall;
2. protein synthesis;
3. nucleic acid synthesis;
4. function of the bacterial cell membrane.

COMPOUNDS THAT AFFECT CELL WALL SYNTHESIS

As described in Chapter 4, the cell wall of a bacterium is essential to maintain the shape and provide structural support for the cell. A major component of the bacterial wall is peptidoglycan, a compound that is unique to bacteria and therefore provides an ideal target for selective toxicity. A number of antibacterials have been found that exert their action by interfering with the synthesis of peptidoglycan. One of the most important of these is **penicillin**, which belongs to a group of antibacterials known collectively as **ß-lactams**. Beta-lactam antibacterials derive their name from the four-membered ß-lactam ring which is present in all these compounds (see Figure 12.1). Bacterial resistance to these compounds is frequently associated with the production by the resistant bacterium of a ß-lactamase enzyme which breaks open this ring and destroys the antibacterial compound. Other members of the group are the cephalosporins, carbapenems and monobactams. (See Figure 12.3.)

The ß-lactams inhibit cell wall synthesis by combining with the transpeptidase enzyme responsible for cross-linking of the peptidoglycan chains. Thus, these drugs are mainly active against growing cells, preventing the formation of a rigid cell wall structure. This results in a cell without the protective support layer and so cell lysis occurs (i.e. a bacteriocidal effect).

Beta-lactam antibacterials are particularly useful because of their low toxicity to humans. However, some people develop an allergy to them due to the formation of a conjugate of the ß-lactam ring with serum proteins that elicits an inflammatory immune response. People who are allergic to penicillin are usually also allergic to most other ß-lactam antibacterials. (See Spotlight box, on this page.)

FIGURE 12.1
THE BETA-LACTAM RING

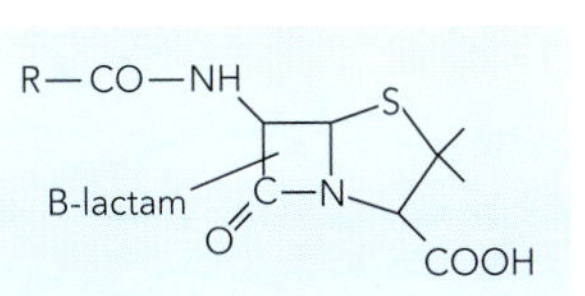

> **SPOTLIGHT**
> **PENICILLIN AND ANAPHYLACTIC SHOCK**
>
> Anaphylaxis due to the parenteral administration of penicillin is a rare but life-threatening occurrence. It has an incidence of about 1 in 200 of all patients receiving penicillin and a mortality of 1 in 5000. Prompt administration of adrenaline (epinephrine) by intramuscular injection is essential.
>
> An allergic (hypersensitivity) reaction to penicillin is a genetically determined reaction associated with the individual's immune system. In some people, exposure to the drug elicits an allergic immune response. The penicillin molecule is broken down and reacts with certain tissue proteins to form a complex that stimulates the immune system to produce IgE antibodies. The antibodies attach to the surface of mast cells and basophils which are distributed throughout the body. These cells are then 'sensitised'. If the patient is exposed to penicillin again, the sensitised cells rapidly release histamine and other active substances that cause anaphylactic reactions ranging from urticaria (rashes), hives and laryngeal oedema to broncho-constriction and hypotension. The most severe form of anaphylaxis is described as anaphylactic shock and can be fatal.
>
> A number of patients report being 'allergic' to penicillin, having reactions that may include symptoms such as a skin rash, but only the anaphylactic response is a major contraindication to its use. It is possible to ascertain whether a patient is hypersensitive to penicillin by the use of a skin test. A positive reaction to the injection of the penicillin complex occurs in 10–15 minutes.
>
> Patients who are hypersensitive to penicillin also exhibit a reaction to the semi-synthetic penicillins as well as to other antimicrobials that have a ß-lactam ring (e.g. the cephalosporins). Usually, vancomycin is used instead of penicillin. However it must be administered by slow intravenous infusion (see Case History 12.1, p. 264).
>
> *Nursing management*
>
> It is essential that all patients be asked whether they have a history of allergy to penicillin before the drug is administered. If patients are unclear about their history or have no memory of having had the drug before, then special precautions must be taken. It is essential that adrenaline (epinephrine) is available when penicillin (or any drug) is administered parenterally. Nurses should check the 'use by' date on the ampoule to ensure the adrenaline is still current.
>
> If penicillin is administered orally, the nurse should observe the patient for any signs of rash, difficulty in breathing, etc.
>
> *Note:* Antihistamines and corticosteroids are *not* effective treatment for penicillin-induced anaphylaxis.

Penicillin

Penicillin is isolated from the mould *Penicillium chrysogenum* and occurs in a number of closely related forms. Of the natural penicillins, penicillin G (benzyl penicillin) was originally found to be extremely effective but it is readily inactivated under the conditions of low pH encountered in the gastric acid in the stomach. It is administered intramuscularly or intravenously as the sodium or potassium salt. Another commonly used natural penicillin, phenoxymethylpenicillin (penicillin V), is acid-stable and can be taken orally although it is not well absorbed and is excreted rapidly. Semi-synthetic penicillins have been developed in an effort to overcome the problems associated with the use of the naturally occurring compounds—problems such as susceptibility to gastric acid; lack of water solubility, short excretion (retention) time; narrow spectrum of activity; and development of resistance.

Table 12.1 lists the major penicillins in use. The naturally occurring penicillins are active mainly against Gram-positive organisms, whereas the newer, semi-synthetic compounds have a broader spectrum of activity. For example, aminopenicillins such as ampicillin and amoxycillin, and the carboxypenicillin, ticarcillin, are also active against Gram-negative organisms. Penicillins that are resistant to ß-lactamase include methicillin and isoxazole penicillins such as flucloxacillin. Chemists are continuing the search for more effective penicillins.

The combination of other compounds, such as clavulanic acid, with penicillin can increase the potency of the drug preparation. Clavulanic acid, which is a naturally occurring compound extracted from a streptomycete, inhibits the action of ß-lactamase, thus preventing inactivation of the penicillin. It does not have significant antibacterial activity on its own. Sodium clavulanate is combined with amoxycillin in Augmentin® and with ticarcillin in Timentin®.

Cephalosporins

Cephalosporins are produced by a species of the marine fungus *Cephalosporium*. They also inhibit synthesis of the peptidoglycan of the cell wall and have a similar structure to the penicillins, containing a ß-lactam ring (Figure 12.2). They are more active against Gram-negative organisms than the penicillins and chemical modification of the side chains of the cephalosporin nucleus has given rise to a series of compounds with increased antibacterial activity, known as second and third generation cephalosporins (see Table 12.2). These are widely used for the treatment of infections in hospitalised patients, the choice of drug being determined by its spectrum of activity and its ability to be absorbed and penetrate to the site of infection.

Carbapenems

Carbapenems are synthetic ß-lactam compounds with a wide spectrum of activity and are stable against a wide range of ß-lactamases. **Imipenem** is rapidly metabolised in the kidney but, if administered in combination with the enzyme inhibitor, cilastin, high concentrations of the drug can be achieved in the urine and serum. Imipemem causes neurological side effects such as convulsions and is being replaced by a new drug, **meropenem**, which is not metabolised by the renal cells.

TABLE 12.1
THE PENICILLINS

PENICILLIN	ROUTE OF ADMINISTRATION	SPECTRUM OF ANTIBACTERIAL ACTIVITY
Natural penicillins		
Benzyl penicillin (Penicillin G)	IV, IM	Streptococci, pneumococci, meningococci
Phenoxymethyl penicillin (Penicillin V)	Oral	Gram-positives, esp. streptococci
Semi-synthetic penicillins		
Ampicillin Amoxycillin Augmentin®	Oral, IM, IV	As for penicillin G plus *E. coli*, *Haemophilus* influenzae
Cloxacillin Flucloxacillin	Oral, IM, IV	Mostly *Staphylococcus aureus*
Ticarcillin Timentin®	IM, IV	Pseudomonads
Piperacillin Azlocillin	IM, IV IV	Gram-negatives Pseudomonads

Note: Methicillin is no longer widely used because of nephrotoxicity.

FIGURE 12.2
CEPHALOSPORINS

Caphalosporins
e.g. cephalexin, cefactor
cefadroxil, cefuroxime
cefamandole, cefotaxime
ceftazidime

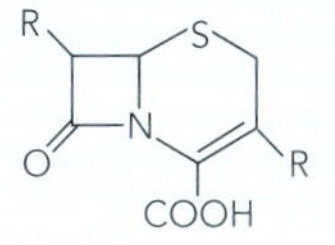

Monobactams

Monobactams are mainly active against aerobic Gram-negative bacteria (except *Pseudomonas*), but anaerobes and Gram-positive organisms are resistant. Monobactams can be used for urinary tract infections, septicaemia and gonorrhoea, and are not inactivated by ß-lactamase enzymes. They are not widely used except in patients who are hypersensitive to the ß-lactams.

Other cell wall inhibitors

The glycopeptides, **vancomycin** and **teicoplan**, are large molecules that interfere with cell wall synthesis by binding to the growing peptide chains that are part of the peptidoglycan molecule, thus preventing further synthesis of the cell wall. Because of their size, these compounds cannot penetrate the Gram-negative outer membrane and so they are active only against Gram-positive organisms. Vancomycin is poorly absorbed from the intestine. It is somewhat toxic and *must* be administered by slow intravenous infusion, in order to prevent histamine release which can lead to cardiac arrest. (See Case History 12.1, p. 264). Because phlebitis is common, vancomycin is usually given via centrally placed catheters. The drug is important for the treatment of methicillin-resistant

FIGURE 12.3
COMPARISON OF THE STRUCTURES OF THE BETA-LACTAM INHIBITORS OF CELL WALL SYNTHESIS

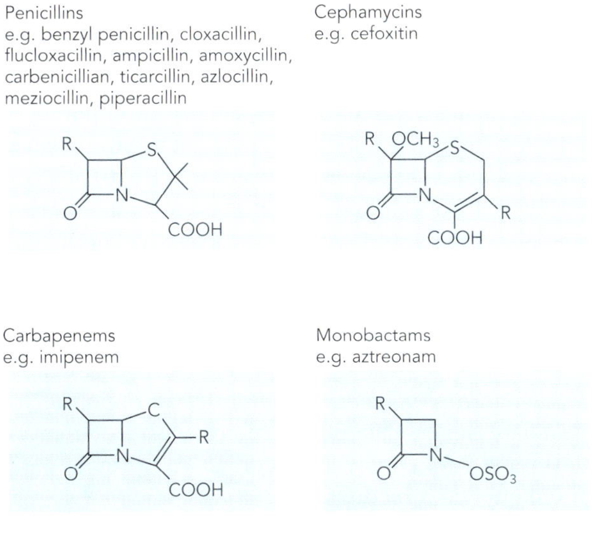

TABLE 12.2
SOME CEPHALOSPORINS AND THEIR DERIVATIVES

CEPHALOSPORIN	ROUTE OF ADMINISTRATION
First generation	
Cephalothin	IM, IV
Cephalexin	Oral
Cephazolin	IM, IV
Second generation	
Cefoxitin	IM, IV
Third generation	
Cefotaxime	IM, IV
Ceftazidime	IM, IV
Ceftriaxone	IM, IV

staphylococcal infections (MRSA), as instances of acquired resistance to vancomycin are extremely rare.

Bacitracin is a polypeptide molecule that is mainly active against Gram-positive bacteria. It inhibits the synthesis of the strands of peptidoglycan by blocking dephosphorylation of the carrier lipid molecule involved in synthesis. Because of its toxicity to humans, its use is limited to topical application for superficial skin infections.

INHIBITORS OF PROTEIN SYNTHESIS

Compounds that inhibit the synthesis of protein in the cell may be bacteriocidal or bacteriostatic. The mechanism of protein synthesis is essentially the same in eucaryotic and procaryotic organisms. However, there are slight differences in the relative sizes and binding properties of the ribosomes in the two types of cell that permit some degree of selective toxicity. Antibacterials that inhibit protein synthesis act by interfering either with the translation of the messenger RNA into protein, or with the binding of the mRNA to the ribosomes. Because the 70S ribosomes in bacterial cells are smaller and less dense than the 80S eucaryotic host cell ribosomes, drugs that target the 70S ribosomes are able to affect the bacterial cells adversely, while not binding significantly to the host ribosomes. However, eucaryotic mitochondria also contain 70S ribosomes, so drugs that inhibit protein synthesis in bacteria can also affect the mitochondria of the host cells.

A number of different groups of antimicrobials affect protein synthesis in bacterial cells. They include the aminoglycosides, the tetracyclines and the macrolides, as well as lincosamides, chloramphenicol, and fusidic acid.

Aminoglycosides

This family of antibacterial agents contains a number of useful drugs, including streptomycin, gentamicin, tobramycin and neomycin (see Table 12. 3). Their action is bacteriocidal as they cause misreading of the messenger

TABLE 12.3
AMINOGLYCOSIDES

AMINOGLYCOSIDE	ROUTE OF ADMINISTRATION	SPECTRUM OF ACTIVITY
Gentamicin Tobramycin Amikacin	IM, IV IM, IV IM, IV	Gram-negative, may be used with penicillins
Streptomycin	IM, IV	TB in combination with other drugs
Neomycin Kanamycin	Topical or oral for 'gut sterilisation'	Gram-positive, coliforms

RNA, leading to substitution of the wrong amino acid into the peptide chain thus forming an inactive protein. **Streptomycin**, isolated from *Streptomyces griseus*, was one of the earliest aminoglycosides identified and initially was extremely useful for the treatment of tuberculosis. It is now used mainly as a second-line drug, as resistance to streptomycin developed rapidly.

Other aminoglycosides (e.g. **gentamicin**) are used commonly in hospitals for the treatment of hospital-acquired infections, especially Gram-negative coliforms and *Pseudomonas* infections. They are often used for their synergistic effect, that is, in combination with another drug to enhance the therapeutic effect. For example, penicillin or ampicillin may be used in combination with gentamicin. The penicillins open up the cell wall allowing greater penetration by the gentamicin. Aminoglycosides are not absorbed from the intestine so are administered intramuscularly or intravenously for systemic infections, and must be monitored carefully for toxic side effects. These include **ototoxicity** (vertigo and deafness) and **nephrotoxicity** (kidney damage). They should be used cautiously in patients with impaired renal function. **Neomycin** is very toxic but is poorly absorbed so is useful in topical preparations.

Tetracyclines

Tetracyclines are a group of broad spectrum bacteriostatic agents that have been isolated from the members of the genus *Streptomyces*. They inhibit protein synthesis by preventing attachment of amino acids to ribosomes. They are active against both Gram-negative and Gram-positive organisms and penetrate cells well, so they are also active against intracellular chlamydiae and rickettsiae. They are useful in the treatment of non-specific urethritis (NSU), when *Chlamydia*, which is not sensitive to penicillin, may be present. They are used to treat psittacosis (*Chlamydia psittaci*) and are also active against mycoplasmas. Doxycycline is a good prophylactic agent for malaria in areas where resistant strains are endemic. It can be used safely for long periods in low doses for the treatment of acne.

Tetracyclines may be administered orally and modification of the side chains (see Figure 12.4) has produced a number of useful compounds that are better absorbed and have longer retention times in the body than the parent compound. Side effects of the tetracyclines are due mainly to their broad spectrum of activity which can cause suppression of the normal flora, leading to a superinfection or overgrowth of undesirable organisms such as *Candida albicans* (thrush). Tetracyclines should not be given to pregnant women as they may affect liver function, or to young children as they deposit in developing teeth, causing permanent yellow discoloration, and may interfere with bone formation. Resistance to tetracyclines develops easily, and their widespread use in animal feeds has been thought to contribute to the transfer of resistant strains of bacteria to humans.

Macrolides

The **macrolides** are a group of antibacterials with a complex structure containing a macrocylic (14-membered) lactone ring (see Figure 12.5). The best known is **erythromycin** which is used extensively as an alternative drug for people who are allergic to penicillin. Its action is bacteriostatic, binding to 50S ribosomes and preventing the release of transfer RNA (tRNA) after peptide bond formation. It is used mainly against Gram-positive organisms as it is unable to penetrate the Gram-negative cell wall. However, it is effective against *Legionella pneumophila* and *Bordetella pertussis* (whooping cough) and is the drug of choice for these diseases. It is also active against mycoplasma and chlamydiae. It is not affected by ß-lactamases and has been used extensively for streptococcal infections, especially in children, as it can be administered orally in a pleasant syrup. However, some resistance has been reported in both streptococci and staphylococci. Clinically, it is used for a variety of respiratory infections, tonsillitis, bronchitis and pneumonia as well as for non-specific urethritis.

Newer macrolides are **azithromycin** and **clarithromycin**. Clarithromycin has a similar spectrum of activity to erythromycin but is also active against *Mycobacterium avium-intracellulare*, an opportunistic infection seen in immunosuppressed patients. Azithromycin is excreted very slowly and is effective in single doses for chlamydial infections.

FIGURE 12.4
TETRACYCLINE STRUCTURE
Tetracyclines are complex molecules consisting of four rings with five different sites for substitution. This gives rise to a family of molecules which differ more in their pharmacological properties than spectrum of activity.

TETRACYCLINE STRUCTURE

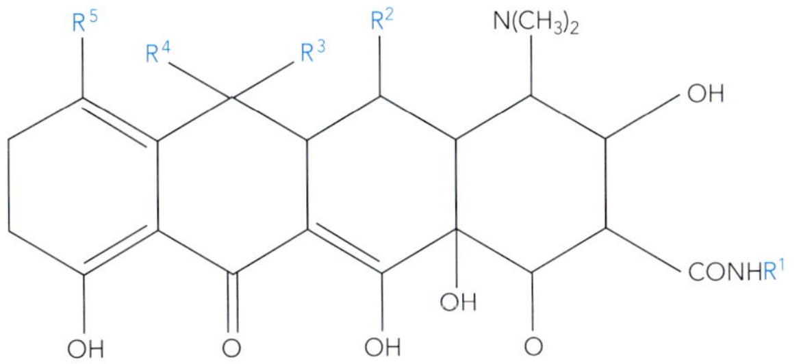

	R^1	R^2	R^3	R^4	R^5
Tetracycline	H	H	CH_3	OH	H
Chlortetracycline	H	H	CH_3	OH	Cl
Oxytetracycline	H	OH	CH_3	OH	H
Doxycycline	H	OH	CH_3	H	H
Minocycline	H	H	H	H	$H(CH_3)_2$

Lincosamides

The chlorinated derivative of lincomycin, **clindamycin** is a drug that has been widely used in hospitals against staphylococci and anaerobes (*Clostridium* spp. and *Bacteroides*). However, it has been implicated as a major factor in the occurrence of pseudomembranous colitis (see Chapter 18) caused by *Clostridium difficile* which is resistant to this drug. Although other antibiotics have also been shown to give rise to this condition, it is particularly frequent following treatment with clindamycin and so the use of clindamycin has been restricted. It penetrates tissue well and is particularly useful for bone and joint infections. It inhibits protein synthesis by binding to the 50S ribosomal subunit and inhibiting peptide bond formation.

Chloramphenicol

Chloramphenicol is a simple compound containing a substituted benzene nucleus (Figure 12.6) and has a wide spectrum of activity against both Gram-positive and Gram-negative organisms. It was originally isolated from *Streptomyces* but is now synthesised chemically because of its simple structure. It is bacteriostatic, inhibiting protein synthesis by binding to the 50S ribosomal subunit and preventing peptide bond formation by the enzyme peptidyl transferase. However, it is also able to bind to human mitochondrial 50S ribosomes which may explain its toxicity to bone marrow. Nitrobenzene, a closely related compound, is a bone marrow suppressant. Toxicity to chloramphenicol is of two types. The first is a reversible suppression of the bone marrow. The other is a rare type of toxicity (1 in 30 000) involving suppression of red blood cell synthesis in the bone marrow, leading to irreversible

FIGURE 12.5
STRUCTURE OF THE MACROLIDE ANTIBIOTIC, ERYTHROMYCIN

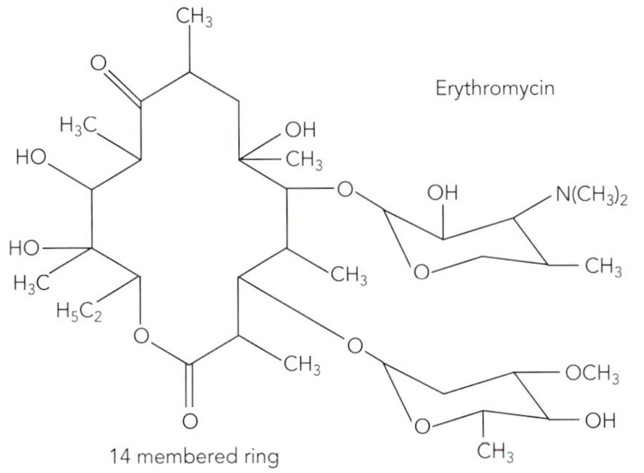

aplastic anaemia. The drug is metabolised in the liver, combining with glucuronic acid to be excreted via the kidneys in an inactive form. It is toxic to neonates because they have immature liver enzyme systems. Because of its toxicity, the use of chloramphenicol has been limited to topical eye preparations. It is sometimes used to treat typhoid fever and, since it penetrates readily into the CSF, can be used for the treatment of some forms of bacterial meningitis.

Fusidic acid

Fusidic acid is a bacteriostatic agent that inhibits protein synthesis by complexing with the growing peptide chain. It is active against Gram-positive cocci and is useful in the treatment of staphylococcal infections that are resistant to the ß-lactams, or in patients allergic to penicillin. Resistance to fusidic acid develops easily so it is usually given in combination with other drugs (e.g. erythromycin).

INHIBITORS OF NUCLEIC ACID SYNTHESIS

Antibacterials that interfere with nucleic acid synthesis can do so either by inhibiting the synthesis of the nucleotide precursors or by inhibiting DNA or RNA replication.

Sulphonamides

As mentioned above, the sulphonamides are a group of synthetic chemical compounds that were found to have antibacterial properties. The most commonly used

FIGURE 12.6
STRUCTURE OF CHLORAMPHENICOL

Chloramphenicol

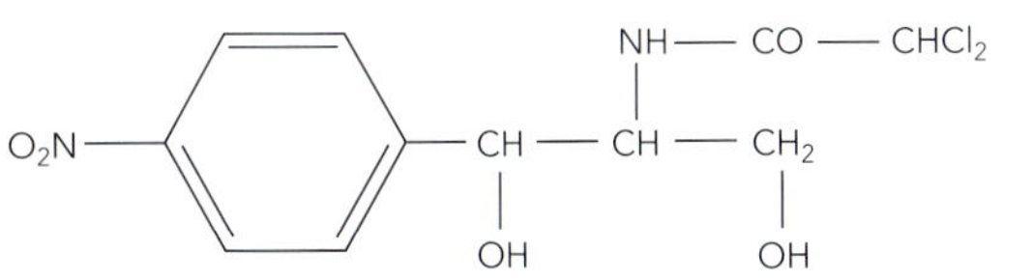

compounds are structural analogues of para-amino-benzoic acid (PABA). They exert their action by competing with PABA in the synthetic pathway of tetrahydrofolic acid (THFA), a substance that is a precursor of the purines and pyrimidines required for nucleic acid synthesis (see Figure 12.7). The basis for the selective toxicity of the sulphonamide drugs is the fact that most bacteria have a pathway of synthesis of THFA, whereas humans are unable to synthesise folic acid and so have a requirement for it in their diet. Drugs that interfere with its synthesis will therefore not affect human cells.

Sulphonamides are broad spectrum bacteriostatic agents active against both Gram-positive and Gram-negative organisms. They can be administered orally and have few toxic side effects, although skin rashes may occur. Because resistance develops readily, they are often used in combination with another drug. A commonly used preparation is **cotrimoxazole**, which combines sulphamethoxazole with trimethoprim. **Trimethoprim** is an analogue of the pyrimidine bases and competes for the enzyme dihydrofolate reductase, which converts dihydrofolic acid to tetrahydrofolic acid (see Figure 12.7). Although the enzyme is also present in human cells, the selective toxicity of the drug depends on the far greater affinity of trimethoprim for the bacterial enzyme than for the human enzyme.

The rationale for using a combination of the two agents, sulphamethoxazole and trimethoprim is based on:

1. the hope that bacterial mutants that are resistant to one drug are unlikely to be resistant to the other; and
2. the fact that, in some cases, the two agents act synergistically; that is, the combined effect is greater than that obtained by a single drug on its own.

Cotrimoxazole is sold in Australia as Bactrim® or Septrim®, and is widely used against a range of urinary tract pathogens, and against *Salmonella typhi*. It has been used successfully for the prevention and treatment of *Pneumocystis carinii* pneumonia in AIDS patients. Trimethoprim alone or in combination with sulphamethoxazole may cause nausea. Sulphonamides, particularly in the elderly, may cause exfoliative dermatitis and may (rarely) be the cause of a fatal bone marrow suppression.

FIGURE 12.7
MECHANISM OF INHIBITION BY SULPHA DRUGS
Sulphonamides and trimethoprim inhibit in series the steps in the synthesis of tetrahydrofolic acid by interacting with key enzymes in the pathway

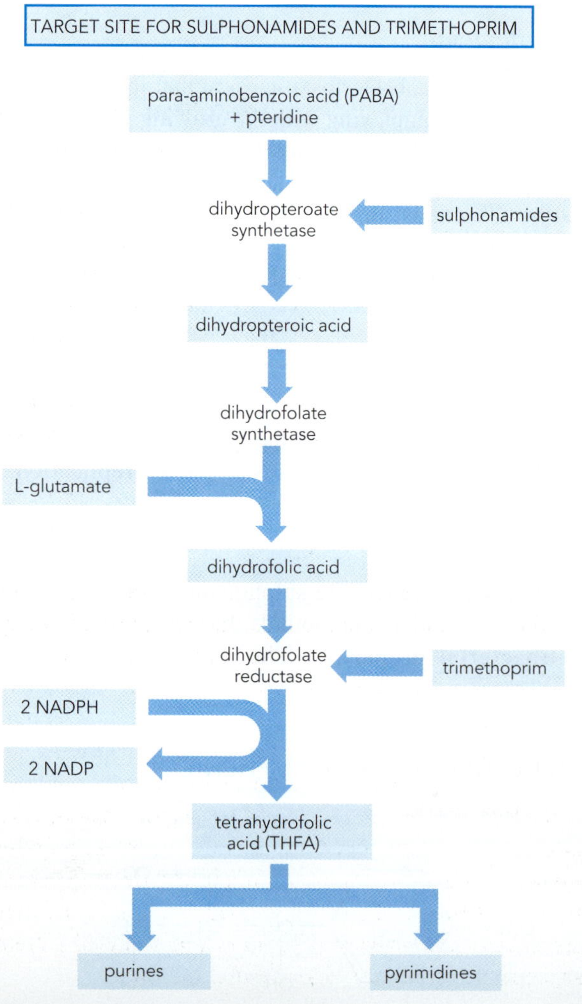

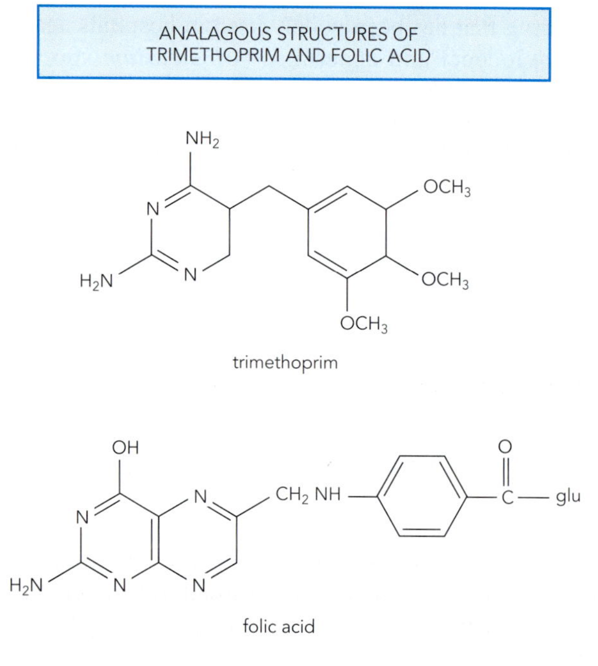

Quinolones

Quinolones are a group of synthetic chemical agents that inhibit the activity of the enzyme, DNA gyrase, which is responsible for the coiling of the bacterial chromosome. Their action is specific to the bacterial enzyme and so is selectively toxic. The earliest compound, **nalidixic acid**, was not very effective; it was not very active and did not reach adequate serum levels to treat systemic infections. The development of the fluoroquinolones has provided a group of compounds with good antibacterial activity. These drugs can be administered orally, they reach good serum concentrations and are well distributed in the body. **Norfloxacin** and **ciprofloxacin** are active against Gram-negative rods and are useful in the treatment of systemic Gram-negative infections and urinary tract infections.

Side effects include nausea, photosensitivity and neurological disturbances. Convulsions have been reported, especially in patients with a history of epilepsy or other predisposing factors to seizures. The absorption of the drug is diminished by concurrent antacid administration.

Rifamycins

Rifampicin is the most important member of the family of **rifamycins** and affects the cell by binding to the enzyme RNA polymerase and blocking the synthesis of mRNA. The basis of the selective toxicity is the greater affinity of the drug for the bacterial enzyme than for the human RNA polymerase. Rifampicin is important in the treatment of mycobacterial infections (e.g. tuberculosis), but is also active against other Gram-positive and Gram-negative organisms, especially staphylococci. It can be administered orally and reaches high concentrations in serum and saliva. It is metabolised in the liver and excreted in body secretions (tears, urine, saliva) which turn red due to the colour of the drug. The main problem with its use is that resistance develops rapidly unless other drugs are used in combination.

INHIBITORS OF CELL MEMBRANE FUNCTION

The cytoplasmic membrane is a selectively permeable barrier surrounding the cytoplasm of all cells. The **polymyxins** are cyclic polypeptides which act as cationic detergents and disrupt the phospholipid bilayer of the membrane. They are especially active against Gram-negative bacteria, such as *Pseudomonas aeruginosa*. They are not readily absorbed if administered orally and are toxic, causing nephrotoxicity and otoxicity. They are used *only* in topical preparations.

Antifungal Drugs

Many common fungal infections are caused by dermatophytes that attack cutaneous or mucocutaneous areas of the body. They include the various forms of tinea (e.g. ringworm, athlete's foot) and, in general, are only mild infections that can be treated by the application of topical antifungal preparations. In recent years, the number of opportunistic fungal infections occurring in immunocompromised patients has increased (see Chapter 6). These infections are potentially life-threatening and require the use of systemic antifungal drugs. Fungal cells are eucaryotic and it is difficult to identify points of selective toxicity. The main target is the synthesis or functioning of the fungal cell membrane which, unlike bacteria, contains sterols.

Imidazoles and **polyenes** are the main type of compounds used for this purpose.

Imidazoles

The **imidazole** group of antifungal drugs includes **clotrimazole**, **miconazole**, **ketoconazole** and **fluconazole**. They inhibit the enzymes involved in sterol biosynthesis, the basis of selective toxicity being the greater affinity of the drug for the fungal enzyme than for the human enzyme.

Polyenes

The **polyene antibiotics** which include **amphotericin B** and **nystatin**, act by combining with ergosterol, a major sterol component of the fungal cell membrane, thereby causing leakage of cell contents and cell death. Both compounds are quite toxic to humans, as they also bind, although less readily, to the cholesterol in human cell membranes.

TREATMENT OF FUNGAL INFECTIONS

Treatment of fungal infections is difficult because of the lack of solubility, toxicity and poor absorption of most of the available drugs. Cutaneous mycoses such as tinea and thrush are mainly treated with topical preparations containing miconazole, clotrimazole or nystatin. Although quite toxic, nystatin is poorly absorbed and so is useful for topical application. Some subcutaneous infections are very persistent and need to be treated with a systemic drug such as **griseofulvin**. This can be administered orally and appears to act specifically by binding to newly formed keratin present in cutaneous cells and inhibiting mitotic division.

Chronic mucocutaneous candidiasis is the most common fungal infection in immunosuppressed patients, followed by infections caused by the yeast *Cryptococcus neoformans*. Severe cryptococcal pneumonia and meningitis are common in AIDS patients. Systemic fungal infections are difficult to treat because of the toxicity of most antifungal drugs. Amphotericin B or ketoconazole are the main antifungal drugs used for systemic infections. Ketoconazole can be taken orally, but amphotericin B must be administered intravenously and is toxic, especially to the kidneys. The newer drug, **fluconazole**, can be taken orally, is better absorbed and is now being used against systemic yeast infections (*Candida* and *Cryptococcus*). Better antifungal drugs are needed, especially as there are increasing numbers of immunocompromised patients susceptible to opportunistic fungal infections.

Antiparasitic Drugs

As we saw in Chapter 6, there are many parasites that can infect the human body. The protozoa are single-celled organisms, some of which have complicated life cycles (e.g. malaria), and it is difficult to find drugs that are selectively toxic against them.

Metronidazole (Flagyl®) is a widely used drug that is active against intestinal protozoa and also against most obligate anaerobic bacteria. It is useful for the treatment of infections due to *Giardia*, *Entamoeba* and *Trichomonas*. There are some side effects associated with its use, such as nausea and alcohol intolerance. Another widely used antiprotozoal drug is tinidazole.

Malaria is caused by four species of the protozoan *Plasmodium*. Derivatives of quinine have been used for years to treat malaria, but quinine itself is now considered too toxic for general use. **Chloroquine** is the main drug used to treat clinical attacks of malaria, although its mechanism of action is unclear. Strains of *Plasmodium falciparum* resistant to chloroquine have developed in some areas and these can be treated with **mefloquine**, although some resistance to this drug has been reported recently. **Quinine** is very toxic and is used only if the infection is due to a resistant strain. **Primaquine** is used to eliminate *P. vivax* and *P. ovale* from the liver once the clinical attack is controlled in order to prevent relapses, which may occur for up to five years after the initial attack. Prophylactic chemotherapy for travellers to endemic areas usually involves the use of chloroquine or **doxycycline**. It is important that travellers to malarious areas consult the Health Department for advice on appropriate antimalarial prophylaxis.

Antihelminthic drugs are discussed in Chapter 6.

Antiviral Drugs

A large number of diseases which afflict humans are caused by viruses. However, because viruses replicate inside the host cell, few antiviral compounds have been found which can kill or inactivate viruses without being severely toxic to the host. Instead, research has focused with some success on the development of vaccines against serious viral diseases. The advent of the human immunodeficiency virus, HIV, which attacks the immune system itself and therefore makes the development of a vaccine particularly difficult, has encouraged the search for antiviral compounds.

For an antiviral drug to be selectively toxic, it must target some point in the cycle of viral replication. This could be, for example, the specific attachment site of the virus to the host cell, or the mechanism of viral uncoating and replication, or a specific viral enzyme synthesised under the direction of the viral genes and required for viral replication. In fact, a number of specific viral enzymes have been identified that can be induced to incorporate nucleotide analogues into the viral DNA, resulting in the production of inactive DNA molecules.

The most successful antiviral drugs are analogues of the purine and pyrimidine bases which are the building blocks of RNA and DNA. They are listed in Table 12.4. Of these, one of the most effective is **acyclovir** which is an analogue of the nucleoside guanosine. It is active against the herpes simplex virus (HSV) types I and II, and varicella zoster virus, VZV (shingles). HSV and VZV contain a virally encoded enzyme, **thymidine kinase**, which is able to phosphorylate acyclovir to the active monophosphate; this is then converted to acyclovir triphosphate and incorporated instead of thymine into the growing chains of viral DNA, where it prevents further elongation. Thymidine kinase is not present in human cells, which means that acyclovir is incorporated only into the DNA of virally infected cells, and so is relatively non-toxic even in high doses.

Acyclovir is used for primary herpes simplex (HSV) infections (oral, genital and conjunctival) as well as the prevention of recurrent genital HSV. It is used mainly in topical applications for HSV, but in severe cases can be taken orally. Its systemic use is usually limited to immunocompromised patients or for severe cases of *Varicella zoster* in adults. An important use is in suspected cases of herpes encephalitis.

Ganciclovir is also a nucleoside analogue of guanosine, but is active against cytomegalovirus as well as HSV and VZV. The mechanism of inhibition is similar to acyclovir, but the drug is more toxic so its use is limited to serious cases of CMV, such as CMV retinitis in AIDS patients. Neutropenia occurs in 25% of patients together with some degree of renal impairment.

Fanciclovir is the latest drug in this group to be released in Australia.

Foscarnet is a pyrophosphate nucleotide derivative that does not require phosphorylation by host or viral enzymes. It has been used as an alternative to ganciclovir

TABLE 12.4
ANTIVIRAL DRUGS

VIRUS	ANTIVIRAL DRUG
HSV Herpes simplex	Acyclovir, idoxuridine (topical)
VZV Varicella zoster	Acyclovir (topical)
CMV Cytomegalovirus	Ganciclovir
HIV AIDS	Zidovudine (AZT) Dideoxycytosine (DDC) Dideoxyinosine (DDI) 3TC
RSV Respiratory syncytial virus	Ribavarin
Influenza A	Amantadine
Hairy cell leukemia	Interferon
Chronic hepatitis B, C	Zidovudine, Interferon

for CMV infections as well as for herpes and varicella zoster.

Amantadine was one of the first antiviral drugs to be used. It is a cyclic amine that is active against influenza A but not influenza B. Its mechanism of action probably involves inhibition of viral uncoating and possibly of other steps in viral synthesis. During influenza epidemics, it can be administered to susceptible people who have not been vaccinated, thus reducing the risk of illness. When used to treat influenza it is most effective if given within the first 48 hours. However, the development of drug resistance is common which means that the resistant virus is then shed by the patient, leading to the spread of drug-resistant strains. It is no longer widely used.

ANTIRETROVIRAL DRUGS

Retroviruses are a particular group of viruses responsible for a number of serious diseases including adult T cell leukaemia and AIDS. They have also been linked to the development of cancers in various animal species. In the search for suitable drugs to treat infections caused by these viruses, scientists have been able to make use of the viruses' unique method of replication (see Chapter 5).

Retroviruses contain RNA and the first step in the replicative process involves the synthesis of DNA from the RNA genome. The DNA 'provirus' is then inserted into the host cell DNA and subsequently directs the synthesis of new viral RNA and protein. The synthesis of DNA is carried out by a specific viral enzyme, an RNA-dependent DNA polymerase called **reverse transcriptase**. This reverse process, which does not occur in human cells, provides a target for antiviral drugs. Various analogues of the nucleosides that are used to synthesise DNA have been tested for their ability to bind to the enzyme, reverse transcriptase. Of these, zidovudine (AZT), an analogue of thymine, was the first to be licensed for the treatment of HIV infection. Although the drug has a high affinity for viral reverse transcriptase, it is also incorporated to some extent into host cell DNA by human DNA polymerase. This leads to occasional depression of bone marrow function and may cause inhibition of mitochondrial DNA synthesis, leading to myopathy. Unpleasant side effects of treatment include nausea, myalgia and headaches.

Other analogues that have been tested include DDI (dideoxyinosine) and DDC (dideoxycytosine). All the analogues block the transcription of viral RNA into DNA by combining with and inhibiting the enzyme, reverse transcriptase, leading to termination of the synthesis of the DNA chain. However, the action of these drugs is virustatic—that is, when the drug is removed viral replication can resume. Various concentrations and combinations of the drugs are still being tested. Investigations are also being carried out to determine the optimum time for administration and the length of treatment in order to maximise the beneficial effects and reduce side effects and development of resistance. Research is continuing for other antiretroviral agents that could kill or inhibit at any of the other steps in the infective and replicative process shown in Figure 12.8.

INTERFERONS

Interferons are a family of small glycoprotein molecules produced by many kinds of mammalian cells (especially lymphocytes, fibroblasts and macrophages), in response to viral infection. The interferons are cell or species specific, not virus specific, and are involved in cell growth and the regulation of immune reactions. Three different classes have been identified—alpha(α), beta(ß) and gamma(γ). Gamma(γ)-interferon is a lymphokine produced by activated T cells in response to viral infection; α- and ß-interferons are produced by many cell types. Virus-infected cells produce interferons that diffuse to neighbouring uninfected cells, where they induce the

FIGURE 12.8
TARGETS OF ANTIVIRAL AGENTS IN THE HUMAN IMMUNODEFICIENCY VIRUS LIFE CYCLE

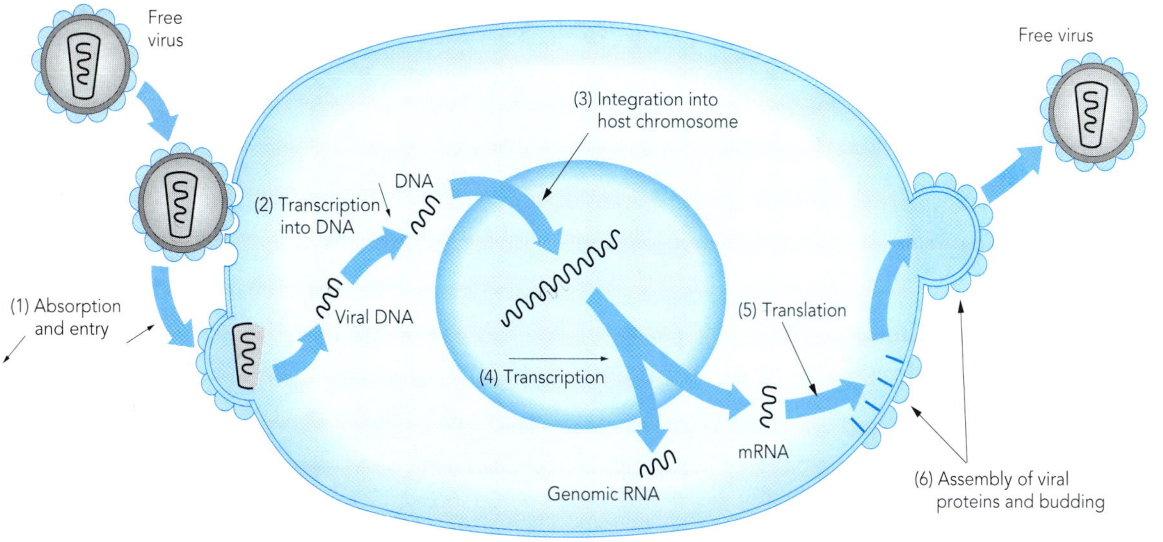

production of enzymes that interfere with further viral replication.

Interferons are species specific, that is, they work only in the species in which they are produced, but they have now been produced commercially by genetic engineering. Alpha-interferon (IFN-α) is being used in the treatment of chronic hepatitis B and C. Studies of results of interferon treatment of chronic hepatitis C patients showed that after an initial response rate of 50%, half the patients relapsed, so the overall response to treatment was 25%. Careful selection of patients for therapy—that is, patients without contributing conditions (e.g. cirrhosis)—may improve the response rate. More clinical trials are required to assess the usefulness of interferon therapy for chronic viral infections. Side effects of the therapy include fever, malaise, headache and myalgia; bone marrow depression may also occur.

PROBLEMS OF ANTIVIRAL THERAPY

The major obstacle to finding effective antiviral drugs is one of selective toxicity. Because viruses replicate inside the host cell, using the host cell machinery, any drug that inhibits the reactions involved in viral replication is also likely to affect similar reactions in uninfected host cells. The available antiviral drugs are **virustatic**; they inhibit viral replication (and relieve the disease symptoms) but they do not eliminate the virus from the body. This is of particular importance in immunosuppressed individuals whose immune system is not able to eliminate the virus. Latent (non-replicating) virus is not affected, so any reservoir of viruses in the body is preserved and can be reactivated later. Genetic mutations are a frequent occurrence during viral replication, giving rise to altered viral proteins with different antigenic properties, so antibodies formed in response to the initial infection may not inactivate the virus. Mutation may also produce enzymes with altered substrate specificity so that the antiviral drugs are no longer effective—that is, the virus becomes resistant.

Antimicrobial Sensitivity Tests

In the previous sections we have described the major chemical compounds that can be used to kill or inhibit the growth of the various types of microorganisms. The choice of the best antimicrobial to use for the treatment of a particular infection is dictated by whether the particular strain of the organism is sensitive to the antimicrobial to be used. For example, although penicillin is effective against actively growing cells of many Gram-positive bacteria, a number of strains of these bacteria have developed mechanisms to resist its action (e.g. ß-lactamase enzymes). To select the most effective antimicrobial drug, it is necessary to test the actual strain of the organism which is causing the infection against a range of possible antimicrobial agents.

There are two main methods for carrying out sensitivity tests in the laboratory; disk diffusion tests, and the minimum inhibitory concentration (MIC) test. In both methods, an appropriate specimen is obtained from the patient and plated out on a suitable medium to obtain single colonies (see Chapter 15). Cells from the colonies are suspended in nutrient medium and tested for susceptibility to a range of antimicrobials. The site of the infection, together with the provisional diagnosis, determines which antimicrobials are tested first. The choice is also based on the susceptibility pattern of the isolates usually encountered in the laboratory, especially for hospital-acquired infections.

DISK DIFFUSION TEST

A lawn of the isolated bacteria is spread on an agar plate and disks impregnated with defined amounts of the drug to be tested are placed on the plate. The drug diffuses into the agar and inhibits the growth of sensitive organisms in a zone around the disk. The **zone of inhibition**, or clear area (in mm) around the disk, represents the sensitivity of the organism to the drug being tested (see Figure 12.9). The amount of drug in the disk is related to the achievable serum concentration of the drug and so is different for each drug tested. In addition, the diameter of the zone of inhibition is related to the ease of diffusion (solubility) of the drug in the agar and so is also different for each drug. This is merely a qualitative method. If no clear zone is apparent, the organism is considered to be resistant to the drug.

MINIMUM INHIBITORY CONCENTRATION TEST

The **minimum inhibitory concentration** (MIC) test is a semi-quantitative procedure which measures the concentration of an antimicrobial that is required to inhibit the growth of a standardised inoculum. This is done in

FIGURE 12.9
DISK DIFFUSION TEST
The diameter of the clear zone around each disk represents the sensitivity of the test organism to the antibacterial drug in the disk. If there is no clearing, the organism is considered resistant to the drugs at that concentration.

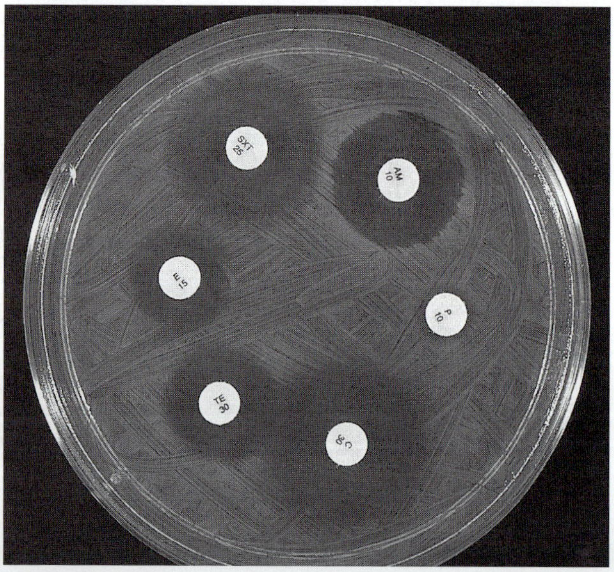

a series of tubes, each containing different concentrations of drug, but with a standardised number of organisms. The method measures the lowest drug concentration (MIC) that will inhibit visible growth. It is a laborious method and is only done in special circumstances where treatment is difficult.

A variation on this method that is useful for busy routine diagnostic laboratories involves the use of **replica plating**. In this, a series of agar plates is prepared, each containing a different concentration of the drug to be tested dissolved in the agar. Cells from the test culture are replica-plated onto each of the plates and the level of growth observed. This method is useful when large numbers of isolates need to be tested.

Results of antimicrobial sensitivity testing can vary from one laboratory to another unless standardised cultures are used as controls.

Therapeutic Use of Antimicrobial Drugs

The availability of compounds that can kill or inhibit the growth of microorganisms has enabled the successful treatment of many diseases that were once likely to be fatal. This is particularly true of bacterial infections. However, many common diseases are caused by viruses and the number of effective antiviral drugs is still very limited. Viruses are responsible for many respiratory tract infections, including the common cold, influenza, RSV, viral pneumonia and viral gastroenteritis. These infections do not respond to treatment with antibacterial drugs, and the unnecessary use of such drugs for illnesses that are primarily viral in nature is one of the contributing factors to the widespread development of resistance to antibacterials.

When an antibacterial drug is used, it may kill or inhibit normal flora as well as any pathogens present. In any bacterial population, a few mutant cells resistant to the drug are likely to arise and they will flourish in an environment where other cells that compete for nutrients have been destroyed. If this happens, the patient may acquire a population of resistant bacteria, even though the original infection was due to a virus. The use of antibacterials is indicated only when secondary bacterial infections such as otitis media or 'strep throat' occur, following invasion of the upper respiratory tract by viruses.

LIMITATIONS OF ANTIMICROBIAL THERAPY

All drugs have some adverse side effects and the nature of the side effects must be weighed against the benefits available from their use. The principle of selective toxicity has already been discussed. Most antimicrobials have some adverse effects on the host and these have been mentioned in the sections dealing with each drug. The most important effects are listed in Table 12.5. The main problems associated with the use of antimicrobials are:

- The suppression or elimination of normal flora, leading to an overgrowth of opportunists such as *Candida albicans* or *Clostridium difficile*.
- The occurrence of adverse side effects such as hypersensitivity, ototoxicity, nephrotoxicity and bone marrow suppression.
- The emergence of strains of pathogens that are resistant to currently available antimicrobial drugs.

TABLE 12.5
SOME ADVERSE EFFECTS OF ANTIMICROBIAL THERAPY

DRUG	ADVERSE EFFECT
Antibacterials	
■ Penicillin (and other ß-lactams)	Hypersensitivity occurs in some people. Occasionally fatal.
■ Aminoglycosides	Ototoxicity (deafness) and nephrotoxicity (renal impairment).
■ Vancomycin	Ototoxicity, nephrotoxicity. Local inflammation—phlebitis. Must be given by slow infusion to avoid histamine release.
■ Quinolones	Nausea, photosensitivity, neurological disturbances.
■ Chloramphenicol	Bone marrow depression—aplastic anaemia.
■ Sulphonamides	Hypersensitivity, skin rashes, agranulocytosis.
■ Tetracyclines	Combine with calcium in developing bones and teeth, causes permanent discoloration of teeth.
Antivirals	
■ Zidovudine	Bone marrow depression, anaemia, nausea, headaches, skin rashes.
Antifungals	
■ Amphotericin	Nephrotoxic.

TREATMENT OF BACTERIAL INFECTIONS

Previous sections have dealt with the various classes of antibacterial drugs that are available for the treatment of infections. The selection is wide and several factors need to be considered before a particular drug is prescribed. The approach taken by the medical practitioner to the treatment of infection may vary, depending on whether the patient is in the community or is hospitalised. The time and cost involved in carrying out a definitive microbiological identification is usually not warranted for most patients in the community. In hospital, patients are often sicker, they may have contributing illnesses, and there is also a greater likelihood of their being infected with resistant organisms. It is therefore usual to collect a specimen, send it to the laboratory for analysis, and start empirical therapy while waiting for the results.

In an ideal situation it would be preferable to delay treatment until sensitivity tests had been carried out but, in practice, by the time patients show obvious signs of infection, they require treatment as soon as possible. Waiting 2 days for definitive laboratory tests to be carried out before prescribing treatment may well jeopardise the health (or life) of the patient. An infection that has just become established can develop into fulminating sepsis in two days.

Usually, the medical practitioner makes a provisional diagnosis, prescribes medication based on the 'best guess' principle and then reviews the prescription when the results of the pathology tests are available. It is important that clinical specimens are collected from the patients *before* any drug therapy is commenced; otherwise, the drug may affect the microorganisms present and incorrect or inconclusive results may be obtained. An appropriate clinical sample of blood, sputum, pus, urine, faeces, CSF or tissue is usually collected. It should be adequate in amount, collected in an aseptic manner, correctly labelled and transported to the laboratory as soon as possible. (See Chapter 15 for methods of specimen collection.)

In deciding which drug to prescribe while awaiting results, the doctor takes into account such factors as:

- the site of the body where the infection is located. This will often indicate the type of organism most likely to be present and the most effective drug to be used.
- whether the infection was acquired in the hospital or community. Many hospital organisms are resistant to antibiotics and the hospital will have developed a prescribing policy to minimise this problem. This often involves the use of two or more antibiotics at the same time.
- the age of the patient. Some drugs are more toxic for children. Some infections are more serious in children and require immediate effective therapy (e.g. meningitis caused by *Haemophilus influenzae* type b).
- other contributing factors such as the immune status of the patient, renal impairment, liver function, etc.

Once the causative organism has been identified, the empirical therapy that was begun can be modified if necessary. Sometimes, the appropriate drug can be selected on the basis of clinical experience. However, it is more usual with hospital-acquired infections to carry out an antimicrobial sensitivity test to determine the sensitivity of the pathogen to the range of antimicrobial agents available. It is essential to carry out sensitivity testing when:

- the organism is of a type that is frequently resistant to drug therapy (e.g. hospital-acquired Gram-negative rods);
- the infection is life-threatening (e.g. meningitis, septicaemia);
- bacteriocidal drugs are preferred (e.g. for immunocompromised patients or in infective endocarditis).

When the doctor has the results of the laboratory tests, there are still a number of factors to be taken into account in order to select the most appropriate therapeutic agent.

1. Absorption—the drug must be able to reach the part of the body where the infection is located. Thus, if the drug is to be given orally, it must be unchanged by gastric acid, be absorbed from the intestine and be able to be transported in the bloodstream to the site of infection. Some drugs must be given parenterally because of their poor absorption from the intestine and so are only suitable for use in hospital.
2. The drug must be able to reach the target tissue. For example, if the infection is in the meninges, a drug must be selected that can cross the blood-brain barrier (although this is sometimes easier when the meninges are inflamed). The drug used to treat a urinary tract infection must be excreted in an active form via the kidneys and must be able to reach a high enough concentration in the urine to kill the microorganisms present in the bladder.
3. Some drugs are not suitable for young children or women during pregnancy and lactation. For example, tetracycline has been shown to bind to calcium and deposit in developing teeth, causing permanent brown staining. It may also interfere with bone development in the foetus.

Other medical conditions that may need to be taken into account include the status of the immune system and the integrity of organ function in the patient. For example, immunocompromised patients should be prescribed bacteriocidal drugs whenever possible, as their immune system is not able to eliminate the microorganisms left after treatment with a bacteriostatic drug. Infective endocarditis must be treated with a bacteriocidal drug, as macrophages are unable to penetrate to the site of the infection to destroy residual bacteria.

Metabolism and elimination of drugs depends on hepatic and renal function. Patients with some degree of renal impairment are not able to excrete drugs effectively via the kidneys. This means that high concentrations of the drug may develop in the bloodstream and thus the prescribed dose needs to be lower. Drugs that affect the kidneys (e.g. the aminoglycosides) are not usually prescribed for patients who already have impaired renal function.

Other factors usually taken into account when selecting the most suitable drug are the likelihood of development of resistance, the risk of interactions between the drug and any other medication being taken by the patient, and the cost of the drug. 'Antibiotic Guidelines' which is published annually by the Victorian Medical Postgraduate Foundation Inc. lists the organisms most commonly found to be responsible for infections in different areas of the body, together with a list of the antimicrobials which are generally recommended for use in Australia.

There is a separate section in the book dealing with recommendations for antibiotic usage in the Northern Territory, where the incidence of infectious diseases, kinds of organisms and levels of resistance to antimicrobials are significantly different from the rest of Australia (see Chapter 14).

Pharmokinetics

The prescribed dosage must be such that an effective concentration of the drug is achieved at the site of infection. Ideally, the antimicrobial agent should be maintained at a reasonably constant concentration in the blood or tissues. The rate of elimination of the drug from the body can be described in terms of **half-life**, that is, the time required for the concentration of the drug in the bloodstream to fall to half its maximum level. The number of times the drug needs to be administered each day will depend on the rate at which the drug is broken down or eliminated from the body (Figure 12.10).

It is also necessary to take into account the therapeutic index of the drug. The **therapeutic index** is the ratio of the effective concentration of the drug required to kill the pathogen to the concentration that would be a lethal dose for the host. The greater the difference between the two figures, the more selectively toxic the drug will be and the less risk there will be of toxic side effects.

Combined therapy

In the hospital it is common for two drugs to be prescribed simultaneously—for the treatment of seriously ill patients; when the cause of the infection is uncertain; or when delay while awaiting the results of conclusive sensitivity tests may be to the detriment of the patient. One advantage of using more than one drug is the efficient treatment of mixed infections following massive trauma. The emergence of resistance can theoretically be significantly retarded by the use of two drugs with different mechanisms of action.

Sometimes, the action of an antimicrobial is potentiated (enhanced) in the presence of another drug or antimicrobial. **Synergism** is the term used to describe the enhancement of one drug in the presence of another. For example, penicillin may be prescribed as well as an aminoglycoside. Penicillin damages the cell wall, allowing better penetration of the aminoglycoside. In systemic fungal infections such as candidiasis or cryptococcosis, amphotericin is used to weaken the cell membrane, allowing uptake of flucytosine. Some infections respond better to the use of two or more drugs. Enterococcal endocarditis responds to a combination of penicillin, or ampicillin, plus gentamicin, vancomycin or streptomycin. Tuberculosis is routinely treated with isoniazid and rifampicin in order to inhibit the development of resistant strains.

Some commercial preparations contain two drugs; for example, cotrimoxazole (Bactrim®, Septrin®) contains sulphamethoxazole and trimethoprim, two drugs which sequentially block the pathway of folate synthesis. Augmentin® contains amoxycillin plus the ß-lactamase inhibitor, clavulanic acid, which prevents inactivation of the amoxycillin.

However, there are some disadvantages to the use of combined therapy. There may be **antagonism** when a reaction occurs between the drugs being used, or when one drug interferes with the action of the other. If bacteriostatic and bacteriocidal drugs are administered simultaneously, the action of both may be affected. For example, tetracycline is bacteriostatic, inhibiting protein synthesis and cell replication. Penicillin is bacteriocidal and is mainly active against dividing cells. If they are used in combination, the tetracycline inhibits cell division

FIGURE 12.10
COMPARISON OF PLASMA DRUG CONCENTRATIONS AFTER DIFFERENT METHODS OF ADMINISTRATION

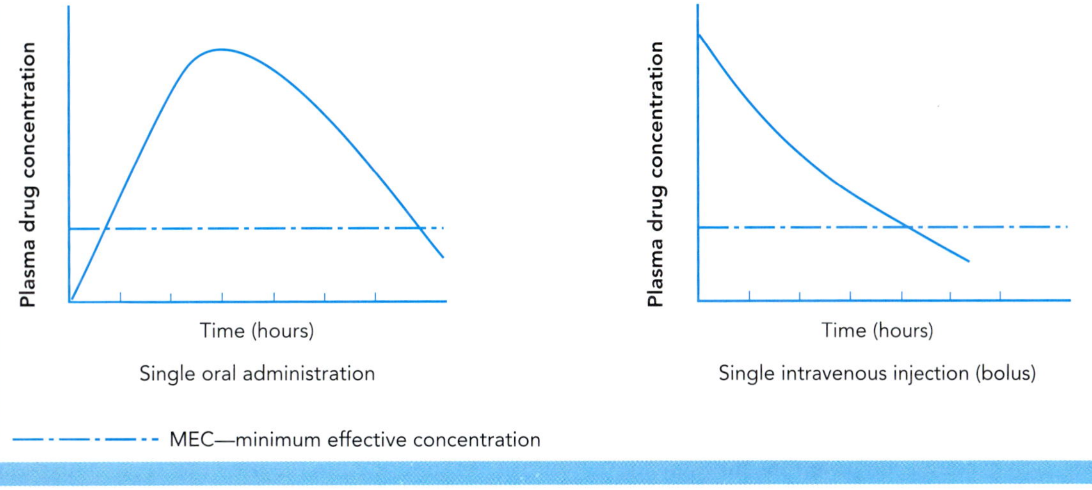

and so the bacteriocidal action of the penicillin is considerably diminished. Some antimicrobials affect the efficacy of other kinds of drugs. Rifampicin stimulates the metabolism (and therefore removal from the body) of oral contraceptives, anticoagulants and corticosteroids.

PROPHYLAXIS

Prophylaxis involves the administration of an antimicrobial drug before there is any evidence of infection, under conditions where the risks of an infection developing are considered to be very high. The risk of a patient acquiring an infection has to be weighed against factors such as toxicity of the drug, the cost, and the risk of superinfection (i.e. an overgrowth by opportunistic pathogens).

Prophylaxis may be considered necessary for some surgical procedures, especially where prosthetic devices are involved. In general, prophylaxis is not so essential if the patient is immunocompetent. However, it is often advisable for patients who are susceptible to infection for other reasons. For example, patients who suffer from rheumatic heart disease involving damage to the heart valves are usually prescribed penicillin following dental surgery. This is to reduce the risk of infection by *Streptococcus viridans* which may enter the bloodstream and infect the damaged valves, causing endocarditis.

Development of Resistance to Antimicrobial Drugs

Although the 20th century has seen the development of drugs able to kill or inhibit many pathogens, one of the major problems confronting medical practice today is the number of microorganisms that are resistant to antimicrobial therapy. Some microorganisms, such as *Pseudomonas*, are naturally less susceptible to many antimicrobial drugs, mainly because of their cellular characteristics, such as an impermeable outer layer. This is regarded as a natural resistance. Of more concern, however, is the fact that, since antimicrobial drugs have been used therapeutically, an increasing number of microorganisms have acquired resistance to the drugs that were previously used effectively against them. Worldwide, there has been the development of multiple drug-resistant strains of organisms such as *Mycobacterium tuberculosis, Neisseria gonorrhoea, Staphylococcus aureus, Streptococcus pneumoniae* and *Enterococcus* species.

Bacteria may exhibit resistance in several ways.

1. By the production of enzymes that are able to destroy or inactivate the drug. For example, the ß-lactamase enzyme produced by many Gram-positive organisms breaks open the ß-lactam ring in the penicillin or cephalosporin molecule, destroying its structure and preventing the drug from binding to its target, which is the enzyme involved in the synthesis of the peptidoglycan molecule.
2. By a change in membrane permeability that results in the drug being unable to penetrate through the membrane into the cell. This may be due to a change in structural protein, a decrease in pore size, or an alteration in the transport system. Alternatively, the rate of efflux of the drug from the cell may be increased so that the drug is not able to attain a sufficiently high concentration inside the cell to cause inhibition. This is the basis of resistance to drugs such as the tetracyclines, which inhibit protein synthesis on the ribosomes inside the cell.
3. By an alteration in the binding sites for the drug in the bacterial cell. Many drugs bind to a specific site in the cell and exert their effect by interfering with enzyme activity or protein synthesis. If the structure of the binding site is altered, the drug no longer fits and so is unable to have any effect on the cell. Aminoglycosides and erythromycin bind to specific sites on the bacterial ribosome and inhibit protein synthesis. An alteration in the structure of the binding sites prevents their action and the cell becomes resistant. Some penicillin-resistant Gram-positive bacteria have altered penicillin-binding proteins, so that penicillin can no longer bind and exert its effect.
4. Some drugs, such as the sulphonamides, exert their effect by inhibiting reactions in essential metabolic pathways. One way in which bacteria develop resistance to these drugs is by the production of other enzymes that have no affinity for the drug and can synthesise the required compounds via an alternate pathway.

The development of these resistance mechanisms involves a change in the genetic properties of the cell. This can occur as the result of a spontaneous mutation. If the cell population is then exposed to an antimicrobial drug, it exerts a selective pressure, killing sensitive organisms and allowing the resistant mutants to multiply. This occurs mostly after a prolonged course of antimicrobial therapy. However, it can also occur when a patient does not complete the full course of a prescribed drug. Resistant mutants will also be selected under these conditions, although the level of drug resistance (i.e the concentration of drug required to kill the cells) may not be quite as high. Without the selective pressure applied by the use of antimicrobial drugs, the population of cells would essentially remain sensitive. The overuse or misuse of antimicrobial drugs can therefore contribute to the development of resistant strains of microorganisms.

Another mechanism whereby the cell can alter its genetic characteristics involves the transfer of resistance genes from resistant to susceptible strains of closely related genera. This is mostly mediated by plasmids during conjugation (see below, and Chapter 4). The extensive use of antimicrobials in animal feed probably contributes to an increase in the numbers of resistant organisms that can be transmitted to humans.

DRUG RESISTANCE IN HOSPITALS

The high usage level of antimicrobial drugs in hospitals provides an atmosphere in which resistant organisms can flourish. As described in the previous section, exposure to antimicrobials creates an environment in which the resistant mutants that arise spontaneously are able to survive and multiply in the presence of the drug. Another phenomenon is the development of cross-resistance, where an organism that has developed a mechanism of resistance to one drug will also be resistant to related drugs. For example, an organism that produces a ß-lactamase enzyme may be resistant to both penicillin and cephalosporin, even though it may have been exposed to only one of the drugs. The enzyme inactivates the drug in both cases by destroying the ß-lactam ring.

The initial appearance of resistance in susceptible bacteria is usually due to a mutation in only one gene. However, the frequency of resistance can be increased if the bacteria acquire additional resistant genes or R-factors from other bacteria. It is now recognised that an important method of spread of resistance is the conjugative transfer of resistance factors on plasmids, not only within species but also between closely related genera (see Chapter 4). Thus, if a patient who is carrying a multi-resistant strain of *E. coli* acquires a sensitive strain of, say, *Shigella,* the resistance genes may be transferred from the related genus, *E. coli,* in the intestine to the *Shigella.* The patient then harbours and excretes a strain of multi-resistant *Shigella* as well as multi-resistant *E. coli*, even though the original *Shigella* has not been exposed to any antimicrobial drugs.

The increase in resistance, especially in hospital isolates of Gram-negative bacteria, is thought to be largely due to the transfer of resistance factors in this manner.

Various strategies are being devised to improve treatment, to control the spread of infections and to limit procedures that may increase the rate of development of antimicrobial resistance. These include:

- hospital policies for prescribing antimicrobials;
- the use of narrow spectrum antimicrobials whenever possible;
- improved surveillance to determine prevalence;
- infection control procedures to prevent hospital-acquired infections;
- the search for vaccines against bacterial infections; for example, the recent successful vaccine against *Haemophilus influenzae* type b (Hib).

Implications for Nursing Practice

Although the microbiologist identifies the organism causing an infection and the doctor prescribes the appropriate antimicrobial, it is usually the nursing staff who are responsible for administering and monitoring the treatment. There are several ways in which good nursing practice can ensure a good outcome for the patient.

SPECIMEN COLLECTION

This is described in detail in Chapter 15. In general, the nurse is responsible for the collection of an appropriate specimen in a sterile container, using aseptic techniques. It should be carefully labelled and transported to the laboratory as soon as possible. Information such as provisional diagnosis, type of sample, site of infection (or sample site), date and time of collection should be included on the request form, together with any other information that might assist the microbiologist. The specimen should be collected *before* any antimicrobial therapy is commenced.

INTERPRETATION OF REPORTS

Nurses need to be familiar with the terms used in microbiology and be able to interpret the reports. Frequently, results are telephoned from the laboratory and the nurse must be able to record results accurately. The nurse is in a position to check that the treatment the patient is receiving is in accord with the diagnostic results.

ADMINISTRATION OF ANTIMICROBIAL THERAPY

This is usually carried out by the nursing staff and, as for any drug, it is important that they are aware of the correct procedures. Before administering any drug, the nurse should take a patient history of any allergies (especially to penicillin). The manufacturer's directions accompanying the antimicrobial drug should be read carefully to ensure that the administration of the drug is by the correct route, at the correct time and that any special precautions are followed. The nurse should check the package for information such as:

- expiry date
- method of reconstitution
- storage condition
- contraindications for use
- method of administration—oral or parenteral.

Oral administration

Ideally, the drug should be maintained at a constant level in the blood or tissues throughout the 24-hour period. For this reason, oral doses are generally given at regular intervals throughout the day, depending on the excretion rate of the drug. Sometimes, this needs to be monitored by taking blood samples to measure the drug level. It is important to note the time the sample is taken after administration of the drug. Other factors may need to be taken into account. The rate of absorption of the drug may be affected by the type of tablet or capsule, the particle size of the drug powder, and the presence or absence of food in the intestine. Some drugs, such as tetracycline, bind to antacids or the calcium in milk, and are then poorly absorbed. Side effects such as nausea can be minimised by the administration of the drug with food. The instructions for administration either before, or with food, are therefore important. Sometimes, other adverse reactions can occur; for example, metronidazole produces alcohol intolerance.

Patients should be educated about the correct way of taking their medication, the need to take it at regular intervals, and the importance of finishing the prescribed course of the antimicrobial so that the drug level is maintained for a sufficient time to eliminate all organisms. It is desirable to explain that the relief or disappearance of clinical symptoms does not mean that all the pathogens have been eliminated from the body and that the full course of the drug should be taken in order to prevent a recurrence of the disease.

Parenteral administration

The correct procedure should be ascertained (intravenous or intramuscular), and calculations for reconstitution and administration checked by another member of staff. Mostly, the drugs are given by slow IV infusion over a period of time. This is important in the case of a number of drugs where a bolus (single injection) can cause histamine release, vasodilation (flushing) and may even lead to cardiac arrest (Case History 12.1).

Monitoring the outcome

After parenteral administration of antimicrobials (especially penicillin) patients should be closely monitored for any adverse reactions, such as local inflammation or difficulty in breathing. Hypersensitivity reactions causing anaphylaxis can occur in patients who are allergic to penicillin and may require the use of resuscitation equipment and injection of adrenaline (see Spotlight box, p. 249).

As with all drugs, the effect of the antimicrobial therapy should be monitored over a period of time and the patient observed for signs of improvement or any side effects (e.g. rashes, ringing in the ears). Suppression of the normal flora may cause an overgrowth of opportunistic organisms such as *Candida albicans*, causing thrush, or *Clostridium difficile*, causing diarrhoea. Some drugs may build up to toxic levels if renal function is impaired, so in these patients blood levels need to be monitored. Careful taking of patient history is important, as factors such as age, weight and hepatic and renal functions affect the action of the drug.

CASE HISTORY 12.1
DRUG ADMINISTRATION

A patient in a Sydney hospital suffered a cardiac arrest and died after receiving a 'bolus' injection of vancomycin to treat an infection by *Staphylococcus aureus*.

A number of common antimicrobials can cause serious, even fatal reactions if they are administered by the wrong method. The administration of a bolus injection can cause reactions such as phlebitis (inflammation), histamine release and even cardiac arrest. The drugs that have been shown to have this effect are vancomycin, quinine, lincosamide and macrolides such as erythromycin.

These drugs must be given by slow intravenous infusion, usually over 30 minutes or longer, to avoid local high concentrations. Because phlebitis is also a problem, they are usually given via a centrally placed line.

Nursing management
Most antimicrobial therapy is administered by nursing staff. It is therefore essential that they read carefully all the literature provided by the manufacturer and follow instructions for the correct usage of the drugs. Hospital microbiologists and pharmacists also provide advice on correct procedures.

Summary

- The idea of finding a chemical to kill the specific microbe responsible for an infection, without damaging the host cells (i.e. a 'magic bullet') was proposed by the chemist Paul Ehrlich in 1908.

THE DEVELOPMENT OF ANTIMICROBIAL CHEMOTHERAPY

- Selective toxicity refers to the ability of a drug to kill or inhibit the microorganism responsible for the disease without damaging the host cells.
- The first successful antimicrobials were the chemically synthesised sulphonamides or sulpha drugs.
- An antibiotic is a chemical, produced by a microorganism, that in small amounts can kill or inhibit another microorganism. Some antibiotics are chemically modified to improve their antimicrobial properties and are called 'semi-synthetic'.
- Antimicrobials are compounds that can kill or inhibit the growth of a microorganism. They include antibacterial, antifungal, antiprotozoal and antiviral drugs.
- Compounds that are active against several different types of microorganisms are broad spectrum drugs; those with a limited range of activity are narrow spectrum drugs.
- Drugs that kill microorganisms have names ending in *-cidal*, while those that inhibit replication end in *-static*.

ANTIBACTERIAL DRUGS

- The main target sites for antibacterial action are the synthesis of the bacterial cell wall, protein synthesis, nucleic acid synthesis and the function of the bacterial cell membrane.
- Peptidoglycan is a compound unique to the bacterial cell wall and therefore provides an ideal target for selective toxicity.
- The ß-lactam antibacterials inhibit cell wall synthesis by combining with the enzyme responsible for cross-linking of the peptidoglycan chains. They include the penicillins, cephalosporins, carbapenems and monobactams.
- Other cell wall inhibitors include the glycopeptides, vancomycin and teicoplan, which interfere with cell wall synthesis by binding to the growing peptide chains of the peptidoglycan molecule.
- Compounds that inhibit the synthesis of protein include the aminoglycosides, the tetracyclines and the macrolides, as well as chloramphenicol, clindamycin and fusidic acid.
- Antimicrobials may inhibit the synthesis of nucleotide precursors, or DNA or RNA replication. They include the sulphonamides, quinolones and rifampicin.
- Polymyxins are cyclic polypeptides which act as cationic detergents and disrupt the phospholipid bilayer of the membrane.

ANTIFUNGAL DRUGS

- The main target of antifungal drugs is the synthesis or function of the fungal cell membrane. They include the imidazoles, which inhibit the enzymes involved in sterol biosynthesis, and the polyene antibiotics, amphotericin B and nystatin.
- Cutaneous mycoses such as tinea and thrush are treated mainly with topical preparations containing miconazole, clotrimazole or nystatin.
- Increasing numbers of immunocompromised patients are susceptible to opportunistic fungal infections.

ANTIPARASITIC DRUGS

- Metronidazole (Flagyl®) is a widely used drug that is active against protozoa.
- Various quinine derivatives are used for the treatment of malaria.
- Prophylactic malaria chemotherapy involves the use of chloroquine or doxycycline.

ANTIVIRAL DRUGS

- For an antiviral drug to be selectively toxic, it must target a unique point in the cycle of viral replication.
- The most successful antiviral drugs are chemically synthesised analogues of the purine and pyrimidine bases.
- Antiretroviral drugs target a specific viral enzyme, called reverse transcriptase.
- The action of these drugs is virustatic (i.e. when the drug is removed, viral replication can resume).
- Interferons are a family of small glycoprotein molecules produced by many kinds of mammalian cells in response to viral infection.

ANTIMICROBIAL SENSITIVITY TESTS

- To be sure of selecting an effective antimicrobial, it is necessary to test the actual strain of the organism causing the infection against a range of possible antimicrobial agents. Two methods are disk diffusion tests, and the minimum inhibitory concentration (MIC) test.

THERAPEUTIC USE OF ANTIMICROBIAL DRUGS

- The use of antimicrobial drugs can lead to suppression of the normal flora, the occurrence of various adverse side effects and the emergence of resistant strains of pathogens.
- Usually, doctors prescribe on the 'best guess' principle and then review the prescription if and when the results of the pathology tests are available.
- The prescribed dosage must be such that an effective concentration of the drug is achieved at the site of infection.
- Two drugs may be prescribed at once to treat mixed infections, or to minimise the risk of resistance.

- Prophylaxis is the administration of an antimicrobial drug before there is any evidence of infection, under conditions where the risks of an infection developing is considered very high.

DEVELOPMENT OF RESISTANCE TO ANTIMICROBIAL DRUGS

- Bacteria may exhibit resistance by the production of enzymes which destroy or inactivate the drug, by a change in membrane permeability, by an alteration in the binding sites for the drug, or by synthesis of the required compounds via an alternate pathway.
- The high usage level of antimicrobial drugs in hospitals provides an environment in which resistant organisms can flourish.
- Strategies to control the spread of antimicrobial resistance include hospital policies for prescribing antimicrobials, use of narrow spectrum antimicrobials, improved surveillance to determine prevalence, infection control procedures to prevent hospital-acquired infections, and a continuing search for vaccines against bacterial infections.

IMPLICATIONS FOR NURSING PRACTICE

- The nurse is responsible for the collection of an appropriate specimen in a sterile, labelled container, using aseptic technique, for arranging transport to the laboratory as soon as possible and for receiving the reports.
- The nurse should be aware of the correct methods of administration of the drugs and any special precautions that apply.
- Patients should be closely monitored for adverse reactions, such as hypersensitivity, which can occur in patients who are allergic to penicillin causing anaphylaxis,.
- The patient must be observed for signs of improvement and for side effects such as an overgrowth of other microrganisms, causing thrush (*Candida albicans*) or diarrhoea (*C. difficile)*.

Study Questions

1. What is meant by the term 'selective toxicity'?
2. Give three examples of ways in which antibacterial drugs can be selectively toxic.
3. Define the terms 'broad spectrum' and 'narrow spectrum' when applied to antimicrobial drugs.
4. Discuss the different ways in which antibacterial drugs can inhibit or damage the bacterial cell.
5. What are some of the major side effects associated with the use of aminoglycosides?
6. Why should tetracyclines not be given to children or pregnant women?
7. Why is chloramphenicol used mainly in topical applications?
8. Discuss the way in which sulpha drugs exhibit selective toxicity.
9. What is the main point of attack of most antifungal drugs?
10. Why is it difficult to design effective antiviral drugs?
11. What are interferons?
12. How is an antimicrobial sensitivity test carried out?
13. Why do doctors prescribe medication before the laboratory results are available?
14. Should specimens for diagnosis of infection be collected before or after the implementation of antimicrobial therapy?
15. What is meant by the half-life of a drug?
16. What is the therapeutic index of a drug?
17. List four ways in which bacteria can resist the action of antibacterial drugs.
18. Why are hospital-acquired infections more likely to be resistant to antibacterial drugs than community-acquired infections?
19. In what situations is the prophylactic use of antimicrobials considered necessary?
20. What are the responsibilities of the nurse in administering and monitoring antimicrobial therapy?

Test Your Understanding

1. Why is it preferable to prescribe bacteriocidal drugs under some conditions, rather than bacteriostatic drugs?
2. Why may bacteria that produce ß-lactamase enzyme exhibit resistance to both penicillins and cephalosporins?
3. What are the advantages of using chemically modified (semi-synthetic) antibiotics?
4. Name two major disadvantages of the indiscriminate use of antimicrobial drugs.
5. Explain why it is more difficult to treat systemic fungal infections than cutaneous infections.
6. Why should travellers to malarious areas seek advice from the Health Department?
7. Explain why analogues of nucleic acid precursors are effective as antiviral agents.
8. Why is it necessary to perform antimicrobial sensitivity tests?
9. What are the advantages/disadvantages of prescribing two drugs simultaneously?
10. Explain how bacteria can become resistant to antimicrobial drugs.

FURTHER READING

'Frontiers in Biotechnology: Resistance to Antibiotics', *Science*, 264, pp. 360–88. (A collection of papers and reports on various aspects of antibiotic resistance).

Simpson, S., 1992, 'Methicillin resistant *Staphylococcus aureus* and its implications for nursing practice: a literature review', *Nursing Practice*, 5, pp. 2–7.

Tomasz, A., 1994, 'Multiple-antibiotic-resistant Pathogenic Bacteria', *The New England Journal Of Medicine*, 330, pp. 1247–51.

Turnidge, J., 1990, 'MRSA—is control worthwhile and feasible?' *Medical Journal of Australia*, 152, pp. 225–26.

Victorian Medical Postgraduate Foundation, Inc., *Antibiotic Guidelines*, 10th edn., 1996.

chapter 13

nosocomial infections

Chapter focus

- *Why are nosocomial infections important?*
- *What factors contribute to the incidence of nosocomial infection?*
- *How does cross-infection occur in hospitals?*
- *What methods are used to control the spread of infection in hospitals?*
- *What are Standard Precautions and Additional Precautions?*
- *Which groups of patients are most susceptible to infection by hospital pathogens?*

The very first requirement in a hospital is that it should do the sick no harm.
Florence Nightingale

A Brief History

The word 'nosocomial' is derived from the ancient Greek words *nosos* meaning 'disease' and *komeion* meaning 'to take care of'. Thus, a **nosocomial infection** is one that is acquired in a hospital or other type of health facility. The term **hospital-acquired infection** (HAI) is also used to describe this type of infection. While most nosocomial infections occur in patients, they can also be acquired by hospital staff, by visitors or by anyone else who has contact with a hospital. Nosocomial infections usually become clinically obvious while the patient is still hospitalised, but sometimes they become apparent only after discharge from hospital. The appearance of hospital-acquired infection after leaving hospital will become more common with the current trend toward earlier discharge (a means of reducing hospital costs). Infections that occur in non-hospitalised people, or that are present or incubating at the time of admission to hospital, are not nosocomial; they are considered to be **community-acquired infections** (CAI).

Nosocomial infections have been a major public health problem since hospitals were first established. In the 18th and early 19th centuries, infections spread rapidly from patient to patient, resulting in mortality rates of 20% or more. To reduce the spread of infection, specialised disease hospitals, such as smallpox hospitals, fever hospitals and tuberculosis sanitoriums, were established. In general hospitals, infection rates and associated mortality rates were always high. For example, in 1869, James Simpson reported that in Britain more than 40% of amputees in large metropolitan hospitals died after surgery, and that this mortality rate was four times higher than for amputations performed by country physicians. He reported that death rates increased with the size of the hospital (see Table 13.1) and that in large hospitals pyaemia (infection) accounted for 60% of the deaths. Another major problem at the time was puerperal fever (childbed fever), a streptococcal septicaemia in women following childbirth. It too was associated with a high mortality rate and was the scourge of maternity hospitals.

The high incidence of morbidity and mortality due to infections in hospitals led several clinicians in the mid-1800s to question their cause and to look for ways of reducing infection. Oliver Wendell Holmes published an essay in 1843 claiming that puerperal fever was contagious. This was at a time when most people believed that miasmas, or toxic emanations from the earth, were responsible for such diseases. At about the same time, the Hungarian physician, Ignaz Philipp Semmelweis, came to a similar conclusion. He demonstrated that when physicians and medical students washed their hands in a chlorinated solution before entering the obstetric ward there was a dramatic decrease in the incidence of maternal mortality following childbirth (see Figure 13.1). He suggested that the cause of post-delivery fever and death was being spread from the corpses in the autopsy room to the labour rooms by doctors and medical students, who moved back and forth between these areas without washing their hands. He was first alerted to this by the smell of cadavers on their hands. Unfortunately, his classic paper was not published until 1860, and then was not accepted by his profession. He was later confined to a mental institution where he died from a streptococcal infection.

Another person who was concerned about the high mortality rates in hospital wards was Florence Nightingale. She is noted for many achievements in nursing, not least for her efforts in English field hospitals in Turkey during the Crimean War. She was sent there in 1854 as Superintendent of Nursing because of a public outcry over the death rate of British soldiers in these hospitals. The

TABLE 13.1
JAMES SIMPSON'S 1869 DATA ON MORTALITY AFTER LIMB AMPUTATION BY SIZE OF HOSPITAL AND DEGREE OF ISOLATION

SIZE OF HOSPITAL	DEATH RATE
300–600 beds	1 in 2.5
100–300 beds	1 in 4
25–100 beds	1 in 5.5
Less than 25 beds	1 in 7
Isolated rooms in country practice	1 in 9

Adapted from R.P. Wenzel (ed.), *Prevention and Control of Nosocomial Infections*, Williams & Wilkins, Baltimore, 1987, p. 8.

FIGURE 13.1
EFFECT OF HYGIENIC HAND DISINFECTION AS INTRODUCED BY SEMMELWEIS IN MAY 1847 ON MATERNAL MORTALITY AT THE VIENNA LYING-IN HOSPITAL

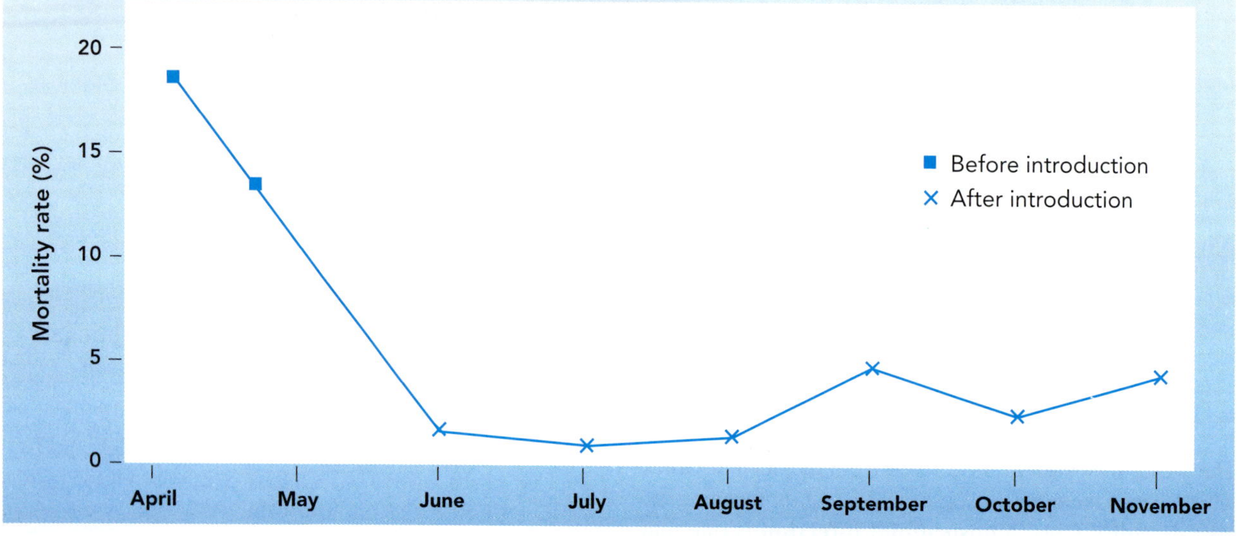

Adapted from R.P. Wenzel (ed.), *Prevention and Control of Nosocomial Infections*, Williams & Wilkins, Baltimore, 1987, p. 4.

conditions in these so-called 'medical facilities' were apalling, and the death rate of over 50% was due mainly to infection. Within six months of her arrival the mortality rate had dropped to under 3%, due to the much improved sanitary measures that she had introduced. Generally, however, infection control measures in hospitals were only slowly adopted. Still concerned 10 years later with infection rates in hospitals, Florence Nightingale wrote that 'in all probability a poor sufferer would have much better chance of recovery if treated at home'.

Joseph Lister, the British surgeon, was concerned with the high infection rate following surgery. In 1867, he introduced the use of carbolic acid to disinfect operating rooms and as an antiseptic in wound dressings, and reported a decrease in mortality after amputation from 46% to 15%. The introduction of antimicrobial drugs led to a great reduction in the mortality rate caused by infection in hospitals. However, this was not matched by a reduction in the number of infections. Despite the many advances in hospital infection control since the mid-1800s, even today 5–10% of patients in hospitals throughout the world develop a nosocomial infection.

The Importance of Nosocomial Infections

Prevalence surveys measure the proportion of patients who have an infection *at a given time*. In the only Australian national survey of nosocomial infections performed to date, an overall prevalence rate of 6.3% was found (McLaws et al)[1]. This compares with a rate of 9.2% found in the National Survey of Infection in Hospitals in England and Wales in 1980, and with a worldwide prevalence rate ranging from 3% to 21% (average 8.7%) reported by the World Health Organization in 1988[2].

Incidence rates give the proportion of patients who develop an infection *within a given period* and thus more closely reflect the true risk of infection, even though they are much more difficult and costly to measure. The incidence of hospital-acquired infection in developed countries is about 5–6%. Because prevalence rates are biased towards patients who are more seriously ill, they are usually higher than incidence rates. It should be recognised that in critical care units the incidence of nosocomial infections is sometimes as high as 20%.

The importance of nosocomial infections should be considered both from the point of view of patient suffering and also in economic terms. It has been estimated that in the United States a hospital-acquired infection, on average, extends the length of hospital stay for the patient by 3 to 4.5 days[1]. In addition, there is the possibility of complications or toxic side effects from the antimicrobial therapy that may be required. Mortality data for nosocomial infections is difficult to interpret. However, one estimate in the United States has the death rate from infection at 1–2%[4]. In economic terms, in 1988, nosocomial infections were estimated to cost Australia around $180 million per year[1]. This figure simply estimated hospital bed costs associated with a prolonged stay. There are many other associated expenses, such as the cost of antimicrobial therapy, the loss of personal income by the patient, the costs to the community of replacing workers, reduced productivity, and claims on medical insurance. Another important consequence is that, once patients are infected, they are an additional source of pathogenic organisms in the hospital.

Types and Causes of Nosocomial Infections

The most common sites of nosocomial infections are the urinary tract, surgical wounds, lower respiratory tract, skin and blood. The frequency of each type of infection varies with the age of the patient, the type of operation in surgical cases, the degree of immunosuppression, the length of time of catheterisation, and a number of other factors. Nevertheless, the relative frequency of infection is remarkably consistent in different studies. Table 13.2 shows the five most common types of infections and their relative frequencies. The most commonly occurring infections are of the urinary tract; many of these are associated with indwelling urinary catheters. Although inconvenient, urinary tract infections do not usually lead to a prolonged stay in hospital. On the other hand, wound infections, pneumonia and septicaemia can be serious, cause significant morbidity and occasionally are fatal. Nosocomial infections may occur as single cases (sporadic) or in outbreaks or clusters of infection (epidemic).

Almost any type of microorganism can cause an infection in hospital, although a few species predominate. Bacteria are responsible for most nosocomial infections, followed by fungi and viruses. Protozoa and worms rarely cause nosocomial infection. The pattern of microorganisms responsible for nosocomial infections has changed over the last 60 years. In the 1920s streptococci, especially *Streptococcus pyogenes,* were the most feared microbes in hospitals. However, with the introduction of sulphonamides in the 1930s, together with improved hygiene and less crowding in hospitals, their importance waned. Within 10 years *Staphylococcus aureus* ('golden staph') had virtually replaced the streptococci as the dominant cause of hospital-acquired infections. Penicillin, the 'wonder drug' introduced in the 1940s, was initially highly effective against staphylococci and streptococci. By the 1950s, however, strains of *Staphylococcus aureus* appeared that were resistant to this drug.

Although methicillin (a derivative of penicillin) was introduced in the early 1960s, strains of **methicillin-resistant *Staphylococcus aureus*** (**MRSA**) soon appeared. Subsequently, strains of *Staphylococcus aureus* emerged that were resistant to methicillin and a number of other drugs and became known as **multi-resistant *Staphylococcus aureus*** (also given the acronym **MRSA**). Since then MRSA has been responsible for numerous epidemics in hospitals and is still a major concern in hospital infection control. MRSA is considered to be endemic in many hospitals throughout the world, including major teaching hospitals in Australia. (See Spotlight box, p. 272)

Gram-negative rods, especially *Escherichia coli* and *Pseudomonas* spp., and to a lesser extent species of *Klebsiella, Proteus, Enterobacter* and other enteric bacteria have always played a prominent role in hospital-acquired infections. The 1980s and 1990s have seen the emergence of a wide spectrum of microorganisms responsible for nosocomial infections. *Staphylococcus epidermidis* and other coagulase-negative staphylococci (organisms commonly found on human skin as normal flora and formerly considered to be non-pathogenic) are now recognised as being responsible for many cases of infection, especially associated with indwelling intravenous lines, cerebrospinal fluid shunts, prosthetic heart valves and other prostheses.

TABLE 13.2
RELATIVE FREQUENCIES OF MAJOR TYPES OF NOSOCOMIAL INFECTIONS

SITE OF INFECTION	RELATIVE FREQUENCY (%)
Urinary tract	30–45
Surgical wound	15–30
Lower respiratory tract	10–25
Skin (especially burns)	5–10
Blood (bacteria)	5–10

In immunocompromised patients, such as AIDS patients or those receiving immunosuppressive drugs or cancer chemotherapy, infections caused by enterococci and mycobacteria have become more common. Fungi like *Candida albicans, Pneumocystis carinii* and *Aspergillus,* and certain viruses like cytomegalovirus and herpes simplex are also being seen with increasing frequency. These opportunists (see Chapter 9) are occurring more frequently because of the increasing use of procedures and medications that lower the resistance of the patient. Not only are immunocompromised patients more susceptible to these previously rare causes of infection, but, once infected, they serve as important reservoirs of these pathogens in hospitals. In specific units or hospitals, other organisms may be important. For example, rotavirus is an important nosocomial pathogen in paediatric hospitals. The common causes and risk factors of nosocomial infections are summarised in Table 13.3.

The Nature of Hospital Pathogens

COMMUNITY VERSUS HOSPITAL STRAINS

Nosocomial infections may be caused by microorganisms that come from either inside or outside the hospital. Those that originate outside are brought into the hospital by patients, staff and visitors, and are regarded as **community strains**. They include the normal flora of these people, as well as any pathogens they may be infected with, or are carrying asymptomatically. In general, these organisms are sensitive to antimicrobial drugs. If these pathogens are shed they can be transmitted to patients or staff. Components of the patient's own normal flora may be the source of the infection—for example, gastrointestinal flora that move to the urinary tract, or *Staphylococcus epidermidis* from the skin that infects an IV catheter insertion site.

Many nosocomial infections are caused by **hospital strains.** As the name implies, these are strains of microorganisms that are found mainly in hospitals or associated with people (patients and staff) who have been in hospitals. Hospital strains differ from community strains by usually having a greater resistance to antimicrobial drugs and some disinfectants. Multi-resistant strains of bacteria like *Staphylococcus aureus* (MRSA), *Staphylococcus epidermidis*, *Pseudomonas, E. coli,*

SPOTLIGHT

MRSA

There is a tendency to forget that more soldiers died during World War I from wound infections than from the actual injuries received in fighting. When it looked as though history would be repeated in World War II, the United States threw its considerable resources behind the commercial development of the new wonder drug, penicillin. Penicillin had been shown by the scientists Fleming, Chain and Florey to be effective in killing the Gram-positive bacteria responsible for many wound infections. These included staphylococci, streptococci and clostridia.

Penicillin was produced in large quantities in the 1940s and many lives were saved. However, the success was short-lived. It was found that some strains of *Staphylococcus aureus* quickly developed resistance to penicillin by producing an enzyme (ß-lactamase) which could break down the penicillin molecule. One of these strains was the particularly virulent phage type 80/81 or 'golden staph', which spread around the world between 1955 and 1965. Golden staph (so named because of the yellow-orange pigment it produces) made headlines in Australia when an epidemic occurred in the neonatal ward of a Sydney hospital in 1953. It then spread rapidly throughout other States, causing major outbreaks of hospital-acquired infections. It was only contained when a number of synthetic derivatives of penicillin, resistant to the ß-lactamase enzyme, were developed. Of these, methicillin became the standard treatment for *Staphylococcus aureus*.

In 1961, the first methicillin-resistant strains of *Staphylococcus aureus* (MRSA) were isolated in Europe. They were first reported in Australia in 1966 in the eastern States, and in the United States in 1968. As well, other strains were identified that had a broad pattern of resistance, not only to methicillin, but also to the aminoglycosides and cephalosporins.

In the 1970s only a small number of methicillin-resistant strains of *Staphylococcus aureus* were isolated (<2%). However, in 1979, a survey in Victoria reported an increase in MRSA infections to 20–40% of all staphylococcal isolates in six of the large teaching hospitals. During 1980–82, the incidence reached 50% in some large hospitals. One 700-bed hospital reported 254 patients infected with MRSA, of whom 30% died. Of special concern was the occurrence of MRSA in the four neonatal special care nurseries in the Melbourne hospitals.

The outbreak was not confined to Melbourne, but also occurred in Sydney and spread to the other Australian states. The ability to phage type (see Chapter 4) strains of staphylococci means that it is possible to trace the spread of a particular strain from hospital to hospital, State to State, or even worldwide.

Although the numbers of MRSA cases have declined since the early 1980s, there continues to be a constant level of MRSA infections reported from most hospitals, with sporadic serious outbreaks of infection. The prevalence survey of McLaws et al.[1] carried out in 1984 reported a surprisingly low incidence of MRSA of 0.3% of total infections, but this may reflect the fact that the survey only measured MRSA infections present at one particular point of time.

Both patients and staff are frequently colonised by MRSA without showing any evidence of infection. MRSA does not seem to be particularly invasive in healthy individuals. The patients who are most at risk are those who are debilitated or have diminished resistance to infection—infants in neonatal intensive care units; cancer and leukaemia patients; patients who are immunodeficient; patients in whom invasive foreign bodies have been inserted, such as heart valves, joint prostheses, IV lines, or catheters; and patients who have undergone extensive surgery.

Patients who are infected with MRSA usually have other serious illnesses. Currently, the only effective drug against MRSA is vancomycin, a very expensive drug with toxic side effects. For superficial infections, a combination of rifampicin and fusidic acid can be used, often with flucloxacillin. One of the major concerns at present is that strains of *Staphylococcus aureus* will appear that are resistant to vancomycin. For this reason careful consideration is given before prescribing the drug since the search for effective alternatives has so far been unsuccessful.

Another major factor is the cost to the health system of vancomycin treatment and the extra hospitalisation needed. Many nursing homes and rehabilitation centres will not accept patients until they have had three consecutive negative swabs for MRSA, so these patients are left to occupy acute care beds for longer periods.

What can be done to contain MRSA?

There have been numerous reports of MRSA outbreaks and of the many different measures taken to contain the organism. Some common factors emerge. Staff who are colonised with MRSA in the nose do not appear to present a significant risk of cross-infection. Even so, opinions vary as to the need to treat them with an antiseptic nasal cream such as mupirocin. On the other hand, staff who are colonised in skin lesions do present a significant risk of cross-infection and should not be assigned to high-risk areas until the MRSA is cleared. Infected patients who are shedding MRSA should be isolated or barrier nursed (isolation is preferable). There are varying opinions about the risks posed by patients who are colonised but not infected.

It has been suggested that outbreaks of MRSA infection are indicative of a general breakdown in infection control procedures, due to such factors as overcrowding, pressure of work, or even complacency on the part of health workers that all infections can be dealt with by the use of antibiotics.

MRSA has been shown to be transported on the hands and is readily removed by effective handwashing between patients. Additional control measures are indicated if a cluster of patients within an institution is found to acquire MRSA, or if an increasing incidence of hospital-acquired infection due to MRSA is observed over a longer period. Some hospitals advocate surveillance (i.e. routine swabbing of staff and patients), but the results of this have to be measured against the cost and the work created for medical, nursing and laboratory staff.

Surveillance may be beneficial in selected situations; for example, monitoring new staff before they are assigned to a high-risk area. Nurses should be aware of the risk they pose if they have been working in the environment of a MRSA patient and are then assigned to a high-risk area where patients are particularly susceptible. This applies especially to agency staff who may move from one hospital to another.

Screening of long-stay surgical patients is often warranted; experience at the St George Hospital in Sydney showed that these patients often had a high level of colonisation and acted as a significant source of infection. Measures taken to control MRSA in the cardiothoracic unit at St Vincent's Hospital in Sydney involved a prospective study to determine the carrier status of all patients entering the unit. Infection control policies were implemented and resulted in a significant reduction in the number of MRSA infections and carriers. Experience at Royal Perth Hospital showed that large outbreaks of MRSA could be avoided by screening all new patients and staff members. This required considerable commitment from the medical, nursing and general administrative staff. All these procedures need to be constantly re-evaluated for cost effectiveness.

Although most strains of MRSA seen in Australia are not nearly as virulent as the golden staph phage type 80/81 of the 1950s, it is still a major cause for concern because of its resistance to all antibiotics except vancomycin. The use of antibiotics has to be monitored carefully at all times as the appearance of resistant strains of other bacteria can be an outcome of the indiscriminate use of antibiotics, both prophylactically and therapeutically. In the United States, vancomycin-resistant enterococci have been isolated, and resistant strains of *Mycobacterium tuberculosis* and *Streptococcus pneumoniae* are being seen more frequently.

It is not possible to rely on antibiotic therapy to cure infections. Rather, it is essential to maintain good infection control practices to prevent the spread of pathogenic microorganisms, of which MRSA is an important example.

TABLE 13.3
COMMON CAUSES AND RISK FACTORS OF NOSOCOMIAL INFECTIONS

INFECTION	COMMON CAUSES	RISK FACTORS
Urinary tract	*E.coli*, *Klebsiella* spp., *Enterococcus* spp., *Pseudomonas aeruginosa*, *Proteus* spp.	Urinary catheter; structural or functional abnormality
Surgical wound	*Staphylococcus aureus*, *Klebsiella* spp., *Streptococcus* spp., *E. coli*, *Pseudomonas aeruginosa*, *Enterococcus* spp., *Enterobacter* spp.	Debility, prosthesis, prolonged surgery, surgery on heavily colonised sites
Pneumonia	*Staphylococcus aureus*, *Klebsiella* spp., *Pseudomonas aeruginosa*, *Candida* spp., *Enterobacter* spp., *Streptococcus* spp., viruses	Underlying disorder, surgery, ventilation
Septicaemia	*Staphylococcus aureus*, *Klebsiella* spp., *E. coli*, *Staphylococcus epidermidis*, *Enterococcus* spp.	Indwelling IV catheter, infection
Skin	*Staphylococcus aureus*, *Candida* spp.	Newborn
Immunocompromised patient	Viruses, *Candida* spp., *Aspergillus* spp.	Transfusion, immunosuppression, immunodeficiency, AIDS

Klebsiella, Enterobacter and *Enterococcus* will cause infections that are difficult to treat, and may even be life-threatening. The major sources of hospital strains are the hospital environment, patients with infections and colonised patients and staff.

COLONISATION

Colonisation refers to the presence and growth of a microorganism on the skin or mucous membrane without any evidence of infection. The organisms that make up a person's own normal flora are the usual colonisers. However, hospital strains can colonise patients within days or even hours of admission. Colonisation may result in the short-term presence of unusual organisms in a particular site, for example, Gram-negative bacteria on the skin or in the oropharynx. Having taken up residence with (or displaced) the normal flora, these hospital strains may then remain there for weeks or months, even after discharge from hospital. The established normal flora are complex and quite resistant to change. However, colonisation with hospital microorganisms becomes increasingly common the longer a person is in hospital, and is favoured if the patient is exposed to antimicrobial drugs. This is because an antimicrobial drug, especially a broad spectrum type, may cause an imbalance in the normal flora of the patient, thus providing the hospital strains with a new niche to colonise. The presence of an antibiotic in the tissues of a patient means, that, if colonisation of that tissue occurs, it will probably be by a drug-resistant strain.

Hospital staff may also be colonised with hospital organisms and are thus carriers of these potential pathogens. These organisms do not usually pose a threat to the carrier unless the resistance of the individual is lowered sufficiently to make them susceptible to infection. Another important aspect is that, once they are colonised with one or more hospital strains, patients and staff add to the number of reservoirs for these troublesome organisms in the hospital. For example, approximately 30% of the general community consistently carry *Staphylococcus aureus* in the nose, while as many as 70% of hospital staff may carry it. Furthermore, some of them may be carrying a multi-resistant, hospital strain and therefore are an important source of this organism.

Burns wounds and surgical wounds are frequently colonised by hospital organisms and often more than one type of organism can be found there. They are ideal sites for microbial growth and multiplication and, if the wound eventually becomes infected, it is probable that one or more of these colonising organisms will be involved. Therefore, burns and surgical wounds, whether infected or not, are important sources of pathogens in hospital cross-infection.

The major sites of colonisation by drug-resistant, hospital organisms are the nose, the skin, the oropharynx, the lower intestine and the urinary tract. The organisms tend to prefer certain sites, as shown in Table 13.4, and it should be remembered that both patients and staff can harbour these organisms.

The High Incidence of Nosocomial Infections: Contributory Factors

MICROBIAL FACTORS

A large proportion of nosocomial infections are caused by hospital strains of bacteria, many of which are drug-resistant. However, it should be recognised that the capacity of a microorganism to cause disease (i.e. its virulence) is *not* directly related to its drug resistance. A strain of a particular organism can be resistant to many drugs but is not necessarily more virulent than a sensitive strain of the same organism. Why then are so many hospital infections caused by resistant strains? The reason is that, in hospitals, where antibiotics are used frequently and in large amounts, sensitive strains are kept in check, so do not provide a significant source of organisms. A resistant strain is more likely to cause infection mainly because it will persist in the hospital despite the use of antibiotics. Resistance to disinfectants used in the hospital, as has been reported in some strains of *Pseudomonas* and MRSA, also facilitates the persistence of these organisms in the hospital.

As explained in Chapters 9 and 10, the outcome of exposure to a microorganism depends on the balance between the virulence of the microbe and the resistance of the host. Generally, the virulence of a microorganism is a vital factor in determining whether infection occurs but, when considering nosocomial infections, an equally important factor is the patient's general resistance. While some hospital pathogens have demonstrated exceptional virulence, such as the 80/81 phage type of *Staphylococcus aureus* that was rampant in the early 1950s, this is not a prerequisite for infection. Many hospital infections are caused by organisms of low virulence (e.g. *Staphylococcus epidermidis*) in patients with compromised body defences.

TABLE 13.4
COLONISATION SITES IN PATIENTS AND STAFF WITH HOSPITAL STRAINS

ORGANISM	COLONISATION SITES
MRSA	Nose Skin—hands, perineum, groin, axillae
E. coli, Klebsiella, Enterobacter	Bowel Oropharynx Urinary tract
Pseudomonas	Bowel Oropharynx
Staph. epidermidis	Skin Urinary tract
Enterococci	Bowel
Candida	Bowel Urinary tract

PATIENT SUSCEPTIBILITY

For a variety of reasons, a high proportion of hospitalised people have lowered resistance to infection and thus can be considered to be immunocompromised (see Chapter 9). Age is an important immunological factor and the newborn are highly susceptible to infection because of the immaturity of their immune system. At the other end of the spectrum, the very old also have a greater risk of infection because of the deterioration of their immune system, or because of impairment to other body functions, such as the blood supply to tissues. Also, immobility in the aged may lead to stasis of body fluids, and hence infection in such organs as the lungs or the bladder.

Lowered resistance may also be associated with some underlying disease. For example, patients with leukaemia are more susceptible to infection because they have inadequate numbers of functional white cells. People with diabetes may have lowered resistance because of vascular changes that cause tissue hypoxia, and because of impaired chemotactic and phagocytic activity in their white cells (see Chapter 9). Infection itself may lower a person's resistance. Thus, patients with an influenza virus infection are more susceptible to bacterial pneumonia. The other obvious and more extreme example is that of HIV infection, which makes the affected person more susceptible to many other infections because of the direct effect of the virus on the immune system.

Many types of medical treatment lower the patient's resistance to infection. Cytotoxic drugs and radiotherapy for the treatment of cancer both severely affect the immune system. Immunosuppressive drugs given to transplant patients to prevent rejection are designed to suppress the immune system, as are anti-inflammatory drugs, especially the corticosteroids. As we saw in Chapter 12, certain antimicrobial drugs can lower a person's resistance to infection by disturbing the balance of normal flora of the body, or by suppression of the bone marrow, such as can occur with the systemic use of chloramphenicol.

Patients with accidental wounds (e.g. road accident victims) are more susceptible to infection because of damage to their protective skin barrier, and because microorganisms may be carried into the tissues when the wound occurs. Patients with burns are also highly susceptible because of loss of skin and lowered body defences (see Chapter 16). Other patients may have breaks in the skin from lesions or from pressure sores.

MEDICAL PROCEDURES

As long as the skin and mucous membranes remain intact they provide very effective barriers against infection (see Chapter 9). However, many diagnostic and therapeutic procedures involve the penetration of these barriers and the introduction of some device into a sterile body area. This provides microorganisms with easy access to susceptible tissues and thus substantially increases the risk of infection. Infections resulting from medical procedures or treatment are termed **iatrogenic infections.** Surgery is an obvious example of a procedure that increases patient susceptibility to infection. Surgical wound infections are the second most common type of nosocomial infection.

Many other procedures also increase the risk of infection. Intravascular and urinary catheters, endotracheal intubation and drainage tubes all allow microorganisms to circumvent the body's external barriers; that is, they open up otherwise protected parts of the body to the outside, allowing microbes to reach, colonise and finally infect these sites. Urinary tract infections are the most common type of nosocomial infection because many hospitalised patients have some condition that requires urinary catheterisation. The microorganisms enter the bladder by travelling either up the outside of the catheter tube, or through the tube itself. They are able to colonise the urethra (outside the tube) because there is not the normal flow of urine to wash away the organisms from the tissue surface. Intraluminal (inside the tube) entry of organisms is usually associated with contamination of the drainage reservoir and then spread via the fluid in the tube to the bladder. The spread of organisms to the bladder via the inside of a catheter tube is reduced by the use of closed drainage systems (see Figure 13.2). Whatever the means of access, the longer a catheter is in place, the greater the risk of infection.

Indwelling intravenous catheters are frequently used to administer fluids, medication or nutrients to patients. These devices also provide organisms with a ready means of entry to the body. The catheter and the skin around the insertion site can easily become colonised from a number of sources and subsequently infected, possibly leading to septicaemia. *Staphylococcus epidermidis*, a normal skin inhabitant, is frequently the cause of such infections. Again, the longer the device is in place, the greater the risk of infection. Very occasionally, the fluid being administered may be contaminated, or the equipment may become contaminated and microorganisms are passed directly into the bloodstream.

Nosocomial lung infections are most often associated with either intubation of the trachea (insertion of a tube into the trachea), or tracheostomy (an opening made into the trachea through the neck). Intubation increases the risk of infection because microorganisms have direct access to lower airways and also because the procedure often causes injury and irritation to the tracheal lining. It is also well recognised that the use of respiratory equipment to administer oxygen or medication deep into the lungs can predispose a patient to infection. Nebulisers, humidifiers and other respiratory equipment provide a moist environment for bacteria to multiply, and are difficult to sterilise.

Many other medical procedures may predispose a patient to infection. The use of endoscopes to examine mucosal passageways and associated organs increases the risk of infection, since endoscopes are difficult to sterilise. They can irritate or break the delicate mucosal linings of the passageways through which they are passed and thereby increase the risk of infection.

The implantation of prostheses such as heart valves or artificial joints comes with a risk of infection, since

FIGURE 13.2
POTENTIAL SITES OF INFECTION ASSOCIATED WITH A URINARY CATHETER. THE DIFFERENCE BETWEEN OPEN AND CLOSED DRAINAGE SYSTEMS

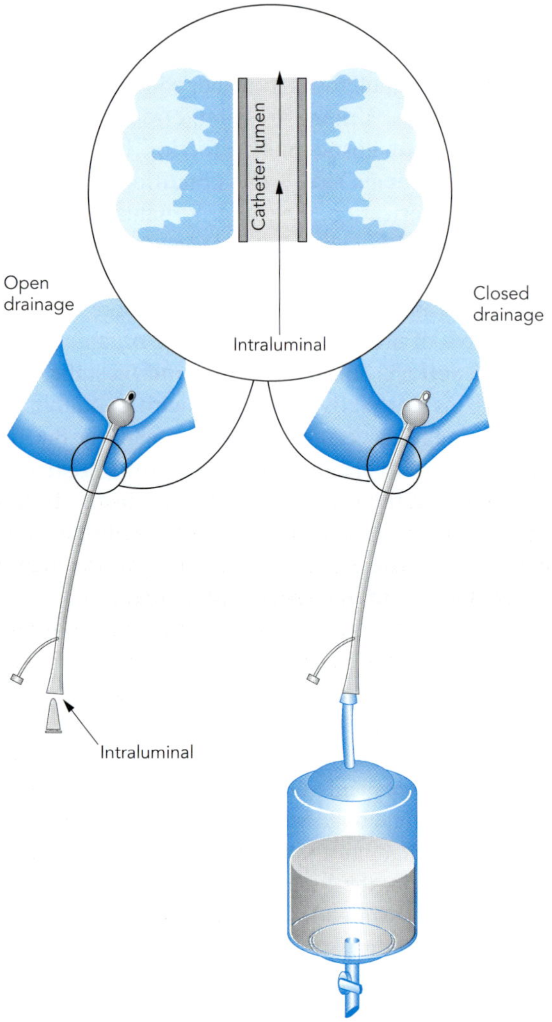

organisms may be introduced at the time of implantation. Foreign bodies such as these may act as sites of colonisation for microorganisms that later enter the bloodstream. Under normal circumstances, low numbers of organisms entering the bloodstream are quickly removed by the body's defences, but inert objects (which do not have a blood supply) provide a site for colonisation that is inaccessible to these defences.

Even the common practice of giving injections using a hypodermic needle brings with it the chance of infection. For such a simple device and common procedure, there are several potential hazards—the needle or syringe may be contaminated, the solution to be injected may be contaminated, or the skin may have been improperly disinfected.

The more severely ill patients are, the more likely they are to acquire an infection, either as a direct result of their clinical condition, or because of the medical or surgical procedures to which they are subjected. The combination of invasive technique and immunosuppressive or antibiotic treatment that is necessary for some patients leaves them with minimal protection against infection. Thus, intensive care units, with severely ill patients, frequently have the highest incidences of infection. As medical science develops, more complex and invasive (lifesaving) procedures are used, with an ever-increasing risk of infection for those subjected to them. The host factors and medical procedures that predispose patients to hospital infection are summarised in Table 13.5.

THE MANY SOURCES OF POTENTIAL PATHOGENS

Another major reason for the high incidence of nosocomial infections is that there are many sources of potential pathogens in hospitals to which the susceptible patient may be exposed. It is customary to classify nosocomial

TABLE 13.5
FACTORS THAT PREDISPOSE PATIENTS TO HOSPITAL INFECTION

FACTOR	SPECIFIC EXAMPLES
Age	The newborn have an immature immune system; the elderly have an immune system that is deteriorating
Underlying disease	Leukaemia, diabetes, cancer, neutropenia
Existing infection	HIV infection; herpes virus lesions can be infected by bacteria (e.g. *Staphylococcus aureus*); viral influenza can lead to bacterial pneumonia
Medicines and treatments	Cancer therapy (cytotoxic drugs, radiotherapy); immunosuppression for transplant patients; anti-inflammatory drugs; antibiotics that alter the normal flora; chloramphenicol (suppresses the bone marrow)
Medical procedures	Surgery; indwelling IV catheters; indwelling urinary catheters; intubation of the trachea; tracheostomy; use of respiratory equipment (which is difficult to sterilise); endoscopes; infections; implantation of prosthesis (e.g. heart valves); dialysis
Accidental wounds	Burns, traffic accident, bed sores

infections according to the source of the causative agent. This can be useful in the epidemiological investigation of outbreaks and for the selection of appropriate methods for infection control in a particular hospital unit. Nosocomial infections can be divided into two general categories based on the source of the causative organism.

1. **Exogenous infections** are infections caused by microorganisms from a source external to the patient, such as the hospital environment, staff, other patients or visitors.
2. **Endogenous infections** are caused by microorganisms that are part of the patient's own normal flora, or are organisms (including hospital strains) that have colonised the patient after admission to hospital. Sometimes they may be organisms that have spread from an infection at another site. They are essentially 'self-infections'.

The distinction between exogenous and endogenous sources may sometimes be useful, but in practice it is often difficult to make.

Exogenous nosocomial infections

There are a large number of exogenous sources of potential pathogens in the hospital. The hospital brings together patients with many different illnesses. Some of them will have infections and will therefore serve as sources of infection for other patients. In a surgical ward, the patient with an infected wound is a potential source of pathogens for any other patient who has just had surgery. Hospital staff may also have an infection and those who have close patient contact are a particularly important source, especially if they have skin lesions on the hands. Infected patients and staff are not the only source, since all people carry a normal flora comprising organisms that can cause infection in a highly susceptible patient. And it is common for hospitalised patients and staff to be colonised with drug-resistant hospital strains, which are capable of causing serious infections, especially in the immunocompromised patient. The transmission of organisms from one person to another, causing infection in the second, is called **cross-infection**. For cross-infection to occur, the human source of the organisms may be infected or merely colonised. This makes control of cross-infection all the more difficult.

The inanimate objects in the hospital environment also carry microorganisms capable of causing infection but are rarely the primary source of pathogenic microorganisms. Mostly they become contaminated with organisms from human sources. Exceptions are organisms such as *Pseudomonas* and *Aspergillus*, which occur in the environment. *Aspergillus* spores are ubiquitous (found everywhere), and *Pseudomonas* is often found associated with soil or flowers, in damp areas such as sinks and pot plants, and sometimes even in disinfectant solutions.

The contribution of the hospital environment to infection is often overstated. While there is plenty of opportunity for the environment to become contaminated, most microorganisms are unable to multiply and do not survive well on clean, dry surfaces such as floors, walls and furniture. Gram-negative rods such as *E. coli*, *Klebsiella* and *Pseudomonas* are susceptible to desiccation and survive for only minutes to hours on dry surfaces. However, the endospores of some bacteria (e.g. *Clostridium*) can survive for long periods and *Staphylococcus aureus* is also resistant to desiccation. It is impossible to know whether a piece of equipment or other part of the environment has been freshly contaminated and is therefore a source of potential pathogens. For this reason, standardised cleaning and disinfection procedures, as prescribed by the hospital, must always be observed.

The situation is very different for moist areas of the hospital environment, which may also have the necessary nutrients (e.g. body fluids or other organic substances) for microbial growth and multiplication to occur. The numbers of organisms in these places may therefore be very high. Items such as fluids for injection, sinks, mops, sponges, respiratory equipment, suction apparatus and humidifiers have all been implicated as potential sources of infection in nosocomial infections (see Figure 13.4). Even disinfectant solutions can sometimes become contaminated, especially if not freshly prepared. Also, some disinfectants are inactivated by organic material such as blood or other tissues (see Chapter 11).

In summary, the most important external sources of infectious organisms are those where microbial multiplication can take place. These include infected patients, human carriers, infected wounds and moist areas of the hospital environment. Dry objects and surfaces in the hospital environment are less important, but should not be ignored as potential sources of infection, particularly if they could have been *recently* contaminated. Figure 13.3 summarises the potential sources of nosocomial infections.

Endogenous nosocomial infections

Although there are many external sources of potential pathogens, the majority of nosocomial infections are endogenous. They consist of the patient's own normal flora, together with any hospital colonisers, and are in an ideal position to cause infection. They are mainly opportunistic pathogens in that they will only cause infection if the patient's resistance is lowered, as is often the case in hospital. There is also the potential for patients who already have an infection to develop another infection elsewhere in the body—the primary infection acts as the source of microorganisms for the second site. The means of transmission may be systemic (through the tissues) or may occur by mechanical transfer via the hands of the patient or staff member. These sources are also summarised in Figure 13.3.

CLOSE CONTACT

A feature of hospitals is the large amount of physical contact that occurs between staff and patients. A nurse or doctor within a given unit or ward may be in contact with every patient in that area several times a day. For example, depending on the size and nature of the unit, a nurse might be required to perform routine procedures

FIGURE 13.3
POSSIBLE SOURCES OF NOSOCOMIAL INFECTIONS

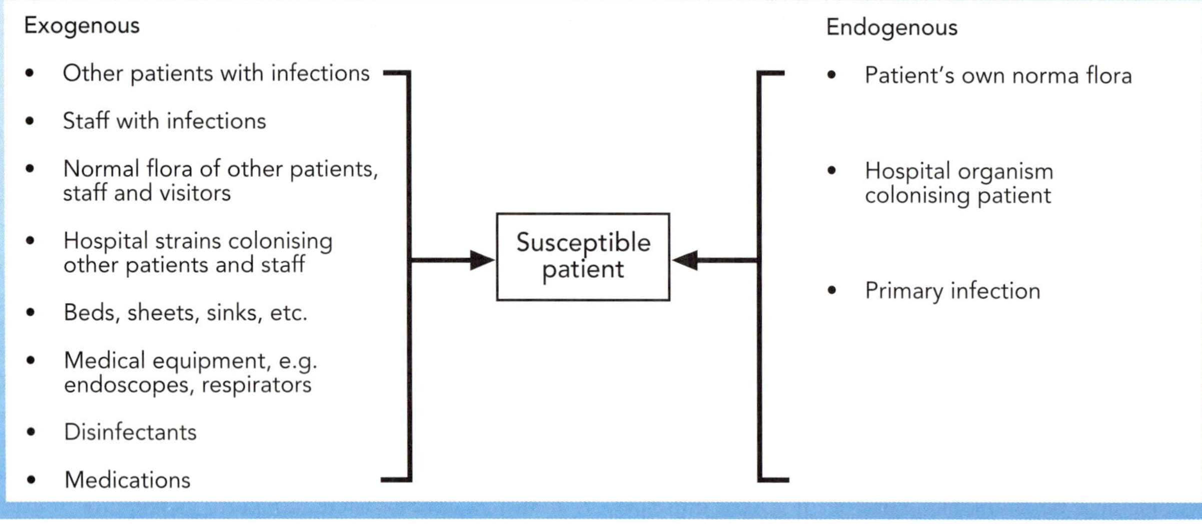

such as temperature, pulse, and blood pressure readings, changing dressings or administering medication for each patient on several occasions during the day. Other health workers may also be attending to these patients as well as to patients in other units throughout the hospital. Thus, not only is there frequent contact between a large number of different hospital staff and a given patient, but also each staff member will have physical contact with many patients, in one or more units throughout the hospital. The contact between patients and staff is thus frequent and varied, enhancing the transmission of microorganisms. Isolation procedures are sometimes instituted to prevent this type of cross-infection.

Cross-infection in Hospitals

As knowledge and understanding of microorganisms and the nature of microbial infections have increased, the methods used to control the spread of pathogens in hospitals have undergone significant change. In the early days of British settlement in Sydney, infectious patients were isolated at the 'Coast Hospital' (now Prince Henry Hospital) at Little Bay, well away from the main settlement at Sydney Cove. Such extreme measures of isolation have now been replaced by a more scientific approach, although travellers and immigrants arriving from overseas and suffering from unidentified infections are still temporarily treated at the Infectious Diseases Hospital at Fairfield in Victoria or in special units in other States.

The main purpose of infection control procedures is to provide high-quality patient care and a safe working environment, by preventing the spread of infection around the hospital or health care facility. Microorganisms can be spread in a variety of ways (Figure 13.5).

1. They can be carried on the hands or clothing of hospital personnel (including doctors, nurses, laboratory technicians, physiotherapists, attendants and cleaners) as well as visitors.
2. Microorganisms present on articles such as keys and patient records, which are handled by a number of different staff, can be picked up and transported around the hospital on their hands.
3. Contaminated equipment or utensils, such as endoscopes and ventilators, which are generally difficult to clean and sterilise, can be the vehicles that transport organisms from one patient to another.
4. Microorganisms can be spread by the incorrect disposal of contaminated material (dressings, body substances, etc.).
5. They can be transmitted via body fluids from asymptomatic carriers, as may occur with hepatitis B, hepatitis C, human immunodeficiency virus (HIV) and cytomegalovirus (CMV).
6. They can be carried on air currents or through air-conditioning or ventilation systems.

Cross-infection involves the infection of a susceptible patient by the transfer of organisms from one patient to another. It should be appreciated that the risk of cross-infection varies significantly from one facility to another, influenced by such factors as:

- the size (number of beds) of the hospital;
- the location of the hospital (e.g. inner city or country); and
- the type of hospital or unit.

For example, the Australian survey carried out by McLaws and co-workers[1], showed a higher incidence of nosocomial infections in the larger teaching hospitals. To a large extent, the incidence is a reflection of the *type* of patient. Patients admitted to a busy accident/emergency unit are likely to be severely traumatised and therefore at greater risk of acquiring infection. Large hospitals usually have intensive care units, specialised burns units and facilities for transplant operations. Patients in these units are particularly susceptible to cross-infection, because of the weakened status of their immune system.

FIGURE 13.4
RESERVOIRS IN HOSPITAL

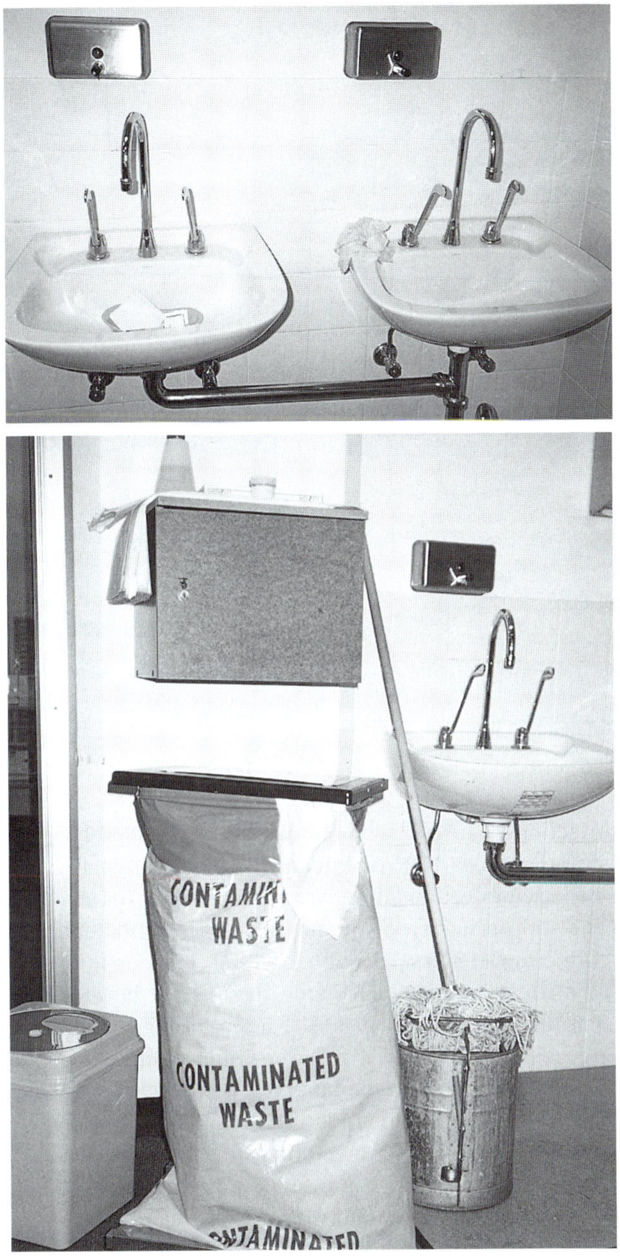

In contrast, geriatric hospitals do not have a population of severely ill patients or patients who are actually infected. There is thus a smaller reservoir of microorganisms present.

All these variables must be taken into account when developing policies and procedures to prevent cross-infection in a hospital.

INFECTION CONTROL COMMITTEES

In the last 30 years in Australia, there has been an increasing awareness of the importance of infection control in our hospitals. The first infection control nurse in New South Wales was appointed at the Prince of Wales Hospital in 1965. Since then infection control programs have evolved to deal with the ongoing problem of nosocomial infections.

In most large city hospitals the policies and procedures for infection control are the responsibility of the Infection Control Committee. This committee usually comprises representatives of the Medical Board, Nursing Administration, Microbiology, Pharmacy, Theatre Staff, Clinical Nurse Consultants and other hospital departments. In practice, the responsibilities and composition of this body will vary considerably depending on the size of the hospital, the resources available and financial considerations. In large city hospitals an infection control team, consisting of one or two Clinical Nurse Consultants, the Microbiologist and Infectious Diseases specialist, is responsible for the daily implementation of infection control policies. In smaller country hospitals the responsibility may rest with one part-time Clinical Nurse Consultant. Infection control personnel are usually responsible for the production of a hospital infection control manual, containing details of procedures for infection control, including cleaning, disinfection and sterilisation that should be followed by all medical and ancillary staff.

Infection control personnel have a range of information services at their disposal. In Australia, the National Health and Medical Research Council (NH&MRC), a statutory authority within the portfolio of the Minister for Health, establishes working parties and publishes guidelines for infection control as well as recommendations on a variety of other health issues (see Chapter 14). These guidelines are interpreted and administered at a State or Territory level by the respective State health departments, who also issue guidelines for hospitals and health practitioners. Individual hospitals and health facilities use these guidelines to develop their own procedures and policies. Advisers within the health departments and hospitals provide advice to practitioners about dealing with particular disease problems. The New South Wales *Nurses Act 1991 Regulation* relating to infection control standards in New South Wales was amended in 1995 to include penalties for improper practice. The Federal Department of Health, Housing and Community Services publishes the fortnightly *Communicable Diseases Intelligence (CDI)* which reports on current outbreaks of infections.

On a worldwide basis, the Centers for Disease Control (CDC) in Atlanta, Georgia, US, publishes the *Morbidity and Mortality Weekly Report (MMWR)*, which details disease outbreaks and the results of surveillance studies, mainly in the United States, but also in other parts of the world that impinge on the United States. They also issue guidelines for infection control policies and warnings about the emergence and distribution of new strains of pathogenic microorganisms (e.g. multi-resistant *Mycobacterium tuberculosis*, which is now a major problem in the United States).

With the increase in worldwide travel, the sharing of this type of information is vitally important in containing the spread of disease. Often, the ideal infection control situation is not achievable because of space, staffing or financial constraints. Alternative procedures may need to be instituted by the Infection Control Committee. Under these circumstances a sound understanding of microorganisms, disease transmission and methods of control can lead to a practical and successful solution. For

FIGURE 13.5
SPREAD OF MICROORGANISMS IN HOSPITAL

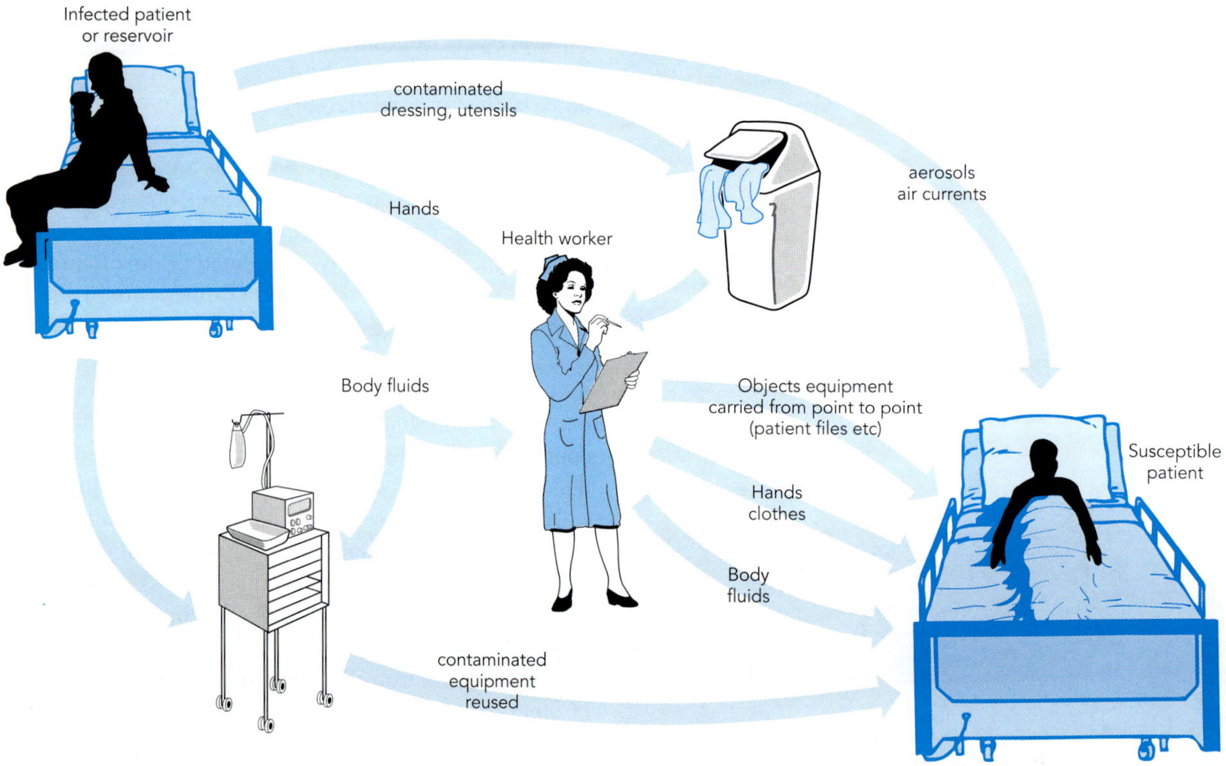

example, in large hospitals, bed pans are routinely cleaned and disinfected in a 'sanitiser', a large automated piece of equipment that kills most organisms by steam treatment. In a smaller hospital without such equipment, a satisfactory, if somewhat more laborious, alternative may be to rinse the bed pan thoroughly and then soak it in a suitable disinfectant solution such as sodium hypochlorite.

Surveillance

One important function of the infection control team is to monitor the incidence of infections within the hospital. Infection control staff are in a position to collect very useful epidemiological data on the type of hospital infections and patterns of antibiotic resistance of isolated organisms. This constant surveillance helps to detect any increase in cases of infection and identifies any outbreak or cluster of similar infections in the hospital, so that measures can be taken to determine the source and means of transmission and thus prevent further cross-infection. This may involve identification and disinfection of contaminated equipment, identification of a procedure that has created a risk, or identification of staff who are shedding the pathogens. Cases of notifiable diseases are recorded and the information is sent to the State or Territory health department. The collected information is published in the *CDI Bulletin* each fortnight (see Chapter 14).

Role of the microbiology laboratory

The microbiology laboratory works closely with the Clinical Nurse Consultant to record the occurrence of infections, particularly those caused by resistant hospital strains such as MRSA. Specimens from patients with a suspected infection are sent to the laboratory for analysis. The appropriate types of specimen and the methods for collection are described in Chapter 15. For a correct identification and subsequent diagnosis it is important that the specimens sent to the microbiology laboratory are collected properly, in an aseptic manner, labelled correctly and sent to the laboratory as soon as possible. The staff of the Microbiology Department are responsible for identifying the pathogen causing the infection and, if necessary, alerting the infection control team so that appropriate infection control measures can be taken.

Education

An ongoing responsibility of the infection control team (usually the Clinical Nurse Consultant) is to conduct information sessions for all hospital staff, to make them aware of the importance of preventing cross-infection and of their own responsibility to observe correct practices. In addition, hospital personnel need to understand the potential health risks to themselves if infection control procedures are not followed, and the importance of compliance with recommended vaccination schedules (see Chapter 14, p. 302).

The potential hazards to health workers vary depending on the type of health facility. In general, staff are at a lower risk of infection than patients unless they have other underlying risk factors, such as depression of the immune system, a broken or weeping skin condition, or pregnancy.

Infection Control Procedures

The actual procedures that are followed may vary from one health care facility to another, but should all be based on sound microbiological principles. Using infection control guidelines published by the National Health and Medical Research Council and State health departments, hospitals develop specific procedures appropriate for their size and the particular types of patient under their care. Procedures common to most health care settings are described below.

HOSPITAL ASEPSIS

Asepsis refers to the absence of all disease-producing organisms. It is a relative term as, in practice, the complete absence of all microorganisms is difficult to sustain for long periods. In hospitals, two levels of asepsis are recognised: medical asepsis and surgical asepsis.

1. **Medical asepsis** refers to practices and procedures that *limit* the number of microorganisms present. It includes practices that are intended to confine microorganisms in a specific area, such as handwashing and good hygiene.
2. **Surgical asepsis** is intended to keep *all* microorganisms away from surgical wounds and tissues exposed during an operation. It requires that all instruments, gloves, surgical drapes, sutures, dressings and other items that come into contact with the patient must be *sterile* (i.e. completely free of all microorganisms and their spores). Surgical asepsis is practised in the operating room and in procedures such as the insertion of intravenous (IV) catheters.

Aseptic technique comprises protective measures designed to prevent infections or the spread of infections.

There is currently a trend towards 'deritualising' many of these procedures. Many practices that have traditionally been carried out have a rather dubious microbiological justification. Education and a thorough understanding of the methods of transmission should lead to more thoughtful and effective procedures being used.

HOSPITAL DISINFECTION AND STERILISATION

The use of disinfectants, antiseptics and different methods of sterilisation are all important in maintaining good aseptic technique. Bacteria do not multiply on clean, dry surfaces. They need a warm, moist environment in which to reproduce. If surfaces and equipment are kept clean, dry and well ventilated, their contribution as a source of infection is greatly reduced. Many hospitals have a central sterilising department (CSD) where equipment and supplies are cleaned and sterilised. The effectiveness of this department is monitored regularly by the microbiology laboratory. Most hospitals now use disposable pre-sterilised instruments, needle syringes, dressing packs and other items.

Medical asepsis can be maintained by the careful cleaning and disinfection of all surfaces and equipment that come into contact with the patient in a non-invasive manner. Careful handwashing and the use of disposable utensils assist in maintaining asepsis.

HOSPITAL CLEANING

Procedures for routine hospital cleaning are established by the hospital Infection Control Committee. In many hospitals most cleaning is carried out a using neutral detergent and water. The use of disinfectants is usually only necessary when contamination (e.g. with blood or body substances) has occurred. Sodium hypochlorite (bleach) is recommended for this purpose. The chlorine in household bleach is effective against HIV, hepatitis B and other viruses. Areas contaminated with blood or body substances should first be washed with soap and water and then treated with a fresh solution of 0.1% sodium hypochlorite. (Household bleach contains 5% available chlorine; a 1:50 dilution gives a 0.1% solution.) The use of gloves is recommended for all cleaning procedures.

Procedures for cleaning, disinfection and sterilisation are described fully in Chapter 11.

PROTECTIVE ASEPSIS

Patients whose immune system is compromised, either from illness or treatment, pose a particular problem in the hospital setting. They are extremely susceptible to infection by the many microorganisms to which they may be exposed, including opportunistic pathogens (i.e. microorganisms that cause infections mainly in immunodeficient hosts). These patients should be cared for using the principles of **protective asepsis**, or **reverse barrier nursing**. This means that an invisible 'barrier' is created between the patient and the rest of the hospital environment so that microorganisms cannot pass through and invade the patient.

However, these procedures do not protect patients from endogeneous infections (i.e. microorganisms derived from their own body or a recurrence of a latent infection). Frequently, these patients already have an infection (e.g. tuberculosis) that would be hazardous if transmitted to hospital personnel and/or other patients. Therefore, measures must also be taken to prevent the spread of this infection by containing it within the patient's environment. Protective asepsis is now generally taken to mean the prevention of the passage of microorganisms *in either direction* across the 'barrier'.

Prevention of Cross-infection

RISK ASSESSMENT

To evaluate the cross-infection risks involved in a particular situation, health workers should consider the following questions:

1. What is the risk of the patient acquiring an infection? It is necessary to assess factors relating to patient susceptibilty, such as the presence of a urinary catheter or IV line, the patient's immune status, underlying or

contributing illnesses, the presence of wounds or pressure sores, etc.

2. Is there a source (reservoir) of microorganisms?
   Potential sources should be identified (see Figure 13.3).
3. What are the risks of transmitting the infection?
   The actual procedures to be carried out when caring for the patient should be examined to assess their potential to spread microorganisms.
4. How can transmission be prevented?
   The protocols developed for the prevention of cross-infection are very similar in all hospitals. The infection control staff implement, modify and advise on procedures when necessary.

HANDWASHING

The oldest, simplest and single most effective method of preventing cross-infection is proper handwashing between each patient contact (see Table 13.6). Handwashing should be carried out immediately *before* and immediately *after* each patient contact. The first washing is to remove microorganisms that may have been picked up from the environment and thus prevent their transfer to the patient. Handwashing after patient contact removes organisms picked up from the patient and prevents their transfer to equipment or to other patients or staff.

Opinion varies considerably in different hospitals and in various parts of the world regarding the most efficient chemical agent to use for handwashing. Many people believe thorough washing with soap and water is satisfactory in most situations. It has been shown to remove transient microorganisms from the hands as well as some of the normal flora. Some hospitals favour the use of antiseptic handwashes, especially those with a residual action (i.e. they continue to act for a significant time after washing), such as chlorhexidine. These are especially useful for surgery, but continual use may sometimes cause skin problems. Damaged skin can then become colonised with potential pathogens and act as a dangerous source of infection.

In Germany, alcohols such as isopropanol, either alone or with chlorhexidine, are widely used. Alcohols have the advantage of drying very quickly but they also dry the skin. Various other antiseptics (e.g. povidone iodine) are also used for skin disinfection.

The most important aspect of handwashing is that staff comply with the guidelines recommended by their hospital or health care facility. Unfortunately, studies have shown that compliance does not always occur, but it is generally agreed that even an abbreviated handwash is preferable to not washing at all. Posters are often used to remind staff about the importance of handwashing.

Gloves are also an important means of reducing cross-infection but their use *does not remove the need for handwashing*. Handwashing should still be performed, preferably before and after using the gloves. *Gloves should also be changed between patients*. The aim is always to protect both the patient and the health care worker. Patients should also be instructed about the importance of handwashing. Many hospital-acquired infections are caused by the patient's normal flora and may actually be transmitted to a wound site (portal of entry) by the patient's own hands.

PROTECTIVE CLOTHING

Protective clothing is used in the hospital to:

- protect health care workers from having their hands, eyes or clothing contaminated by microorganisms from an infected patient;
- prevent microorganisms on health care workers' hands, clothing or body (respiratory tract) being transferred to a susceptible patient.

Protective clothing may comprise gloves, masks, gowns, goggles or eye protection, face shields, plastic aprons and overshoes.

Microorganisms are transported around the hospital on the clothing of the health care worker. Clean, freshly laundered clothing carries very few microorganisms. However the current practice is for hospital staff to 'live out' and to wear their uniforms outside the hospital environment—on public transport for example. The responsibility therefore lies with the health professionals for the cleanliness of their clothing and person. Inevitably, the uniforms will be contaminated with organisms derived from the environment outside the hospital. To a large extent these organisms are likely to be antibiotic-sensitive community strains. Their transmission can be largely prevented by the use of protective gowns or plastic aprons supplied by the hospital.

Gowns can also be used to limit the transfer of organisms from an infectious patient to the clothing of the health worker, and their subsequent spread around the hospital. The use of protective gowns and aprons therefore contributes to the practice of protective asepsis, that is, creating a barrier between the source of an infection and a susceptible host. However, it is important that the gowns are used correctly, that they are put on and removed so that other clothing is not contaminated. Also, if they have been used while caring for an infectious patient, they must be left in the infectious area or put in the appropriate laundry container and not worn around the hospital. If a gown becomes wet, the protective effect is lost, as microorganisms can pass through wet material.

The use of gowns has obvious benefits, but there is considerable discussion about the usefulness of masks in the prevention of cross-infection. Masks are used routinely in surgery and for other procedures where there is thought to be a risk of microorganisms from the nose/throat of the health worker being transmitted to the patient. Masks can also guard against microorganisms from an infectious patient entering the respiratory tract of the health worker, although they are not very effective in preventing staff from exposure to TB. In practice, most masks have been shown to be somewhat ineffective as bacterial filters, especially when moist. The universal habit of continually adjusting masks may in fact transfer microorganisms to the hands of the health worker, where they are potentially

TABLE 13.6
HAND WASHING TECHNIQUES

TYPE	TECHNIQUE (HOW)	DURATION	DRYING	EXAMPLE (WHEN)
Routine hand wash	Wet hands thoroughly and lather vigorously using neutral pH soap. Rinse under running water. Do not touch taps with clean hands —if elbow or foot controls are not available, use paper towel to turn taps off.	10–15 seconds	Pat dry using paper towel	Before eating or smoking After going to the toilet Before significant contact with patients e.g. physical examination, emptying a drainage reservoir (catheter bag) Before injection or venipuncture Before and after routine use of gloves After handling any instruments or equipment soiled with blood or body substances.
Hand wash prior to aseptic procedures (non-surgical)	Wash hands thoroughly using an anti-microbial soap or skin cleanser. Rinse carefully. Do not touch taps with clean hands —if elbow or foot controls are not available use paper towel to turn taps off.	1 minute	Pat dry using paper towel	Before any non-surgical procedures which require aseptic techniques (such as inserting intravenous catheters)
Surgical wash	Wash hands, nails and forearms thoroughly and apply an anti-microbial skin cleanser (containing 4% w/v chlorhexidine or detergent based povidone iodine containing 0.75% available iodine). Rinse carefully, keeping hands above the elbows. No-touch techniques apply.	First wash for the day 5 minutes and subsequent washes 3 minutes	Dry with sterile towels	Before any invasive surgical procedure (operating room procedures)

Source: NH&MRC, Infection Control in the Health Care Setting, April 1996.

more hazardous. There is considerable discussion about the value of protective clothing, especially masks, in the prevention of cross-infection. Overshoes have largely been discarded and it may be that the use of gowns could also be rationalised. In general, when selecting the type of protective attire to be used, consideration should be given to the probability of exposure to infection, especially from blood and other body substances. The selection of appropriate protection (disposable or reusable gowns, gloves, masks, goggles, etc.) is determined by the *risk* of exposure and the *amount* of body fluids likely to be encountered. This is discussed further in the next section.

The use of protective clothing by staff is sometimes seen as creating a psychological problem for patients, who are already feeling isolated in a strange environment. For this reason, health workers should ensure they use only the appropriate clothing and explain its use to the patient.

UNIVERSAL PRECAUTIONS

Before the outbreak of HIV/AIDS, hospitals had a number of different procedures to prevent the transmission of various types of organisms. These were based on the guidelines proposed by the Centers for Disease Control (CDC) in 1983. These guidelines recommended that hospitals should adopt one of two systems.

1. **Category-specific isolation precautions**, which included:

- Strict Isolation
- Respiratory Isolation

- Enteric Precautions
- Contact Isolation
- Tuberculosis Isolation
- Drainage Secretion Precautions
- Blood/Body Fluid Precautions.

Within these categories, specific diseases were listed, together with the secretions, excretions, body fluids and tissues that are, or might be, infective for each disease.

2. **Disease-specific isolation precautions**, which allowed for a more specific set of instructions to be implemented for each disease.

Hospitals were free to implement appropriate infection control procedures using the CDC guidelines. Generally, hospitals in Australia adopted infection control procedures similar to those recommended by the CDC.

In 1987, the CDC issued a document, *Recommendations for Prevention of Transmission of HIV in Health Care Settings*. This document recommended that Blood and Body Fluid Precautions be used for all patients *regardless of their infection status*. The extension of these precautions to *all* patients was referred to as **Universal Blood and Body Fluid Precautions.** Under the CDC Universal Precautions, blood and *certain* body fluids of all patients are considered potentially infectious for HIV, hepatitis B virus (HBV) and other blood-borne pathogens. A report from CDC in June 1988 listed the body fluids included in Universal Precautions and outlined other infection control measures for blood-borne pathogens.

The discovery of the human immunodeficiency virus (HIV), a hitherto unknown deadly virus that is found in blood and body fluids, drew attention to the fact that there could be many other viruses and microorganisms with the potential to cause disease, but which have not yet been described. Even more importantly, there are many situations where patients may be infectious despite being asymptomatic (i.e. they show no evidence of infection). This is true during the incubation period or when a person is a carrier of the disease. Hepatitis C has now been placed in the same category as hepatitis B and HIV—that is, viruses that are transmitted by contact with blood or other body substances from infected carriers.

AUSTRALIAN GUIDELINES

In Australia, the Universal Precautions recommended by CDC were extended to include 'all blood, body fluids and body substances', and the National Health and Medical Research Council (NH&MRC) and the Australian Council on AIDS (ANCA) issued a joint document on infection control in 1993 (NH&MRC, 1993). However, due to the changing patterns of health care, professional responsibiities and perceived risks of infection, there was a need to review the guidelines. The NH&MRC and ANCA established a working party to carry out the review, resulting in the publication of the joint document, *Infection control in the health care setting—Guidelines for the prevention of transmission of infectious diseases* (NH&MRC, April 1996).

This document provides current technical information on best practice for infection control, and aims to establish a nationally accepted minimum standard for infection control. The implementation of the guidelines is the responsibility of individual health care establishments.

The following is an extract from the Australian Guidelines. They set out to provide:

> 'A practical approach to health care involving risk assessment and risk management, based on strategies which minimise the risk of infection for both patients and health care workers. Risk minimisation strategies historically included the adoption of "Universal Precautions", a concept defined in Australia as work practices which assumed that all blood and body substances were a potential risk of infection, independent of perceived risk.
>
> However, in Australia it was perceived that the term "Universal Precautions" was ambiguous, resulting in some confusion and a false sense of security in its application. Some health care workers appeared to consider the use of gloves to be a substitute for hand washing, and there was concern that this mistaken perception could increase the risk of nosocomial transmission of infection.
>
> As an alternative to the term "Universal Precautions" the NH&MRC council and ANCA recommends adoption of the terms 'Standard Precautions" (applied as the first line approach to infection control) and "Additional Precautions" where Standard Precautions may be insufficient to prevent transmission of infection particularly via the airborne route. This change in terminology reflecting a two-tiered approach based on modes of disease transmission, is in line with changes in terminology adopted by the US Centers for Disease Control and Prevention.'
>
> NH&MRC, April 1996 page 1.

The recommendations are set out in Spotlight box, p. 286.

Health care workers should be aware that these guidelines may need to be updated from time to time.

STANDARD PRECAUTIONS

Universal Precautions were originally developed to protect the health worker from the risk of transmission of blood-borne pathogens from a patient. However, these procedures are designed to also prevent staff-to-patient transmission as well as patient-to-patient transmission. The current Australian guidelines cover all pathogens that are likely to be present in *any type of body fluid or substance*. Standard Precautions, therefore, should also protect against the transmission of pathogens such as cytomegalovirus (CMV) in urine or saliva as well as pathogens that may be present in the body fluids of an asymptomatic patient. However, the pathogens of most concern are HIV, hepatitis B and hepatitis C.

There is a slight, but real, risk of transmission of blood-borne pathogens (such as hepatitis B or HIV) from an infected health worker to a patient. CDC have published guidelines dealing with this situation and the Australian health departments, both Federal and State, have also issued

STANDARD PRECAUTIONS

Standard Precautions are work practices required for the basic level of infection control. They include good hygiene practices, particularly washing and drying hands before and after patient contact, the use of protective barriers which may include gloves, gowns, plastic aprons, masks, eye shields or goggles, appropriate handling and disposal of sharps and other contaminated or infectious waste, and use of aseptic techniques. Standard Precautions include 'Enteric Precautions'.

Standard Precautions are recommended for the treatment and care of all patients, regardless of their perceived infectious status, and in the handling of:

- blood;
- all other body fluids, secretions and excretions (excluding sweat), regardless of whether they contain visible blood;
- non-intact skin; and
- mucous membranes.

Standard Precautions also apply to dried blood and other body substances, including saliva.

ADDITIONAL PRECAUTIONS

Additional Precautions are used for patients known or suspected to be infected or colonised with epidemiologically important or highly transmissible pathogens that can cause infection.

- by air-borne transmission (e.g. *Mycobacterium tuberculosis*, measles virus, chickenpox virus); or
- by droplet transmission (e.g. mumps, rubella, pertussis, influenza); or
- by direct or indirect contact with dry skin (e.g. colonisation with MRSA), or with contaminated surfaces; or
- by any combination of these routes.

Additional Precautions are designed to interrupt transmission of infection by these routes and should be used in addition to Standard Precautions when transmission of infection might not be contained by using Standard Precautions alone. Additional Precautions may be specific to the situation for which they are required, or may be combined where microorganisms have multiple routes of transmission.

Source: NH&MRC, Infection Control in the Health Care Setting, April 1996.

statements. Dental patients are considered to be at greatest risk because of the invasive nature of dental treatment and the risk of injury to the dentist as well as patient. The Dental Registration Board in each State has regulations for registration of dentists and recommends vaccination for hepatitis B and the use of an autoclave for the sterilisation of all instruments.

These regulations are also designed to protect against the transmission of other pathogens that may be present in blood or other body fluids of a person who is already infected, is incubating a disease, is a carrier, or is asymptomatic.

There has so far been only one documented case of HIV transmission from health worker to patient worldwide, but a case of transmission of HIV from one patient to another due to a breakdown in surgical aseptic technique was recorded in Australia in 1993. In many cases, it is very difficult to establish definitely the source of an infection and it may be that instances of transmission of HIV infection are more frequent. Health departments require all health practitioners to know their own status with regard to the blood-borne pathogens, HIV, HBV and HCV, to follow infection control guidelines, to exercise the duty of care and, if they are a carrier of HIV, HBV or HCV, to refrain from carrying out exposure-prone procedures.

ADDITIONAL PRECAUTIONS

The implementation of Standard Precautions is the primary strategy for the successful control of nosocomial and iatrogenic infections. However, it should be remembered that Additional precautions may be required for a patient with a suspected or confirmed infection which is carried by the airborne or droplet route. Respiratory infections such as tuberculosis are difficult to contain unless the patient is isolated. A private room with appropriate ventilation and the wearing of masks by susceptible people may be necessary. Additional precautions should also be used where patients are colonised by epidemiologically significant pathogens such as MRSA. Similarly, an infection involving excessive shedding of skin cells may also require isolation. Infections such as diarrhoea or viral gastroenteritis which are transmitted by the faecal-oral route may require a single room with dedicated toilet facilities.

Ideally, it is preferable to care for a patient with an infectious disease in a single room. However, for a variety of reasons, this may not always be possible or desirable. With a thoughtful approach to infection control it is often possible to create an effective 'barrier' between the source of the infection and the environment. The implementation of the barrier will depend on the type of infection and the way it is transmitted as well as an analysis of perceived risk factors.

The current approach to infection control requires that the infection control procedures to be implemented are assessed individually for each patient. Standard Precautions should be applied to all patients whether a symptomatic infection is present or not. The need to contain an infection means that patients may be cared for differently, depending on such factors as their dependence on staff, whether they are losing excessive blood or other fluids, their ability to comply with personal hygiene, whether they are mobile and other relevant factors. For example, during a seasonal outbreak of an infection, it may be possible to nurse 'in cohort'; that is, patients with the same infection can be accommodated in the same room.

Patients with a highly communicable disease, such as active tuberculosis or MRSA, should be kept in isolation until they are deemed not to pose a significant risk to other patients or personnel. For identifiable bacterial diseases that can be treated with antibiotics, the patient is not considered infectious once therapy is established and symptoms are alleviated. For viral infections there is usually no effective therapy, so patients are considered to be infectious until asymptomatic. Obviously, a patient suffering from an unknown infection should be isolated until a diagnosis is made or symptoms disappear. It should be remembered, however, that in some diseases (e.g. typhoid fever), carriage or shedding of the organisms can occur well after clinical recovery. In such cases, patients continue to be a source of infection even though they may be asymptomatic.

Specific Problems in Infection Control

Although the general principles of transmission and cross-infection (described above) apply to all areas of the hospital, there are various situations where additional precautions need to be taken. In these situations, patients are particularly susceptible to infections because of the nature of their treatment, the state of their immune system or the type of microorganisms to which they are exposed (see Spotlight Box on MRSA, pp. 272–73). One important consideration is that some units of the hospital are more likely than others to harbour a population of resistant organisms. These tend to be units where there are seriously ill or compromised patients and thus an associated high level of antibiotic usage. Staff working in these units are much more likely to be nasal carriers of resistant organisms with the potential to spread them around the hospital. Continual surveillance of hospital staff would help to prevent this kind of cross-infection. We now look at some specific examples.

OPERATING THEATRES/SURGICAL PATIENTS

Operating theatres are a potential source of infection as the patient's external defences are breached during surgery. In general, there are two types of surgical patients:

1. Patients undergoing elective surgery.
   When these patients enter hospital, they are colonised by their own normal flora. The longer their stay in hospital, either preoperatively or postoperatively, the greater the possibility that some of their own (mainly antibiotic-sensitive) population of normal flora will be replaced by the (largely antibiotic-resistant) hospital organisms. These patients have what are generally regarded as 'clean' wounds—that is, wounds where infection would not be expected unless they became contaminated during surgery.
2. Patients undergoing surgery because of some trauma or accident.
   These patients may already have injuries or breaks in their skin which have allowed microorganisms to breach the body's defences and enter the tissues. These microorganisms could be derived from the patient's normal flora, but may also include exogenous microorganisms from the environment. The wound site may be contaminated or an infection may already be established. If the site of injury is already infected, the surgery is considered to be 'dirty'. Patients with dirty wounds are usually given prophylactic antibiotics prior to surgery (see Chapter 12).

Patients may develop postsurgical infections at the site of the wound. These may be caused by bacteria from their own body (elective surgery), bacteria from their own skin *and* from the environment (in the case of accident/trauma surgery), or bacteria derived from the air or personnel in the operating theatre (in both types of surgery). As many as 50% of hospital personnel carry *Staphylococcus aureus* in the nose or on broken skin, and *Clostridium perfringens* (the most important cause of gas gangrene) is commonly carried in the human intestine. Both these organisms can be regularly found in the air of operating theatres. Occasionally, wounds can become contaminated by exposure to non-sterile surfaces or equipment.

Reduction of wound infection rates

The risk of surgically acquired infections can be reduced by various methods. Operating theatres are cleaned after each operation or as indicated by the nature of the medical risk involved. All personnel wear sterile gowns, masks and gloves. Medical and nursing staff scrub hands and arms with antiseptic wash before gloving. All equipment, drapes, sutures and dressings that come into contact with the patient are sterilised. However, the value of some of the procedures used to reduce the traffic of microorganisms from the outside environment into the operating theatre on trolleys or on the clothing and shoes of theatre personnel, has been questioned, as it is thought they do not contribute significantly to hospital-acquired infection. Some hospitals use a filtered air flow system into the operating suites, and overnight disinfection with UV light to minimise the number of microorganisms in the air space.

Patients should be carefully monitored after surgery for any sign of wound infection. Inflammation, drainage from the suture line, purulent discharge and fever are all indicators of infection. If the wound is infected, a swab is taken and sent to the microbiology laboratory for identification of the causative organism and determination of antibiotic sensitivities.

Reduced hospital stay

Wound infections are potentially more serious, even life-threatening, when the infection is due to a resistant hospital organism. One way in which this problem has been addressed is by minimising the patient's stay in hospital, especially preoperatively. Previously, patients undergoing major operations (e.g. open heart surgery) were admitted two to three days before the operation in order to carry out tests and stabilise the patient. However, it was found that this allowed time for patients to become colonised with resistant hospital organisms, replacing their own normal flora. If wound contamination occurred, the outcome was often quite serious. Patients for major surgery are now admitted as close as possible to the time of surgery, to minimise exposure to hospital strains.

Prophylactic antibiotics

The use of prophylactic antibiotics in all surgical cases has been widely discussed. Their use for surgery of previously contaminated sites is obviously indicated. They are also useful for surgery on the bowel or genital tract where there is already a large population of resident normal flora that may be released into the body cavity. However, widespread use of antibiotics for all types of surgery creates a dilemma—it has the potential to lead to an increase in resistant bacterial strains that pose a threat, not only to the individual patient, but also to the hospital environment; on the other hand, the medical profession is increasingly aware of the risks of litigation if preventive treatment is not given (see Chapter 12).

THE BURNS UNIT

The survival rate of patients with extensive burns has improved in recent years, partly because of improved infection control practices, as well as new treatments. Burns vary in their degree of severity, depending on the cause of the burn and the area of the body that is affected. A large percentage of children admitted to accident and emergency are suffering from burns caused by boiling water, which can cause extensive damage to children's delicate skin. Inhalation burns from smoke or fire damage the epithelial lining of the lungs and may predispose to pneumonia.

Patients suffering from burns to a large part of their body are at an increased risk of infection since one of the primary body defences (an intact skin) has been destroyed (see Chapter 9). Shock and fluid loss mean that the patient may also be receiving IV fluids, which creates another possible point of entry for microorganisms. The burn site itself provides a moist area, full of nutrients, ideal for the growth of organisms. In addition, the nature of the tissue damage means that phagocytic cells and antibodies are unable to reach the damaged area and prevent bacterial multiplication from taking place.

When burns become infected, it is difficult to treat them with systemic antibiotics because damage to the vascular tissue around the burn site prevents the antibiotics from reaching the infection. Similarly, topical application of antibiotics is not always successful because of large quantities of dead tissue. The two most common organisms found in infected burns are *Pseudomonas aeruginosa* and *Staphylococcus aureus*. Both of these pathogens have strains which are resistant to many antibiotics and some disinfectants. It is therefore very important to maintain asepsis in a burns unit.

As the burns unit can be such a significant source of antibiotic-resistant microorganisms, staff should exercise appropriate infection control precautions when moving from burns units to areas of the hospital that have particularly susceptible patients (e.g. transplant units, oncology and ICU).

INTENSIVE CARE UNITS

Patients in intensive care units (ICUs) are usually seriously ill and so their body defences are highly compromised. The invasive nature of their treatment, which may involve procedures such as intubation and the use of ventilators and monitoring equipment, renders patients in ICUs very susceptible to hospital-acquired infections.

Usually, patients in ICUs are receiving a number of different medications, administered for convenience via a central venous catheter. A recent study in Australia (Collignon 1994) showed that these catheters are associated with a high level of sepsis, which, in other countries, has been correlated with high rates of morbidity and mortality. Central vein catheters carry a much higher risk of causing infection than peripheral vein catheters. Sepsis associated with peripheral vein catheters can be reduced by adhering to strict infection control protocols. Control of sepsis in central catheters is more difficult because the patient is usually seriously ill and the catheter may need to be in place for a longer period. The length of time the catheter is in place affects the likelihood of infection and opinions vary about the optimum time for replacement of catheters.

The most common organisms associated with infections are *Staphylococcus aureus* and coagulase negative staphylococci. Sepsis due to *Candida albicans* is found with central catheters but is not common with peripheral vein catheters. Unfortunately, due to the high antibiotic usage in ICUs, many of the infections acquired there are caused by resistant organisms. Staff who work in these units are also often colonised by antibiotic-resistant pathogens. Handwashing, the maintenance of strict aseptic technique and the use of protective clothing (gowns) are essential to minimise the risk of infection. Special care should be taken when handling intravenous catheters.

TRANSPLANT AND ONCOLOGY WARDS

Patients in transplant and oncology wards, in addition to being critically ill, are usually being treated with immunosuppressive drugs. These wards are thus important areas of the hospital where opportunistic infections and resistant organisms can flourish, and patients require special care to prevent cross-infection.

MATERNITY WARDS

Patients in a maternity ward are often thought of as 'well' because their hospitalisation is not due to an illness. However, there are significant infection risks associated with childbirth. These include infections that may occur at the site of a caesarean section, or in the perineal area where tearing or tissue damage may occur. A significant number of women carry potentially pathogenic microorganisms (e.g. *Streptococci* spp.) in the normal flora of the vagina and these can readily invade damaged tissue. Faecal bacteria can also contaminate the wound. *Streptococci* are usually responsible for puerpural or childbed fever which, until the 1930s, carried a 10% mortality rate; it is now relatively uncommon in developed countries.

Care of the patient involves education about personal hygiene and careful monitoring for any signs of infection (e.g. fever, inflammation, pus). Patients should also be instructed about breast care, as cracked nipples can lead to mastitis (infection of the milk glands). Although these infections are often caused by normal flora there is a real risk that hospital strains can be transported to the mother, either on the nurse's hands or on the baby which has been handled in a communal nursery. Standard Precautions should be observed for all blood and body substances.

Neonatal infections

All women carry a population of normal flora in the vagina. Most of these organisms do not pose any infection risk to either mother or baby. However, sometimes the mother is carrying opportunistic pathogens in the vagina, or has acquired a sexually transmitted disease. Babies born to infected mothers are at risk of being infected either transplacentally or during passage through the birth canal. These infections include organisms such as *Candida albicans* (thrush), herpes simplex virus, Group B *Streptococci*, *Chlamydia*, *Mycoplasma*, *Neisseria gonorrhoea*, *Treponema pallidum* (syphilis), hepatitis B and HIV/AIDS.

All of these infections are very serious for the neonate whose immune system is immature and who may not have maternal antibodies for protection. Some of these infections are highly contagious and can be transmitted to other babies in the nursery, usually on the hands of hospital staff. Organisms can enter through the eyes, umbilicus or any breaks in the skin. Infections such as herpes are easily transmitted; babies must be isolated if possible and the mothers instructed about the disease and ways to prevent transmission.

Neonates are also at risk of acquiring hospital infections caused by *E. coli, Staphylococcus aureus* and many other pathogens. Neonates should be regarded as particularly susceptible because of their immature immune system, and the constant handling they receive. Isolation, handwashing, and careful hygiene procedures when handling nappies, are essential to prevent the spread of infection.

A SPECIAL PROBLEM WITH CHILDREN

Everything we have said about the prevention of cross-infection applies to paediatric wards, but there are some additional factors to be considered. Children are highly mobile. Adults can usually be expected to stay in one place but children are very active and are therefore more likely to spread an infection around a ward. Spills and injuries often occur when staff have to control struggling, frightened children. In particular, needlestick (sharps) injuries and body fluids and substance exposures are likely to be more common, and staff must be encouraged to report all incidents. It is often more difficult with children to contain faeces, vomitus and other excreta. Small children tend to put articles such as toys in their mouth and this facilitates the spread of organisms that may be present in the saliva or respiratory secretions. Unless careful infection control procedures are followed, respiratory infections and gastrointestinal infections, such as rotavirus, can easily spread.

During epidemic outbreaks of diseases such as RSV (respiratory syncytial virus) in the winter months, hospitals may be besieged with cases. Isolation may not be possible and it may be necessary to nurse 'in cohort' (i.e. place patients with the same infection in the same ward) or with other patients who are immune.

Occasionally, children may develop an infectious disease such as chickenpox after admission for some other procedure. It is then necessary to identify all susceptible patients and staff and take steps to protect them from this highly contagious disease. A vaccine for chickenpox will soon be available in Australia and would be advisable for non-immune staff. Leukaemia patients are particularly susceptible to infection and need to be protected from contact with people who may be infectious. Each situation needs to be assessed carefully by the infection control team.

Occupational Exposure for Hospital Staff

The hospital environment may be hazardous, not only for patients, but also for staff, so all health workers need a good understanding of the potential risks involved in the work they do. In general, hospital staff are healthy and thus have very low susceptibility when exposed to the many pathogens found in hospital. However, they should be up to date with the immunisation schedule recommended by the Department of Health for tuberculosis and hepatitis B, as well as for the usual childhood diseases. Exposure to blood-borne pathogens such as hepatitis B and C and HIV poses a significant risk and all staff should be educated about observing Standard Precautions. This is particularly important for staff responsible for the disposal of contaminated waste.

NEEDLESTICK INJURIES

A major risk factor is the occurrence of needlestick injuries; that is, when a health worker is accidentally cut or pricked by a sharp object, usually a needle, that has been contaminated by blood or body substance. Hospital guidelines require that needles should *not* be resheathed and that all sharps should be disposed of in a sharps container. In paediatric wards, injuries may be caused by safety pins used for nappies, or by biting and scratching by struggling children. The use of non-pin nappy fasteners is one way to reduce this risk.

Nevertheless, many health workers still receive needlestick injuries and they should always be reported. Each hospital has its own procedures for assessing the situation, and the worker may be offered prophylactic treatment if the injury is known to have been caused by a sharp from a patient with hepatitis B or HIV. It should be noted here that health workers should be immunised against hepatitis B. If injury does occur and the staff member is not immunised, hyperimmune anti-hepatitis B globulin can be administered.

In the case of HIV, antiretroviral (zidovudine) therapy is available, but to be effective should be initiated within hours of injury. Data on the protective efficacy of administration of this drug are still limited, and staff are usually counselled at the time of injury before deciding to undertake the therapy, which has some side effects. At present, there is no treatment for hepatitis C.

TUBERCULOSIS

Another major risk to health workers is exposure to tuberculosis (TB), which is an increasing problem. After its virtual eradication in Australia in the 1950s by a mass X-ray screening and immunisation campaign, there has been a resurgence of the disease. This is due partly to travellers bringing in the disease from Asian countries where it is endemic. Patients who are immunodeficient are particularly susceptible to infection or reactivation of latent TB and thus can act as a potent reservoir of the organism in the hospital environment.

Most staff are tested for previous exposure to TB (Mantoux test) and if negative are advised to have the BCG vaccination against TB. There is some difference of opinion regarding the value of vaccination and recommendations vary in different States (see Chapter 14). At present, the multi-resistant strains that are common in the United States have not reached Australia.

RISKS ASSOCIATED WITH PREGNANCY

Health care workers who are pregnant should be aware of the possible congenital effects of some infections. Rubella is most likely to be found in children and all health workers (male and female) who are working with chidren are advised to be immunised.

Cytomegalovirus (CMV) is a mild infection in children or adults but can cause severe infections in immuno-compromised patients. Women contracting CMV during pregnancy risk serious damage to the foetus (see Chapter 19). CMV infection, which may often be asymptomatic, is transmitted in body fluids and so staff can minimise risks by following Standard Precautions, especially for urine and saliva.

Chickenpox can be a serious illness in pregnancy and workers who are not immune should avoid contact with children. Staff can discuss the occupational exposure risks associated with pregnancy with the infection control team.

Summary

- Nosocomial infections (hospital-acquired infections) are infections acquired by patients in a hospital or other health facility.
- Infections that are acquired in non-hospitalised people are called community-acquired infections.

THE IMPORTANCE OF NOSOCOMIAL INFECTIONS

- The incidence of hospital-acquired infection in hospitals is generally around 5–6%, but in critical care units can be as high as 20%.
- Nosocomial infections increase patient suffering, prolong the length of hospital stay and increase the cost of medical care.

TYPES OF NOSOCOMIAL INFECTIONS

- The most common sites of nosocomial infections are the urinary tract, surgical wounds, lower respiratory tract, skin and blood.

CAUSATIVE AGENTS

- Bacteria are the most common cause of nosocomial infections, followed by fungi and viruses.
- In immunocompromised patients, organisms such as enterococci, mycobacteria, fungi and certain viruses frequently cause infections.
- Methicillin-resistant *Staphylococcus aureus* (MRSA) emerged in the mid-1970s in Australia and is still a major concern in hospital infection control.

THE NATURE OF HOSPITAL PATHOGENS

- Community strains are organisms that originate from outside the hospital and are generally sensitive to most antimicrobial drugs.
- Hospital strains originate from within the hospital and can be difficult to treat because they are frequently resistant to antimicrobial drugs and disinfectants.

COLONISATION

- Colonisation refers to the presence and growth of a microorganism on the skin or mucous membrane without infection. Major sites are the nose, skin, oropharynx, lower intestine and urinary tract.
- Colonisation with hospital strains can occur after admission and becomes more likely the longer the stay in hospital. Exposure to antimicrobial drugs also favours colonisation.
- Hospital staff are frequently colonised by hospital organisms and are thus carriers of these potential pathogens.
- Patients with lowered resistance (e.g. surgical or burns patients) may be infected by a multi-resistant hospital strain, and then become an important reservoir of these organisms.
- The transmission of organisms from one person to another, causing infection in the second, is called cross-infection.

THE HIGH INCIDENCE OF NOSOCOMIAL INFECTIONS: CONTRIBUTORY FACTORS

- Drug-resistant strains of microorganisms are more likely to persist in a hospital where large amounts of antimicrobial drugs are used.
- Many hospital patients have lowered resistance to infection due to age (young or old), immobility, underlying disease or infection, or surgical or traumatic wounds.
- Medical treatments can lower a patient's resistance to infection: these include cancer therapy, immuno-suppressive drugs, anti-inflammatory drugs and some antimicrobial drugs.
- Diagnostic and therapeutic procedures (e.g. injections, the use of intravascular and urinary catheters, endotracheal tubes and drainages, and endoscopes) involve the penetration of the protective skin and mucous membrane barriers.
- Infections that are brought about by some medical procedure or treatment are called iatrogenic infections.
- Implanted prostheses are favoured sites of colonisation by microorganisms.
- Nosocomial infections may be exogenous (derived from outside the patient's body, e.g. from other patients or staff or the hospital environment) or endogenous (derived from the patient's own body).
- Clean, dry surfaces are not a significant source of microorganisms unless freshly contaminated, but the numbers of microorganisms contaminating moist areas or objects may be very high.

CROSS-INFECTION IN HOSPITALS

- Cross-infection involves the infection of a susceptible patient by the transfer of organisms from another patient. The risk of cross-infection varies among hospital facilities.
- Microorganisms can be spread on hands, clothing, equipment and utensils, air currents and contaminated material.
- In most large city hospitals the policies and procedures for infection control are the responsibility of the Infection Control Committee.
- The infection control team monitors the incidence of infections within the hospital and conducts information sessions for hospital staff.
- The Microbiology Department is responsible for identifying the pathogen causing the infection and informing the infection control team, so that appropriate infection control measures can be taken.

INFECTION CONTROL PROCEDURES

- Asepsis refers to the absence of all disease-producing organisms.

- Medical asepsis refers to practices and procedures that *limit* the number of microorganisms present.
- Surgical asepsis is intended to keep *all* microoganisms away.
- Aseptic technique comprises protective measures designed to prevent infections or the spread of infections.
- Methods for cleaning, disinfection and sterilisation are contained in each hospital's infection control manual.
- Patients whose immune system is compromised need to be protected from infection.

PREVENTION OF CROSS INFECTION

- The health worker needs to evaluate the risks of transmission for each patient.
- Handwashing is the most effective method of preventing cross-infection.
- Gloves are an important means of reducing cross-infection but their use does not remove the need for handwashing.
- Various kinds of protective clothing are worn to prevent the spread of microorganisms.
- Standard Precautions are a set of procedures to be followed to prevent patient-to-staff, staff-to-patient and patient-to-patient transmission of pathogens present in blood or any body substances, especially HIV, HBV, HCV, and CMV.
- Additional precautions may be required for a patient with an infection carried by the air-borne route, such as pulmonary tuberculosis.
- Infection control procedures should be used for all patients until they are deemed to be no longer infectious.

SPECIFIC PROBLEMS IN INFECTION CONTROL

- Patients in some units of the hospital are more susceptible to infection than others (e.g. surgical patients, because their defences have been breached).
- Various methods have been introduced to reduce the incidence of postoperative wound infections, such as attention to sterilisation and disinfection, reduced hospital stays and the use of prophylactic antimicrobial drugs.
- Other patients who are particularly susceptible to infection are those with burns, those in intensive care units, the immunocompromised, and those who are susceptible because of the nature of the treatment they require.
- Infection risks in maternity and neonatal wards include post-partum infections of the mother as well as the baby.
- There are special risk factors associated with paediatric wards, because of the nature of children.

OCCUPATIONAL EXPOSURE FOR HOSPITAL STAFF.

- Hospital staff are at risk of becoming infected via needlestick injuries and exposure to respiratory diseases such as TB.
- Staff should be fully immunised.
- Pregnant staff should be aware of the infection risks associated with pregnancy.

Study Questions

1. Differentiate between nosocomial infections and community-acquired infections.
2. What was the major contribution of Ignaz Semmelweis to hospital infection control?
3. List the common types of nosocomial infections.
4. What is MRSA?
5. What is an important difference between hospital strains of bacteria and community strains?
6. What is meant by colonisation in relation to microorganisms and the human body?
7. What factors favour colonisation?
8. List the factors that can make a patient immunocompromised.
9. What is a iatrogenic infection? Give three examples.
10. Define the terms 'exogenous infection', 'endogenous infection' and 'cross-infection'.
11. What are the important sources of organisms that cause exogenous infections in hospitalised people?
12. Dry objects and surfaces do not generally support the growth of microorganisms, but can still act as a source of infection. Explain.
13. List the common ways that microorganisms can be spread in the hospital.
14. What are the major responsibilities of a hospital's Infection Control Committee?
15. Define the terms 'asepsis' and 'aseptic technique'?
16. What is meant by the term 'protective asepsis'?
17. Handwashing at the appropriate times is an extremely important means of reducing cross-infection in hospitals. When are the appropriate times? Explain your answer.
18. Describe the basic principles of Standard and Additional Precautions, and explain why they are necessary.
19. What procedures are followed in Standard Precautions?
20. Describe the major ways by which the incidence of surgical wound infections can be reduced?
21. List the types of patients that are particularly susceptible to hospital-acquired infections.
22. What procedures are used to reduce the incidence of needlestick injuries?
23. What types of infections are particularly serious if contracted while pregnant?

Test Your Understanding

1. Why do drug-resistant strains of microorganisms cause so many hospital infections?
2. Why are hospital-acquired infections often more serious than those acquired in the community?
3. Explain why patients in the burns unit are particularly susceptible to infection.
4. Explain the difference between medical asepsis and surgical asepsis.
5. What special precautions should be used when caring for a patient who is immunocompromised?
6. Discuss the merits of the various types of protective clothing that can be worn by health workers.

REFERENCES

1. McLaws, M., J. Gold, K. King, L.M. Irwig & G. Berry, 1988, 'The prevalence of nosocomial and community acquired infections in Australian hospitals'. *Medical Journal of Australia*, 149, pp. 582–590.
2. Mayon-White, R.T., G. Ducel, T. Kereselidze & E. Tikomirov, 1988, 'An international survey of the prevalence of hospital acquired infection'. *Journal of Hospital Infection*, 11, (suppl. A) pp. 43–48.
3. Haley, R.W., D.R. Schaberg & K.B. Crossley, 1981, Extra charges and prolongation of stay attributable to nosocomial infections: a prospective interhospital comparison. *American Journal of Medicine*, 70:51–58.
4. Wenzel, R.P. (ed), 1987, *Prevention & Control of Nosocomial Infections*. Baltimore: Williams & Wilkins.

FURTHER READING

CDC: 1987, Recommendations for the prevention of transmission of HIV in health-care settings. *MMWR* 6: Suppl. 25:1S-18S.

CDC: Update: 1988, Universal precautions for prevention of transmission of human immunodeficiency virus, hepatitis B virus and other blood-borne pathogens in health care settings. *MMWR* 37:377–388.

CDC Guidelines, 1983, *Infection Control* 4: 249–325.

Collignon, P.J., 1994, Intravascular catheter associated sepsis. *Medical Journal of Australia*, 161:374-378. (This article reports on a study of data from 15 hospitals throughout Australia to estimate the number of episodes of intravascular catheter associated sepsis that occur per year.)

Faoagali, J.L., M.L. Thang & D. Grant, 1992, Ten years' experience with methicillin-resistant Staphylococcus aureus in a large Australian hospital. *Journal of Hospital Infection*, 20:113–119. (This articles reports the occurrence of MRSA in Royal Brisbane Hospital from 1979 to 1989.)

Mallon, D.F.J., W. Shearwood, S.A. Mallal, M.A.H. French & R.L. Dawkins, 1992, Exposure to blood borne infections in health care workers. *Medical Journal of Australia*, 157:592–595. (This article reports on the incidence and nature of occupational exposures to blood and body fluids in health care workers in a large Australian hospital.)

National Health and Medical Research Council and Australian National Council on AIDS, 1993, *Management Guidelines for the Control of Infectious Disease Hazards in Health Care Establishments*. Canberra: Australian Government Publishing Service.

National Health and Medical Research Council and Australian National Council on AIDS, 1996, *Infection control in the health care setting—Guidelines for the prevention of transmission of infectious diseases*. Canberra: Australian Government Publishing Service. (This comprehensive document replaces the guidelines from 1993, and introduces new terminology for methods of infection control. It details the types of infections that can be transmitted in health care establishments, the modes of transmission of infectious diseases, risks assessment, and methods for prevention of cross infection.)

Selwyn, S., 1991, Hospital infection: the first 2500 years. *Journal of Hospital Infection*, 18 (suppl. A):5–64. (This review article examines the history of hospital infection and the development of infection control procedures over time.)

chapter 14

issues in public health

Chapter focus

- *How is information about the incidence and prevalence of infectious diseases in Australia collected and distributed?*
- *Which aspects of primary health care are concerned with the prevention of infectious diseases?*
- *What are the particular challenges facing the provision of health care in rural and remote areas of Australia?*
- *How do public health issues in New Zealand differ from those in Australia?*

The Australian Health Scene

The 20th century has seen remarkable improvements in the standard of health and health care. This is particularly true in developed countries such as Australia, which has one of the highest standards in the world. Nevertheless, even in developed societies with a high standard of living, there may be major inequalities in health status and quality of health care between different groups in the population. We discuss this later in the chapter.

One of the most dramatic changes has been in the number of deaths attributable to infectious diseases. At the beginning of the century more than 60% of all deaths were due to infections. In the 1990s, less than 5% of deaths are directly caused by microorganisms. However, although no longer fatal, many of the diseases are still part of our everyday lives and contribute to serious morbidity and significant expense in the health system.

The decline in mortality due to infectious diseases has largely been due to three factors.

1. The ability to isolate and identify the microorganisms responsible for causing infections has enabled scientists and health professionals to develop and implement procedures to prevent or control the spread of many diseases. This has resulted in an improvement in general standards of hygiene, sanitation facilities, housing and quality of water supply, all of which contribute to an improved standard of living and a decrease in the incidence of disease.
2. The 1940s saw the discovery of antibiotics, which were hailed as 'magic' drugs able to selectively kill the bacteria responsible for many life-threatening illnesses (see Chapter 12).
3. The availability of vaccines has dramatically reduced mortality from the so-called 'childhood diseases', and mortality from 'adult' diseases such as influenza and pneumococcal disease has also been reduced. However, vaccine coverage in many at-risk groups still remains poor (see pp. 304–307.) In addition, vaccines are a valuable preventive measure against viral infections, which are difficult to treat with antibiotics for reasons we have discussed in Chapters 5 and 12. The use of vaccines and the principles of immunisation are discussed more fully later in this chapter.

The responsibility for the delivery of health care in Australia rests with a number of government bodies at Commonwealth, State and Territory level, as well as with the private sector. At the local level, each State or Territory is organised into Area or District Health Services which report to the State Health Department on matters of public health.

The Commonwealth Department of Human Services and Health has the responsibility of providing direction and information in regard to health policies of national importance. The National Health and Medical Research Council (NH&MRC) is a statutory authority within the portfolio of the Minister for Health, and its objective is to 'advise the Australian community on the achievement and maintenance of the highest practicable standards of individual and public health and to foster research in the interests of improving those standards'. This involves the publication of recommendations covering areas such as immunisation schedules, child health, communicable diseases, infection control, nutrition, mental health and other health issues. Another function of the NH&MRC is to advise the government on funding of competitive grants for medical and public health research.

An important function of the various health authorities is to collect epidemiological data (see Chapter 8) and carry out surveillance of the occurrence of communicable diseases. Information supplied by doctors, laboratories, hospitals and health services to local, State and Commonwealth authorities is used to develop policies to control the spread of disease. The control of infectious diseases is one area of public health for which there are intervention strategies of proven efficacy. Immunisation is available to prevent previously fatal childhood diseases and to protect against primarily adult illnesses such as influenza and hepatitis B. Antimicrobial therapy is a valuable tool for treatment and prevention of infection. Hospital infection control programs based on a knowledge of the aetiology (cause) and transmission of disease can also reduce the incidence of hospital acquired (nosocomial) infections.

Notifiable Diseases

A number of communicable diseases are required by law to be notified to the health authorities when diagnosed in a patient. The National Notifiable Diseases Surveillance System (NNDSS) was established in 1990 under the auspices of the Communicable Diseases Network,

Australia. The NNDSS coordinates the adoption of the NH&MRC list of diseases for notification and the reporting of notifiable diseases at a Commonwealth level. Sources of surveillance data include doctors, hospitals and laboratory notifications. Methods of surveillance vary somewhat among the States and Territories, as does the list of notifiable diseases. However, a 'core' group of notifiable diseases has been agreed upon which includes all vaccine-preventable childhood diseases.

When the diagnosis can be made largely by symptoms, the responsibility for notification rests with the local general practitioner. Diagnostic microbiology and serology laboratories are required to notify any cases of communicable diseases that they identify. The chief executive officers of hospitals and general managers of health services have the responsibility of coordinating notifications of diseases in hospitalised patients, although, in practice, this often consists of direct notification from a hospital doctor or laboratory to the identified State or Territory surveillance centre.

The data collected for each notification include an identification number, the State or Territory, sex and age of the patient, date of onset, date of notification, Aboriginality or ethnicity and post code. This information is important for epidemiological studies and for identification of epidemics. It is collected and published by the Commonwealth Department of Human Services and Health in the fortnightly bulletin, *Communicable Diseases Intelligence (CDI)*, together with case reports and comments on outbreaks of disease. The data are analysed on the basis of age, sex, geographical distribution and seasonal variation, and presented in table form with cumulative data for each year. An annual report is also published. These publications provide a valuable resource for health practitioners.

Notifications compiled by the NNDSS should be interpreted with some caution. They are influenced by a number of factors. For example, diagnostic laboratories are not always able to distinguish between incidence and prevalence statistics (see Chapter 8)—they may test the same patient more than once and record the disease each time they carry out the test, even though only one patient is involved. In addition, a disease that is rare or severe is more likely to be notified. A proportion of cases of some diseases, such as rubella or hepatitis C, may be asymptomatic and so the number of cases reported may significantly underestimate the true incidence.

Although the NH&MRC has recommended a uniform list of diseases and case definitions, each State or Territory health authority determines which diseases are actually required to be notified, using its own criteria. For example, *Chlamydia* is notifiable in the Northern Territory but not in New South Wales; gastrointestinal infections due to *Shigella* and *Campylobacter* are identified in most States, but in New South Wales they are listed as food-borne gastroenteritis. In Tasmania, rubella is notified only if congenital rubella syndrome occurs.

Other surveillance schemes coordinated through CDI include those for specific diseases caused by *Mycobacterium tuberculosis*, meningococci, gonococci and *Salmonella*. The National Influenza Surveillance derives data from several different schemes and this is also coordinated through CDI. HIV and AIDS surveillance is coordinated by the National Centre in HIV Epidemiology and Clinical Research (NCHECR) in collaboration with the various government authorities.

In addition, there are two laboratory reporting schemes: the Virology and Serology Reporting Scheme, LABVISE, which began in 1977, and the Laboratory Database of Organisms from Sterile Sites (LABDOS) begun in 1992, also coordinated through CDI. As with the NNDSS, the data reported by these schemes is subject to variation, depending on its source from the different laboratories and States.

An extension of the surveillance system is the use of chickens as an early warning of an increased incidence of arbovirus activity, in particular Murray Valley encephalitis virus, Barmah forest virus and Kunjin virus. By monitoring the appearance of antibodies in sentinel chicken flocks (that is, the animal host), it is possible to anticipate an outbreak of arbovirus infection and take steps to implement mosquito control programs.

In all, it can be seen that a large amount of data is collected and published. Even though it may not represent the 'total' number of cases, it gives a very good indication of the incidence and distribution of the important infectious diseases in Australia.

ANNUAL REPORT OF THE NNDSS

The annual report of the NNDSS is published each year in the *CDI* bulletin. The data in this section are extracted (with permission) from the 1994 report, published in October 1995. The total number of notifications for each of 42 diseases in each State in 1994 is listed in Table 14.1. It provides a useful overview of the major infectious diseases and their distribution in Australia.

As in previous years, the highest *number* of notifications came from Queensland, but the highest *rate* of notifications (i.e. notifications per 100 000 population) came from the Northern Territory (see Table 14.2), reflecting the high incidence of communicable diseases in the susceptible Aboriginal population in that part of Australia. This is discussed later in this chapter. Changes, from year to year, in the number of notifications of certain diseases, such as hepatitis B and C, may reflect a change in reporting procedures.

Australia is free of some diseases that present major problems in other parts of the world. This is either because there are no reservoirs of infection for the microorganisms or the appropriate vector is not found in Australia. This situation may change with increasing travel. No cases of poliomyelitis, rabies, plague, botulism, yellow fever or other haemorrhagic fevers were reported. There was a drop in the number of cases of dengue fever from 690 in 1993 to only 17 in 1994. This reflects the epidemic outbreak that occurred in Queensland in 1993. All index cases of dengue fever were known to be imported cases

TABLE 14.1
NATIONAL NOTIFIABLE DISEASES SURVEILLANCE SYSTEM REPORTS, 1994, BY STATE OR TERRITORY AND DISEASE

DISEASE	ACT	NSW	NT	QLD	SA	TAS	VIC	WA	TOTAL
Arbovirus									
Ross River virus infection	1	337	312	3141	28	–	58	97	3974
Dengue[1]	0	0	6	3	1	–	6	1	17
NEC[2]	0	46	34	457	0	24	17	9	587
Botulism	0	–	NN	NN	0	0	0	NN	0
Brucellosis	0	4	0	27	0	0	3	0	34
Campylobacteriosis[3]	308	–	324	2109	2318	503	3479	1076	10 117
Chancroid	0	0	0	0	NN	0	0	0	0
Chlamydial infection (NEC)	93	NN	722	2524	732	295	1306	847	6519
Cholera	0	0	0	2	0	0	1	0	3
Diphtheria	0	0	0	0	0	0	0	0	0
Donovanosis	0	NN	68	30	NN	0	0	19	117
Gonococcal infection[4]	8	358	736	708	156	8	154	843	2971
Haemophilus influenzae type b infection	1	63	1	38	19	4	32	11	169
Hepatitis A	17	561	68	803	54	10	154	227	1894
Hepatitis B	–	81	26	49	34	2	96	39	327
Hepatitis C—incident[5]	6	33	–	–	4	–	–	–	43
Hepatitis C—unspecified[5]	428		301	3177		53[8]	3523	1416	8898
Hepatitis (NEC)	0	5	0	15	4	0	18	NN	42
Hydatid infection	2	20	1	8	3	1	19	2	56
Legionellosis	0	62	5	21	26	1	44	20	179
Leprosy	0	3	1	2	0	0	3	2	11
Leptospirosis	1	13	2	59	5	3	40	0	123
Listeriosis	1	8	0	13	3	0	8	1	34
Lymphogranuloma venereum	0	NN	0	0	NN	0	2	NN	2
Malaria	24	188	40	297	31	13	83	27	703
Measles	114	1484	402	2483	70	32	177	133	4895
Meningococcal infection	7	142	5	92	19	5	58	55	383
Mumps[6]	5	10	3	NN	7	NN	62	7	94
Ornithosis	1	NN	0	3	19	3	57	2	85
Pertussis	19	1516	138	1937	982	26	447	568	5633
Plague	0	0	0	0	0	NN	0	0	0
Poliomyelitis	0	0	0	0	0	0	0	0	0

(continued)

TABLE 14.1 Continued

DISEASE	ACT	NSW	NT	QLD	SA	TAS	VIC	WA	TOTAL
Q fever	0	267	0	286	29	0	77	8	667
Rabies	0	NN	0	0	0	0	0	0	0
Rubella[7]	51	123	49	2053	81	0	211	747	3315
Salmonellosis (NEC)	44	1053	475	1450	488	119	1055	599	5283
Shigellosis[3]	8	–	127	148	63	2	87	289	724
Syphilis	16	1016	451	549	43	2	143	104	2324
Tetanus	0	4	0	0	8	0	1	2	15
Tuberculosis	9	409	31	113	57	14	309	82	1024
Typhoid	1	17	3	2	2	2	7	16	50
Viral haemorrhagic fever (NEC)	0	0	0	0	0	0	0	0	0
Yellow fever	0	0	0	0	0	0	0	0	0
Yersiniosis (NEC)[3]	0	–	1	291	97	1	21	3	414
Total	1165	7823	4332	22 890	5450	1123	11 758	7252	61 726

NN Not notifiable.
NEC Not elsewhere classified.
– Elsewhere classified
1. Western Australia: notifiable since 24 June 1994.
2. Tasmania: includes Ross River virus infection and dengue.
3. New South Wales: only as 'foodborne disease' or 'gastroenteritis in an institution'.
4. Northern Terrritory, Queensland, South Australia and Victoria: includes gonococcal neonatal ophthalmia.
5. States and Territories reported notifications of incident cases only and/or all notifications.
6. Northern Territory: compiled since September 1994 and notifiable since 22 December 1994.
7. Tasmania: congenital rubella syndrome only.
8. A further 241 cases of unspecified hepatitis C were notified in Tasmania but not reported to the NNDSS for incorporation into the national dataset.

Source: Communicable Diseases Intelligence 19, 30 October 1995, p. 545.

in travellers. There were over 700 notifications for malaria but, again, these occurred in people who had contracted the disease outside Australia; the situation highlights the need for better preventive measures. Both malaria and dengue fever have the potential to become established in Australia as the appropriate mosquito vectors are found here.

The data reveal marked differences between the incidence of various diseases in different parts of Australia. Health workers should be aware that, if they choose to work in rural or remote areas, the diseases and health problems they are likely to encounter will be quite different to those in a big city hospital. For example, the Northern Territory has diseases that are rarely seen in the southern States (see p. 310). Diseases such as hydatids (dog tapeworm) are seen mainly in rural areas where dogs are fed raw offal, and Q fever occurs mainly in cattle-raising areas.

The distribution of diseases is also influenced by climate and environmental factors. Where a vector such as a tick or mosquito is required for transmission, the disease is confined to areas where the vector is found. In addition, seasonal variations occur, often linked to breeding seasons

TABLE 14.2
NATIONAL NOTIFIABLE DISEASES: ANNUAL RATE OF NOTIFICATION (CASES PER 100 000 POPULATION)

	1993	1994
ACT	371.9	387.2
NSW	160.2	129.3
NT	2161.9	2531.4
QLD	678.1	716.0
SA	399.0	366.2
TAS	418.1	237.7
VIC	248.5	262.7
WA	377.8	426.1
Total	344.0	345.9

Source: Data derived from *Communicable Diseases Intelligence* 19, 30 October 1995, p. 546.

for vectors such as mosquitoes. For example, Ross River fever occurs in most parts of the country, with the highest rates in the Murray region of South Australia, the Mallee in Victoria and also in North Queensland, but is most common in late summer when the mosquito population is high (Figure 14.1).

The highest number of notifications for any disease, in 1994, was for campylobacteriosis (10 117), followed by unspecified hepatitis C (8898) and chlamydial infections (6519). The actual rate for chlamydia may be much higher as it is not a notifiable disease in New South Wales. Contrary to media reports of an 'epidemic of hepatitis C', the high number of notifications actually represents the availability of a diagnostic test for hepatitis C rather than a real increase in infection rate. This test has only been available since 1990, so many people with asymptomatic hepatitis C are now being identified when their blood is tested for other reasons. Blood donations and samples for other tests can now be screened for hepatitis C. The presence of antibodies to hepatitis C is often detected without the person having any knowledge of prior exposure to the disease.

In future years the NNDSS will introduce incidence surveillance (i.e. disease symptoms) as well as prevalence statistics (i.e. presence of antibodies).

Among the most common illnesses notified were gastrointestinal infections due to *Campylobacter* (85.8 per 100 000), *Shigella* (6.1 per 100 000) and *Salmonella* (29.6 per 100 000). These data do not include gastrointestinal infections caused by these organisms in New South Wales.

For sexually transmitted diseases, the highest rate of notification was in the Northern Territory and the Kimberley region of Western Australia. In these regions there was a recorded incidence of *Chlamydia* of 421 per 100 000 population, and gonorrhoea of over 400 per 100 000 (see Figure 14.2), compared with average figures for the whole of Australia of 55 per 100 000 and 16 per 100 000 respectively.

A number of diseases are preventable by vaccination but a significant number of cases of some of them still occur, sometimes with serious outcomes. The actual incidence of vaccine-preventable diseases recorded in 1994 was 27.4 per 100 000 for measles, 31.6 per 100 000 for pertussis and 18.6 per 100 000 for rubella, but the real incidence is probably greater. This is unacceptably high in a country like Australia where a free childhood vaccination program is available to all (see p. 301).

As mentioned previously, LABVISE records the incidence of diseases that are diagnosed by serological techniques. These are mainly viral diseases, but other organisms such as *Chlamydia*, which are slow or difficult to grow in the laboratory and for which there is a specific antibody test available, are also diagnosed in this way. Outbreaks of viral diseases tend to occur mainly in the winter months. The 20 most commonly reported infectious agents from this surveillance data are shown in Figure 14.3. Herpes simplex type 1 and type 2 accounted for a large number of notifications. Hepatitis C notifications are also high.

Among the viruses that affect mainly children, the highest incidence of infections was due to respiratory syncytial virus (RSV). Rotavirus, which causes serious gastroenteritis, was the most commonly reported viral infection in the 1–4 year old age group.

FIGURE 14.1
ROSS RIVER FEVER
(a) Annual rate of notification of Ross River virus infection per 100 000 population, 1994, by statistical division of residence; (b) Notifications of Ross River virus infection with onset dates in 1994, by month of onset.

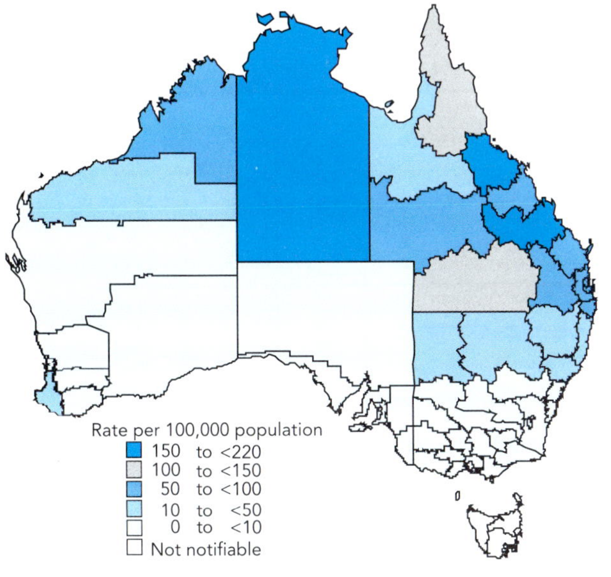

(a)

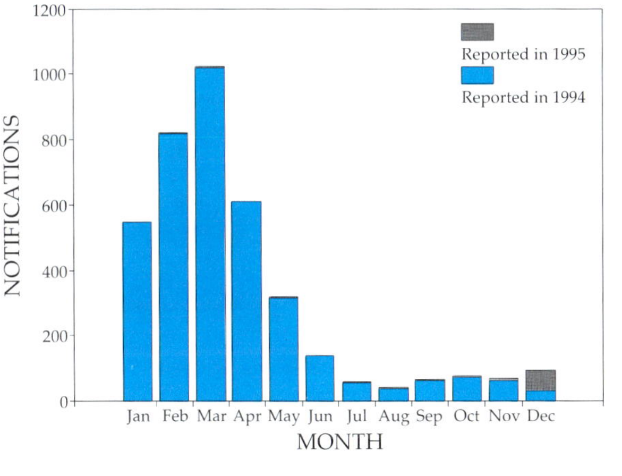

(b)

Source: Communicable Diseases Intelligence 19, 30 October 1995, pp. 548, 549.

FIGURE 14.2
INCIDENCE OF GONORRHOEA
Annual rate of notification of gonococcol infection per 100 000 population, by statistical division of residence.

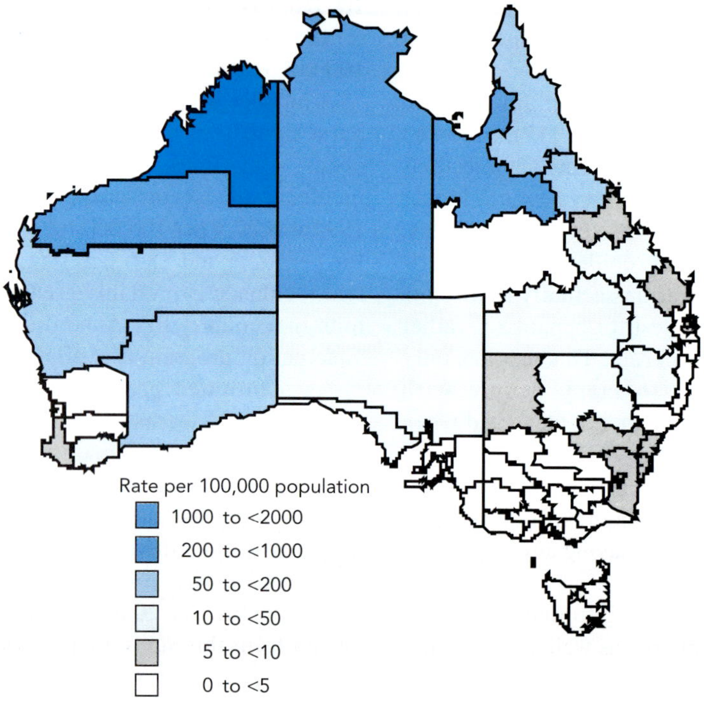

Source: Communicable Diseases Intelligence 19/23, 30 October 1995, p. 554.

FIGURE 14.3
LABVISE REPORT MOST COMMON INFECTIONS
The twenty most commonly reported agents, 1994 and 1991–93 average, as % of total reports for the period.

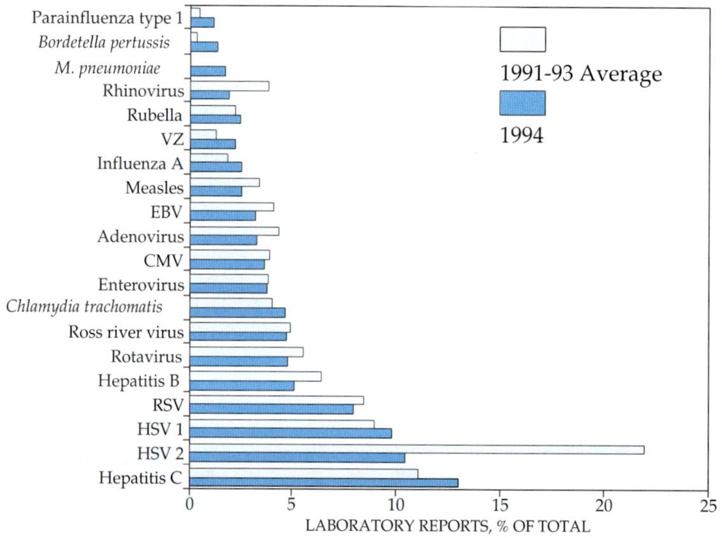

Source: Communicable Diseases Intelligence 19/23, 30 October 1995, p. 594.

An important aspect of surveillance data is the information that is obtained about risk factors. Unfortunately, these data are often incomplete, but an analysis of the information provided in the LABVISE report is useful. Figure 14.4 shows the major risk factors associated with the diseases diagnosed by serological methods. As can be seen, injecting drug users are at substantial risk of acquiring serious infectious diseases, making up over 43% of all notifications. Patients whose immune system is compromised are also at risk (e.g. HIV-positive people (7.8%) and transplant recipients(8.6%)). More sensitive indicators such as ethnicity (Aboriginality) and poverty are harder to obtain.

FIGURE 14.4
RISK FACTORS

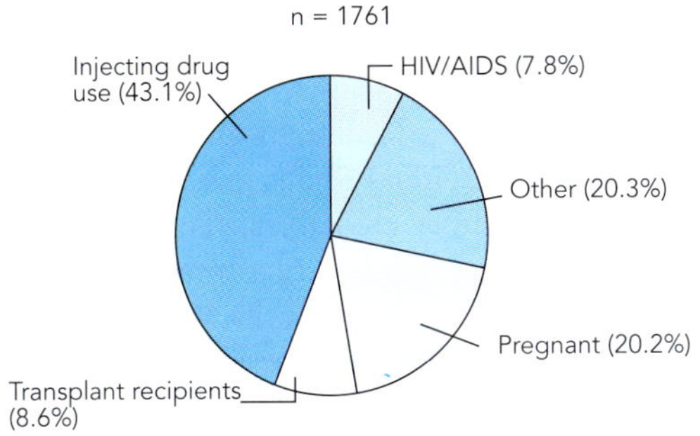

Source: Communicable Diseases Intelligence 19/23, 30 October 1995, p. 598.

Primary Health Care

Primary health care, in its broadest sense, is a philosophy of promoting equal health care at all levels of the social system. It involves the provision of services on the basis of the needs of the population, the provision of health education and the development of a balanced system of health promotion, disease prevention and treatment of illness.

In Australia there is evidence that, despite an overall high standard of health, there are in the community disadvantaged groups of people whose health status is poor. For example, Aborigines and Torres Strait Islanders have a much lower general standard of health than the rest of Australia, due partly to the poor standard of housing and physical environment in which many of them live. We examine the infectious diseases that affect Aborigines later in this chapter.

The major factors that influence health are socio-economic conditions. Other factors such as marital status, sex, ethnicity, level of education and place of dwelling (urban or rural) also affect health.

Some of the social circumstances that can cause inequalities in health status are:

- level of education;
- level of economic resources;
- living conditions, including quality of housing, clean water supply, air pollution, hazardous environments;
- working conditions;
- availability of social support.

Numerous studies show that people in the lowest socioeconomic groups, with low levels of education have the poorest health. They tend to delay seeking treatment, so their illnesses have often become severe by the time they present to the hospital or health service. Other untreated, underlying illnesses often contribute to morbidity. They are also less likely to seek out preventive services such as screening and immunisation.

Two aspects of primary health care which can directly affect the level of infectious diseases in the community are immunisation and preventative screening programs. There are other activities of primary health care that are beyond the scope of this text, but should be kept in mind as being essential for good health. They include:

- basic education, including health education;
- provision of adequate food and nutrition;
- provision of a safe water supply and proper sanitation;
- control of endemic diseases;
- provision of maternal and child care, and family planning information;
- provision of appropriate medication and treatment.

Immunisation

The development of vaccines and the implementation of immunisation programs are among the major reasons for the improvement in health in this century. One of the great success stories of vaccination campaigns is the worldwide eradication of the dreaded disease, smallpox. In many developed countries, polio has been virtually eliminated. During the polio epidemics in Australia in the 1940s and 1950s, there were up to 1000 cases of paralytic disease and 100 deaths each year. The introduction of the **Salk vaccine** (a killed preparation) and later the **Sabin vaccine** (an attenuated virus) saw a dramatic fall in the occurrence of the disease. The last recorded case of polio in Australia was in 1986. There were no other cases in the 1980s and only 14 in the 1970s.

The principles behind the development of immunity to an infectious disease are fully described in Chapter 9. To summarise: when a person is exposed to a foreign organism, the body responds by producing antibodies, activated lymphocytes and long-term memory cells against that organism. If the person is subsequently exposed to the same organism, the preformed antibodies and memory cells (which produce more antibodies and activated T lymphocytes) combine to kill or remove the invading organism before disease can occur. The person is said to be *immune* to that disease. Immunity is specific for each disease and sometimes even for each different strain of a pathogenic organism. Thus, if the organism is slightly different (due to a mutation, such as occurs with the influenza virus) then the person may not be immune to the altered form of the pathogen.

The possibility of producing immunity by artificial means was recognised as far back as 1796 when EDWARD JENNER noticed that milkmaids who had suffered from cowpox, a mild disease with lesions similar to smallpox, appeared to be immune to smallpox. He first used a preparation derived from cowpox (caused by *Vaccinia* virus, hence the word 'vaccine') to immunise people successfully against smallpox. The milder cowpox virus also induced immunity to smallpox.

Jenner's work laid the basis for our modern immunisation programs. In practice, the terms 'vaccination' and 'immunisation' are used interchangeably. However, **vaccination** is used by some people in a general sense to denote the administration of any vaccine without regard to whether the recipient is made immune. **Immunisation** is a more specific term, denoting the process of inducing or providing immunity artificially. It may be active or passive.

Active immunisation is the administration of a vaccine in order to stimulate the body's immune system to produce both specific antibodies and cellular immunity to the antigens contained in the vaccine.

Passive immunisation is the provision of temporary immunity by the administration of preformed antibodies derived from another person or animal. They may be in the form of pooled, non-specific human immunoglobulin, specific antitoxins (e.g. tetanus) or specific antibody preparations (e.g. hepatitis B immunoglobulin). These products are used mainly when a person has been exposed to a serious disease and has no immunity. The antibodies circulate only for a short time (weeks to months) before being degraded by normal body processes.

Maternal antibodies that cross the placenta in the late stages of pregnancy are a natural type of passive immunisation which protects the infant from infection during the first months of life. At birth the neonate has a range of maternal IgG antibodies which represent the exposure of the mother to previous infectious diseases. Premature infants (less than 32 weeks) have not yet received maternal IgG transplacentally and so are at a significantly higher risk of infection. Further passive protection is afforded by the IgA present in colostrum and breast milk, especially against gastrointestinal infections.

As the immune system develops, the maternal antibodies are destroyed and the infant builds up its own immunity to the various microorganisms to which it is exposed. The development of protective immunological memory in early childhood can be stimulated by the administration of appropriate vaccine preparations, before significant risks of exposure to the infectious agents occur. This is called **artificial active immunity**.

VACCINATION SCHEDULES

Until the widespread introduction of childhood immunisation, many children died from infectious diseases. However, the last 50 years has seen a dramatic decrease in infant mortality due to vaccine-preventable diseases (see Table 14.3).

The Australian Health Department provides free vaccination for most childhood diseases. The current recommended childhood vaccination schedule is shown in Table 14.4. Health professionals should be aware of variations among individual States and Territories (see, e.g. the Northern Territory guidelines, Table 14.9, p. 315). The Northern Territory also recommends an adult immunisation schedule (see Table 14.10, p. 316). There are also differences between Australia and other countries—for example, New Zealand (see Table 14.15, p. 321). The schedule is continually modified to include new vaccines and to take into account new knowledge and changes in the prevalence of various diseases.

The NH&MRC publishes up-to-date comprehensive information on immunisation procedures and recommendations for administration. Vaccines should be administered by the correct route and at the optimal site (for injections).

The age at which vaccines are administered is also important. Maternally derived antibodies (IgG) seem to affect the infant's response to live (attenuated) vaccines, but do not interfere with the response to the non-replicating (killed) vaccines. For this reason, DTP (triple antigen: diphtheria, tetanus, pertussis) can be given as early as two months of age, but the live MMR (measles, mumps, rubella) vaccine is better delayed to 12 months. Since premature infants are lacking in maternal antibodies, immunisation should begin at the chronological age and not be delayed because of prematurity.

ADULT IMMUNISATION

Although the major emphasis in all vaccination campaigns is on childhood vaccination, there is a large number of adults who, for various reasons, are not fully immunised. This may be because they are recent immigrants from countries where vaccination is not readily available, or it may be

TABLE 14.3

DECREASE IN MORTALITY DUE TO VACCINE-PREVENTABLE DISEASES

Deaths (in decades) from vaccine-preventable infectious diseases, Australia, 1926 to 1985.

YEARS	DIPHTHERIA	PERTUSSIS	TETANUS	POLIOMYELITIS	MEASLES	AUSTRALIAN POPULATION (AVERAGE MILLIONS)
1926–35	4073	2808	879	430	1102	6.6
1936–45	2791	1693	655	613	822	7.2
1946–55	624	429	625	1013	495	8.6
1956–65	44	58	280	123	210	11.0
1966–75	11	24	82	2	117	13.8
1976–85	2	14	31	2	62	14.9
1986–94	2	8	19	0	29	17.1

TABLE 14.4
THE NH&MRC STANDARD CHILDHOOD VACCINATION SCHEDULE

AGE	DISEASE	VACCINE
2 months	Diphtheria, tetanus and pertussis Poliomyelitis *Haemophilus influenzae* type b (Hib) (Schedule 1 or 2)**	DTP—'Triple antigen' OPV— Sabin vaccine Hib vaccine (a or b or c)*
4 months	Diphtheria, tetanus and pertussis Poliomyelitis Hib (Schedule 1 or 2)**	DTP—'Triple antigen' OPV—Sabin vaccine Hib vaccine (a or b or c)*
6 months	Diphtheria, tetanus and pertussis Poliomyelitis Hib (Schedule 1 only)**	DTP—'Triple antigen' OPV—Sabin vaccine Hib vaccine (a or b)*
12 months	Measles, mumps and rubella Hib (Schedule 2 only)**	MMR Hib vaccine (c)*
18 months	Diphtheria, tetanus, and pertussis Hib (Schedule 1 only)**	DTP—'Triple antigen' Hib vaccine (a or b)*
Prior to school entry (4–5 years)	Diphtheria, tetanus, and pertussis Poliomyelitis	DTP—'Triple antigen' OPV—Sabin vaccine
10–16 years	Measles, mumps and rubella	MMR
Prior to leaving school (15–19 years)	Diphtheria and tetanus Poliomyelitis	ADT—Adult diphtheria and tetanus OPV—Sabin vaccine

* Abbreviations for Hib vaccines—(a) is HbOC ('HibTITER'); (b) is PRP-T ('Act-HIB'); (c) is PRP-OMP ('PedvaxHIB').

** There are 2 different schedules for Hib vaccines. Schedule 1 Hib vaccination applies to the use of HbOC and PRP-T. The selected vaccine is given at 2, 4, 6, and 18 months. Schedule 2 Hib vaccination refers to the use of PRP-OMP. This vaccine is given at 2, 4, and 12 months.

Note that a 4th Hib vaccine (PRP-D; ProHIBit') is approved for use as single injection for children over 18 months of age.

All of the vaccines in the standard schedule, except OPV, are given by deep subcutaneous or intramuscular injection. OPV is given orally. OPV should never be injected.

Source: Australian Immunisation Procedures Handbook, 5th edition, 1994, p. 16.

because of their age and the previous unavailability of vaccines. There is significant morbidity and mortality among adults from vaccine-preventable diseases and there is a need to develop a national strategy aimed at immunising adults. The Northern Territory has developed an adult immunisation schedule (see Table 14.10, p. 316).

TYPES OF VACCINES

Obviously, it would not be safe to administer live pathogens in order to promote an immune response. It has been necessary to develop suitable preparations which contain the specific immunogenic groups (antigens) of the pathogen but which are unable to cause disease (see Chapter 9). Table 9.3 (p. 199) lists the properties of vaccines in common use. Some (e.g. measles, mumps, rubella, Sabin polio) consist of live, attenuated (weakened) forms of the pathogen. They have the advantage of being able to multiply in the host, producing a high level (titre) of antibody formation from a single dose of vaccine, but do not cause disease (Figure 14.5(a)). There is always a very slight risk that these preparations may revert to a virulent (disease-producing) strain, but this is extremely rare.

Toxoids are inactivated forms of bacterial toxins that retain their immunogenicity. Toxoids are used when the disease symptoms are due mainly to the formation of a toxin; for example, tetanus toxoid and diphtheria toxoid. Some vaccines contain killed, whole cells of the pathogen. Pertussis vaccine is currently the only preparation of this type in use in the childhood immunisation schedule. Occasionally it produces side effects (see p. 307). An effective cell-free pertussis vaccine which causes fewer local reactions has been developed and used in Japan and the United States, but is not yet available in Australia.

The safest vaccines are preparations that consist only of that part of the pathogenic organism that induces effective immunity. They do not contain any nucleic acid, so replication (and disease) is not possible. For example,

FIGURE 14.5
ANTIBODY FORMATION IN RESPONSE TO VARIOUS TYPES OF VACCINES
(a) The use of living organisms in a vaccine gives rise to a high antibody titre after only one dose; (b) multiple doses of vaccine prepared from non-replicating antigens are required to build up immunity.

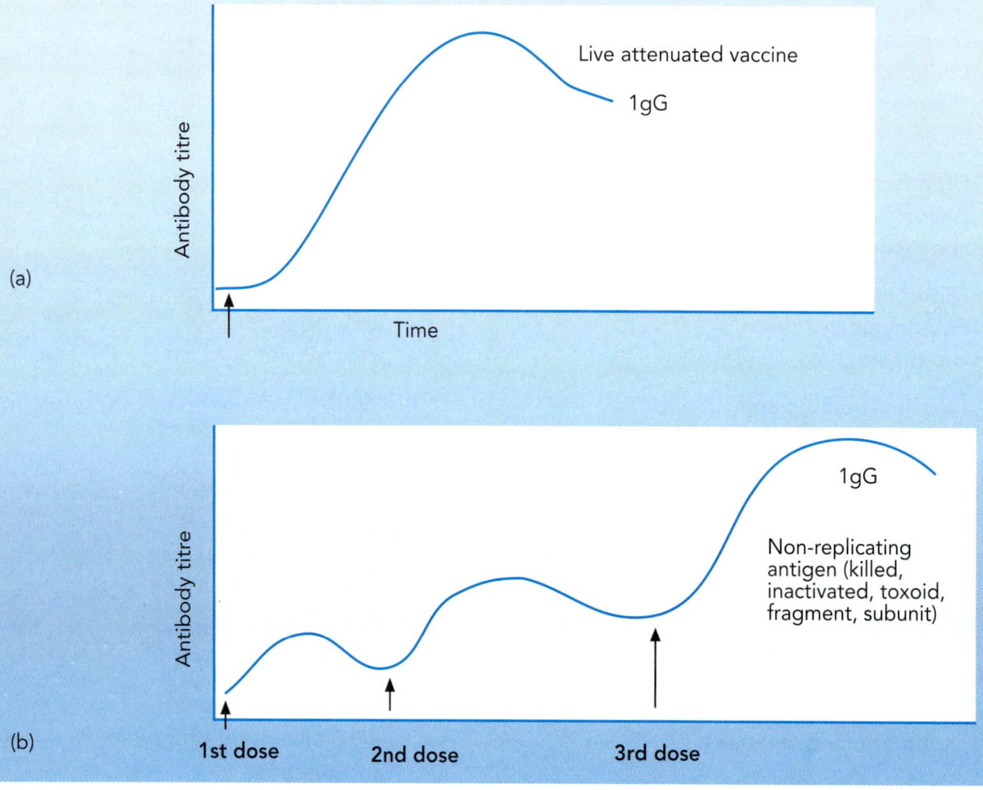

the vaccine for hepatitis B consists of the surface antigen HBsAg from the outer layer of the virus. It is produced by placing the viral gene for HBsAg into cells of the yeast, *Saccharomyces cerevisiae*, inducing the synthesis of large quantities of the antigen, which is then extracted and purified for use in the vaccine. The recently licensed vaccine against *Haemophilus influenzae* type B (Hib) is a **conjugate vaccine,** consisting of the antigenic polysaccharide from Hib, bound to a protein carrier.

Vaccines containing non-replicating antigens require the administration of several doses to build up adequate levels of immunity (Figure 14.5(b)). Theoretically, live vaccines should require only one dose, but some of the newer attenuated viral vaccines have only been available since the 1970s and are still being evaluated in order to determine how long the artificially acquired immunity will last. In many cases (e.g. rubella, hepatitis B), antibody titres are known to fall over time. Measurements of antibody titre at various time intervals after immunisation sometimes show wide variations among individuals, and it is not known whether this represents a lowered level of immunity. At present, it is recommended that women intending to become pregnant should have their rubella antibody level checked; if seronegative they should be vaccinated or, if their antibody titre is low, have a booster dose of vaccine. This should be done at least three months before becoming pregnant. Since it is a live vaccine, its use close to, or during pregnancy, is not advised, although there are no reports of congenital abnormalities due to vaccine use.

To achieve control over measles in Australia, a two-dose vaccination schedule (given in the combined measles-mumps-rubella, MMR, preparation) is now recommended. The first MMR is given at 12 months (9 months for Aboriginal children) and the second dose at 10 to 14 years.

Haemophilus influenzae type B (Hib) is responsible for the invasive diseases meningitis and epiglottitis in young children, with an overall fatality rate of 2–5%. Sequelae to Hib meningitis, ranging from mild hearing loss to neurological impairment, occur in 20–30% of cases. In 1992, a Hib vaccine suitable for children aged 18 months to 5 years was approved for use in Australia; in 1993, vaccines suitable for infants of 2 months were licensed and included in the routine immunisation schedules. The result has been a dramatic decrease in the incidence of Hib (see Figure 14.6). In children under 5 years there was a 76% reduction in the number of notifications between 1992 and 1994.

COMPLIANCE WITH IMMUNISATION

The success of immunisation programs in developed countries has meant a dramatic reduction in infant morbidity and mortality. However, to maintain this situation it is essential that parents continue to have their children immunised. An important factor in maintaining a community free of disease is the proportion of individuals in the community who are immune to a particular disease. This is described as group or **herd immunity**. As we saw in Chapter 8, to control the spread of disease the

FIGURE 14.6

INCIDENCE OF Hib

Haemophilus influenzae type b notifications by age group and month of onset, january 1991 to November 1994.

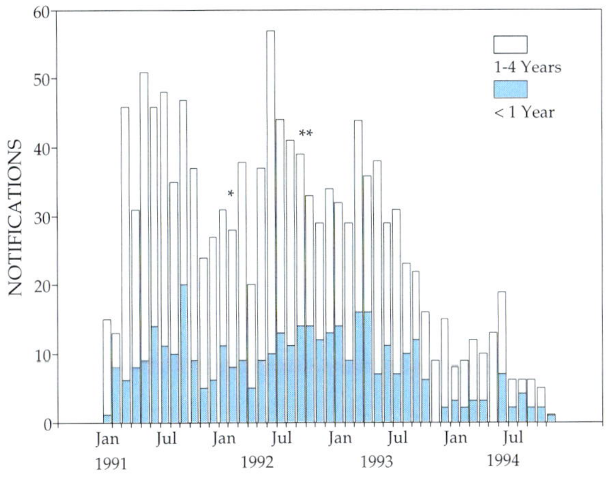

Source: Communicable Diseases Intelligence 18/13, 27 June 1994, p. 672.

reservoirs of infection must be eliminated, in this case by immunisation. If the number of immune individuals is high, then the disease can affect only a few susceptible people and so the likelihood of exposure of unimmunised individuals—and therefore transmission of the disease—is low. Thus a high group immunity protects not only the immunised members, but also the susceptible ones (see Figure 14.7).

This is particularly important for a disease like pertussis (whooping cough). Older children and adults suffer a severe but usually non-fatal illness. However, for babies under six months pertussis is often fatal. If the older children and adults are immunised, they do not contract the disease and so the susceptible babies are protected because they have less chance of being exposed to an infected person.

It is necessary to understand the concept of herd immunity in order to realise the importance of continuing vaccine programs after the incidence of a disease has declined (e.g. polio). If a person with polio (e.g. a traveller from a country where the disease is still prevalent) enters a largely unvaccinated community, there is the potential for an epidemic to occur. This will continue to be the case until the disease is eradicated completely (see Spotlight box, p. 306).

Not all vaccines are 100% effective. For example, the measles vaccine produces immunity in only 90–95% of people vaccinated. If there is also a low compliance with immunisation programs, then the level of protection can fall as low as 50% in the community. In fact, figures from the Australian Bureau of Statistics for the period 1989–90 show that, overall, only 52.9% of children under six years were *fully* immunised, although the level of immunisation for individual diseases was much higher (Table 14.5).

FIGURE 14.7

HERD IMMUNITY

The greater the percentage of immune persons in a population, the less likely a susceptible individual is to be exposed to the disease.

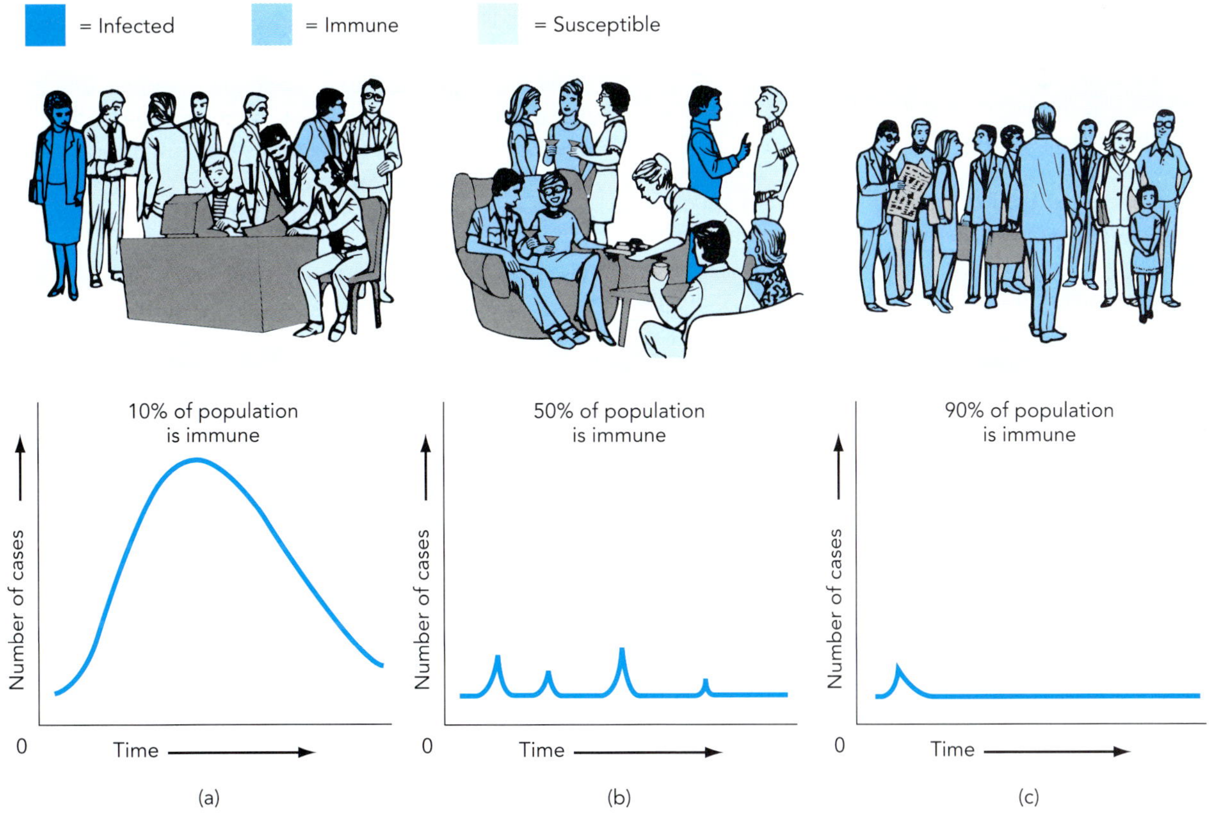

TABLE 14.5
COMPLIANCE WITH IMMUNISATION IN CHILDREN AGED 0–6 YEARS, 1989–90 (%)

IMMUNISATION CONDITION	NSW	VIC	QLD	SA	WA	TAS	NT	ACT	AUST.
Diphtheria/Tetanus	84.9	85.2	90.2	87.1	85.6	89.1	87.5	88.2	86.3
Whooping cough	70.2	69.2	73.6	70.0	71.2	77.0	69.3	75.4	70.9
Polio	72.3	69.9	75.5	72.3	73.6	67.5	59.9	80.1	72.1
Measles	84.6	87.1	87.6	85.3	87.4	82.3	81.6	87.4	86.0
Mumps	78.2	83.4	83.2	80.4	80.6	76.8	57.8	83.9	80.5
Fully immunised	51.6	51.0	56.1	53.1	56.4	48.9	46.4	64.3	52.9

Source: ABS, 1992.

SPOTLIGHT
DIPHTHERIA EPIDEMIC IN RUSSIA

Newspaper headlines in August 1993 announced that Moscow was in the grip of a diphtheriaa epidemic. It occurred because, in 1966, the then Soviet Union announced that it had not recorded any cases of diphtheria in the previous year and so concluded that the Socialist State had wiped out the disease. In Moscow, 774 cases of diphtheria, mainly among children, were recorded in the first six months of 1993, with 33 deaths. Health authorities were faced with the need to implement a program to vaccinate millions of unprotected residents. Although there were adequate supplies of vaccine, drugs for treatment of the disease were in short supply.

The epidemic has continued in areas of the former USSR and the World Health Organisation has estimated that a further 150 000 to 200 000 cases can be expected. The incidence of the disease has been as high as 30 per 100 000 in Russia, with a fatality rate of 2–3%, but as high as 20% in other areas. One in four people who contracted the disease were left with some level of permanent disability.

Comment: This kind of tragedy can easily happen if immunisation programs are not maintained. The unvaccinated population is particularly vulnerable to infections carried into the country by travellers. Although vaccines are available, it is difficult to carry out mass immunisation campaigns after an epidemic has started.

This lack of full immunisation greatly increases the risk of epidemics, as is shown by a number of recent outbreaks of measles in Australia (see Figure 14.8(a)). The epidemic of measles that began in 1992 continued into 1994 with 4895 cases being reported. Measles can be a serious and sometimes fatal disease; it also has a rare post-viral complication—subacute sclerosing panencephalitis (SSPE)—which is usually fatal (see Chapter 5). In the United States, measles vaccination is required before entry to school or college and there has been a dramatic reduction in the number of measles cases. Immunisation of all schoolage children provides herd immunity which also protects susceptible children under 15 months.

Measles and pertussis (Figure 14.8(b)) illustrate the importance of maintaining herd immunity to prevent epidemics. There are various reasons why people do not comply with immunisation recommendations, including:

- ignorance or complacency about the serious nature of vaccine-preventable diseases;
- fear of complications of vaccination;
- lack of correct information about side effects and/or contraindications.

RISKS AND COMPLICATIONS OF VACCINATION

In the past there have been instances of adverse reactions, even some deaths, following administration of vaccines. The standard of vaccine production and administration is now very high. Health professionals should be familiar with the contraindications for vaccination. Children with immunodeficiencies require special consideration. Chapter 3 of the *Australian Immunisation Procedures Handbook 1994* (5th edition) contains complete information about the use of the recommended vaccines together with a description of adverse reactions that might be expected and contraindications for use.

MMR vaccine is a combined measles-mumps-rubella vaccine which protects against three serious diseases. The first of these, measles, is an acute, highly infectious, viral illness. Acute encephalitis occurs in 2–10 people per 10 000 reported cases of measles, with a mortality rate of 10–15%. About 15–40% of survivors have permanent brain damage. Mumps is an unpleasant but less serious infection, and permanent adverse sequelae are rare. Orchitis may occur in up to 20% of post-pubertal males, but subsequent sterility is rare. Rubella is a mild, often subclinical infection. However, when contracted during the first 8–10 weeks of pregnancy it results in foetal damage in up to 90% of pregnancies.

Vaccination with the combined measles-mumps-rubella (MMR) vaccine is recommended at 12 months and again at 10–14 years. Malaise, fever and a rash may occur 7–10 days after MMR vaccination. Febrile convulsions occur in about 0.1% of children. Symptoms can be alleviated with paracetamol.

FIGURE 14.8

(a) MEASLES OUTBREAK

Notifications of measles by month of onset, January 1992 to November 1994.

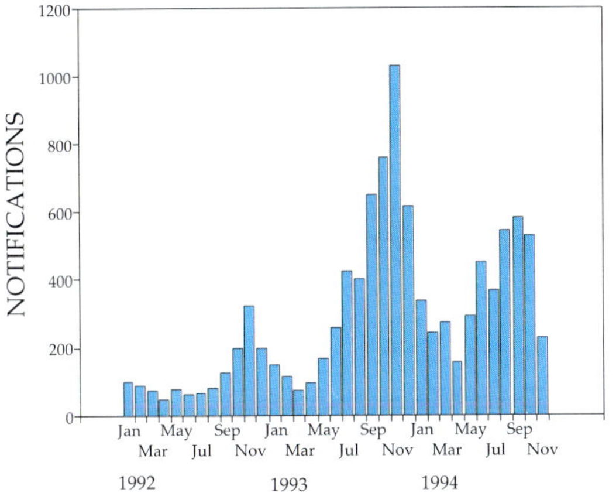

(b) PERTUSSIS OUTBREAK

Notifications of pertussis by month of onset, January 1992 to November 1994.

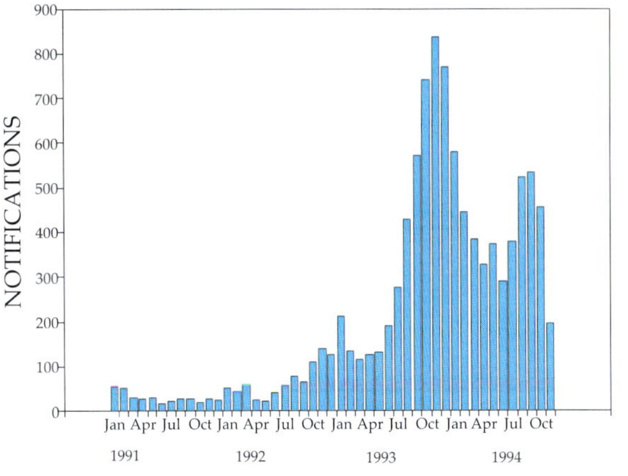

Source: *Communicable Diseases Intelligence* 18/13, 27 June 1994, p. 673.

The DTP or triple antigen (TA) vaccine contains diphtheria and tetanus toxoid and killed *Bordetella pertussis*. Pertussis (whooping cough) is a serious, sometimes fatal, respiratory infection that is particularly serious in infants under six months of age (fatality rate in Australia is 0.5%). The vaccine is very effective in reducing the incidence of the disease. Much publicity has focused on the side effects of the pertussis vaccine. It is common for infants to be feverish and crying after the DTP vaccination and there may be swelling at the site of the vaccination in 20% of infants. This can be relieved with non-prescription drugs such as paracetamol. A small number of children experience a stronger reaction to the vaccine which may require medical attention. Effects include fever over 40.5°C, convulsions (0.05%), hypotonic or hypoconvulsive episodes (0.05%), severe local reactions and prolonged screaming (1%).

Although the DTP vaccine has been blamed for serious brain damage, *several large controlled case studies have failed to show any permanent neurological damage that was directly attributable to the pertussis vaccine*. For comparison, encephalopathy in patients who contract pertussis disease occurs in 1.1% of all infants under six months of age. There were nearly 4000 cases of pertussis notified in Australia in 1993. Acute neurological complications from an attack of whooping cough occur in 2–7% of unimmunised individuals, which is significantly higher than any of the side effects from vaccination.

These figures make it obvious that the risks from immunisation are much less than the risks from having the disease. More importantly, as we explained before, a high level of immunisation in the community protects not only the immunised individuals, but also the infants who are not old enough to have been immunised. Thus, the process of immunisation has wider implications for the community than merely protecting the health of the individual.

The NH&MRC has issued recommendations regarding the attendance at school and day-care centres of children who are not adequately immunised. Victoria, the ACT and New South Wales have enacted legislation requiring the provision of immunisation certificates prior to school entry. Children who are not vaccinated against particular diseases will be excluded from school when an outbreak of one of the diseases occurs.

IMMUNISATION AGAINST OTHER DISEASES

As discussed previously, it is important that adults as well as children are fully immunised against the vaccine-preventable diseases. There are other, less common, diseases that are also preventable by vaccines, but immunisation is usually only recommended for high-risk groups. Table 14.6 lists vaccines that are available for special purposes and the groups who are most at risk. Other vaccines are required only by travellers to countries where a particular disease is endemic. Travellers should consult their State health departments for current recommendations for vaccination.

Immunisation for health professionals

Due to the nature of their work, health professionals are at significantly higher risk of encountering infectious diseases. Health workers are advised to be vaccinated against hepatitis B and tuberculosis (BCG). The value of the BCG vaccine in offering partial protection against tuberculosis is a controversial area. Some States recommend vaccination for all health workers, but others favour regular Mantoux testing, followed by antibiotic prophylaxis if required. In some institutional facilities, vaccination for hepatitis A may be advisable.

People working with children should ensure they have adequate immunisation against all the 'childhood diseases', especially as some of these diseases are much more severe in adults. Immunisation is also necessary in order to protect susceptible children (and adults) such as those suffering from leukaemia, who are particularly vulnerable to infection.

TABLE 14.6
VACCINES FOR SPECIAL PURPOSES

DISEASE	RECOMMENDED USAGE
Hepatitis A	(i) High-risk groups include: • Travellers to areas of high endemicity; • Staff in child-care centres. (ii) Others at risk through occupational exposure: • Staff, teachers of intellectually disabled; • Health workers in paediatric and infectious diseases wards; • Sewerage workers. (iii) Homosexual men. (iv) Individuals with chronic liver disease. (v) Recipients of blood products.
Hepatitis B	(i) Infants and young children born to carrier mothers or belonging to ethnic groups with high carriage rate. (ii) Individuals who are sexual partners or close contacts of Hepatitis B carriers. (iii) Health workers at occupational risk of exposure. (iv) Individuals at risk because of lifestyle.
Note: Hepatitis B vaccine is being used more widely to protect any person likely to come in contact with blood or body fluids.	
Influenza	(i) Individuals over 65 years of age, especially those with contributing illness such as chronic cardiac or lung disease. (ii) Aborigines and Torres Strait Islanders (ASTIC) over age 50. (iii) Other at-risk individuals, including: • Staff of nursing homes; • Staff caring for immunosuppressed patients; • Individuals with chronic debilitating disease.
Meningococcal infections	(i) Travellers to Nepal or other endemic areas. (ii) Control of outbreaks of meningococcal disease (serogroups A,C,W135,Y).
Pneumococcal infection	(i) Individuals in ASTIC communities over age 50. (ii) Individuals with other underlying illnesses.
Q fever	(i) Persons at risk from contact with infected animals or meat: • Abattoir workers; • Veterinarians; • Laboratory personnel.
Tuberculosis	(i) In children who are: • ATSIC neonates in regions of high incidence; • Children under five who are travelling to live in countries of high incidence. (ii) In household contacts of: • Recent immigrants from areas of high endemicity; • Patients with active TB. (iii) Health workers who are at high risk of occupational exposure.
Note: There is considerable divergence of opinion about the value of the BCG vaccination. Consult the Handbook.	
Chickenpox	(i) Immunosuppressed children. (ii) Health workers caring for children or immunosuppressed patients.
Note: Clinical trials are taking place in Australia.	

Source: Data derived from *The Australian Immunisation Procedures Handbook* 5th edition, 1994.

A vaccine for chickenpox is being tested and is desirable for all non-immune paediatric nurses.

Homoeopathic immunisation

'The NH&MRC childhood immunisation schedule has been shown to prevent tetanus, diphtheria and poliomyelitis and give a high level of protection against whooping cough, measles, mumps and rubella. Homoeopathic "immunisation" has not been shown to be effective. The NH&MRC warns that homoeopathic "immunisation" is useless and leaves children unprotected against serious and potentially fatal disease.'
(NH&MRC Statement from November 1990.)

Screening Procedures

Another important aspect of primary health care is the implementation of screening programs for the detection of infectious diseases. Early detection often allows intervention which can reduce or prevent morbidity and mortality.

ANTENATAL SCREENING TESTS

Among the most useful screening programs are antenatal screening tests. Some infections that are transmitted from mother to baby are not apparent in the mother and can affect the outcome of the pregnancy. If infection can be detected during pregnancy, appropriate treatment can be given. Useful serological screening tests during pregnancy are for the detection of susceptibility to infection (e.g. the presence or absence of rubella antibody), or the diagnosis of infection in which the presence of antigen or antibody indicates chronic infection (e.g. hepatitis B (HBV), syphilis, human immunodeficiency virus (HIV) infection). For most diseases, the presence of specific IgG antibodies indicates past infection and the absence of IgG antibodies indicates susceptibility. The presence of specific IgM antibody suggests recent infection.

Routine screening is only recommended if there is a suitable sensitive test available and there is significant risk of damage to the foetus or infant, *which is preventable*.

One of the most important screening procedures is the investigation of pregnant women to determine their status with respect to immunity to rubella. Rubella is a mild disease in adults, but is known to cause serious congenital defects if contracted during the first trimester of pregnancy. Antenatal screening identifies women who are not immune and who should therefore be advised to avoid exposure to people who have the disease. Measurement of the woman's immune status also enables the risk to the foetus from exposure to rubella during pregnancy to be determined. Vaccination of pregnant women is not advised but postnatal immunisation is offered to women who are not immune. Mass immunisation of the whole population with MMR vaccine at 12 months and again at 10–14 years is recommmended, as well as screening.

Screening for hepatitis B is particularly useful. Mothers who are chronic hepatitis B carriers have a high risk of their baby being infected at term or during delivery. Babies who are likely to be exposed to the virus can be identified by maternal screening during pregnancy, allowing prophylactic treatment to be given. The baby is given anti-hepatitis B immunoglobulin at birth, followed by a course of vaccination. This treatment breaks the chain of vertical transmission.

If syphilis infection is detected early during pregnancy, treatment with antibiotics (penicillin) can be given to the mother to prevent birth defects which do not usually occur until after 20 weeks' gestation.

Babies are also at risk of infection during passsage through the birth canal with organisms present in the vagina. Of thcsc, Group B streptococci (GBS) are the commonest cause of neonatal sepsis (about 1–2 cases per 1000 live births). Detection of GBS in the vagina by screening at 26–28 weeks allows for intra-partum anti-bacterial prophylaxis for high-risk women (administration of antibacterials just before and during labour).

TUBERCULOSIS

The **Tuberculin skin test (TT)**, or **Mantoux test (Mx)**, consists of a simple skin test to determine whether a person has been exposed to and infected by the tubercle bacillus. It does not reveal the state of the infection but allows follow-up investigations to be carried out. The test looks for a delayed hypersensitivity reaction to the intradermal injection of a small dose of purified protein from *Mycobacterium tuberculosis*. The injection site is examined after 48–72 hours and the diameter (in mm) of the resulting **induration** (inflammation) measured as an estimate of the strength of the reaction.

A Mantoux test may be positive if the person has a latent infection or active disease, has recovered from active disease, or has been vaccinated against tuberculosis with the BCG (Bacille Calmette Guerin) vaccine. It may also give a positive result if the person has been infected with a non-tuberculous mycobacterium (e.g. leprosy). The majority of Mantoux-positive persons have a latent infection, and do *not* have active disease when investigated further.

Preventive treatment may be offered to those with a latent infection. Individuals who are infected with the human immunodeficiency virus have a high risk of reactivation of a latent TB infection.

SCREENING OF BLOOD PRODUCTS

In Australia all blood and blood products supplied by the blood bank are screened for the presence of infectious agents. These include the human immunodeficiency virus (HIV), hepatitis B virus (HBV) and hepatitis C virus (HCV), *Treponema pallidum* (syphilis) and human T cell leukaemia virus I (HTLVI). Blood is not usually accepted from donors who are classified as 'high-risk' on the basis of their medical history or sexual preference, who are intravenous drug users or who have had previous blood transfusions. Although there is always the possibility of as yet undiscovered viruses or infectious agents being present, current screening procedures ensure that the supply of blood and blood products is as safe as possible.

CERVICAL CANCER DETECTION

Sexually mature women are advised to have regular cervical smear tests (Pap smears) to detect any changes in the cells of the cervix which may lead to invasive carcinoma. Although this is not strictly an infection, many cases of cervical cancer have been associated with prior infection by the human papilloma virus (HPV). Regular screening can detect early cellular changes so that treatment can be given to minimise the risk of progression to cancer (see Spotlight box, p. 102).

Health Care in Rural and Remote Areas

The challenges of the provision of health care in remote areas of Australia are often quite different to those encountered in large city hospitals. Various factors influence the type and severity of the infectious diseases encountered. They include:

- Climate and environmental conditions that favour some microorganisms not commonly found in other parts of Australia;
- Socioeconomic factors such as education, unemployment and lifestyle, as well as availability of good housing, sanitation and clean water supplies;
- Availability and access to health services and the level of compliance with public health measures such as immunisation.

There are many areas of rural Australia where certain diseases occur with a frequency above the national average. This is particularly true in the unique tropical northern regions of Australia, which include the Northern Territory, North Queensland and the Kimberley region of Western Australia. The range and incidence of infectious diseases vary between regions and are significantly different to the rest of Australia. These areas have a wide range of vegetation and a tropical climate, and are the habitat for organisms not usually found in other parts of Australia. When humans disturb the natural ecology of these regions they may be exposed to new microorganisms.

The special health problems faced by the people in the northern parts of Australia are the subject of a number of ongoing research projects at the Menzies School of Health Research in Darwin. As well, the Northern Territory Department of Health and Community Services collects and coordinates the publication of reports of infectious diseases in the monthly *Northern Territory Communicable Diseases Bulletin*.

ABORIGINAL HEALTH

The northern tropical areas of Australia have a larger proportion of Aborigines and Torres Strait Islanders than other regions. There have been numerous studies and reports dealing with the health status of Aborigines. They highlight the disparity in general health and incidence of infectious diseases that exists between Aboriginal and non-Aboriginal people. Aborigines have a lower life expectancy, up to 20 years less than other Australians, which is largely noticeable in the high mortality rate in young adults (20–40 years). The mortality rate for Aborigines is between two and four times the rate for the Australian population as a whole. Although many deaths are due to circulatory diseases, hypertension, chronic heart disease, diabetes, alcohol abuse and trauma, there are also significant differences in the morbidity and mortality rates for infectious diseases (see Figure 14.9).

Approximately 25% of Aborigines and Torres Strait Islanders live in remote areas, mainly the Northern Territory, including the Top End and Central Australia. While many Aborigines living in urban environments experience poorer health and lower socioeconomic conditions than other Australians, Aborigines in the north are also exposed to a number of unique tropical diseases. The overall notification rate for communicable diseases from the Northern Territory is six times the national average and this reflects the increased burden of disease in the Aboriginal population.

There are significant differences in the incidence of infectious diseases between Central Australia and the Top End, and between Aboriginal and non-Aboriginal people in each region (Tables 14.7, 14.8). The differences between the Top End and Central Australia are explained, in part, by the differences in the climate and socioeconomic conditions. Notification data are often incomplete, so these

TABLE 14.7
COMPARISON OF RATES OF NATIONALLY NOTIFIABLE DISEASES BY ETHNIC ORIGIN BETWEEN THE TOP END AND CENTRAL AUSTRALIA

ETHNIC ORIGIN	TOP END RATES	CENTRAL RATES	TOTAL NT RATES
Aboriginal	3908** (3670–4150)	7232 (6790–7680)	5030 (4810–5250)
Non-Aboriginal	282** (250–314)	1025 (912–1140)	448 (413–484)
Total	1847 (1770–1920)	2894 (2740–3050)	2108 (2040–2180)

(95% confidence intervals)
** 46.6% of the data from the Top End is missing and therefore these are the minimum rates.
Source: A. Ruben, Master of Applied Epidemiology thesis, ANU, 1994.

FIGURE 14.9
DIAGRAM OF ABORIGINAL HEALTH

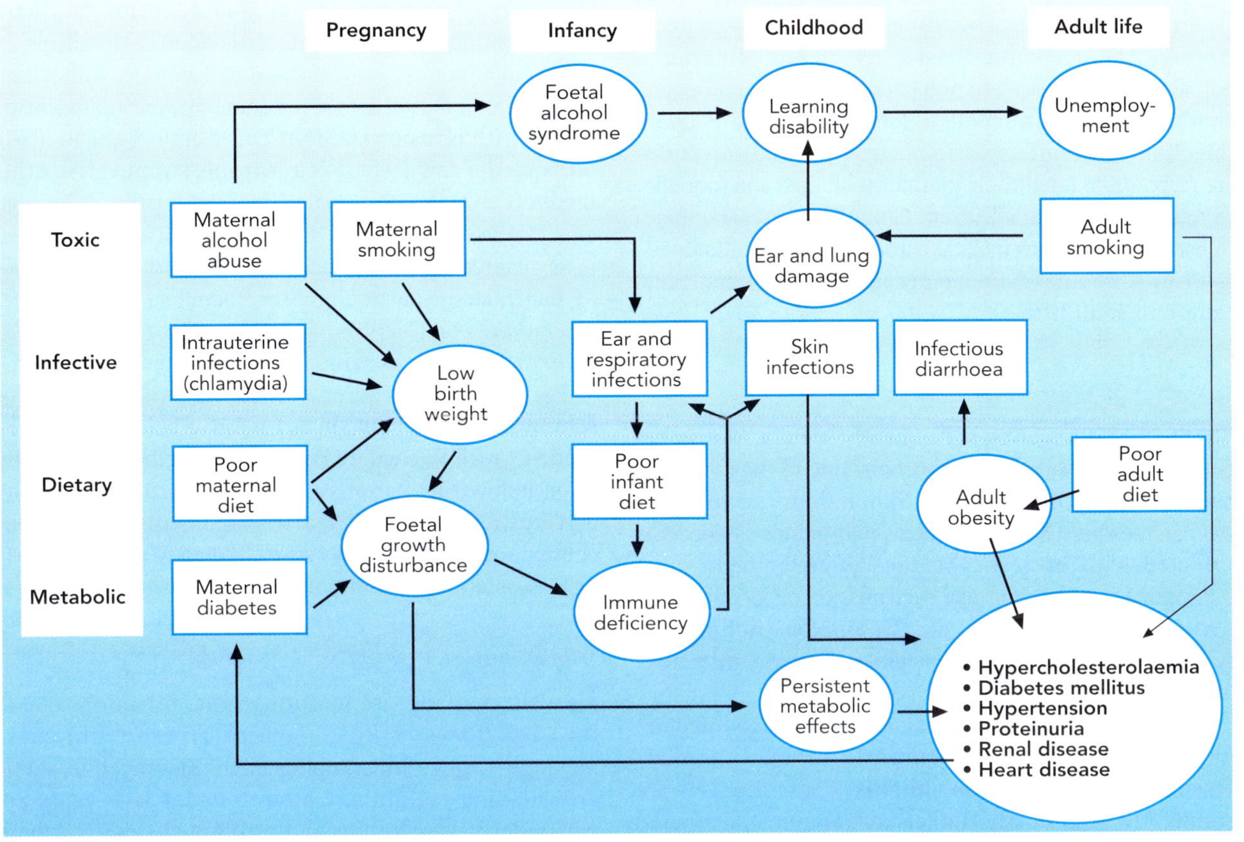

Source: Mathews, J. et al, *Aboriginal Health*, Menzies School of Health Research, Darwin, reproduced with permission from *Today's Life Science*, (1995) 7(8):24.

TABLE 14.8
RATE RATIOS OF NORTHERN TERRITORY NATIONALLY NOTIFIABLE DISEASES; AUSTRALIAN RATES AS REFERENCE

LOCATION AND ETHNIC ORIGIN	RATE RATIO AUSTRALIA = 1
Top End Aboriginal	11.1**
Top End non-Aboriginal	0.8**
Top End total	6.9
Central Aboriginal	20.6
Central non-Aboriginal	2.9
Central total	8.3
Total Northern Territory Aboriginal	14.3**
Total Northern Territory non-Aboriginal	1.9**
Total Northern Territory	6.0

** 46.7% of the data from the Top End is missing and therefore these are the minimum rate ratios
Source: A. Ruben, Master of Applied Epidemiology thesis, ANU, 1994.

figures are probably an underestimate of the true incidence of infections.

At all stages of their lives, Aborigines experience poorer health than non-Aborigines. Despite improvements in recent years, the infant mortality rate (in the first year of life) is still two to three times higher than the rest of Australia. Disorders of growth and nutrition are prevalent among Aboriginal people. Infants are often malnourished and vulnerable to a range of infections and other diseases. In all age groups, there are serious diseases that occur more commonly in Aboriginal than in non-Aboriginal people. They include diabetes, circulatory disorders, eye and ear infections, and other communicable diseases. Many of these are directly related to deficiencies in nutrition, lifestyle and housing. Among the communicable diseases, Aborigines have a much higher incidence of sexually transmitted diseases and tuberculosis than the rest of Australia.

To improve Aboriginal health, there is general agreement on the need to coordinate services at the community level, with community-controlled health services and Aboriginal health workers taking a prominant role in the delivery of primary health care and the implementation of specific programs. It is important that health professionals have a good understanding of the culture of the people for whom care is being provided.

INFECTIOUS DISEASES IN THE ABORIGINAL POPULATION

Overcrowded living conditions and poor hygiene in Aboriginal communities lead to a high rate of bacterial colonisation. The carriage of bacteria by infants and young children provides a reservoir of infection and allows cross-infection and reinfection to occur. Bacterial infections are responsible for chronic morbidity (illness) and mortality in many Aboriginal children. Complications (sequelae) of bacterial infections include chronic bronchitis, blindness, infertility, deafness, rheumatic heart disease and renal failure in adult life.

Group A Streptococcus pyogenes (GAS)

Streptococcal impetigo is frequently seen in Aboriginal children. A number of factors contribute to the existence and persistence of skin sores. Skin lesions due to minor trauma, mosquito bites and scabies infestations can become infected with bacteria. Scabies is endemic in most Aboriginal communities and transmission occurs via close body contact, bed linen, etc. Continuous itching and scratching of scabies allow secondary bacterial infections with GAS to occur.

Various sequelae (outcomes) are attributed to infection with GAS, including **rheumatic fever** and **post-streptococcal glomerulonephritis**. These diseases are commonly seen in Aboriginal communities, attributed largely to overcrowded living conditions. Such diseases are rarely seen in developed countries if streptococcal infections are well managed.

Rheumatic fever may cause damage to the aortic and mitral valves of the heart due to immunogenic reactions to streptococcal antigens. The weakened heart valves are susceptible to further infection and disease later in life (see Chapter 20).

Epidemics of **acute post-streptococcal glomerulonephritis (APSGN)** occur at regular intervals in Aboriginal communities in the Northern Territory and far North Queensland. However, **glomerular haematuria** and/or **proteinuria** (blood and protein in the urine) are also common in non-epidemic circumstances (the incidence is 20% in schoolage children), and patients with infected skin sores are more likely to have evidence of renal impairment. The incidence of end stage renal failure is about 100 times greater for Bathurst and Melville Islanders than for other Australians, and rates for other Northern Territory Aborigines are about 10 times the national average. The contribution that persistent childhood infections with GAS makes to chronic renal disease is uncertain as other factors, including diabetes, obesity and hypertension, also play a role.

Otitis media

Chronic otitis media (OM) (middle ear disease) and associated hearing loss are prevalent among Australian Aborigines. About 50–80% of schoolage children have been shown to be affected, as well as a significant proportion of adults. Studies have shown the presence of perforated ear-drums in up to 40% of infants aged less than 12 months. Recent studies in the Northern Territory have shown that otitis media develops in Aboriginal infants below the age of 3 months with a high prevalence of non-inflamed but immobile ear-drums, **otitis media with effusion** (**OME**). This can progress to **acute otitis media** and develop into **chronic suppurative otitis media (CSOM)** with associated loss of hearing. The rapid and early onset of otitis media in Aboriginal children is associated with early nasal colonisation by a number of bacteria, in particular *Streptococcus pneumoniae, Haemophilus influenzae,* and *Moraxella (Branhamella) catarrhlis*, which are able to spread to the middle ear.

Ear infections leading to hearing impairment have serious educational outcomes for the affected individuals. Students with fluctuating hearing loss are likely to exhibit poor behaviour patterns and to experience learning difficulties. Lack of hearing and subsequent poor communication skills may cause children to perform poorly or to stop attending school altogether.

Haemophilus influenzae type b (Hib) infections

As well as giving rise to otitis media, infections due to invasive *Haemophilus influenzae* type b (Hib) cause meningitis, epiglottitis, septicaemia, osteomyelitis, septic arthritis and cellulitis. Children under five years are particularly susceptible and children in the Northern Territory, especially Aboriginal children, used to have among the highest rates of Hib infection in the world. The recent introduction of Hib vaccine has seen a dramatic fall in the incidence of Hib disease in the Northern Territory as well as the rest of Australia (see Figure 14.6).

Streptococcus pneumoniae

As well as causing otitis media in children this organism is a significant cause of pneumonia and meningitis in children and adults. In the Northern Territory, invasive pneumococcal disease is responsible for 40% of community-acquired bacterial pneumonia in adult Aborigines admitted to hospital, with a mortality rate of 21%.

Gastrointestinal infections

The rates in the Northern Territory for enteric diseases caused by *Shigella*, *Salmonella*, *Campylobacter* and hepatitis A are all significantly higher than in other parts of Australia. The highest incidence occurs in children under five years of age, and the ratio of Aboriginal to non-Aboriginal infections is as high as 30:1. Shigellosis is the most infectious of the bacterial enteric diseases. Seasonal outbreaks of gastroenteritis due to the protozoan *Cryptosporidium parvuum* have been reported from Alice Springs.

Hepatitis A

A seroprevalence study of Aboriginal children in the Top End has shown that over 95% have been exposed to hepatitis

A by the age of five years. Similar data are not available for non-Aboriginal children in the Northern Territory.

Hepatitis E

At present, Hepatitis E is rarely seen in Australia. One case of probable hepatitis E, apparently acquired in the Northern Territory, was reported in 1994. However, all other cases have been acquired overseas. Hepatitis E is endemic in Asia and Africa.

Tuberculosis

The Northern Territory has the highest incidence of notifications of new cases of tuberculosis in Australia—there were 26 new cases, or 15.36 per 100 000, in 1994 compared with a national total of 944 new cases, giving an average of 5.35 per 100 000 for the rest of Australia. Although there is a high level of TB in the Aboriginal population, two-thirds of all notifications in Australia are for foreign-born individuals.

Leprosy

Eleven new cases of leprosy were notified in 1994 but only one was in the Northern Territory. The rest were spread among the other States. In 1993, the highest rate was in the Kimberley region of Western Australia. In previous years, the highest incidence of leprosy was in the Northern Territory and there are several people still under supervision for leprosy, although only a few require treatment. Early diagnosis and use of the WHO recommended multi-drug therapy can help to prevent serious neurological damage.

Sexually transmitted diseases

Sexually transmitted diseases (STDs) account for over 50% of all notifications of communicable diseases from the Northern Territory. They occur mainly in the 15–50 age group, with a higher frequency in Central Australia than in the Top End, which may reflect the higher proportion of Aboriginal people in Central Australia. Syphilis, gonorrhoea and chlamydia are the most commonly notified STDs, followed by genital herpes, non-specific urethritis (NSU) and donovanosis. Donovanosis is common in the Northern Territory, although it is rarely seen in the southern parts of Australia (see Figure 14.10). The high level of STDs in the Northern Territory is of concern because of the possibility of the spread of AIDS. STDs that have ulcerative lesions, such as syphilis and donovanosis, provide an increased risk factor for transmission of the AIDS virus.

UNUSUAL DISEASES OF RURAL AND REMOTE AREAS

Melioidosis is the most common cause of fatal, community-acquired bacterial pneumonia in the Northern Territory. It is caused by a soil organism, *Burkholderia pseudomallei* (formerly *Pseudomonas pseudomallei*), which gains entry to the body through breaks in the skin during

FIGURE 14.10
DISTRIBUTION OF DONOVANOSIS
Annual rate of notification of donovanosis per 100 000 population, 1993, by statistical division of residence.

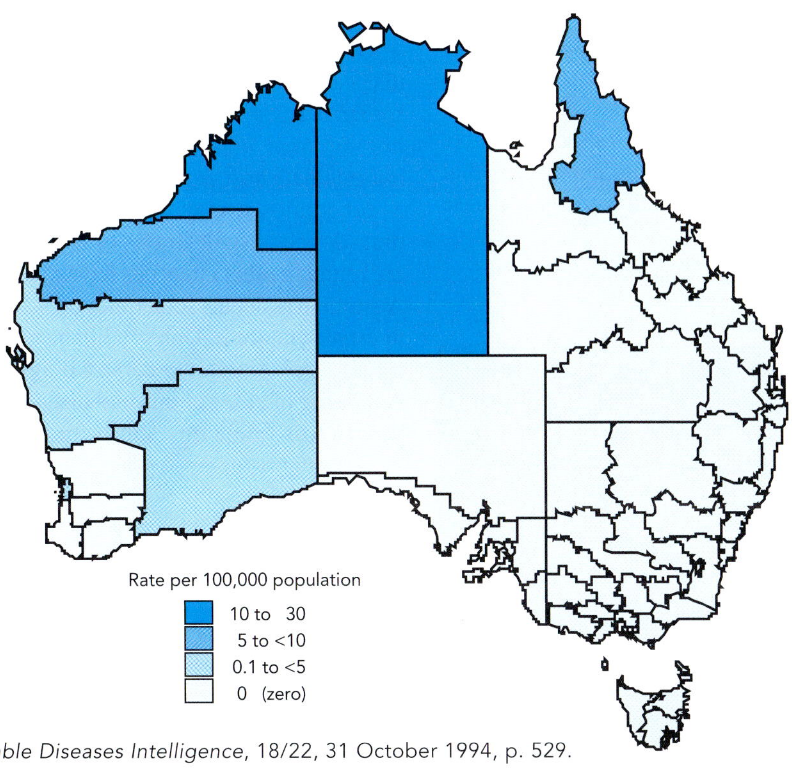

Source: Communicable Diseases Intelligence, 18/22, 31 October 1994, p. 529.

exposure to soil or water, especially during the wet season. In the last three wet seasons there have been a total of 82 cases of melioidosis, with 21 deaths (Currie 1995). Melioidosis can cause fulminant sepsis or subclinical infections which may reactivate years later. It can also cause abscesses in skin and deep tissue and in body organs (Figure 14.11). Prompt diagnosis and treatment is required to prevent fatal outcomes. The organism is resistant to penicillin and gentamicin but sensitive to third generation cephalosporins.

Leptospirosis occurs mainly in rural Victoria, Queensland and the Northern Territory. *Leptospira interrogans* is the organism responsible for causing **Weil's disease**, an acute renal failure with a 5–10% fatality rate. Symptoms include headache, chills, myalgia, rash and, sometimes meningitis, haemolytic anaemia, haemorrhage, and liver and kidney failure. Transmission is by ingestion of the organism which is present in the urine of infected animals. The disease is usually a result of occupational exposure to animals and animal urine, but can be contracted by recreational exposure to contaminated water (e.g. in national parks). Reservoirs include domestic and native rodents, bandicoots, rabbits, cattle and feral pigs. Although not common in Australia, there have been several cases reported in recent years.

A number of other diseases are more common in remote or rural areas than in the rest of Australia. They include diseases such as **Q fever** which occurs mainly in cattle-raising areas, although it is not seen in the Northern Territory.

The tropical climate of Northern Queensland favours the mosquito *Aedes aegypti*, which can act as a vector for dengue fever. Although the dengue virus is not endemic in Australia, cases of the disease imported by travellers from overseas can cause an epidemic if the mosquitoes are not controlled (see p. 317).

IMPLICATIONS FOR HEALTH CARE

The range and severity of infectious diseases seen in remote areas, together with the socioeconomic conditions that prevail, pose special challenges to health workers. Because of the distances involved, many people living in these areas often do not seek medical care until the disease is well advanced. In addition, underlying illnesses may contribute to the severity of the disease and make diagnosis more difficult. Health workers also need to be aware of the customs and taboos of the indigenous people. Protocols have been developed specifically for these areas and health workers should be aware of their existence and use them to optimise the treatment and control of infectious diseases. They include:

- Specific immunisation schedules (see Tables 14.9, 14.10);
- Additions to the list of notifiable diseases (e.g. the Northern Territory includes donovanosis and invasive pneumococcal disease);
- Treatment protocols for use by health workers;
- Antibiotic guidelines for Central and North Australia;
- The Central Australian Rural Practitioners Standard Treatment Manual and the Northern Territory and Top End Standard Treatment Manual.

FIGURE 14.11
LESION OF MELIOIDOSIS

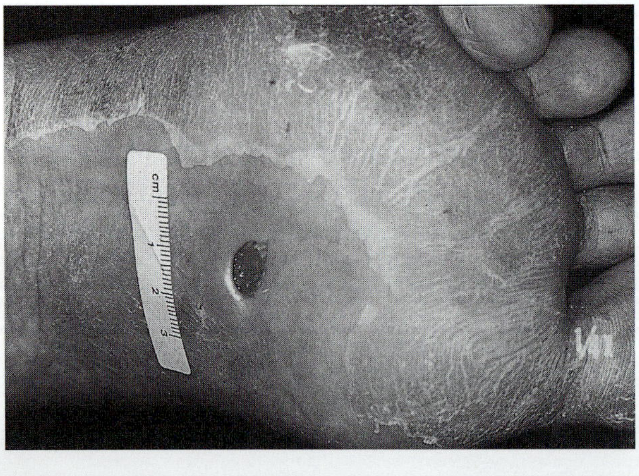

Infectious Diseases from Outside Australia

Australia is fortunate in that, being an island, it is free from some of the infectious diseases that occur in other parts of the world. However, there is always the risk that some of these diseases may be imported into Australia, carried by travellers, tourists, students or immigrants. As more people undertake overseas travel and more tourists and students visit Australia, the potential for the spread of microorganisms and/or their vectors is increased. The entry of illegal immigrants who have not undergone health screening prior to their arrival poses an additional health risk. In this section we look briefly at some of the diseases that are potential health problems.

Occasionally, a person suffering from one of these diseases may enter Australia, but the disease will not be spread because of the lack of an appropriate vector, or will not become established because of the lack of an intermediate host or animal reservoir. Other diseases, such as tuberculosis, may already occur in Australia, but the multidrug-resistant strains of the causative organism that are found in other countries have not yet reached Australia. Australian residents sometimes present to their doctors with unusual symptoms. Unless a full history, including overseas travel, is obtained, the correct diagnosis may be missed. A number of cases of unusual diseases are diagnosed each year in Australian travellers returning from overseas.

TUBERCULOSIS

Prior to 1945 the incidence of active tuberculosis in Australia was more than 45 per 100 000 population. A national TB campaign of mass chest X-rays, BCG vaccinations and treatment resulted in a large decline in the rate of notifications. Since 1987, the notification rate for the whole country has averaged about 5.5 per 100 000 population. Although this rate compares favourably with

TABLE 14.9
NORTHERN TERRITORY CHILDHOOD VACCINATION SCHEDULE
Immunise your child at these important ages.

AGE	VACCINE	ROUTE
Birth	Hepatitis B Vaccine (HBV) * Hepatitis B Immunoglobulin * BCG	IM IM Intradermal
1 month	HBV	IM
2 months	Diphtheria, pertussis, tetanus (DPT) Oral polio vaccine (OPV) Haemophilus influenzae type b (Hib)	IM Oral IM
4 months	DTP OPV Hib	IM Oral IM
6 months	DTP OPV HBV	IM Oral IM
9 months (Aboriginal)	Measles, mumps, rubella (MMR)	IM
12 months (non-Aboriginal) 12 months	MMR Hib	IM IM
18 months	DPT	IM
4–5 years	DPT OPV	IM Oral
10 years (rural areas)	Tuberculin skin test	Intradermal
10 years	MMR	IM
1st year High School (urban areas)	Tuberculin skin test	Intradermal
15 years, and then at 10 year intervals 15 years	Adult diphtheria, tetanus (ADT) OPV	IM Oral

PRP-OMP (PedvaxHIB)

* Specified risk groups only

other countries, it is still a cause for concern. The rate varies from over 18 per 100 000 in the Northern Territory to 2 per 100 000 in Tasmania. Two-thirds of all notifications are in foreign-born people, mainly from Indo-China.

The NH&MRC working party has identified a number of issues that affect the incidence and management of TB in Australia. These include:

- the pattern of immigration and travel;
- the increased worldwide incidence of TB;
- the emergence of multidrug-resistant strains;
- the interaction of TB and HIV infection.

Tuberculosis is a highly infectious disease that is readily transmitted from person to person on aerosol droplets. The bacterium lodges in the body, usually in the lungs. It may remain latent for many years or it may develop into active TB (see Chapter 17). People infected with HIV are particularly susceptible to reactivation of latent TB infection as well as to new infections. Although immigrants are screened prior to entry to Australia, it is possible they may develop TB by reactivation of a prior infection. In the United States there is an increasing incidence of the disease caused by multidrug-resistant strains of *Mycobacterium tuberculosis* (MDR-TB).

At present, these strains are not common in Australia but it is possible they can be transported to Australia by returning travellers. In 1992, 12.4% of isolates were resistant to one antibiotic, but only 1% (six isolates) were resistant to two or more antibiotics. These infections did not occur in HIV-positive patients so, at present, the HIV and MDR-TB link is not established in Australia. However, there is concern that all these factors may combine to cause a serious epidemic in a population that is largely non-immune.

The **BCG vaccine** offers some protection against infection by *Mycobacterium tuberculosis*, but does not guarantee immunity. It is currently recommended for health care workers in some States, for children in high-risk groups (e.g. Northern Territory Aborigines) and for young travellers to high-risk areas. A disadvantage of BCG vaccination is that it interferes with the Mantoux or Tuberculin test which is used to identify whether exposure to TB has occurred and whether preventive treatment is necessary.

TABLE 14.10
NORTHERN TERRITORY ADULT IMMUNISATION SCHEDULE

ALL ADULTS	
AGE	**VACCINE**
15 years, and then every 10 years throughout life	Adult diphtheria, tetanus (ADT)
15 years	OPV, MMR (if not received in year six)
50 years (Aboriginal)	Pneumococcal Influenza (yearly thereafter)
65 years (non-Aboriginal)	Pneumococcal Influenza (yearly thereafter)
SPECIAL GROUPS	
IMMUNOCOMPROMISED	**VACCINE**
Anatomlc or functional asplenia	Meningococcal, pneumococcal, influenza (yearly) and Hib
Diabetes and malignant diseases Chronic: alcoholism lung and cardiac disease renal failure	Pneumococcal, influenza (yearly)
HIV infection	Meningococcal, pneumococcal, influenza (yearly) and Hib
Haemodialysis or transplant recipients	Pneumococcal, influenza (yearly), hepatitis B and Hib
Chronic liver disease	Pneumococcal, influenza (yearly), hepatitis A and hepatitis B
LIFESTYLE	**VACCINE**
Homosexally active men Injecting drug users	Hepatitis A and hepatitis B
Multiple sexual partners and/or sexually tranmissible diseases	Hepatitis B
Women considering pregnancy	Check Rubella antibody titre. If negative MMR two months before conception
TRAVELLERS	**VACCINE**
Vaccine requirements will depend on individual itineraries	Consult Health Department

MALARIA

Malaria is the most important of the disease carried by insect vectors (see Chapter 20). It is endemic in the tropical regions north of Australia, especially Papua New Guinea and the Pacific Islands. The cause of malaria, the protozoan *Plasmodium*, is carried by the Anopheles mosquito which is found in many parts of Australia, especially in the north (see Figure 14.12). As we said in Chapter 8, for the disease to spread there has to be a reservoir or pool of infected people, and conditions suitable for the appropriate vector to breed and transmit the disease. Although there has not been a recorded case of transmission occurring in Australia for many years, there is always a real possibility of the reintroduction of malaria, especially in Northern Australia where there is a large number of mosquitoes, many of the dwellings are open and there is an influx of immigrants, tourists and students from high-risk endemic areas. Control of the mosquito vector is the most effective way to prevent reintroduction of the disease.

Australian travellers to endemic areas are at risk of contracting malaria. In 1992 there were 712 cases of malaria reported in Australia and three deaths. This is a huge increase in the number of cases compared to 20 years ago and reflects an increase in travel by Australians to endemic areas. As well, strains of *Plasmodium* resistant to the antimalarial drug chloroquine have appeared in many areas. Although several trials are in progress there

FIGURE 14.12
WORLD DISTRIBUTION OF MALARIA

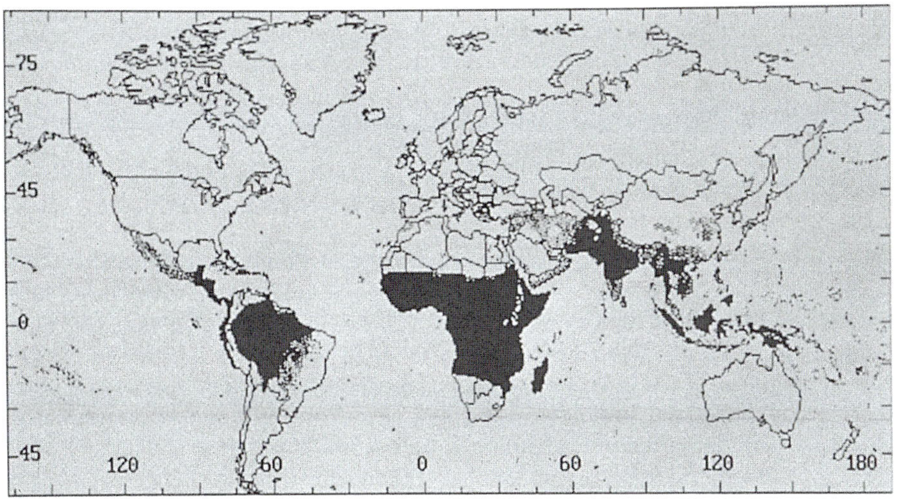

is currently no vaccine against malaria, and travellers should consult their health department to obtain up-to-date information on appropriate medication for the areas they intend to visit.

It is important to use preventive strategies to avoid mosquito bites: insect repellant, long-sleeved clothing, mosquito nets and screens. Travellers should be aware that they may contract malaria, despite taking medication, if the particular strain of the organism is drug-resistant, or if the medication is not appropriate or not taken for long enough. Malaria should be suspected in any person who has recently returned from a malarious area and who is suffering intermittent bouts of fever, headaches and nausea. Microscopic examination of blood films can give a correct diagnosis. Malaria can be treated successfully if diagnosed early in the course of the disease, but delay can have fatal consequences.

DENGUE FEVER

Dengue fever is a mosquito-borne viral disease occurring mainly in northern parts of Australia. It is carried by the vector *Aedes aegypti*, which is found in some areas of Queensland and Western Australia. Outbreaks of dengue occur from time to time, usually associated with good mosquito-breeding conditions. The last major outbreak occurred in Queensland in 1992. The symptoms of dengue fever include acute headache, joint pain, rash and fever, but occasionally haemorrhagic fever and dengue shock syndrome may occur, especially in young children. The occurrence of haemorrhagic dengue fever appears to be due to a second infection with a different serotype of the virus in people who have a prior history of dengue disease. Dengue fever has been known for many years but has only become a major health problem since there has been extensive movement of people, which has led to the circulation of the four serotypes. Control of the vector *Aedes aegypti* is important in preventing outbreaks of dengue.

YELLOW FEVER

Yellow fever is an acute viral disease, transmitted by mosquitoes. It is found in Africa and parts of South America, but does not occur in Australia. A vaccine is available and travellers entering Australia from endemic areas are required to have been vaccinated or to undergo quarantine.

MENINGOCOCCAL MENINGITIS

This is a serious, sometimes fatal, disease caused by *Neisseria meningitidis*. Although the bacterium is endemic in Australia, outbreaks are very infrequent. However, the rate of notification has been steadily increasing in recent years. In 1994 there were 216 notifications, mainly types B and C. A vaccine for types A, C, W-135 and Y is available, but its widespread use is not usually considered to be warranted. Travellers to areas where it is endemic (e.g. Nepal) are advised to be vaccinated. The change in climatic conditions, together with the climbing activities that most tourists undertake, render them more susceptible to the disease. In New Zealand, epidemics of meningococcal disease have occurred in recent years, mainly in children under five years of age (see p. 319).

SHISTOSOMIASIS

Shistosomiasis is a chronic parasitic infection caused by trematodes, or flukes. Their complex life cycle involves a larval form, the free-swimming **cercariae**, which are released from the intermediate host, a freshwater snail. Infection of humans occurs when the cercariae penetrate the skin, usually when the person is working, swimming or wading in contaminated water. A number of cases of shistosomiasis have been recorded in travellers returning to Australia; for example, in a rugby team that had visited Zimbabwe and been white water rafting on the Zambezi river. Other travellers had been swimming in Lake Malawi.

When correctly diagnosed, shistosome infections can be treated with praziquantel. Travellers should be aware of areas where shistosomiasis is endemic. As long as the particular species of freshwater snail that is needed as the intermediate host is not imported into Australia, people who are infected will not pose a health risk to other Australians.

GASTROINTESTINAL DISEASES

Gastrointestinal infections are commonly acquired by travellers. Vaccines are available against typhoid and hepatitis A and should be considered for travellers to areas where these diseases are endemic. Another viral cause of acute hepatitis, hepatitis E, is endemic in Asia, Africa and Mexico. One cases of hepatitis E was reported in the Northern Territory in 1994 and there have been suspected cases in people who have been travelling overseas. It is transmitted by the faecal-oral route and so could easily be spread, once imported into Australia.

Public Health Issues in New Zealand

Many infectious diseases occur throughout the world, while others are restricted to certain regions. Each country produces its own statistics for the incidence of diseases, and develops policies and regulations appropriate for their control that may differ from their neighbours. Although New Zealand is geographically close to Australia, its climate and population are different. In this section, we examine some of the public health issues that are unique to New Zealand.

The population is about 3.5 million of whom 13% are Maori, 5% are from the Pacific Islands and the remaining 82% are of mainly European origin with an increasing number of people from Asia. The Pacific Islands population living in New Zealand is heterogeneous, consisting of people of the Samoan, Tongan, Cook Islands, Tokelauan, Niuean, Fijian and Tuvaluan ethnic groups. as well as people from Papua New Guinea, Vanuatu and the Solomon Islands. The lifestyles and health problems of the three major groups are different and contribute to the variations in incidence statistics for the various diseases.

COMMUNICABLE DISEASES IN NEW ZEALAND

A monthly communicable diseases report, the *New Zealand Public Health Report (NZPHR)*, is prepared by the Institute of Environmental Science and Research (ESR) and published jointly by the Ministry of Health and the ESR. The list of notifiable diseases includes those required by the World Health Organization, as well as other infections for which a public health intervention is required or for which the incidence needs to be monitored (see Table 14.11). A revised schedule of notifiable diseases came into effect in June 1996, one of the main changes being the addition of vaccine preventable diseases. The figures presented here should be interpreted with caution, as they do not necessarily represent the total number of cases of the disease. For example, only an estimated 10–25% of food-borne infections are notified. Table 14.12 shows the incidence of selected notifiable diseases and compares it with data from Australia and the United States.

Comparison of rates of notification of infectious diseases in Australia and New Zealand

Several diseases in New Zealand have a higher rate of notification than in Australia. They include tuberculosis, meningococcal meningitis and rheumatic fever, and the less common diseases, leptospirosis and listeriosis.

TABLE 14.11
NOTIFIABLE DISEASES IN NEW ZEALAND

Number and rate of notified cases of selected communicable diseases 1988–93

	NUMBER OF NOTIFICATIONS			*RATE PER 100 000*		
	1991	1992	1993	1991	1992	1993
Food and water-borne illness						
Hepatitis A	223	290	258	6.6	8.6	7.6
Listeriosis	26	16	12	0.8	0.5	0.4
Typhoid	9	12	12	0.3	0.4	0.4
Food poisoning	228	370	660	6.8	11.0	19.6
Shigellosis	141	120	124	4.2	3.6	3.7
Salmonellosis	1209	1215	1331	35.8	36.0	39.4
Campylobacteriosis	4111	5138	8026	121.8	152.3	237.9
Other diseases						
Meningococcal disease	71	153	201	2.1	4.5	6.0
Hepatitis B	227	221	114	6.7	6.6	3.4
Leptospirosis	55	71	109	1.6	2.1	3.2
Legionellosis	14	11	24	0.4	0.3	0.7
Rheumatic fever	91	70	78	2.7	2.1	2.3
Malaria	36	29	47	1.1	0.9	1.4

Source: Our Health, Our Future 1994, New Zealand Ministry of Health.

TABLE 14.12
NOTIFIABLE DISEASES IN NEW ZEALAND COMPARED WITH AUSTRALIA AND THE UNITED STATES

International comparisons of reported cases of selected communicable diseases, rates per 100 000

DISEASE (RATE PER 100 000)	NZ 1992	AUSTRALIA 1991	USA 1990
Campylobacteriosis	152.3	75.8	
Salmonellosis	36.0	31.4	19.5
Shigellosis	3.6	7.9	10.9
Listeriosis	0.5	0.3	
Hepatitis A	8.6	12.7	12.6
Hepatitis B	6.6	21.1	8.5
Hepatitis C	2.2	29.0	
Leptospirosis	2.1	1.0	
Meningococcal disease	4.5	1.6	
Hib	5.4	3.5	
Hib age < 5years	46.2		11.0*
Tuberculosis	9.5	3.4	10. 3
AIDS	10.8	18.0	16.7*

Key: Hib *Haemophilus influenzae* b disease. * = 1991.

Source: Our Health, Our Future 1993, New Zealand Ministry of Health.

TABLE 14.13
NOTIFIED CASES OF SELECTED COMMUNICABLE DISEASES IN NEW ZEALAND BY ETHNICITY

DISEASE	RATE PER 100 000 1988-92 M	PI	E + O
Hepatitis A	10.5	5.9	4.7
Listeriosis	0.2	0.5	0.4
Typhoid	0	2.8	0.3
Food poisoning	0.3	1.3	2.6
Shigellosis	4.9	18.2	3.4
Salmonellosis	20.5	37.5	42.0
Campylobacteriosis	24.3	22.9	131.6
Meningococcal disease	5.8	7.3	1.4
Hepatitis B	17.1	12.2	6.0
Leptospirosis	1.8	0.4	2.5
Legionellosis	0.3	0.3	0.8
Rheumatic fever	9.4	21.6	0.6
Malaria	0.1	1.4	0.9
1993			
DISEASE	M	PI	A
Hepatitis A	15.9	10.5	5.6
Listeriosis	—	1.3	0.3
Typhoid	—	4.6	0.1
Food poisoning	3.9	2.0	14.6
Shigellosis	0.7	7.8	3.6
Salmonellosis	20.7	21.6	39.9
Campylobacteriosis	51.1	37.9	262.6

Key: M = Maori, A = all other ethnic groups, PI = Pacific Islands people, U = unknown.

Source: Our Health, Our Future 1993, New Zealand Ministry of Health.

The higher incidence of **tuberculosis** in New Zealand occurs mainly in the Maori and Pacific Islander population (see p. 321). The incidence of drug-resistant strains is low: only 4 of 417 isolates of TB were multidrug-resistant (1%) in 1993.

Meningococcal disease is a serious illness caused by *Neisseria meningitidis*. There are three major serogroups—A, B and C—and two minor groups—Y and W-135. A tetravalent vaccine is available for serogroups A, C, W-135 and Y. In 1985–87, there was an epidemic of meningococcal disease, serogroup A, in New Zealand. The number of cases then declined, but has risen again since 1992 (see Figure 14.13). In 1994, the notification rate was 6.2 per 100 000 population. Of these, 75% of cases were due to serogroup B, for which no vaccine is available. When the cases are due to a vaccine-preventable serogroup, a vaccination program for children is instigated. Meningococcal disease presents as meningitis, septicaemia and other diseases. Children under five years are most at risk, especially Maori and Pacific Island children. In 1994 there were 208 cases, with 11 deaths, an overall 6.3% mortality rate.

Compared with other developed countries, New Zealand has high rates of post-streptococcal disease such as **rheumatic fever**. The disease presents as arthritis and carditis, affecting the aortic and mitral valves of the heart, and sometimes causing residual damage to the valves of the heart. The person is susceptible to further streptococcal infections and damage to the heart valves. Rheumatic fever is a notifiable disease in New Zealand and a register of patients was set up in 1986. The incidence is highest among Maori and Pacific Island children. In Australia the incidence of rheumatic heart disease is highest among the Aborigines.

Although the number of cases has decreased since 1980, the rate of notification of **leptospirosis** in New Zealand is still almost double the rate for Australia. Leptospirosis is a zoonotic bacterial infection that occurs mainly in young adults, often agricultural workers or people associated with meat or animals.

Listeriosis is a food-borne illness caused by the bacterium *Listeria monocytogenes*. The rate of notification of the disease in New Zealand, although not high, is still higher than in Australia. *Listeria* is important because it can infect pregnant women causing abortion, preterm delivery or infection of the baby. Overall death rates sometimes approach 30%, with the highest incidence in the newborn. It may cause only mild illness in healthy people but can cause severe illness in immunocompromised people, those with diabetes or renal transplants. Infections are usually associated with contaminated food—milk, soft cheese, meat or fish.

FIGURE 14.13
EPIDEMIC OF MENINGOCOCCAL MENINGITIS IN NEW ZEALAND

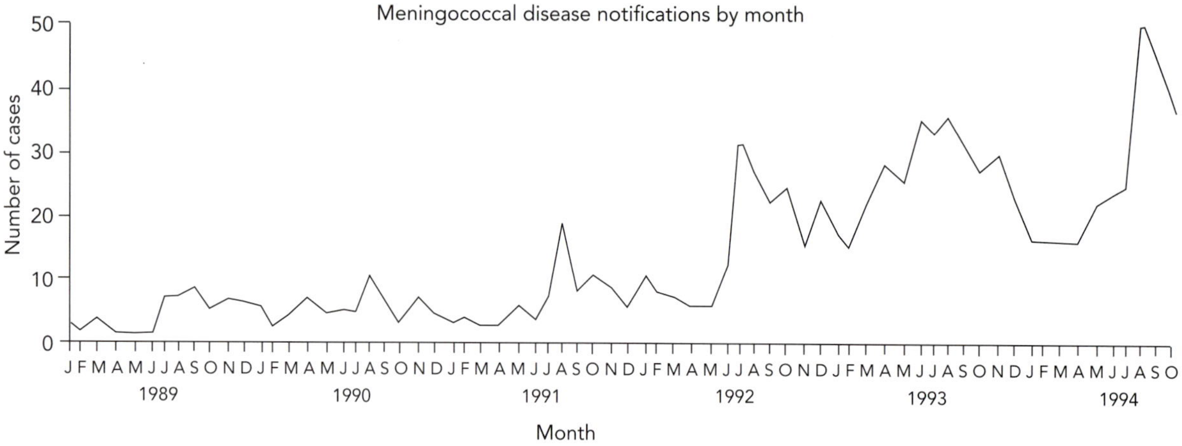

Source: Our Health, Our Future 1993, New Zealand Ministry of Health.

THE HEALTH STATUS OF DIFFERENT ETHNIC GROUPS

The health status of different groups within the community is affected by socioeconomic conditions as well as ethnicity. Various measurements are used to determine the relative health status of the different ethnic groups that make up the New Zealand population. These include general health, prevalence of disease or disability, the infant mortality rate, incidence of infectious diseases, and death rates. At the turn of the century, a series of epidemics of infectious diseases (influenza, whooping cough, measles), a high mortality rate and land wars drastically reduced the population of Maoris. The situation was addressed by public health measures such as improvement in hygiene, sanitation, water supplies and vaccination. The 1994 report of the Public Health Commission of New Zealand, together with the 1994 report on the Health of the Pacific Islands people in New Zealand, identify differences which still exist in health, incidence of infections and outcome of diseases for the major ethnic groups in New Zealand. Some examples from these reports are presented here.

Infant mortality rate

Indicators such as the infant mortality rate are often regarded as sensitive to social conditions and health services. There has been an overall decline in infant mortality in New Zealand in the last 15 years, but the rate for Maoris is still almost twice that for Europeans. The rate for Pacific Islanders is similar to that for Europeans. Of the Maori infant mortality rate, 50% is attributed to sudden infant death syndrome (SIDS).

Infectious diseases

Table 14.13 compares the rate of notification of selected diseases in the period 1988–92 for Maoris, Pacific Islanders, Europeans and people of other ethnic origin.

Of the gastrointestinal infections, Maoris had higher rates of **hepatitis A**, but **Campylobacteriosis** was higher among Europeans. Of concern is the high incidence of meningococcal disease in Maoris and Pacific Islanders, compared with Europeans. The incidence of hepatitis B in New Zealand is quite high, mainly in young adults and injecting drug users. Maoris have a high rate of infection, and a greater chance of subsequent **hepatitis B** carriage, leading to chronic hepatic disease.

The incidence of **rheumatic fever** in Pacific Islanders was 20 times that for Europeans and double the incidence for Maoris. Hearing loss resulting from **otitis media** affects 6–10% of New Zealand schoolchildren. It is more likely to occur in children under seven and is more common among males and Maori children (15%). Pacific Island children have a similar rate to Maori children.

Tuberculosis has declined in most developed countries but there is concern that the incidence will increase as the number of immunosuppressed people rises and there is spread of multi-resistant strains. In New Zealand, there is a marked difference between the incidence of TB in different ethnic groups (see Table 14.14). For Europeans the rate was 1.9 per 100,000, Maoris 9.3 per 100 000, Pacific Islanders 19.6 per 100 000, and other ethnic origins 29.7 per 100,000. Of all reported cases (1990–92), 17.9% had been in New Zealand for less than five years (Table 14.14). New guidelines for tuberculosis control in New Zealand were published in 1992.

IMMUNISATION

The New Zealand Department of Health recommended vaccination schedule (Table 14.15), is contained in the handbook, *Immunisation*. This is continually revised and health professionals should ensure they are aware of the most recent schedule.

Up to now vaccine-preventable diseases have not been notifiable in New Zealand so it is not possible to assess the success of the vaccination campaign or the level of compliance with the vaccination schedule. A survey carried out in 1992 indicated that less than 60% of all children and only 42% of Maori children had been fully immunised by their second birthday. (To prevent outbreaks it is considered that a level of coverage of 85–95% in the community is required.) A survey based on the number of people submitting claim forms for health benefits associated with immunisation in 1994 showed an increase in the percentage coverage for the second year of life compared with 1992 data.

The occurrence of vaccine-preventable diseases has a similar pattern to Australia. In order to improve the compliance with vaccination, a new schedule was issued in February 1996 (see Table 14.15). Children now have to attend on only five separate occasions (instead of eight with the old schedule) in order to receive all their vaccinations. An additional dose of pertussis has been added to the schedule to be given at 15 months with the first dose of MMR.

Note: Hepatitis B vaccine is recommended for all children.

TABLE 14.14
NUMBER OF NOTIFIED CASES OF TUBERCULOSIS IN NEW ZEALAND 1990–92, BY YEAR AND ETHNICITY

	1990	1991	1992	AGGREGATED (3 YEARS)
Numberof notifications	337	311	318	966
Rate per 100 000	10.0	9.2	9.4	9.5
Confirmed cases	156	245	136	537
Rate per 100 000	4.6	7.3	4.0	5.3

	1990–92 ETHNICITY			
	M	PI	E	O
Number of notifications	243	163	285	248
Rate per 100 000	18.6	35.5	3.6	83.3
Confimed cases	144	93	182	111
Rate per 100 000	11.0	20.3	2.3	37.3

Key: M = Maori, PI = Paclfic Island, E = European, O = People of other ethnic origin.
Source: NZCDC.

TABLE 14.15
NEW ZEALAND VACCINATION SCHEDULE

	6 WEEKS	3 MONTHS	5 MONTHS	15 MONTHS	11 YEARS
Hepatitis B	✓	✓	✓		
DTPH*	✓	✓	✓	✓	
Polio	✓	✓	✓		✓
MMR				✓	✓
Td**					✓

* *DTPH = Combined Diphtheria, Tetanus Pertussis, Haemophilus influenzae type b (Hib).*
** *Td = Combined Diphtheria, Tetanus.*
Source: NZ Public Health Report Vol. 3, No. 2, February 1996.

Summary

- The decline in mortality from infectious diseases in the 20th century has been due to an improved standard of hygiene, the discovery of antibiotics and the development of vaccines.
- Responsibility for the delivery of health care in Australia rests with various State, Territory and Federal authorities.

NOTIFIABLE DISEASES

- A core group of communicable diseases is required by law to be notified to the health authorities when diagnosed in a patient.
- The NNDSS coordinates the adoption of the NH&MRC list of diseases for notification and the reporting of notifiable diseases at a Commonwealth level.
- The annual report of the NNDSS is published in the *CDI* bulletin.

PRIMARY HEALTH CARE

- Primary health care involves the provision of services such as health education, health promotion, disease prevention and treatment of illness.
- In Australia the major factors that influence health status are socioeconomic conditions.
- The Aborigines and Torres Strait Islanders have a much lower general standard of health than other Australians.

IMMUNISATION

- Major reasons for the improvement in health in the 20th century are the development of vaccines and the implementation of immunisation programs.
- Active immunisation is the administration of a vaccine to stimulate the body's immune system to produce both specific antibodies and cellular immunity.
- The Australian Health Department provides free vaccination for most childhood diseases.
- The NH&MRC publishes information on immunisation procedures and recommendations for administration.
- The most effective type of vaccine consists of live, attenuated (weakened) forms of the pathogen. Some vaccines consist of toxoids, some contain killed, whole cells of the pathogen, others consist of fragments of the pathogen.
- The principle of herd immunity means that, for a population to be protected from a disease, a certain percentage must be immunised against that disease.
- In Australia, compliance with immunisation schedules is not complete and there have been epidemics of measles and pertussis.
- The risks from immunisation are much less than the risks from having the disease.
- Children who are not vaccinated against a particular disease will be excluded from school when an outbreak of the disease occurs.
- Vaccines are available for travellers and health workers.
- The NH&MRC warns that homoeopathic 'immunisation' is useless and leaves children unprotected against serious and potentially fatal disease.

SCREENING PROCEDURES

- Screening of women during pregnancy is useful to detect the presence of, or susceptibility to, pathogens that may cause congenital defects.
- The Tuberculin Skin Test (TT), or Mantoux test (Mx), is a skin test that can determine whether a person has been exposed to and infected by the tubercle bacillus.
- In Australia all blood and blood products supplied by the blood bank are screened for the presence of infectious agents such as the human immunodeficiency virus (HIV), hepatitis B virus (HBV) and hepatitis C virus (HCV), *Treponema pallidum* (syphilis) and human T cell leukaemia virus I (HTLVI).
- Pap smears can detect changes in the cells of the cervix that may lead to invasive carcinoma.

HEALTH CARE IN RURAL AND REMOTE AREAS

- Factors such as climate, socioeconomic conditions and access to health services affect the incidence of infectious diseases in remote areas.
- The Northern Territory Department of Health and Community Services collects and coordinates the publication of reports of infectious diseases in the monthly *Northern Territory Communicable Diseases Bulletin*.

ABORIGINAL HEALTH

- There is a disparity in general health and incidence of infectious diseases between Aboriginal and non-Aboriginal people.
- The overall notification rate for communicable diseases from the Northern Territory is six times the national average.
- The infant mortality rate is 2–3 times higher than the rest of Australia.
- Aborigines have a much higher incidence of sexually transmitted diseases and tuberculosis than the rest of Australians.
- Overcrowded living conditions and poor hygiene in the Aboriginal communities lead to a high rate of disease and cross-infection.
- Complications (sequelae) of bacterial infections include chronic bronchitis, blindness, infertility, deafness, rheumatic heart disease, and renal failure in adult life.
- Skin infections with Group A *Streptococcus pyogenes* (GAS) may have outcomes such as post-streptococcal glomerulonephritis and rheumatic fever.
- Chronic otitis media (OM) and associated hearing loss are prevalent among Australian Aborigines.
- *Haemophilus influenzae* type b (Hib) infections can cause meningitis, epiglottitis, septicaemia, osteomyelitis, septic arthritis and cellulitis.

- The introduction of the Hib vaccine has reduced the incidence of Hib disease in the Northern Territory as well as in the rest of Australia.
- The incidence of gastrointestinal infections is significantly higher in the Northern Territory than in other parts of Australia.

UNUSUAL DISEASES OF RURAL AND REMOTE AREAS

- Melioidosis is the most common cause of fatal, community-acquired bacterial pneumonia in the Northern Territory.
- *Leptospira interrogans* is the cause of Weil's disease, an acute renal failure with a 5–10% fatality rate. Other unusual diseases include Q fever and dengue fever.

IMPLICATIONS FOR HEALTH CARE

- There are special procedures to be implemented for health care in remote areas—specific immunisation schedules, additional notifiable diseases, antibiotic guidelines for Central and North Australia, and special protocols for treatment.

INFECTIOUS DISEASES FROM OUTSIDE AUSTRALIA

- Diseases that are not endemic in Australia may be imported by travellers.
- Two-thirds of all notifications of active tuberculosis in Australia are in foreign-born people, mainly from Indo-China.
- Multidrug-resistant strains of *Mycobacterium tuberculosis* (MDR-TB) occur in the United States. At present these strains are not common in Australia.
- Australian travellers to endemic areas are at risk of contracting malaria.
- Dengue fever is an imported viral disease, occurring usually in northern parts of Australia where the vector *Aedes aegypti* is found.
- Yellow fever is an acute viral disease, transmitted by mosquitoes. It is found in Africa and parts of South America, but does not occur in Australia. A vaccine is available.
- *Neisseria meningitidis* is endemic in Australia, but outbreaks are very infrequent. Travellers to endemic areas (e.g. Nepal), should be vaccinated.
- In New Zealand, epidemics of meningococcal disease have occurred in recent years.
- Cases of shistosomiasis have been recorded in travellers returning to Australia from Africa.

PUBLIC HEALTH ISSUES IN NEW ZEALAND

- Some public health issues are unique to New Zealand, because of its different climate and population.

COMMUNICABLE DISEASES IN NEW ZEALAND

- A monthly communicable diseases report, the *New Zealand Public Health Report* (*NZPHR*), is prepared by the Institute of Environmental Science and Research (ESR) and published jointly by the Public Health Commission, the Ministry of Health and the ESR. The list of notifiable diseases includes those required by the World Health Organization, as well as other infections for which a public health intervention is required or for which the incidence needs to be monitored.
- The health status of the different ethnic groups within the community is affected by socioeconomic conditions as well as ethnicity.
- The infant mortality rate for Maoris is almost twice that for Europeans; 50% of it is attributed to sudden infant death syndrome (SIDS). The infant mortality rate for Pacific Islanders is similar to that for Europeans.
- The incidence of several infectious diseases varies among the different ethnic groups.
- Vaccine-preventable diseases are not notifiable in New Zealand.
- Compliance with vaccination schedules improved from 60% in 1992 to over 85% in 1994.

Study Questions

1. What is meant by a 'notifiable' disease?
2. Who is responsible for the notification of infectious diseases?
3. Where can you find information about the incidence of infectious diseases in Australia?
4. What are the functions of the NH&MRC?
5. What are some of the public health strategies for the prevention and control of infectious diseases?
6. How does immunisation protect a person from a particular disease?
7. What are the current recommended schedules for childhood vaccination?
8. Why do some vaccines require more than one dose?
9. Why is vaccination for rubella particularly important for pregnant women?
10. What is homoeopathic immunisation—does it work?
11. Why are antenatal screening tests carried out for some infectious diseases?
12. What information can be gained from a Mantoux test?
13. What is a Pap smear?
14. What are some of the major differences between the health of Aboriginal Australians and other Australians?
15. What are some of the infectious diseases that particularly affect Aboriginal people in the Northern Territory?
16. Describe some of the unusual infectious diseases that are seen mainly in remote or rural areas?
17. Name two diseases that are not presently endemic in Australia and describe how they could become established.
18. How does the incidence of infectious diseases in New Zealand differ from that in Australia?

Test Your Understanding

1. Why is it important to have comprehensive data on the incidence and prevalence of infectious diseases?
2. What is meant by herd immunity?
3. What are the dangers of non-compliance with vaccination schedules?
4. What are some of the advantages of screening programs?
5. Why should all sexually mature women have regular Pap smears?
6. What are some of the challenges for the provision of health care in remote areas?
7. Why is Australia free of some serious diseases? How could this change?

REFERENCES

Annual Report of the CDI Virology and Serology Reporting Scheme 1994, *Communicable Diseases Intelligence*, 19, 13 November 1995, p. 590.

Annual Report of the Notifiable Diseases Surveillance System 1994, *Communicable Diseases Intelligence*, 19, 30 October 1995, p. 542.

Department of Human Services and Health, *Communicable Diseases Intelligence Bulletin* (published fortnightly), Canberra: Australian Government Publishing Service.

'Enough to make you sick': How Income and Environment affect Health, National Health Strategy Research Paper No. 1, Canberra, 1992

Menzies School of Health Research, Darwin, Annual Reports 1991–1995.

New Zealand Department of Health, *HIV-AIDS: Information for Health Professionals*, Wellington, 1993.

New Zealand Department of Health, *Guidelines for Tuberculosis Control in New Zealand*, Tuberculosis Working Party, Auckland, 1992.

New Zealand Ministry of Health, *Immunisation Handbook*, Wellington, 1996.

New Zealand Public Health Commission, *A Strategic Plan for Maori Public Health*, Wellington, 1994–1995.

New Zealand Public Health Commmission, *Our Health—Our Future: The state of the public health in New Zealand*, Wellington, 1994.

New Zealand Public Health Commission, *The Health of Pacific Islands People in New Zealand*, Wellington 1994.

NH&MRC, *The Australian Immunisation Procedures Handbook*, 5th edn., Canberra: Australian Government Publishing Service, 1994.

Northern Territory Department of Health and Community Services Disease Control Unit, *Northern Territory Communicable Diseases Bulletin* (published monthly), Darwin.

Ruben, A., *Thesis, Masters of Applied Epidemiology*, National Centre for Epidemiology and Population Health, ANU, Canberra, 1994.

FURTHER READING

Brown, G.V., 1993, 'Chemoprophylaxis of Malaria', *Medical Journal of Australia*, 159, p. 187.

Currie, B., 1993, 'Medicine in Tropical Australia', *Medical Journal of Australia*, 158, p. 609.

Desovitz, R.S., *The Malaria Capers—Tales of Parasites and People*, New York: Norton & Co., 1991.

Kemp, D., I. Bastian, F. Bowden, S. Hutton, A. Haase & B. Currie, 1995, 'Oddball infectious diseases of the Top End', *Today's Life Science*, 7, No. 8, pp. 38–40.

Mathews, J., T. Weeramanthri & P. D'Abbas, 1995, 'Aboriginal Health', *Today's Life Science* 7, No. 8, 1995.

Public Health Association of Australia, 'TB: A Global Emergency', Proceedings of National Tuberculosis Conference, 1994.

Walker, J., 1995, 'Malaria? Not in my backyard', *Today's Life Science* 7, No. 11, p. 36.

Wass, A. (ed.), *Promoting Health: The Primary Health Care Approach*, Sydney: Harcourt Brace & Co., 1994.

unit IV

infections of body systems

chapter 15

microbiological techniques

for diagnosis of infection

Chapter focus

- *What methods are used in the microbiology laboratory to diagnose infections?*
- *What types of specimens are collected for microbiological analysis?*
- *What are the important considerations in the proper collection and transport of specimens for microbiological analysis?*

The main function of the clinical microbiology laboratory is to assist in the diagnosis of infectious diseases. Relatively few infectious diseases can be accurately diagnosed solely on clinical grounds. For an accurate laboratory diagnosis it is essential that an appropriate specimen be properly collected. To achieve this, one must have a good understanding of the pathogenesis and possible cause of infection. If it is suspected that a patient has an infectious disease, certain laboratory tests should be requested, based on the nature of the symptoms and the likely causative agent. One or more specimens may have to be collected and the doctor, nurse or other qualified health care worker must perform the collection procedure properly. The specimen must then be transported promptly to the laboratory for processing. Laboratory findings should be conveyed back to the ward as soon as possible to facilitate the prompt diagnosis and appropriate treatment of the disease.

A number of different methods are used in the laboratory for the diagnosis of infections. The appropriate method in a given situation is determined by the nature of the likely causative agent. Generally, laboratory tests are designed to detect either (1) the microorganism itself or a component of it in a specimen from the patient, or (2) evidence of an immune response, usually antibodies, to the causative organism in the blood of the patient. Four main types of methods are employed.

1. *Direct microscopic examination of a specimen.* Microscopy is a fundamental technique in microbiology laboratories. A direct microscopic examination of a specimen can provide a very rapid presumptive diagnosis in certain situations. It may also provide information about the host cells present in the specimen, which can indicate the probable type of infection (e.g. viral versus bacterial) as well as the quality of the specimen (e.g. a mucoid versus a purulent sputum).
2. *Culture and isolation of microorganisms from patient material.* A specimen from the patient is used to inoculate appropriate microbiological media and, after incubation, the cultures are examined for the presence of pathogens. In some cases (e.g. urinary tract infections), the number of bacteria in the specimen is estimated. When the causative agent is bacterial, the organism's sensitivity to antibiotics can also be determined. Unfortunately, not all pathogens are able to be cultured (especially some viruses and protozoa). Another major disadvantage is that culture results are not usually available for 18 hours or more for many bacteria, and much longer for viruses. Thus, faster diagnostic methods are continually being sought.
3. *Identification of infection using serologic (or immunologic) reactions.* This involves either the detection of specific antibodies to a microorganism in the serum or other body fluid of a patient, or the use of specific antibodies to identify the presence of a particular microorganism or a component of it in patient material. A serologic method is generally used when culture of the pathogen is not possible or too difficult, or when culture takes too long (e.g. viruses, protozoa, some bacteria).
4. *Identification of microorganisms using techniques to identify microbial nucleic acids.* A gene sequence that is specific for a particular microorganism can be detected in patient material by the use of a DNA probe. This method, in conjunction with DNA amplification techniques such as the polymerase chain reaction (PCR), is likely to be increasingly used in the clinical microbiology laboratory. The immense interest in these DNA techniques stems mainly from their potential speed in identifying microorganisms that are difficult to isolate by cultural methods.

Time and accuracy are the two key factors in the laboratory diagnosis of infectious diseases. The earlier a laboratory report becomes available, the sooner steps can be taken to ensure appropriate management of the patient. Not all the methods outlined above are suitable or available for all infections; and the fastest methods are not always the most accurate. The time frames for microscopic, cultural and serological methods, currently the most commonly used, are summarised in Figure 15.1. It should be noted that the times given are for typical organisms, and that there are many exceptions to those shown in the figure. There are also many specific methods for specific organisms that are not shown in the figure.

Microscopic Techniques

Direct microscopic examination of certain specimens can sometimes provide a presumptive diagnosis within an hour, although several hours may be required for more complex staining and microscopic methods. Generally speaking, direct microscopy using a simple light microscope is most useful in the following circumstances:

- When the site of infection is a normally sterile part of the body. For example, in a case of meningitis, a Gram stain of cerebrospinal fluid (CSF) can provide rapid and vital information about the likely cause. The three most common causes of acute bacterial meningitis are *Neisseria meningitidis* (a Gram-negative coccus),

FIGURE 15.1
LABORATORY DIAGNOSIS OF INFECTIOUS DISEASES

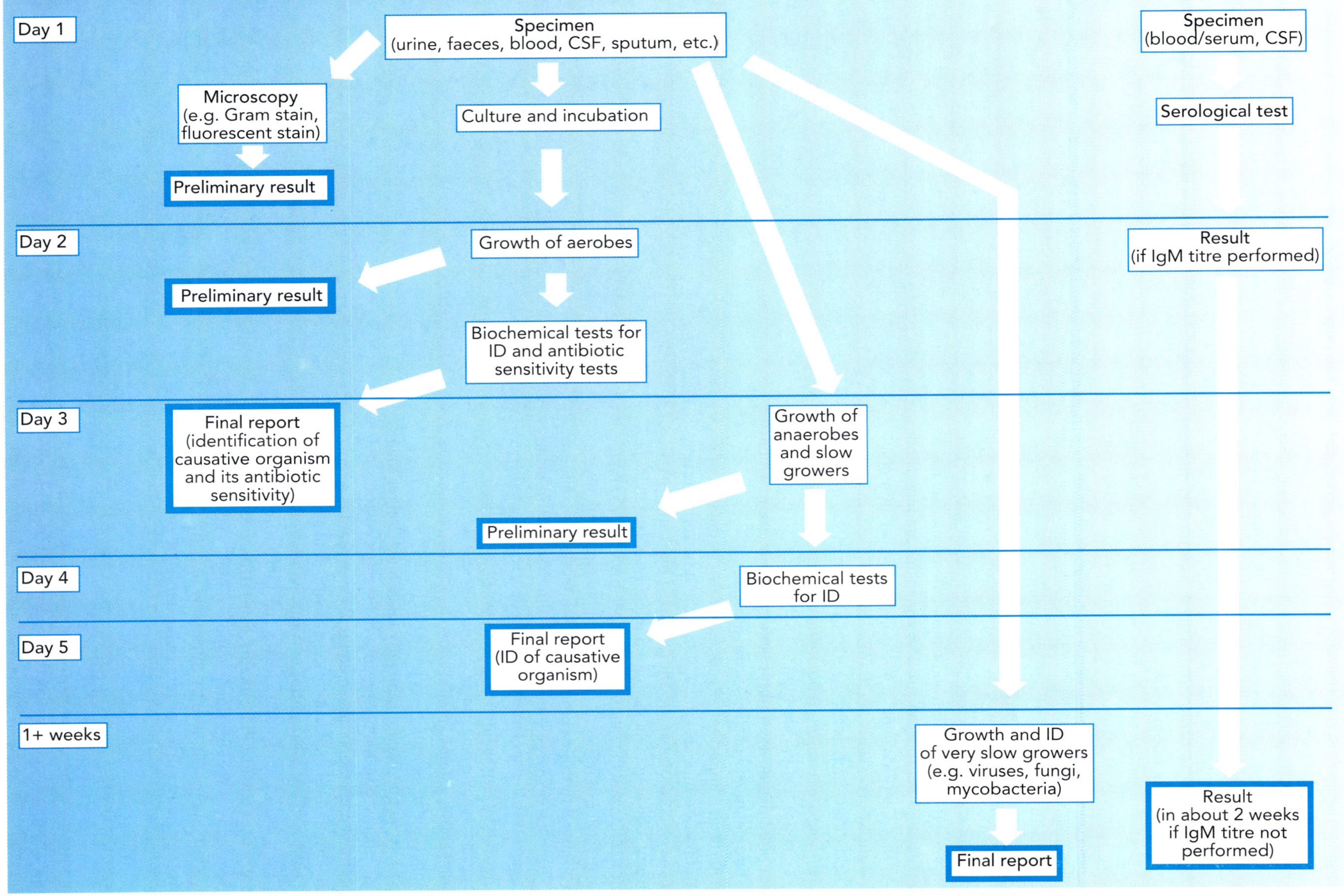

Haemophilus influenzae (a Gram-negative rod) and *Streptococcus pneumoniae* (a Gram-positive coccus), all of which can be distinguished in a Gram stain (see Figure 15.2).

- When the pathogen is morphologically distinguishable under the microscope. Certain intestinal parasites can be readily identified in a wet mount of faeces or other specimen—for example, *Giardia* (a protozoan) and *Ascaris lumbricoides* (a roundworm), as shown in Figure 15.3. Malaria is diagnosed by microscopic examination of a blood smear. In the case of parasites such as these, microscopy is often crucial, since culture of these organisms is not possible.
- When the pathogen can be differentially stained so that it can be specifically identified under the microscope. For example, mycobacteria (causing tuberculosis) can be identified in a Ziehl-Neelsen stained (acid-fast stain) smear of sputum. *Cryptococcus neoformans* is identified in CSF using an India ink stain (see Figure 20.3, p. 479). Another particularly useful staining technique involves the use of fluorescent dyes attached to antibody molecules specific for a particular microorganism. The organisms are identified if they fluoresce under a microscope using an ultraviolet light source. This technique can be used in many situations, such as for the identification of *Legionella*, *Chlamydia* and for *Treponema pallidum* in fluid from a genital lesion (see Figure 15.4). It is also useful as a rapid diagnostic tool for acute viral infections when large numbers of viruses are present.

A further important advantage of direct microscopic examination of a specimen is that the host cells present in the specimen can be identified. This can provide information about whether or not infection exists, the type of infection and the quality of the specimen. For example, the presence of pus cells (polymorphonuclear leukocytes) in a sample of urine is indicative of infection (see Figure 15.5), whereas large numbers of epithelial cells in urine suggest that the specimen was improperly collected (i.e. not a mid-stream sample). The presence of pus cells in CSF suggests an acute bacterial infection, whereas lymphocytes indicate that a non-bacterial cause (e.g. virus, fungus) or a tuberculous meningitis is more likely.

Electron microscopy generally takes much longer than light microscopy, mainly because of the more complicated specimen preparation that is required. However, it is a most valuable tool for the identification of viruses in specimens, as well as from virus cultures. Virus culture takes days or even weeks, and some viruses can't be cultured at all (e.g. rotaviruses). The major limitation of electron microscopy is that the microscope is a highly specialised piece of equipment, usually affordable only by specialist virology laboratories or research establishments.

Specimen Collection for Culture

An infectious disease is most accurately diagnosed when the causative agent is isolated and identified from patient material. The specimen is cultured on appropriate microbiological media and then an identification of the causative organism is made. This is usually based on its colony morphology, and/or its biochemical properties, and/or its antigenic properties (see p. 339). The microbiological analysis in the laboratory is only as reliable as the quality of the specimen allows. Thus, the correct selection, timing, collection and transport of patient specimens is of the utmost importance. When specimens are not properly collected and handled:

FIGURE 15.2
GRAM STAINS OF THE THREE MOST COMMON CAUSES OF BACTERIAL MENINGITIS
(a) *Neisseria meningitidis;* (b) *Haemophilus influenzae;* and (c) *Streptococcus pneumoniae*

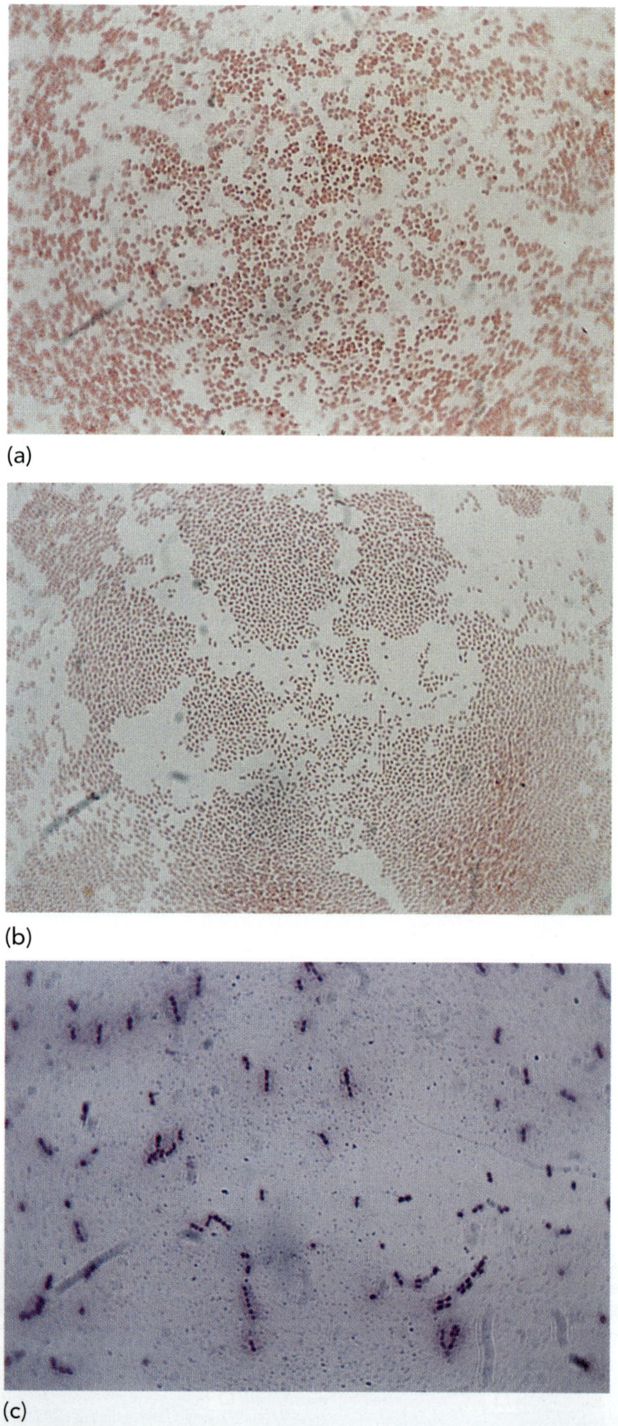

FIGURE 15.3
EGG OF *ASCARIS LUMBRICOIDES* AS SEEN IN A LIGHT MICROSCOPE

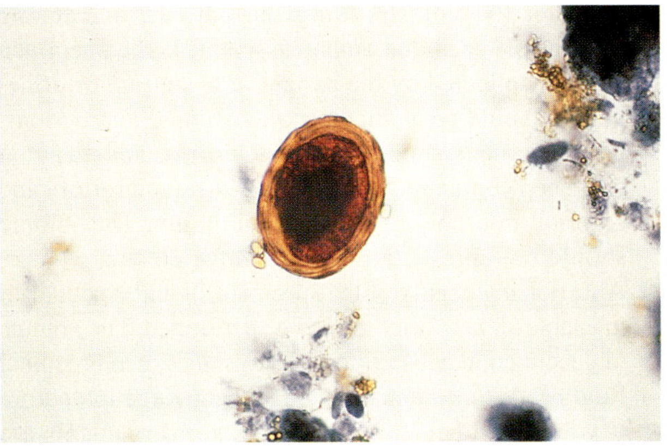

FIGURE 15.4
THE FLUORESCENT ANTIBODY TECHNIQUE
(a) Fluorescent antibody stain results of *Treponema* and an unrelated microorganism in a specimen;
(b) photomicrograph of treponemes fluorescing.

(a)

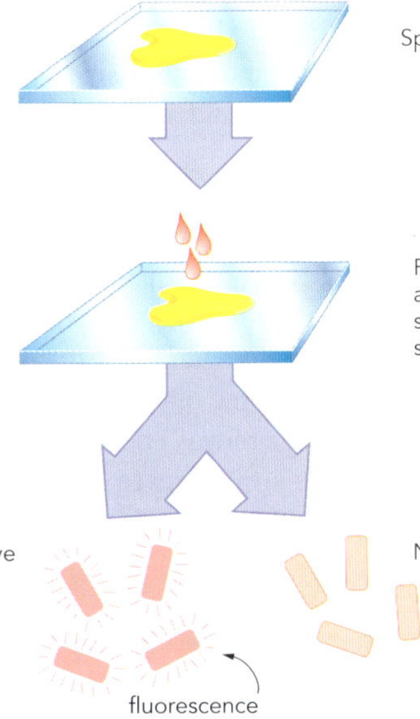

(b)

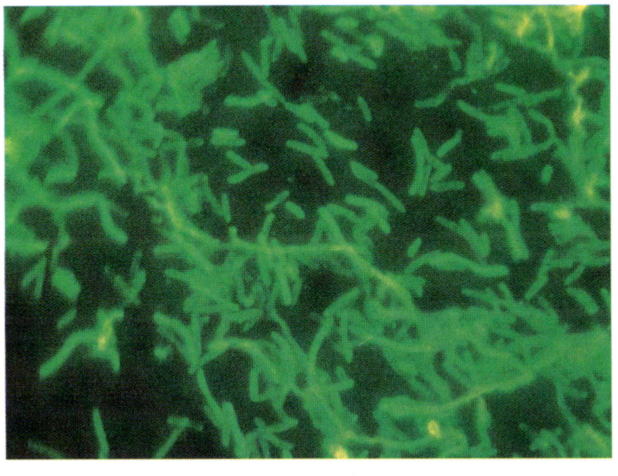

FIGURE 15.5
DIRECT MICROSCOPIC EXAMINATION OF URINE
(a) Pus cells (polymorphonuclear leukocytes) in urine are indicative of infection; (b) epithelial cells suggest poor specimen collection.

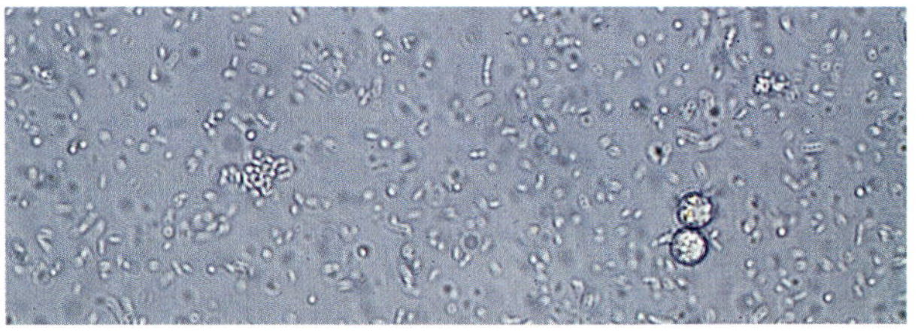

(a)

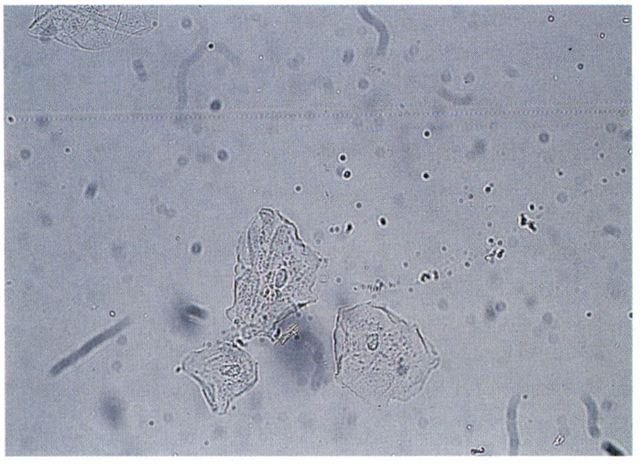

(b)

- the causative organisms may not be present in the specimen at all; or
- the organisms may die if subjected to adverse conditions; or
- the causative organisms may be overgrown by indigenous microbial flora also present in the specimen.

As stated earlier, a major disadvantage of cultural methods is the length of time required for a result. It should be recognised that results of culture can take up to 18 hours, or even much longer (e.g. as long as 1–2 weeks for blood cultures). Then another 5–24 hours may be required for antibiotic sensitivity results. Preliminary results from direct microscopic examination (Gram stain) of the specimen may be obtained within 15 minutes.

SPECIMEN SELECTION

Many different types of specimens are sent to the laboratory for culture, including blood, urine, faeces, sputum, pus and swabs from sites of infection. These specimens are generally readily obtained. However, for some infections, tissues or body fluids from less accessible sites may have to be collected, such as fluid from a deep abscess, bone marrow, cerebrospinal fluid or peritoneal exudate. The selection of the most appropriate specimen type(s) to be collected should be based on the nature of the infection and the suspected sites of organism persistence. That is, the specimen should be collected from a site where the organism is most likely to be found. For example, a patient with urinary frequency and pain during urination should have a specimen of urine collected for microscopy and culture. Similarly, a patient with respiratory symptoms and a productive cough should have sputum collected for examination. However, it is not always so straightforward. For instance, *Salmonella typhi*, the cause of typhoid fever, is most likely to be isolated from blood in the first two weeks of infection, but then from faeces or urine in the next two weeks. A good knowledge of the course of the infection is obviously necessary.

TIMING OF SPECIMEN COLLECTION

It is important that, wherever possible, specimens for laboratory culture are collected before antibiotic therapy is initiated. Once antibiotic therapy has begun the likelihood of culturing the causative organism from the specimen is lessened. Antibiotics may not only quickly reduce the numbers of pathogenic microorganisms in the tissues, but they may also interfere with the growth of the organisms in culture. In certain situations, however, it may not be possible to delay antibiotic therapy until a specimen is collected. For example, in a case of meningitis, which can be life-threatening, antibiotic therapy may have to be initiated before a lumbar puncture for CSF collection can be performed.

A knowledge of the usual clinical course of a given infection, combined with a careful observation of the patient's signs and symptoms, should indicate the appropriate time for specimen collection. For most infections, the collection of the specimen should simply be done as soon as possible but, for some, more precise timing is required. For example, early morning sputum specimens should be collected for the diagnosis of tuberculosis to maximise the chance of finding organisms. Correct timing of the collection of blood samples for culture is critical because organisms may only be intermittently released from the infection source. In septicaemia, chills followed by fever represent the showering of microorganisms into the bloodstream. Cultures are most likely to be positive when they are collected during such episodes. For most infections, if the responsible pathogen is to be recovered, specimens must be collected during the acute rather than convalescent stage of disease (see Chapter 7).

PROPER COLLECTION OF SPECIMENS

The proper collection of specimens is vital for three main reasons: (1) to obtain an appropriate and useful specimen; (2) to prevent contamination of the specimen during collection; and (3) to prevent cross-infection during specimen collection. The following general procedures should be observed.

- Hospital Standard Precautions guidelines should be followed at all times. All specimens should be treated as potentially hazardous.
- Sterile, leak-proof containers of an adequate size to hold the specimen should generally be used. Care should be taken not to contaminate the external surface of the collection container and its accompanying paperwork. If contamination of the container or paperwork does occur, appropriate steps for their disinfection or disposal must be taken.
- Specimen collection should be performed with care and tact to avoid harming the patient, or causing discomfort or undue embarrassment. If the specimen is to be collected by the patient (e.g. sputum or urine) he/she should be given clear and detailed instructions.
- All specimens should be collected in a manner that will keep contamination by commensal microflora and external microorganisms to a minimum. The sample should be representative of the infected site.
- A sufficient quantity of the specimen should be obtained to enable all necessary tests to be performed. The volume of specimen may be critical. For instance, cerebrospinal fluid needs to be concentrated by centrifugation before it is cultured because the numbers of organisms are often low.
- The specimen container must be properly labelled and accompanied by the appropriate laboratory requests on the requisition. The label should identify the patient and the source of the specimen, and the date and time of collection to indicate to the laboratory the transit time. Any information that will aid the laboratory in performing the appropriate analyses should be included on the requisition form.
- Specimen containers should always be sterile. Faecal specimen containers are an exception since faeces has a very high microbial load and is plated on highly selective media.
- Certain specimen types, especially swabs, require special transport systems for protection of pathogens from drying and overgrowth by commensals.

Swabs are frequently used to collect specimens for microbiological analysis. There is a tendency to take a swab of an infected site, rather than some other type of specimen (e.g. a volume of pus or a tissue biopsy) because the former is easier to collect. In some situations (e.g. pharyngitis) a swab may be the only possible type of specimen, but in other situations it is less than ideal. The main problems with swab specimens are that only a limited amount of material can be collected, and specimens are highly susceptible to dessication leading to reduced viability of microorganisms. After collection, swabs should be placed into a transport medium for transport to the laboratory.

SPECIMEN TRANSPORT

Specimens should be delivered promptly to the laboratory so that microbiological examination can begin as soon as possible. Also, it is important that the results of the analysis accurately represent the microbiological population present in the specimen at the time of collection. If delivery is delayed, some fragile pathogens may die; and if the specimen is from a site in the body with an indigenous microflora, the more hardy or faster-growing members of the flora may overgrow the pathogens.

While it is most desirable to submit specimens to the laboratory quickly and in an unaltered state, this is not always possible. Therefore certain specimens should be sent to the laboratory in a transport device, containing a

transport medium. This is a liquid or semi-liquid, designed to prevent the specimen from drying and to maintain microorganism viability, while retarding their growth prior to culture. It is designed to maintain the microbial population in the specimen as close as possible to its composition at the time of collection. Not all specimens need to be transported in transport medium, but it is strongly recommended for specimens that could easily dry out, such as swabs and small amounts of fluid, tissue or biopsy material. For some specimens (e.g. a small amount of biopsy material) the medium may simply be 0.85% NaCl. There is a variety of commercial or laboratory prepared specialised devices, such as swab transport systems, anaerobe transport systems and viral transport media.

It should always be remembered that clinical specimens for culture are collected and sent to the laboratory because they may contain pathogenic microorganisms. Careless handling of the specimen during collection or transport could result in contamination of the outside of the container and the accompanying paperwork. Anyone who handles these (e.g. nurse, orderly, laboratory technologist) may then be exposed to any pathogens present.

Common Specimen Types for Culture

BLOOD CULTURES

A blood culture is usually performed in the investigation of a patient with fever or other manifestations of systemic infection. The blood is collected taking care to avoid contamination with skin flora. It is usually inoculated into one or two bottles of culture medium (depending on the commercial system being used). In two-bottle systems one bottle is for growth of aerobes and one is for anaerobes. In one-bottle systems both aerobes and anaerobes grow in the same bottle. Less than one bacterial cell may be present in a millilitre of blood, even in serious illness. Thus, the volume of blood collected for culture is critical. In infants and children with bacteraemia the concentration of organisms in the blood is often higher than in adults, so less blood is required. The volumes usually collected for culture are:

- children: 1–5 mL of blood
- adults: 10–30 mL of blood

Because the number of microorganisms is often low, and because they may be shed into the bloodstream only intermittently, three sets of separately collected blood cultures are usually obtained over a 24–48 hour period. A single blood culture may miss intermittently occurring bacteraemia. Also, a differentiation between pathogens and contaminants is possible if more than one sample is collected. Timing of the collections is important because intermittent bacteraemia usually coincides with the onset of fever or chills, although these symptoms may occur as much as an hour after the organisms are shed into the bloodstream.

It is essential that blood for culture is collected aseptically. This is done by first cleansing the venipuncture site with 70% alcohol (isopropyl or ethyl alcohol) and then by applying an appropriate antiseptic solution (e.g. 10% povidone-iodine or 70% alcohol). The antiseptic should be left on the skin for at least one minute. The intended venipuncture site should not then be touched except with similarly disinfected gloved fingers. After the venipuncture, any residual antiseptic should be removed with an alcohol pad. The stoppers of the culture bottles or collection tubes should be disinfected with alcohol prior to their inoculation. Optimally, the blood should be inoculated directly into the culture bottles with the same syringe and needle at the bedside of the patient. Figure 15.6 shows blood culture bottles inoculated with blood.

In the laboratory, cultures are incubated and examined either macroscopically for evidence of growth or by use of an instrument for the detection of evolved carbon dioxide. Cultures are examined later on the day of collection and daily thereafter for 7–14 days, or until growth occurs. Clinically significant bacteria are recovered within this period in the majority of cases.

INTRAVASCULAR CATHETERS

Intravascular catheters may become colonised and serve as a source of microorganisms in septicaemia. Culturing of a catheter tip may help to determine if there is a relationship between the catheter and infection. A distal segment of the catheter (approximately 5 cm) should be obtained by aseptically clipping off the end of the catheter directly into a screw-cap, sterile container at the time the catheter is removed. This specimen should be sent immediately to the laboratory before excessive drying occurs. The number and type of viable bacteria in the catheter specimen may then be determined.

SPECIMENS FOR URINARY TRACT INFECTIONS

Bladder urine is normally sterile. However, it is usually contaminated during urination by the normal microflora of the urethra. Contamination can be reduced by collecting a 'clean-catch' or mid-stream urine specimen. If this method is properly performed, the urethra is flushed out with the first portion of urine and the middle portion is collected for urinalysis.

Proper instruction of patients on how to collect a mid-stream specimen of urine (MSU) is critical to ensure the collection of a good specimen and hence the accuracy of laboratory results. An understanding by nursing personnel of the proper methods for obtaining urine specimens from bedridden patients is also very important. If the patient is collecting the specimen, he/she should be given detailed instructions, including diagrams.

To collect an MSU specimen from a female

1. The urethral opening and vaginal vestibule are cleansed with soapy water or clean gauze pads soaked with liquid soap.
2. The area is rinsed well with sterile water or wet gauze wipes.
3. The labia are held apart during voiding.

FIGURE 15.6
BLOOD CULTURE BOTTLES INOCULATED WITH BLOOD FROM A PATIENT

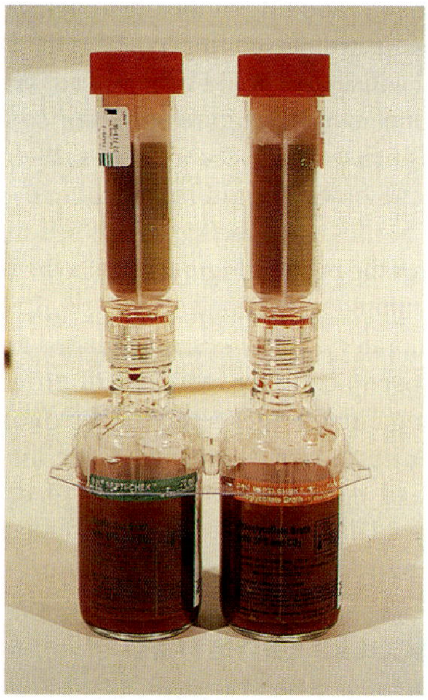

4. A few millilitres of urine are allowed to pass. The flow of urine should not be stopped.
5. The mid-stream portion of urine is collected into a sterile container.

To collect an MSU specimen from a male

1. The foreskin is retracted (if not circumcised) and the penis is washed with soapy water.
2. The area is then well rinsed with sterile water.
3. With the foreskin still retracted, a few millilitres of urine are allowed to pass. The flow of urine should not be stopped.
4. The mid-stream portion of urine is collected into a sterile container.

Soap rather than disinfectants should be used for cleaning the urethral area, because disinfectants introduced into the urine during collection may inhibit the growth of microorganisms.

Urine is an excellent growth medium for microorganisms. If a urine sample is left standing at room temperature, contaminating bacteria may increase from low to high numbers. In large numbers they may inhibit the growth of the pathogen, or be mistaken for the pathogen. Specimens should be sent to the laboratory within one hour of collection. If this is not possible, they should be labelled with the time of collection and refrigerated.

Urine is cultured quantitatively for bacteria, since the number of viable bacteria or colony-forming units (CFU) per litre is of major importance in the interpretation of urine cultures. A urinary tract infection is indicated if the number of bacteria in a clean-catch MSU exceeds 10^8 organisms per litre, and if increased numbers of white cells are present. Lower numbers of organisms may be considered significant in certain situations (e.g. if antibiotic therapy has been commenced, or in a patient with high urine output). Chapter 21 gives a more detailed description of how urinalysis is interpreted.

Contamination of the urine by urethral or vaginal bacterial flora may be avoided by suprapubic aspiration. This involves the collection of urine directly from the bladder by needle aspiration. It may be used for patients with clinical evidence of urinary tract infection but in whom bacterial counts in MSU specimens are low and indeterminate. It is also useful for neonates and young infants, and for other patients who can't produce an MSU and in whom catheterisation is contraindicated.

In patients with indwelling urethral catheters attached to a closed drainage system, urine is collected by disinfecting the wall of the catheter at its juncture with the drainage tube and puncturing it with a needle attached to a syringe (see Figure 15.7). The connection between the catheter and the drainage tube should not be broken for specimen collection, and the material in the drainage bag, which may have been standing for several hours, must not be used. Urine may also be collected for culture during the course of cystoscopy or retrograde pyelography.

SPECIMENS FOR CENTRAL NERVOUS SYSTEM INFECTIONS

In a case of suspected meningitis, cerebrospinal fluid (CSF), obtained by lumbar puncture, is investigated. A lumbar puncture must be performed under conditions of strict asepsis to protect the patient. Also, if contamination of the specimen occurs, the isolation and identification of the true causative agent may be impaired. The skin should be disinfected with an antiseptic such as povidone-iodine. Specimens should be collected in sterile containers that are sealed with a screw cap to prevent leakage and loss, or contamination of the contents. Usually, three tubes are collected for microbiology, cytology and biochemistry testing. The most turbid (cloudy) tube should be sent to microbiology. If only one tube of CSF is obtained, it should be submitted to the microbiology laboratory first so that it can be opened aseptically.

Rapid transport of CSF specimens to the laboratory is essential, since fragile organisms such as *Haemophilus influenzae, Streptococcus pneumoniae* and *Neisseria meningitidis* may not survive storage or variations in temperature. Also, meningitis is a life-threatening infection, warranting rapid diagnosis and treatment. Blood cultures should also be collected from patients suspected of having meningitis.

SPECIMENS OF OTHER BODY FLUIDS

Apart from blood, urine and CSF, other normally sterile body fluids that may be collected include pleural, peritoneal and synovial fluids. These are usually collected by percutaneous needle aspiration using strict aseptic technique. The numbers of microorganisms in these specimens may be low, primarily because of their dilution by fluid accumulation at the site. It is therefore necessary to collect as large a specimen sample as possible and to transport it immediately to the laboratory.

FIGURE 15.7
COLLECTION OF A CATHETER SPECIMEN OF URINE
A needle is inserted just below the junction between the catheter and collection tube.

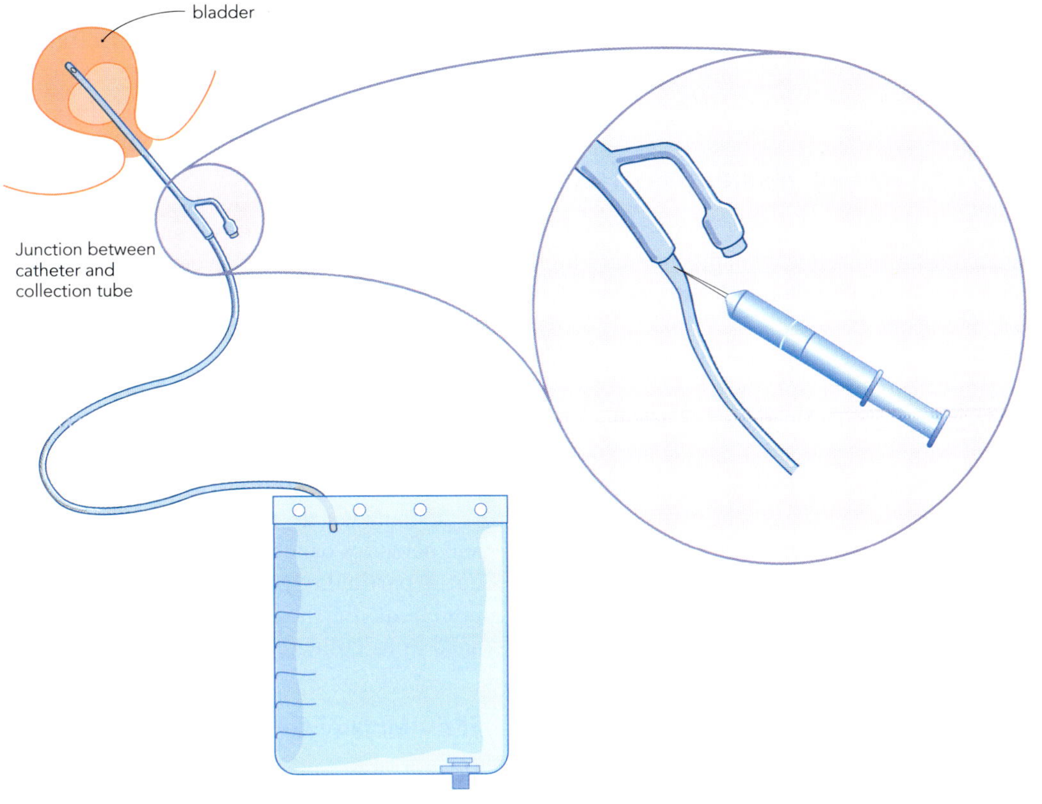

SPECIMENS FOR UPPER RESPIRATORY TRACT INFECTIONS

A number of different types of specimens may be collected from the upper respiratory tract, including throat, nasal and nasopharyngeal swabs, nasopharyngeal fluid, and nasal washings. The type of specimen is determined by the type of organism suspected.

Throat swabs (pharyngeal specimens) are collected primarily for the detection of infection by Group A streptococci (*Streptococcus pyogenes*), *Neisseria gonorrhoeae* (in pharyngeal gonorrhoea), *Candida albicans* (thrush) and *Haemophilus influenzae* (e.g. epiglottitis in children). The procedure involves:

1. Depressing the tongue gently with a tongue depressor;
2. Extending a sterile swab between the tonsillar pillars and behind the uvula (avoiding contact with the cheeks, tongue, uvula or lips);
3. Sweeping the swab back and forth across the posterior pharynx, tonsillar areas, and any inflamed or ulcerated areas to obtain sample (see Figure 15.8).

A throat sample should not be collected if the epiglottis is inflamed, as sampling may cause serious respiratory obstruction.

Nasal swabs are collected primarily for the detection of carriers of *Staphylococcus aureus*. The procedure involves:

1. Inserting a sterile swab into one nostril until resistance is met at the level of the turbinates;
2. Rotating the swab against the nasal mucosa;
3. Repeating the process on the other nostril using the same swab.

Nasopharyngeal suction is performed for the detection of carriers of Group A streptococci, *Neisseria meningitidis, Corynebacterium diphtheriae* and *Bordetella pertussis*. Material is suctioned from the nasopharynx and collected into a sterile container.

Nasopharyngeal swabs are collected primarily for the detection of carriers of *Neisseria meningitidis* and to diagnose *Bordetella pertussis* infections. In this procedure a flexible wire swab is carefully inserted through the nose into the posterior nasopharynx. The swab is rotated, keeping it near the septum and floor of the nose.

Nasal washings are collected primarily for culture of viruses. The patient should be instructed not to swallow during the procedure. With the patient's head hyper-

FIGURE 15.8
COLLECTION OF A THROAT SWAB

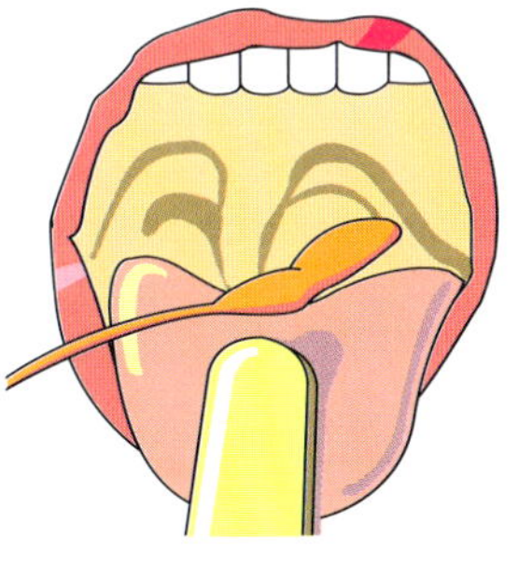

extended (about 70° angle), approximately 5 mL of sterile isotonic saline is instilled into each nostril. To collect the material, the head is tilted forward and the fluid allowed to run out of the nares into a sterile container; or the fluid is aspirated using a rubber bulb syringe. The nasal washings are placed in an equal volume of viral transport medium, or transported in a sterile container.

SPECIMENS FOR LOWER RESPIRATORY TRACT INFECTIONS

The specimen most often collected in the investigation of lower respiratory infection is sputum. Health care personnel should be aware of the need for a fresh, clean specimen produced from a deep cough. They should also realise that the specimen must be transported to the laboratory promptly. Sputum is frequently contaminated with oropharyngeal flora, many of which are potential pathogens. Delayed transport to the laboratory can allow overgrowth of the pathogen by more hardy members of the normal flora. This makes it difficult to determine which of the organisms isolated is responsible for the infection. For this reason, culture of sputum often does not yield clear-cut results.

Some of these problems can be minimised by assessing the quality of the specimen by Gram stain. Sputum specimens with excessive squamous epithelial cells are judged to be unsatisfactory because such specimens are likely to be significantly contaminated with oropharyngeal flora. In some laboratories such specimens may not be cultured at all.

A better specimen may be obtained by bronchial aspiration through a bronchoscope, or by inserting a needle into the trachea below the glottis (trans-tracheal aspiration). Needle biopsy of the lungs may be necessary for the diagnosis of infections in which there is no productive cough (e.g. fungal and viral infections).

If tuberculosis is suspected, extreme care should be exercised in handling the sputum specimen because the organism can be transmitted from the specimen to the health care worker. Specimens for TB culture may be refrigerated for several hours without significant loss of viability.

SPECIMENS FOR GASTROINTESTINAL TRACT INFECTIONS

Faeces (stools) may be collected for the culture of bacteria causing gastroenteritis, or for the detection of protozoa, helminths or viruses. The proper collection and preservation of faeces are frequently neglected, but are important requirements for the isolation of microorganisms responsible for intestinal infections.

A stool specimen can be effectively obtained by:

- passing the stool directly into a sterile, wide-mouth, leak-proof container with a tight-fitting lid; or
- passing the stool into a clean, dry bedpan, and then transferring it into a sterile leak-proof container with a tight-fitting lid.

Toilet paper should not be used to collect the stool because it may be impregnated with barium salts, which are inhibitory for some faecal pathogens. The specimen should be transported to the laboratory promptly, or refrigerated if a delay is unavoidable. If a stool specimen cannot be processed within several hours of collection, it may be mixed with a suitable transport medium. Deterioration of parasites (protozoa and helminths) in stool samples may be prevented by the use of appropriate fixatives, which preserve the morphology of the protozoa and helminths.

In selected circumstances, such as in the detection of rectal gonorrhoea, a rectal swab may be necessary. The swab should be passed beyond the anal sphincter, carefully rotated, and withdrawn. The swab should be placed in a screw-cap tube containing a preservative such as Cary-Blair medium and transported to the laboratory.

Other specimens that may be required include gastric aspirates for certain parasites (e.g. *Giardia, Cryptosporidium*) and gastric biopsies (for detection of *Helicobacter pylori*).

A single negative stool culture or examination for eggs and parasites cannot be regarded as sufficient for ruling out a particular gastrointestinal pathogen. For many infectious diarrhoeas, up to three stool specimens may need to be collected and examined.

SPECIMENS FOR GENITAL TRACT INFECTIONS

Genital tract specimens are submitted mainly for the detection of such pathogens as *Neisseria gonorrhoeae, Chlamydia trachomatis,* herpes simplex virus, genital wart virus, *Trichomonas, Haemophilus ducreyi,* Group B streptococci, *Candida albicans* and certain anaerobic bacteria.

In females, a number of specimens may be collected depending on the site of infection. For example:

- cervical swab;
- vaginal swab;
- urethral swab;
- amniotic fluid;
- rectal swab;
- vesicle fluid (e.g. on vulva).

In males typical specimens include:

- urethral swab;
- fluid or swab from penile lesion;
- rectal swab.

SPECIMENS FROM INFECTED WOUNDS AND TISSUE

There are two important principles that apply to specimens collected from infected wounds and tissues:

1. Specimen quality is important, and tissue or fluid is generally superior to a swab specimen;
2. In general, the more specimen the better.

Tissue and biopsy specimens should be placed into a sterile, screw-cap container and transported immediately to the laboratory. If the specimen is small, it should be immersed in sterile isotonic saline to prevent it from drying out. From an infected wound a volume of pus should be collected if possible. There are circumstances, however, when only a swab specimen can be obtained. In such cases, the swab should be used to sample as much of the lesion as possible. Swabs should be transported to the laboratory in transport medium.

SPECIMENS FOR ANAEROBIC BACTERIA

Anaerobic bacteria can cause a variety of infections in humans, including appendicitis, cholecystitis, periodontal infections, endocarditis, endometritis, osteomyelitis, peritonitis, empyema, salpingitis, sinusitis, and wound infections following bowel surgery or trauma. These bacteria may be overlooked or missed if the specimen is not properly collected and transported to the laboratory and then subjected to appropriate laboratory procedures. Anaerobes vary in their sensitivity to oxygen, but a brief exposure of less than 10 minutes to atmospheric oxygen is enough to kill the more fastidious organisms. If anaerobes are suspected, the laboratory request form should indicate it, and the specimen should be exposed to air for as brief a time as possible.

One of the best specimens for anaerobic culture is pus, obtained by using a needle and syringe. In a volume of pus the bacteria are somewhat protected from oxygen and drying. The material, however, should *not* be transported in the needle and syringe. Needle transport is very unsafe because there is the potential risk of a needlestick injury, and syringe transport poses a risk because the specimen may be expelled during transport, creating a threat to people and the environment. So, aspirated material should be transferred to an anaerobic transport vial. Large volumes of purulent material may be transported in a sterile, screw-cap container.

Tissue samples and biopsy samples are also very good specimens for anaerobic culture. After collection they should be placed into an anaerobic transport device, or a sterile tube or petri dish, which is then placed into a sealable plastic bag that generates an anaerobic atmosphere. Large pieces of tissue can be transported in a sterile jar. When a swab must be used to collect a specimen, one of a number of commercially available anaerobe swab systems should be used.

Extremes of heat or cold should be avoided. If delays are unavoidable, the specimens should be held at room temperature until processing.

SPECIMENS FOR FUNGAL CULTURE

A variety of specimens may be collected for the culture of fungi, depending on the site of infection. For superficial infections, skin scrapings, hair or nail clippings from the site of infection are most appropriate. For subcutaneous infections, possible specimens include sputum, blood and pus. Specimens for the culture of fungi should be collected aseptically, placed in sterile containers, and delivered to the laboratory within several hours. Swabs are the least suitable, but specimens from certain body sites, such as the ear canal, nasopharynx, throat, vagina and cervix, are not readily collected by other means.

Specimens should be transported in sterile, humidified, leak-proof containers. Only dermatological specimens should be transported in a dry container. Transport medium should not be used unless the specimen can be easily and completely retrieved from the medium.

SPECIMENS FOR VIRAL CULTURE

For the laboratory diagnosis of any infection, the specimen should reflect the target organ whenever possible. With many viral infections, the clinical symptoms frequently identify the target organ(s) and suggest the appropriate specimen(s) to collect. Typical specimens for viral culture are listed in Table 15.1. In addition to a specimen from the clinical site of infection, blood, throat washings and faeces are also often collected. Specimens should be collected as soon after onset of symptoms as possible. The chance of virus recovery is best if the specimen is collected within three days of the onset of symptoms; for many viruses it is greatly reduced beyond five days. Specimens other than fluids should be placed in a sterile, leak-proof container with viral transport medium.

Culturing Bacteria and Fungi

CULTURE MEDIA

A nutrient composition prepared for the growth of microorganisms is called a **culture medium**. When microbes are grown on a culture medium the growth is

TABLE 15.1
SPECIMENS REQUIRED FOR VIRAL CULTURE

CLINICAL DISEASE	SPECIMENS REQUIRED
Measles (rubeola)	Blood, urine, nasopharyngeal secretions
German measles	Throat and nasal swabs, blood, urine
Chickenpox	Vesicle fluid
Respiratory syncytial virus	Nasal washings
Herpes simplex—skin lesions	Vesicle fluid
Herpes simplex—encephalitis	Cerebrospinal fluid, brain biopsy
Diarrhoea (e.g. rotavirus infection)	Faeces, rectal swab

called a **culture**. It is possible to grow the majority of bacteria and fungi in artificial (chemically prepared) culture media, but there is no single medium in which all of them are able to grow. Some bacteria have very special nutrient requirements. For example, *Streptococcus pyogenes* can grow only if red blood cells are supplied in the medium, and *Neisseria gonorrhoea* can grow only if the blood is heated (to release the nutrients) before being added to the medium. Microorganisms that require special growth factors, such as these, are said to be **fastidious**, requiring **enriched media**. There are some bacteria that are so fastidious they can't be grown in culture media at all; for example, *Treponema pallidum* and *Mycobacterium leprae*, and others, such as the chlamydia and rickettsia, can't be grown in artificial media but can be grown in cell cultures (cultures of living animal cells).

Some culture media are designed to allow the growth of certain microorganisms, while inhibiting the growth of others. For example, Sabouraud dextrose medium has a low pH and high sugar content, which inhibits bacteria but allows fungi to grow. MacConkey medium contains bile salts which inhibit non-enteric bacteria. These are called **selective media**. MacConkey medium is also an example of what are termed **differential media**, because certain bacteria can be differentiated from others by the particular nature of their growth on the medium (see Figure 15.9).

FIGURE 15.9
DIFFERENTIAL GROWTH MEDIUM
Differentiation of (a) *E. coli* and (b) *Pseudomonas aeruginosa* on MacConkey agar.

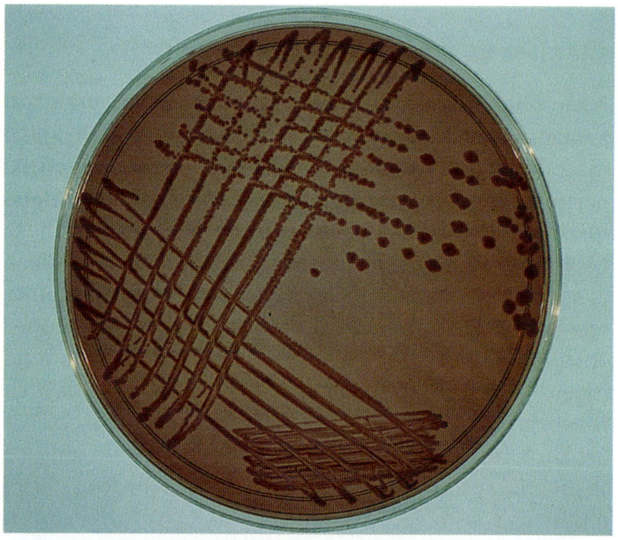

(a)

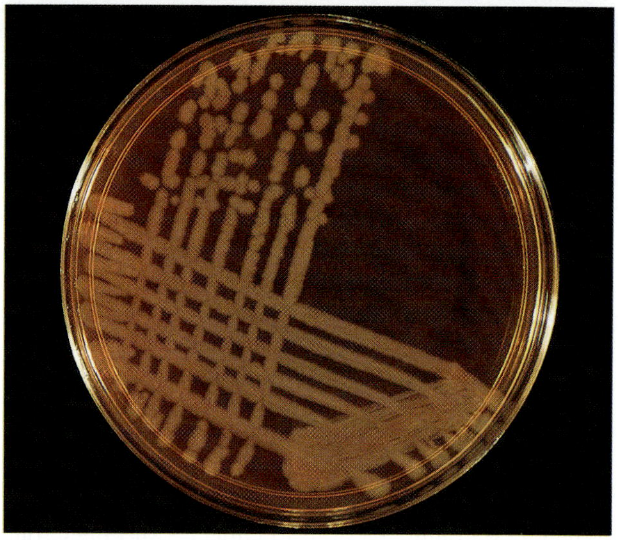

(b)

PURE CULTURES

Culture media may be liquid, but most of the time they are made solid by the addition of a gelling agent, called agar. A solid medium contained in a petri dish (a circular plastic or glass dish) is called an **agar plate**. Solid media are often used because bacteria and fungi can grow on the surface of the media, forming colonies, composed of millions of cells, derived from a single cell implanted on the surface. All the cells in a colony are identical because they are the progeny of a single cell. If a single colony is transferred to a fresh agar plate, and spread over the surface, numerous colonies will grow on the plate, and all the colonies will be comprised of the same species of organism. This is called a **pure culture**. In order to perform any tests on a microorganism it is essential to have a pure culture, so that the test results reflect the attributes of that organism alone.

The way in which pure cultures are usually prepared is called the **streak plate method**. Bacteria are picked up by a sterile wire loop and, as the loop is moved lightly over the surface of the agar in lines (or streaks), they are deposited on the surface of the plate on the lines. The loop is sterilised by flaming between different areas of streaking, resulting in fewer and fewer bacteria being deposited. This has a diluting effect and results in single bacterial cells being deposited in the areas that are streaked last. When the plate is incubated, a separated, single colony will grow where each cell is deposited (see Figure 15.10).

Streak plating to obtain pure cultures is necessary because the majority of clinical specimens contain mixtures of microorganisms, particularly if the specimen has been taken from a body site which has a normal microbial flora. Streak plating allows the separation of different organisms and their subsequent purification.

Sometimes, liquid media are used first to increase the numbers of organisms, followed by culture on solid media. This process is used for culture of blood, because the numbers of bacteria in a sample of blood may be very small.

INCUBATION

The majority of bacteria and some fungi (yeasts) grow from single cells to macroscopic colonies on an agar plate in 18–24 hours, although anaerobes usually require 48 hours. Some bacteria (e.g. Mycobacteria) and moulds grow much more slowly and can take several days and sometimes weeks to form visible colonies.

FIGURE 15.10

THE STREAK PLATE METHOD FOR OBTAINING PURE CULTURES

(a) Organisms are picked up on a sterile wire inoculating loop and lightly streaked across the agar in region 1; the loop is sterilised by flaming and more streak lines are made in region 2; the loop is sterilised again and the streaking is repeated in region 3; after incubation, well-separated colonies of bacteria appear on streak lines, especially in region 3; (b) a streak plate after incubation.

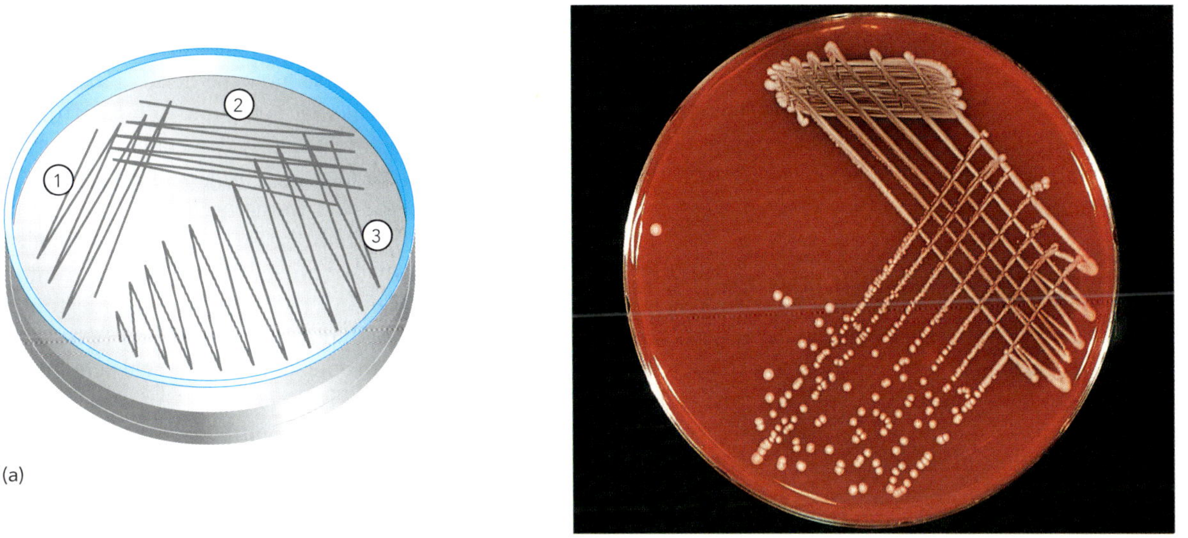

(a)

(b)

IDENTIFICATION OF CULTURED ORGANISMS

Once a culture of a pathogenic bacteria is obtained, various criteria and tests are used to establish the identity of the organism. Different criteria are needed to identify different organisms, but a presumptive identification is usually based on:

- Gram reaction (see Chapter 4);
- cell morphology (i.e. the shape and arrangement of the cells);
- colony morphology (i.e. the characteristics of the colonies on solid culture media);
- ability to grow aerobically (in the presence of oxygen), or anaerobically, or both;
- specialised growth requirements.

To confirm the identity of an organism other properties usually need to be examined, such as:

- the production of special enzymes (e.g. coagulase by *Staphylococcus aureus*);
- biochemical activities (e.g. the ability to metabolise different sugars);
- its motility (ability to swim through liquid);
- its ability to form endospores.

The biochemical profile is usually performed using commercially available multi-test systems, such as that shown in Figure 15.11. These require incubation for 4–24 hours, depending on the type of kit used. In recent years a number of automated bacterial identification systems have been developed, aimed at achieving a more rapid identification.

Fungi are usually identified on the basis of their colony appearance (e.g. colour) and the microscopic morphology of their cells and reproductive structures (see Chapter 6). A biochemical analysis is used for some yeasts.

Overall, for most bacteria and yeasts, culture results are usually available 24–48 hours from the time of arrival at the laboratory. However, slow-growing bacteria and moulds can take up to several weeks to culture.

ANTIBIOTIC SENSITIVITY TESTS

Bacteria isolated in pure culture may also have their sensitivity to different antibiotics determined. This is required for organisms whose antibiotic sensitivity pattern

FIGURE 15.11

MULTI-TEST SYSTEMS ARE USED TO PERFORM MULTIPLE BIOCHEMICAL TESTS ON A MICROORGANISM SIMULTANEOUSLY

Shown here is the commercially prepared API 20E system being used to distinguish between three different bacteria.

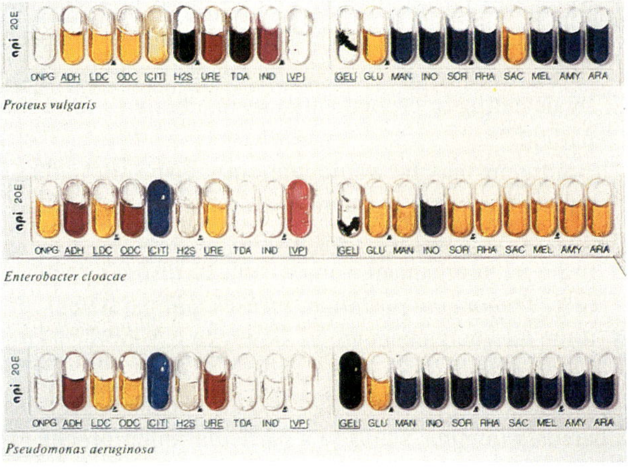

cannot be predicted. Many of the bacteria that cause hospital-acquired infections certainly fall into this category. Antibiotic sensitivity testing is generally performed on agar plates, using filter paper discs impregnated with antibiotics, as described in Chapter 12. Briefly, colonies from a culture of the test bacterium are used to seed the whole surface of a plate, and antibiotic discs are then placed on the plate. During incubation, growth of the bacterium is inhibited around the discs containing the antibiotics to which it is sensitive. Thus, antibiotic sensitivity testing requires a further overnight incubation period, although a number of automated sensitivity testing instruments can now give some results in 3–6 hours.

Culture of Other Microorganisms

Viruses and the bacteria belonging to the genera *Chlamydia* and *Rickettsia* are obligate intracellular parasites and must therefore be grown in cell or tissue cultures, as described in Chapter 5. Growth in cell cultures usually requires a minimum of several days.

Cultured viruses are identified by the cytopathic effect the virus has on the cells that it has been grown in, and/or by electron microscopic examination of the cultured viruses. Although virus isolation gives the most accurate diagnosis of infection, in most clinical settings it is not practical. The culture of viruses (and *Chlamydia* and *Rickettsia)* is time-consuming and involves highly specialised techniques, so alternative diagnostic methods (especially serology) are generally used by clinical microbiology laboratories. Culture is done mainly by specialist virology or research laboratories.

Very few protozoa and helminths can be cultured *in vitro*. Thus, laboratory diagnosis of parasitic infections is usually done by non-cultural methods. Many parasites can, in fact, be quickly identified on morphological grounds by microscopic examination of the specimen. Infections caused by other parasites are usually diagnosed by immunological methods (see next section).

Serology (Immunologic Diagnosis)

The study of antigen-antibody reactions in the laboratory is called **serology**. A serologic diagnosis of infectious disease may be carried out in two ways:

1. by examination of body fluids and detection of antibodies against certain antigens of an infectious agent; or
2. by detecting microbial antigens in a body fluid of the patient.

The antigens may be whole microorganisms, or parts of them, such as viral coats, or bacterial walls, flagella or toxins. Serological tests are useful:

- if the microorganism is impossible or difficult to grow (e.g. *Treponema pallidum*, viruses and parasites); or
- if the microorganism grows slowly (e.g. *Cryptococcus*, *Legionella* and viruses).

The detection of antibodies can also be used to assess a person's immune status to a particular microorganism. For instance, immunity to rubella in pregnant women is determined by measurement of antibodies to the virus in serum. Serological techniques are also used in non-microbiological tests, such as in blood banks for typing blood, for typing tissue before transplant operations and for typing of immunoglobulins in certain immunological disorders.

Most serologic diagnoses are based on antibody measurements. These have the disadvantage that usually two to four weeks or more must elapse from the time of infection before a clearly detectable antibody response is produced. Another drawback is that a positive test only represents exposure to the organisms at some time and not necessarily active disease (see Chapter 9). For a positive diagnosis it is most desirable to demonstrate **seroconversion** in a patient—that is, a fourfold increase in antibody content in sera collected two weeks apart (usually termed acute and convalescent sera—see clinical stages of disease, p. 147ff).

The patient's serum antibody titre is determined by adding the microbial antigens to serial dilutions of the patient's serum; for example, tube 1 = 1/20, tube 2 = 1/40, tube 3 = 1/80, tube 4 = 160, tube 5 = 320, etc. (see Figure 15.12). The greatest dilution that shows a positive reaction is the antibody titre of the patient's serum. These titrations are frequently performed in microtitre plates (see Figure 15.13), which can be automated and which use only small volumes of materials. An antibody titration can also be performed on other body fluids (e.g. urine, CSF).

In contrast, assays that detect the presence of antigen in patient blood or other tissues do not depend on the host immune response and may be positive early in infection. For example, cryptococcal antigen can be detected in the CSF of patients with cryptococcal meningitis early in the infection. Antigens of the human immunodeficiency virus (HIV) can be detected in blood during the antibody negative (window) period, which can exceed three months in some people (see Chapter 19). These methods utilise specific antibodies to identify fragments of the organism in patient material.

A number of methods are available to determine the amount of antibody in an individual's serum. The method used depends mostly on whether the antigen is a whole cell, a toxin, a cell component or a virus. Because all antibodies have two or more antigen-binding sites (see Chapter 9), a reaction between antibody and antigen forms a latticework (or aggregate) of many antigen-antibody molecules that becomes quite large in appropriate conditions. If the antigen is on particulate material, such as a bacterial cell or latex particles, the end result is a clumping of the particles, or **agglutination.** If the particles are red cells the positive reaction is called a **haemagglutination**.

Other methods measure the gain or loss of a certain property of the antigen. An example of this is a reaction between antibodies and a bacterial toxin, resulting in neutralisation of the toxin; such antibodies are given the general name **antitoxin**. A similar principle is used in

FIGURE 15.12

THE PROCEDURE FOR MAKING SERIAL DILUTIONS OF A PATIENT'S SERUM IN AN AGGLUTINATION TEST

The titre is the last tube that shows a positive reaction (clumping), which in this example is 160.

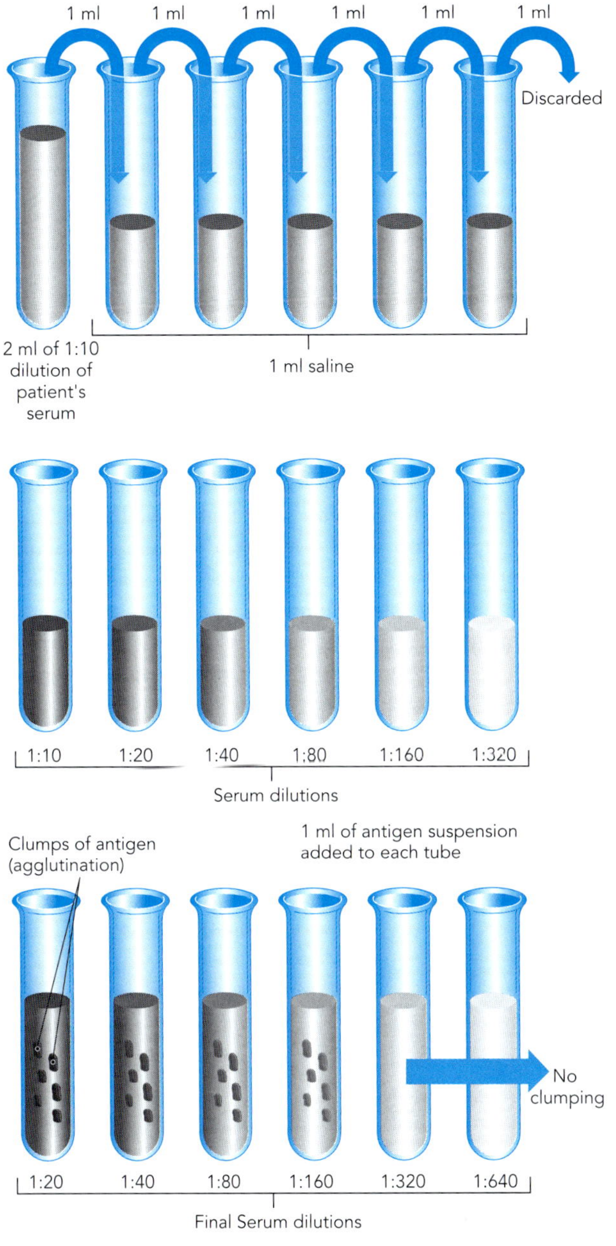

tests that use antibodies to neutralise viruses, thus preventing the viruses from infecting cells.

Other commonly used assays are the complement fixation test, the fluorescent antibody test and the enzyme linked immunosorbent assay (ELISA).

IgM testing

A major drawback of serological diagnosis of infection is the need to demonstrate an increase in antibody titre in paired sera (acute and convalescent). For this reason a serological diagnosis is usually retrospective. This can be overcome if specific IgM antibodies can be detected. As we saw in Chapter 9, IgM is present early in infection, and only for a limited time. It is therefore indicative of active, rather than past infection, permitting a diagnosis to be made from a single specimen. The technology to test for specific IgM antibodies has been developed for only some diseases.

FIGURE 15.13

SEROLOGICAL ASSAY PERFORMED IN A MICROTITRE PLATE

Serial dilutions of patients' serum are made in horizontal rows; in this haemagglutination test, a diffuse layer of cells in the bottom of the well represents a positive reaction, whereas a small button of cells is a negative reaction.

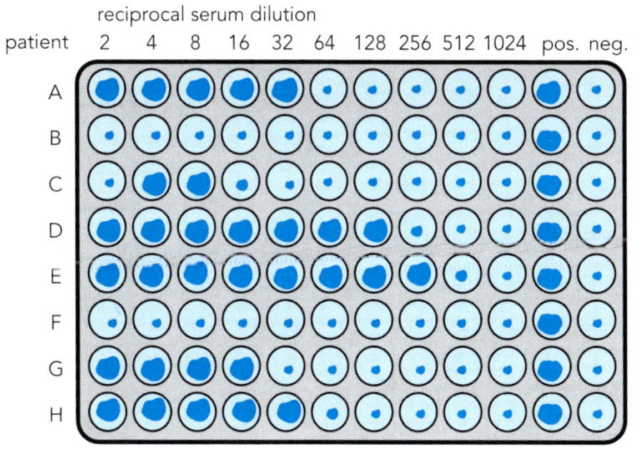

Detection of Microorganisms Using Molecular Techniques

Molecular-based techniques have been proclaimed by many people to be the most significant development in diagnostic microbiology in decades. Techniques such as the use of genetic probes and the polymerase chain reaction can greatly reduce the time required for identification of certain microorganisms by the laboratory. While there are relatively few commercial kits available for laboratory use at present, these and other molecular-based techniques will probably become common procedures in the clinical microbiology laboratory in the next decade or two. They also promise to play vital roles in cancer diagnosis, human genetics, forensic science and archaeology.

NUCLEIC ACID PROBES

If a microbe itself cannot be detected in a specimen, or a culture of the specimen, its DNA may be identifiable with the use of a nucleic acid probe. Virtually all microorganisms contain some unique nucleotide sequence in their genome which, in theory, can be utilised as a fingerprint for rapid identification. A nucleic acid probe is a single-stranded segment of DNA or RNA that is complementary to the nucleic acid that is to be detected. The probe binds to a complementary nucleic acid sequence, if present, to form a novel duplex molecule (see Figure 15.14). The binding of labelled probe with the target nucleic acid is called hybridisation. Probes are labelled with

FIGURE 15.14

USE OF A DNA PROBE TO IDENTIFY A PARTICULAR DNA SEQUENCE

(a) A sample of double-stranded DNA for testing; (b) separation of the DNA segment; (c) binding of the labelled probe DNA to the sample DNA, thereby identifying it.

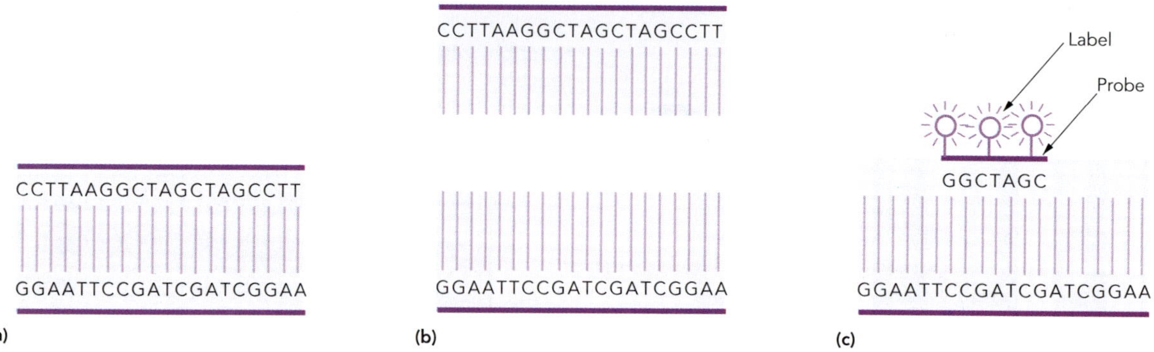

radioisotopes (such as ^{32}P), enzymes, or substances that give colour reactions, so that the formation of duplex molecules can be readily detected. Probes can be made that are specific to the genus, species, or even strain, by varying the nucleotide sequence that is used.

A probe can be used to identify unknown organisms growing in culture. For example, gene probes for *Mycobacterium tuberculosis* and *M. avium-intracellulare* have reduced the time required to identify cultures of these organisms from weeks to hours. To date, a limited number of commercially available probes have been produced for culture confirmation, but many more will undoubtedly follow.

Another use for probes is in the detection of pathogens in a specimen. The direct detection of microbial nucleic acid in a clinical sample is the most exciting potential for probes because it has the advantage of speed and specificity. Probes for enterotoxins of *Escherichia coli* or cholera toxin have been applied directly to faeces. A commercially available ^{125}I-labelled DNA probe directed against sequences specific for *Mycoplasma pneumoniae* has been used successfully to detect the organism in sputum specimens.

Other probes for direct use on clinical specimens, such as for *Neisseria gonorrhoeae* and *Chlamydia trachomatis* from cervical or urethral specimens, and *Legionella pneumophila* in sputum, are at present mainly research tools. Overall, there are few probes available for current use but they will be increasingly developed for diagnostic purposes.

There are limitations to this technology. First, positive specimens must still be cultured for antibiotic susceptibility testing. Second, gene probes are generally unable to detect low numbers of organisms (few copies of the gene) in clincal specimens. Gene amplification methods (e.g. the polymerase chain reaction) may be a possible answer to this problem.

CASE HISTORY 15.1

HERPES SIMPLEX ENCEPHALITIS

A 10-year-old girl who was previously well presented with a nine-day illness, characterised by fevers and headache. On the day before her admission her temperature was noted to be 'very high'. She had rigors, seemed delirious with abnormal speech and was becoming increasingly drowsy. By the day of admission, she was agitated, abusive and incomprehensible. She was admitted to a base hospital where investigations were all normal, except for a CT scan which showed left uncal haemorrhage.

The CSF taken on the day of admission contained 100×10^6/L red blood cells, 400×10^6/L lymphocytes, 100×10^6/L polymorphs, 3.7 mmol/L glucose, 0.88g/L protein, intracranial pressure 13–15 cm.

Polymerase chain reaction (PCR) for herpes simplex virus (HSV) DNA was positive. Serum taken on Day 2 of admission was negative for HSV IgM and low positive for IgG.

A second CSF was taken on Day 3 of admission, containing 420×10^6/L red blood cells, 550×10^6/L lymphocytes, 24×10^6/L polymorphs, 2.8 mmol/L glucose, 0.8 g/L protein. The CSF was sterile for both bacteria and viruses, was negative for HSV IgM and IgG, and was again positive by PCR. A third CSF taken eight days after admission had borderline HSV IgM and positive HSV IgG, but was negative by PCR.

When the PCR results were known, ceftriaxone therapy was ceased and acyclovir treatment was continued for a total of 14 days.

Questions on this case are posed in the 'Test Your Understanding' section at the end of this chapter.

Adapted from J. Montanaro, 'Early detection of herpes simplex encephalitis by polymerase chain reaction', *Communicable Diseases Intelligence* 16/4, 24 February 1992, pp. 76–77.

POLYMERASE CHAIN REACTION

As stated above, a major limitation of probe technology is its low sensitivity; that is, its inability to detect very small amounts of nucleic acid. The polymerase chain reaction (PCR) is a technique that can increase the quantity of a specific nucleotide sequence contained within a sample by a process of directed DNA synthesis. The PCR is an amplification and detection technique that can result in the production of millions of copies of DNA or RNA from even a single molecule of the nucleic acid in a very short time.

At present, a major limitation to the routine use of PCR in diagnostic microbiology is the risk of false positive results due to contamination with DNA from other sources. PCR has already been applied to a variety of specimens to diagnose infections and this versatile technique will undoubtedly be developed for wider clinical applications. It shows great promise for the detection of organisms that are difficult to culture, and in other medical areas such as the amplification of genes associated with genetic diseases like cystic fibrosis and haemophilia. It is also expected to be useful in the examination of museum and archaeological specimens.

Molecular-based techniques are not suitable for the diagnosis of all infections. In certain situations they may be used as rapid alternatives to cultural methods. However, if antibiotic sensitivity is required, culture of the causative agent must still be performed. Other limitations are that they do not distinguish between viable and non-viable organisms, and they are less effective in identifying an infection caused by multiple organisms. At present, their cost and availability are also limiting factors. When developed, they will be most useful for the identification of organisms that grow slowly *in vitro*, such as *Mycobacterium tuberculosis*, *Chlamydia trachomatis* and viruses, and for organisms that can't be readily cultured, like *Mycobacterium leprae* and *Treponema pallidum*.

Summary

- The main function of the clinical microbiology laboratory is to assist in the diagnosis of infectious diseases.
- For an accurate laboratory diagnosis it is essential that an appropriate specimen is properly collected and transported promptly to the laboratory for processing.
- Laboratory tests are designed to detect either (1) the microorganism itself or a component of it in a specimen from the patient, or (2) evidence of an immune response to the causative organism in the blood of the patient.

MICROSCOPIC TECHNIQUES

- Direct microscopic examination of certain specimens can sometimes provide a presumptive diagnosis within an hour.
- A major advantage of direct microscopic examination of a specimen is that the host cells present in the specimen can be identified; this can provide information about whether infection exists, the type of infection and the quality of the specimen.

SPECIMEN COLLECTION FOR CULTURE

- An infectious disease is most accurately diagnosed when the causative agent is isolated and identified from patient material.
- The specimen is cultured on appropriate microbiological media and then an identification of the causative organism is made.
- Microbiological analysis in the laboratory is only as reliable as the quality of the specimen allows.
- A major disadvantage of cultural methods is the length of time required for a result; this may be up to 18 hours and, for some specimens, as long as several weeks.
- Many different types of specimens can be sent to the laboratory for culture: blood, urine, faeces, sputum, pus and swabs from sites of infection.
- The selection of the most appropriate specimen type(s) to be collected should be based on the nature of the infection and the suspected sites of organism persistence.
- Wherever possible, specimens for laboratory culture are collected before antibiotic therapy is initiated.
- Proper collection of specimens is vital for three main reasons: (1) to obtain an appropriate and useful specimen; (2) to prevent contamination of the specimen during collection; and (3) to prevent cross-infection during specimen collection.
- These general procedures should be followed when collecting specimens:
  - Hospital standard precautions guidelines should be followed at all times.
  - Sterile, leak-proof containers of adequate size should be used. Care should be taken not to contaminate the external surface of the collection container or its accompanying paperwork.
  - Specimen collection should be performed with care and tact to avoid harming the patient, or causing discomfort or undue embarrassment.
  - When specimens are collected by patients they should be given clear and detailed instructions.
  - All specimens should be collected in a way that will minimise contamination by commensal microflora and external microorganisms.
  - A sufficient quantity of the specimen should be obtained to enable all necessary tests to be performed.
  - The specimen container must be properly labelled and accompanied by the appropriate laboratory requests on the requisition.
- Specimens should be delivered to the laboratory promptly so that microbiological examination can begin as soon as possible.
- Certain specimens, such as swabs and small amounts of tissue or fluid, should be sent to the laboratory in a transport medium.

COMMON SPECIMEN TYPES FOR CULTURE

BLOOD CULTURES

- A blood culture is usually performed when investigating a patient with fever or other manifestations of systemic infection.
- The blood is collected, taking care to avoid contamination with skin flora, and is usually inoculated into one or two bottles of culture medium (depending on the commercial system being used).
- Usually, three separate sets of blood cultures are collected over a 24–48 hour period.
- Timing of the collections is important because intermittent bacteraemia usually coincides with the onset of fever or chills.
- In the laboratory, cultures are examined later on the day of collection and daily thereafter for 7–14 days, or until growth occurs.

INTRAVASCULAR CATHETERS

- Intravascular catheters may become colonised and serve as a source of microorganisms in septicaemia.
- Culturing of a catheter tip may help to determine if there is a relationship between the catheter and infection.

SPECIMENS FOR URINARY TRACT INFECTIONS

- Bladder urine is normally sterile, but urine usually becomes contaminated with the normal microflora of the urethra during urination.
- Contamination of urine can be reduced by collecting a 'clean-catch' or mid-stream specimen of urine (MSU).
- Urine is an excellent growth medium for micro-organisms, so specimens should be sent to the laboratory within 1 hour of collection, or labelled with the time of collection and refrigerated.
- A urinary tract infection is indicated if the number of bacteria in a clean-catch MSU exceeds 10^8 organisms/L, and if increased numbers of white cells are present.

- Suprapubic aspiration of urine directly from the bladder may be used for neonates and young infants, and for other patients who can't produce an MSU.
- In patients with indwelling urethral catheters attached to a closed drainage system, urine is collected by disinfecting the wall of the catheter at its juncture with the drainage tube, and puncturing it with a needle attached to a syringe.
- Urine may also be collected for culture during the course of cystoscopy or retrograde pyelography.

SPECIMENS FOR CENTRAL NERVOUS SYSTEM INFECTIONS

- In a case of suspected meningitis, cerebrospinal fluid (CSF), obtained by lumbar puncture, is investigated. A lumbar puncture must be performed under conditions of strict asepsis.
- Usually, three tubes of CSF are collected for microbiology, cytology and biochemistry testing. Rapid transport of CSF specimens to the laboratory is essential.
- Blood cultures should also be collected from patients suspected of having meningitis.

SPECIMENS OF OTHER BODY FLUIDS

- Other normally sterile body fluids that may be collected include pleural, peritoneal and synovial fluids; they are usually collected by percutaneous needle aspiration.

SPECIMENS FOR UPPER RESPIRATORY TRACT INFECTIONS

- Several different types of specimens may be collected from the upper respiratory tract—throat, nasal and nasopharyngeal swabs; nasopharyngeal fluid; nasal washings.

SPECIMENS FOR LOWER RESPIRATORY TRACT INFECTIONS

- The specimen most often collected in the investigation of lower respiratory infection is sputum.
- Sputum specimens with excessive squamous epithelial cells are unsatisfactory, because such specimens are likely to be significantly contaminated with oropharyngeal flora.
- Other specimens which may be obtained include bronchial aspiration through a bronchoscope, transtracheal aspiration, or needle biopsy of the lungs.
- If tuberculosis is suspected, extreme care should be exercised in handling the sputum specimen.

SPECIMENS FOR GASTROINTESTINAL TRACT INFECTIONS

- Faeces (stools) may be collected for the culture of bacteria causing gastroenteritis, or for the detection of protozoa, helminths or viruses.
- The specimen should be transported to the laboratory promptly, or refrigerated if a delay is unavoidable.
- Other specimens that may be required for certain infections include rectal swabs, gastric aspirates and gastric biopsies.

SPECIMENS FOR GENITAL TRACT INFECTIONS

- In females, specimens that may be collected include a cervical swab, vaginal swab, urethral swab, amniotic fluid, rectal swab and vesicle fluid.
- In males, typical specimens include a urethral swab, fluid or a swab from penile lesions, and a rectal swab.

SPECIMENS FROM INFECTED WOUNDS AND TISSUE

- Two important principles apply to specimens collected from infected wounds and tissues: (1) tissue or fluid is always superior to a swab specimen; and (2) in general, the more specimen the better.
- Tissue and biopsy specimens should be placed into a sterile, screw-cap container and transported immediately to the laboratory.
- From an infected wound a volume of pus should be collected if possible.
- When only a swab specimen can be obtained, the swab should be used to sample as much of the lesion as possible and transported to the laboratory in transport medium.

SPECIMENS FOR ANAEROBIC BACTERIA

- Anaerobic bacteria can cause a variety of infections in humans.
- If anaerobes are suspected, the laboratory request form should indicate it, and the specimen should be exposed to air for as brief a time as possible.
- One of the best specimens for anaerobic culture is pus, obtained by using a needle and syringe, and transferred to an anaerobic transport vial.
- Tissue samples and biopsy samples are very good specimens for anaerobic culture.
- When a swab must be used to collect a specimen, one of the commercially available anaerobe swab systems should be used.

SPECIMENS FOR FUNGAL CULTURE

- For superficial infections, skin scrapings, hair or nail clippings from the site of infection are most appropriate.
- Specimens for the culture of fungi should be collected aseptically, placed in sterile containers, and delivered to the laboratory within several hours.

SPECIMENS FOR VIRAL CULTURE

- In addition to a specimen from the clinical site of infection, blood, throat washings and faeces are also often collected.
- Specimens should be collected as soon after onset of symptoms as possible.
- Specimens other than fluids should be placed in a sterile, leak-proof container with viral transport medium.

CULTURING BACTERIA AND FUNGI

CULTURE MEDIA

- A nutrient composition prepared for the growth of microorganisms is called a culture medium.
- When microbes are grown on a culture medium, the growth is called a culture.
- Some bacteria have very special nutrient requirements and are said to be fastidious.

- Some bacteria can't be grown in culture media at all.
- Some culture media are designed to allow the growth of certain microorganisms while inhibiting the growth of others; they are called selective media.
- Differential media are so called because certain bacteria can be differentiated from others by the nature of their growth on such media.

PURE CULTURES

- Culture media may be liquid, but most are made solid by the addition of a gelling agent, called agar.
- A solid medium contained in a petri dish is called an agar plate.
- Solid media are used because bacteria and fungi can grow on the surface of the media, forming colonies.
- All the cells in a colony are identical because they are the progeny of a single cell.
- A pure culture is one in which all the colonies comprise the same species of organism.
- Pure cultures are usually prepared by the streak plate method. Streak plating is necessary to obtain pure cultures because most clinical specimens contain mixtures of microorganisms.
- Streak plating allows the separation of different organisms and their subsequent purification.

INCUBATION

- Most bacteria and some fungi (yeasts) grow from single cells to macroscopic colonies on an agar plate in 18–24 hours.

IDENTIFICATION OF CULTURED ORGANISMS

- Once a culture of a microorganism is obtained, various criteria and tests are needed to identify different organisms.
- For most bacteria and yeasts, culture results are available in 24–48 hours; slow-growing bacteria and moulds can take up to several weeks to culture.

ANTIBIOTIC SENSITIVITY TESTS

- Bacteria isolated in pure culture may have their sensitivity to different antibiotics determined.

CULTURE OF OTHER MICROORGANISMS

- Viruses, and the bacteria of the genera *Chlamydia* and *Rickettsia*, are obligate intracellular parasites and must therefore be grown in cell or tissue cultures.
- Growth in cell cultures usually requires a minimum of several days.
- Cultured viruses are identified by the cytopathic effect the virus has on the cells that it has been grown in, and/or by electron microscopic examination of the cultured viruses.

SEROLOGY (IMMUNOLOGIC DIAGNOSIS)

- Serology is the study of antigen-antibody reactions in the laboratory.
- A serologic diagnosis of infectious disease may be carried out in two ways: (1) by examination of body fluids and detection of antibodies against certain antigens of an infectious agent; or (2) by detecting microbial antigens in a body fluid of the patient.
- Serological tests are useful if the microorganism is impossible or difficult to grow, or if it grows slowly.
- The detection of antibodies is also used to assess a person's immune status to a particular microorganism.
- For a positive diagnosis of infection it is most desirable to demonstrate seroconversion in a patient.
- A patient's serum antibody titre is determined by adding the microbial antigens to serial dilutions of the patient's serum; the greatest dilution that shows a positive reaction is the antibody titre of the patient's serum.
- IgM specific antibody is present early in infection and is indicative of active infection.

DETECTION OF MICROORGANISMS USING MOLECULAR TECHNIQUES

- Molecular-based techniques can greatly reduce the time needed for identification of certain microorganisms by the laboratory.
- Molecular-based techniques promise to play vital roles in clinical microbiology, cancer diagnosis, human genetics, forensic science and archaeology in the future.

NUCLEIC ACID PROBES

- If a microbe itself cannot be detected in a specimen, or a culture of the specimen, it may be possible to identify its DNA with the use of a nucleic acid probe.
- A nucleic acid probe is a single-stranded segment of DNA or RNA that is complementary to the nucleic acid that is to be detected.
- A probe can be used to identify unknown organisms growing in culture.
- The direct detection of microbial nucleic acid in a clinical sample has the advantage of speed and specificity.

POLYMERASE CHAIN REACTION

- The polymerase chain reaction (PCR) is a technique that can increase the quantity of a specific nucleotide sequence contained within a sample.
- The PCR is an amplification and detection technique that can result in the production of millions of copies of DNA or RNA from even a single molecule of the nucleic acid.

Study Questions

1. What are the major advantages of a direct microscopic examination of patient material where possible?
2. How does one determine what type of specimen should be collected for the diagnosis of a particular infection?
3. Why should specimens be collected prior to commencement of antibiotic therapy where possible?
4. List the important procedures which should be followed when collecting a specimen for microbiological examination.
5. Although swabs are commonly collected for microbiological analysis, they are not always the most appropriate specimen to collect. Explain.
6. What is a 'transport medium' and why is it used?
7. Why are three samples of blood often collected over a 24 to 48 hour period from a patient suspected of having a septicaemia?
8. What is a 'mid-stream specimen of urine' and why is this the preferred specimen for the diagnosis of urinary tract infections?
9. What is the main problem associated with the delayed transport (several hours) of urine to the microbiology laboratory?
10. What is the main problem associated with the delayed transport (several hours) of sputum to the microbiology laboratory?
11. What are the important principles which should be considered when collecting a specimen from an infected wound?
12. In general, what are the best specimens to collect for the diagnosis of anaerobic infections?
13. What, in microbiological terms, is a 'culture'?
14. Explain the purpose of the streak plate method in microbiology.
15. What type of organisms cannot be grown on agar plates?
16. What is 'serology'?
17. What are detected in serological tests?
18. What is meant by the term 'seroconversion'?
19. Define the terms 'agglutination' and 'haemagglutination'.
20. What are 'nucleic acid probes'? What are their potential uses in microbiology?
21. What is PCR and what are its potential clinical applications?

Test Your Understanding

Case History 15.1: Herpes simplex encephalitis

1. What is the advantage of PCR in this case?
2. Why were antibody tests initially negative?
3. How is PCR able to detect infection so early?

FURTHER READING

Balows, A., W.J. Hausler, K.L. Herrman, H.D. Isenberg & H.J. Shadomy (eds), *Manual of Clinical Microbiology*, 5th edn, Washington: American Society for Microbiology, 1991. (This clinical laboratory manual gives a detailed coverage of specimen collection and handling, diagnostic methods used in the clinical laboratory, characteristics of microorganisms and the role of the clinical laboratory in hospital- and community-acquired infections.)

Hall, G.S., 1992, 'Probe technology for the clinical laboratory', *Archives of Pathology and Laboratory Medicine* 117, p. 578. (This review article examines the value of nucleic acid probes in the clinical microbiology laboratory.)

Isenberg, H.D. (ed.), *Clinical Microbiology Procedures Handbook*, Washington: American Society for Microbiology, 1992. (This clinical laboratory manual also gives a detailed coverage of specimen collection and handling, and diagnostic methods used in the clinical laboratory.)

Matthews, R.C. & J.P. Burnie, 1992, 'Clinical applications of molecular biology to diagnostic microbiology' *Journal of Clinical Pathology* 45, p. 465. (This brief review article outlines the major advantages and disadvantages in the use of molecular biology techniques in diagnostic microbiology laboratories.)

Mims, C.A., J.H.L. Playfair, I.M. Roitt, D. Wakelin & R. Williams, *Medical Microbiology*, St Louis: Mosby, 1993. (A general text of medical microbiology that covers specimen collection and handling, and diagnostic methods in a brief but comprehensive fashion.)

chapter 16

skin, wound and eye infections

Chapter focus

- *What microorganisms cause infections of the skin?*
- *What are the clinical features and important infection control considerations of skin infections ?*
- *What are the common causes and clinical features of surgical wound infections and burns wound infections?*
- *What infection control procedures prevent infections of surgical and burns wounds?*
- *What are the common causes and clinical features of eye infections?*

The skin accounts for approximately 15 per cent of body weight. Except when damaged, the skin provides an effective barrier against invasion by most microorganisms. It acts as a structural barrier and has various chemical factors that inhibit microorganisms, such as a low pH, high salt concentration, lysozyme and fatty acids (see Chapter 9). Although the skin is a relatively inhospitable place for microorganisms, it does have a normal flora that helps to defend against potential pathogens. The flora includes a variety of aerobic and anaerobic organisms such as staphylococci, micrococci, diphtheroids and propionibacteria. Many other organisms, such as streptococci and Gram-negative enteric bacteria (e.g. *Escherichia coli*, *Proteus* spp.), may transiently colonise the skin. The moister areas of skin, such as the axilla (armpit) and groin support relatively large numbers of organisms.

The eye is also exposed to the outside world and is therefore vulnerable to microorganisms and other foreign particles. It too has a number of highly effective defences which generally keep it free of infection. The exposed surface of the eye and the interior surface of the eyelid are covered by the conjunctiva, a thin, mucus-secreting epithelial membrane. As described in Chapter 9, mucous membranes are armed with both non-specific and specific defences. In addition, tears mechanically flush the eye and contain the inhibitory substance lysozyme. The eye has a sparse normal flora, similar in composition to the skin.

Infections of the Skin

Tissue damage is the most common factor leading to infection of the skin, although in some situations apparently normal skin is infected. Minor trauma, such as abrasions, small cuts or cracks, can lead to infection of the skin. More severe trauma, such as that due to surgery, puncture wounds or burns, can lead to serious skin infection, often with involvement of underlying soft tissue. In addition, there are some systemic infections in which organisms are carried in the bloodstream and localise in skin tissue. A skin rash may be the major manifestation of these infections, such as occurs in measles, rubella and chickenpox. The terms used in dermatology to describe different types of lesions on skin are listed and described in Table 16.1.

TABLE 16.1
DERMATOLOGICAL TERMS FOR SKIN LESIONS

Erythema	Area of redness due to vasodilation
Macule	A circumscribed, flat area of altered skin colour
Papule	A circumscribed, elevated area of skin, less than 1 cm in diameter
Nodule	A circumscribed, elevated area of skin, larger than 1 cm in diameter
Vesicle	A small blister containing clear fluid, less than 0.5 cm in diameter
Bulla	A large blister containing clear fluid, more than 0.5 cm in diameter
Pustule	A vesicle or bulla containing cloudy fluid
Wheal/Urticaria	A raised, often itchy erythematous lesion
Erosion	A superficial, circumscribed loss of epidermis, which heals without scarring
Ulcer	An area of tissue loss, varying in depth; an ulcer may involve skin only, or may extend more deeply
Excoriation	An area of skin, denuded of epidermis by scratching
Scale	An abnormal accumulation of keratin; scaling may occur on normal skin, but more often forms on abnormal skin
Crust ('scab')	The dried exudate from an erosion or ulcer
Petechia	A small flat haemorrhage
Purpura	Numerous petechiae

BACTERIAL SKIN INFECTIONS

Folliculitis, boils and carbuncles

Staphylococcus aureus is a common cause of skin infections because it is often present on the skin and mucous membranes, particularly the nasal mucosa. Thus, the staphylococci that cause a skin infection often come from a person's own flora, or from another person's skin flora. Infection can occur when the organism invades a hair follicle, causing **folliculitis**, also referred to as a **pimple** or **pustule**. These occur mostly on the scalp, face or limbs and are often precipitated by some irritation or dermatitis. When the deeper areas of a hair follicle are affected, a larger, deeper, pus-filled nodule develops, called a **furuncle** or **boil**. Usually, a boil continues to expand slowly, eventually coming to a head on the surface of the skin. Nasal carriers of virulent *S. aureus* may suffer recurrent boils anywhere on the skin.

Boils may discharge to adjacent areas of skin, resulting in multiple abscesses, called a **carbuncle.** Carbuncles tend to develop at particular sites, such as on the neck, upper back and buttocks. In addition to the abscesses, there are often systemic symptoms such as fever, malaise and lymphadenopathy. Septicaemia may complicate even simple lesions, especially in the immunocompromised. Boils and carbuncles are encapsulated abscesses, representing the body's attempt to localise the infection (see Chapter 9).

Diagnosis is usually made on clinical grounds, but a laboratory confirmation of the causative organism is readily achieved by culture of pus. In general, antibiotics enter abscesses poorly, and, when they do enter, are inactivated by neutrophil enzymes. For this reason, treatment of these infections usually requires surgical drainage of the lesions.

Impetigo

Impetigo is a highly infectious, pyogenic (pus-forming) infection caused by staphylococci, streptococci, or both (Figure 16.1). It occurs predominantly in young children, where minor skin damage due to insect bites, eczema and scabies is the usual predisposing factor. Lesions often start on the face around the nose and may then spread to other sites of the body. Scratching and other abrasions can result in new lesions, as well as transmission of the organism to others in close contact. It is readily spread on hands, toys and furniture, and can be spread through schools and day-care centres.

There are two main forms of impetigo—the bullous form, caused mainly by *Staphylococcus aureus*, and the non-bullous form caused by staphylococci and/or Group A streptococci (especially *Streptococcus pyogenes*). The non-bullous form usually occurs on the face and is characterised by small vesicles which rupture easily, resulting in weeping, honey-coloured crusts that dry and self-resolve. Bullous lesions are larger, with clear fluid that later becomes cloudy and yellow. After rupture, brownish crusts form. Bullous lesions are most common on the buttocks and limbs but can occur anywhere on the body. There is generally no systemic illness unless deeper tissues are involved.

Laboratory diagnosis is based on culture of a swab of the lesions under the crusts.

Scalded skin syndrome is caused by strains of *S. aureus* that produce a toxin called **exfoliatin**. It can occur as a complication of minor skin lesions or impetigo. Exfoliatin causes layers of cells in the epidermis to separate, and sheets of skin are shed, leaving large areas of skin that have the appearance of being scalded. The neonatal form is sometimes referred to as Ritter's disease.

Erysipelas

Erysipelas is an infection that begins as a small, raised, rubbery lesion, often on the face, and spreads rapidly. Typically, it develops into a bright red, swollen lesion with a sharply demarcated edge (Figure 16.2), followed by bullae that rupture and weep. Systemic symptoms of fever, headache and vomiting often precede the cutaneous signs. Erysipelas is usually caused by Group A streptococci, although other bacteria such as *S. aureus* or *Haemophilus influenzae* are occasionally responsible. It occurs most

FIGURE 16.1
IMPETIGO
A highly contagious disease characterised by vesicles on the skin which break down to a crust form.

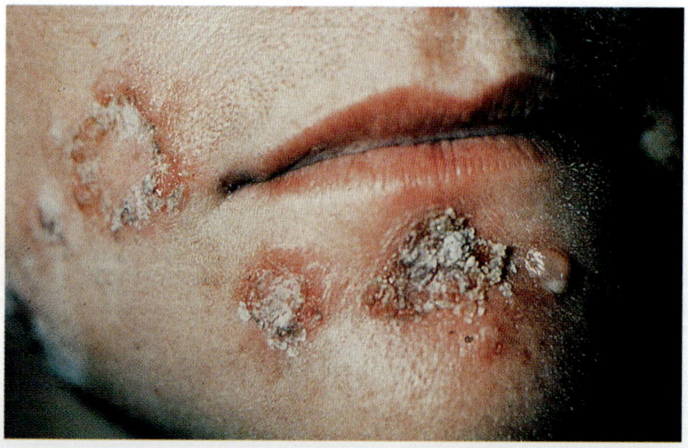

FIGURE 16.2
A SEVERE CASE OF ERYSIPELAS

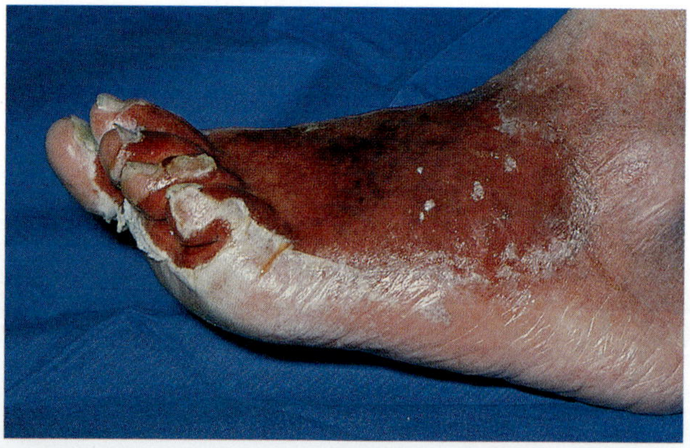

often in young children and the elderly. The streptococci usually enter through a break in the skin, but sometimes there is no apparent predisposing lesion. Without appropriate antibiotic treatment the organisms may spread through the lymphatics and cause nephritis, septicaemia, pneumonia and even gangrene.

The diagnosis is usually based on clinical appearance, but the causative agent can be confirmed by culture of fluid from the edge of the lesion.

Cellulitis

Cellulitis is an acute bacterial infection of the skin that spreads to subcutaneous tissues. The infected tissue becomes hot, painful, red and swollen. Fever, chills, bacteraemia and local lymph node enlargement may be present. It may occur following a superficial skin infection or after skin trauma. Following trauma, streptococci are usually responsible, but other organisms such as *S. aureus*, *Pseudomonas aeruginosa* and *Streptococcus pneumoniae* may be involved. *Haemophilus influenzae* type b is most likely in young children. *Clostridium perfringens* and other anaerobes can cause cellulitis in poorly oxygenated tissue, especially after deep wounds and fractures.

Culture of aspirates of the leading edge of the lesion, or skin biopsy, are the usual means of laboratory diagnosis. Blood cultures should also be taken.

Bairnsdale ulcer

Bairnsdale ulcer is a chronic, relatively painless cutaneous ulcer caused by *Mycobacterium ulcerans*. This infection was first reported in 1948 in a group of six patients in Australia, five of whom came from the Bairnsdale district of Victoria. It is a rare condition found mostly in Australia, Papua New Guinea and Africa. It is thought that the organism is associated mainly with waste and drainage water. Infection occurs when the bacterium enters the skin through minor cuts or abrasions, leading to a progressive ulcer which does not respond to normal antibiotics.

FIGURE 16.3
RUBELLA
The patient shows the macular rose-pink spots typical of this disease.

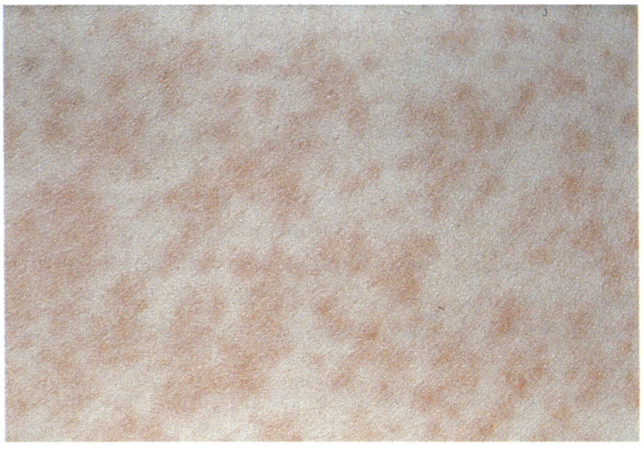

Treatment of bacterial skin infections

For small, minor skin infections, local measures, particularly wound drainage and gentle debridement of crusted lesions, are often all that is necessary. Sometimes, treatment with topical antibiotics and bathing with antiseptics are required as an adjunct to drainage. In general, systemic antibiotic therapy is given when there are systemic symptoms, such as fever, or when the infection is severe or widespread, or involves deeper tissue. Underlying skin disease, scabies infection or eczema should also be treated. Impetigo and other streptococcal infections are highly contagious and are usually treated with oral penicillin, or erythromycin in allergic people. Patients with severe infections (especially children) should be isolated until the infection is under control.

VIRAL SKIN INFECTIONS

Some viruses cause skin lesions by localising in and infecting cutaneous tissue. The wart viruses and most poxviruses are the major groups of this type. Other viruses cause skin lesions as well as infecting other body sites. The common systemic viral diseases that produce skin lesions as the major manifestation are herpes simplex infections, chickenpox, measles and rubella.

Rubella

Rubella, or **German measles**, is one of several systemic human viral diseases that cause a skin rash. It is caused by a togavirus spread mainly by the air-borne route from infected individuals. It is highly contagious for about a week before and a week after the rash appears. Despite the availability of an effective vaccine (see below), the

FIGURE 16.4
A SEVERE CASE OF MEASLES
The disease is characterised by small, raised maculopapular lesions.

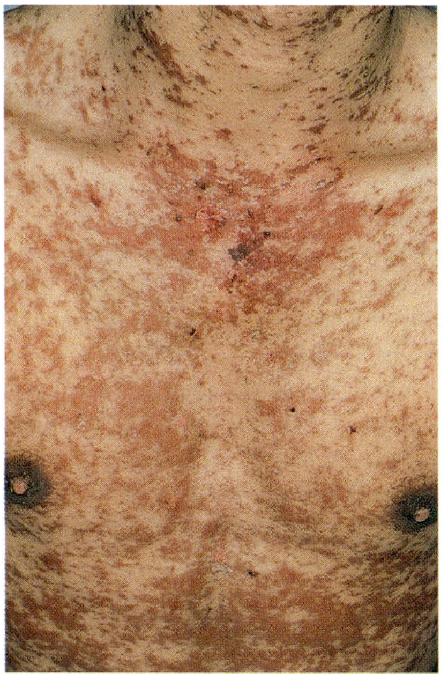

CASE HISTORY 16.1
CELLULITIS

A 3-year-old-girl was taken to a casualty department with a red, swollen left forearm. Her doctor had diagnosed her as having chickenpox four days earlier. Vesicular and pustular lesions were still present over the whole of her body, with older crusted lesions in certain parts. Her temperature was 39.5°C. A white cell count showed her to have a marked leukocytosis with a predominance of neutrophils. It was suspected that she had a cellulitis of the forearm.

Comment:
Cellulitis is potentially a very severe disease because of possible invasion of the bloodstream and subsequent systemic infection.

National Notifiable Diseases Surveillance System reported an epidemic level of rubella activity in 1992 to 1994, with over 3000 cases notified in each of those years.

Except for the congenital form (described below), rubella is generally a mild, often subclinical disease. Many infected individuals do not have a rash but are still able to transmit the virus to others. The incubation period is 2–3 weeks. In adults, a short period of mild fever, malaise and upper respiratory symptoms may occur first. The rash is the main symptom of rubella, and it appears first on the face or trunk, but quickly spreads to the rest of the body. The lesions are macular with a light rose-pink colour (Figure 16.3). Lymph nodes are usually enlarged and in severe cases conjunctival infection may be marked. The rash usually disappears after three days.

Congenital rubella syndrome results from infection of a developing foetus when the virus crosses the placenta from the mother's circulation. The effect on the foetus varies with the gestational age at the time of maternal infection. The virus slows cell replication and differentiation, so the most severe damage occurs if the woman is infected in the first trimester, when foetal organ systems are developing. The most severe effects of congenital rubella include stillbirth, microcephaly, deafness, eye defects, cardiac abnormalities, hepatomegaly, splenomegaly, pneumonitis and low birth weight. Major abnormalities are rare if infection occurs after the 16th week of pregnancy. The link between rubella infection in early pregnancy and congenital defects in infants was first suggested in 1941 by Norman Gregg, an ophthalmologist working at the Royal Alexandra Hospital for Children in Sydney.

Rubella cannot be reliably diagnosed by clinical means, so when the diagnosis must be confirmed (e.g. in a pregnant woman or someone in contact with a pregnant woman, or in an affected neonate), serological tests are required. Serology is also used to assess the immunity of pregnant women in prenatal screening tests.

A live, attenuated rubella vaccine was licensed in Australia in 1970 and a mass vaccination program commenced in 1971. It is now a component of the MMR

CASE HISTORY 16.2
CONGENITAL RUBELLA

A 32-year-old shop owner was pregnant for the first time. She could not recall having received rubella vaccination at school, but remembered that her mother always said that vaccinations were a waste of time. At her first visit to the obstetrician (about six weeks after becoming pregnant), blood was taken for rubella serology and she was found to have no detectable antibodies. Three weeks later she became ill with what she thought was a cold and conjunctivitis. She did not recall having any rash.

Her son was born at full term, but his birth weight was 2450 g, and his Apgar scores were 9 at 1 minute and 10 at 5 minutes (i.e. normal). The paediatrician made a diagnosis of congenital rubella syndrome based on clinical findings, including micropthalmia and a cataract in the right eye and profound deafness, and on the mother's history.

(measles-mumps-rubella) vaccine offered to children from 12 months of age. Vaccination has been extremely successful, resulting in a significant reduction in congenital rubella. A second immunisation is recommended for girls and boys 10–16 years of age. Vaccination of adolescents usually induces lifelong immunity, but antibody levels may fall with the passage of time. Low levels of antibody may not protect against infection. Since it is a live vaccine, it is not recommended for pregnant women.

Measles

Measles, or **rubeola**, is caused by a paramyxovirus, and has a worldwide distribution. In Australia, in 1992 and 1993, there was an epidemic level of measles with over 4500 notifications in each of those years. This was three times the rate of the two previous years. The highest rates of notification were in the age groups under 20 years. It is a highly infectious disease, spread mainly by the air-borne route via respiratory secretions of infected people. An acute case of measles is infectious from just before the onset of symptoms and as long as fever is present.

After an incubation period of 9–14 days symptoms of fever, runny nose, dry cough and watery eyes typically develop. After 3–4 days, **Koplik's spots**, which are areas of white necrosis on a reddened mucosa, may appear in the mouth. They may also appear on other mucosa such as the conjunctiva. Usually, within another two days, a dusky red, maculopapular rash develops, often starting behind the ears, and then spreading to the face and thence down the body, eventually reaching the lower extremities (Figure 16.4). The Koplik's spots disappear shortly after the rash appears. The rash fades in several days, starting from the top of the body, and progressing in a way similar to its appearance. There is usually a generalised, but minor lymph node enlargement. If the virus invades the lungs, kidneys or brain, especially in the immunocompromised, the disease is often fatal.

CASE HISTORY 16.3
MEASLES

An outbreak of measles occurred in a primary school in Canberra between January and March 1992. Concerned individuals within the community alerted health authorities to the outbreak. Once the outbreak was identified, a standardised questionnaire was devised to survey the whole school population, as the opportunity existed for a vaccine efficacy study.

There were 151 children in seven grades. One hundred and two fully completed questionnaires were returned. The ages of the children in the school ranged from 4 to 12 years. The majority of respondents were not vaccinated (60 children).

A case was defined as a child considered to have measles by doctors, parents or teachers. There were 38 cases of measles, with the majority occurring in the 5–9 year age group. No case occurred in those who had a history of measles vaccination (42 children). Four children were 'vaccinated' by alternative homoeopathic methods; two of these developed measles.

Adapted from D. Cheah, 'An estimate of measles vaccine efficacy in a Canberra school', *Communicable Diseases Intelligence* 16/14, 13 July 1992, p. 294

Measles is potentially a very serious disease. **Measles encephalitis** is the most serious complication, occurring in approximately one patient per 1000. Most of these patients recover without problem, but some become comatose and may die. In approximately 1 patient in 200 000, the virus is not completely cleared from the body, but persists in the brain. Six to eight years later, **subacute sclerosing panencephalitis (SSPE)** develops, and is nearly always fatal. It is due to viral destruction of nerve cells, with progressive mental deterioration, muscle rigidity and coma. In some less developed areas of the world, such as Africa, mortality rates due to measles or its complications can be as high as 10–20%. Other less serious complications of measles are secondary bacterial bronchopneumonia and middle ear infections.

Measles is usually diagnosed clinically by the initial catarrhal symptoms and dry cough, followed by a rash. It can also be diagnosed serologically by detection of specific IgM antibodies in serum. Treatment is limited to alleviating symptoms and dealing with complications. Secondary, bacterial, infections can be effectively treated with antibiotics.

The availability of measles vaccine now prevents major epidemics in many developed countries. It is usually used in the form of the MMR vaccine (containing attenuated viruses of measles, mumps and rubella). Measles vaccination should occur at around 12 months of age. Encephalitis is a very rare complication of measles vaccination (one in 1 million doses), much rarer than in natural infection. Although an effective measles vaccine has been available in Australia since 1969, there is still an unnecessarily high incidence of this disease, due to poor acceptance and uptake of the vaccine. Deaths due to measles infection still occur in this country. Outbreaks of measles can be contained by the prompt vaccination of susceptible (non-vaccinated) children and children with doubtful immunity (uncertain vaccination history) who have been in contact with an infected case.

Since measles vaccine comprises living viruses, it should not be used in immunocompromised people or pregnant women. Immunoglobulin is available for such cases.

Chickenpox and shingles

The varicella zoster virus (VZV), a member of the herpes family, causes both chickenpox (varicella) and shingles (zoster). Chickenpox is a common, highly infectious disease, transmitted by the air-borne route from the respiratory secretions or saliva of infected people, or by direct contact with skin lesions. Like other herpes viruses, VZV enters sensory nerve endings during primary infection and becomes latent in sensory ganglia. After remaining latent there for decades, it can be reactivated to cause shingles.

Chickenpox is usually a mild disease, but it is more severe in adults. Sometimes there may be a short period of fever and malaise, but usually the rash is the first sign of infection. The rash comprises different types of lesions at different stages of development, from macules to papules to vesicles and pustules. The lesions dry and crust over in a few days. They appear in crops over several days as the virus goes through cycles of replication. They start on the scalp and trunk and spread to the face and limbs, sometimes to the mouth, throat and vagina. More severe infection and complications can occur, particularly in adults. Complications include interstitial pneumonia, secondary bacterial pneumonia and meningitis. Infection can be severe in women who are pregnant and in neonates infected after birth.

In **shingles**, clusters of painful, vesicular lesions like those of chickenpox develop. The lesions are usually confined to one side of the body, following the unilateral location of affected sensory nerves (Figure 16.5). This infection is most common in the elderly, in whom the immune system is becoming less effective. It is also common in immunocompromised patients, who can suffer widespread infections, sometimes involving internal organs, that can be fatal. Some people experience recurrent attacks, often marked by pain but with no skin lesions. Chronic infections can occur in patients with HIV infection.

When reactivated, the virus spreads from a ganglion along the pathway of its associated nerve or nerves. The rash may be preceded by a burning sensation or severe pain in the area of the nerves. The lesions are localised in certain areas and may be minor to severe. The rash can be accompanied by headache, fever and malaise. Most patients experience background pain with intermittent sharp stabs, although some are pain-free. Lesions often appear on the trunk but may also occur on the face or eye. As in chickenpox, the lesions are rich in virus particles and therefore highly infectious. Neuralgia, which can last several months, is a common sequela of shingles.

FIGURE 16.5
SHINGLES RASH

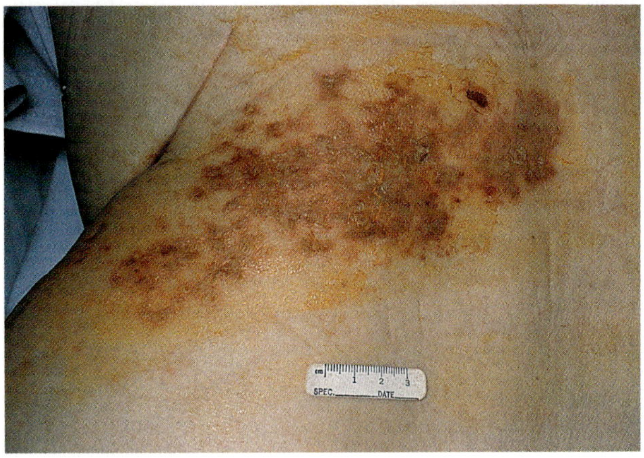

Diagnosis of chickenpox and shingles is generally based on clinical signs and symptoms. Laboratory confirmation is rarely required, but in uncertain cases serology or microscopy of culture of fluid from lesions can provide a definitive diagnosis. Therapy consists of supportive care, such as calamine lotion and soothing baths to relieve itchiness and scratching in chickenpox, and analgesics to relieve the pain in shingles. Acyclovir may be used for shingles, especially in immunocompromised patients, to prevent spread of infection and complications. It is very effective if given within a few days of diagnosis and may prevent recurrent attacks. Zoster immune globulin should be given to those in whom varicella may be life-threatening and who have been exposed to the virus—for example, immunosuppressed people, pregnant women, neonates and premature babies.

Warts

Warts are caused by human papillomaviruses (HPV), of which there are over 50 different types. HPV specifically attack skin and mucous membranes, but different types tend to infect different body sites. For example, HPV 2, 3 and 10 typically cause the common warts seen on fingers and knees, whereas HPV 6, 12, 16, 18, 31, 33 and 35 cause genital warts. It is thought that infection lasts a lifetime and, when warts disappear or are removed, the virus still remains dormant in the cells of surrounding tissue.

HPV are transmitted by direct contact, usually between humans, or via fomites. Dermal warts occur when the virus enters the skin through abrasions. The virus replicates slowly, stimulating the cells to divide in an uncontrolled way to form a benign mass which protrudes above the skin surface. The incubation period varies from one week to 12 months for dermal warts. Genital warts, which are sexually transmitted, are discussed in Chapter 21.

Warts vary in appearance in different areas of the body. On normal skin, warts develop as small, painless nodules. Often several in number, they occur in areas of friction or minor trauma. Some may be hardly visible. Plantar warts occur in the thick skin on the soles of the feet, level with the skin surface, but with deeper underlying growth. Pressure on them when walking can cause severe discomfort. Warts in moist areas such as the mouth or genital tract are more papillary and profuse. Dermal warts usually regress spontaneously, all at the same time, presumably when the immune system gains control, although this may take several years. There appears to be an association of some HPV with cancer, particularly serotypes 16 and 18 with cervical cancer.

Wart viruses have not been cultured in the laboratory, so diagnosis is based on clinical observation. Warts can be removed by local freezing of the tissue with liquid nitrogen or by curetting, cautery or laser. Topical treatments include podophyllin and salicylic acid. Recurrences after treatment are common.

Herpes simplex

Primary infection with herpes simplex type 1 virus usually involves the skin around the mouth or nose. Occasionally it affects other sites, such as the genitalia, cheeks or forehead. Herpes simplex type 2 virus predominantly involves the genitalia, but sometimes other sites, including the mouth. Genital herpes infections are dealt with in Chapter 21.

Most primary infections are minor or subclinical in immunocompetent people, but may be severe in the immunocompromised. In fact, severe herpes infections often indicate underlying immune disorder. Herpes skin lesions (cold sores) usually begin as areas of tender erythema, followed by the development of closely grouped vesicles (Figure 16.6) which ultimately progress through pustular and crusting stages. Large amounts of virus are present in the lesions. In patients with impaired cellular immunity (see Chapter 9) due to corticosteroids, cytotoxic drugs or HIV infection, the lesions may be more extensive and spread into the mouth, and progress and resolve more slowly. Primary infection can sometimes occur at other sites such as the finger (called herpetic whitlow), the conjunctiva (keratoconjunctivitis) or areas of the face subject to frequent rubbing (e.g. 'scrum pox' in rugby footballers).

During primary infection, herpes viruses enter sensory nerve endings and travel to the sensory ganglion, where they remain latent. The virus remains in the sensory ganglion for life. The virus can be reactivated by many

FIGURE 16.6
COLD SORES CAUSED BY HERPES SIMPLEX VIRUS

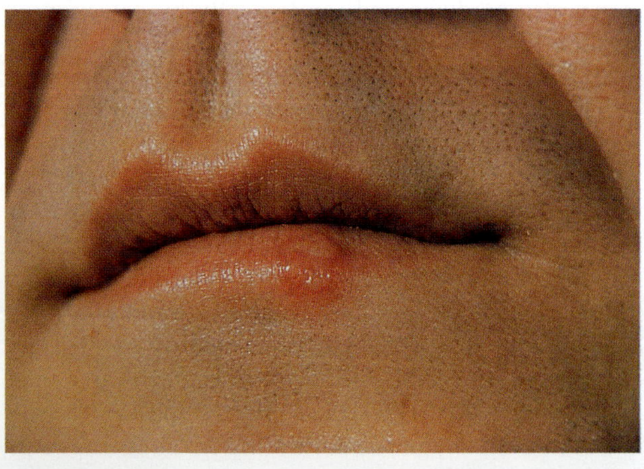

stimuli, such as sunlight, trauma, viral respiratory infection, menses, stress or immunosuppression, and it then travels back down the same sensory nerves to cause lesions at the same site. The interval between recurrences of symptoms can vary from several months to a year, or there may be no recurrence at all.

The infection is readily recognised clinically, so a laboratory diagnosis is often not necessary. A Tzanck smear of cells from the base of a lesion showing multinucleated giant cells is diagnostic. Microscopy or culture of lesion fluid can identify the virus, but are rarely performed because of the need for highly specialised methods and equipment.

In the immunocompetent, lesions usually resolve spontaneously in 4–5 days. Treatment with saline bathing, peroxide or other astringents may help. In the immunocompromised, treatment is usually with oral acyclovir, or intravenously if lesions are disseminated. Secondary infection of herpes lesions by *Staphylococcus aureus* or streptococci may occur.

Molluscum contagiosum

Molluscum contagiosum is a common viral infection, with worldwide distribution, caused by viruses of the pox group. It is transmitted from person to person by direct contact, or indirectly, via clothing, gym equipment or swimming pools, for example. The infection is characterised by clusters of small (2–5 mm), flesh-coloured papular lesions scattered over the skin. The lesions are disseminated to other areas by scratching. The virus infects epidermal cells, causing epidermal hyperplasia.

Diagnosis is made by the clinical appearance or by electron microscopic examination of biopsy material. Spontaneous resolution usually occurs within 6–9 months, but therapy is desirable to prevent spread of infection. Treatment is best achieved by superficial curettage, although a trichloroacetic acid paint or cryotherapy are sometimes used.

FUNGAL SKIN INFECTIONS

Tinea (ringworm)

The fungi that infect keratinised tissue, causing **tinea** (or **ringworm**), are called **dermatophytes**. Fungal skin infections are called **dermatomycoses.** These diseases can be caused by any one of several organisms from three genera: *Epidermophyton, Microsporum,* and *Trichophyton*. They cause the disease commonly referred to as athlete's foot and tinea of the skin, nails, scalp, beard and groin. Different species have a preference for different body sites.

Tinea is spread by contact with arthrospores of the fungi, which may be acquired directly from another person, or indirectly from communal bathrooms, dressing sheds or swimming pools. Superficial abrasions or wounds increase the risk of infection. The fungi are keratin-loving and invade skin, nails and hair. The characteristic lesion of tinea is an annular (hence the name 'ringworm', although a worm is not involved), scaling patch of dry skin with a red, raised margin. In hairy parts of the body, the hair might be lost where the lesions develop. The lesions are often, but not always, itchy. Dermatophytes occasionally invade subcutaneous tissues, after invading follicles, and cause severe pustular lesions.

In **tinea pedis**, or **athlete's foot**, infection usually starts between the toes as a result of maceration from sweating and occlusive footwear. It produces dry, scaly lesions between and under the toes, and subsequently causes the skin to crack and peel (Figure 16.7). The toenails are often infected (**tinea unguium**, tinea of the nails) and may become discoloured, thickened and brittle. Secondary infection by bacteria or *Candida* leads to itchy, soggy, white areas between the toes.

Tinea corporis (tinea of non-hair-bearing parts of the body) is characterised by one or more annular, scaly lesions, often on the trunk. **Tinea cruris** (tinea of the groin) occurs in skin folds in the pubic region, and sometimes extends down the thighs. **Tinea capitis** (tinea of the scalp) is most common in children. There are a number of different forms, depending on the organism involved. At least some hair loss and scaling of the skin are typical.

Laboratory diagnosis of tinea is made by direct microscopic examination of skin scrapings or nail or hair clippings. Sometimes, culture of these specimens is performed, but this can take up to two weeks. Some species of dermatophytes fluoresce under ultraviolet light and can be seen when the light is shone onto the infected skin. Treatment generally involves the use of a topical, antifungal cream, powder or ointment and/or a keratolytic agent such as Whitfield's ointment (benzoic acid compound). If lesions are widespread or involve nails or hair, oral griseofulvin (or ketoconazole if resistant) is used. Prevention of athlete's foot depends on maintaining healthy, clean, dry skin and avoidance of contact in communal facilities.

Candidiasis

Candida albicans, an oval, budding yeast, is present among the normal flora of the digestive, respiratory and urogenital tracts of humans. It can cause **candidiasis** (or **moniliasis**) in a number of body sites. Superficial infection of mucous membranes appears as **thrush**, milky white patches of inflammation on mucous membranes, especially in infants, diabetic, debilitated patients, and those receiving prolonged antibiotic therapy. It can also cause **vaginitis**.

Candida skin infections generally occur in areas of warmth, moisture and maceration, such as in skin folds and under tight clothing. *Candida albicans* is an opportunistic pathogen (see Chapter 7), usually requiring some predisposing factor such as diabetes mellitus or antibiotic therapy to cause infection. Obesity also predisposes to *Candida* skin infection, the moist skin folds providing an ideal site for the yeast to grow. Skin infection is characterised by areas of moist erythema with an irregular, soft, white edge. Satellite areas of infection in the form of red papules or pustules are usually present. If the lesions become generalised, an underlying immune disorder may be present.

In immunocompromised individuals, *Candida* can invade the lungs, kidneys and heart. Candidiasis is the

FIGURE 16.7
TINEA PEDIS, OR ATHLETE'S FOOT, CAUSED BY FUNGI CALLED DERMATOPHYTES

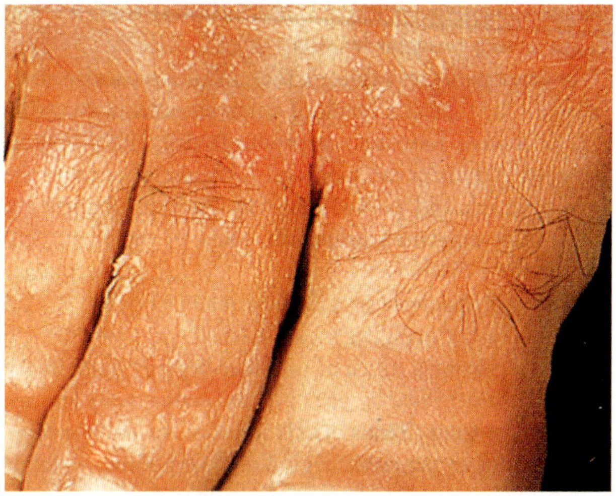

most commonly seen fungal infection in hospitalised patients with serious disease such as tuberculosis, leukaemia or AIDS.

Diagnosis is usually based on clinical examination. A laboratory diagnosis is made by microscopy and culture of a swab of the lesion. Treatment usually involves the use of antifungal antibiotic creams or ointments, such as nystatin or imidazole. Systemic therapy may be necessary in severe infections.

Tinea versicolor (pityriasis versicolor)

Tinea versicolor is a common, superficial infection caused by the yeast *Malassezia furfur*. The trunk is most often affected, but there may be spread to other areas including the upper arms, neck and abdomen. The lesions are small, sharply demarcated, scaling macules. The organism interferes with pigment production—on white skin the lesions are dark, and on dark skin they are lighter, hence the name 'versicolor'. The infection is basically cosmetic, causing little irritation, but can persist for years if untreated.

Treatment consists of topical applications for several weeks of selenium sulphide shampoos or topical imidazole antifungal agents. Pale areas will repigment, but may take many months to do so. Recurrence is common, often because patients do not use the applications for sufficient time.

FIGURE 16.8
CANDIDA ALBICANS INFECTION OF THE SKIN
The infection is characterised by areas of moist erythema.

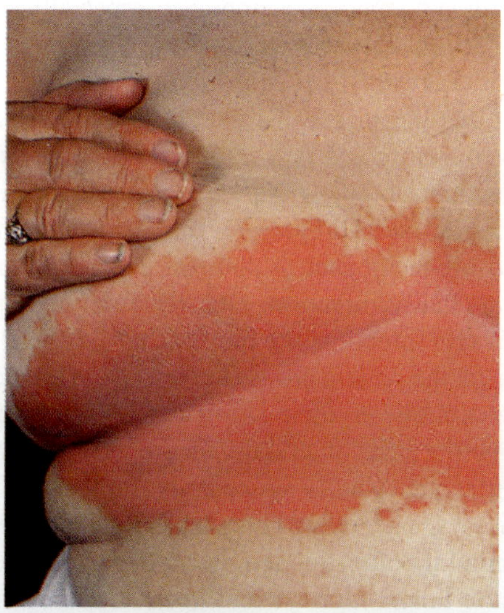

ARTHROPOD INFESTATIONS

Scabies

Scabies is caused by the mite *Sarcoptes scabiei* var. *hominis*. The adult female is about 0.4 mm in length, just visible to the naked eye. Mites most commonly infest the hands and wrists, elbows, feet and ankles, penis and scrotum, buttocks and axillae. The female mite burrows in the epidermis, laying eggs as she goes (Figure 16.9(a)). The typical scabies lesion is the burrow, but papules, pustules and nodules are also usually seen (Figure 16.9(b). Itchiness, representing a sensitisation to mites, eggs and faeces in

FIGURE 16.9
(a) AN ADULT SCABIES MITE; (b) SCABIES INFECTION

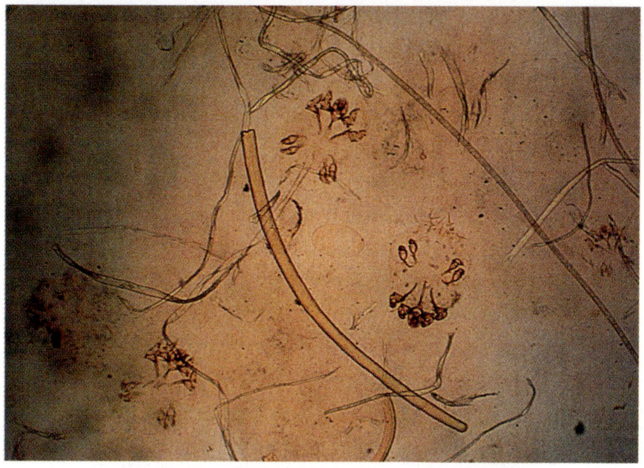

(a)

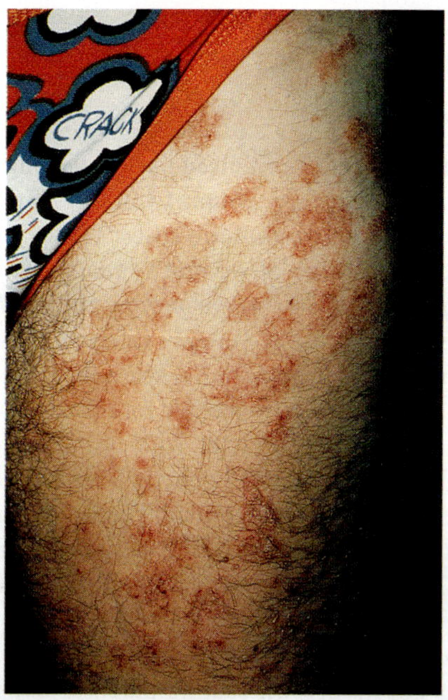

(b)

the skin, is severe, and is often worse at night. Secondary infection of the lesions by streptococci or staphylococci is a common complication when they are scratched.

Norwegian (crusted) scabies is characterised by formation of thick crusts on the face, scalp, hands, feet and pressure-bearing areas. It is typically found in patients who are either immunologically or neurologically impaired, such as AIDS patients, transplant patients receiving immunosuppressive agents, patients with leukaemia and individuals with trisomy 21. In this form, the host may be harbouring thousands of mites, and their epithelial debris may be highly infectious.

The mites are spread by close personal contact. In adults, the usual source is a sexual partner. Because scabies is a highly contagious disease, outbreaks can occur in hospitals and nursing homes. It can be spread directly from patient to patient, or via health care personnel, visitors and fomites.

Diagnosis is based on clinical examination and microscopic demonstration of mites or eggs in a skin burrow, scraped with a needle point. A number of scabicides, such as permethrin, provide effective treatment. Although scabies rarely seems to be transmitted by clothing, towels or bedding, dry cleaning or machine washing in hot water of these items is recommended. Patient contacts should also be evaluated for infestation.

Pediculosis

Pediculosis, or lice infestation, may involve the scalp, the pubic area or the body. Three species of lice infest these different sites: *Pediculus humanus capitis* (head louse), *Pediculus humanus corporis* (body louse) and *Phthirus pubis* (crab louse). The major symptoms of pediculosis are itching and a maculopapular rash. Scratching can cause crusting and secondary bacterial infection. Enlarged lymph nodes are common.

Head lice infestation mainly affects young schoolchildren. The head louse (Figure 16.10) lays her eggs (called nits) at the base of hairs, to which they are firmly attached. After 8–10 days the eggs hatch, leaving translucent shells fixed to the hair. Pink or white dots can be seen near the scalp. Transmission is by hair to hair contact, brushes or hair apparel.

FIGURE 16.10
THE HEAD LOUSE, *PEDICULUS HUMANUS CAPITIS*

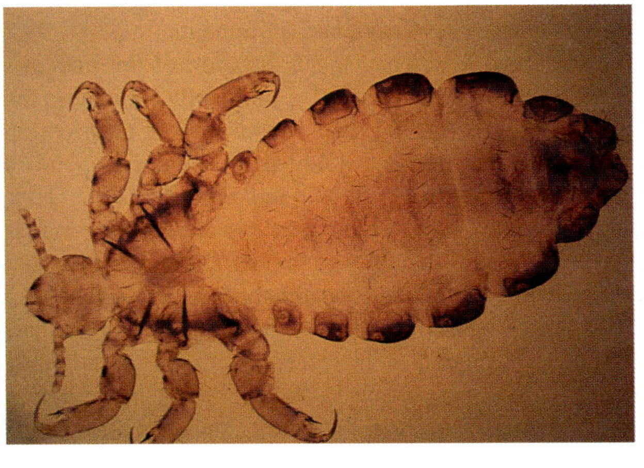

Body lice infestation is generally related to poor hygiene, especially when clothes are infrequently laundered. The body louse lives on the clothing, depositing eggs there, and then travels to the body to feed.

Louse infestation of the pubic area (sometimes called 'the crabs') is usually sexually transmitted. Many patients with this infestation have another sexually transmitted disease, such as gonorrhoea. *P. pubis* prefers the pubic area, but can infest other sites such as the perianal area, thighs and trunk.

Lotions or shampoos of permethrin or other insecticides kill lice and nits, which can then be removed with a fine-tooth comb. Clothes and linen should be dry cleaned or washed in hot water.

Wound Infections

Wound infections result from microbial invasion of severe cutaneous lesions. The common types are listed in Table 16.2. Some people are hospitalised because of wounds (trauma or burns), and many people in hospital suffer wounds from surgery, intravascular catheters or pressure sores, all of which increase their risk of infection. Most wounds contain a serous exudate which, together with any dead tissue, provides an excellent culture medium for bacteria. Organisms that enter the site can colonise it, and sometimes this leads to infection. Since wounds are often colonised, it is sometimes difficult to determine whether an infection exists or not. Inflammation is not always due to infection, but local signs of erythema (redness), pain, oedema, wound odour, and especially a purulent exudate, are suggestive of infection.

SURGICAL WOUND INFECTIONS

Infections of surgical wounds are one of the more common nosocomial infections (see Chapter 13) and are a major cause of morbidity in patients following surgery. About 5–6% of all surgical wounds become infected, but the infection rate varies considerably with the type of surgery, the body site involved, and patient susceptibility.

When an operation has been completed, the wound almost always contains some bacteria. Infection in many cases, therefore, depends on a balance between host resistance and the numbers and virulence of the microbes introduced during surgery. Infection of clean, closed wounds is most likely to be due to organisms introduced during surgery, since in most closed wounds the skin edges are sufficiently sealed within several hours to prevent the entry of microorganisms during postoperative care. However, in situations where skin closure is delayed, microorganisms acquired postoperatively become more important. If surgery involves a site that is normally heavily colonised, such as the colon, the number of organisms which contaminate the wound can be very large, and there is a much greater risk of infection. Thus, in bowel surgery, for example, part of the preoperative preparation may involve the reduction of this microbial load with antimicrobial drugs.

TABLE 16.2
TYPES OF WOUND INFECTIONS AND THE COMMON CAUSATIVE ORGANISMS

TYPE OF WOUND	COMMON CAUSES
Surgical wounds (clean)	*Staphylococcus aureus* Gram-negative enterobacteria
Surgical wounds (dirty)	As above, plus anaerobes and enterococci
Burns	*Pseudomonas aeruginosa* *Staphylococcus aureus* Gram-negative enterobacteria Enterococci
Intravascular catheters	*Staphylococcus aureus* Coagulase negative staphylococci Gram-negative enterobacteria *Corynebacterium jeikeium*
Pressure sores	*Staphylococcus aureus* Group A streptococci Gram-negative enterobacteria Enterococci
Dog/cat bites	*Pasteurella multicoda* *Capnocytophaga canimorsus* Oral anaerobes
Accidental wound (soil or faecal contamination)	Clostridia *Pseudomonas aeruginosa*

The most common causes of postoperative wound infections are bacteria, particularly *Staphylococcus aureus* (including MRSA—multi-resistant *Staphylococcus aureus*), *Escherichia coli* and other Gram-negative enterobacteria, *Pseudomonas aeruginosa,* enterococci and various anaerobes (e.g. *Bacteroides* spp.). However, the common causative agents vary from one hospital setting to another. Most surgical wound infections become apparent within several days of the surgery, and some can be extremely quick, occurring within hours.

Epidemiology of surgical wound infections

Most surgical wound infections are probably acquired at the time of the operation. Possible sources of the organisms include:

- the operating room environment;
- the hands of operating personnel;
- other body parts of operating room personnel; and
- the patient's own body.

Strict environmental control and stringent sterilisation and disinfection practices help to reduce infection, as do preoperative scrubbing with an antiseptic with residual action and the use of surgical gloves. Dermatitis on the hands of surgical personnel increases the risk because of the heavy colonisation of these lesions by bacteria. Other areas of skin of personnel can be important sources of infection. Materials used for gowns and drapes may not be effective barriers for bacteria, especially if they become moist, since microbes on underlying skin may then penetrate the gown and enter the operative field.

The major source of organisms in surgical wound infections is thought to be the patient's own skin and mucosal membranes. These include the patient's normal flora as well as any organisms that the patient may have been colonised with since entering hospital. As explained in Chapter 13, hospital organisms can be resistant to antibiotics, and thus the infections they cause can be difficult to treat.

Factors that increase the risk of surgical wound infection

Whether or not a surgical wound becomes infected depends on (1) the number of microorganisms delivered to the site, (2) the virulence of those organisms, and (3) the health of the person's immune system. A number of factors can influence these critical requirements.

It has been shown that the duration of the patient's preoperative stay in hospital significantly influences the risk of acquiring a surgical wound infection. Infection rates are approximately doubled if the patient spends a week, as opposed to a day, in hospital prior to surgery, and approximately trebled after two weeks. The longer patients are in hospital, the greater the possibility that they will be colonised by pathogenic hospital bacteria.

If the patient already has an infection in another part of the body, there is an increased risk of the wound being infected. When organisms have access to the bloodstream, their spread to the surgical wound site is facilitated.

The duration of the operation is a major risk factor for surgical wound infection. Longer procedures are thought to have a higher risk of wound colonisation because of the length of time the tissues are exposed. Longer procedures also usually involve greater amounts of tissue and more extensive damage.

Other factors that increase the risk of infection are:

- age, due to the waning of the immune system;
- the presence of underlying debilitating disease in the patient, such as diabetes or cancer; and
- obesity, because a large amount of fat tissue can prolong the operation.

Classification of surgical wounds

It is common to classify operations into one of four types. A typical scheme is detailed in Table 16.3. This allows the risk of infection for different types of surgery to be estimated. Actual infection rates can then be assessed.

Preventive measures

Given the usual sources of infecting organisms and the factors that increase the risk of infection, the major measures for preventing surgical wound infections are:

- reducing the preoperative hospitalisation of patients;
- eradication of other infections prior to surgery, where possible;
- appropriate prophylactic use of antimicrobial drugs;
- washing of the skin and the application of antiseptics at the incision site; and
- strict aseptic technique when changing dressings, especially for open wounds.

Laboratory diagnosis

The most common specimen collected for the identification of the cause of surgical wound infection is a swab. The swab should be used to collect as much purulent material as possible from the base of the wound, and transported to the laboratory in transport medium. Where large amounts of pus are present, this should be collected into a syringe and then transferred to an anaerobic transport vial. Where anaerobes are suspected, a tissue specimen should be collected and sent in a sterile container. These procedures are described more fully in Chapter 15. Blood cultures should be collected if the patient is febrile.

Cultures of wound specimens are often difficult to interpret. The main reasons are that pathogenic organisms can simply colonise a wound without causing infection, and that common colonisers (e.g. coagulase negative staphylococci) can sometimes cause infection. Also, mixed infections are common, and pathogens and colonisers may be difficult to differentiate. Poor specimen quality and insufficient clinical information on request forms can add to the problem.

Treatment

Superficial infections rarely require antimicrobial therapy; local measures, including drainage, debridement and irrigation are often adequate. However, antimicrobial drugs are generally used when the infection is extensive or involves deeper tissues, or if the patient has impaired immune defences. In these situations, empirical therapy is usually commenced when the clinical diagnosis is made, and then modified, if necessary, when the sensitivity of the causative agent has been determined. Local measures should accompany this treatment, since pus and necrotic tissue can prevent antimicrobial drugs from reaching the organisms, and can also inactivate the drugs.

BURNS WOUND INFECTIONS

Burns wounds are highly susceptible to infection for a number of reasons. First, they are moist and full of nutrients and necrotic tissue, ideal for microbial growth and proliferation. Second, not only has the skin barrier been lost, but other defences may be impaired. Extensive and deep wounds lead to depressed immune system function, with both humoral and cellular defences affected. There

TABLE 16.3
CLASSIFICATION OF SURGICAL WOUNDS—A TYPICAL SCHEME

CLASSIFICATION	DESCRIPTION
■ Clean	■ No infection encountered ■ Gastrointestinal, respiratory and genital tracts not entered ■ No break in aseptic technique
■ Clean-contaminated	■ Gastrointestinal, respiratory or genital tract entered ■ Minimal spillage of contents
■ Contaminated	■ One of above tracts is entered with significant spillage of contents ■ Or acute inflammation without pus encountered ■ Or surgery involving a minimally contaminated traumatic wound ■ Or a major break in aseptic technique
■ Dirty	■ Pus encountered ■ Or perforated viscus found ■ Or heavily contaminated traumatic wound involved

is evidence that cytotoxic T cell activity can be suppressed, serum immunoglobulin and complement levels may be reduced, and neutrophil activity impaired (see Chapter 9). Even functional defence cells have difficulty in reaching the infection because of the damage to the vascular system. In addition, blood-borne antimicrobial drugs do not readily reach the infection site.

Patients who survive severe burns may suffer fatal infections while in hospital. Infections commonly occur in patients with burns affecting more than 30% of the body surface. The vast majority of burns wounds become infected after the patient is admitted to hospital, and are therefore appropriately regarded as hospital-acquired infections.

The thick crust or scab that forms over a burn is called an **eschar**. Microbes growing in or on the eschar are usually not a problem but, if they multiply and reach sufficiently large numbers to invade beneath the eschar, infection of adjacent tissue occurs. If they then enter the blood vessels, septicaemia, with a potentially high mortality, ensues.

Causative organisms, sources and transmission

Like surgical wounds, burns wounds are generally colonised by bacteria, some of which may cause infection. *Staphylococcus aureus* and a variety of Gram-negative organisms, particularly *Pseudomonas aeruginosa* and enterobacteria, are the most common causes of burn infections. Bacteria are the main cause, but *Candida albicans* and filamentous fungi, such as *Aspergillus* spp., cause a significant number of infections. In a given burns unit, certain organisms tend to predominate, but the predominant types may vary over time.

Patients are a major source of burns wound pathogens. Burns quickly become colonised, and usually contain large numbers of organisms. Burns wounds thus constitute a huge reservoir of microbes for cross-contamination to other patients. Organisms may be transmitted from patients with old burns to new patients by hands, clothing, other fomites and air. The gastrointestinal tracts of patients contain many potential pathogens and may also be important sources of infection, especially in wounds where faecal contamination is likely to occur (e.g. burns involving the groin, buttocks or upper thigh).

Hospital staff can carry pathogens on their hands and are also an important reservoir of organisms in burns infections. In addition, their hands are important vectors for the transmission of microbes from other sources to the wound. Hands of staff may become contaminated directly from contact with a patient, or indirectly from contaminated environmental surfaces. This emphasises the importance of proper handwashing immediately before and after contact with a patient.

Diagnosis and treatment

A wound biopsy is the preferred specimen for the diagnosis of burns wound infection, because a quantitative culture can be performed and histologic evidence of infection (as opposed to colonisation) can be obtained. However, the invasiveness of the technique and the time taken for collection and processing of this specimen means that swabs or excised necrotic tissue are most often collected. Blood cultures should be collected if systemic symptoms are present.

Antimicrobial therapy has only a supportive role in the treatment of infected burns wounds. Debridement or surgical excision of dead tissue is the most important aspect of treatment, and this will also aid in the delivery of antimicrobial drugs to the infected site.

Prevention of burns wound infections

Prevention of burn infections is difficult, even when patients are maintained within specialised hospital burns units. Prevention involves prompt excision of dead tissue, skin graft closure of the wound, good wound care, the use of topical antimicrobials to suppress the multiplication of organisms on the wound surface, and strict environmental control. Environmental control includes strictly enforced handwashing, the use of good barrier nursing techniques, and gowns and gloves, and fastidious sterilisation and disinfection of fomites.

NECROTISING INFECTIONS

Necrotising infections (sometimes called **gangrenous infections**) are infections of the soft tissue below the dermis (the superficial fascia), resulting in extensive tissue necrosis. **Necrotising fasciitis** is the name for the inflammation that develops in this tissue. Necrotising infections usually occur in tissue following trauma, surgery, ischaemia or other causes of tissue damage. These infections progress rapidly and can quickly be fatal without appropriate treatment.

Most necrotising infections are caused by multiple organisms. Since there is often local hypoxia due to the tissue damage, anaerobic bacteria—especially *Bacteroides* spp. or *Peptostreptococcus* spp.—are usually involved, in combination with facultative anaerobes such as streptococci or Gram-negative enterobacteria (e.g. *E. coli*, *Enterobacter*, *Klebsiella* or *Proteus*). However, there are two types of necrotising infections caused by a single bacterial species. Streptococcal gangrene is usually caused by Group A streptococci, while gas gangrene (or clostridial myenonecrosis) is most often caused by *Clostridium*

CASE HISTORY 16.4
GANGRENE

A 78-year-old woman was admitted to hospital with cellulitis of her lower leg. She recalled being jabbed by a thorn in that leg two days earlier when doing some gardening. She was immediately given intravenous antibiotics, but on the next day she complained of severe pain. On examination it was observed that the tissue above her ankle was discoloured, and there were several blisters containing a dark fluid. She was then taken to theatre for surgical debridement of the wound. *Clostridium perfringens* was isolated from a sample of the necrotic tissue excised during surgery.

perfringens or occasionally by other clostridial species such as *C. novyi*, *C. septicum* and *C. bifermentans*.

Gas gangrene can occur within hours of tissue damage or surgery. Spores of clostridia are found in soil and in human and animal faeces, and can be introduced into tissues by accidental puncture wounds, or during surgery if improperly sterilised instruments are used, or faecal contamination of the wound occurs. In tissue that is damaged and hypoxic, the spores germinate and the bacteria multiply rapidly, producing toxins that kill more tissue cells, thereby extending the anaerobic environment in which they can grow. The major toxin, alpha toxin, is a lecithinase which hydrolyses lipids in cell membranes, causing cell lysis and death. This allows the organism to invade deeper into the muscle tissue. As the organisms grow they produce bubbles of gas, which further distort the tissue. This crepitant (rattling) tissue sometimes makes a popping sound when the patient moves, and the bubbles of gas can sometimes be seen in the wound. As the infection progresses, the tissue becomes black and clearly dead. Symptoms include the sudden onset of pain, high fever and shock.

Diagnosis is usually based on clinical findings. Because of the infection's rapid progression and potentially fatal outcome, treatment is commenced before laboratory test results are available. Wide debridement of the affected area is mandatory, and penicillin (or metronidazole) is administered. Amputation of badly infected limbs may sometimes be necessary to prevent the spread of infection. Gas gangrene can be prevented by adequate cleansing and debridement of wounds to remove dead and damaged tissue and by the use of prophylactic antibiotics for surgery when faecal contamination of tissues is likely to occur.

Management of all necrotising infections is based on debridement of devitalised tissue plus appropriate antibiotic therapy as above.

Infections of the Eye

Infections of the eye most often involve the conjunctiva, resulting in inflammation, or **conjunctivitis**. It can occur in people of all ages but is most common in children. There is a wide variety of other causes of conjunctivitis, including the long-term use of eye medications and irritation due to the presence of particulate matter, but the majority have an infectious or allergic basis. Of the infectious causes, bacteria are the most common, followed by viruses. The infection may be confined to the conjunctiva, or may additionally involve the cornea (**keratoconjunctivitis**) or the eyelid (**blepharoconjunctivitis**).

BACTERIAL CONJUNCTIVITIS

Common causative agents

A wide range of bacteria comprise the normal flora of the eye, including *Staphylococcus epidermidis*, *Propionibacterium*, streptococci and corynebacteria. Some of these organisms can cause conjunctivitis, but usually only in the immunocompromised. Bacterial conjunctivitis primarily affects infants and young children. The most common causes of bacterial conjunctivitis are *Haemophilus influenzae*, *Streptococcus pneumoniae*, *Moraxella catarrhalis* and *Staphylococcus aureus*. *H. influenzae* is the most frequent cause in children.

Patients with conjunctivitis usually experience watery eyes due to irritation, a feeling of grittiness in the eyes, a burning or stinging sensation and photophobia. In the early stages there may be a watery discharge, but this usually becomes mucopurulent or purulent. On awakening the eyelids can be stuck together by the discharge. Even without treatment, many patients will recover completely without permanent sequelae. Conjunctivitis is extremely contagious, especially among children, and can spread rapidly through schools and day-care centres. Children rub itchy, running eyes and transfer organisms to their playmates.

Contact lens related conjunctivitis can be caused by *Pseudomonas* or other Gram-negative bacteria, especially in individuals using extended-wear soft lenses.

Neisseria gonorrhoeae infections

In Australia and other developed countries *Neisseria gonorrhoeae* is now an uncommon cause of conjunctivitis. In the past it was recognised as a potentially serious problem in neonates, who usually acquired the infection from their mother during passage through the birth canal. Thus it is an important cause of **ophthalmia neonatorum.** Early in this century, 20–40% of children in European institutions for the blind had suffered from this disease. In underdeveloped countries the disease is still prevalent. The infection is still regarded as a very serious disease, requiring prompt treatment, because it can cause **keratitis** (inflammation of the cornea); this can progress rapidly to ulceration and scarring of the cornea, and even perforation leading to blindness. Perforation can occur within three days of onset of infection.

Nowadays the most common means of transmission is by auto-inoculation from infected genitalia. Penicillin

FIGURE 16.11
TRACHOMA
A conjunctivitis caused by *Chlamydia trachomatis*. Note the follicles on the conjunctival membrane.

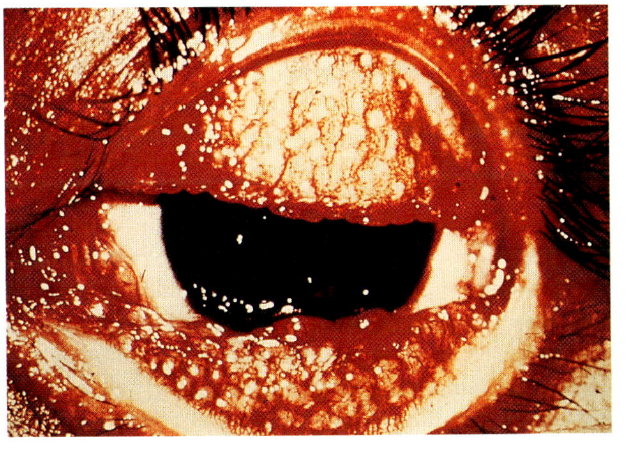

was once the treatment of choice, but resistant strains have developed, and tetracycline is now used. Tetracycline has the advantage of also being effective against chlamydia, which often coexist with *N. gonorrhoeae*. Preventive measures have almost eradicated the disease in developed countries. Formerly, a 1% solution of silver nitrate in the eyes of neonates was used to prevent infection, but this preventive measure has been replaced by the use of antimicrobial drugs such as penicillin, tetracycline or erythromycin.

Chlamydia trachomatis infections

Chlamydia trachomatis serotypes D to K are able to cause conjunctivitis. Patients with chlamydial conjunctivitis often have a concomitant genital infection (see Chapter 21), and thus transmission is usually from genital secretions. Transmission has also been reported to occur from person to person and via unchlorinated swimming pools.

Trachoma (Figure 16.11), from the Greek word meaning 'pebbled' or 'rough', is caused by *Chlamydia trachomatis* serotypes A to C. It is the leading cause of preventable blindness worldwide; it is estimated that 500 million people are infected, and over 20 million are already blind. The disease is widespread in parts of Asia, Africa and South America, in some areas affecting 90% of the population. It is especially prevalent in arid conditions and in communities with poor hygiene. It is still common in some remote Aboriginal communities. Flies are important mechanical vectors, and close mother-child contact facilitates transfer.

Trachoma is a chronic follicular conjunctivitis, with follicles being more prominent on the upper eyelid. In chronic infection, fibrosis may occur, which can cause contraction of the eyelid tissue and a turning under of the eyelashes. The lashes abrade the cornea, leading to blindness.

Laboratory diagnosis and treatment

An accurate diagnosis of bacterial conjunctivitis is best achieved by culture of scrapings of the conjunctival surface. A swab may be used and rolled firmly several times across the conjunctiva to obtain conjunctival cells. A swab of conjunctival exudate does not generally reveal the causative agent because the organisms attach to and invade the epithelial cells. As stated above, many cases of acute bacterial conjunctivitis are self-limiting and antimicrobial therapy is not always required. However, appropriate treatment will shorten the course of infection, relieve patient discomfort, and limit the spread to other individuals. Topically applied antimicrobials, such as chloramphenicol, are the main form of treatment for bacterial conjunctivitis, except for chlamydial infections. Children should not return to school until their infection is cleared.

Laboratory diagnosis of chlamydial infection usually involves microscopic examination of conjunctival scrapings, using a fluorescent antibody to identify the organism. Isolation of the organism by cell culture provides a definitive diagnosis but is a very difficult technique and rarely performed in most laboratories. Commercial DNA probes are available. Treatment is with oral tetracyclines or cotrimoxazole; in chlamydial conjunctivitis, treatment may also need to be provided for the patient's sexual partner, because of possible sexual transmission.

VIRAL CONJUNCTIVITIS

Viruses are the second most common cause of infectious conjunctivitis. Adenoviruses cause the overwhelming majority of these infections, but other viruses such as the herpes simplex virus, varicella zoster virus, enteroviruses, coxsackie viruses and cytomegalovirus can also be involved. Viruses usually cause a follicular conjunctivitis, characterised by smooth, clear, dome-shaped lesions on the conjunctiva.

Adenovirus infections

Epidemic keratoconjunctivitis (EKC) is caused by adenovirus serotypes 8, 19 and 37. After an incubation period of around a week, the conjunctiva become inflamed and painful, followed by foreign body sensation, watery eyes and photophobia. In contrast to bacterial conjunctivitis, the discharge usually remains watery. Within days the infection spreads to the corneal epithelium and sometimes to deeper corneal tissue.

Direct contact with infected individuals or contaminated fomites is the most common form of transmission. EKC has often been transmitted in epidemic form in eye clinics and ophthalmologists' offices via contaminated equipment or hands. Particular care should be taken in washing hands and disinfecting instruments. The virus has been found to be still infectious after two months on unsterilised equipment. The patient should be informed of the extremely contagious nature of this disease.

Another less common disease, caused by adenovirus serotypes 3 and 7, is pharyngoconjunctival fever. This disease mainly affects children less than 10 years of age, and is characterised by pharyngitis, fever and conjunctivitis. This is also a highly contagious, person-to-person contact disease.

There is no effective treatment for adenovirus infections; symptomatic relief is all that can be provided. Infections normally resolve spontaneously within 2–6 weeks.

Herpes simplex conjunctivitis

Ocular herpes infections are most often due to herpes simplex type 1 virus. It can produce a number of different clinical manifestations, the most serious being a keratitis, which can result in severe visual impairment. The peak incidence is in children between the ages of 1 and 10 years, who have not previously been exposed to the virus and lack protective antibodies. Inoculation of the conjunctiva usually results from direct contact with a person who is shedding the virus from skin or mucous membrane lesions, or by self-inoculation from a primary infection elsewhere in the body.

As with other herpes simplex infections, there is the chance of recurrence due to the latency of the virus in a nerve ganglion, and factors that cause suppression of the immune system (e.g. HIV infection) increase the risk of recurrence. Herpes simplex type 2 virus can also cause conjunctivitis and is most commonly associated with congenital and neonatal disease after acquisition from the mother's genital tract.

Treatment of herpes conjunctivitis is with topical antiviral agents, such as idoxuridine or vidarabine.

Diagnosis of viral conjunctivitis

Viral isolation methods are difficult and are generally performed only by specialist virus laboratories. Giemsa staining of conjunctival smears can enable bacterial and viral causes to be distinguished. Polymorphonuclear cells (neutrophils) are prevalent in bacterial infections while lymphocytes are seen with viruses.

OTHER EYE INFECTIONS

As we have seen, **keratitis**, or inflammation of the cornea, can result in permanent damage and vision impairment. Normally, the cornea is quite resistant to infection, but a number of factors such as trauma, contact lens wear, and topical corticosteroid use can predispose to keratitis. Keratitis can be caused by various fungi, viruses and protozoa, but bacteria are the most common cause. A wide variety of bacteria can be involved, including all the common causes of conjunctivitis. *Pseudomonas* spp. and the protozoan *Acanthamoeba* are important causes associated with contact lens use. *Acanthamoeba* is ubiquitous in soil and water (including tap water) and therefore commonly contaminates lens cases and solutions. Corneal thinning and perforation are potential threats of severe infection.

Blepharitis, or inflammation of the eyelid margin, is predominantly caused by *Staphylococcus aureus*. Other possible causes include herpes simplex virus and the crab louse, *Phthirus pubis*. **Endophthalmitis** is an inflammation of the fluid behind the cornea and usually follows intraocular surgery when bacteria are exogenously introduced. **Retinitis**, inflammation of the retina, can occur following congenital infection or in immunocompromised patients. Cytomegalovirus retinitis is one of the more common AIDS-associated infections.

A summary of infections of the eye is presented in Table 16.4.

TABLE 16.4
EYE INFECTIONS

TYPE OF INFECTION	COMMON CAUSES
Bacterial conjunctivitis (inflammation of conjunctiva)	*Haemophilus influenzae* *Streptococcus pneumoniae* *Moraxella catarrhalis* *Staphylococcus aureus*
Trachoma (chronic follicular conjunctivitis)	*Chlamydia trachomatis*
Viral conjunctivitis	Adenovirus Herpes simplex virus types 1 & 2
Keratitis (inflammation of cornea)	All causes of bacterial conjunctivitis *Pseudomonas* spp. Herpes simplex virus *Acanthamoeba*
Blepharitis (inflammation of eyelid margin)	*Staphylococcus aureus*
Endophthalmitis (inflammation of fluid behind cornea)	*Staphylococcus aureus* *Pseudomonas aeruginosa* Enterobacteriaceae
Retinitis (inflammation of retina)	Cytomegalovirus Human immunodeficiency virus
Preseptal cellulitis (cellulitis of eyelid)	*Staphylococcus aureus* Streptococci *Haemophilus influenzae*
Orbital cellulitis (cellulitis of orbit)	*Staphylococcus aureus* Streptococci *Haemophilus influenzae*

Summary

- Except when it is damaged, the skin provides an effective barrier against invasion by most microorganisms.
- The normal flora of the skin includes a variety of aerobic and anaerobic organisms such as staphylococci, micrococci, diphtheroids and propionibacteria.
- The eye also has a number of highly effective defences which generally keep it free of infection.
- The eye has a sparse normal flora, similar in composition to that of the skin.

INFECTIONS OF THE SKIN

- Tissue damage is the most common factor which leads to infection of the skin.
- Severe trauma, such as that due to surgery, puncture wounds or burns, can lead to serious skin infection, often with involvement of underlying soft tissue.
- In some systemic infections (e.g. measles, rubella and chickenpox), a skin rash may be the major manifestation of infection.

BACTERIAL SKIN INFECTIONS

Folliculitis, boils and carbuncles

- *Staphylococcus aureus* is a common cause of skin infections.
- Infection can occur when the organism invades a hair follicle, causing folliculitis (a pimple or pustule).
- When the deeper areas of a hair follicle are affected, a larger, deeper, pus-filled nodule develops, called a furuncle or boil.
- Nasal carriers of virulent *S. aureus* may suffer recurrent boils.
- Boils may discharge to adjacent areas of skin, resulting in multiple abscesses, called a carbuncle.
- Diagnosis is usually made on clinical grounds, but a laboratory confirmation of the causative organism is readily achieved by culture of pus.
- Treatment of these infections usually requires surgical drainage of the lesions.

Impetigo

- Impetigo is a highly infectious, pyogenic (pus-forming) infection caused by staphylococci, streptococci, or both.
- Impetigo occurs predominantly in young children, and minor skin damage is the usual predisposing factor.
- Lesions often start on the face around the nose and may then spread to other sites of the body.
- Laboratory diagnosis is based on culture of a swab of the lesions under the crusts.
- Scalded skin syndrome is caused by strains of *S. aureus* that produce a toxin called exfoliation.

Erysipelas

- Erysipelas is an infection that begins as a small, raised, rubbery lesion, and then develops into a bright red, swollen lesion with a sharply demarcated edge, followed by bullae that rupture and weep.
- Erysipelas is usually caused by Group A streptococci.
- Without treatment the organisms may spread through the lymphatics and cause nephritis, septicaemia, pneumonia and gangrene.
- Diagnosis is usually based on clinical appearance.

Cellulitis

- Cellulitis is an acute bacterial infection of the skin that spreads to subcutaneous tissues. The infected tissue becomes hot, painful, red and swollen.
- Following trauma, streptococci are usually responsible. *Haemophilus influenzae* type b is most likely in young children. *Clostridium perfringens* and other anaerobes can cause cellulitis in poorly oxygenated tissue.
- Culture of aspirates of the leading edge of the lesion or skin biopsy are the usual means of laboratory diagnosis.

Treatment of bacterial skin infections

- Wound drainage and debridement of crusted lesions are often all that is necessary for minor skin infections.
- Impetigo and other streptococcal infections are highly contagious and are usually treated with oral penicillin, or erythromycin.

VIRAL SKIN INFECTIONS

Rubella

- Rubella (German measles) is caused by a togavirus spread mainly by the air-borne route from infected individuals.
- A rash is the main symptom of rubella. The patient is highly contagious for about a week before and a week after the rash appears.
- Congenital rubella syndrome results from infection of a developing foetus when the virus crosses the placenta from the mother's circulation. The most severe damage occurs if the woman is infected in the first trimester.
- The most severe effects of congenital rubella include stillbirth, microcephaly, deafness, eye defects, cardiac abnormalities, hepatomegaly, splenomegaly and pneumonitis.
- Laboratory diagnosis of rubella is by serological testing.
- A live, attenuated rubella vaccine is a component of the MMR (measles-mumps-rubella) vaccine offered to children from 12 months of age. A second immunisation is recommended for girls and boys 10–16 years of age.

Measles

- Measles, or rubeola, is caused by a paramyxovirus.
- Measles is a highly infectious disease, spread mainly by the air-borne route via respiratory secretions of infected people.
- After an incubation period of 9–14 days, typical symptoms are fever, runny nose, dry cough and watery eyes. Usually, a dusky red, maculopapular rash develops.

- Measles encephalitis is the most serious complication of measles infection.
- Measles can be diagnosed serologically by detection of specific IgM antibodies in serum.
- Treatment is limited to alleviating symptoms and dealing with complications.
- Measles vaccine prevents major epidemics and is usually given in the form of the MMR vaccine.
- Measles vaccine should not be used in the immunocompromised or in pregnant women.

Chickenpox and shingles

- The varicella zoster virus (VZV) causes both chickenpox and shingles.
- Chickenpox is a highly infectious disease transmitted by the air-borne route from the respiratory secretions of infected people, or by direct contact with skin lesions.
- The rash in chickenpox comprises different types of lesions, from macules to papules to vesicles and pustules.
- VZV enters sensory nerve endings during primary infection and becomes latent in sensory ganglia. After remaining latent for decades, it can be reactivated to cause shingles.
- In shingles, clusters of painful, vesicular lesions develop; they resemble those of chickenpox, but are usually confined to one side of the body.
- Shingles occurs usually in the elderly and in the immunocompromised.
- The lesions in chickenpox and shingles are highly infectious.
- Diagnosis of chickenpox and shingles is generally based on clinical signs and symptoms.
- Therapy consists of supportive care to relieve itchiness in chickenpox and analgesics to relieve the pain of shingles.
- Acyclovir may be used for shingles, especially in immunocompromised patients.
- Zoster immune globulin may be given to people in whom varicella may be life-threatening and who have been exposed to the virus.

Warts

- Warts are caused by human papillomaviruses (HPV), which specifically attack skin and mucous membranes.
- HPV are transmitted by direct contact or via fomites.
- Genital warts are sexually transmitted.
- Plantar warts occur in the thick skin on the soles of the feet, level with the skin surface, but with deeper underlying growth.
- Dermal warts usually regress spontaneously, presumably when the immune system gains control.
- There appears to be an association of some HPV, particularly serotypes 16 and 18, with cervical cancer.
- Diagnosis is based on clinical observation.
- Warts can be removed by local freezing of the tissue with liquid nitrogen or by curetting, cautery or laser. Topical treatments include podophyllin and salicylic acid. Recurrences after treatment are common.

Herpes simplex

- Primary infection with herpes simplex type 1 virus usually involves the skin around the mouth or nose.
- Herpes simplex type 2 virus predominantly involves the genitalia.
- Most primary infections are minor but may be severe in the immunocompromised.
- Herpes skin lesions (cold sores) usually begin as areas of tender erythema, followed by the development of closely grouped vesicles which ultimately progress through pustular and crusting stages. Large amounts of virus are present in the lesions.
- During primary infection, herpes viruses enter sensory nerve endings and travel to the sensory ganglion, where they remain latent.
- The virus can be reactivated by many stimuli; it then travels back down the same sensory nerves to cause lesions at the same site.
- Treatment with saline bathing, peroxide or other astringents may help. In the immunocompromised, treatment is usually with acyclovir.

Molluscum contagiosum

- Molluscum contagiosum is a common viral infection caused by pox viruses.
- It is transmitted from person to person by direct contact, or indirectly.
- The infection is characterised by clusters of small, flesh-coloured papular lesions scattered over the skin.
- Diagnosis is made by the clinical appearance or by electron microscopic examination of biopsy material.
- Spontaneous resolution usually occurs within 6–9 months, but therapy is desirable to prevent spread of infection. Treatment is best achieved by superficial curettage.

FUNGAL SKIN INFECTIONS

Tinea (ringworm)

- The fungi that infect keratinised tissue, causing tinea (ringworm), are called dermatophytes.
- Fungal skin infections are called dermatomycoses and can be caused by any one of several organisms from three genera: *Epidermophyton*, *Microsporum* and *Trichophyton*.
- Tinea is spread by contact with arthrospores of the fungi.
- The characteristic lesion of tinea is an annular, scaling patch of dry skin with a red, raised margin.
- In tinea pedis, or athlete's foot, infection usually starts between the toes as a result of maceration from sweating and occlusive footwear.
- Tinea corporis is characterised by one or more annular, scaly lesions, often on the trunk.
- Tinea cruris occurs in skin folds in the pubic region.
- Tinea capitis (tinea of the scalp) is most common in children.

- Laboratory diagnosis of tinea is made by direct microscopic examination of skin scrapings or nail or hair clippings.
- Treatment generally involves the use of a topical, antifungal cream, powder or ointment and/or a keratolytic agent such as Whitfield's ointment.
- If lesions are widespread or involve nails or hair, oral griseofulvin or ketoconazole is used.

Candidiasis

- *Candida albicans*, a yeast, is present among the normal flora of the digestive, respiratory and urogenital tracts of humans. It can cause candidiasis in a number of body sites.
- Superficial infection of mucous membranes appears as thrush—milky-white patches of inflammation on mucous membranes.
- *Candida* skin infections generally occur in areas of warmth, moisture and maceration; they are characterised by areas of moist erythema with an irregular, soft, white edge.
- *Candida albicans* is an opportunistic pathogen, usually requiring some predisposing factor in order to cause infection.
- Diagnosis is usually based on clinical examination. A laboratory diagnosis is made by microscopy and culture of a swab of the lesion.
- Treatment usually involves the use of antifungal antibiotic creams or ointments, such as nystatin or imidazole.

Tinea versicolor (pityriasis versicolor)

- This is a common superficial infection caused by the yeast *Malassezia furfur*. The trunk is most often affected.
- The lesions are small, sharply demarcated, scaling macules; on white skin the lesions are dark, and on dark skin they are lighter.
- Treatment consists of topical applications of selenium sulphide shampoos or imidazole antifungal agents.

ARTHROPOD INFESTATIONS

Scabies

- Scabies is caused by the mite *Sarcoptes scabiei* var. *hominis*.
- The female scabies mite burrows in the epidermis, laying eggs; the typical scabies lesion is the burrow.
- Itchiness, representing a sensitisation to mites, is severe, and is often worse at night.
- Secondary infection of the lesions by streptococci or staphylococci is a common complication.
- Norwegian (crusted) scabies is characterised by formation of thick crusts on the face, scalp, hands, feet and pressure-bearing areas.
- In Norwegian scabies the host may be harbouring thousands of mites, and their epithelial debris may be highly infectious.
- The mites are spread by close personal contact.
- Outbreaks can occur in hospitals and nursing homes.
- Diagnosis is based on clinical examination and microscopic demonstration of mites or eggs in a skin burrow.
- A number of scabicides, such as permethrin, provide effective treatment.

Pediculosis

- Three species of lice infest different sites: *Pediculus humanus capitis* (head louse), *Pediculus humanus corporis* (body louse) and *Phthirus pubis* (crab louse).
- The major symptoms of pediculosis are itching and a maculopapular rash.
- Head lice infestation primarily affects young schoolchildren. The head louse lays eggs (called nits) at the base of hairs.
- Body lice infestation is generally related to poor hygiene.
- Louse infestation of the pubic area is usually sexually transmitted.
- Lotions or shampoos of permethrin or other insecticides kill lice and nits.

WOUND INFECTIONS

- Most wounds contain a serous exudate which, together with any dead tissue, provides an excellent culture medium for bacteria.
- Since wounds are often colonised, it is sometimes difficult to determine whether an infection exists or not.
- Local signs of erythema, pain, oedema, wound odour, and especially a purulent exudate, are suggestive of infection.

SURGICAL WOUND INFECTIONS

- Infections of surgical wounds are one of the more common nosocomial infections. About 5–6% of all surgical wounds become infected.
- Infection of clean, closed wounds is most likely to be due to organisms introduced during surgery.
- In situations where skin closure is delayed, microorganisms acquired postoperatively become important.
- When surgery involves a site that is normally heavily colonised, the number of organisms contaminating the wound can be very large.
- The most common causes of postoperative wound infections are *Staphylococcus aureus*, *Escherichia coli*, other Gram-negative bacteria and various anaerobes.

Epidemiology of surgical wound infections

- Most surgical wound infections are probably acquired at the time of the operation.
- Dermatitis on the hands of surgical personnel increases the risk because of the heavy colonisation of these lesions by bacteria.
- The major source of organisms in surgical wound infections is thought to be the patient's own skin and mucosal membranes.

Factors that increase the risk of surgical wound infection

- Whether or not a surgical wound becomes infected depends on the number of microorganisms delivered to the site, the virulence of those organisms, and the health of the patient's immune system.
- The longer patients are in hospital preoperation, the greater their risk of acquiring a surgical wound infection.
- If the patient already has an infection in another part of the body, there is an increased risk of the wound being infected.
- Longer surgical procedures have a higher risk of wound colonisation.
- Other factors that increase the risk of infection are age, underlying debilitating disease and obesity.

Classification of surgical wounds

- It is common to classify operations into types to allow the risk of infection from surgery to be estimated.

Preventive measures

- The main ways of preventing surgical wound infections are (1) reducing preoperative hospitalisation, (2) eradicating other infections before surgery, (3) appropriate prophylactic use of antimicrobial drugs, (4) washing the skin and applying antiseptics at the incision site, and (5) strict aseptic technique when changing dressings.

Laboratory diagnosis

- A swab should be used to collect as much purulent material as possible and should be transported to the laboratory in transport medium.
- Where possible, large amounts of pus should be collected into a syringe and then transferred in an anaerobic transport vial.
- Blood cultures should be collected if the patient is febrile.

Treatment

- For superficial infections, drainage, debridement and irrigation are often adequate.
- Antimicrobial drugs are used in addition to these local measures when the infection is extensive or involves deeper tissues, or if the patient has impaired immune defences.

BURNS WOUND INFECTIONS

- Burns wounds are highly susceptible to infection. Most become infected after the patient is admitted to hospital.

Causative organisms, sources and transmission

- Burns wounds are generally colonised by bacteria, some of which may cause infection.
- *Staphylococcus aureus* and a variety of Gram-negative organisms are the most common causes of burn infections.
- Burns wounds constitute a huge reservoir of microbes for cross-contamination to other patients.
- Hospital staff can carry pathogens on their hands and are also an important reservoir of organisms in burns infections.

Diagnosis and treatment

- Swabs or excised necrotic tissue are the specimens most often collected for the diagnosis of burns wound infections, although wound biopsy is the preferred specimen.
- Blood cultures should be collected if systemic symptoms are present.
- Debridement or surgical excision of dead tissue is the most necessary aspect of treatment.

Prevention of burns wound infections

- Prevention involves prompt excision of dead tissue, skin graft closure of the wound, good wound care, the use of topical antimicrobials and strict environmental control.

NECROTISING INFECTIONS

- Necrotising infections are infections of the soft tissue below the dermis. They usually occur following trauma, surgery, ischaemia or other damage.
- Most necrotising infections are caused by multiple organisms, especially anaerobic bacteria in combination with facultative anaerobes.
- The two types of necrotising infections are caused by a single bacterial species: streptococcal gangrene, caused by Group A streptococci; and gas gangrene, caused by *Clostridium perfringens*.
- The alpha toxin of *C. perfringens* hydrolyses lipids in cell membranes, causing cell lysis and death. As the infection progresses, the tissue becomes black.
- Management of all necrotising infections is based on debridement of devitalised tissue plus appropriate antibiotic therapy.

INFECTIONS OF THE EYE

- Infections of the eye most often involve the conjunctiva, resulting in conjunctivitis.
- There are many causes of conjunctivitis, but most have an infectious or allergic basis.
- The infection may be confined to the conjunctiva, or may involve the cornea (keratoconjunctivitis) or the eyelid (blepharoconjunctivitis).

BACTERIAL CONJUNCTIVITIS

Common causative agents

- Bacterial conjunctivitis primarily affects young children.
- The most common causes of bacterial conjunctivitis are *Haemophilus influenzae*, *Streptococcus pneumoniae*, *Moraxella catarrhalis* and *Staphylococcus aureus*.
- Patients with conjunctivitis usually experience watery eyes, a feeling of grittiness in the eyes, a burning or stinging sensation and photophobia.
- Conjunctivitis is extremely contagious and can spread rapidly through schools and day-care centres.

Neisseria gonorrhoeae infections

- *Neisseria gonorrhoeae* conjunctivitis can be acquired by babies during passage through the birth canal. It is an important cause of ophthalmia neonatorum.
- The infection can cause keratitis, and ulceration and scarring of the cornea, leading to blindness.
- Tetracycline is the treatment of choice.

Chlamydia trachomatis infections

- Chlamydia trachomatis serotypes D to K cause conjunctivitis.
- Patients with chlamydial conjunctivitis often have a concomitant genital infection.
- Trachoma, caused by *Chlamydia trachomatis* serotypes A to C, is the leading cause of preventable blindness worldwide.
- Trachoma is a chronic follicular conjunctivitis.

Laboratory diagnosis and treatment

- An accurate diagnosis of bacterial conjunctivitis is best achieved by culture of scrapings of the conjunctival surface.
- Topically applied antimicrobials, such as chloramphenicol, are the main form of treatment for bacterial conjunctivitis, except for chlamydial infections.
- Laboratory diagnosis of chlamydial infection involves microscopic examination of conjunctival scrapings.
- Treatment of chlamydial infections is with oral tetracyclines or cotrimoxazole.

VIRAL CONJUNCTIVITIS

- Adenoviruses cause most viral conjunctival infections.
- Viruses usually cause a follicular conjunctivitis, characterised by smooth, clear, dome-shaped lesions on the conjunctiva.

Adenovirus infections

- Epidemic keratoconjunctivitis (EKC) is caused by adenovirus serotypes 8, 19 and 37.
- In EKC the conjunctiva become inflamed and painful, followed by foreign body sensation, watery eyes and photophobia.
- Direct contact with infected individuals or contaminated fomites is the most common form of transmission of EKC.
- The patient should be informed of the extremely contagious nature of this disease.
- Pharyngoconjunctival fever is a highly contagious disease caused by adenovirus serotypes 3 and 7.
- Symptomatic relief is all that can be provided. Infections normally resolve spontaneously in 2–6 weeks.

Herpes simplex conjunctivitis

- Ocular herpes infections are most often due to herpes simplex type 1 virus.
- Eye infection with herpes simplex can produce a number of different clinical manifestations, the most serious being a keratitis.
- Inoculation of the conjunctiva usually results from direct contact with a person who is shedding the virus or by auto-inoculation.
- Recurrent infections are possible because of the latency of the virus in a nerve ganglion.
- Treatment of herpes conjunctivitis is with topical antiviral agents.

Diagnosis of viral conjunctivitis

- Giemsa staining of conjunctival smears can enable bacterial and viral causes to be distinguished.

OTHER EYE INFECTIONS

- Factors such as trauma, contact lens wear, and topical corticosteroid use can predispose to keratitis.
- Keratitis can be caused by fungi, viruses and protozoa, but bacteria are the most common cause.
- *Pseudomonas* spp. and the protozoan *Acanthamoeba* are important causes of keratitis associated with contact lens use.
- Corneal thinning and perforation are potential threats of severe infection.
- Blepharitis (inflammation of the eyelid margin) is caused mainly by *Staphylococcus aureus*.
- Endophthalmitis is an inflammation of the fluid behind the cornea and usually follows intra-ocular surgery.
- Retinitis, inflammation of the retina, can occur following congenital infection or in immunocompromised patients.

Study Questions

1. What are the characteristics of skin that make it such an effective barrier against infection?
2. What defences does the eye have to protect it from infection?
3. Name the common causes and describe briefly the clinical features of (a) a boil, (b) a carbuncle, (c) impetigo, (d) erysipelas and (e) cellulitis.
4. What are the important infection control considerations for patients with impetigo or erysipelas?
5. Why is the spread of rubella difficult to control in an outbreak?
6. What is the congenital rubella syndrome?
7. How is rubella prevented?
8. What serious complication can result from measles infection?
9. Why do outbreaks of measles infection still occur in Australia despite the availability of an effective vaccine?
10. What are the contraindications for the use of measles vaccine? Explain.
11. What infections are caused by the varicella zoster virus?
12. Explain the implications of latency of the varicella zoster virus.
13. What are the causative agents of warts and what is their link with cancer?
14. What are the common sites of infection of the herpes simplex 1 and 2 viruses?
15. How does the herpes simplex 1 virus cause recurrent infections?
16. What is a dermatomycosis and what are the causative organisms?
17. How is tinea diagnosed?
18. What is thrush, and what are the common predisposing factors for this infection?
19. What is scabies?
20. Why is Norwegian scabies potentially very contagious?
21. What is pediculosis and how is it transmitted?
22. Why are wounds so readily colonised by microorganisms?
23. What are the signs that indicate a wound is infected?
24. List the factors that can increase the risk of surgical wound infection.
25. List the procedures that are implemented to prevent infection of surgical wounds.
26. How should pus be collected and transported to the laboratory for diagnosis of wound infection?
27. How are wound infections treated?
28. What are the common causes of burns wound infections and what are their usual sources?
29. What specimens are appropriately collected for the laboratory diagnosis of infected burns?
30. List the procedures that help to prevent infection of burns wounds.
31. What are necrotising infections?
32. What pathogenic mechanisms are utilised by *Clostridium perfringens* to cause gas gangrene?
33. What is conjunctivitis and what are the common causes?
34. What is ophthalmia neonatorum?
35. What is trachoma and what causes this infection?
36. What specimens are appropriate for the laboratory diagnosis of conjunctivitis?
37. What is epidemic keratoconjunctivitis and how is it transmitted?
38. Define the terms: keratitis, blepharitis, endophthalmitis and retinitis.

Test Your Understanding

Case History 16.1: Cellulitis

1. What is the most likely reason for this girl developing cellulitis?
2. What specimen(s) should be collected in this case?
3. What important infection control considerations are there in this case?

Case History 16.2: Congenital rubella

1. What does this case indicate about the effectiveness of the rubella vaccine?
2. Why was the woman not vaccinated once she was found to be antibody negative?
3. How could the doctor's diagnosis of congenital rubella be confirmed?
4. Why are the effects of infection so severe in this infant?

Case History 16.3: Measles

1. What does this case suggest about the efficacy of the measles vaccine?
2. There are a number of possible biases in this study that should be noted. What are they?
3. What does this case indicate about the transmissibility of measles?
4. It is thought that a vaccination rate of at least 90% is required to provide herd immunity. What does this mean?

Case History 16.4: Gangrene

1. What are the possible reasons for failure of the initial therapy with antimicrobial drugs?
2. What are the possible sources of the clostridia in this case?
3. How could a simple wound caused by a thorn lead to this potentially serious infection?

FURTHER READING

Andrew, J. & D. Grando, 1992, Clinical Microbiology Update Programme, *No. 33 Laboratory Diagnosis of Eye Infection*, Sydney: University of New South Wales. (A comprehensive description of eye infections with an emphasis on their diagnosis.)

Collignon, P., R. Munro & W. Pryor, 1993, Clinical Microbiology Update Programme, *No. 37 Laboratory Diagnosis of Wound and Soft Tissue Infections*, Sydney: University of New South Wales. (A comprehensive discussion of the nature of wound infections and their diagnosis.)

Hogan, D.J., L. Schachner & C. Tanglertsampan, 1991, 'Diagnosis and treatment of childhood scabies and pediculosis', *Pediatric Dermatology* 38(4), p. 941. (Describes the epidemiology, pathogenesis and treatment of scabies and pediculosis.)

Jackson, W.B., 1993, 'Differentiating conjunctivitis of diverse origins', *Survey of Ophthalmology* 38 (suppl.), p. 91. (Describes the causes, pathogenesis and nature of both infectious and allergic conjunctivitis.)

Meers, P., W. Jacobsen and M. McPherson, *Hospital Infection Control for Nurses,* London: Chapman & Hall, 1992. (Has a section on wound infections and their prevention in hospitals.)

Sippe, J.R.A., 1991, 'Common skin infections' *Australian Family Physician* 20(6), p. 783. (Describes the skin infections that are commonly seen in general practice.)

chapter 17

respiratory tract infections

Chapter focus

- *What are the main factors that predispose people to respiratory tract infections?*
- *What are the major types of upper respiratory tract infections and what are their common causes?*
- *How are upper respiratory tract infections diagnosed and treated?*
- *What are the major types of lower respiratory tract infections and what are their common causes?*
- *How are lower respiratory tract infections diagnosed and treated?*
- *What microoranisms cause chronic infection of the lower respiratory tract?*
- *How are chronic infections of the lower respiratory tract diagnosed and treated?*

Each day thousands of litres of air pass into and out of the respiratory tract of an adult. This air can contain thousands of microorganisms per cubic metre. Given the numbers of microbes present in the air we breathe, it is not surprising that respiratory infections are among the most common that afflict humans. Most of the microbes in air are harmless, but the respiratory tract is nevetheless a major route of entry into the body of potentially pathogenic microorganisms.

Respiratory pathogens may be expelled in enormous numbers as a result of coughing or sneezing. In addition, a number of potentially pathogenic microbes form part of the normal flora of the upper respiratory tract (see Table 17.1). These microbes are continually suppressed by other normal flora organisms, but can cause infection when the host becomes more susceptible, or when they are transferred to another individual who is immunocompromised in some way. Most pathogens that enter the body via the respiratory tract infect only the respiratory tract, but the respiratory system is also a route of entry for some organisms that infect other parts of the body, such as measles, mumps and rubella viruses.

In order to resist the constant threat of microbial invasion, the respiratory system has a number of important defence mechanisms for preventing organisms infecting the upper parts of the tract, and reaching and infecting the lower regions. These defences (summarised in Table 17.2) are responsible for keeping the lungs free of microorganisms and other foreign particles. The importance of these defences is clearly illustrated in individuals who have a defect in one or more of these mechanisms, or in whom some defences are bypassed, for example, by an endotracheal tube. The incidence of respiratory infection in such people is greatly increased.

A number of factors predispose people to respiratory infections. The most important are:

- *Young age.* Young children are much more susceptible because their immune system is not fully developed, and because their narrower airways are more easily obstructed.
- *Old age.* Pulmonary defences in the elderly are compromised by (1) reduced effectiveness of the cough reflex, due to loss of elastic recoil in the lung and reduced respiratory muscle strength, (2) a waning immune system, (3) other chronic diseases and their treatments, and (4) declining mobility.
- *Cigarette smoking.* Smoking inhibits ciliary action in the respiratory tract, increasing the risk of infection as well as its severity.
- *Chronic obstructive pulmonary disease (COPD).* The major types of COPD are asthma, chronic bronchitis and emphysema. Cystic fibrosis and bronchiectasis are less common, but nevertheless important, forms. Lower respiratory infection is a common complication of COPD, due to reduced mucociliary clearance,

TABLE 17.1
NORMAL FLORA OF THE UPPER RESPIRATORY TRACT

Commonly present	Viridans streptococci *Neisseria* spp. *Moraxella catarrhalis** *Branhamella* spp. *Staphylococcus aureus** *Staphylococcus epidermidis* Corynebacteria (avirulent strains) *Bacteroides* spp.* *Vellionella* spp. *Candida albicans** *Streptococcus mutans* *Haemophilus influenzae** *Candida albicans*
Occasionally present	*Streptococcus pyogenes** *Streptococcus pneumoniae** *Neisseria meningitidis* *Corynebacterium diphtheriae** *Klebsiella pneumoniae** *Pseudomonas* spp.* *Escherichia coli**

* Potentially pathogenic in the respiratory tract.

TABLE 17.2
DEFENCES OF THE RESPIRATORY SYSTEM

DEFENCE MECHANISM	ACTION
Normal flora of upper respiratory tract	Inhibit the establishment of potential pathogens by blocking their adherence to the mucosal surface
Nasal hairs	Trap large particles in air
Mucus secretions	Trap particles in air and prevent organisms attaching to tissue surface
Ciliated epithelium lining the larynx, trachea and bronchi	Moves mucus and particles trapped in it upwards away from the lungs, to be swallowed or expelled Together with mucus it is termed the **mucociliary escalator**
Non-specific antimicrobial substances in secretions (e.g. lysozyme, lactoferrin)	Destroy microbes or prevent their establishment in the respiratory tract
Secretory IgA antibodies	Present in secretions protecting against a variety of pathogens
Cough and sneeze reflexes	Expel large particles and purulent or excessive secretions from central airways and the larynx
Alveolar macrophages	Phagocytosis of foreign materials and microbes that reach the lungs
Tonsils and lymph nodes	Line the respiratory tract and provide specific humoral and cellular immunity against organisms that enter the tissues

diminished effectiveness of cough reflex because of reduced air flow and respiratory muscle fatigue, the effects of cigarette smoking or other factors.

- *Poor living standards*. Low socioeconomic standards, including pre-existing illness, poor health care facilities and crowded living conditions, are major factors. Thus, chronic upper respiratory disease is almost universal in the children of many rural Aboriginal communities. This, and the higher incidence of bacterial pneumonia in these groups, contributes to the high prevalence of chronic airway disease seen in adults.
- *Alcoholism*. Alcohol intoxication and liver disease interfere with virtually all respiratory tract defences, including cough reflex, ciliary motility, glottic reflex, and alveolar macrophage and NK cell activity.
- *Immunosuppression*. Immunosuppression can predispose a person to unusual and severe infections, the prime example being pneumocystosis (caused by *Pneumocystis carinii*) in people with AIDS. This organism is ubiquitous in nature, but rarely causes infection in immunocompetent individuals.
- *Cancer*. Pneumonia is one of the common causes of death in patients with malignancy. Respiratory tract defences may be compromised by the malignancy itself, by associated chronic diseases, or as a result of cancer treatments that cause immunosuppression.

Acute respiratory infections are major causes of illness throughout the world. They are the most common form of illness in developed countries, the most common cause for consultation of general practitioners, and a major reason for hospital admission of children. Although the respiratory system is a continuous tract from the mouth and nose to the lungs, it is convenient to consider it in two parts: the upper respiratory tract and the lower respiratory tract (see Figure 17.1).

In this chapter, we consider first infections of the upper respiratory tract. This region is colonised by normal flora organisms and infections there are generally not life-threatening (although, as will be shown, there are exceptions). In contrast, the lower respiratory tract, especially the lungs, is normally free of microorganisms, and infections there are often serious. Pneumonia, especially in infants and the elderly, is one of the leading causes of death worldwide, and is still responsible for a large number of deaths in developed countries. While the incidence of upper respiratory tract infections is similar throughout the world, the incidence of lower respiratory infections, especially pneumonia, is more than 10 times greater in undeveloped regions of the world than in industrialised countries.

Most acute respiratory infections are caused by viruses, but the more severe diseases are generally caused by bacteria. Fungi and protozoa are important causes of pneumonia, but tend to be restricted mainly to immuno-compromised people. The main reservoirs of respiratory pathogens are people with infections, although for some lower respiratory infections the source may be the normal flora of the upper respiratory tract. Respiratory infections

FIGURE 17.1
SITES OF INFECTION IN THE RESPIRATORY TRACT

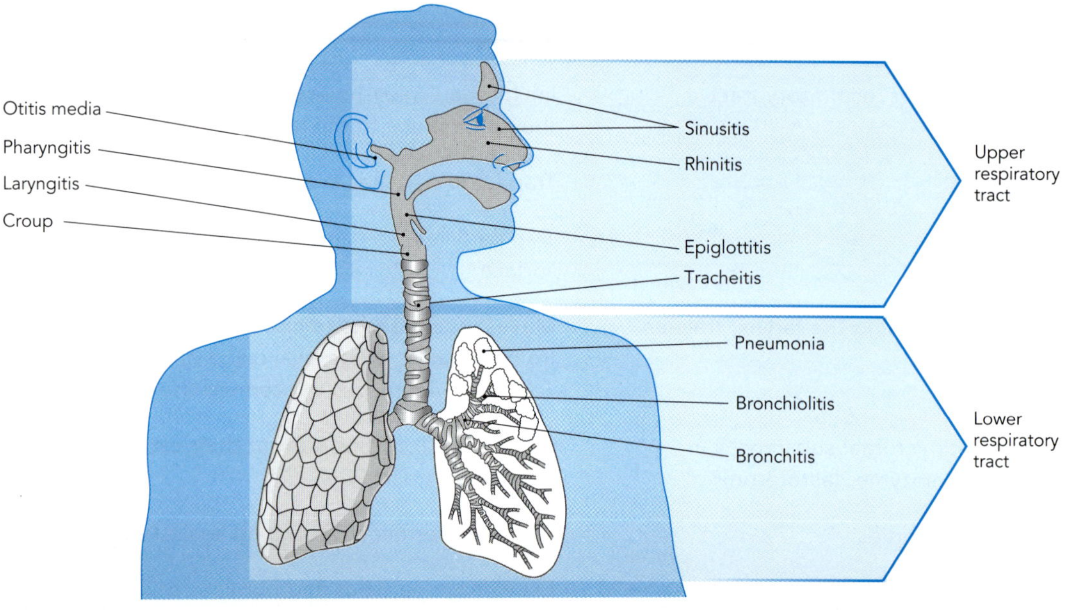

are spread mainly via the air-borne route through coughing and sneezing. In addition, some organisms can be readily transferred from the eyes and nose of infected people by hands or on contaminated fomites. A few diseases, such as Q fever and ornithosis, are acquired from animals. In the case of legionellosis, environmental sources are responsible (see pp. 385–386).

Upper Respiratory Tract Infections

The upper respiratory tract consists of the nose, throat (pharynx), sinuses, eustachian (auditory) tubes and middle ear. They are all closely interconnected, enabling infection to spread readily from one site to another. Generally, the epiglottis, larynx and trachea are also considered to be part of the upper respiratory tract. The majority of upper respiratory infections are due to viruses, and most are self-limiting, mild infections, especially in adults. The infections of the upper respiratory tract are summarised in Table 17.3.

THE COMMON COLD

The common cold is a normally mild and brief illness, lasting less than a week. It involves mainly infection and inflammation of the nasal passages (called **rhinitis** or **coryza**) and the oropharynx (**pharyngitis**). There are a variety of causes, but rhinoviruses are the most common, followed by coronaviruses (see Table 17.4). Other causes include picornaviruses, myxoviruses, adenoviruses, paramyxoviruses and many other viruses. Rhinoviruses have great antigenic diversity, with over 100 serotypes found. The large number of colds that people, especially children, can suffer is due largely to the fact that infection with one serotype of the virus does not confer protection against another. In addition, immunity to rhinoviruses appears to wane with time. Coronaviruses also show marked antigenic variation. Despite this, immunity to cold viruses does appear to accumulate, since colds occur most frequently in childhood and progressively less often in adulthood.

Colds generally occur more frequently in colder weather, but the exact reason for this is not known. The most likely explanations appear to be that closer, indoor contact in winter promotes transmission, or that people may, for some as yet unknown reason, be more susceptible in winter.

A cold is characterised by a blocked or runny nose with excessive nasal discharge and sneezing. A sore throat, headache and cough may also occur. Infected humans are the only known reservoir of cold viruses, and their nasal secretions contain large numbers of virus particles. It has long been assumed that cold viruses are transmitted by coughing and sneezing, but it is now recognised they are also readily transmitted by hands and objects (e.g. door knobs, money, telephones) that have become contaminated with nasal secretions. Touching of the nose or eyes with contaminated fingers enables the viruses to enter the body.

Rhinoviruses first attach to specific receptors on respiratory epithelial cells, invade the cells, and then spread to adjacent epithelial cells. They cause little damage to the epithelium, but induce excessive mucus production and the other symptoms of colds by stimulating the release and local action of inflammatory mediators such as bradykinin. Coronaviruses have a similar effect on respiratory epithelium, although they can cause some damage to the cells lining the nose and trachea. Apart from discomfort, most colds are mild and resolve within a week. Secondary bacterial infection of the paranasal sinuses and middle ear are possible complications of a cold when the sinuses or middle ear become blocked by the inflammatory exudate. Other possible complications are the exacerbation of chronic bronchitis or asthma.

TABLE 17.3
COMMON INFECTIONS OF THE UPPER RESPIRATORY TRACT

DISEASE	CAUSATIVE AGENT(S)	MODES OF TRANSMISSION
Common cold	Rhinoviruses, coronaviruses, adenoviruses, plus other viruses	Respiratory secretions—air-borne, via fomites
Otitis media	*Streptococcus pneumoniae, Haemophilus influenzae, Moraxella catarrhalis, Proteus* spp., *Pseudomonas aeruginosa,* viruses (?)	Direct, as a complication of other upper respiratory infections
Acute sinusitis	As for otitis media	As for otitis media
Pharyngitis and tonsillitis	Adenoviruses, E-B virus, rhinoviruses, other viruses, *Streptococcus pyogenes*	Respiratory secretions
	Neisseria gonorrhoeae	Genital secretions
	Candida albicans	Part of normal flora, after antibiotic therapy or immunosuppression
Diphtheria	*Corynebacterium diphtheriae*	Respiratory secretions—cases and carriers
Acute epiglottitis	*Haemophilus influenzae*	Respiratory secretions—cases and carriers
Laryngotracheitis (croup)	Parainfluenza viruses, respiratory syncytial virus, influenza virus	Respiratory secretions

TABLE 17.4
CAUSES OF THE COMMON COLD

VIRUS	TYPES INVOLVED
■ Rhinovirus	More than 100 serotypes
■ Coronavirus	Several types
■ Parainfluenza virus	Types 1–4
■ Respiratory syncytial virus	One type
■ Influenza virus	Several types
■ Adenovirus	Up to 10 types
■ Other viruses	Many

The common cold is usually diagnosed by clinical findings alone. Because the illness is generally mild and self-limiting with no effective treatment, laboratory tests are usually not performed. Treatment with decongestants and analgesics may help to reduce symptoms, but antibiotic therapy for colds represents a misuse of these drugs, unless secondary bacterial infection is present. There is no effective vaccine for the prevention of colds, essentially because of the large number of possible causes, and the serologic diversity of the major causes, the rhinoviruses.

MIDDLE EAR INFECTIONS

Infections involving the middle ear are called **otitis media**. They occur most often in infants and small children. It is thought that the diameter and shape of the eustachian tube in young children gives nasopharyngeal bacteria greater access to the middle ear. Blockage of the eustachian tube due to viral respiratory infection or allergy may interfere with normal mucociliary expulsion of upper respiratory bacteria. The resultant proliferation of bacteria then causes further inflammation and blockage. Many children have only occasional episodes of otitis media, but some can have recurrent and severe disease.

Otitis media can be caused by almost any bacterium present in the upper respiratory tract, but *S. pneumoniae* and *H. influenzae* are the most common causes in all age groups, followed by *Moraxella catarrhalis*. Viruses are also thought to be possible causes. Chronic middle ear infections tend to be caused by organisms such as *Pseudomonas aeruginosa* and *Proteus* spp., as well as *S. pneumoniae*. Otitis media can also be associated with swimming in contaminated water and with head trauma.

Some cases of otitis media are asymptomatic, but usually earache and fever are present. The ear-drum becomes inflamed and swollen due to increased pressure in the middle ear. If untreated, perforation of the ear-drum may occur. In some children, non-specific symptoms of fever, diarrhoea and vomiting occur. Laboratory diagnosis is not usually performed because of the pain associated with middle ear aspiration and because the infection is usually successfully treated empirically with antibiotics such as amoxicillin or penicillin. Nasal administration of a vasoconstrictor, such as ephedrine, may also be used to reduce congestion.

Even with appropriate therapy, fluid can persist in the middle ear (called 'glue ear'), impairing hearing for weeks or even months. Perforation of the ear-drum may also lead to later problems with hearing. Impaired hearing has often led to children being wrongly labelled as inattentive or disobedient, and can lead to poor speech development.

ACUTE SINUSITIS

The major causes of acute sinusitis are *S. pneumoniae* and *H. influenzae*. Viruses or environmental allergens or pollutants probably play a role in many cases of sinusitis by inducing inflammation and increased mucus production and congestion of the nasopharyngeal mucosa. Clinical features include facial pain, due to pressure caused by blockage and fluid accumulation in sinuses, a nasal discharge that is often purulent, and headache. It may be possible to identify the causative bacteria by microscopy and culture of pus aspirated from the sinus, but sinus puncture is not often carried out. The patient is usually treated empirically with ampicillin or amoxycillin, plus an analgaesic for the pain, and a nasal vasoconstrictor to reduce congestion.

PHARYNGITIS AND TONSILLITIS

Cause, pathogenesis and clinical features

Pharyngitis, or an inflamed, sore throat, is a common condition that can be caused by many different organisms, although viruses are the usual causes (see Table 17.3). When the tonsils are affected, it is called a **tonsillitis**. A sore throat may be due to infection restricted to the throat, or may be one of the early symptoms of a cold, influenza or certain systemic infections. Apart from a sore throat (especially when swallowing), the patient may have a fever, chills, enlarged lymph nodes in the neck, and a headache. Otitis media and sinusitis are possible complications.

Adenoviruses are particularly common causes of sore throat, and may infect the conjunctiva as well, causing what is known as pharyngo-conjunctival fever. Epstein-Barr (EB) virus causes a pharyngitis as part of the syndrome called infectious mononucleosis, or glandular fever (see Chapter 19). Other viral causes include rhinoviruses, coronaviruses, herpes simplex virus and coxsackie A virus. Bacteria are less common causes of pharyngitis and tonsillitis, but the infections they cause can be very serious. The most important bacteria are:

- *Streptococcus pyogenes* (Group A streptococci), the cause of streptococcal sore throat;
- *Corynebacterium diphtheriae*, the cause of diphtheria (see p. 377);
- *Haemophilus influenzae* type b, is the major cause of severe epiglottitis (see p. 377); and
- *Neisseria gonorrhoeae*, in pharyngeal gonorrhoea (see Chapter 21).

The yeast, *Candida albicans*, is an important cause of pharyngitis in immunosuppressed patients.

Acute pharyngitis caused by *S. pyogenes* is commonly referred to as a 'strep sore throat'. It occurs predominantly in children. The oropharynx of humans is the natural reservoir of this organism. It can be found in low numbers in the throat and nose of normal people, and in large numbers in the throat of infected people. It is spread primarily by coughing and sneezing and can persist for long periods in dried mucoid material and dust. Although this organism causes less than 10% of cases of acute pharyngitis, it is important because of the possibility of more serious complications (see below). Some strains of *S. pyogenes* also produce an erythrogenic toxin, which causes the erythematous skin rash characteristic of **scarlet fever**.

Laboratory diagnosis and treatment

In most cases, the clinical condition of pharyngitis or tonsillitis is not serious enough to warrant a laboratory diagnosis and, because the vast majority are caused by viruses, no specific therapy exists. Bacterial infections can usually be readily identified by culture of a throat swab (see Chapter 15). When bacteria are suspected, a laboratory diagnosis may be warranted because of their potential seriousness and because they can be treated with antibiotic therapy. *S. pyogenes* is almost universally sensitive to penicillin. Infectious mononucleosis is diagnosed by serological means (see Chapter 19).

Possible sequelae of streptococcal sore throat

Two non-infectious complications of streptococcal sore throat occasionally occur. **Rheumatic fever** is an indirect complication of streptococcal sore throat in which antibodies, formed against antigens in the streptococcal cell wall, cross-react with the sarcolemma (muscle cell membrane) of human heart, and other tissues. Rheumatic heart disease, representing damage to the heart valves by these antibodies, can result from repeated infections.

Acute glomerulonephritis develops when antibodies combine with certain streptococcal antigens to form circulating immune complexes. These complexes can be deposited in glomeruli, resulting in local inflammation and kidney disease.

Rheumatic fever and acute glomerulonephritis occur in only a minority of people, but are, nevertheless, potentially serious consequences of streptococcal sore throat. They are common diseases in some rural Aboriginal communities in Australia where the rate of streptococcal infection is high. In people prone to suffering from either of these sequelae, each episode of untreated streptococcal sore throat will lead to an episode of rheumatic fever or acute glomerulonephritis. Therefore, prompt diagnosis and treatment of streptococcal sore throat in susceptible individuals are essential for the prevention of these sequelae. In severe cases, prophylactic antibiotics to prevent streptococcal infection may be warranted. Rheumatic fever is discussed in detail in Chapter 19.

DIPHTHERIA

Cause, pathogenesis and clinical features

Diphtheria is an acute infectious disease caused by toxin-producing strains of *Corynebacterium diphtheriae*. The infection was once a major cause of death throughout the world, but is now rare in developed countries due to the availability of an effective vaccine (see Figure 17.2). It is still common in many developing countries where the vaccine is not so readily available or administered. In Australia, less than 40 cases per year are currently reported, although sporadic outbreaks in non-immunised people still occur.

Non-toxigenic strains can exist as part of the normal flora of the pharynx, but only toxigenic strains cause infection, mainly of the pharynx and larynx. *C. diphtheriae* can also infect the skin, but usually only in people with poor skin hygiene living in the tropics. The organism infects existing skin lesions, causing poorly healing ulcerations covered by a grey membrane.

The organism is usually transmitted by the air-borne route from infected people or asymptomatic carriers. Once it is established in the respiratory tract, usually on the pharynx, it secretes a toxin that destroys the epithelial surface, forming an ulcer. A sore throat and fever are the first symptoms to develop. The ulcer becomes covered by a greyish membrane, consisting of dead tissue cells, bacteria and inflammatory exudate (called a **pseudo-membrane**). In severe cases the membrane can block the airway. Removing the membrane exposes a raw bleeding ulcer that will eventually be re-covered by another membrane. If the larynx is infected, a life-threatening respiratory obstruction is more likely.

The bacteria multiply locally without invading deeper tissues or spreading to other sites in the body, but the toxin is absorbed into the bloodstream, killing cells in the heart, kidneys and nervous system by interfering with protein synthesis. The toxin is highly potent—10 ug is sufficient to kill a healthy adult. Cardiac failure and death can result from the action of the toxin on the heart. Partial paralysis of the soft palate, face or laryngopharyngeal tract can occur when the nervous system is affected.

FIGURE 17.2
ANNUAL RATE OF NOTIFICATIONS OF DIPHTHERIA IN AUSTRALIA, 1917–91

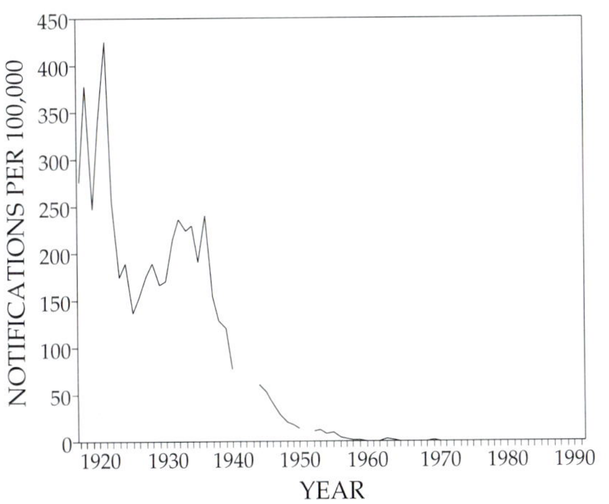

Source: *Communicable Diseases Intelligence* 17/11, 31 May 1993.

Diagnosis and treatment

Diphtheria is a life-threatening disease requiring urgent diagnosis and treatment. A diagnosis of diphtheria is confirmed by the isolation and identification of toxin-producing corynebacteria in a swab from under the membrane. As soon as the diagnosis is suspected clinically, treatment with antitoxin, to neutralise the toxin, should be commenced. Penicillin or erythromycin is given in conjunction with antitoxin to eliminate the infection and prevent further toxin production. Diphtheria of the larynx may require a tracheostomy. Antitoxin is produced in horses, and delayed hypersensitivity reactions to the foreign animal proteins may occur a week or so later.

Close contacts should be tested for carriage of toxigenic *C. diphtheriae* and have their immunisation status checked. Non-immunised contacts should be given penicillin or erythromycin as a prophylactic measure, and be vaccinated.

Prevention

Diphtheria has almost disappeared from developed countries, due to immunisation of children with the diphtheria vaccine. The vaccine consists of formaldehyde-inactivated diphtheria toxin, which stimulates production of antitoxin. It is currently incorporated in the diphtheria, tetanus and pertussis (DTP) triple vaccine and the combined diphtheria and tetanus (CDT) vaccine. For children over eight years, and adults who have not been vaccinated, the lesser dose adult diphtheria and tetanus (ADT) vaccine is used.

ACUTE EPIGLOTTITIS

The epiglottis is a flap of cartilage that prevents food and fluids from entering the larynx. **Epiglottitis**, inflammation of the epiglottis, is most often seen in young children, and is almost always caused by *Haemophilus influenzae* type b. It has a peak incidence in children 2–4 years old. It is one of the more serious types of upper respiratory infection. The organism probably extends from an initial focus of infection in the nasopharynx. Bacteraemia is usually present and the patient is usually toxic and febrile. A swollen, red epiglottis may be seen when the child's mouth is opened.

There may be respiratory distress because of obstruction of the airway, which can be fatal if it becomes completely obstructed. The infected child often adopts a characteristic posture with the neck hyperextended and the chin pushed forward, to maximise airway diameter. Forcing the child to adopt another posture is not advisable as this may precipitate complete airway obstruction. It is a rapidly

CASE HISTORY 17.1
EPIGLOTTITIS

Timothy, a 3-year-old, had been suffering from symptoms of a cold for two days. His crying woke his parents in the middle of the night and they observed that he was feverish and having some difficulty breathing. They immediately took him to the casualty department of the local hospital.

On examination, his epiglottis was red and swollen, confirmed by X-ray of the neck. A diagnosis of epiglottitis was made and Timothy was immediately taken to theatre to have an endotracheal tube inserted. Blood cultures were taken and treatment with cefuroxime was commenced. In four days he had completely recovered.

progressive disease which can result in death within a few hours. Older children and adults may be affected, but usually only if immunocompromised. Obstruction is not a prominent feature in these groups because of their greater airway diameter.

Patients with epiglottitis must be treated as a medical emergency. An endotracheal tube is usually inserted as a prophylactic measure and treatment is begun immediately with antibiotics, such as cefuroxime. The clinical diagnosis is confirmed by isolating bacteria from blood and possibly the epiglottis. Extreme care must be taken when examining the throat, since the swollen epiglottis can be sucked into the oedematous airway and cause total obstruction. Treatment with antibiotics is usually effective.

Epiglottitis is the second most common infection caused by *H. influenzae* type b (Hib), after meningitis. Conjugate Hib vaccines have been available in Australia since 1992 and have been part of the standard childhood vaccination schedule since 1993. The vaccines have already resulted in a significant reduction in incidence of Hib disease. Hib vaccines are discussed in more detail in Chapter 20.

LARYNGOTRACHEITIS

Viral infections of the upper respiratory tract may spread downwards to involve the larynx and the trachea. **Laryngotracheitis** (inflammation of the larynx and trachea), or **croup**, is characterised by stridor (noisy respiration), hoarseness and a resonant cough, often described as 'barking' or 'brassy'. These manifestations are due to partial obstruction of the larynx, resulting from inflammatory oedema and spasm. In most cases, the symptoms become no more serious than this and recovery occurs within a week. However, in some children, respiratory failure can occur, precipitated by such factors as emotional distress.

Croup is most common in children under four years old because of the narrowness of their larynx, and the ease with which it can be partially obstructed by inflammation. There is often a preceding cold, pharyngitis or cough. Some children suffer repeated episodes of croup, perhaps because of hyperreactive airways. Laryngeal or tracheal infection in adults (**laryngitis** or **tracheitis**) causes hoarseness and a burning pain on breathing in and out, usually without obstruction of the larynx.

Laryngotracheitis is usually caused by viruses, especially the parainfluenza group, but sometimes respiratory syncytial virus or influenza virus may be involved. *H. influenzae* (epiglottitis) and *C. diphtheriae* (diphtheria) are rare causes. Croup can also be caused by the inhalation of a foreign body, and airway obstruction.

The diagnosis of viral croup is based on clinical and radiologic examination. Patient management involves humidification to soften mucus and soothe the inflamed mucosa, and oxygenation to reverse hypoxaemia. Intubation or tracheostomy may be performed if complete obstruction is likely. Antibiotics are administered if a bacterial cause is demonstrated.

Lower Respiratory Tract Infections

In contrast to the upper respiratory tract, the lower respiratory tract is normally sterile and so infections involving it are potentially more serious. Lower respiratory tract infections include a spectrum of diseases ranging from acute bronchitis to pneumonia. The major syndromes that will be discussed here are whooping cough, bronchitis, bronchiolitis, influenza and pneumonia. Chronic infections of the lower respiratory tract are dealt with later in the chapter (see p. 388).

Pathogenic microorganisms may reach the lower respiratory tract in a number of ways:

- inhalation of organisms suspended in air (aerosols or dust);
- aspiration of oropharyngeal contents (and sometimes gastrointestinal contents) when asleep, intoxicated or unconscious;
- spread of infection from the upper respiratory tract;
- via the bloodstream, from a primary site of infection elsewhere in the body.

PERTUSSIS

Causative agent and pathogenesis

Pertussis (**whooping cough**) is a severe, sometimes fatal, disease caused by the Gram-negative coccobacillus, *Bordetella pertussis*. Affecting mainly children, it is a highly infectious disease that is spread from person to person by air-borne droplets (see Figure 17.3). Its incidence in developed countries has been markedly reduced through immunisation, but in developing countries where immunisation is lacking, infection rates are high. Despite the availability of a vaccine, not all parents have their children vaccinated. As a result, epidemics tend to occur every 3–4 years. In non-epidemic years, less than 1000 cases are usually reported, but this can increase fivefold when epidemics occur.

The organism has specific adhesins that allow it to attach to the ciliated respiratory mucosa. It multiplies in the epithelial cells but does not invade further. The

FIGURE 17.3
ANNUAL RATE OF NOTIFICATION OF PERTUSSIS PER 100 000 POPULATION IN AUSTRALIA IN 1993 BY AGE GROUP AND SEX

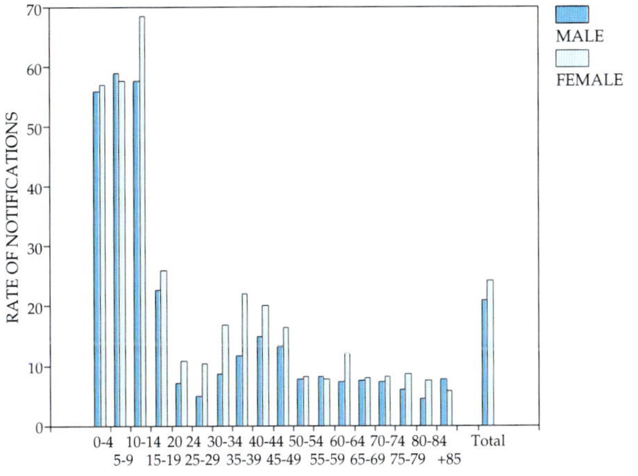

Source: *Communicable Diseases Intelligence* 18/22, 31 October 1996.

organism produces several toxins, which combine to produce the symptoms of disease. The exact activity of pertussis toxin is not clear, but it appears to enter phagocytes and impair their chemotaxis and killing power. It may also be partly responsible for the increase in respiratory secretions and mucus production characteristic of whooping cough. Adenylate cyclase toxin also appears to inhibit vital functions of neutrophils such as chemotaxis, phagocytosis and killing activity, and may also be involved in inducing the inflammatory response. Tracheal cytotoxin is a cell wall component that specifically kills tracheal epithelial cells, thereby partially immobilising the mucociliary escalator and causing an accumulation of mucus in the airway. No exact role for pertussis endotoxin has been established but, like the endotoxin of other Gram-negatives, it may be involved in the production of fever and inflammation. The major activities of *B. pertussis* toxins are illustrated in Figure 17.4.

Clinical features

After an incubation period of 7–10 days, there is an initial catarrhal illness that resembles a cold, characterised by runny nose, infrequent cough and mild fever. This is the most infectious period. The cough, caused by an accumulation of mucus in the airway, gradually becomes more irritating and paroxysmal (abrupt, short attacks) over the next 1–2 weeks. A paroxysm is characterised by a series of short coughs productive of copious mucus, followed by a 'whoop'—a characteristic sound produced by a gasp of air at the end of a coughing episode. The whoop represents the rush of air through the narrowed airway. Frequent coughing episodes can cause exhaustion of a young child. The characteristic whoop may be absent in some patients, particularly in very young infants, older children and adults. Despite the severity of the cough, the symptoms are confined to the respiratory tract. Coughing episodes may persist for 1– 6 weeks.

Possible complications include cerebral hypoxia, bronchopneumonia and secondary pneumonia due to invasion of the damaged respiratory tract by other bacteria (e.g. *Staphylococcus aureus*). Death, due to hypoxia, occurs in up to 0.5% of infants. Infection in adults is often asymptomatic or mild. Adults can become infected if never immunised, or once their vaccine-induced immunity has waned.

Diagnosis

The organisms can be isolated from throat swabs or on 'cough plates', but they are extremely fastidious and do not survive well outside the body, making them difficult to culture. The specimen must be quickly inoculated onto the culture medium. A direct fluorescent antibody test

FIGURE 17.4
PROPOSED MECHANISMS OF ACTION OF THE TOXINS OF *BORDETELLA PERTUSSIS*

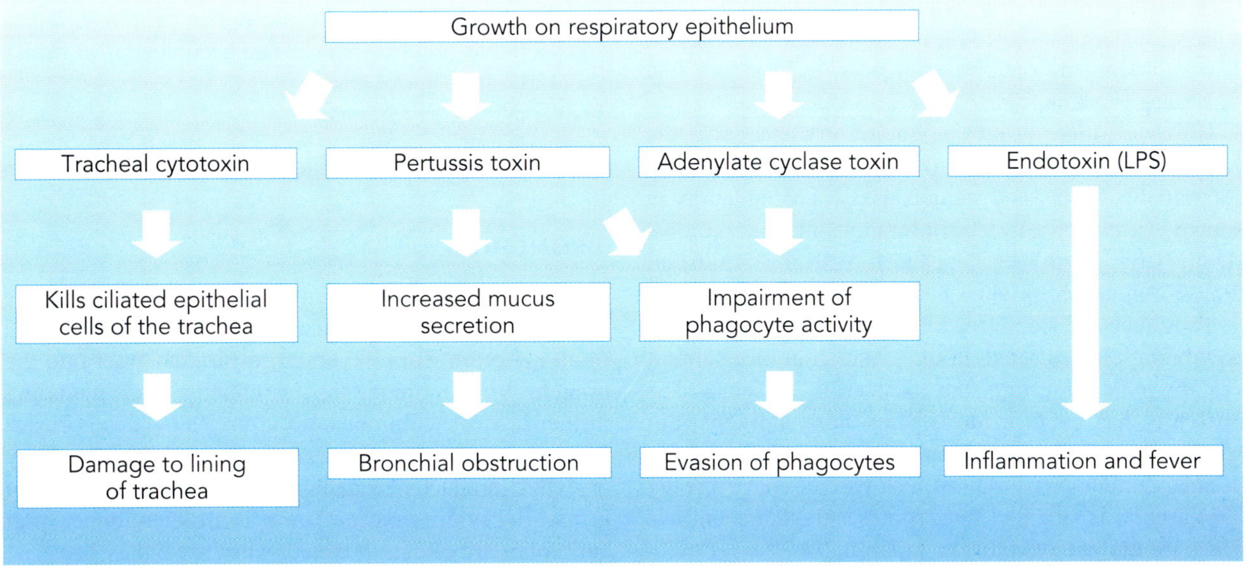

to detect the organism in nasopharyngeal aspirates is commonly used.

Treatment

Supportive care, including oxygen and suctioning, is of prime importance. Antibiotics do not appear to reduce the severity or duration of infection. However, erythromycin reduces the numbers of organisms in the throat, and is thus useful in helping to control the spread of infection. Erythromycin prophylaxis of close contacts of active cases may prevent infection or reduce the severity of subsequent infection. Maternal antibodies do not appear to be highly protective, so infants are very susceptible prior to immunisation.

Prevention

The National Health and Medical Research Council of Australia recommends immunisation against pertussis from two months of age, unless there are contraindications such as a current acute illness, or significant reaction following a previous dose. Immunisation is effective in reducing the incidence and severity of pertussis. A whole cell vaccine consisting of a killed suspension of *B. pertussis* cells has been used for many years. It is usually combined with diphtheria and tetanus toxoids and administered as **DTP** or **triple antigen**. Although pertussis vaccine offers complete protection in only about 80% of people, and protection wanes after several years, it has nevertheless been very effective in reducing the number of infections (up to 90% reduction) in countries where uptake has been high.

In recent years there have been major concerns about the possible side effects of the vaccine, leading to its reduced uptake, and subsequently a marked increase in incidence and some major epidemics (e.g. in the UK and Japan). Possible complications of vaccination include:

- a short episode (1–2 days) of mild fever, malaise, and swelling and redness at the injection site (occurs in 20–50% of infants);
- convulsions(in about 0.05%), high-pitched, unusual screaming (in 0.1%) or prolonged crying (in 1%), none of which appears to cause any long-term effects;
- encephalopathy or febrile seizures, in less than 1 in 100 000 vaccinations (< 0.001%).

However, there is no convincing evidence that the vaccine causes these neurological disorders. By comparison, pertussis disease causes encephalopathy in approximately 1% of cases in infants under six months. Deaths from pertussis still occur in Australia, almost all in non-immunised infants.

To reduce the side effects of vaccination, efforts are now being concentrated on the production of a subunit vaccine containing only the 'protective' antigens. The difficulty has been in identifying those antigens, but combinations of inactivated pertussis toxin and filamentous haemagglutinin have promise; such vaccines have already been used in Japan, the United States and other countries. They are not yet available in Australia.

CASE HISTORY 17.2
WHOOPING COUGH

A 5-week-old, fully breast-fed boy, SG, was admitted to a country hospital for investigation of failure to thrive. He remained in hospital for a week and began to gain weight after being changed to bottle feeding. Two days before he was discharged, a 6-month-old infant with suspected whooping cough was admitted to the cot opposite.

At home, seven days after his whooping cough contact, SG began to develop a frequent cough. After 3–4 days he was vomiting mucus with the cough, going blue or purple with paroxysms of coughing, and was not breathing during the attacks. He had no whoop. A pernasal swab grew *Bordetella pertussis.*

Both SG's parents developed a ticklish, intermittent cough. The mother's cough woke her at night, causing retrosternal pain and vomiting of phlegm, and was associated with a loud whoop. The father had a sore throat, mild cough but no whoop.

SG was readmitted to the country hospital. He had a clear nasal discharge and paroxysmal cough without whoop but with apnoea and cyanosis. His peripheral white blood cell count was 14.1 x 10^9/L with 77% lymphocytes. The paroxysms became increasingly frequent and were associated with arterial oxygen desaturation to 85%. Transport was requested, and SG was transferred by ambulance to intensive care at the Royal Alexandra Hospital for Children. He appeared well, vigorous and afebrile between coughing paroxysms, had a respiratory rate of 40 per minute and his chest was clear. Chest X-ray was normal. Initially he was maintained in head-box oxygen but was having paroxysms of cough with apnoea and cyanosis every 1–2 minutes. He was, therefore, muscle-relaxed, intubated and ventilated. SG and both parents were given a 14-day course of oral erythromycin.

Meanwhile, a nurse at the referring hospital had developed coryza followed by a paroxysmal cough, and was eventually recognised as having pertussis. She had continued working in the newborn nursery. It was decided to offer erythromycin prophylaxis to all 52 infants with whom she had been in contact from six days after her exposure.

Adapted from D. Isaacs, 'Nosocomial Whooping Cough', *Communicable Diseases Intelligence* 16/25, 14 December 1992.

BRONCHITIS

Acute bronchitis represents an inflammation of the tracheobronchial tree, and is usually a result of the spread of an infection from the upper respiratory tract into the bronchi. Viruses are the most common causes, including influenza virus, common cold viruses and adenoviruses. *Mycoplasma pneumoniae* can also be responsible. A dry or slightly productive cough is the major feature. Treatment is mainly symptomatic. There is little evidence that antibiotics are effective, except when secondary bacterial infection occurs. In otherwise healthy individuals, there is usually a speedy recovery with few sequelae.

Chronic bronchitis is a condition in which there is a chronic or recurrent cough and excessive secretion of mucus. It appears to result from a combination of factors, which may include infection, cigarette smoking, inhalation of pollutants, and a genetic predisposition. Infection with rhinoviruses or influenza virus may precipitate relapses, and bacteria such as *S. pneumoniae*, *H. influenzae* and *M. catarrhalis* may be involved in acute exacerbations. Further spread of bacteria into the lungs can result in pneumonia.

Antibiotics, such as amoxycillin or cotrimoxazole, are used for the treatment of associated bacterial infections.

BRONCHIOLITIS

Cause and epidemiology

Bronchiolitis is predominantly a disease of childhood and usually occurs in children less than two years old. The bronchioles of a young child are so narrow that, if their lining cells are swollen by inflammation, the passage of air to and from the alveoli may be severely restricted. Infection results in necrosis of the epithelial cells that line the bronchioles, and the infection may spread into the lung tissue and cause pneumonia. Most of these infections are caused by respiratory syncytial virus (RSV), although other viruses (e.g. influenza and parainfluenza viruses) and *Mycoplasma pneumoniae* may be involved.

RSV is highly infectious and can cause community and hospital outbreaks in winter. It is a frequent cause of lower respiratory tract infections in infants, but rarely produces significant illness in adult contacts. Its surface spikes are fusion proteins (not haemagglutinins or neuraminidases) which fuse host cells to form **syncytia** (multi-nucleated masses of fused cells—hence the name, respiratory syncytial virus). The infection is transmitted by droplets and to some extent via hands. The only known reservoir is infected humans.

Clinical features

In children and adults the virus is restricted to the upper respiratory tract, causing a mild, common cold-type illness. However, infection in infants can be severe if the virus invades the lower respiratory tract. Typical symptoms include fever, coryza (rhinitis—inflammation of the nasal passages with nasal discharge), a cough, and respiratory obstruction resembling asthma, possibly leading to respiratory distress and cyanosis, especially in infants with some other underlying disorder. Viral pneumonia can develop in some patients. Most cases begin to resolve within a few days, but some children, even a year or two later, may continue to show depressed pulmonary function or wheezing. Recurrent infections are common although they are generally less severe.

Diagnosis and treatment

RSV-specific antigens in nasopharyngeal washings are detectable by immunofluorescence or ELISA. As bronchiolitis is caused mainly by viruses, antimicrobial drugs are generally unhelpful, but the antiviral agent ribavirin, given by aerosol, is effective in some severe cases.

INFLUENZA

Influenza epidemics occur worldwide and cause significant morbidity and mortality. Influenza viruses cause a range of clinical conditions that affect all levels of the respiratory tract.

Causative agents

The causative agents are the influenza viruses (myxoviruses), whose structure is shown in Figure 17.5. Influenza A viruses cause epidemics, and occasionally pandemics, and infect a variety of animals and birds, as well as humans. Influenza B viruses cause epidemics but do not involve an animal host. Generally, one or more outbreaks of type A or B influenza occur each year. Approximately every 10 years a type A pandemic occurs.

The envelope of an influenza virus has two surface glycoprotein antigens, the haemagglutinin (H) and neuraminidase (N) spikes. Protective antibodies are made to both these antigens in infected people, but influenza viruses can vary these antigens over time by 'antigenic drift' and 'antigenic shift' (see Chapter 10). Antigenic drift represents small, constantly occurring mutations, affecting the H and N antigens. If the changes occur in areas where antibodies bind to these antigens, the antibodies may not bind as well, allowing the virus to reinfect communities repeatedly over time, even though the individuals have immunity due to previous flu infections.

Antigenic shift represents a sudden, major change in the H or N antigens based on recombination between different virus strains when they infect the same cell. This major change in H or N antigens results in completely different antigen structures, enabling the new strain to spread through populations in epidemic form. Major shifts have resulted in pandemics of Asian flu in 1957, Hong Kong flu in 1968 and Russian flu in 1977. Only type A strains undergo antigenic shift.

FIGURE 17.5
ELECTRON MICROGRAPH OF THE INFLUENZA VIRUS

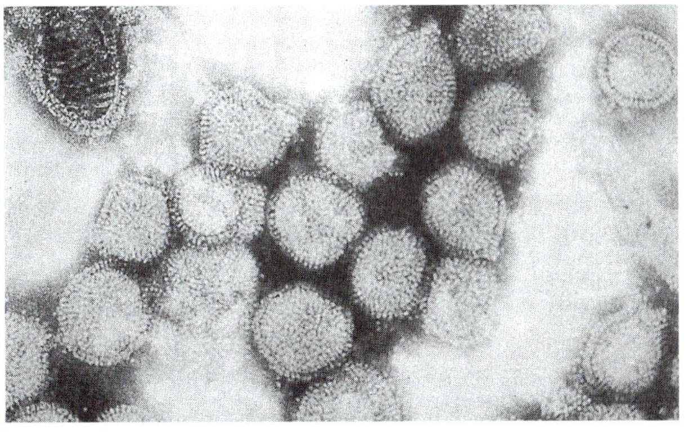

Transmission of influenza is by droplet inhalation and fomites, and infectivity can be very high (up to 30% attack rate generally, and over 50% in epidemics). Influenza occurs throughout the world and, except in the tropics, is almost entirely restricted to the coldest months of the year. This is largely because, during cold weather, people spend more time inside buildings, favouring transmission via aerosols and fomites.

Pathogenesis and clinical features

The virus enters the respiratory tract via droplets and attaches to receptors on respiratory epithelial cells via the H spikes on its envelope. One to three days after infection, symptoms such as fever, chills, malaise and muscle pain develop, due mainly to cytokines liberated from damaged cells and infiltrating leucocytes. As the virus spreads, symptoms of runny nose, sore throat and dry cough may occur. Subclinical or mild infections resembling a cold are common. Recovery usually occurs within 1–3 weeks, although the infection can be severe enough to develop into bronchitis or pneumonia. Secondary bacterial infection may occur—especially in people with COPD (chronic obstructive pulmonary disease)—caused by staphylococci, pneumococci, *H. influenzae* or other organisms.

The life-threatening form of influenzal pneumonia, which caused tens of millions of deaths in the 1918–19 pandemic, and which still occurs occasionally, is usually due to a mixed influenza and bacterial (e.g. staphylococcal) infection.

Mortality is highest in the elderly and the debilitated, especially in developing countries, and is usually due to secondary bacterial pneumonia or exacerbation of chronic cardiac or respiratory disease. Meningeal symptoms occur rarely, but appear to be due to indirect immunopathological complications rather than invasion of the CNS by the virus.

Diagnosis

A specific diagnosis can be made by serological means, by detection of viral antigen in respiratory samples, or by isolating the virus. In most cases, these methods are impractical and unnecessary for an individual patient, but may be important for public health authorities when following infection with a new virus strain.

Treatment and prevention

Rest, fluids and analgesics form the basis of treatment, and recovery is usually within a week. Antibiotics are required if secondary bacterial infection occurs. Amantadine and rimantadine can be used prophylactically to prevent outbreaks in elderly, non-immunised residents of institutions such as nursing homes. These drugs are effective only against influenza A.

Influenza virus vaccine, when given before the epidemic season arrives, offers partial protection, but only against those strains covered by the vaccine. The vaccines are multivalent, directed against several strains of the virus.

CASE HISTORY 17.3
INFLUENZA

On 17 August 1993 the Infectious Diseases Program of Health and Community Services, Victoria, was contacted by the director of nursing from a Melbourne metropolitan nursing home. She was concerned about an outbreak among residents and staff of a febrile illness with upper respiratory symptoms; approximately half the residents became ill over a 2-week period.

Sera were collected from six acutely ill residents and four acutely ill staff, as well as from those who had been acutely ill during the previous five days. Convalescent sera were collected three weeks after the acute sera. All samples were tested for antibodies to influenza A and B. Seroconversion to influenza A virus was demonstrated in most cases.

The mean age of all residents was 83 years, and of staff, 43 years. There were 34 cases in total, of which 18 were staff and 16 were residents. The mean age of affected residents was 82 years, and the mean age of affected staff was 44 years. The index case (a member of staff) occurred on 6 August 1993, and there was a subsequent outbreak among residents that peaked on August 12. The last case occurred on August 29.

The mean duration of illness was 12 days, with a range of 3–28 days. Fever, malaise, cough, rhinorrhoea, muscle aches, headache and sore throat were the most commonly reported symptoms. There were three deaths, four hospitalisations for pneumonia or chest infection (with eventual recovery), and four cases with respiratory complications not requiring hospitalisation. All complications and deaths occurred in residents.

INFLUENZA CASES AT THE NURSING HOME BY DATE OF ONSET AND PATIENT TYPE

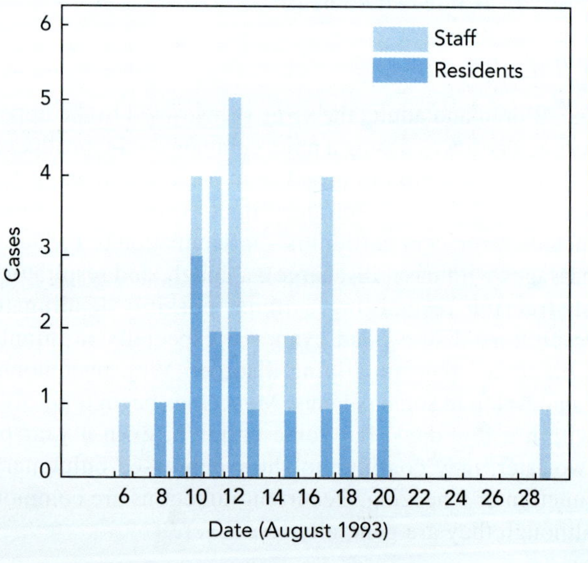

Source: R. MacIntyre, C. Mansell, P. Lynch and J. Rich, 'An outbreak of influenza A, at a Victorian nursing home', *Communicable Diseases Intelligence* 18/2, 24 January 1994, p. 32.

The composition of annual vaccines is based on the anticipated pattern of active influenza A and B viruses, determined by worldwide surveillance coordinated by the World Health Organization. In Australia, we usually get the current flu strain six months after the European winter, so we often have the right vaccine ready when the epidemic strikes. Vaccination is recommended for high risk individuals, such as the elderly and debilitated (e.g. residents of nursing homes and chronic care facilities), and people with chronic cardiopulmonary disease.

PNEUMONIA

Pneumonia is an infection and inflammation of the lungs. It is a major cause of death throughout the world, especially in the elderly in developed countries, and in children and the malnourished living in crowded and unhygienic conditions. Worldwide, as many as five million people are thought to die each year from pneumonia.

A wide variety of microorganisms are capable of causing pneumonia. Bacteria and viruses cause most cases, but fungi (e.g. *Aspergillus* and *Pneumocystis carinii*) can also be responsible, especially in the immunocompromised. The common causative agents of pneumonia are listed in Table 17.5. The cause will depend on a number of risk factors such as age, underlying disease and particular exposure to pathogens through occupation, travel or contact with animals. Pneumonia is the most commonly fatal type of nosocomial infection. As many as 15% of all deaths in hospitals may be attributed to a hospital-acquired pneumonia. Most of these occur in postsurgical patients or patients in intensive care.

Clinical features

Patients with pneumonia usually present with a fever, cough and chest pain. The cough is generally unproductive at first, but later may become purulent and sometimes blood-stained. As the disease progresses, the patient experiences increasing breathlessness and shallow, rapid breathing. Inspiratory rales (crackling sounds) are usually heard over the affected area of the lung. Some infections result in symptoms confined mainly to the chest, whereas others, such as Legionnaires' disease, have a much wider systemic involvement and the patient may present with mental confusion, diarrhoea, and evidence of renal or liver dysfunction. A chest X-ray confirms the presence and distribution of shadows in the lung, indicating consolidation. Severe pneumonia can quickly lead to respiratory failure, requiring ventilation and intensive care. Antibiotics have greatly reduced the mortality rate, but deaths still occur, despite appropriate treatment.

Complications of infection include spread of the infecting organisms directly to extra-pulmonary sites such as the pleural space, giving rise to empyema, or indirectly via the bloodstream to other parts of the body.

Pathogenesis

Microorganisms may reach the lungs by inhalation of fine, aerosolised particles, or by the downward movement of mucus, which carries normal flora organisms or pathogens from the upper respiratory tract. Micro-aspiration of oropharyngeal and gastric secretions may also occur, especially in the critically ill, because of their supine position or use of nasogastric tubes. The mucociliary

TABLE 17.5
COMMON CAUSES OF PNEUMONIA: COMMUNITY-ACQUIRED VERSUS HOSPITAL-ACQUIRED INFECTIONS

COMMUNITY-ACQUIRED		HOSPITAL-ACQUIRED	
Organism	**% of cases**	**Organism**	**% of cases**
Streptococcus pneumoniae	30–40	*Pseudomonas aeruginosa*	15–30
Mycoplasma pneumoniae	10–20	*Staphylococcus aureus*	10–30
Haemophilus influenzae	5–10	*Klebsiella* species	5–15
Influenza viruses	5–10	*Escherichia coli*	5–15
Legionella species	5	*Enterobacter* species	5–10
Chlamydia pneumoniae	5	*Acinetobacter* species	5
Staphylococcus aureus	< 5	*Proteus* species	5
Moraxella catarrhalis	< 5	*Streptococcus pneumoniae*	< 5
Parainfluenza virus	< 5	*Candida* species	< 5
		Legionella species	< 5
		Moraxella catarrhalis	< 5

escalator normally functions to move mucus, foreign material and microorganisms trapped in it upwards away from the lungs, but this function can be impaired in people with an upper respiratory viral infection, and in those with damaged cilia due to inhalation of pollutants (e.g. cigarette smoke), alcoholism or the presence of a tumour or foreign body. Sometimes, the lungs become infected by organisms that have spread, via the bloodstream, from another infected site in the body.

In response to infection or the action of microbial toxins, inflammation occurs, resulting in the filling of the affected alveoli—first with a serous exudate, and then later with pus cells and sometimes red blood cells. Once the alveoli fill with infectious exudate, an overflow of the fluid occurs and there is a progressive spread of infection to adjacent alveoli.

Pneumonia has traditionally been classified into types according to differences in clinical signs and radiological findings. **Lobar pneumonia** is an infection and consolidation (solidification of the tissue due to inflammatory exudate in the alveoli) confined to one or two lobes of the lung. Most cases are caused by *Streptococcus pneumoniae*. **Bronchopneumonia** is a more diffuse, patchy inflammation of the lungs with numerous, small foci of consolidation occurring throughout the lungs. A large variety of bacteria, such as *S. pneumoniae*, *Staphylococcus aureus*, *Mycobacterium tuberculosis* and *Haemophilus influenzae*, or viruses, can be responsible.

Outcomes common to both types of pneumonia are respiratory distress resulting from the interference with air exchange in the lungs, and systemic effects typical of any severe infection. A **pleural effusion** occurs if the inflammatory exudate enters the space between the lung tissue and pleural membranes. **Empyema** is the term used to describe infection of the pleural space, and **pleurisy** means an inflammation of the pleural membranes.

Bacterial causes

Pneumococcal pneumonia. The most common bacterial cause (approximately 30% of cases) of community-acquired pneumonia is *Streptococcus pneumoniae* (the 'pneumococcus'), a normal inhabitant of the upper respiratory tract of some people. Pneumococcal pneumonia is still a cause of significant morbidity and mortality throughout the world, and is an important infection and cause of death in patients post-splenectomy. The virulence of the organism is due to an extracellular polysaccharide capsule, which makes it resistant to phagocytosis (see Chapter 4). There are at least 83 different serotypes of pneumococcus, but most infections are caused by a limited number of these serotypes. Pneumococcal pneumonia is a common complication of AIDS.

Usually, a chest X-ray is performed when pneumonia is suspected. This may indicate that infection and inflammation exist, but laboratory investigations are required to identify the causative organism. Making a specific laboratory diagnosis of pneumonia is often a problem, because of the variety of causes, and the different requirements for their identification. Blood and sputum culture are the main methods for diagnosing bacterial pneumonias, although there are doubts about the sensitivity of both procedures. More invasive techniques, such as transtracheal aspiration, bronchoscopy and broncho-alveolar lavage, and open lung biopsy, may yield more useful results. However, collection of sputum and blood are relatively simple and non-invasive, and are therefore most often collected. Both should be collected before antibiotic therapy is started. Sputum samples are best collected in the morning, because sputum tends to accumulate while the patient is lying in bed, and before breakfast, to reduce contamination by food particles and bacteria from food. It is critical that the specimen collected is truly sputum and is free of oropharyngeal contamination, since some oropharyngeal flora can cause pneumonia, and may be incorrectly identified as the cause.

Examination of a Gram-stained smear of sputum can give a presumptive diagnosis of pneumococcal pneumonia within minutes if it demonstrates polymorphs and Gram-positive diplococci characteristic of *S. pneumoniae* (see Figure 17.6). Other rapid non-cultural techniques have also been applied successfully to the diagnosis of pneumococcal pneumonia. Detection of pneumococcal antigen by agglutination of antibody-coated latex particles (see Chapter 18) can be used both on sputum and urine specimens (antigen is excreted in the urine). Use of this technique means the result is available within an hour of receipt of the specimen, but antibiotic susceptibility tests cannot be performed unless the organisms are isolated.

First-line treatment of pneumonia before results are available is usually with ampicillin and/or erythromycin, but treatment failure is possible because of the wide range of potential causes and their differing drug sensitivities. The standard treatment for pneumococcal pneumonia is penicillin, but strains with high-level resistance have recently emerged and caused some concern. The patient with pneumonia may also require oxygen, and physiotherapy should be given if there is significant sputum.

FIGURE 17.6
A GRAM STAIN OF A SMEAR OF SPUTUM CAN PROVIDE A RAPID PRESUMPTIVE DIAGNOSIS
This slide shows Gram-positive diplococci and pus cells suggestive of *Streptococcus pneumoniae* infection.

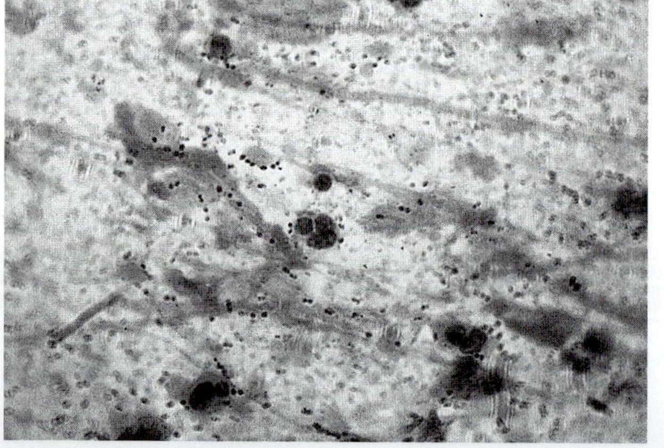

In the severely ill, direct suction with an endotracheal tube may be necessary. Even with appropriate antibiotic therapy, pneumonia can be fatal, usually because of rapidly progressive disease, or because of its interaction with some other underlying disorder.

A polyvalent vaccine containing 23 of the most common or most virulent polysaccharide capsular antigen types of *S. pneumoniae* is available and recommended for people at high risk—for example, prior to splenectomy, in those with sickle-cell disease or malignancy, and in those with chronic, underlying illnesses such as chronic lung disease, nephrotic syndrome, cardiac failure or liver disease. It is also recommended for adults, especially those over the age of 50, in communities with high attack rates (e.g. some Aboriginal and Torres Strait Islander communities).

Staphylococcus aureus. Staphylococcal pneumonia is most common as a complication of viral respiratory infection, such as influenza or measles. Intravenous drug users may develop a staphylococcal endocarditis and pneumonia, following use of a contaminated needle or syringe. Elderly people, the immunocompromised, and patients with diabetes or cystic fibrosis are also susceptible. Diagnosis is by sputum culture and possibly blood culture (as for pneumococcal pneumonia).

Gram-negative enterobacteria. Gram-negative enterobacteria, such as *Escherichia coli*, *Pseudomonas aeruginosa*, *Klebsiella* spp. and *Serratia marcescens*, are particularly associated with pneumonia acquired in hospital, but can also cause community infections in the elderly, alcoholics and the immunocompromised. These organisms can colonise the upper respiratory tract of hospitalised people, especially after antibiotic therapy, and then be aspirated into the lower airways. Ventilators and humidifiers provide the necessary moisture for these organisms to persist and are well recognised as potential sources of infection in hospitals. Mechanical ventilation is a major risk factor for patients in intensive care, because an endotracheal tube bypasses upper airway defences. These organisms can also infect the lungs via the bloodstream, from infectious foci in the genitourinary or gastrointestinal tracts. The endotoxins in the cell wall of these bacteria are potent inducers of inflammmation.

The diagnosis of pneumonia caused by Gram-negative bacteria is based on culture of sputum and sometimes blood (see pneumococcal pneumonia for general principles). Appropriate antibiotic therapy is based on the culture results and sensitivity testing. Drug resistance is a problem in hospital-acquired infections, especially in Gram-negative enterobacteria.

Haemophilus influenzae. Haemophilus influenzae causes pneumonia, often as an exacerbation of epiglottitis, chronic bronchitis, brochiectasis, septicaemia or meningitis. Like *S. pneumoniae*, *H. influenzae* is a frequent cause of severe pneumonia in children in developing countries and Australian Aboriginal communities. In general, type b strains of *H. influenzae* cause most cases, but it is now recognised that non-type b strains are also important causes. *H. influenzae* mainly affects children under the age of four years because of a lack of protective antibodies. Diagnosis is based on culture of blood and sputum (see pneumococcal pneumonia).

Infections caused by *H. influenzae* have classically been treated with ampicillin, but the emergence of resistant strains has led to increased use of third generation cephalosporins (e.g. cefotaxime or ceftriaxone). Effective *H. influenzae* vaccines have been available in Australia since 1992 (see p. 377).

Pneumonia in cystic fibrosis. Several of the organisms described above are involved in recurrent or chronic lung infections in patients with cystic fibrosis (CF). The organisms most often encountered are *H. influenzae*, *S. aureus*, *S. pneumoniae*, *P. aeruginosa* and other *Pseudomonas* species. Of these, *P. aeruginosa* is the most important, causing a chronic lung infection that is almost impossible to eradicate in most CF patients. Over time, the infection and, more particularly, the inflammation it induces leads to permanent lung damage and often death. The predisposition of CF patients to lung infections appears to be related to the production of overly viscid bronchial secretions, and the suppressive effect this has on mucociliary clearance. Once established, the *Pseudomonas* protects itself against other defence mechanisms and antibiotics by growing in microcolonies coated with a film of alginate, a mucoid barrier through which many substances cannot pass.

Legionnaires' disease. Legionella pneumophila (serogroups 1–6) and other species, particularly *L. longbeachae*, *L. bozemanii* and *L. micdadei*, cause a pneumonia referred to as **Legionnaires' disease** (or **legionellosis**). *L. pneumophila* causes the majority of infections. These aerobic, Gram-negative, rod-shaped organisms are widely distributed in warm, wet habitats, especially in air-conditioning cooling towers. The organism is spread in air-borne droplets from cooling towers, taps, shower heads and contaminated environmental sources (e.g. creeks, lakes and soil).

Dispersion from cooling towers can lead to outbreaks of infection as occurred in the first recognised incident, involving 182 people (29 deaths) at a conference of the American Legion (war veterans) in Philadelphia in 1976. The high fatality rate in that outbreak was due partly to the delay (six months) in identifying the causative agent, because of its fastidious growth requirements and the difficulty in culturing it.

Person-to-person transmission of legionellosis does not appear to occur. In Australia there are on average less than 200 cases per year, with the highest rates of notification in the over 60 age groups (see Figure 17.7).

The incubation period of Legionnaires' disease is usually 2–10 days. Together with symptoms of pneumonia, there may be: systemic manifestations, including diarrhoea; abdominal pain; neurological signs, such as clouded consciousness and ataxia; and renal failure, with blood and protein in the urine.

FIGURE 17.7
ANNUAL RATE OF NOTIFICATION OF LEGIONELLOSIS IN AUSTRALIA PER 100 000 POPULATION IN 1994, BY AGE GROUP AND SEX

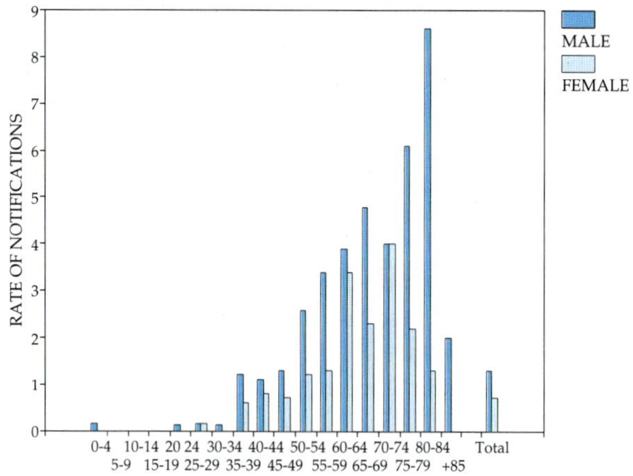

Source: Communicable Diseases Intelligence 19/22, 30 October 1995.

The cough in Legionnaires' disease is usually only slightly productive, if at all. Fever is almost always present. The disease is more likely to affect the elderly, but other major risk factors are cigarette smoking, underlying respiratory disease (e.g. chronic obstructive pulmonary disease—asthma, chronic bronchitis or emphysema), immunosuppression (e.g. malignancy, corticosteroid use) and excessive alcohol intake. However, legionellosis can occur in apparently healthy people of all ages. **Pontiac fever** is a mild form of *Legionella* infection, characterised by myalgia, fever, malaise and headache.

Nosocomial legionellosis can occur when water supplies in hospitals become contaminated, particularly when hot water lines are kept at low temperatures (less than 55°C). Below this temperature *Legionella* are able to survive and multiply in water supplies, and can be spread from shower roses and taps, as well as from cooling towers. *Legionella* have also been isolated from humidifiers and vaporisers. An important factor in hospitals is that they contain many people who are very susceptible and at high risk of infection. Mortality rates in the immunosuppressed can be very high.

For the diagnosis of Legionnaires' disease, culture of sputum or induced sputum (induced by inhalation of hypertonic saline) and serology, demonstrating a fourfold increase in antibody titre, are the definitive methods. Culture is not always successful because the cough is often non-productive. Another disadvantage of culture is that it takes 3–5 days for growth to occur. A direct fluorescent antibody test (DFA) on sputum can provide a rapid laboratory diagnosis of Legionnaires' disease, but it lacks sensitivity, tending to be positive only in severe cases. There is a urinary antigen test that is fairly sensitive and specific for *L. pneumophila* serogroup 1. Erythromycin usually provides effective treatment; it is sometimes used in conjunction with rifampicin.

The contamination of cooling systems and hot water supplies by legionellae has been the subject of intense study, and regulations are now in force to provide guidance for maintenance engineers.

Atypical pneumonia. Several bacteria cause what is sometimes referred to as an **atypical pneumonia**, so named not because it is uncommon, but because of its diffuse, patchy nature and an unresponsiveness to the normally effective antibacterials, sulphonamides and penicillin. The major causes are *Mycoplasma pneumoniae* and *Chlamydia pneumoniae*.

M. pneumoniae is transmitted in air-borne droplets. It affects mainly the upper respiratory tract, but causes clinical pneumonia in 3–30% of infected people. It occasionally causes epidemics of pneumonia. *C.*

CASE HISTORY 17.4
LEGIONNAIRES' DISEASE

The Western Sector Public Health Unit in North Parramatta, New South Wales, was notified of two cases of Legionnaires' disease on 16 January 1995. Over the next two weeks it was notified of a further nine cases of Legionnaires' disease. All 11 cases were due to *Legionella pneumophila* serogroup 1.

The date of onset of disease for the first notified case was 7 January 1995, and for the last notified case it was 25 January 1995. There were nine males and two females. The mean age of cases was 65 years (range: 45–75 years). Nine cases were confirmed by sputum culture, and the remaining two cases by serology.

Most cases were current cigarette smokers (eight), two were past smokers, and one had never smoked. Three of ten cases had a history of chronic obstructive airway disease. None of the cases was on immunosuppressives, and only one case was taking steroids.

All 11 cases were admitted to hospital, and seven cases were treated in an intensive care unit. There were three deaths (two males and one female).

In the environmental assessment, 49 premises were investigated and a total of 50 cooling towers were sampled. A cooling tower was classified as contaminated if ≥ 100 cfu/mL of *Legionella* organisms were detected in the water sample. Seventeen cooling towers (34%) were contaminated.

Seven cases either lived close by, or had been in the vicinity of one contaminated cooling tower in a shopping mall (1500 cfu/mL of total *Legionella* organisms). Two other cases had been to premises that housed another contaminated cooling tower (1600 cfu/mL of total *Legionella* organisms). The remaining two cases were reported not to have been anywhere near the above-mentioned contaminated cooling towers. Each, however, had visited other unrelated premises with contaminated cooling towers.

Adapted from B. Jalaludin, I. Goldthorpe, C. Chow, J. Liddle, N. Shaw and A. Capon, 'Legionnaires' disease outbreak in Western Sydney', *Communicable Diseases Intelligence* 19/5, 6 March 1995, p. 114.

pneumoniae has recently been recognised as an important pathogen of both the upper and lower respiratory tracts. It is not a new organism, but the recognition of its association with respiratory disease is recent. It is probably transmitted from person to person by the respiratory route, and causes as many as 10% of community-acquired pneumonia.

Mycoplasma can be cultured in the laboratory, but they are very slow-growing and can take up to two weeks to form visible colonies. Thus, diagnosis is usually based on serological tests. Culture of *Chlamydia* is also difficult, so serological tests are also used for infections caused by this organism. It is now possible to detect *C. pneumoniae* directly in a smear of sputum, using fluorescent-labelled antibodies (see Figure 17.8). Tetracyclines are used for the treatment of mycoplasmal and chlamydial pneumonia.

FIGURE 17.8
CHLAMYDIA PNEUMONIAE IDENTIFIED WITH A FLUORESCENT-LABELLED ANTIBODY

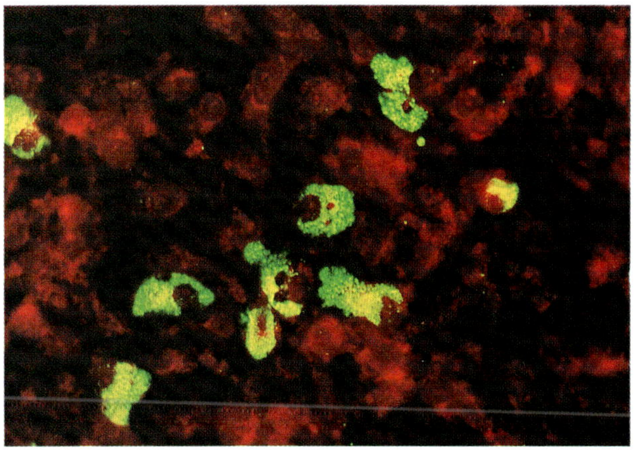

Q fever. The bacterium *C. burnetii* is the cause of **Q fever**, a pneumonia in which chronic infection of the liver, heart valves and other organs may also occur. It was originally recognised in the 1930s in Australia, when it was found to be infecting workers in a Brisbane abattoir. It was given the name Q (for query) fever, because the cause was unknown until Sir Frank Macfarlane Burnet identified the causative agent as a rickettsia. The organism is found in a variety of wild animals, in sheep, and especially in cattle, and is spread from animal to animal via ticks. It is shed in faeces, milk and urine of infected animals. Humans acquire Q fever mainly by consumption of unpasteurised milk or by inhalation of aerosols generated in dairy barns or abattoirs. Farmers can also become infected via contact with contaminated placental material from an infected cow. The organism is very resistant to drying and can be spread by dust or on wool, animal hides and straw. Generally, there are 500–1000 notifications per year in Australia, with highest rates of notification usually in Queensland and New South Wales. *C. burnetii* is removed from milk by pasteurisation.

Many cases of Q fever are asymptomatic. It has an incubation period of 1–4 weeks, and produces an influenza-like illness of severe headache, fever and muscle pain lasting 1–2 weeks. Pneumonia or mild hepatitis may subsequently develop. Endocarditis, which may occur years later, is one of the more serious possible complications.

C. burnetii can be grown in cell culture, but diagnosis is usually by serological means. Treatment with tetracyclines is generally effective. A Q fever vaccine, consisting of killed organisms, is available and recommended for those at risk (e.g. abattoir workers and veterinarians). Severe reactions to this vaccine can occur in individuals already immune, so a person's immunity and skin sensitivity to the vaccine antigens should first be tested.

Ornithosis. Sir Frank Macfarlane Burnet also identified *C. psittaci* in the 1930s, in Australian parrots. This bacterium causes a pneumonia called **ornithosis** (or **psittacosis**), acquired by inhalation of dust particles from bird droppings, especially parrots, but also budgerigars, pigeons, ducks and other birds. Sometimes, the birds themselves also suffer from a diarrhoeal or respiratory illness. Infections in humans are found mainly in people who keep birds as pets. Ornithosis is notifiable throughout Australia, except in New South Wales. There are 100–150 cases reported per year, with no clear geographical or seasonal trend. Most cases are mild and self-limiting, but severe pneumonia occurs in some patients.

Diagnosis of ornithosis is usually by serological testing or by antigen detection in sputum using a fluorescent antibody technique. Tetracyclines are generally effective in the treatment of ornithosis.

Melioidosis. **Melioidosis** is caused by the soil organism *Burkholderia pseudomallei*. It is a disease found mainly in tropical areas, including South-East Asia and northern Australia. Most cases in Australia come from the Northern Territory and Queensland. In the Northern Territory, 76 cases (20 deaths) were reported in the four years between 1989 and 1993[1].

Humans become infected via skin lesions or inhalation, and possibly by ingestion of organisms. The most common form of illness is pneumonia, but the organism can spread via the bloodstream to almost any organ of the body. Abscesses can form in the skin, spleen, prostate and other organs. Mortality is usually associated with certain other factors, particularly alcoholism and diabetes.

Laboratory diagnosis is by culture of sputum, blood, or other specimen from the likely site of infection, although growth can take up to six days. Ceftazidime is the drug of choice, followed by maintenance therapy with doxycycline or cotrimoxazole for three months to prevent relapse.

Viral causes

A number of viruses can cause pneumonia. Adenoviruses and influenza viruses are occasional causes of pneumonia, when they spread from their usual sites of infection higher up in the respiratory tract. Similarly, RSV and parainfluenza viruses occasionally cause pneumonia in infants when infection extends beyond the bronchioles. Viruses tend to cause an interstitial pneumonia—that is, one that involves the interstitium of the lung. Some viruses do not themselves cause pneumonia but may, by damaging tissues and defences, predispose the patient to secondary bacterial pneumonia.

Measles virus can cause pneumonia in individuals with impaired immune defences, or, under certain circumstances, cause enough damage to predispose the person to secondary bacterial pneumonia. In children in developing countries, secondary bacterial pneumonia is a frequent complication of measles infection. Cytomegalovirus does not normally cause respiratory illness, but in immunocompromised patients (e.g. transplant recipients and AIDS patients) it can give rise to an interstitial pneumonia. Measles and cytomegalovirus infections are discussed more fully in Chapters 16 and 19, respectively.

Chronic Infections of the Lower Respiratory Tract

TUBERCULOSIS

Tuberculosis, or consumption, as it was formerly called, has plagued the world since ancient times, and is still one of the major diseases affecting humans. In the developing world, it still ranks as one of the most common causes of death due to a single infectious agent.

Incidence

Approximately 8 million new cases occur in the world each year, with 2–3 million deaths. In developed countries, the incidence has declined significantly this century (see Figure 17.9), but in some countries there is a recent, disturbing trend of increased occurrence, linked partially to infection with the human immunodeficiency virus. In the United States, the annual incidence of tuberculosis has been rising since 1985, increasing by 17% between 1987 and 1991. In the United Kingdom and Europe there have also been reports of rises in incidence.

In Australia, about 1000 cases of tuberculosis are reported each year. The notification rate in Australia has not been increasing in recent years, and the overall rate of less than 6 cases per 100 000 population per year compares favourably with those from other countries. The highest rates of infection are in the northern parts of the country (see Figure 17.10), reflecting the high incidence in the Aboriginal and Islander populations. Other high-risk groups include people born overseas (especially those from China, Vietnam, Cambodia, other South-East Asian countries and the Philippines), the homeless, and people infected with the human immunodeficiency virus (HIV).

Lung disease is the most common form of tuberculosis, but the organism may infect other sites (e.g. the lymphatic system, meninges, bones and joints) and sometimes cause a generalised infection ('miliary' tuberculosis). It can affect the apparently healthy as well as being a serious disease of the immunocompromised. Tuberculosis is one of the more common opportunistic infections associated with HIV infection.

Apart from its persistence worldwide, the other main concern with tuberculosis is the emergence of strains that are resistant to more than one standard anti-tuberculous drug—referred to as multidrug-resistant tuberculosis (MDR-TB). In the United States, there have been a number of outbreaks of MDR-TB, affecting patients and health care workers in hospitals and inmates and guards in prisons. At present, most of these strains are resistant to two drugs (isoniazid and rifampicin), but some have been found to be resistant to as many as seven drugs. In Australia, less than 2% of isolates are currently found to be resistant to isoniazid and rifampicin.

Cause and transmission

Tuberculosis is caused mainly by the rod-shaped, acid-fast bacterium *Mycobacterium tuberculosis*, but other species of mycobacteria, *M. bovis* and *M. africanum*, can also be responsible. The usual source of infection is a person with pulmonary or laryngeal tuberculosis, who can emit enormous numbers of mycobacteria when coughing. The organisms are passed on in aerosols or dust. They can survive for long periods in air and dust because of their waxy outer coat that allows them to resist drying. Generally, people with tuberculosis of other organs (e.g. bone marrow or kidneys) are unlikely to be contagious, except during surgery or autopsy procedures, when there may be contact with infected tissues or aerosolisation of organisms in the tissues.

M. tuberculosis grows very slowly, with a generation time of 20 hours or more, compared with 20–30 minutes for most bacteria.

Pathogenesis

In primary infection, the organisms are engulfed by the alveolar macrophages. However, the bacteria can both survive and multiply in these cells because of their resistance to intracellular killing. This appears to be based either on resistance to phagocytic enzymes or an ability of the bacterium to escape the phagolysosome. The macrophages eventually carry the bacteria via the

FIGURE 17.9
ANNUAL RATE OF NOTIFICATIONS OF TUBERCULOSIS IN AUSTRALIA 1917–91

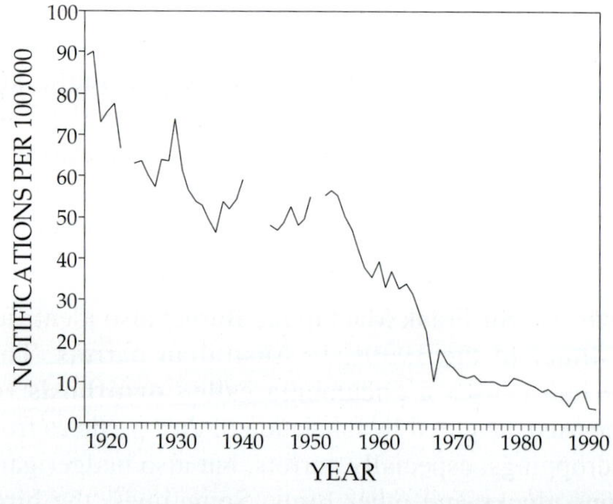

Source: Communicable Diseases Intelligence 17/11, 31 May 1993.

FIGURE 17.10
ANNUAL RATE OF NOTIFICATION OF TUBERCULOSIS IN AUSTRALIA PER 100 000 POPULATION IN 1993, BY STATISTICAL DIVISION OF RESIDENCE

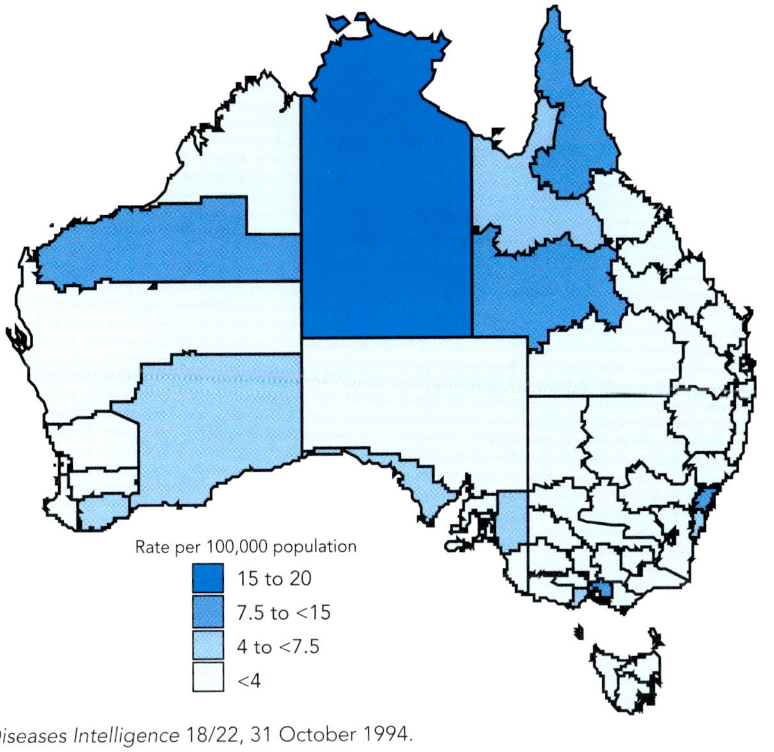

Source: Communicable Diseases Intelligence 18/22, 31 October 1994.

lymphatics to the local lymph nodes, where an immune response, predominantly cell-mediated immunity (CMI), is stimulated. The CMI response acts to prevent the spread of the bacteria by causing the release of lymphokines from sensitised T cells, which activate macrophages and increase their ability to destroy the bacteria. In addition, an infiltration of cells (lymphocytes, macrophages and epithelioid cells) to the sites of infection serves to contain the organisms within **tubercles**, small granulomas consisting of epithelioid cells and giant cells. This type of lesion in the lung, plus the enlarged lymph nodes, is called the **Ghon** (or primary) **complex**.

After a time, the material within the granuloma becomes necrotic and caseous (cheesy). In people who are otherwise healthy, the tubercles may heal spontaneously, become fibrotic or calcified and persist as such for a lifetime. They will show up years later on a chest X-ray. However, in a small percentage of people with primary infection, particularly in the immunocompromised, the mycobacteria are not destroyed or contained within the tubercles. Instead, they invade the bloodstream and cause a potentially fatal disseminated disease (called **miliary tuberculosis**). Tubercles may then form in many organs, including the liver, spleen, kidneys and meninges.

In some people, the activated macrophages never completely eliminate these extremely hardy bacteria, even though the patients recover clinically from the primary infection. It appears that the mycobacteria produce substances that interfere with macrophage activation by lymphokines. The bacteria can remain dormant within granulomas for many years because the macrophages have controlled their multiplication but not killed them.

Secondary tuberculosis occurs in a small percentage of people, often many years later; this is due to reactivation of dormant mycobacteria, usually as a consequence of impaired immune function resulting from factors such as malnutrition, infection (e.g. AIDS), chemotherapy for treatment of malignancies, or corticosteroids for treatment of inflammatory diseases. Obviously, anything that compromises either T cell or macrophage function can lead to reactivation. Reactivation usually occurs in the apex of the lungs, fitting more closely the classical form of tuberculosis. This site is more highly oxygenated and allows the mycobacteria to multiply more rapidly. The pathogenesis of tuberculosis is illustrated in Figure 17.11.

Clinical features

Primary tuberculosis is completely asymptomatic in most immunocompetent people, in whom there may be only a small lesion in the periphery of the lung and minor enlargement of draining lymph nodes. In the symptomatic, the onset of symptoms is often insidious, infection proceeding for some time before the patient develops fever, weight loss and malaise, and becomes sufficiently ill to seek medical attention. Without treatment, pneumonia-like symptoms often develop, with production of blood-stained sputum. The infection can resolve spontaneously or the organisms may spread locally to cause pleurisy or bronchopneumonia, or via the bloodstream to cause meningitis or disseminated disease.

In miliary tuberculosis, numerous small granulomas (resembling millet seed, hence the name) develop in a variety of tissues. The prognosis is poor in this form of

FIGURE 17.11
THE PATHOGENESIS OF TUBERCULOSIS

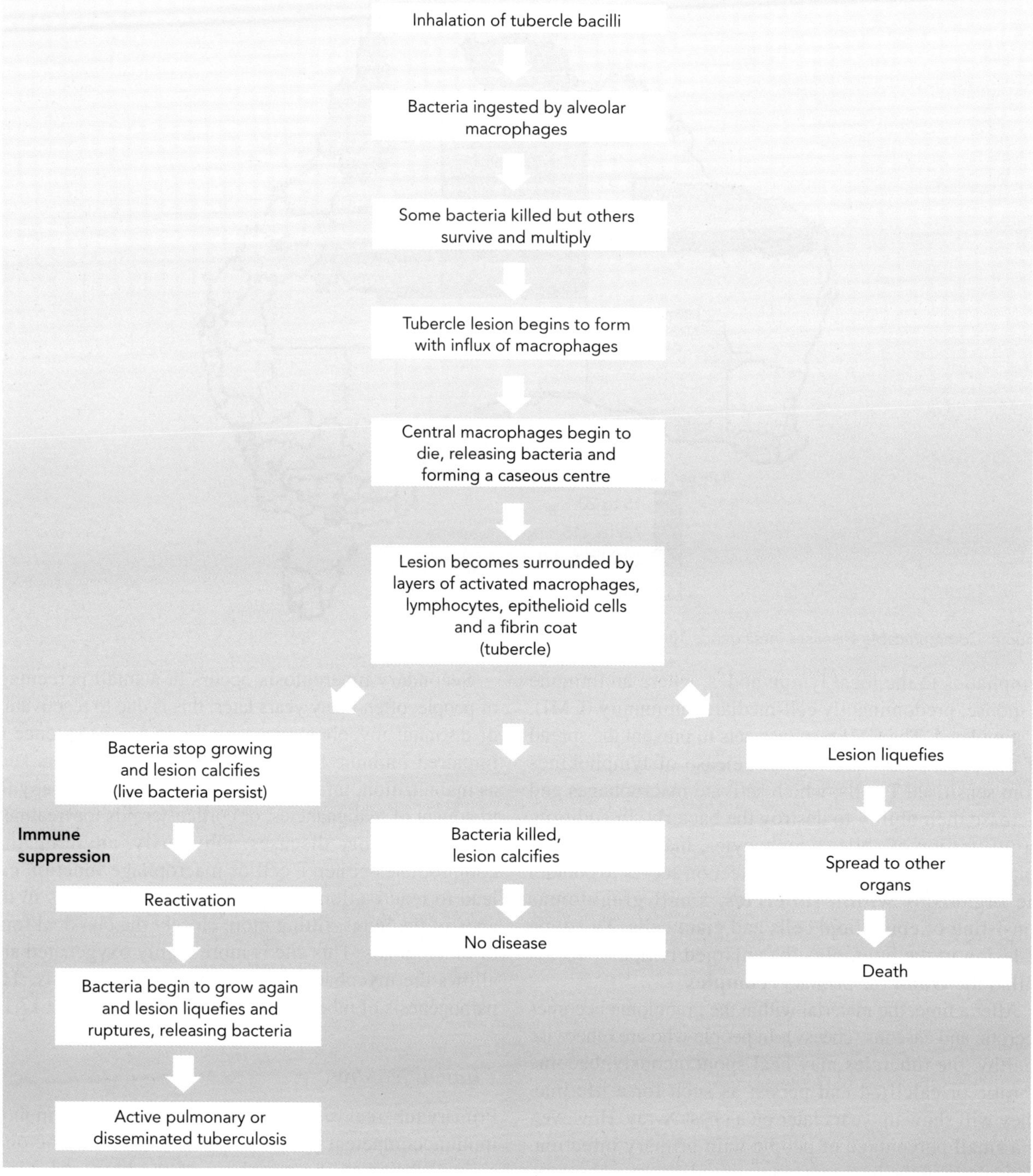

the disease. Infection may be confined to the abdominal viscera, especially in *M. bovis* infection or in *M. tuberculosis* infection acquired by ingestion. Factors that increase the probability of a person becoming symptomatic include co-infection with HIV, immunosuppression, alcoholism, renal failure and diabetes mellitus.

Secondary infection may occur in virtually any organ because the mycobacteria have the ability to colonise almost any site in the body. The clinical manifestations are variable: fatigue, weight loss, weakness and fever are all associated with tuberculosis. When infection occurs in the lungs there is characteristically a chronic cough productive of sputum, which may be blood-stained as a result of tissue destruction.

Diagnosis

A diagnosis of tuberculosis is usually made by the clinical signs and symptoms, supported by chest X-ray findings and a positive tuberculin (Mantoux) skin test (see below). Confirmation is by demonstration of acid-fast rods in sputum stained by Ziehl-Neelsen's method (see Figure 17.12), and culture of *M. tuberculosis* from sputum. With microscopic examination of a smear of sputum, a result

FIGURE 17.12

ZIEHL-NEELSEN STAIN OF SPUTUM

Acid-fast (pink) rods of *Mycobacterium tuberculosis* against a blue background.

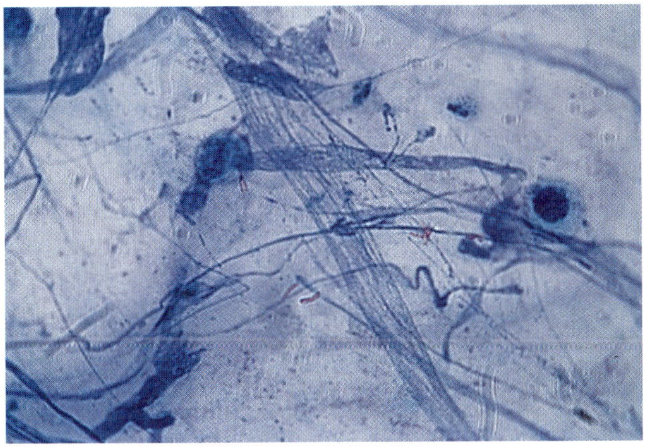

FIGURE 17.13

PNEUMOCYSTIS CARINII (FLUORESCENT ANTIBODY STAIN)

Found by microscopic examination of sputum, lung biopsy or bronchial alveolar lavage

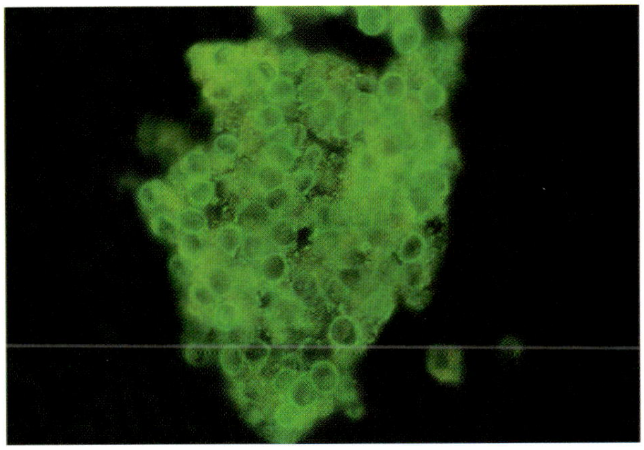

CASE HISTORY 17.5
TUBERCULOSIS

In 1979, a 57-year-old man was admitted to hospital with fever and rapidly increasing breathlessness. He had been treated with cytotoxic drugs three months earlier, after a bronchial biopsy had shown that he had a small cell carcinoma in the left lung. There was some improvement initially but he soon became much more dyspnoeic, and radiotherapy to the upper part of his body was begun two weeks before his final admission to hospital.

Consolidation of the left lung was obvious on both physical examination and chest X-ray. No likely pathogens were isolated from sputum or blood cultures, and the patient died after three days of intensive treatment with antibiotics.

At autopsy on the following day, the primary tumour could not be found although the pathologist cut numerous sections through the lung. Macroscopically, the consolidation was thought to be due to carcinomatous infiltration rather than to infection. Ten days later, routine histology revealed its tuberculous nature and very many acid-fast bacilli were demonstrated. Miliary tubercules were also found in the spleen.

A group of 48 newly enrolled third-year medical students attended the autopsy demonstration on this patient. Following the usual practice at the University of Sydney, these students were scheduled to have Mantoux tests during their first term, so that those with negative results could complete BCG vaccination before they began their clinical training in the hospitals. The risk of students being exposed to tuberculosis during the weekly autopsy demonstrations in this early part of their Paraclinical Science course had been regarded as remote because the total number of deaths from tuberculosis in New South Wales was less than 40 per year; that is, less than 0.1% of all deaths.

One week after the autopsy, Mantoux tests were performed by the Student Health Service on all the third-year medical students. These tests were read on the same day as the histological examination of the autopsy specimen was taking place. Although some students were given BCG vaccination that day, when the histology result became available, the other vaccinations were withheld while the situation was assessed.

It was found that 13 of the students in the exposed group were already Mantoux positive, eight because of previous BCG vaccinations. None subsequently developed clinical evidence of active tuberculosis. When Mantoux tests were repeated two months later, 13 of the 35 students who had previously tested negative had converted to positive. Five of these 13 were among those who had received BCG vaccine 'on the spot', before the Department was notified of the histology result.

That is, of the 35 Mantoux-negative students at risk:

- Twenty-two had no evidence of infection two months later. They were then vaccinated with BCG.
- Five had inadvertently received BCG soon after exposure. They were kept under clinical surveillance. All had normal chest X-rays in July 1981.
- Eight had presumptive evidence of infection. They were advised to take isoniazid prophylactically, and chest X-rays were taken after six months and two years.

Although some did not take isoniazid, seven of the eight remained well, with no evidence of active tuberculosis. One who had elected to take isoniazid developed a minimal radiological lesion in the upper zone of the right lung and acid-fast bacilli were detected in one gastric aspirate six weeks after exposure. Culture yielded *M. tuberculosis*. He was treated with standard therapy and the radiological lesion resolved.

Adapted from D. Wilkins, A.J. Woolcock & Y.E. Cossart, 'Tuberculosis: medical students at risk', *Medical Journal of Australia*, 160, 1994, p. 395.

can be obtained within an hour of receipt of the specimen by the laboratory. This is important because *M. tuberculosis* can take up to six weeks to form visible colonies in culture. Culture enables drug sensitivity testing to be performed. A PCR (polymerase chain reaction) diagnostic kit has recently been developed for the detection of *M. tuberculosis* in sputum and bronchial alveolar lavage specimens.

Tuberculin (Mantoux) skin test

A skin test is performed by intradermal injection of tuberculin, a purified protein derivative (PPD) of *M. tuberculosis*, and examination 48–72 hours later for a reddening and thickening (induration) of the skin at the site of injection. This is a delayed hypersensitivity reaction to the antigen (see Chapter 9). A strongly positive tuberculin skin test is suggestive of active or recent infection. A weak reaction may reflect past infection or vaccination. A negative reaction may exclude infection, although positive reactions can become negative when a person's cellular immunity is depressed by immunosuppressive therapy, other infection, or by tuberculosis itself. The skin test is most useful as an indicator of infection if a baseline test before exposure is available for comparison.

Treatment

The basis of treating drug-sensitive tuberculosis is the use of three or four drugs in combination therapy (usually isoniazid, rifampicin, pyrazinamide and ethambutol). *M. tuberculosis* rapidly develops resistance to anti-tuberculosis drugs, but this is minimised with combination therapy, which is continued until the patient has been completely cured. Treatment is usually continued for at least six months after sputum tests become negative for tuberculosis bacilli, because the bacteria can remain hidden in intracellular locations for long periods and be difficult to reach with antibiotics. With good compliance, the cure rate of drug-sensitive tuberculosis approaches 100%, usually without serious side effects of treatment. However, patient compliance for prolonged therapy can be difficult to achieve, especially after they start to feel well. Failure to complete the full drug treatment can result in incomplete elimination of the organism and the development of resistance.

If the organism is multidrug-resistant (i.e. resistant to isoniazid and rifampicin and possibly other drugs), a course of treatment with more toxic second-line drugs, such as ofloxacin, ciprofloxacin, ethionamide and kanamycin, is needed. Treatment for as long as 24 months may be required and the cure rate falls below 50% in the immunocompetent, and much lower in the immunosuppressed.

Prevention

Prevention of tuberculosis in areas of low prevalence is based on case finding and effective treatment, and contact tracing and chemoprophylaxis with isoniazid. The BCG (Bacille Calmette et Guerin) vaccine, a suspension of live, attenuated *M. bovis*, was developed in the 1920s by the French bacteriologists Albert Calmette and Alphonse Guerin of the Pasteur Institute. In high-risk areas, BCG vaccination of children should be considered. It is also recommended for children under the age of five who are going to live in countries of high incidence, for Aboriginal and Torres Strait Islander children in areas of high incidence, and for neonates born to women with leprosy (to protect against leprosy—see Chapter 20). Its general use in low risk areas is no longer recommended because of its variable efficacy (reported to be 0–80%). Furthermore, in low-risk countries it is considered to be a disadvantage, because it interferes with the use of the tuberculin test to identify recent infection and hence with the use of chemoprophylaxis to prevent active infection.

In hospitals, patients with active tuberculosis should be isolated from non-tuberculous patients in a well-ventilated room. Patients should be educated to cover their mouths when coughing or sneezing, and on the careful disposal of sputum. Other people entering the room should wear a mask.

Certain health care workers have a high risk of exposure, particularly nurses and doctors, staff of chest clinics and tuberculosis wards, physiotherapists, autopsy room staff and microbiology laboratory staff. Such people, if Mantoux negative, should have routine tuberculin skin tests. The use of BCG in these people is controversial and the National Health and Medical Research Council currently suggests that the decision to vaccinate should be made by local public health authorities[2].

Rapid diagnosis and treatment of infected patients and properly implemented infection control procedures are important approaches, since the greatest risk in hospitals comes from undiagnosed cases. The incidence of *M. bovis* infections is controlled by pasteurisation of milk, and screening and eradication of infected cattle.

Atypical mycobacteria infections

In the last decade, the role of other species of *Mycobacterium* in causing tuberculosis-like illnesses has been recognised. *M. avium* and *M. intracellulare*, often referred to as the *Mycobacterium avium* complex (MAC) or *M. avium-intracellulare*, are the most important of these, but there are other species, including *M. kansasii*, *M. fortuitum*, *M. chelonei* and *M. scrofulaceum*. MAC has come to prominence as a result of the AIDS epidemic but, curiously, it is not very common in people immunosuppressed by factors other than the human immunodeficiency virus. It is also rare in immunocompetent people.

In people without AIDS, MAC most often causes a pulmonary infection, usually in association with an underlying lung disorder. In people with AIDS, the gastrointestinal tract is often the primary site of infection, but disseminated disease is common in the end stages of AIDS. The diagnosis is difficult because MAC is ubiquitous in the environment (water, soil, dust) and is sometimes isolated from clinical specimens in the absence of infection. Blood culture is the most reliable method for diagnosis. These mycobacteria are atypical in being resistant to most anti-tuberculous drugs. Many of the drugs used to treat the infection are toxic, and the ideal regimen has yet to be determined.

FUNGAL PNEUMONIA

A variety of fungal spores is usually present in air, but these organisms are much less frequent causes of lower respiratory tract infection than bacteria and viruses. In the main, fungi are opportunistic pathogens, and so most infections are seen in immunosuppressed patients. Given the increasing number of people who are immunosuppressed as a result of treatment (e.g. chemotherapy, corticosteroids, radiotherapy), infection (e.g. AIDS) and other diseases (e.g. cancer), the number of infections has also increased significantly over the last two decades. Several fungi can cause a chronic type of pneumonia.

Pneumocystis pneumonia

Pneumocystis carinii is a ubiquitous organism that was originally classified as a protozoan, but is now recognised to be more closely related to fungi. This organism has come to prominence with the AIDS epidemic. It is the most common infectious complication of AIDS and a major cause of death in those patients. It can also infect other immunocompromised individuals, as well as infants and the elderly.

P. carinii infects the tissue surrounding the alveoli, in which a foamy exudate forms, containing large numbers of the thick-walled cyst form of the organism. Typical symptoms include fever, dyspnoea and cyanosis. Laboratory diagnosis is by microscopic demonstration of the organism in a specimen from the patient (Figure 17.13). Sputum is rarely positive, so lung biopsy or bronchial alveolar lavage may be necessary. The organism is usually sensitive to cotrimoxazole, but treatment frequently fails because of the associated immune deficiency. Strains resistant to cotrimoxazole have been isolated in other countries (e.g. the United States and in Europe).

Cryptococcal pneumonia

Cryptococcus neoformans is an encapsulated yeast that is widely distributed in nature. A number of serotypes exist, belonging to two subspecies: *C. neoformans* var. *neoformans* and *C. neoformans* var. *gatti*. Like other fungi, these organisms mainly cause infection in the immunocompromised, especially in patients with HIV infection. The major route of infection is the respiratory tract, where these organisms cause pneumonia. However, in most patients, the organisms quickly spread to the brain and thus the presenting symptoms often reflect a meningitis, rather than pneumonia. In lung infection, the organism can be observed in sputum. A microscopic examination of the specimen treated with India ink stain shows the yeast cell with its characteristic large capsule. Chapter 20, on central nervous system infections, has further information on *C. neoformans*.

Other causes

A number of other fungi can cause pneumonia. Exposure of immunosuppressed individuals to the widespread, airborne spores of *Aspergillus fumigatus* can result in pulmonary infection. Similarly, exposure to spores of *Rhizopus* and *Mucor* can also lead to infection. Other possible causes are listed in Table 17.5.

PARASITIC INFECTIONS OF THE LUNG

Various parasitic infections may involve the lung. Certain nematodes, namely *Ascaris* and some hookworms, transiently infect the lungs as their larvae migrate through the body on their way to the intestine. The tapeworm, *Echinococcus granulosus*, can infect the lungs, and form hydatid cysts in the lung tissue. The cysts can become quite large and cause considerable respiratory dysfunction. These helminth infections are discussed more fully in Chapter 18.

Summary

- Respiratory infections are among the most common that afflict humans.
- Respiratory pathogens may be expelled in enormous numbers by coughing and sneezing.
- Several potentially pathogenic microbes form part of the normal flora of the upper respiratory tract.
- Factors that predispose people to respiratory infections include young age, old age, cigarette smoking, chronic obstructive pulmonary disease, poor living standards, alcoholism, immunosuppression, and cancer.
- Most acute respiratory infections are caused by viruses, but the more severe diseases are generally caused by bacteria.
- Fungi and protozoa are important causes of pneumonia, but are restricted mainly to immunocompromised people.

UPPER RESPIRATORY TRACT INFECTIONS

- Most upper respiratory infections are due to viruses, and most are self-limiting, mild infections.

THE COMMON COLD

- The common cold mainly involves infection and inflammation of the nasal passages (rhinitis or coryza) and the oropharynx (pharyngitis).
- Rhinoviruses are the most common causes, followed by coronaviruses.
- A cold is characterised by a blocked or runny nose with excessive nasal discharge and sneezing, and a sore throat.
- Cold viruses are transmitted by coughing and sneezing, and by hands and objects that have become contaminated with nasal secretions.
- The illness is generally mild and self-limiting with no effective treatment.

MIDDLE EAR INFECTIONS

- Infections involving the middle ear are called otitis media. They occur most often in infants and small children.
- *S. pneumoniae* and *H. influenzae* are the most common causes.
- Chronic middle ear infections are due to bacteria such as *Pseudomonas aeruginosa*, *Proteus* spp., and *S. pneumoniae*.
- Earache and fever are the usual symptoms.
- The infection is usually successfully treated empirically with antibiotics such as amoxicillin or penicillin.

ACUTE SINUSITIS

- The major causes of acute sinusitis are *S. pneumoniae* and *H. influenzae*.
- Clinical features include facial pain, a nasal discharge that is often purulent, and headache.
- The patient is usually treated empirically with ampicillin or amoxycillin.

PHARYNGITIS AND TONSILLITIS

- Pharyngitis, or sore throat, is a common condition caused by many different organisms, but usually viruses.
- When the tonsils are affected, it is called tonsillitis.
- Apart from a sore throat, the patient may have a fever, chills, enlarged lymph nodes in the neck, and a headache.
- Adenoviruses are particularly common causes of sore throat.
- Epstein-Barr (EB) virus causes a pharyngitis in the disease called glandular fever.
- The most important bacterial causes are *Streptococcus pyogenes*, *Corynebacterium diphtheriae* (diphtheria), *Haemophilus influenzae* type b (epiglottitis), and *Neisseria gonorrhoeae* (pharyngeal gonorrhoea).
- *Candida albicans* is an important cause of pharyngitis in the immunosuppressed.
- *S. pyogenes* causes less than 10% of cases of acute pharyngitis, but is important because of the possibility of the serious complications of rheumatic fever and acute glomerulonephritis.

DIPHTHERIA

- Diphtheria is an acute infectious disease caused by toxin-producing strains of *Corynebacterium diphtheriae*.
- Cases in developed countries occur mainly in non-immunised people.
- The organism is usually transmitted by the air-borne route from infected people or asymptomatic carriers.
- *C. diphtheriae* secretes a toxin in the respiratory tract that destroys the epithelial surface; an ulcer forms and becomes covered by a greyish membrane.
- The bacteria multiply locally without invading deeper tissues or spreading to other sites in the body, but the toxin is absorbed into the bloodstream.
- Cardiac failure and death can result from the action of the toxin on the heart.
- Diphtheria is a life-threatening disease requiring urgent diagnosis and treatment.
- A diagnosis of diphtheria is confirmed by the isolation and identification of toxin-producing corynebacteria in a swab from under the membrane.
- Immediate treatment with antitoxin should be commenced, and penicillin or erythromycin given in conjunction.
- Diphtheria vaccine is currently incorporated in the diphtheria, tetanus and pertussis (DTP) triple vaccine and the combined diphtheria and tetanus (CDT) vaccine.

ACUTE EPIGLOTTITIS

- Epiglottitis, inflammation of the epiglottis, is most often seen in young children, and is almost always caused by *Haemophilus influenzae* type b.
- Bacteraemia is usually present and the patient is usually toxic and febrile.
- There may be respiratory distress because of obstruction of the airway.
- Epiglottitis is a medical emergency. An endotracheal tube is usually inserted and antibiotic treatment begun immediately.

- The clinical diagnosis is confirmed by isolating bacteria from blood and possibly the epiglottis.
- *H. influenzae* vaccines have been part of the standard childhood vaccination schedule since 1993.

LARYNGOTRACHEITIS

- Laryngotracheitis (inflammation of the larynx and trachea), or croup, is characterised by stridor, hoarseness and a resonant cough, due to oedema and spasm of the larynx.
- Croup is most common in children under four, because of the narrowness of their larynx.
- In adults, laryngotracheitis causes hoarseness and a burning pain during breathing, usually without obstruction of the larynx.
- Laryngotracheitis is usually caused by viruses, especially the parainfluenza group.
- The diagnosis of viral croup is based on clinical and radiologic examination.
- Patient management is based on humidification to soften mucus and soothe the inflamed mucosa, and oxygenation. Intubation or tracheostomy may be performed if complete obstruction is likely.

LOWER RESPIRATORY TRACT INFECTIONS

- Because the lower respiratory tract is normally sterile, infections involving it are potentially serious.
- Pathogenic microorganisms may reach the lower respiratory tract by inhalation, aspiration or spread of infection from the upper respiratory tract or via the bloodstream.

PERTUSSIS

- Pertussis (whooping cough) is a severe disease caused by the Gram-negative coccobacillus, *Bordetella pertussis*.
- A highly infectious disease that affects mainly children, pertussis is spread from person to person by air-borne droplets.
- Its incidence in developed countries has been markedly reduced by immunisation.
- The organism multiplies in respiratory epithelial cells but does not invade further.
- The organism produces several toxins, which combine to produce the symptoms of disease.
- There is an initial catarrhal illness, characterised by runny nose, infrequent cough and mild fever. The cough, caused by an accumulation of mucus in the airway, gradually becomes more irritating and paroxysmal.
- A paroxysm is a series of short coughs followed by a 'whoop'.
- Possible complications include cerebral hypoxia, bronchopneumonia and secondary pneumonia.
- The organisms can be isolated from throat swabs or on 'cough plates'.
- A direct fluorescent antibody test to detect the organism in nasopharyngeal aspirates is commonly used.
- Supportive care, including oxygen and suctioning, is of prime importance.
- Antibiotics are useful to help reduce the spread of infection to others.
- Immunisation against pertussis is recommended from two months of age.
- Pertussis vaccine is usually combined with diphtheria and tetanus toxoids and administered as DTP or triple antigen.

BRONCHITIS

- Acute bronchitis represents an inflammation of the tracheobronchial tree.
- Viruses are the most common causes, including influenza virus, common cold viruses and adenoviruses.
- The syptoms of chronic bronchitis are chronic or recurrent cough and excessive secretion of mucus.

BRONCHIOLITIS

- Bronchiolitis occurs mainly in children less than two years old.
- Most infections are caused by the respiratory syncytial virus (RSV).
- RSV is highly infectious and causes community and hospital outbreaks in winter.
- Infection in infants can be severe if the virus invades the lower respiratory tract.
- Typical symptoms include fever, coryza, cough and respiratory obstruction.
- Most cases begin to resolve within a few days, but recurrent infections are common.
- RSV-specific antigens in nasopharyngeal washings are detectable by immunofluorescence or ELISA.

INFLUENZA

- Influenza viruses (myxoviruses) cause a range of clinical conditions affecting all levels of the respiratory tract.
- Influenza A viruses cause epidemics, and occasionally pandemics. Influenza B viruses cause epidemics.
- The envelope of an influenza virus has two surface glycoprotein antigens: the haemagglutinin (H) and neuraminidase (N) spikes.
- Over time, influenza viruses can vary their H and N antigens by antigenic drift and antigenic shift.
- Transmission of influenza is by droplet inhalation and fomites.
- One to three days after infection, symptoms such as fever, chills, malaise and muscle pain develop. Recovery usually occurs within 1–3 weeks.
- Secondary bacterial infection can occur, especially in those with chronic obstructive pulmonary disease.
- Mortality is highest in the elderly and the debilitated and is usually due to secondary bacterial pneumonia or exacerbation of chronic cardiac or respiratory disease.
- Rest, fluids and analgesics form the basis of treatment.
- Amantadine and rimantadine can be used prophylactically to prevent outbreaks in the elderly.

- Influenza virus vaccine, when given before the epidemic season arrives, offers partial protection, but only against strains covered by the vaccine.
- Vaccination is recommended for high-risk individuals, such as the elderly and debilitated, and people with chronic cardiopulmonary disease.

PNEUMONIA

- Pneumonia is an infection and inflammation of the lungs and is a major cause of death throughout the world.
- Bacteria and viruses cause the vast majority of cases, but fungi can also be responsible, especially in the immunocompromised.
- Pneumonia is the most commonly fatal type of nosocomial infection.
- Patients with pneumonia usually present with a fever, chest pain and cough.
- Lobar pneumonia is an infection and consolidation confined to one or two lobes of the lung.
- Bronchopneumonia is a more diffuse, patchy inflammation of the lungs, with numerous, small foci of consolidation throughout the lungs.
- The outcome common to both types of pneumonia is respiratory distress.
- A pleural effusion occurs if the inflammatory exudate enters the space between the lung tissue and pleural membranes.
- Empyema is the term used to describe infection of the pleural space, and pleurisy means an inflammation of the pleural membranes.

Bacterial causes of pneumonia

- A chest X-ray and blood and sputum culture are the main methods for diagnosing most bacterial pneumonias.
- First-line treatment of pneumonia, before results are available, is usually with ampicillin and/or erythromycin.
- Even with appropriate antibiotic therapy, pneumonia can be fatal, usually because of rapidly progressive disease or interaction with another, underlying disorder.
- The most common bacterial cause of community-acquired pneumonia is *Streptococcus pneumoniae*.
- The standard treatment for pneumococcal pneumonia is penicillin, but strains with high-level resistance have emerged.
- A polyvalent vaccine *S. pneumoniae* is recommended for those at high risk.
- Staphylococcal pneumonia, due to *Staphylococcus aureus*, is most common as a complication of viral respiratory infection.
- Gram-negative enterobacteria are particularly associated with pneumonia acquired in hospital.
- *Haemophilus influenzae* causes pneumonia, often as an exacerbation of epiglottitis, chronic bronchitis, brochiectasis, septicaemia or meningitis.
- *H. influenzae* mainly affects children under four.
- Several organisms are involved in recurrent or chronic lung infections in patients with cystic fibrosis (CF). *P. aeruginosa* causes a chronic lung infection in most CF patients that is almost impossible to eradicate.
- The predisposition of CF patients to lung infections appears to be related to the production of overly viscid bronchial secretions, and suppression of mucociliary clearance.
- *Legionella pneumophila* and other species of *Legionella* cause a pneumonia referred to as Legionnaires' disease (or legionellosis).
- *Legionella* are spread in air-borne droplets from cooling towers, taps, shower heads and contaminated environmental sources. Person-to-person transmission of legionellosis does not appear to occur.
- Legionnaires' disease is characterised by symptoms of pneumonia, and sometimes diarrhoea, fever, abdominal pain, neurological signs and renal failure.
- Major risk factors of Legionnaires' disease are old age, cigarette smoking, underlying respiratory disease, immunosuppression and alcoholism.
- For the diagnosis of Legionnaires' disease, culture of sputum and serology are the definitive methods.
- Erythromycin usually provides effective treatment for Legionnaires' disease.
- Atypical pneumonia is characterised by diffuse, patchy lesions and an unresponsiveness to normally effective antibacterials.
- The major causes of atypical pneumonia are *Mycoplasma pneumoniae* and *Chlamydia pneumoniae*. Serological tests are the usual means of diagnosing infections caused by *Mycoplasma* and *Chlamydia*, and tetracyclines are used for treatment.
- The bacterium *Chlamydia burnetii* is the cause of Q fever.
- Humans acquire Q fever mainly by drinking unpasteurised milk or by inhaling aerosols generated in dairy barns or abattoirs.
- A Q fever vaccine, consisting of killed organisms, is recommended for those at risk.
- *Chlamydia psittaci* is a bacterium that causes a pneumonia called ornithosis (or psittacosis), acquired by inhaling dust particles from bird droppings. Most cases of ornithosis are mild and self-limiting.
- Melioidosis is caused by the soil organism, *Burkholderia pseudomallei*. Humans become infected with *B. pseudomallei* via skin lesions or inhalation, and the most common form of illness is pneumonia.
- Laboratory diagnosis of melioidosis is by culture of sputum, blood, or other specimen from the likely site of infection; ceftazidime is the drug of choice.

Viral causes of pneumonia

- Adenoviruses and influenza viruses are occasional causes of pneumonia.
- RSV and parainfluenza viruses occasionally cause pneumonia in infants.
- Viruses tend to cause an interstitial pneumonia.

CHRONIC INFECTIONS OF THE LOWER RESPIRATORY TRACT

TUBERCULOSIS

- In the developing world tuberculosis is still one of the most common causes of death.
- In developed countries, tuberculosis has declined significantly, but there is increasing occurrence, partially linked to infection with the human immunodeficiency virus.
- Lung disease is the most common form of tuberculosis.
- A major concern is the emergence of multidrug-resistant strains.
- Tuberculosis is caused mainly by *Mycobacterium tuberculosis*, but other species of mycobacteria can also be responsible.
- The usual source of infection is the person with pulmonary or laryngeal tuberculosis, who can emit enormous numbers of mycobacteria when coughing.
- The organisms can survive for long periods in air and dust.
- In primary infection, an infiltration of cells to the sites of infection serves to contain the organisms within tubercles—small granulomas consisting of epithelioid cells and giant cells.
- In otherwise healthy people, the tubercles may heal spontaneously.
- In a small percentage of people with primary infection, particularly the immunocompromised, the mycobacteria invade the bloodstream and cause a potentially fatal disseminated disease called miliary tuberculosis.
- Primary tuberculosis is asymptomatic in most immunocompetent people.
- Secondary tuberculosis occurs in a small percentage of people and is due to reactivation of dormant mycobacteria, usually as a consequence of impaired immune function.
- A diagnosis of tuberculosis is usually made by the clinical signs and symptoms, supported by chest X-ray findings and a positive tuberculin (Mantoux) skin test; confirmation is by demonstration of acid-fast rods in sputum and culture.
- A skin test is performed by intradermal injection of tuberculin, a purified protein derivative of *M. tuberculosis*, and examination 48–72 hours later for induration of the skin at the site of injection.
- A strongly positive tuberculin skin test is suggestive of active or recent infection.
- The basis of treating drug-sensitive tuberculosis is the use of three or four drugs in combination therapy, usually isoniazid, rifampicin, pyrazinamide and ethambutol.
- Treatment is usually continued for at least six months after sputum tests become negative.
- If the organism is multidrug-resistant, a course of treatment with more toxic second-line drugs is necessary.
- Prevention of tuberculosis in areas of low prevalence is based on case finding and effective treatment, and on contact tracing and chemoprophylaxis with isoniazid.
- In high-risk areas, BCG vaccination should be considered.
- In hospitals, patients with active tuberculosis should be isolated in a well-ventilated room.
- Health care workers with a high risk of exposure should have routine tuberculin skin tests.
- Other species of *Mycobacterium* cause a tuberculosis-like illness, and are referred to as atypical mycobacteria.

FUNGAL PNEUMONIA

- Fungi are mainly opportunistic pathogens, and so most infections occur in immunosuppressed patients.
- *Pneumocystis carinii* is the most common infectious complication of AIDS and a major cause of death in AIDS patients.
- Typical symptoms of *Pneumocystis* pneumonia include fever, dyspnoea and cyanosis.
- Laboratory diagnosis of *Pneumocystis* pneumonia is by microscopic demonstration of the organism in a specimen from the patient.
- *Cryptococcus neoformans* is a yeast that causes infection mainly in the immunocompromised. A microscopic examination of the specimen treated with India ink stain shows the yeast cell with its characteristic large capsule.

PARASITIC INFECTIONS OF THE LUNG

- Certain nematodes and some hookworms transiently infect the lungs as their larvae migrate through the body on their way to the intestine.
- The tapeworm, *Echinococcus granulosus*, can infect the lungs and form hydatid cysts in the lung tissue.

Study Questions

1. List the major defences of the respiratory tract.
2. List the important factors that predispose people to respiratory infections.
3. What type of microorganisms are responsible for the majority of upper respiratory infections?
4. Why do people suffer repeatedly from the common cold?
5. What is otitis media and what are the common causes?
6. What are the common causes of pharyngitis?
7. Why is *Streptococcus pyogenes* an important cause of pharyngitis?
8. What is the cause of diphtheria and what are the major features of this disease?
9. Describe the treatment for diphtheria.
10. How is diphtheria prevented?
11. Why is acute epiglottitis a potentially life-threatening disease?
12. What is croup?
13. How do microorganisms gain access to the lower respiratory tract?
14. Name the cause and describe the pathogenesis of whooping cough.
15. Explain the importance of vaccination against whooping cough, and also describe the disadvantages.
16. What is acute bronchitis and what are the common causes?
17. What is bronchiolitis and what is the usual cause?
18. What is meant by antigenic drift and antigenic shift in influenza viruses?
19. How can people be protected against influenza and who should be protected?
20. What is pneumonia?
21. Distinguish between lobar pneumonia and bronchopneumonia.
22. Define the terms: pleural effusion, pleurisy, empyema.
23. What virulence factor enables *Streptococcus pneumoniae* to cause pneumonia?
24. What specimen(s) is/are commonly collected for the laboratory diagnosis of pneumonia?
25. What is Legionnaires' disease?
26. What are the major risk factors associated with Legionnaires' disease?
27. What is atypical pneumonia and what are the major causes?
28. What is Q fever and how is it acquired by humans?
29. What is ornithosis and how is it acquired by humans?
30. What viruses most commonly cause pneumonia?
31. What are the common clinical features of pneumonia?
32. What are the major aspects of patient management for a person with pneumonia?
33. In which groups in Australia is tuberculosis most commonly found?
34. What sites in the body does *Mycobacterium tuberculosis* infect?
35. Define the terms: tubercle, miliary tuberculosis, secondary tuberculosis.
36. How is tuberculosis diagnosed?
37. What is a Mantoux test and what does it detect?
38. How is tuberculosis treated?
39. What is the greatest risk factor for atypical mycobacteria infection?
40. What is the cause of pneumocystis pneumonia and what is the major risk factor?
41. In a patient with fungal pneumonia, what is the most likely predisposing factor?

Test Your Understanding

Case History 17.1: Epiglottitis

1. Why did Timothy have an endotracheal tube inserted?
2. Why were blood cultures collected from Timothy?
3. *H. influenzae* typically causes infections in children less than four years old. Why is this age group so susceptible?

Case History 17.2: Whooping cough

1. What does this case demonstrate about the transmissibility of whooping cough?
2. Why was SG at high risk of infection?
3. How could SG's infection have been prevented?
4. What does this case demonstrate about the susceptibility of adults to whooping cough?

Case History 17.3: Influenza

1. What evidence confirmed this as an outbreak of influenza?
2. How could this outbreak of influenza have been prevented?
3. Why is influenza infection so important in nursing home residents, and what makes staff infections so important?
4. Why does influenza vaccination have to occur annually?

Case History 17.4: Legionnaires' disease

1. Are the people involved in this outbreak typical of those usually affected by Legionnaires' disease?
2. How is Legionnaires' disease usually acquired?
3. Why are the sources of infection in Legionnaires' disease often difficult to identify?

Case History 17.5: Tuberculosis

1. What was the most likely means of transmission of infection in this outbreak of tuberculosis?
2. What are the advantages and disadvantages of BCG vaccination?
3. What infection control procedures are necessary to prevent the spread of tuberculosis in hospital?
4. What is it about tuberculosis that makes it so difficult to control in a population?

REFERENCES

1. Currie, B., 1993, 'Is melioidosis increasing in tropical Australia?', *The Northern Territory Communicable Diseases Bulletin*, 1(10), p. 1.
2. National Health and Medical Research Council, *The Australian Immunisation Procedures Handbook*, 5th edn., Canberra: Australian Government Publishing Service, 1994.

FURTHER READING

A'Court, C. & C.S. Garrard, 1992, 'Nosocomial pneumonia in the intensive care unit: mechanisms and significance', *Thorax* 47, p. 465. (A summary of the factors that predispose critically ill patients to acquiring pneumonia.)

Hosker, H.S.R., G.M. Jones & P. Hawkey, 1994, 'Management of community-acquired lower respiratory tract infection', *British Medical Journal* 308, p. 701. (A review article detailing the epidemiology, causes, clinical signs and management of patients with lower respiratory tract infections.

Kayser, F.H., 1992, 'Changes in the spectrum of organisms causing respiratory tract infections: a review', *Postgraduate Medical Journal* 68 (suppl. 3), p. S17. (Details the common causative agents of respiratory tract infections, including nosocomial pneumonia.)

Krause, V.L. & W.J. Britton, 1993, 'Tuberculosis in the tropics', *Medical Journal of Australia* 159, p. 412. (This article outlines the extent of the tuberculosis problem in Australia and the rest of the world.)

Skerrett, S. J., 1994, 'Host defences against respiratory infection', *Medical Clinics of North America* 78, p. 941. (A detailed description of the defences of the respiratory tract and some of the common defects that can occur in these defences.)

Yu, V. L., 1993, 'Legionnaires' disease: new understanding of community-acquired pneumonia', *Hospital Practice*, 30 October, p. 63. (A review article that outlines the epidemiology, pathogenesis and treatment of Legionnaires' disease.)

chapter 18

gastrointestinal tract infections

Chapter focus

- *What microorganisms cause acute diarrhoeal disease in humans?*
- *What is the role of microorganisms in peptic ulcer disease?*
- *What microorganisms cause typhoid and paratyphoid fevers?*
- *What helminths are associated with gastrointestinal infections?*
- *What viruses cause hepatitis?*
- *What are the common modes of transmission of gastrointestinal infections?*
- *What are the important clinical features of gastrointestinal infections?*
- *How are gastrointestinal infections treated and how may they be prevented?*

The gastrointestinal tract (GIT) is a portal of entry into the body for numerous microorganisms. Most foods and beverages contain large numbers of organisms, but relatively few of these microbes are capable of taking up residence in the GIT. To establish and cause infection, microbes have to be ingested in sufficient numbers, and be able to circumvent a variety of highly effective antimicrobial defences, which include:

- gastric acidity;
- digestive enzymes;
- bile salts;
- intestinal motility;
- the normal flora of the intestine; and
- specific immune defences provided by the lymphoid tissues of the GIT.

These defences are described in detail in Chapter 9. It should be noted that the gastrointestinal tract is a hostile environment for most microorganisms, the majority of which are killed by the acid of the stomach, and do not even reach the intestine alive. Certain pathogens, however, have properties that enable them to survive these defences.

Most intestinal pathogens remain localised in the gastrointestinal tract, multiplying and/or producing toxins there, and causing local symptoms. There are some, however, that cause more generalised symptoms by invading intestinal tissues and then spreading to other parts of the body. Other microbes cause gastrointestinal disease by growing and secreting toxins (exotoxins) in the food before it is consumed. These diseases have a very short incubation period, because symptoms are produced soon after the preformed toxins are ingested and absorbed.

Most gastrointestinal infections manifest as an acute diarrhoeal disease. In this chapter we will first consider the major causes of acute diarrhoeal disease, which include bacteria, viruses and protozoa. Other forms of gastrointestinal infection in which diarrhoea is not a major symptom include *Helicobacter pylori* infections (gastritis and peptic ulcers) and helminth (worm) infections. Other infections discussed in this chapter are the enteric fevers, typhoid and paratyphoid fever, caused by bacteria that invade the GIT and spread to other parts of the body, and hepatitis, an infection of the liver caused mainly by viruses.

The terminology used to describe infections of the gastrointestinal tract can be very confusing. Some terms are used interchangeably, and some terms are given different meanings by different authors. In this text, **food poisoning** (or **food-borne illness**) is used in a general sense to refer to any gastrointestinal disease related to the consumption of food, including microbial and non-microbial factors. A **gastrointestinal infection** is a disease of the gastrointestinal tract caused by the establishment and multiplication of microorganisms in the gastrointestinal tract. **Food intoxication** is used for diseases caused by the presence of preformed toxins (microbial or non-microbial) in food. Other terms in common use and their meanings as applied in this text are given in Table 18.1.

Acute Diarrhoeal Diseases

A range of microbial pathogens is capable of producing symptoms of diarrhoeal disease. They include those that multiply in the GIT, as well as those that secrete toxins in food (food intoxications). The latter group is discussed separately within this section because of differences in the symptoms they produce and their different modes of pathogenesis. Gastrointestinal pathogens are acquired mainly by the faecal-oral route, from contaminated food, fluids or hands. The major symptom of infection is **acute diarrhoea**, a sudden disruption in bowel habits in which normally formed stools are replaced by more frequent, liquefied movements. Diarrhoea is the result of increased secretion of fluid and electrolytes into the lumen of the intestine, and represents a non-specific response of the intestine to a number of different factors, including infection, the action of toxins, sensitivity to drugs, and ischaemia. However, the most common causes are microbial infections, due to bacteria, viruses or protozoa. Some helminths can cause diarrhoea, but usually only in chronic infections.

Acute diarrhoeal infections can result in a wide range of illnesses, from a mild attack of loose stools lasting one to several days, to a severe illness with considerable fluid loss, which may be fatal. Overall, they are extremely common throughout the world, second only to upper respiratory infections.

TABLE 18.1
COMMON TERMS USED TO DESCRIBE GASTROINTESTINAL INFECTIONS

TERM	DEFINITION
Food poisoning or food-borne illness	Gastrointestinal disease related to the consumption of food containing pathogenic microorganisms or their toxins, or other non-microbial toxins
Gastrointestinal infection	A disease of the gastrointestinal tract caused by the establishment and multiplication of microorganisms in the gastrointestinal tract
Food intoxication	Gastrointestinal disease caused by the consumption of food containing toxins (microbial or non-microbial)
Gastroenteritis	Inflammation of the gastrointestinal tract, including the stomach and intestine
Gastritis	Inflammation of the mucosa of the stomach
Diarrhoea	A disruption in bowel habits characterised by more frequent passage of loose and watery stools
Dysentery	An inflammatory disorder of the gastrointestinal tract characterised by severe diarrhoea with blood and pus in the stools

In developing countries, diarrhoeal diseases are a major cause of morbidity and mortality. It has been estimated that they may be responsible for up to 4.5 million infant and childhood deaths per year. Diarrhoeal disease also contributes to the malnutrition that is prevalent in the children of Third World countries. The magnitude of the problem of diarrhoeal disease in developed countries has declined with economic and public health improvements, but this type of disease is still a common complaint. In the latter context it is, however, usually mild and self-limiting, except in the very young, the elderly, and immunocompromised patients.

THE EPIDEMIOLOGY OF ACUTE INFECTIOUS DIARRHOEA

Acute infectious diarrhoea is usually acquired through ingestion of pathogenic microorganisms. Common sources of the organisms include:

- food or water contaminated with faeces;
- faecally contaminated hands;
- food contaminated with faecal organisms spread by flies.

Many pathogens of the intestinal tract are able to survive for at least a short time in the environment and on the surface of fomites. Some can survive for long periods in polluted natural water courses.

The highest incidence of acute diarrhoeal disease is in areas of the world where there are poor facilities for sanitation and sewage disposal. Transmission is mainly via contaminated food or water. In developed countries, food-borne transmission is the most common (e.g. in campers, or in people who have eaten at a restaurant or bulk catering facility), but acute diarrhoeal disease also occurs in international travellers, hospitalised people, and those people with AIDS. Outbreaks sometimes occur in hospital nurseries and day-care centres. Certain microbes tend to be associated with each of these epidemiological settings (see Table 18.2).

Food-borne gastroenteritis

Food-borne gastroenteritis is a common cause of acute infectious diarrhoea. The majority of cases are due to bacteria, but viruses and parasites can also be involved. Food-borne illness can occur when contaminated meats or seafood are eaten raw or are undercooked, or when food is improperly preserved, allowing significant multiplication of organisms in the food before its consumption. Generally, slightly contaminated food poses little risk if cooked properly and eaten fresh. Different foods tend to harbour certain types of organisms, as shown in Table 18.2.

Most cases of food-borne gastroenteritis are self-limiting, resolving in a few days with supportive care only. However, in certain situations, severe and even life-threatening disease can occur. Young children, the elderly and the immunosuppressed are particularly susceptible. Children can dehydrate very rapidly, and may require hospitalisation and intravenous fluids.

Hospital nurseries

Many pathogens can cause diarrhoeal disease in neonates. The infant can become infected by bacteria or viruses during passage through the birth canal, or after birth, from parents, siblings, hospital personnel or from contaminated formula or water. Because of the immaturity of their immune system, they are highly susceptible to any potential pathogens encountered. Some infections can be very serious and represent a potential danger to other infants in the nursery. Nursery outbreaks sometimes occur, often initiated by an asymptomatic infant shedding the organism.

TABLE 18.2
EPIDEMIOLOGICAL ASSOCIATIONS WITH MICROBES THAT CAUSE DIARRHOEA

EXPOSURE	COMMON ORGANISMS
■ Food-borne:	
beef and pork	*Salmonella, Staphylococcus aureus, E. coli Clostridium perfringens, Campylobacter, Yersinia*
poultry	*Salmonella, Staphylococcus aureus, Clostridium perfringens*
milk and cheese	*Salmonella, E. coli, Campylobacter, Yersinia*
vegetables	*Clostridium botulinum, Salmonella, Shigella, Bacillus cereus*
shellfish	Vibrios, Norwalk virus, Norwalk-like virus, hepatitis A
water	*E. coli*, vibrios, *Shigella, Giardia, Cryptosporidium*
■ Schools, nurseries and day-care centres	*Shigella*, rotavirus, *Campylobacter, Giardia, Cryptosporidium, Salmonella, Aeromonas, Plesiomonas*
■ Travellers	*E. coli, Shigella, Campylobacter, Giardia, Aeromonas, Salmonella, Entamoeba histolytica, Vibrio cholerae*
■ Hospitalised patients receiving antibiotics	*Clostridium difficile*
■ Immunocompromised (e.g. AIDS)	*Cryptosporidium, Isospora, Salmonella, Microsporidium*

Day-care centres

In Australia and other developed countries, there is increasing demand for child care, including day-care centres. It has been reported that the incidence of diarrhoeal disease in children attending day-care centres may be twice as high as that in children at home. Factors promoting spread include the presence of non-toilet trained children, oral exploration of objects, contamination of hands, close contact and lack of appropriate infection control measures. *Shigella* spp., *Giardia intestinalis*, rotavirus and *Cryptosporidium* have frequently been associated with outbreaks. These organisms typically require only a low inoculum in order to cause infection in infants.

Faecal-oral spread and environmental contamination are the most common means of transmission. The most important interventions to prevent outbreaks of infection are good hygiene and handwashing practices.

Traveller's diarrhoea

This is the name given to acute diarrhoea that frequently occurs in people visiting a foreign country. Travellers may be exposed to unfamiliar organisms, for which they have no specific immunity, and which may cause an episode of acute diarrhoea. Some pathogens are contracted by consumption of faecally contaminated food or water, especially when visiting countries with poor sanitation and sewage disposal, or by eating unwashed fruit and vegetables in areas where sewage is used as a fertiliser. Certain countries in Asia, the Middle East, Africa and South America are well recognised as destinations where there is a high risk of developing gastroenteritis. Enterotoxigenic *E. coli* is the predominant cause of traveller's diarrhoea; other common causes are shown in Table 18.2.

Traveller's diarrhoea is generally a benign, self-limiting disease, although some of the more virulent agents may cause severe illness, such as a bloody dysentery (e.g. *Shigella*) or a chronic diarrhoea (e.g. *Giardia*).

Hospitalised patients

Diarrhoea can sometimes develop in hospitalised people. Mild diarrhoea is a common side effect of antibiotic therapy, but a more serious form, also associated with antibiotic therapy, is due to the bacterium *C. difficile*. Broad spectrum antibiotics can predispose a patient to a pseudomembranous colitis, caused by *C. difficile*, by altering the intestinal microbial flora that normally inhibit its establishment in the intestine.

People with AIDS

Almost all AIDS patients experience at least one episode of diarrhoea during their illness. The suppression of their immune system makes them susceptible to some unusual, opportunistic organisms, as shown in Table 18.2.

CLINICAL FEATURES OF ACUTE DIARRHOEAL DISEASE

It is difficult to differentiate between causative agents of acute diarrhoea on the basis of signs and symptoms alone. The majority of acute diarrhoeal infections have an incubation period of 1–4 days, but shorter or longer incubations can occur (see Table 18.3). Most diarrhoeal infections are self-limiting, but the illness can be as short as one day or as long as three weeks, depending on the cause. Infectious diarrhoea can be divided into one of two syndromes based on the nature of the diarrhoea produced:

1. non-inflammatory diarrhoea—characterised by watery stools without blood, mucus or pus;
2. inflammatory diarrhoea (or dysentery)—characterised by stools containing blood, mucus and pus.

In general, inflammatory diarrhoeas are more severe than the non-inflammatory types and require more intensive evaluation and treatment, although non-inflammatory diarrhoea, on occasions, can be very serious. The characteristics of these two forms of diarrhoea are summarised in Table 18.4.

Inflammatory diarrhoeas are caused by invasive microorganisms or by organisms that liberate toxins. Mainly the colon is affected, resulting in disruption of the mucosal lining. Damage to the colonic lining leads to the oozing of red cells, serous fluid and white cells into the lumen of the intestine. Typically, the patient has a small-volume, bloody diarrhoea, often with mucus. The patient also frequently complains of tenesmus (straining without passing stools), faecal urgency (inability to delay passing stools) and abdominal cramps. Also, the patient usually has a fever. Microscopic examination of the stool reveals the presence of numerous leucocytes. Some organisms may initially cause a watery diarrhoea before invading the mucosa, but later produce the typical inflammatory form when invasion occurs. The microorganisms that usually cause an inflammatory diarrhoea are listed in Table 18.4.

Non-inflammatory diarrhoeas are caused by microorganisms that primarily affect the small intestine. They may adhere to the intestinal epithelium, secrete toxins or even invade the cells, but they generally don't cause significant damage to the tissue. They produce diarrhoea by causing excessive secretion of fluids from the lining cells. Typically, the patient has a profuse, watery, non-bloody diarrhoea and often experiences nausea and abdominal cramping as well. With viral causes, vomiting may also be a major symptom. Leucocytes and red cells are not generally found in the stools, because of the absence of mucosal destruction and therefore leakage of cells from the bloodstream. Typical causes are listed in Table 18.4.

BACTERIAL CAUSES OF ACUTE DIARRHOEA

Campylobacter

Campylobacter species are comma-shaped Gram-negative rods. Since the mid-1980s they have emerged as the most common causes of diarrhoea in humans in many developed countries. Currently, in Australia, about 9000 cases are reported annually to the National Notifiable Diseases Surveillance System, with the highest rates occurring in the Northern Territory. The group most commonly affected are children under four years old (see Figure 18.1). Several species are associated with human disease, but *C. jejuni* is by far the most common.

A large reservoir of *Campylobacter* exists in animals such as cattle, sheep, poultry and wild birds. Human infections are thus usually acquired by consumption of contaminated and poorly cooked foods of animal origin, especially poultry, red meat and milk.

Campylobacter enteritis is due to ulceration and inflammation of the mucosal surface in the jejunum, ileum and colon, suggesting an invasive process. Several toxins of *C. jejuni* have been identified, but their role in the pathogenesis of infection has not been elucidated. Invasion and bacteraemia can occur, especially in neonates and

TABLE 18.3
DIARRHOEAL DISEASES: INCUBATION PERIOD AND DURATION OF DISEASE

PATHOGEN	INCUBATION PERIOD	DURATION OF ILLNESS
Staphylococcus aureus	1–6 hours	12–24 hours
Bacillus cereus	1–24 hours	12–48 hours
Clostridium perfringens	6–24 hours	12–24 hours
Norwalk virus	1–2 days	24–48 hours
Campylobacter spp.	1–2 days	3 days to 3 weeks
Salmonella spp.	1–2 days	2–7 days
Vibrio parahaemolyticus	1–2 days	1–3 days
Vibrio cholerae	1–3 days	5–7 days
Enterotoxigenic *E. coli*	1–3 days	5–10 days
Shigella spp.	1–4 days	1–3 days
Yersinia enterocolitis	4–7 days	1–2 weeks
Giardia intestinalis	2 weeks	weeks to months

TABLE 18.4
THE DIFFERENCES BETWEEN INFLAMMATORY AND NON-INFLAMMATORY DIARRHOEA

CHARACTERISTIC	INFLAMMATORY DIARRHOEA	NON-INFLAMMATORY DIARRHOEA
Leucocytes in stools	Present	Absent
Blood in stools	Present	Rare
Mucus	Present	Rare
Stool volume	Small (normal)	Greatly increased
Abdominal pain	Severe—lower left quadrant	None to slight
Body temperature	May be elevated	Usually normal
Site of infection	Colon	Small intestine
Common causes	*Shigella*, *Salmonella*, *Yersinia*, *Campylobacter*, *Clostridium difficile*, invasive and enterohaemorrhagic *E. coli*, *Entamoeba histolytica*, *Vibrio parahaemolyticus*, *Aeromonas*	Viruses, *Vibrio cholerae*, *Giardia*, enterotoxigenic and enteropathogenic *E. coli*, *taphylococcus aureus*, *Bacillus cereus*, *Clostridium perfringens*, *Cryptosporidium*, *Isospora Cyclospora*

FIGURE 18.1
RATE OF NOTIFICATIONS OF *CAMPYLOBACTER* INFECTIONS PER 100 000 POPULATION IN AUSTRALIA IN 1994, BY AGE GROUP AND SEX

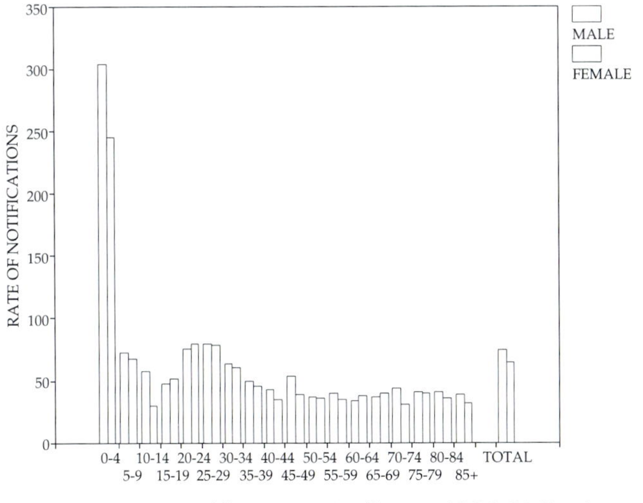

Source: *Communicable Diseases Intelligence* 19/22, 30 October 1995.

debilitated adults. Some infected people excrete the organism asymptomatically.

Salmonella

In developed countries, salmonellae are second only to *Campylobacter* as a major cause of diarrhoea. In Australia, 4000–5000 cases are reported annually. Highest rates of notifications occur in children under four years of age, and in the northern parts of the country (see Figure 18.2). There are numerous serovars (serotypes) of *Salmonella* that cause gastroenteritis, the most common being *S. typhimurium*. Other serotypes commonly encountered in Australia include *S. virchow*, *S. saintpaul*, *S. newport*, *S. chester*, *S. birkenhead* and *S. heidelberg*.

The major source of diarrhoea-causing salmonellae is the intestinal tract of animals. In developed countries, the organisms are transmitted to humans mainly via contaminated foods, especially poultry and eggs, meats such as pork, lamb and beef, and dairy products. Typically, salmonellae are found contaminating poultry products and animal meats and cause infection when the food is improperly stored and/or cooked. Take-away chickens and foods containing eggs, such as baby formulas, have caused outbreaks of infection. Salmonellae can also be transmitted from infected people and asymptomatic carriers to other people. Transmission by food handlers who are carriers and do not observe proper hygiene standards is particularly important.

Salmonellae invade the intestinal mucosa of the ileum and colon to produce disease. They replicate in the lamina propria, causing diarrhoea with blood and mucus. Most cases of salmonellosis are self-limiting diarrhoeal diseases. After clinical recovery, many patients become asymptomatic carriers for some weeks to months, and continue to act as potential sources of infection. In some cases, especially in the young, elderly and immunosuppressed, the organisms invade mesenteric lymph nodes from which they can spread via the bloodstream to cause arthritis, osteomyelitis, pneumonia or meningitis.

Escherichia coli

Some strains of *Escherichia coli* are harmless members of the normal GIT flora in humans and animals (see Chapter 3), whereas other strains possess virulence factors which enable them to cause infection in the intestinal tract. The strains that cause diarrhoeal disease have been classified

FIGURE 18.2

RATE OF NOTIFICATIONS OF *SALMONELLA* INFECTIONS (EXCLUDING ENTERIC FEVERS) PER 100 000 POPULATION IN AUSTRALIA IN 1994, BY STATISTICAL DIVISION OF RESIDENCE

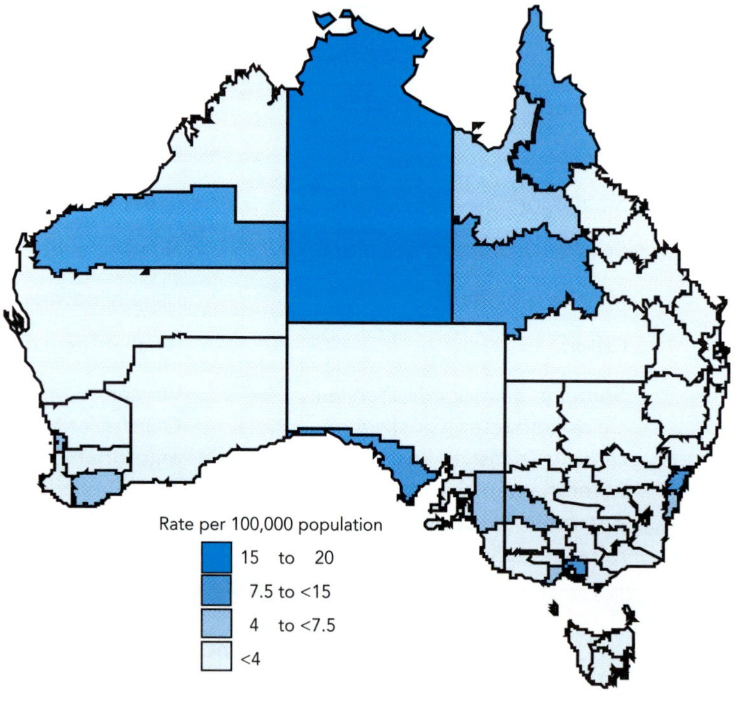

Source: Communicable Diseases Intelligence 19/22, 30 October 1995.

into four main groups according to their different pathogenic mechanisms.

1. Enterotoxigenic *E. coli* (ETEC) bind to specific receptors on the intestinal cell membranes where they produce potent enterotoxins. The heat-labile toxin (LT) of ETEC has a similar mechanism to that of cholera toxin (see Chapter 10). Both cause an increase in levels of cyclic AMP in intestinal epithelial cells, resulting in a massive outflow of water and electrolytes into the lumen of the intestine, manifested as profuse diarrhoea. In addition, ETEC have heat-stable toxins (ST) that also cause diarrhoea by similar mechanisms. ETEC are a major cause of diarrhoea in children in developing countries and travellers to those regions.
2. Enterohaemorrhagic *E. coli* (EHEC) include a number of different serotypes which have become recognised as important causes of haemorrhagic colitis and which can sometimes lead to **haemolytic uraemic syndrome (HUS)**. This is a serious complication, characterised by a haemolytic anaemia, uraemia and thrombocytopaenia, and renal failure, which can occur within the first few days of onset. Renal failure causes death in some patients. HUS can occur in any age group, but is most common in children under four.

   EHEC produce a verotoxin (VT), which causes destruction of the colonic epithelium and haemorrhage. HUS follows when other toxins cause small blood vessel damage in various sites including the kidney. Red cells are fragmented when passing through these damaged vessels, resulting in anaemia. Platelets, which cluster in the vessels, are destroyed, causing a thrombocytopaenia. The diagnosis of EHEC infections can be difficult because the organisms are rarely present in stools after the initial diarrhoeal phase. The need for treatment of HUS is urgent and may involve intensive care treatment, haemodialysis and prolonged hospitalisation.

   Sporadic cases of HUS associated with EHEC have been reported in Australia, but the first outbreak due to a common source was recorded in South Australia in early 1995 (see Spotlight box, p. 407). Large outbreaks have occurred in the United States and other developed countries.
3. Enteropathogenic *E. coli* (EPEC) were the first group of this species to be identified as intestinal pathogens. These organisms appear to adhere intimately to enterocytes and cause destruction of the brush border at that site. The events within the enterocytes that lead to diarrhoea are presently unknown. Diarrhoea caused by EPEC remains common in children in developing countries, but also occurs occasionally in developed areas of the world.
4. Enteroinvasive *E. coli* (EIEC) cause a gastrointestinal disease that is similar to the dysentery caused by *Shigella* spp. EIEC actively invade epithelial cells of the large intestine and spread laterally to adjacent cells, causing cell death, ulceration of the mucosa, and consequently inflammation. The inflammatory response causes an outpouring of pus, blood and mucus into the lumen.

SPOTLIGHT
HAEMOLYTIC URAEMIC SYNDROME

In December 1994 to January 1995, an outbreak of disease caused by enterohaemorrhagic *Escherichia coli* serotype O111 and, perhaps, other unidentified serotypes was associated with mettwurst produced by a smallgoods manufacturer in South Australia. The outbreak was declared after three children with haemolytic uraemic syndrome (HUS) had been reported to the Communicable Disease Control Unit of the South Australian Health Commission by Adelaide Women's and Children's Hospital between 25 December 1994 and 16 January 1995.

Active surveillance was initiated for cases of HUS and other disease, such as bloody diarrhoea, which may have been related to the outbreak. Epidemiological investigations were undertaken in South Australia in an attempt to identify the source of the infections, and laboratory investigations were performed on the patients and on suspect food sources.

By 23 January, a total of nine children had been identified with HUS. Eight were in South Australia and one had been to South Australia over the Christmas period and was being managed in Sydney. By 3 February, a total of 18 cases of dialysis-requiring HUS in children (aged between 5 months and 14 years) and two cases of thrombotic thrombocytopaenic purpura in adults had been identified. One 4-year-old girl had died. Onset dates ranged from 25 December 1994 to 29 January 1995.

Escherichia coli O111 was identified in faeces from most of the cases. All but two of the cases had a history of consumption of mettwurst or a related product. One of the others was an infant whose mother ate mettwurst, and the other lived in a household in which there had been mettwurst. Thirteen of the cases identified had eaten mettwurst from one manufacturer. The implicated mettwurst with 'use by dates' between 26 January and 12 April were recalled by the manufacturer, as were all its other uncooked fermented meat products.

Sporadic cases of HUS associated with enterohaemorrhagic *E. coli* have previously been reported in Australia, but this was the first documented outbreak. Large outbreaks have been recorded in the United States, linked with consumption of undercooked minced beef, roast beef, raw milk and apple cider.

Adapted from S. Cameron, C. Walker, M. Beers, N. Rose & E. Anear, 'Enterohaemorrhagic *Escherichia coli* outbreak in South Australia associated with the consumption of mettwurst', *Communicable Diseases Intelligence* 19/3, 6 February 1995.

Cholera

Cholera is an acute infection of the gastrointestinal tract caused by the comma-shaped Gram-negative bacterium *Vibrio cholerae*. Cholera is endemic in South-East Asia, parts of Africa and much of Central and South America (see Figure 18.3). Several pandemics of cholera occurred during the 19th century, originating in the Indian subcontinent. Australia is considered to be free of cholera, except for imported cases; less than 100 cases have been reported since 1917.

V. cholerae causes infection only in humans. Symptomatic people and asymptomatic carriers are the reservoirs of infection. The organism is able to survive for long periods in water and thus occurs most frequently in areas where clean drinking water and adequate sewage disposal are not available. Transmission via food (e.g. seafood) contaminated with human faeces also occurs. The disease is often associated with natural disasters (e.g. floods, earthquakes) as well as situations of social unrest and upheaval. More than 7000 people died from cholera in Rwanda in 1994, associated with the civil crisis in that country.

The symptoms of cholera are due to the action of the enterotoxin of *V. cholerae*. Essentially, the toxin causes the levels of cyclic AMP in intestinal epithelial cells to increase, resulting in a massive outflow of water and electrolytes into the lumen of the intestine, manifested as profuse diarrhoea. Chapter 10 gives a more detailed description of its action. Many cases are mild or asymptomatic. In severe cases, the patient may lose up to 30 litres of fluid in a day, and the stools are primarily a mixture of water and mucus, having the classic appearance of 'rice water stools'. Without fluid and electrolyte replacement, mortality can be as high as 40–60 percent.

A heat-killed, whole-cell vaccine for cholera is available. However, it is protective in only about 50% of recipients, and the duration of protection is only 3–6 months. Because of this, it is no longer recommended by Australian health authorities or by the World Health Organization for routine use, even for travellers to cholera-endemic areas. Ensuring consumption of clean food and water is considered to be of greater importance. Oral vaccines are currently being developed, and it is hoped these will be more effective.

Shigella

Shigella diarrhoea is also known as bacillary dysentery. There are four species—*Shigella sonnei* causes mostly mild infections, *S. flexneri* and *S. boydii* usually cause moderate disease, and *S. dysenteriae* is the most serious. *Shigella* infections are most common in children under 10 years, and are often reported in schools and day-care centres. Day-care staff and family members may also become infected. Shigellosis is more common in disadvantaged communities, and is much more prevalent among Aboriginal children than other Australian children. Around 700 cases of shigellosis are notified annually in Australia, with the highest rate occurring in children under four years of age.

Shigella are strictly human pathogens, so the source of infection is always a symptomatic person or carrier of the organisms. Faecal-oral spread is the major mode of transmission. Prolonged excretion of *Shigella* may occur in some patients for several weeks after recovery. Handwashing and good hygiene are considered to be the

FIGURE 18.3
COUNTRIES IN WHICH CHOLERA WAS REPORTED IN 1991 AND 1992

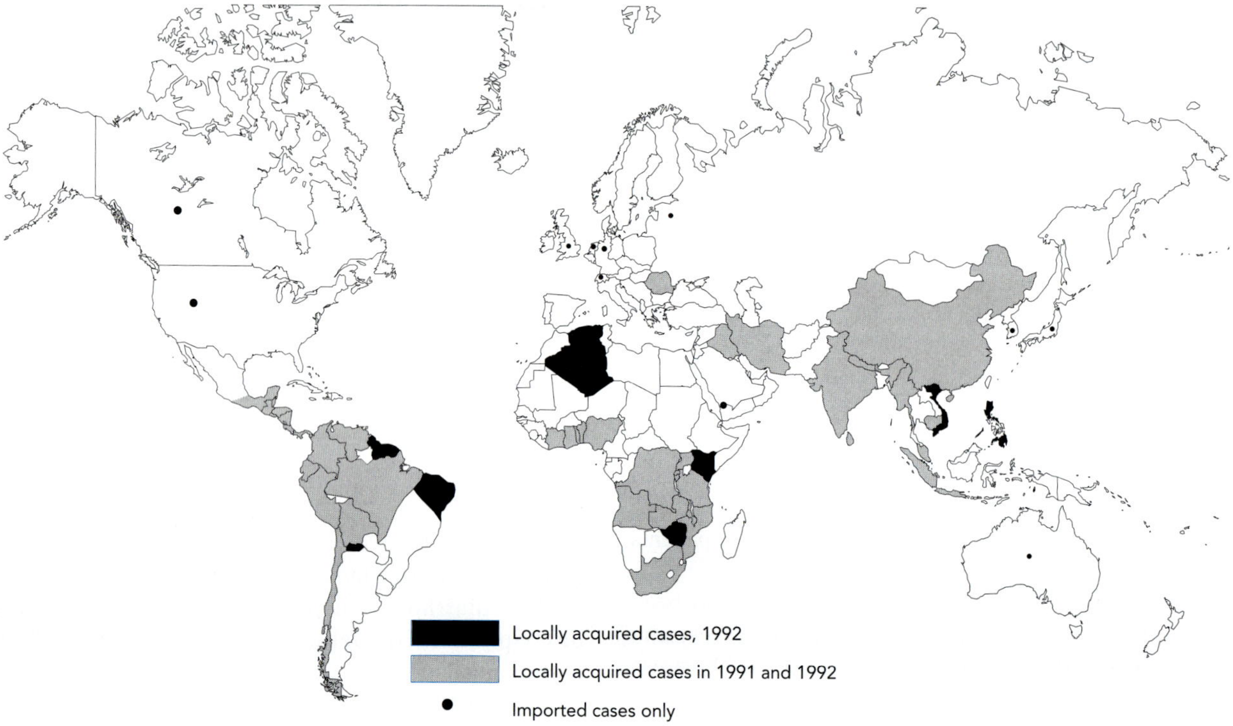

Source: Communicable Diseases Intelligence 17/19, 20 September 1993, p. 425.

most important means of preventing transmission of these organisms.

Shigella are readily transmitted and highly virulent —as few as 10–100 organisms may cause disease. Their pathogenesis is due to their enteroinvasive properties as well as their secretion of the Shiga toxin. In the intestine, the bacteria are phagocytosed by colonic epithelial cells. They then lyse the phagocytic vesicle, multiply intracellularly, and invade adjacent cells. The Shiga toxin acts by cleaving ribosomal RNA in colonic cells, halting protein synthesis and killing the cell. The Shiga toxin is also thought to damage endothelial cells and in some cases causes haemolytic uraemic syndrome similar to the enterohaemorrhagic *E. coli*.

CASE HISTORY 18.1
SHIGELLOSIS

In 1993, in a small town south of Cairns, *Shigella sonnei* was isolated from a young Aboriginal child who had recently visited the Northern Territory. Ultimately, four members of the child's extended family became infected, and two were hospitalised in Cairns. In the hospital, another child in the same ward and a nurse became infected.

Comment:
This case clearly illustrates the ease with which shigellosis can be transmitted.

Adapted from *Communicable Diseases Intelligence* 17/17, 23 August 1993, p. 374.

Clostridium difficile (antibiotic-associated colitis)

Diarrhoea can arise whenever the normal intestinal flora is disrupted or altered. When antimicrobial drugs, particularly broad spectrum agents, are used in the treatment of infectious diseases, they can affect the normal flora, as well as the pathogen. A change in the balance of the normal flora can lead to a mild diarrhoea. Since the late 1970s, it has been recognised that antibiotic therapy can sometimes lead to much more serious gastrointestinal disease, characterised by severe diarrhoea and a form of inflammation in the colon that results in the formation of yellow-white raised plaques or pseudomembranes on the colonic mucosa. The Gram-positive anaerobic rod, *Clostridium difficile*, is the cause of this pseudomembranous colitis, not the antibiotics. The normal colonic flora of adults and children over the age of 12 months effectively prevents colonisation by *C. difficile*, but antibiotics can disrupt the flora, allowing *C. difficile* to become established, multiply and produce disease. Infection with *C. difficile* may present in a variety of ways, ranging from mild diarrhoea without abdominal discomfort to the potentially life-threatening pseudomembranous colitis.

C. difficile spores are ubiquitous. The organism is able to survive for long periods in the hospital environment, because of its spores. It has been cultured from floors, toilets, bedding, mops and furniture and also from the hands of hospital personnel. Heavy contamination can be found in rooms that have been occupied by infected patients. Thus, transmission of the organism to an individual who is susceptible because of antibiotic therapy can readily occur. It is now recognised as an important type of nosocomial infection.

Although pseudomembranous colitis was initially related to clindamycin usage, almost all broad spectrum antibiotic agents have now been implicated in this disease, but the main offenders are clindamycin, ampicillin, cephalosporins and aminoglycosides. While the use of antibiotics is recognised as the major predisposing factor, anything that disrupts the intestinal flora of the gut, including another gastrointestinal infection, can lead to *C. difficile* infection.

C. difficile produces two exotoxins, but an enterotoxin (called toxin A) is the main pathogenic factor. One of the distinctive features of toxin A is its ability to induce a local inflammatory response with the activation of macrophages and mast cells, the mobilisation of neutrophils and destruction of the mucosa. A pseudomembrane, consisting of necrotic tissue debris, mucus, and neutrophils and monocytes, forms over the mucosa. Perforation of the colon, abscess formation and vascular thrombi are possible late complications. *C. difficile* infection should be considered in any patient receiving antimicrobial drugs and who develops diarrhoea while in hospital. Non-toxigenic strains of *C. difficile* exist, but their role in disease is uncertain.

Vibrio parahaemolyticus

Vibrio parahaemolyticus is a Gram-negative, halophilic (salt-loving) organism commonly found in seafood such as crabs, oysters and fish. In Japan and South-East Asia, where seafoods are often consumed uncooked, this bacterium is responsible for a large number of cases of food-borne illness. The mechanism of pathogenesis is still unclear, but there is evidence to suggest that the organism invades the epithelial cells of the small intestine. A number of other vibrios cause diarrhoeal disease, including *V. fluvialis*, *V. mimicus* and *V. hollisae*.

Yersinia

Yersinia enterocolitica is a Gram-negative rod that is a member of the family Enterobacteriaceae. The organism is found in a large variety of animals, especially pigs and cows. As a result, many cases of yersiniosis are traced to meat and dairy products. *Yersinia* is also sometimes found in domestic animals, and transmission to humans from pet dogs has been reported. Faecal-oral spread between humans also occurs, enhanced by the possible faecal excretion of the organism for weeks after infection. Most infections occur in young children. In Australia, about 500 cases of yersiniosis are reported each year.

The pathogenesis of *Y. enterocolitica* stems mainly from its ability to invade the mucosa of the terminal ileum and replicate in the Peyer's patches, producing an inflammatory diarrhoea. The disease may be confused with an appendicitis, especially in children. The organism also secretes an exotoxin, but its role in virulence is unclear. Another species, *Y. pseudotuberculosis,* is also associated with diarrhoeal disease in humans.

Aeromonas and Plesiomonas

The bacterium *Aeromonas hydrophila* and the closely related *Plesiomonas shigelloides* (formerly *Aeromonas shigelloides*) are now recognised as causes of diarrhoeal disease, especially in paediatric patients. They are also possible causes of traveller's diarrhoea. Disease can be very serious in debilitated or immunosuppressed patients.

Clostridium perfringens

Clostridium perfringens is associated with diarrhoeal disease when a threshold number of bacteria are ingested in contaminated food, followed by *in vivo* secretion of an enterotoxin. This organism produces two different food-borne illnesses. Type A organisms cause a self-limiting diarrhoeal illness, which occurs in developed countries, and type C organisms cause a potentially life-threatening syndrome known as 'enteritis necroticans' in under-developed tropical areas.

Type A clostridial food poisoning is typically associated with meat and poultry products in which there is a long delay between cooking and serving of the food. Clostridial spores, which are widely present in human and animal faeces and uncooked meats and vegetables, can survive cooking temperatures and can germinate and multiply when meat products are allowed to stand at 15–60°C for several hours or more. The food must be heavily contaminated for infection to occur. This food-borne illness is usually associated with situations where bulk food preparation occurs, such as in institutions and fast food outlets.

Enteritis necroticans is ususally due to the consumption of ß-toxin-producing type C strains of *C. perfringens* in undercooked pork. In healthy individuals this toxin is inactivated by trypsin and other intestinal proteases. However, people with malnutrition may have a deficiency in proteases, and the toxin is not destroyed and can cause necrosis of the intestinal wall. It is traditionally associated with ritual pig-feasting by the natives of highland New Guinea, where it is known as 'pig-bel'. This syndrome has also been reported in other countries such as Thailand, Nepal and China. *C. perfringens* also causes gas gangrene in wounds and soft tissue (see Chapter 16).

VIRAL CAUSES OF ACUTE DIARRHOEA

Viruses are responsible for more cases of diarrhoeal illnesses in developed countries than any other organisms, and they affect particularly infants under the age of three years. Rotaviruses are the most important in this age group, but enteric adenoviruses, small round viruses (including

Norwalk virus and Norwalk-like viruses) and caliciviruses also cause disease in this and other age groups. Enteric viruses survive well in the environment and are somewhat resistant to sewage treatment processes and post-treatment chlorination.

Rotavirus

Rotaviruses, first identified in 1973 by the Melbourne scientists Ruth Bishop and Ian Holmes, are a major cause of gastroenteritis in infants. Five distinct antigenic groups of rotaviruses have subsequently been recognised. Group A rotaviruses are the major human pathogens, while groups B to E are associated primarily with animals. Rotaviruses (Figure 18.4) are the most common cause of severe watery diarrhoea in young children throughout the world. In Australia, about 2000 notifications of rotavirus infection are received annually.

Most infections occur within the first two years of life, and are potentially life-threatening due to severe dehydration. Intravenous fluids may be urgently required. Older children and adults are less susceptible, presumably because of antibodies developed early in life. Rotavirus infections in the day-care setting are common, and are generally attributed to faecal-oral transmission and contamination of fomites. Epidemics are sometimes seen in hospital nurseries.

Very large numbers of virus particles (> 10^{12} particles per gram) are shed in faeces. Cross-infection readily occurs since the infective dose in a child is thought to be only 10–100 particles. The virus infects enterocytes at the villous tips in the small intestine, causing lysis of the cells and destruction of the villous tip epithelium, but there is no inflammation or loss of blood. Transport mechanisms in the intestine are disrupted and the loss of water and electrolytes results in diarrhoea.

Other viruses

Norwalk virus and Norwalk-like viruses have not yet been cultivated *in vitro*, and are often referred to as 'small round structured viruses' (SRSVs). They are important food-borne pathogens in many countries, including Australia, the United Kingdom and Japan. Infection is most common in older children and adults, and typically occurs through a common source rather than by person-to-person contact. The foods most commonly implicated are poorly cooked or raw shellfish. For example, Sydney rock oysters have been implicated in a number of outbreaks of gastroenteritis, resulting in the introduction of compulsory purification of oysters in tanks of clean water. Contaminated drinking water and natural waters used for swimming have also been implicated. Antibody to Norwalk virus does not appear to be protective against reinfection.

Enteric adenoviruses (serotypes Ad40 and Ad41) cause gastroenteritis and are thought to be major causes of acute diarrhoea in paediatric patients. Adenoviruses appear to infect enterocytes, causing them to rupture, with the development of villous stunting.

Caliciviruses have been found to cause diarrhoea in children in day-care centres, and typically affect children aged three months to six years. Prolonged excretion of these viruses by symptomatic and asymptomatic individuals can make control extremely difficult.

Astroviruses mainly affect children less than four years of age, and are rare in adults.

PROTOZOAL CAUSES OF ACUTE DIARRHOEA

The three main protozoal pathogens in diarrhoeal disease are *Giardia intestinalis, Entamoeba histolytica* and *Cryptosporidium parvum.* In most cases infection depends on contact with faecally contaminated material, infection flourishing where low standards of hygiene and sanitation, poverty and overcrowding exist.

Giardia intestinalis

The first intestinal parasite to be seen under a microscope was *Giardia intestinalis* (also called *G. lamblia* and *G. duodenalis*), when in 1681 Anton van Leeuwenhoek peered through the simple microscope he had just made and saw the moving 'animalcules' in a preparation of his own faeces. *G. intestinalis* are now recognised as flagellated protozoa (Figure 18.5) that have a worldwide distribution.

In developing countries, infections are associated with overcrowding, poor sanitary conditions and poor water quality. In endemic areas, people often become reinfected within months of treatment. In developed countries, where prevalence rates range between 2 and 7%, faecal-oral transmission is most common, and children are most likely to be infected. *Giardia* is readily spread in day-care centres, from child to child, and from children to other family members. In Australia, high rates of infection have been reported in some remote Aboriginal communities. A high prevalence of the parasite has also been found in domestic cats and dogs in Australia, but whether they act as a reservoir for human infection remains uncertain. Direct transmission of *Giardia* among homosexual men is increasingly being found.

Giardia has a simple life cycle with two forms: the flagellate trophozoite and the resistant cyst. The trophozoites live in the upper portion of the small intestine, attaching to the mucosa, and rapidly multiplying there. Cyst formation occurs at regular intervals, and they are passed out in stools. These resistant structures are the infective form and can survive for months in the environment when conditions are suitable. They are also somewhat resistant to chlorine, so can survive some water purification procedures. Infection occurs when cysts are ingested, with as few as 10–25 being able to establish infection. Once in the small intestine they develop into the trophozoite form. Attachment of the parasite to the mucosa and resultant physical damage is thought to be part of the disease process, but the role of other factors such as toxins is unclear.

Many cases of giardiasis are asymptomatic, but when illness occurs it is characterised by diarrhoea, nausea, a foul flatulence and fatigue. It is usually self-limiting

FIGURE 18.4
ROTAVIRUS—WHEEL-SHAPED VIRUSES THAT CAUSE DIARRHOEA

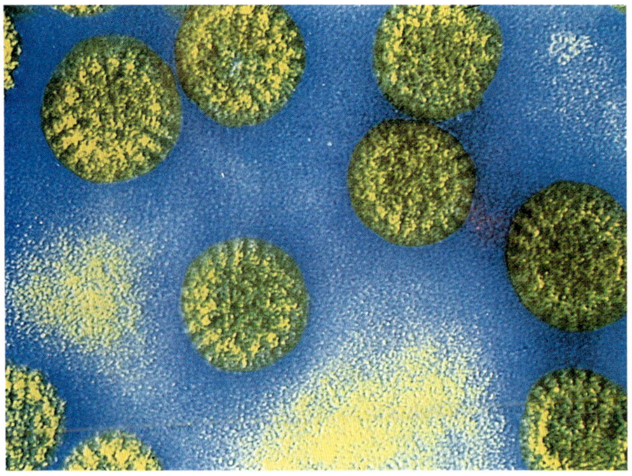

(resolving within a week), but may persist for months. Chronic infection is typically manifested as periodic episodes of these symptoms, between periods without symptoms. In children in developing countries or from disadvantaged groups (e.g. Australian Aborigines), the major concern is the possibility of worsening malnutrition and retardation of growth and development.

Entamoeba histolytica

Entamoeba histolytica is an enteric protozoan with a worldwide distribution. It is thought to infect as much as 10% of the world's population. It is endemic in many areas, including Mexico, India and Africa, where as many as 50% of the high-risk population may be infected. Infection is transmitted by faecal contamination of food or drink by infected food-handlers or as a result of inadequate sanitation. Obviously, travellers to these areas are at high risk of infection.

FIGURE 18.5
GIARDIA INTESTINALIS
A flagellated protozoan that causes diarrhoea in humans.

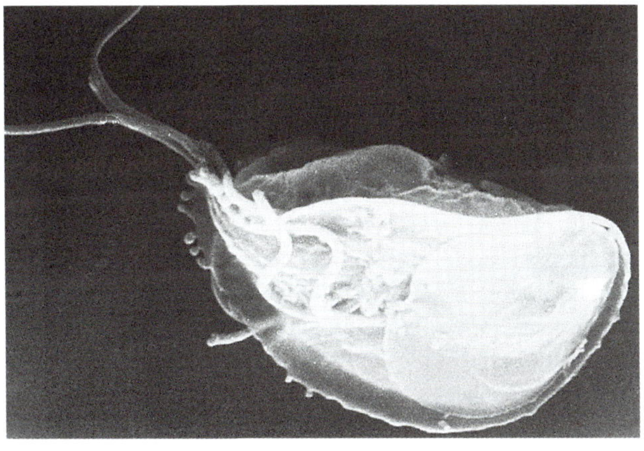

Trophozoites of some low-virulence strains of *E. histolytica* live on the mucosal surface of the large intestine, frequently as harmless commensals. They replicate there, periodically forming resistant cysts that are excreted in faeces. These cysts can survive in the external environment and act as the infective stages. Most infected people are asymptomatic cyst passers or have only mild to moderate diarrhoeal symptoms. However, other strains cause invasive disease, ulcerating the bowel wall and spreading to remote sites, especially the liver, resulting in hepatic abscess. Production of small, localised ulcers in the colon causes a mild diarrhoea, whereas the formation of deep, confluent ulcers leads to the classic inflammatory diarrhoea called **amoebic dysentery**.

Cryptosporidium parvum

Cryptosporidium parvum was first recognised as a cause of diarrhoea in humans in 1976. The advent of the AIDS epidemic focused attention on its capacity to produce disease and its widespread distribution. Prevalence rates of 1–3 % of patients with diarrhoea is reported in developed countries, including Australia, and 5–10% in Africa and Asia. Transmission is possible by a variety of routes, including faecally contaminated food, water and hands, and from pets. A number of outbreaks in day-care centres have been reported, often with day-care workers and family contacts also being affected. The organism has been recently recognised as an important cause of traveller's diarrhoea and of outbreaks associated with swimming pools, especially when filters are not routinely checked.

An important feature of *C. parvum* is its thick-walled oocyst (see Figure 18.6), which is resistant to many disinfectants, including hypochlorite (hence its association

FIGURE 18.6
CRYPTOSPORIDIUM PARVUM
A Zeihl-Neelsen stain of oocysts.

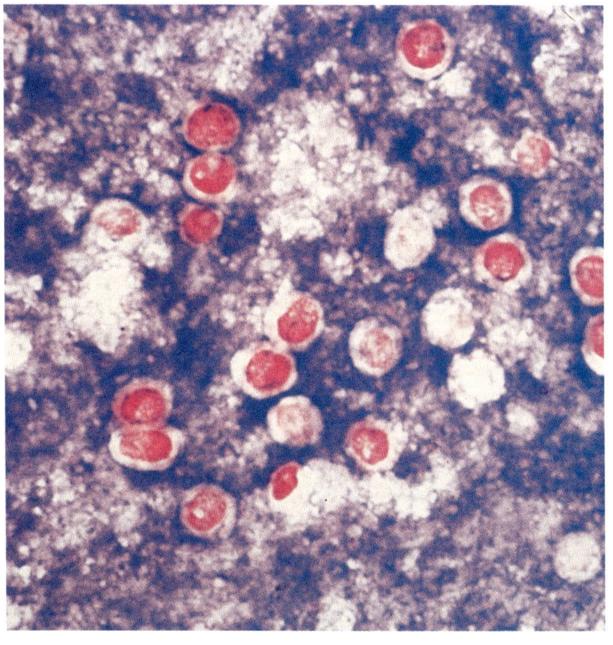

CASE HISTORY 18.2
CRYPTOSPORIDIOSIS

In November 1994, the supervisor of a child day-care centre in North Queensland advised the Tropical Public Health Unit in Cairns of an outbreak of diarrhoea in the centre. She was concerned that seven of the eight infants in the nursery (aged less than 15 months) had symptoms.

Faecal samples were collected from all eight infants in the nursery, and *Cryptosporidium parvum* oocysts were identified in the faeces of all the symptomatic children. The asymptomatic child had been away from the centre during the previous two weeks. The children at the centre drank only boiled water. There was no paddling pool or pets at the centre.

The diarrhoea persisted in all children for at least seven days, and for several weeks in some of them.

Comment:
Cryptosporidium infection is commonly acquired via water-borne or zoonotic transmission, but in this outbreak these modes would seem to be unlikely.

Adapted from J. Hanna & D. Brookes, 'Cryptosporidiosis in a child day-care centre', *Communicable Diseases Intelligence* 19/1, 9 January 1995, p. 6.

with swimming pool outbreaks). Another feature is its low infective dose and ease of transmission.

In the small intestine the organism invades the epithelial cells, where it undergoes sexual reproduction, eventually forming oocysts which are excreted in faeces. A watery diarrhoea occurs approximately five days after ingestion of oocysts, and lasts several days to two weeks. In young children, the diarrhoea may persist for more than three weeks, and in immunodeficient hosts the disease may be severe and chronic, and sometimes fatal.

Isospora belli

Isospora belli is another protozoan that, as a result of the AIDS epidemic, has been identified as an important cause of diarrhoeal disease. It is endemic in South America, Africa and South-East Asia and is probably transmitted by faecally contaminated food or water. Sporozoites invade the mucosa of the small intestine, destroying the microvilli. It can cause diarrhoea in travellers, but its highest prevalence is in immunocompromised people. It has been reported to be responsible for up to 4% of diarrhoeal infections in AIDS patients in Australia. Clinically, it is similar to cryptosporidial infection.

Cyclospora

Protozoa of the genus *Cyclospora* have been confirmed as causes of diarrhoea in developing countries, and in travellers and patients with AIDS. The life cycle, pathogenic mechanisms and epidemiologic features of *Cyclospora* are largely unknown.

Blastocystis hominis

Blastocystis hominis is a frequently identified protozoan in the gastrointestinal tract of humans. However, the pathogenicity of this parasite remains uncertain. Some people with this organism and no other identifiable pathogen have mild diarrhoeal disease, but many are asymptomatic. No pathogenic mechanisms have been fully described.

FOOD INTOXICATIONS

These illnesses are characterised by the rapid onset of nausea, vomiting and abdominal pain, usually within 6–8 hours of ingestion of contaminated food. Fever and diarrhoea can occur but are less common. The major causes are the enterotoxins (see Chapter 10) of *Staphylococcus aureus*, *Bacillus cereus* and *Clostridium botulinum*, preformed in food. Thus, they are food intoxications, rather than infections. The fact that the toxins are preformed in the food is the reason why the incubation period is so short in comparison to infections. In these intoxications the organisms do not have to multiply in the intestine to produce disease; instead, the toxin must simply be absorbed. The toxin of *C. botulinum* is absorbed in the intestine and enters the bloodstream, eventually reaching and acting on peripheral nerve synapses, causing a flaccid paralysis. Since the botulinum toxin blocks nerve transmission rather than causing gastrointestinal disease, botulism is discussed in Chapter 20.

Staphylococcus aureus intoxication

Foods rich in protein, salt and sugar (e.g. ham, creamy cakes, salads with mayonnaise), and which have been inadequately refrigerated, favour the growth of staphylococci. If an enterotoxin-producing strain is involved, consumption of the food can result in gastrointestinal symptoms. Foods usually become contaminated by resident staphylococci in the nose or on the skin of food-handlers. Skin lesions colonised by staphylococci are a particularly dangerous source. Symptoms occur rapidly, typically 1–6 hours after consumption of the contaminated food.

There are five distinct enterotoxins (A–E) produced by strains of *S. aureus*, with enterotoxin A the most commonly implicated. The exact mechanism of action of the enterotoxins has not been determined, but they cause increased secretion of water and electrolytes in animal models, and are thought to induce vomiting by stimulating enteric autonomic sensory neurons.

Bacillus cereus

Bacillus cereus is an aerobic, Gram-positive rod that is resistant to moderate cooking temperatures because of the production of heat-resistant spores. If the cooked food is allowed to cool for an extended period at room temperature, the spores germinate and the vegetative cells then produce a heat-stable enterotoxin in the food. Ingestion of preformed toxin in the food causes an acute onset of

CASE HISTORY 18.3
STAPHYLOCOCCAL GASTROENTERITIS

Six guests who had been to a noon wedding attended Casualty at the local hospital between 3 and 5 pm the same afternoon. All were complaining of diarrhoea, vomiting and abdominal cramps. Public health authorities were notified and the other 60 guests and the owner of the wedding reception venue were subsequently contacted.

Overall, 19 of the guests experienced gastrointestinal symptoms, all within 2–5 hours of the lunch. Faecal specimens were collected from each of the 10 people who ultimately attended the hospital. Enterotoxin-producing *Staphylococcus aureus* was cultured from four of these specimens.

An examination of the kitchen of the wedding reception house revealed a physically clean kitchen. None of the food served at the wedding remained for testing. The only food consumed by all the ill guests was cold chicken pieces, and it was assumed that this was the source of the staphylococcal food poisoning.

nausea, vomiting, abdominal pain, without diarrhoea, within 1–6 hours. This emetic (vomiting-inducing) form of the disease is frequently associated with rice dishes, especially fried rice. The practice in restaurants of cooking a large amount of rice and allowing it to cool slowly over several hours, and then to flash fry it just before serving, is believed to be the major reason for the disease's association with this food in particular.

Less commonly, *B. cereus* causes another form of disease when vegetative cells, rather than toxin, are ingested and a different enterotoxin is formed in the intestine. This disease usually occurs 8–16 hours after ingestion of contaminated food, with diarrhoea and abdominal cramps the main symptoms. This diarrhoeal form has been associated with a wide variety of foods.

LABORATORY DIAGNOSIS

Generally, it is not possible to distinguish between the different causes of diarrhoeal disease solely on clinical grounds. Information on the patient's recent food consumption and/or travel history is often helpful, but a precise diagnosis can only be achieved by laboratory investigations. For most patients with mild to moderate diarrhoea, the illness will be self-limiting and will require no evaluation other than a clinical one. However, for severe or persistent illness, or in the investigation of an outbreak, a definitive diagnosis is necessary. A number of laboratory tests can be used to provide such a diagnosis. Microscopic examination of a stool specimen enables a differentiation to be made between inflammatory and non-inflammatory diarrhoeal disease. While this test indicates the pathological process occurring in the intestine and the likely causative agents, it does not identify the cause of infection.

Stool culture is the standard method for the diagnosis of most bacterial causes of diarrhoea. Fresh stool specimens (at least 5 g or 5 mL) should be sent immediately to the laboratory in a sterile, wide-mouth container with a firmly fitting screw lid. If transport is delayed, refrigeration is recommended. Special media are required for cultivation of some bacteria, such as vibrios and *Y. enterocolitica*, so the request form accompanying the specimen should provide adequate information about the patient's history and food consumption and an indication that such organisms are suspected.

For suspected *C. difficile* infections, anaerobic culture on special selective media and the detection of cytotoxin in faeces are the standard diagnostic procedures. In staphylococcal or *Bacillus* food intoxications, the organisms are often not present in faeces and are not able to be cultured, but culture of vomitus may be more productive. In all cases of bacterial food-borne illness, culture of the suspect food may be attempted, particularly in the investigation of an outbreak.

Culture of enteric viruses is not routine in diagnostic clinical laboratories. Laboratory confirmation of viral gastroenteritis is usually based on the demonstration of viral particles or antigens in stools by serologic or electron microscopic means. However, these tests are not always available in routine laboratories, and are not highly sensitive. Thus, the diagnosis of viral gastroenteritis is often made on the patient history and clinical grounds.

Diagnosis of protozoal infections usually involves the microscopic identification of cysts or trophozoites in stool specimens. Collection of three stool specimens on alternate days is recommended to improve the likelihood of organism detection. Highly sensitive and reliable ELISA and fluorescein-labelled antibody tests have recently been developed for detecting antigens of some protozoa (e.g. *Giardia*) in stools. The diagnosis of liver abscess caused by *E. histolytica* is based on a CT scan or ultrasound scan of the liver, plus stool examination and serological testing for circulating antibodies. The use of DNA probes, polymerase chain reaction and antigen detection techniques are promising, but not yet sufficiently developed.

MANAGEMENT OF PATIENTS WITH DIARRHOEAL DISEASE

The major problem of infectious diarrhoea, irrespective of the cause, is loss of fluid and dehydration. Therefore, for any patient with acute diarrhoea, fluid and electrolyte replacement is essential, and can be lifesaving in severe cases. In mild disease, oral intake of fluids is usually adequate, but in cases of moderate to severe fluid loss, and especially in young infants, intravenous hydration with isotonic fluids containing dextrose may be necessary.

Most patients with acute diarrhoea do not require specific antimicrobial therapy. In fact, antibiotic therapy should be avoided if possible, because in some cases it may prolong the carriage and excretion of an organism (e.g. *Salmonella*) by the patient, increasing the risk of transmission to others. Also, the risk of increasing microbial resistance to antibiotics is not warranted in self-limiting diseases. There is no effective antimicrobial treatment for viral causes, and antibiotics are not warranted in food intoxications because disease is caused by preformed toxins, not multiplication of the bacterium in the intestine.

There are some situations, however, where antibiotic therapy is justified; for example:

- to reduce faecal excretion, environmental contamination and spread of infection (e.g. in *Shigella* infections);
- to resolve persistent infections (e.g. giardiasis);
- to resolve serious and life-threatening infections (e.g. amoebiasis and antibiotic-associated colitis); and
- to hasten recovery in special groups (e.g. travellers).

In the case of *Shigella* infections, an antimicrobial agent such as cotrimoxazole may be administered to shorten the duration of symptoms and to prevent the spread of infection. Antibiotic-associated colitis caused by *C. difficile* may be resolved by discontinuation of the antibiotic, but severe cases may require treatment with vancomycin or metronidazole. Relapse of disease often occurs with the termination of treatment, requiring a second course of the drug. Enteropathogenic *E. coli* can cause severe and protracted diarrhoea, especially in hospital nursery and paediatric ward outbreaks. When the organism is hospital-acquired, it may be highly resistant to antibiotics, making antibiotic sensitivity testing of the isolate necessary. Although cholera is potentially fatal, most cases can be adequately treated with oral rehydration and electrolyte replacement. In severe cases, or to prevent transmission, furazolidone is generally used.

Treatment of protozoal infections is often with metronidazole, because of its broad activity. For confirmed *G. intestinalis* infection, quinacrine or furazolidone (in infants) are often used. Treatment of *E. histolytica* infections is with drugs such as iodoquinol or paromomycin for asymptomatic cyst passers, or metronidazole for invasive infections. In cases of disseminated infection that do not respond to therapy, surgical drainage is usually required. There is currently no proven effective treatment for infections caused by *Cryptosporidia* or *Cyclospora*. Treatment of *Isospora* infections is with cotrimoxazole or metronidazole.

During a diarrhoeal illness, the patient's diet should also be modified. The intestinal tract has difficulty in processing complex materials, and starch foods are recommended. A number of non-specific drugs may be used to reduce the symptoms. Mostly, these are adsorbents (e.g. kaolin) to reduce the liquidity of stools, or anti-motility drugs (e.g. loperamide) to inhibit intestinal motility and enhance fluid absorption, thereby reducing the number of stools passed.

PREVENTION

Prevention of diarrhoeal disease essentially involves avoidance of the organisms. In the case of food-borne illness and traveller's diarrhoea, this means proper food processing, proper cooking of foods, the non-consumption of high-risk foods (especially raw) and beverages, and the sterilisation of drinking water where appropriate. In day-care centres, strict handwashing practice, good general hygiene, sanitary food preparation, use of disposable gloves when contact with faecal matter is possible, and exclusion of symptomatic children are important measures (see Chapter 14).

In hospitals and other institutions, people with severe diarrhoea are a potential source of infection for other patients. Enteric precautions and strict handwashing after contact with these patients is essential. While the use of disposable gloves is strongly recommended, this *does not* obviate the need for strict handwashing practices.

Other Gastrointestinal Diseases

HELICOBACTER PYLORI INFECTION

The initial suggestions made in the early 1980s by Barry Marshall and Robin Warren in Western Australia, that the spiral-shaped bacterium, *Helicobacter pylori* (Figure 18.7), might be responsible for duodenal ulcer were treated with great scepticism. However, since then, much evidence has accumulated linking the organism not only with peptic ulcers but also with gastric carcinoma. *H. pylori* is now recognised as the main cause of gastritis (inflammation of the stomach mucosa) and a major factor in the develop-ment of most cases of duodenal and gastric ulcers. Its causal role in gastric cancer has not been firmly established, but it appears likely to be a contributing factor in at least some cases.

In developed countries, more than 20% of the population may be infected with *H. pylori*, but many cases are asymptomatic. The prevalence of infection is higher in lower socioeconomic groups, and especially high in developing countries. The organism is most probably acquired by oral-oral transmission.

How *H. pylori* establishes in the hostile environment of the gastric mucosa and causes gastritis is not clearly known. Studies have indicated that motility and adhesins are probably important in the organism's ability to colonise the gastric epithelium. Also, it seems likely that the large amounts of the urease enzyme produced by the bacterium may be involved in its pathogenesis. This enzyme, by breaking down urea in the stomach, might generate a 'cloud' of ammonia there, protecting the organism from the gastric acidity. Once a person becomes infected with *H. pylori*, the organism appears able to persist in the stomach for many years, and perhaps for life. Only in some people is the inflammation induced by the bacterium severe enough to produce symptoms. Severe and prolonged inflammation of the gastric mucosa appear to be major requirements for ulceration and carcinogenesis. *H. pylori* may play an important role in the initiation of gastric cancer, but other factors, such as diet, also appear to be important.

A laboratory diagnosis of *H. pylori* infection is by histological examination of biopsy specimens taken during endoscopy. A rapid urease test and culture may also be performed on these specimens. A non-invasive test has recently been developed in which radio-labelled carbon dioxide is detected in the breath of an infected person

FIGURE 18.7
ELECTRON MICROGRAPH OF HELICOBACTER PYLORI

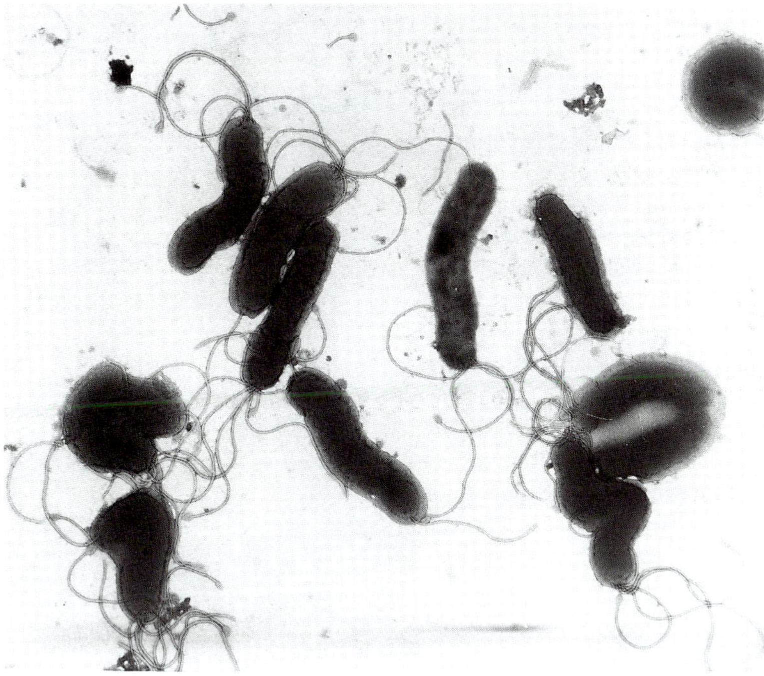

after ingestion of an isotopically labelled solution of urea. Triple therapy with a bismuth salt, tetracycline and metronidazole is effective in more than 90% of cases.

ENTERIC FEVERS: TYPHOID AND PARATYPHOID

Causative agents and transmission

Salmonella typhi and *S. paratyphi* types A, B and C, all cause enteric fevers, although *S. typhi* is responsible for the vast majority of infections. These species are restricted to humans, and are usually spread via faecally contaminated food or water. Infections are most common in developing countries with poor standards of water supply and sewage disposal. In Australia, there are less than 100 new cases of enteric fever reported each year, and most of these are established as having been acquired overseas.

Pathogenesis

After ingestion, many of the salmonellae are killed by the acidity of the stomach but, if the infecting dose is high enough, some bacteria enter the small intestine. There they penetrate the intestinal mucosa, where they are quickly ingested by macrophages. A major feature of these organisms is their ability not only to survive, but to actively multiply inside macrophages. They are transported by these cells to the mesenteric lymph nodes where they continue to multiply. Eventually they reach the thoracic duct and then the bloodstream. Once in the blood, they can seed many organs, especially the spleen, bones and the liver. After further multiplication, there is reinvasion of the blood, which marks the end of the incubation period and the beginning of clinical illness.

This second phase of bacteraemia leads to invasion of other organs, such as the kidney. The gall bladder becomes infected either from the blood or from the liver. The organism grows actively in the bile, and enters the intestine for a second time. Most of the symptoms caused by *S. typhi* can be attributed to the inflammation induced by its lipopolysaccharide. It does not have any recognised exotoxins.

Clinical features

After an incubation period of 10–14 days, the early symptoms of fever, headache and respiratory symptoms (typically a dry cough) appear. Mild abdominal discomfort with either diarrhoea or constipation occurs. Without treatment, the fever increases in a stepwise fashion and the patient may eventually lapse into a stupor. Other common symptoms are rose spots (pink macular spots which blanch on pressure), bradycardia and splenomegaly. Without treatment, an uncomplicated infection lasts 4–6 weeks. A serious complication is secondary invasion of the intestine from the gall-bladder. In a small proportion of patients this can lead to inflammation and then perforation or haemorrhage of the intestine. Death occurs in approximately 15% of untreated cases.

Many patients continue to excrete *S. typhi* in the faeces for several weeks after recovery. In up to 3% of infected people, the organism persists in the gall bladder, and bacteria continue to be shed in faeces for years. Such chronic carriers are a major public health problem. In countries with inadequate sewage disposal, it may mean continued contamination of water supplies. In developed countries, chronic carriers can become a major hazard if they are employed in food handling. Mary Mallon

('Typhoid Mary'), a cook in New York City in the early 1900s, is the classic example. As a carrier, she caused many outbreaks of the disease and was ultimately imprisoned for life for refusing to stop working as a cook.

Laboratory diagnosis

The diagnosis of enteric fever relies on the isolation of *S. typhi or S. paratyphi* from the patient. Blood cultures generally become positive at the onset of symptoms, and in many patients remain positive over the next two weeks (see Figure 18.8). Faeces and urine should also be cultured, especially at 2–4 weeks after onset of symptoms, when seeding of the kidneys and secondary infection of the intestine occurs. Asymptomatic chronic carriers are also diagnosed by positive cultures from faeces and urine. Serum antibodies to the organisms can be detected by an agglutination test (the Widal test), but positive results must be interpreted with care where past exposure or vaccination are a possibility. A fourfold rise in titre between acute and convalescent sera is diagnostic.

FIGURE 18.8
THE ISOLATION OF TYPHOID BACTERIA FROM DIFFERENT SPECIMENS OVER THE COURSE OF THE DISEASE

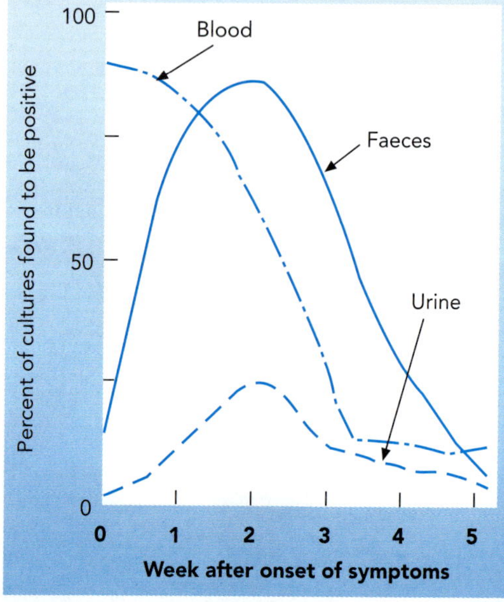

Treatment and prevention

Oral treatment with chloramphenicol, ampicillin, cotrimoxazole or ciprofloxacin is generally effective and should be maintained for 14 days to reduce the possibility of relapse. Strains of *S. typhi* resistant to one or more of the above agents have been reported, particularly on the Indian subcontinent. For chronic carriers, long-term therapy with ampicillin or ciprofloxacin may be effective but, if not, cholecystectomy (removal of the gall bladder—the site of carriage) may be warranted.

In developing countries, prevention of infection depends on good personal hygiene, adequate sewage disposal and a clean water supply. In the developed world, outbreaks of enteric fever are rare. Typhoid carriers are a particular concern and should be treated or excluded from employment that involves food handling. A killed vaccine against *S. typhi* is available, and is recommended for travellers to developing countries, but it is only 70–90% effective, and protects for several years only. Adverse effects of vaccination are common and include painful local reaction, fever, malaise and headache. Attenuated, oral vaccines are currently being tested.

Helminth Infections of the Gastrointestinal Tract

The types and characteristics of helminths (worms) are described in Chapter 6. Briefly, there are three major groups:

- nematodes (roundworms);
- cestodes (tapeworms); and
- trematodes (flukes).

The nematodes are further subdivided into roundworms, hookworms and threadworms (pinworms).

Parasitic helminths continue to be a major cause of morbidity in humans, particularly in the tropics and subtropics, and where there is poor sanitation. Worldwide, more than one billion people are estimated to be infected with an intestinal helminth. In Australia, helminth infections occur mostly in the northern (tropical) parts of the country, and are predominantly due to nematodes. Intestinal nematodes are found particularly in northern Aboriginal communities with poor sanitation and inadequate medical facilities. Fortunately, some of the more serious helminth infections, such as schistosomiasis, river blindness and filariasis (elephantiasis), which are endemic in other parts of the world, do not occur in this country. The common helminth infections in Australia are listed in Table 6.3 (p. 126); all are nematodes except the beef tapeworm (*Taenia saginata*), the cause of hydatid cysts (*Echinococcus granulosus*), and the tapeworm, *Hymenolepis nana*.

The real incidence of helminth infections in Australia is difficult to determine. The most common is undoubtedly the pinworm (or threadworm) *Enterobius vermicularis*, which is found throughout the country. The least common is probably hydatid disease, of which there are 30–40 reports each year.

The helminths listed in Table 6.3 are acquired in two distinct ways. *Ancylostoma duodenale* and *Necator americanus* (the hookworms) and *Strongyloides stercoralis* infect humans by penetration of the skin by infective larvae, whereas all the others are acquired by ingestion of the infective eggs of the helminths. All specifically inhabit the bowel except for *E. granulosus* (liver and lungs), and *S. stercoralis*, which can spread from the bowel to cause disseminated infection.

In nematode infections, the severity of disease is largely a function of the number of worms in the body. Increasing the worm load generally requires repeated exposure to the infectious larvae or eggs, since all except *Strongyloides* do not multiply in the host. Thus, travellers and immigrants from non-endemic areas are likely to have mild, if any, symptoms, whereas residents of endemic areas are more likely to be reinfected frequently and to suffer a more severe disease.

ENTEROBIUS VERMICULARIS

In contrast to other nematodes, *Enterobius vermicularis* is prevalent in temperate as well as tropical regions. Tens of thousands of Australians are believed to harbour this worm, but it does not cause serious illness. Adult pinworms (approximately 1 cm in length) pass out of the anus at night, depositing eggs in the perianal area. Many people are asymptomatic but, when symptoms do occur, anal pruritis (itching), especially at night, is the classic sign. Transmission usually occurs directly from fingers contaminated by scratching, but the eggs are also light enough to be carried in dust. After hatching, the worms mature entirely in the intestine.

The eggs of *Enterobius* are rarely present in faeces, but can be identified by applying adhesive tape to the perianal skin when the patient wakens, followed by microscopic examination of the tape. Infections are effectively treated with mebendazole or pyrantel.

ASCARIS LUMBRICOIDES

Adult worms are 15–35 cm long, hence the common name of giant roundworm (Figure 18.9). The females lay an enormous number of eggs into the intestine (about 200 000 in a day), which are passed in faeces. The eggs can remain infective in soil for many weeks or months, depending on the conditions. The infection is usually transmitted by faecal-oral passage of eggs via contaminated hands.

After ingestion, the eggs hatch in the intestine, releasing the larvae. The larvae penetrate the gut wall and are carried via the blood through the liver to the lungs. From there they work their way up the bronchi and trachea and are swallowed, and once again enter the intestine. The adult worms live freely in the gut lumen, feeding on intestinal contents. Most people with a small worm load are asymptomatic or experience only mild abdominal discomfort. Most only become aware of their infection when they pass a worm in their stools.

In some cases, the migration of the larvae through the lungs can cause severe respiratory distress (pneumonitis). With large worm loads, and especially in children, intestinal obstruction may occur. Even a single worm can cause harm, if it migrates into the hepatobiliary tree and occludes the ducts, causing acute biliary colic, cholangitis and cholecystitis.

Diagnosis is based on the microscopic examination of faeces. The eggs of *Ascaris* and many other helminths are characteristic, and readily recognised in a fresh stool specimen. Ideally, the specimen should be transported to the laboratory so that it can be examined within 30 minutes of collection, or else preserved with a fixative to maintain the egg structures. Three or more specimens may have to be collected in some cases, because of low numbers or intermittent shedding. A variety of antihelminthic drugs are available for treatment of intestinal nematodes (e.g. mebendazole, pyrantel).

HOOKWORMS

Hookworms are a serious cause of long-term morbidity in developing countries, because of the anaemia and hypoproteinaemia that result from heavy infection. Adult hookworms, *Ancylostoma duodenale* and *Necator americanus* (approximately 1 cm in length), attach to the intestinal mucosa by specialised mouth structures (Figure 18.10). They rupture capillaries and suck blood, and lay thin-coated eggs that are passed in faeces into the environment. The eggs mature and hatch in soil, and infection of a new host takes place when larvae come into contact with unprotected skin of a person (sometimes swallowed in the case of *Ancylostoma*). They penetrate the skin, migrate via the blood to the lungs, climb the trachea and are swallowed, maturing into adult worms in the small intestine.

Most people with light worm loads are asymptomatic. Heavy infections may cause abdominal pain, flatulence, a bloody diarrhoea, and an iron deficiency anaemia in children or in anyone with existing malnutrition. Hookworm infections are diagnosed and treated in a similar way to *Ascaris* infections.

An unusual outbreak of enteritis occurred in Townsville, Queensland, in the 1980s. This area is free of human hookworm, but all cases were closely associated with dogs, and a dog hookworm was suggested as the cause. All patients were successfully treated with antihelminthic drugs.

STRONGYLOIDES STERCORALIS

The tiny adult worms (2–3 mm in length) dwell just beneath the intestinal mucosa, where they lay their eggs. These eggs hatch in the intestine and are passed in the faeces. *Strongyloides* infection occurs when larvae in faecally contaminated soil or fomites penetrate the skin or mucous membranes. They then enter the bloodstream, and break into the alveoli in the lungs. Like the hookworms, they ascend the bronchi and trachea, are swallowed, and reach the small intestine where maturation is completed. This worm, however, is unlike any other intestinal nematode in its ability to multiply in the host. In some cases, the internally generated larvae can then penetrate the intestinal mucosa or the perianal skin and migrate via the lungs back to the small intestine, in what is essentially an 'auto-infection cycle'. This cycle is most likely to occur in the immunocompromised, or in patients with malnutrition or other debilitating disease. Infection may persist for decades. In uncontrolled infections larvae may infect other organs, including the urinary tract, liver and brain.

People with low worm burdens are often asymptomatic. With greater numbers of worms, there may be non-specific gastrointestinal symptoms of abdominal pain, intermittent diarrhoea and nausea. Heavy intestinal infection causes a persistent and profuse diarrhoea, with dehydration and

FIGURE 18.9
ASCARIS LUMBRICOIDES, THE GIANT ROUNDWORM
Female worms can lay as many as 200 000 eggs in a day in the gut of an infected person.

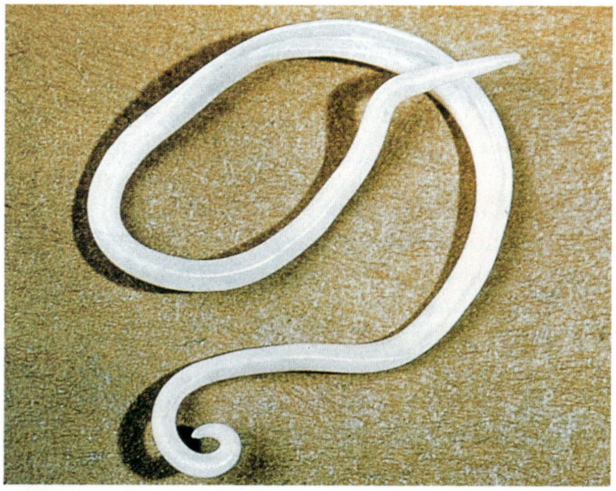

electrolyte imbalance. Invasion of other body sites by large numbers of auto-infective larvae can be fatal. Asymptomatic immigrants from endemic areas such as South-East Asia, especially those with unexplained eosinophilia, are often found to be infected with *Strongyloides*. It is also found in some Aboriginal communities, and was common in Australian soldiers held in Asian prisoner of war camps.

Strongyloides infection is difficult to diagnose, but can be done by finding larvae in fresh stools. Many stool specimens may have to be examined before larvae are found. Serological tests for *Strongyloides* are available, but do not distinguish between past and current infection. Infections are usually treated with thiabendazole, but eradication of the worm is not always achieved, especially in the immunosuppressed. Repeated, short courses of treatment may be necessary to keep the worm load at a low level.

HYDATID DISEASE

Hydatid disease is caused by the tapeworm *Echinococcus granulosus*. The parasite's definitive host is the dog, but it can be transmitted to other animals, particularly sheep. Other dogs then become infected when fed on the viscera of infected sheep. Humans act as accidental hosts when the eggs of the parasite are ingested, usually as a result of contact with the fur or tongue of an infected dog. Young children of sheep-farming families are at greatest risk. Recent evidence indicates that the parasite is also found in certain wildlife species, such as dingoes, wallabies, kangaroos and foxes; these animals could therefore be additional sources of infection. Currently, in Australia, there are less than 50 notifications of hydatid infection each year, with an average of three deaths per year due to this infection.

After ingestion of eggs, the larvae emerge and migrate through the gut and then the bloodstream, and eventually localise in organs such as the liver, lungs and brain. In these organs they form fluid-filled sacs, called cysts, which contain thousands of developing worms and can reach the size of a grapefruit. Residence within these sacs enables the worms to evade host defence mechanisms (see Chapter 10). Symptoms result from the local pressure of the cyst on the organ. Bursting of the cyst can lead to seeding of other organs with the worms and, in some people, a life-threatening anaphylactic reaction to hydatid antigens.

Diagnosis of hydatid cysts is by radiologic demonstration of a cystic lesion, supported by positive serology. Treatment may be achieved with the drug albendazole, but surgical removal of the cysts is often necessary.

FIGURE 18.10
ANCYLOSTOMA DUODENALE
This worm attaches to the intestinal mucosa by specialised mouth structures.

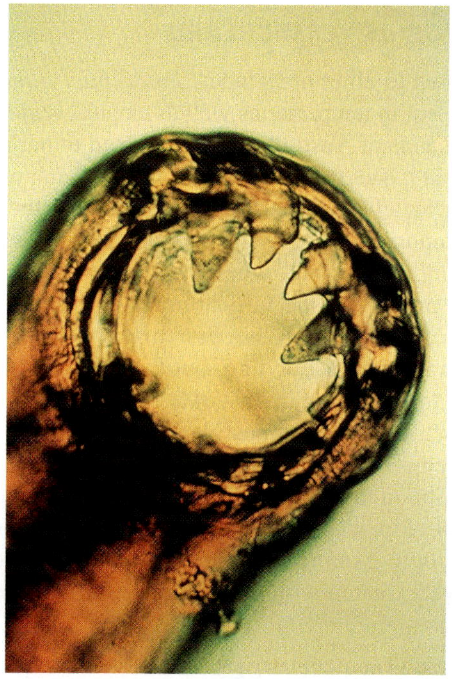

TAENIA SAGINATA

The beef tapeworm attaches by its head to the intestinal mucosa. Most patients are asymptomatic or experience only mild abdominal discomfort. The most obvious sign of infection is the passing of white, motile proglottids, or long segments of a worm. Infections are diagnosed in a similar way to *Ascaris* infections. Treatment is usually with praziquantel or niclosamide.

TRICHURIS TRICHIURA

Adult worms are 3–4 cm in length. The worms remain within the large bowel, attaching to the epithelial layer. As with all intestinal worms, children are the members of the community most heavily infected with this parasite, acquiring eggs from contaminated soil or vegetation. Most infections are asymptomatic, but moderate to heavy worm loads, especially in children, can cause abdominal pain and diarrhoea, occasionally leading to prolapse of the rectum. Impaired nutrition and retarded growth of children may result. Infections are diagnosed and treated in a similar way to *Ascaris* infections.

HYMENOLEPIS NANA

Hymenolepis nana is a tapeworm (2–4 cm long) that causes an asymptomatic infection in most patients. In heavy infections it can cause diarrhoea, abdominal pain and loss of appetite. There are thought to be many millions of people worldwide infected with this parasite. Infections are diagnosed and treated in a similar way to *Ascaris* infections.

Hepatitis

The term **hepatitis** refers to injury and inflammation of the liver. Viruses are major causes of hepatitis, but other microorganisms, alcohol, drugs and various other disorders (e.g. biliary obstruction) may also be responsible (see Table 18.5). A number of important viruses, including cytomegalovirus, Epstein-Barr virus (infectious mononucleosis) and rubella virus, can infect the liver and cause hepatitis as part of a systemic infection. These are dealt with in Chapter 19. Here we will focus on the viruses that infect mainly the liver. These are the hepatitis viruses A, B, C, D and E. Each of these belongs to a different virus family, and they have little in common except the target organ they affect. The characteristics of the different hepatitis viruses are outlined in Table 18.6.

Viral hepatitis is a major cause of morbidity and mortality throughout the world. Hepatitis A virus (HAV) and hepatitis E virus (HEV) are spread mainly by faecal-oral means; and the other three—hepatitis B virus (HBV), hepatitis C virus (HCV) and hepatitis D virus (HDV)—are spread principally by exposure to blood, although transmission via other body fluids, especially genital secretions for HBV, also occurs.

Hepatitis viruses produce acute inflammation of the liver. This may result in a clinical illness with variable

TABLE 18.5
CAUSES OF HEPATITIS

Viruses
Hepatitis viruses A, B, C, D, E
Cytomegalovirus
Epstein-Barr virus (infectious mononucleosis)
Herpes simplex virus
Rubella virus
Yellow fever virus

Other infections
Syphilis
Tuberculosis
Toxoplasmosis
Q fever
Amoebiasis

Non-infectious causes
Biliary obstruction
Primary biliary cirrhosis
Drug toxicity
Drug hypersensitivity
Alcohol abuse

TABLE 18.6
CHARACTERISTICS OF HEPATITIS VIRUSES

	HEPATITIS A	HEPATITIS B	HEPATITIS C	HEPATITIS D	HEPATITIS E
Family	Picornaviridae	Hepadnaviridae	Flaviviridae	(unclassified)	Caliciviridae
Genome	ssRNA	dsDNA	ssRNA	ssRNA	ssRNA
Mode of transmission	Faecal-oral	Blood; sexual; mother to child	Blood; ? sexual; ? mother to child	Blood; sexual	Faecal-oral
Incubation period	2-6 weeks	1-6 months	2-26 weeks	2-9 weeks	2-9 weeks
Acute mortality rate	0.2%	0.2%	0.2%	2-20%	0.2%
Infectious period	2 weeks before onset to 1 week after symptoms subside	Many weeks before onset to life in carriers	1 or more weeks before onset to life in carriers	Not known, but maximal just before onset	Not known
Chronicity	None	5–10%	50–70%	2–20%	None
Vaccine	Yes	Yes	No	No	No

features (see Table 18.7), including gastrointestinal symptoms such as anorexia, nausea and vomiting, fever, malaise and jaundice (yellowing of the skin and whites of the eyes). In more serious cases, liver function can fail. Marked increases in serum concentrations of the liver enzymes, alanine aminotransferase (ALT) and aspartate aminotransferase (AST), are characteristic of acute viral hepatitis. Generally, the different types of hepatitis cannot be distinguished by their signs and symptoms. The patient's history and risk factors may indicate the likely type(s), but specific laboratory tests are required for a definitive diagnosis.

At present there is no effective treatment for acute viral hepatitis, although α-interferon (see Chapter 9) has been used with limited success in chronic hepatitis B and C. Vaccines are currently available only for hepatitis A and B.

TABLE 18.7
COMMON CLINICAL FEATURES OF VIRAL HEPATITIS

- Jaundice
- Anorexia, nausea, vomiting
- Diarrhoea or constipation
- Abdominal pain
- Fever, malaise
- Myalgia, arthralgia
- Fatigue, weakness
- Anaemia
- Increased serum alanine aminotransferase (ALT)
- Increased serum aspartate aminotransferase (AST)

HEPATITIS A

HAV is a small RNA virus, belonging to the family of picornaviruses. The virus was first isolated in cell culture in 1979, and is still the only hepatitis virus that has been propagated *in vitro*. In Australia there are about 2000 notifications of hepatitis A annually. However, it is thought that a large number of asymptomatic (not notified) infections occur in northern parts of the country.

Transmission

Transmission of HAV is primarily by the faecal-oral route because it is excreted in large amounts in faeces. However, transmission by other means, such as intravenous drug use and sexual contact (especially in homosexual men), is also possible. It is spread mainly from person to person by contact (hands) or by contamination of food or water. Once transferred to fomites from unwashed hands, the virus can persist on surfaces for several days.

Contamination of food or water can lead to sudden, explosive epidemics of hepatitis A. Poor personal hygiene, poor sanitation and close personal contact (e.g. household or sexual contact) facilitate transmission of the virus. Hepatitis A is endemic in many tropical and subtropical regions of the world and in most rural Aboriginal communities in Australia, with most infections occurring in young children. Because its spread is due primarily to poor hygiene, it was formerly referred to as 'infectious hepatitis'. It may also be transmitted via shellfish from polluted waters, especially if eaten raw.

HAV infection often occurs in institutional settings, and has been reported in health care workers caring for infected patients. In Australia, there have been several reports of hepatitis in nursing staff, particularly in paediatric wards in hospitals in northern and central parts of the country, where there is a high incidence of infection among Aboriginal children. Failure to wear gloves when contact with faeces occurred, or to wash hands thoroughly before eating have been suggested as the major faults in these cases. Lack of good sanitation and hygiene can lead to outbreaks in schools, camps and day-care centres.

Outbreaks of hepatitis A among injecting drug users have been reported, including one in Sydney[1], but it is believed they were more likely to have been due to faecal contamination of drugs or injecting materials, or poor hygiene and close contact among abusers, than to blood-borne transmission. In recent years, there has been an increased incidence of hepatitis A among male homosexuals, possibly related to oral-anal sexual practices.

Pathogenesis and clinical features

After infection, the virus is believed to replicate initially in intestinal cells. This is followed by a brief period of viraemia (viruses in the blood) and then spread to the liver. The incubation period ranges from 2 to 6 weeks, with an average of about 25 days. During this lengthy incubation period, liver cells are damaged, possibly by immune mechanisms rather than direct viral action.

Hepatitis A varies considerably in its presentation. The illness is usually not apparent in children less than four years old, but it becomes progressively more severe with increasing age. When symptomatic, it is generally a mild to moderate disease, with typical manifestations of fever, anorexia, nausea, vomiting, fatigue, liver pain and sometimes jaundice, due to impaired liver function. Complete recovery occurs in most cases in 4–6 weeks; there is no carrier state, and chronic infection does not generally occur. However, shedding of the virus may continue for up to six months in asymptomatic neonates.

Laboratory diagnosis

Since the clinical presentation of any type of hepatitis is not definitive, laboratory tests are required for the diagnosis. HAV is not routinely cultured, and the other hepatitis viruses have not yet been cultured, so diagnosis of hepatitis, in general, is based on serological tests. The diagnostic tests for all the hepatitis viruses are summarised in Table 18.8.

The standard method for diagnosing hepatitis A is by detection of anti-hepatitis A antibodies in the patient's serum. Anti-HAV IgM is usually detectable approximately

TABLE 18.8
ROUTINE SEROLOGIC TESTS FOR THE DIAGNOSIS OF HEPATITIS

	HEPATITIS A	HEPATITIS B	HEPATITIS C	HEPATITIS D	HEPATITIS E
Antigens detected	HAAg	HBsAg, HBeAg	None available	None available	None available
Antibodies detected	Anti-HAV Anti-HAV IgM	Anti-HBs Anti-HBc Anti-HBc IgM Anti-HBe	Anti-HCV	Anti-HDV Anti-HDV IgM	None available

CASE HISTORY 18.4
HEPATITIS A

In February 1994, two registered nurses working in a 48-bed district hospital became unwell within 10 days of each other. Both were subsequently diagnosed as having acute hepatitis A. Neither nurse had children or any contact with a child-care facility, neither had recently been overseas, and neither had any known contact with a recent case of hepatitis A outside the hospital.

When interviewed, both nurses recalled caring for a 22-month-old Aboriginal child at the same time. The child had profuse diarrhoea, and on one occasion one of the nurse's uniforms was grossly soiled with the child's faeces, and the other nurse had assisted with the clean-up. The child's discharge diagnosis was 'acute gastroenteritis'. She was never jaundiced. The child was later tested and found to be hepatitis A IgM positive. It was assumed that she was the source of infection for the two nurses.

Comment

Hepatitis A is a frequently asymptomatic infection common in many rural Aboriginal communities in Australia. Hospital-acquired hepatitis A is not common, but can occur when adequate cross-infection procedures are not observed.

Adapted from J. Hanna, 'Hospital-acquired hepatitis A', *Communicable Diseases Intelligence* 18/13, 27 June 1994, p. 312.

25–30 days after infection, and indicates current or recent infection. The anti-HAV test measures total antibody against HAV and includes IgM and IgG. IgG is present in the patient's serum for years after recovery, and so a single anti-HAV titre does not differentiate between current and past infection. Therefore, with this test, a rise in titre in paired serum samples must be demonstrated to diagnose infection. Serum concentrations of liver enzymes are usually markedly increased during infection.

Treatment and prevention

As for many viral infections, there is no specific cure for hepatitis A. Symptomatic treatment is all that is available. Prevention relies on good hygiene and the prophylactic use of gammaglobulin after suspected exposure. Gammaglobulin is a pooled serum preparation from normal blood donors that contains antibodies to hepatitis A virus and other common diseases. Gammaglobulin must be given within 7–10 days of exposure to prevent infection. It can also be given to provide short-term protection (4–6 months) to travellers to endemic areas. An inactivated HAV vaccine has recently been developed and licensed for use in Australia.

School-based outbreaks are often attributed to inadequate toilet facilities. Improvement of facilities and thorough handwashing are the most important interventions for preventing infections in schools.

HEPATITIS B

Hepatitis B is caused by a hepadna (hepatitis DNA) virus. As shown in Figure 18.11 the HBV has an outer coat containing an antigen called the hepatitis B surface antigen (HBsAg). This was formerly called the 'Australia antigen' because it was originally identified in the serum of an Australian Aborigine. The inner component is called the hepatitis core antigen (HBcAg) and inside this is the viral DNA (HBV-DNA) and the viral enzyme, DNA polymerase. A third hepatitis B antigen is the hepatitis Be antigen (HBeAg). The HBeAg is a secreted product of the core antigen, and its presence in blood is indicative of active viral replication. The whole virus particle is called a Dane particle, named after the scientist who first saw it by electron microscopy. HBV has not been isolated or propagated in cell culture.

Hepatitis B has a worldwide distribution. There are thought to be more than 300 million carriers throughout the world, and approximately one million deaths each year. High carrier rates (up to 25%) are found in some populations, such as in some Asian and African countries, in some Pacific islands and in some Australian Aboriginal communities.

Transmission

Hepatitis B virus can be found in the blood and body fluids of acutely infected people or carriers. Blood and blood products have the highest concentrations of HBV and are the most common sources of transmission, but other body fluids, especially semen, vaginal secretions and serous fluids, can also transmit the virus. Since the number of infectious particles in blood can be extremely high (up to a million infectious doses per microlitre), very small amounts of blood can be infectious. The virus is fairly stable and can survive for days in dried blood contaminating the surface of an object. The virus has been found in saliva, urine and faeces, but infrequently and in lower concentrations. It is therefore only rarely transmitted via these body substances, but it is important to recognise them as potential sources of infection.

Most cases in developed countries now occur in homosexual and bisexual males, IV drug abusers and people with multiple sexual partners (homosexual and heterosexual). Babies born to mothers with hepatitis B have a high risk of infection. Perinatal transmission occurs primarily as a result of the infant's exposure to infected blood or genital secretions during delivery. Health care workers may be exposed to HBV via needlestick injuries, or when contaminated blood comes into contact with mucous membranes (e.g. the splashing of blood into the eyes) or with skin cuts or abrasions. Doctors, nurses and dental workers are at particularly high risk. There has been much debate as to whether HBV is spread by mosquitoes or other biting insects. The evidence to date suggests that, if this does occur, it does so very infrequently.

FIGURE 18.11
HEPATITIS B VIRUS
The complete virion (called a Dane particle) and different forms of HBsAg as seen by electron microscopy in the serum of infected people.

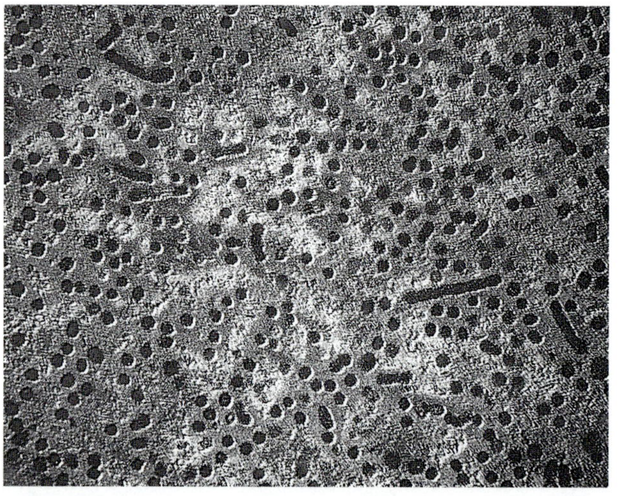

Pathogenesis and clinical features

Replication of the hepatitis B virus in the liver results in cell damage but the virus does not directly kill hepatocytes. Much of the pathology is due to immune mechanisms, including destruction of infected liver cells by cytotoxic T cells. The virus replicates prolifically in the liver, but assembly of components to form complete virions is very inefficient (see Figure 18.11). As a result, large numbers of virus particles are released into the bloodstream, but only a small fraction of these are complete viruses. Large amounts of antigenic viral components are released, and these, and antibodies to them, can be detected in the blood in diagnostic laboratory tests.

The incubation period of hepatitis B is 4–26 weeks (average 75 days). Acute hepatitis B is clinically similar to hepatitis A, although usually more severe. In some patients there is an initial, brief illness with rash and arthralgia due to the formation of immune complexes between HBsAg and anti-HBsAg antibodies, and their deposition in the skin and joints (see Chapter 9). A large proportion of cases are anicteric (without jaundice). In otherwise healthy adults, 90% will spontaneously recover within six months of the onset of the illness. In 1% or less of patients, acute **fulminant hepatitis** occurs. This is a clinical syndrome in which there is severe impairment or necrosis of liver cells, liver failure and death in about 80% of those affected. Acute hepatitis B has a mortality rate of around 0.2%.

When people recover completely from acute HBV infection, they do so because of the destruction of all infected lymphocytes by primed cytotoxic T cells. However, in about 5–10% of infected individuals, complete elimination of the virus does not occur and they develop **chronic hepatitis**, becoming chronic carriers of the virus. Chronic hepatitis is defined as the persistence of viral antigens in the bloodstream for at least six months. Vertical transmission (from mother to baby) is very serious, because it is associated with an extremely high rate of chronicity. More than 90% of perinatally infected infants become chronically infected.

Many people with chronic hepatitis B infection are asymptomatic, but may remain lifelong carriers of HBV without knowing it, whereas others with chronic active hepatitis can suffer a severe illness due to marked liver dysfunction. It is not known why some people are silent carriers, while others have active disease. However, both forms are serious because both are associated with an increased likelihood of developing hepatic cirrhosis (fibrosis) and/or hepatocellular carcinoma later in life (10–30 years later), although patients with active persistent infection are much more likely to develop these sequelae. The cirrhosis occurs because of long-term inflammation of the liver.

The mechanisms involved in oncogenesis have not been fully elucidated, but the integration of the viral DNA into the host cell's genome has been demonstrated. Hepatitis B is thought to be responsible for as much as 80% of all cases of liver cancer in the world, resulting in 1–2 million deaths per year.

Laboratory diagnosis

Diagnosis of hepatitis B is by examination of serum for evidence of various viral antigens and antibodies to those antigens (see Figure 18.12). HBsAg appears in the blood during the incubation period and implies ongoing infection, either acute or chronic. HBsAg levels generally fall and finally disappear during recovery, but HBsAg remains in the blood of carriers. Persistence of HBsAg in the blood for more than six months indicates chronic infection. As

FIGURE 18.12
THE TYPICAL COURSE OF ACUTE HEPATITIS B INFECTION AND THE ASSOCIATED SEROLOGICAL EVENTS

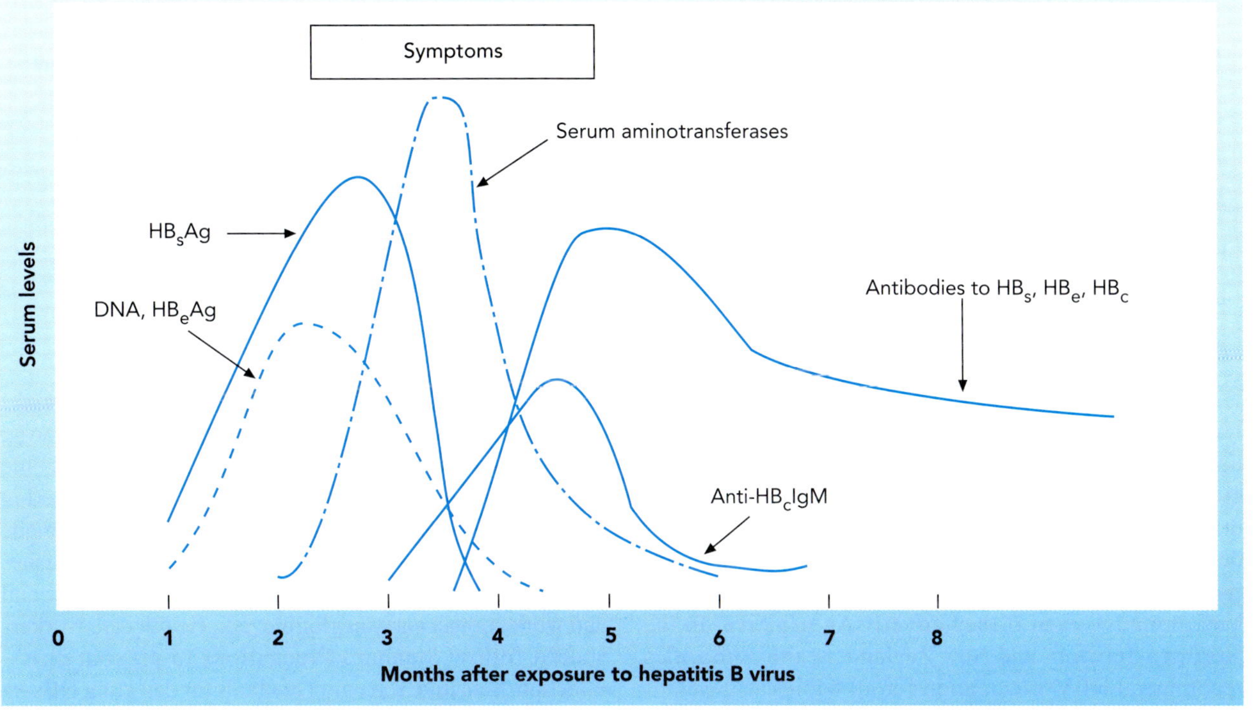

HBsAg disappears, anti-HBs antibody becomes detectable. Anti-HBs antibodies are present for years in the serum of people who have fully recovered and are not carriers. Anti-HBs antibodies are the only serologic marker in people immunised with the hepatitis vaccine.

HBeAg is found in serum early during acute infection and in chronic infections. Detection of HBeAg indicates there are large amounts of virus in the blood, and thus high infectivity. HBeAg is not detected in serum that is negative for HBsAg, but HBeAg negativity in patients with detectable HBsAg may indicate low levels of viral replication. The appearance of anti-HBe antibody and disappearance of HBeAg signals a cessation of viral replication and resolution of disease.

HBV-DNA can be detected in serum during acute and chronic infection. It is considered to be the best evidence of viral replication and infectivity in patients, and is often positive in patients with low-grade viraemia who are negative for HBeAg. The loss of HBV-DNA from serum indicates resolution of disease.

During the illness, antibodies to the core antigen, HBcAg, appear. These antibodies represent an immunologic response to infection, but are not indicative of disease resolution.

The interpretation of the serologic tests for hepatitis B is summarised in Table 18.9.

Treatment and prevention

As with hepatitis A, there is no fully effective therapy for hepatitis B. Hydration and anti-nauseants are the basic forms of symptomatic treatment. Alpha-interferon, which appears to have both antiviral and immunomodulatory effects, has been used for the treatment of chronic hepatitis B with some success. In approximately one-third of patients with chronic HBV infection, treatment with α-interferon results in a suppression of HBV replication and clinical improvement, but discontinuation of the drug results in a relapse in many of these people. A large number of possible side effects are associated with α-interferon use, especially with the first dose and high doses. The severity of side effects ranges from fever, chills, fatigue and muscle aches to vascular collapse, coma, cyanosis, congestive heart disease and bone marrow depression. Thus, the safety and relative benefit of interferon therapy for hepatitis B and other hepatitis viruses are still somewhat unclear.

Both passive and active immunisation are available for prevention of hepatitis B. Hepatitis B immunoglobulin (HBIG) is used to provide immediate post-exposure protection to unimmunised people following needlestick injury or high-risk sexual encounter, or to neonates born to HBsAg positive mothers. HBIG is prepared from plasma donated through routine blood bank collection and selected on the basis of containing high antibody titres to HBsAg.

The best way to prevent hepatitis B infection is with the HBV vaccine. This is a safe, effective vaccine consisting of genetically engineered HBsAg produced in yeast cells. Three doses of vaccine generally give good protection (efficacy around 95%), and vaccination is recommended, especially for those frequently exposed to blood or blood products, such as surgeons, nurses, dentists, and other health professionals, multiply-transfused or dialysed patients, and intravenous drug abusers. It is essential that the vaccination schedule be completed for full protection, and advisable that the antibody titre is checked, since not all people seroconvert.

TABLE 18.9
INTERPRETATION OF SEROLOGICAL ASSAYS FOR HEPATITIS B

	NO INFECTION PAST OR PRESENT	ACUTE INFECTION	CHRONIC INFECTION	PAST, RESOLVED INFECTION	PREVIOUS IMMUNISATION
HBsAg	–	+	+	–	–
Anti-HBc	–	+	+	+	–
Anti-HBc IgM	–	+	–	–	–
HBeAg	–	+	+/–	–	–
Anti-HBeAg	–	–	+/–	+/–	–
Anti-HBsAg	–	–	+/–	+	+

Administration of both HBIG and HBV vaccine to neonates within 12 hours of birth is recommended if the mother is HBsAg positive, to prevent transmission of infection to the baby. Neonatal infection is so serious that HBV vaccine is often given to babies born to 'high-risk mothers' (i.e. IV drug users or those of certain ethnic backgrounds), even if they are HBsAg negative. In the Northern Territory and New Zealand, health authorities recommend HBV vaccination for all babies.

The World Health Organization Expanded Programme on Immunization recommended that countries with an HBV carrier rate of 8% or more include HBV vaccine in their routine immunisation programs by 1995, and all other countries by 1997. Rare hepatitis B mutants causing infection in patients with antibodies to the present vaccine have been reported, but their significance, at present, is uncertain.

CASE HISTORY 18.5
HEPATITIS B

A 27-year-old bank clerk went to Casualty at a local hospital because he had been feeling ill for several days. His illness was marked by fever, nausea and right abdominal pain. He thought he had flu, but noticed that morning that his eyes were quite yellow. He had never experienced any severe illness, although he recalled that he had experienced similar symptoms several years earlier. The symptoms then had been milder, so he hadn't seen a doctor. He admitted to using drugs occasionally, but said he never used a needle that someone else had used. He stated that he had a very active sex life, although he didn't have a permanent girlfriend.

Liver function tests revealed an AST (aspartate aminotransferase) level of 60 IU/L (normal range: 10–45 IU/L), an ALT (alanine transaminase) level of 56 IU/L (normal range: 5–45 IU/L), and a total bilirubin level of 27 µmol/L (normal: 0–18 µmol/L). Serology for hepatitis viruses was performed. Positive results were found for HBsAg and HBeAg, and the anti-HBc was negative.

Sexual transmission can be prevented by the use of barrier contraceptive measures. People with acute or chronic hepatitis B should be warned about the risk of infecting sexual partners who are not immune. They should be made aware that some practices, like the sharing of toothbrushes or razors, carry a risk, but that ordinary domestic, social and work contact carry negligible risk. Health care workers should follow Standard Precautions to prevent cross-infection. Sensitive screening methods for detecting HBsAg are now employed by blood banks in Australia.

HEPATITIS C

The existence of a third hepatitis virus became apparent in 1975, when new diagnostic tests for hepatitis A and hepatitis B used on stored serum samples revealed that many cases of transfusion-associated hepatitis were not due to either HAV or HBV. Most cases of what was formerly called non-A, non-B (NANB) hepatitis have now been attributed to the hepatitis C virus. The HCV genome was cloned in 1989 and viral protein produced. Soon after, antibody assays were developed and HCV was established as the cause of 80–95% of cases of transfusion-associated non-A, non-B hepatitis. Australian blood banks began screening blood for anti-HCV antibody in early 1990. The virus itself has not been isolated, and was only recently tentatively visualised by electron microscopy. It is an RNA virus that is related to the flaviviruses and pestiviruses.

HCV has a worldwide distribution. In Australia, about 0.5% of blood donors are found to be HCV positive, and it has been estimated that more than 100 000 Australians may be infected by the virus. It is difficult to determine accurately the rates of HCV infection, because many cases are asymptomatic, and because current tests do not differentiate between acute, chronic and past infection. The highest number of infections is in the 25–44 years age group, with a preponderance in males.

Transmission

Transmission of HCV is predominantly via contaminated blood; that is, by receipt of blood or blood products and by intravenous drug abuse. IV drug use is now the greatest risk factor in countries where screening of blood donors is routine. The prevalence of HCV among intravenous drug users is reportedly about 60%. Occupational acquisition of infection after needlestick injury has been clearly demonstrated. It appears that sexual transmission and perinatal transmission (from mother to baby) of HCV can occur, but they are not common modes of infection. There appear to be other, as yet unknown, modes of transmission, because many cases occur in people with no known risk factor (see Figure 18.13).

Pathogenesis and clinical features

The incubation period of hepatitis C appears to be quite variable, ranging from 14 to 180 days (average 50 days). Most cases of acute HCV infection are asymptomatic. When symptomatic, the disease is usually mild, with jaundice occurring in a minority of cases and liver enzymes only minimally to moderately elevated. The liver disease appears to be due to the ability of the virus to kill hepatocytes directly. The host's T cells, attempting to eliminate virus-infected cells, may also have a role in hepatic damage. Clinically, it is indistinguishable from other forms of acute viral hepatitis.

Despite the mild nature of acute infection, at least 60% of cases progress to chronic infection. This is a much higher rate than occurs with acute hepatitis B infection. As with chronic hepatitis B infections, the majority of chronic infections are asymptomatic. In symptomatic cases, there are often only mild symptoms of fatigue, weakness and a tender liver. But whether asymptomatic or not, the virus causes relentless damage to hepatocytes, and more than 20% of patients eventually develop hepatic cirrhosis (within 10 years) and/or hepatocellular carcinoma (within 20–30 years).

FIGURE 18.13
RISK FACTORS FOR HEPATITIS C INFECTION
Note that in many cases the mode of transmission is not known.

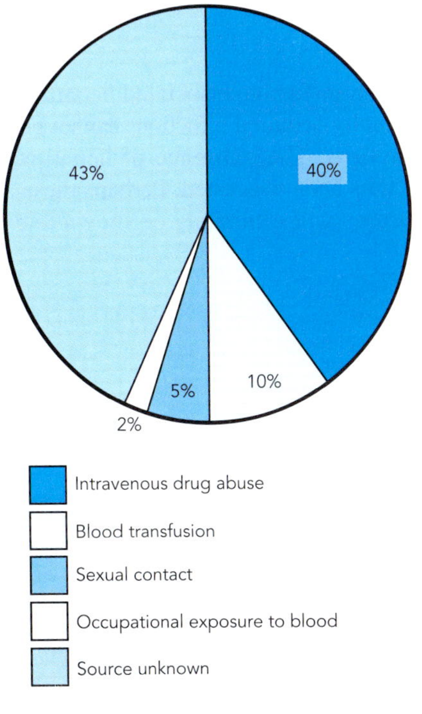

Laboratory diagnosis

Laboratory diagnosis of hepatitis C is based on the detection of antibodies in the serum of the patient. Unfortunately, the time from infection to seroconversion can be anywhere between two and nine months. This long 'window period' means that many cases of potentially infectious HCV may be missed by antibody tests. Furthermore, the current assays do not differentiate acute, chronic or past infection. Direct demonstration of the virus itself is achieved by detection of viral RNA in serum, using the polymerase chain reaction (PCR) technique. However, this methodology is available only in specialist laboratories, and there is some doubt about its reliability, since both false positives and false negatives occur with currently available kits.

Treatment and prevention

Supportive care, as for other types of hepatitis, should be provided. There is no strong evidence that gammaglobulin offers significant protection. Treatment of chronically infected patients with α-interferon has been encouraging, more so than with HBV or HDV infection. It normalises serum transaminases and reduces viraemia in about 50% of treated patients; although relapses occur in half the patients within several months of discontinuation of therapy, the remainder appear to be cured. Another drug, ribavirin, has also produced some favourable results in preliminary studies.

Transmission via blood transfusion has been significantly reduced by the routine testing of donors for antibody to hepatitis C. Vaccines for HCV are currently under investigation.

HEPATITIS D

In the late 1970s a new hepatitis virus was discovered in hepatitis B carriers in Italy. It was originally called the delta virus, but is now known as the hepatitis D virus. This virus has a very small RNA genome and is a defective virus, because it requires a coexisting, active hepatitis B infection to be able to complete its own replicative cycle. When it buds from the surface of an HBV-infected liver cell it is coated with the hepatitis B surface antigen, HBsAg, and it is this hepatitis B coat that enables it to attach to, and infect, other hepatocytes. Thus, a person cannot contract an HDV infection unless simultaneously infected with HBV (i.e. a co-infection), or unless already infected with HBV (i.e. an HDV superinfection).

HDV is found throughout the world, but its highest prevalence is in Central and South-East Asia, the Middle East, Africa and South America. Hepatitis D is currently not notifiable in Australia, and is relatively uncommon in this country.

Transmission

Blood and blood products are the major sources of HDV. The primary routes of transmission are believed to be similar to those of HBV and HCV. People who are drug abusers or who have received multiple blood transfusions are at highest risk. Perinatal transmission has been reported, but is rare.

Pathogenesis and clinical features

The incubation period varies from 2–9 weeks, being shorter in HBV carriers superinfected with HDV than when co-infection with both viruses occurs. In co-infection, the disease is often indistinguishable from hepatitis B alone but, when HDV superinfects a chronic carrier of HBV, the infection is usually severe and can lead to cirrhosis and hepatic failure, with a high mortality. Furthermore, chronic hepatitis develops in 1–3% of co-infections and 70–80% of superinfections. The majority of patients with chronic HBV/HDV hepatitis develop hepatic cirrhosis, and almost 25% of these die of liver failure.

Laboratory diagnosis

The laboratory diagnosis is based on serological tests for HDV antigen (HDVAg) or for antibody to HDVAg. Anti-HDV IgM levels are high in the acute stage of infection, and are suggestive of acute infection. Anti-HDV (total anti-HDV) detects both IgM and IgG classes of antibody. It tends to be low and transient in acute infection, but high in chronic infection.

Treatment and prevention

There is no effective treatment, other than physiologic support in rehydration and anti-nauseants. There is no HDV vaccine, but vaccination against hepatitis B prevents hepatitis D infection.

HEPATITIS E

Hepatitis E is caused by a small RNA virus that is a member of the calicivirus family. The virus has not been grown in cell culture but, in 1990, its genome was cloned, and then some of its antigens were synthesised by recombinant DNA technology. The virus is shed in faeces and spread by the faecal-oral route, but it appears to be less readily transmitted than HAV.

HEV appears to have a restricted distribution of Central and South-East Asia, Africa, the Middle East and Central America. It is best known for causing water-borne epidemics but is also responsible for a large proportion of sporadic hepatitis in countries where it is endemic. It is the cause of occasional cases of hepatitis in travellers to endemic areas. The first case of locally acquired HEV in Australia was reported in 1994 in the Northern Territory.

The incubation period ranges from 2 to 9 weeks, with a mean of about 40 days. Clinically, HEV infection is similar to HAV infection. Hepatitis E is generally a mild to moderate disease (mortality rate of 0.2–1%), but initial illness may be severe and fatal when associated with the malnutrition or other medical problems that are typical of its Third World victims. It can also cause severe infection in pregnant women, in whom the mortality rate can reach as high as 20% if infected in the third trimester. The virus is eliminated from the body on recovery, and appears not to cause chronic infection or long-term sequelae.

Serological tests for HEV have recently become available, but their validity and interpretation is presently unclear. HEV infection should be suspected in a patient who has travelled to an endemic region and exhibits signs of hepatitis, but who has negative test results for other hepatitis viruses. Prevention of infection after exposure can be attempted with gammaglobulin, but gammaglobulins prepared in non-endemic countries are unlikely to be protective, simply because of the lack of HEV and thus anti-HEV in those populations. Locally produced immunoglobulin (i.e. in the country where infection was acquired) may be of value, but this remains to be confirmed.

The risk of infection when travelling in endemic countries may be minimised by practising rigorous hygiene, drinking only appropriately treated water, and care in food consumption.

OTHER HEPATITIS VIRUSES

Up to 10% of transfusion-associated hepatitis and up to 5% of community-acquired infections cannot be attributed to a known virus. The existence of hepatitis F and G viruses has thus been suggested. Perhaps these and other hepatitis viruses will ultimately be shown to exist.

Summary

- The gastrointestinal tract (GIT) is a portal of entry into the body for numerous microorganisms.
- Food poisoning (food-borne illness) is a general term that refers to any gastrointestinal disease related to the consumption of food, including microbial and non-microbial factors.
- A gastrointestinal infection is a disease caused by the establishment and multiplication of microorganisms in the gastrointestinal tract.
- Food intoxication is a disease caused by the presence of preformed toxins (microbial or non-microbial) in food.

ACUTE DIARRHOEAL DISEASES

- Gastrointestinal pathogens are acquired mainly by the faecal-oral route, from contaminated food, fluids or hands.
- The major symptom of gastrointestinal infection is acute diarrhoea.
- Diarrhoea is the result of increased secretion of fluid and electrolytes into the lumen of the intestine.
- In developing countries, diarrhoeal diseases are a major cause of morbidity and mortality, and also contribute to malnutrition.

THE EPIDEMIOLOGY OF ACUTE INFECTIOUS DIARRHOEA

Food-borne gastroenteritis

- Food-borne gastroenteritis is a common cause of acute infectious diarrhoea.
- Food-borne illness can occur when contaminated meats or seafood are eaten raw or are undercooked, or when food is improperly preserved.

Hospital nurseries

- Infants can become infected by bacteria or viruses during passage through the birth canal or after birth.
- Nursery outbreaks of acute diarrhoea sometimes occur.

Day-care centres

- Factors promoting spread of diarrhoeal disease include the presence of non-toilet trained children, oral exploration of objects, contamination of hands, close contact and lack of appropriate infection control measures.
- *Shigella* spp., *Giardia intestinalis*, rotavirus and *Cryptosporidium* have frequently been associated with outbreaks. These organisms typically require a low inoculum.

Traveller's diarrhoea

- Traveller's diarrhoea is the acute diarrhoea that frequently occurs in people visiting a foreign country.
- Certain countries in Asia, the Middle East, Africa and South America are well recognised as high-risk destinations for gastroenteritis.
- Enterotoxigenic *E. coli* is the predominant cause of traveller's diarrhoea.

Hospitalised patients

- Mild diarrhoea is a common side effect of antibiotic therapy.
- Broad spectrum antibiotics can predispose a patient to pseudomembranous colitis caused by *Clostridium difficile*.

People with AIDS

- Almost all AIDS patients experience at least one episode of diarrhoea during their illness.

CLINICAL FEATURES OF ACUTE DIARRHOEAL DISEASE

- Most acute diarrhoeal infections have an incubation period of 1–4 days.
- Most diarrhoeal infections are self-limiting.
- Infectious diarrhoea can be divided into:
  - non-inflammatory diarrhoea, characterised by watery stools; and
  - inflammatory diarrhoea, characterised by stools containing blood, mucus and pus.

BACTERIAL CAUSES OF ACUTE DIARRHOEA

Campylobacter

- *Campylobacter* species are comma-shaped Gram-negative rods that are common causes of diarrhoea.
- Infections are usually acquired by consumption of contaminated and poorly cooked foods of animal origin.
- *Campylobacter* enteritis is due to ulceration and inflammation of the mucosal surface of the jejunum, ileum and colon.

Salmonella

- Numerous serovars of *Salmonella* can cause gastroenteritis, the most common being *S. typhimurium*.
- In developed countries the organisms are transmitted to humans mainly via contaminated foods, especially poultry and eggs, meats and dairy products.
- Salmonellae invade the intestinal mucosa of the ileum and colon to cause diarrhoea with blood and mucus.
- Most cases of salmonellosis are self-limiting diarrhoeal diseases but, after clinical recovery, many patients become asymptomatic carriers.

Escherichia coli

- Enterotoxigenic *E. coli* (ETEC) bind to specific receptors on the intestinal cell membranes where they produce potent enterotoxins.
- The heat-labile toxin of ETEC causes an increase in levels of cyclic AMP in intestinal epithelial cells, resulting in a massive outflow of water and electrolytes into the lumen of the intestine.
- Enterohaemorrhagic *E. coli* (EHEC) include a number of serotypes that are important causes of haemorrhagic colitis, and sometimes haemolytic uraemic syndrome (HUS).

- EHEC produce a verotoxin which causes destruction of the colonic epithelium and haemorrhage.
- HUS is a serious complication, characterised by a haemolytic anaemia, uraemia and thrombocytopaenia, and renal failure.
- Enteropathogenic *E. coli* (EPEC) adhere intimately to enterocytes and cause destruction of the brush border.
- Enteroinvasive *E. coli* (EIEC) actively invade epithelial cells of the large intestine, causing cell death, ulceration of the mucosa and inflammation.

Cholera

- Cholera is an acute infection of the gastrointestinal tract caused by the comma-shaped Gram-negative bacterium *Vibrio cholerae*.
- Cholera is endemic in South-East Asia and parts of Africa and Central and South America.
- The symptoms of cholera are due to the action of an enterotoxin that causes the levels of cyclic AMP in intestinal epithelial cells to increase, resulting in a massive outflow of water and electrolytes into the lumen of the intestine.
- Without fluid and electrolyte replacement, mortality can be as high as 40–60%.

Shigella

- *Shigella* diarrhoea is also known as bacillary dysentery.
- *Shigella* infections are most common in children under 10 years.
- Faecal-oral spread is the major mode of transmission.
- Handwashing and good hygiene are the most important means of preventing transmission of these organisms.
- *Shigella* are readily transmitted since as few as 10–100 organisms may cause disease.
- The pathogenesis of *Shigella* is due to their enteroinvasive properties and the Shiga toxin.
- The Shiga toxin acts by cleaving ribosomal RNA in colonic cells, halting protein synthesis and killing the cell.

Clostridium difficile (antibiotic-associated colitis)

- Antibiotic therapy can sometimes lead to serious intestinal disease, characterised by severe diarrhoea and the formation of plaques or pseudomembranes on the colonic mucosa.
- The Gram-positive anaerobic rod, *Clostridium difficile*, is the cause of pseudomembranous colitis.
- The normal colonic flora effectively prevents colonisation by *C. difficile*, but broad spectrum antibiotics can disrupt the flora, allowing *C. difficile* to become established.
- Infection with *C. difficile* may range from mild diarrhoea to the potentially life-threatening pseudomembranous colitis.

Vibrio parahaemolyticus

- *Vibrio parahaemolyticus* is a Gram-negative organism commonly found in seafood, such as crabs, oysters and fish.
- This bacterium is responsible for many cases of food-borne illness in countries where seafoods are eaten uncooked.

Yersinia

- *Yersinia enterocolitica* is a Gram-negative rod found in a large variety of animals.
- Many cases of yersiniosis are traced to meat and dairy products.
- Most of infections occur in young children.
- The pathogenesis of *Y. enterocolitica* stems mainly from its ability to invade the ileum.

Aeromonas and Plesiomonas

- *Aeromonas hydrophila* and *Plesiomonas shigelloides* are causes of diarrhoeal disease, especially in paediatric patients.
- Disease can be serious in debilitated or immunosuppressed patients.

Clostridium perfringens

- *Clostridium perfringens* causes diarrhoeal disease when the bacteria are ingested in contaminated food.
- Type A organisms cause a self-limiting diarrhoeal illness, and type C organisms cause a potentially life-threatening syndrome known as 'enteritis necroticans'.

VIRAL CAUSES OF ACUTE DIARRHOEA

Rotavirus

- Rotaviruses are the most common cause of severe watery diarrhoea in young children worldwide.
- Very large numbers of rotavirus particles are shed in the faeces of infected people.
- The infective dose in a child is thought to be only 10–100 particles.
- The virus infects enterocytes at the villous tips, causing lysis of the cells and destruction of the villous epithelium.

Other viruses

- Norwalk virus and Norwalk-like viruses are important food-borne pathogens in poorly cooked or raw shellfish.
- Enteric adenoviruses (serotypes Ad40 and Ad41) are thought to be major causes of acute diarrhoea in paediatric patients.
- Caliciviruses and astroviruses have been found to cause diarrhoea in children.

PROTOZOAL CAUSES OF ACUTE DIARRHOEA

Giardia intestinalis

- *Giardia intestinalis* is a flagellated protozoan with a worldwide distribution.
- In developing countries, infections are associated with overcrowding, poor sanitary conditions and poor water quality.
- In developed countries, faecal-oral transmission is most common, and children are most likely to be infected.

- Trophozoites live in the small intestine, attaching to the mucosa and multiplying rapidly.
- Cyst formation occurs at regular intervals, and they are passed out in stools. These resistant structures are the infective form and can survive for months in the environment.
- Many cases of giardiasis are asymptomatic.
- When illness occurs, it is characterised by diarrhoea, nausea, a foul flatulence and fatigue.

Entamoeba histolytica

- *Entamoeba histolytica* has a worldwide distribution and is thought to infect as much as 10% of the world's population.
- Infection is transmitted by faecal contamination of food or drink.
- Most infected people are asymptomatic cyst passers or have only mild symptoms.
- Some strains cause invasive disease, ulcerating the bowel wall and spreading to remote sites, especially the liver.

Cryptosporidium parvum

- *Cryptosporidium parvum* is responsible for 1–3% of cases of diarrhoea in developed countries.
- Transmission is by faecal contamination of food, water and hands, and from pets.
- It causes traveller's diarrhoea and outbreaks associated with swimming pools and day-care centres.
- *C. parvum* has a thick-walled oocyst that is resistant to many disinfectants.
- A watery diarrhoea occurs about five days after ingestion of oocysts, and lasts several days to two weeks.
- In immunodeficient hosts the disease may be severe, chronic and sometimes fatal.

Isospora belli

- *Isospora belli* is endemic in South America, Africa and South-East Asia and is probably transmitted by faecally contaminated food or water.
- Sporozoites invade the mucosa of the small intestine, destroying the microvilli.
- Its highest prevalence is in immunocompromised people.

Cyclospora

- Protozoa of the genus *Cyclospora* cause diarrhoea in developing countries, and in travellers and patients with AIDS.

Blastocystis hominis

- *Blastocystis hominis* is a frequently identified protozoan in the gastrointestinal tract of humans, but its pathogenicity remains uncertain.

FOOD INTOXICATIONS

- Food intoxications are characterised by the rapid onset of nausea, vomiting and abdominal pain.
- The major causes are the enterotoxins of *Staphylococcus aureus*, *Bacillus cereus* and *Clostridium botulinum*, preformed in food.

Staphylococcus aureus intoxication

- Foods usually become contaminated by staphylococci from the nose or skin of food-handlers.
- Symptoms usually occur 1–6 hours after consumption of the contaminated food.

Bacillus cereus

- *Bacillus cereus* is an aerobic, Gram-positive rod that is resistant to moderate cooking temperatures because of the production of heat-resistant spores.
- If cooked food is allowed to cool for an extended period, the spores germinate and the vegetative cells produce a heat-stable enterotoxin in the food.
- Ingestion of toxin in the food causes acute onset of nausea, vomiting and abdominal pain within 1–6 hours.

LABORATORY DIAGNOSIS

- In most patients with mild to moderate diarrhoea, the illness will be self-limiting and requires no evaluation other than a clinical one.
- Stool culture is the standard method for the diagnosis of most bacterial causes of diarrhoea.
- Fresh stool specimens should be sent immediately to the laboratory in a sterile container with a firmly fitting screw lid.
- For suspected *C. difficile* infections, culture and the detection of cytotoxin in faeces are the standard diagnostic procedures.
- In staphylococcal and *Bacillus* food intoxications, the organisms are often not present in faeces and cannot be cultured.
- The diagnosis of viral gastroenteritis is often made on the patient history and clinical grounds.
- Diagnosis of protozoal infections usually involves the microscopic identification of cysts or trophozoites in stool specimens.

MANAGEMENT OF PATIENTS WITH DIARRHOEAL DISEASE

- For any patient with acute diarrhoea, fluid and electrolyte replacement is essential.
- Antibiotic therapy should be avoided where possible, because it may prolong the carriage and excretion of an organism by the patient.
- Treatment of protozoal infections is often with metronidazole.

PREVENTION

- In the case of food-borne illness and traveller's diarrhoea, prevention involves proper food processing and cooking, the non-consumption of high-risk foods and beverages, and the sterilisation of drinking water where appropriate.
- In day-care centres, strict handwashing practice, good general hygiene, sanitary food preparation, use of disposable gloves when contact with faecal matter is possible, and exclusion of symptomatic children are important measures.

- In hospitals, enteric precautions and strict handwashing after contact with patients is essential.

OTHER GASTROINTESTINAL DISEASES

HELICOBACTER PYLORI INFECTION

- *Helicobacter pylori* is recognised as the main cause of gastritis and a major factor in the development of most cases of duodenal and gastric ulcers; it also has a possible role in gastric cancer.
- Once a person becomes infected with *H. pylori*, the organism appears able to persist in the stomach for many years.
- Only in some people is the inflammation induced by the bacterium severe enough to produce symptoms.
- A laboratory diagnosis of *H. pylori* infection is by histological examination of biopsy specimens taken during endoscopy.
- Therapy with a bismuth salt, tetracycline and metronidazole is effective in most cases.

ENTERIC FEVERS: TYPHOID AND PARATYPHOID

Causative agents and transmission

- *Salmonella typhi* and *S. paratyphi* types A, B and C, all cause enteric fevers, although *S. typhi* is responsible for most infections.
- These species are usually spread via faecally contaminated food or water.
- Infections are most common in developing countries with poor standards of water supply and sewage disposal.

Pathogenesis

- A major feature of these organisms is their ability to survive and multiply inside macrophages.
- The salmonellae are transported by macrophages from the intestine to the lymphatic system and then into the bloodstream, from where they seed many organs.
- Most of the symptoms caused by *S. typhi* can be attributed to the inflammation induced by its lipopolysaccharide.

Clinical features

- After an incubation period of 10–14 days, the early symptoms of fever, headache and a dry cough appear. Diarrhoea or constipation occurs.
- Infection lasts 4–6 weeks; death occurs in about 15% of untreated cases.
- Many patients continue to excrete *S. typhi* in the faeces for several weeks after recovery.
- In some people, the organism persists in the gall bladder, and bacteria are shed in faeces for years.

Laboratory diagnosis

- Blood cultures generally become positive at the onset of symptoms.
- Faeces and urine should also be cultured.
- Serum antibodies to the organisms can be detected by the Widal test.

Treatment and prevention

- Oral treatment with chloramphenicol, ampicillin, cotrimoxazole or ciprofloxacin is generally effective.
- For chronic carriers, long-term therapy with ampicillin or ciprofloxacin may be effective; if not, cholecystectomy may be warranted.
- A killed vaccine against *S. typhi* is available, and recommended for travellers to developing countries, but it is only 70–90% effective.

HELMINTH INFECTIONS OF THE GASTROINTESTINAL TRACT

- Parasitic helminths are a major cause of morbidity in humans.
- Helminth infections are acquired either by penetration of the skin by larvae, or by ingestion of the eggs of helminths.
- All helminths except *E. granulosus* and *S. stercoralis* specifically inhabit the bowel.
- The severity of disease is largely a function of the number of worms in the body.

ENTEROBIUS VERMICULARIS

- Adult pinworms (*Enterobius vermicularis*) pass out of the anus at night, depositing eggs in the perianal area.
- Many people are asymptomatic but, when symptoms do occur, anal pruritis (itching), especially at night, is the classic sign.
- Transmission usually occurs directly from fingers contaminated by scratching.
- The eggs of *Enterobius* can be identified by applying adhesive tape to the perianal skin and microscopic examination of the tape.
- Infections are effectively treated with mebendazole or pyrantel.

ASCARIS LUMBRICOIDES

- Adult worms are 15–35 cm long, hence the name 'giant roundworm'.
- The infection is usually transmitted by faecal-oral passage of eggs via contaminated hands.
- After ingestion, the eggs hatch in the intestine, the larvae penetrate the gut wall and are carried via the blood through the liver to the lungs. They work their way up the bronchi and trachea, are swallowed, and again enter the intestine.
- Most people with a small worm load are asymptomatic or have only mild abdominal discomfort.
- With large worm loads, intestinal obstruction may occur.
- Diagnosis is based on the microscopic examination of faeces.
- A variety of antihelminthic drugs are effective, including mebendazole and pyrantel.

HOOKWORMS

- Hookworms are a serious cause of long-term morbidity in developing countries due to the anaemia and hypoproteinaemia that result from heavy infection.
- Adult hookworms, *Ancylostoma duodenale* and *Necator americanus*, attach to the intestinal mucosa by specialised mouth structures. They rupture capillaries and suck blood, and lay thin-coated eggs that are passed in faeces into the environment.
- The eggs mature and hatch in soil. Infection of a new host takes place when larvae come into contact with unprotected skin of a person. They penetrate the skin, migrate via the blood to the lungs, climb the trachea and are swallowed, maturing into adult worms in the small intestine.
- Heavy infections may cause abdominal pain, flatulence, a bloody diarrhoea, and an iron deficiency anaemia in children or in anyone with existing malnutrition.
- Hookworm infections are diagnosed and treated in a similar way to *Ascaris* infections.

STRONGYLOIDES STERCORALIS

- *Strongyloides* infection occurs when larvae in faecally contaminated soil or fomites penetrate the skin or mucous membranes. They then enter the bloodstream, and break into the alveoli in the lungs. They ascend the bronchi and trachea, are swallowed, and reach the small intestine where maturation is completed.
- This worm is unlike any other nematode in its ability to multiply in the host.
- Heavy intestinal infection causes a persistent and profuse diarrhoea, with dehydration and electrolyte imbalance.
- *Strongyloides* infection can be diagnosed by microscopic examination of fresh stools.
- Infections are usually treated with thiabendazole.

HYDATID DISEASE

- Hydatid disease is caused by the tapeworm *Echinococcus granulosus*.
- Humans act as accidental hosts when the eggs of the parasite are ingested, usually as a result of contact with an infected dog.
- After ingestion of eggs, the larvae migrate through the gut and then the bloodstream, and eventually localise in organs such as the liver, lungs and brain. In these organs they form fluid-filled sacs, called cysts, which contain thousands of developing worms.
- Symptoms result from the pressure of the cyst on the organ.
- Bursting of the cyst can lead to seeding of other organs with the worms, and, in some people, a life-threatening anaphylactic reaction to hydatid antigens.
- Diagnosis of hydatid cysts is by radiologic demonstration of a cystic lesion, supported by positive serology.
- Treatment may be achieved with the drug albendazole, but surgical removal of the cysts is often necessary.

TAENIA SAGINATA

- The beef tapeworm attaches by its head to the intestinal mucosa.
- Most patients are asymptomatic or experience only mild abdominal discomfort.
- Infections are diagnosed in a similar way to *Ascaris* infections.
- Treatment is usually with praziquantel or niclosamide.

TRICHURIS TRICHIURA

- The worms remain within the large bowel, attaching to the epithelial layer.
- Most infections are asymptomatic, but moderate to heavy worm loads can cause abdominal pain and diarrhoea.
- Infections are diagnosed and treated in a similar way to *Ascaris* infections.

HYMENOLEPIS NANA

- *Hymenolepis nana* is a tapeworm that causes an asymptomatic infection in most patients.
- In heavy infections it can cause diarrhoea, abdominal pain and loss of appetite.
- Infections are diagnosed and treated in a similar way to *Ascaris* infections.

HEPATITIS

- The term 'hepatitis' refers to injury and inflammation of the liver.
- Viruses are major causes of hepatitis, but other microorganisms, alcohol, drugs and various other disorders may also be responsible.
- The hepatitis viruses produce acute inflammation of the liver; this may result in a clinical illness with variable features, including anorexia, nausea and vomiting, fever, malaise and jaundice. In more serious cases, liver function can fail.
- Marked increases in serum concentrations of the liver enzymes, alanine aminotransferase (ALT) and aspartate aminotransferase (AST), are characteristic of acute viral hepatitis.

HEPATITIS A

- Hepatitis A virus (HAV) is a small RNA virus, belonging to the family of picornaviruses.

Transmission

- Transmission of HAV is primarily by the faecal-oral route.
- Once transferred to fomites, the virus can persist on surfaces for several days.
- Poor personal hygiene, poor sanitation and close personal contact facilitate transmission.
- Hepatitis A is endemic in most rural Aboriginal communities in Australia, with most infections occurring in young children.

- Lack of good sanitation and hygiene can lead to outbreaks in schools, camps and day-care centres.
- There is an increased incidence of hepatitis A among male homosexuals.

Pathogenesis and clinical features

- The virus is believed to replicate initially in intestinal cells, followed by a brief period of viraemia and then spread to the liver.
- The incubation period ranges from 2 to 6 weeks.
- The illness is usually inapparent in children less than four years old, but it becomes progressively more severe with increasing age.
- Complete recovery occurs in most cases within 4–6 weeks, there is no carrier state, and chronic infection does not generally occur.

Laboratory diagnosis

- The standard method for diagnosing hepatitis A is by detection of anti-hepatitis A antibodies in the patient's serum.

Treatment and prevention

- Symptomatic treatment is all that is available.
- Prevention relies on good hygiene and prophylactic use of gammaglobulin after exposure.
- An effective HAV vaccine has recently been developed.

HEPATITIS B

- Hepatitis B virus (HBV) has an outer coat containing the hepatitis B surface antigen (HBsAg). The inner component is called the hepatitis core antigen (HBcAg) and inside this is the viral DNA (HBV-DNA). A third antigen is the hepatitis Be antigen (HBeAg).
- The whole virus particle is called a Dane particle.
- There are thought to be more than 300 million carriers throughout the world, and about one million deaths each year.

Transmission

- Blood and blood products are the most common sources of transmission, but other body fluids, especially semen, vaginal secretions and serous fluids, can also transmit the virus.
- Very small amounts of blood can be infectious.
- The virus can survive for days in dried blood.
- Most cases in developed countries now occur in homosexual and bisexual males, IV drug abusers and people with multiple sex partners.
- Babies born to mothers with hepatitis B have a high risk of infection.
- Health care workers may be exposed to HBV via needlestick injuries, or when contaminated blood comes into contact with mucous membranes, cuts or abrasions.

Pathogenesis and clinical features

- Much of the pathology is due to immune mechanisms, including destruction of infected liver cells by cytotoxic T cells.
- The virus replicates in the liver and large numbers of virus particles are released into the bloodstream.
- Acute hepatitis B is clinically similar to hepatitis A, although usually more severe.
- Most healthy adults recover spontaneously within six months.
- Acute fulminant hepatitis is a clinical syndrome in which there is severe impairment of liver cells, liver failure and death in about 80% of those affected.
- In 5–10% of infected individuals, complete elimination of the virus does not occur; they develop chronic hepatitis and are chronic carriers of the virus.
- Transmission from mother to baby results in an extremely high rate of chronicity.
- Many people with chronic hepatitis B infection are asymptomatic; others with chronic active hepatitis can suffer marked liver dysfunction.
- Chronic hepatitis is associated with an increased likelihood of developing hepatic cirrhosis and/or hepatocellular carcinoma.

Laboratory diagnosis

- Diagnosis of hepatitis B is by examination of serum for antibodies and viral antigens.
- HBsAg in serum implies ongoing infection, either acute or chronic.
- Persistence of HBsAg in the blood for more than six months indicates chronic infection.
- HBeAg is found in serum early during acute infection and in chronic infections, and indicates high infectivity.
- HBV-DNA detected in serum is the best evidence of viral replication and infectivity in patients.

Treatment and prevention

- There is no fully effective therapy for hepatitis B.
- Hydration and anti-nauseants are the basic forms of symptomatic treatment.
- Hepatitis B immunoglobulin (HBIG) is used to provide immediate protection to unimmunised people following exposure.
- The HBV vaccine is safe and effective.
- Sexual transmission can be prevented by the use of barrier contraceptives.

HEPATITIS C

- Most cases of what was formerly called non-A, non-B (NANB) hepatitis have been attributed to the hepatitis C virus (HCV).

TRANSMISSION

- Transmission of HCV is mainly via contaminated blood.
- The prevalence of HCV among intravenous drug users is reportedly about 60%.

Pathogenesis and clinical features

- Most cases of acute HCV infection are asymptomatic. When symptomatic, the disease is usually mild.
- At least 60% of cases progress to chronic infection.

- Most chronic infections are asymptomatic, but more than 20% of patients eventually develop hepatic cirrhosis and/or hepatocellular carcinoma.

Laboratory diagnosis

- Laboratory diagnosis of hepatitis C is based on the detection of antibodies in serum.
- The time from infection to seroconversion can be anywhere between 2 and 9 months.

Treatment and prevention

- Treatment of chronically infected patients with α-interferon is effective in some cases.
- Transmission via blood transfusion has been significantly reduced by the routine testing of donors for antibody to hepatitis C.

HEPATITIS D

- The hepatitis D virus (HDV) is a defective virus, requiring a coexisting, active hepatitis B infection to be able to complete its own replicative cycle.
- A person cannot contract an HDV infection unless simultaneously infected with HBV, or already infected with HBV.
- Blood and blood products are the major sources of HDV.
- When HDV superinfects a chronic carrier of HBV, the infection is usually severe and can lead to cirrhosis and hepatic failure, with a high mortality.
- The laboratory diagnosis is based on serological tests for HDVAg or for antibody to HDVAg.
- There is no effective treatment, other than physiologic support in rehydration and anti-nauseants.
- There is no HDV vaccine, but vaccination against hepatitis B prevents hepatitis D infection.

HEPATITIS E

- Hepatitis E virus (HEV) is shed in faeces and spread by the faecal-oral route.
- HEV appears to have a restricted distribution of Central and South-East Asia, Africa, the Middle East and Central America.
- Clinically, HEV infection is similar to HAV infection.
- It can cause severe infection with high mortality in pregnant women.
- The virus appears not to cause chronic infection.
- Serological tests for HEV exist, but their significance is currently unclear.

Study Questions

1. What is the physiological basis of diarrhoea?
2. What microorganisms are commonly associated with outbreaks of diarrhoeal disease in day-care centres?
3. Describe the differences between inflammatory and non-inflammatory diarrhoea.
4. How are *Salmonella* diarrhoeal infections usually acquired?
5. How do enterotoxigenic *E. coli* cause diarrhoea?
6. What is haemolytic uraemic syndrome and what is the major cause?
7. Why is cholera a potentially fatal disease?
8. Why is cholera vaccine no longer recommended for routine use in travellers?
9. What is bacillary dysentery?
10. Why is shigellosis so readily transmitted from person to person?
11. What is the basis of antibiotic-associated colitis?
12. List the viruses that commonly cause diarrhoea and indicate their usual sources.
13. What is amoebic dysentery?
14. What characteristics of *Cryptosporidium parvum* enable it to be easily spread?
15. What is a food intoxication?
16. How are diarrhoeal diseases usually diagnosed?
17. What are the major aspects of treatment of a patient with diarrhoea?
18. What important diseases are thought to be caused by *Helicobacter pylori*?
19. How is *Helicobacter pylori* infection diagnosed?
20. What important virulence factor is possessed by *Salmonella typhi*?
21. Explain how *Salmonella typhi* causes the symptoms that are commonly associated with typhoid fever.
22. What specimens are required for the laboratory diagnosis of typhoid fever?
23. What are the typical symptoms of *Enterobius vermicularis* infection and how is the infection diagnosed?
24. What specimens are required for the laboratory diagnosis of worm infestation of the intestine?
25. Describe the life cycle of *Ascaris lumbricoides*.
26. Describe the life cycle of hookworms.
27. What is the major difference between *Strongyloides stercoralis* and other nematodes that cause intestinal infection?
28. What is the cause of hydatid disease? Describe its main features.
29. Define hepatitis and list the possible causes.
30. Draw up a table to show the cause, common modes of transmission, important diagnostic tests, treatment and prevention of each of the five major types of viral hepatitis.
31. In which types of viral hepatitis is chronic infection possible, and what are the major problems associated with chronic viral hepatitis?

Test Your Understanding

Case History 18.1: Shigellosis

1. What important infection control procedures have perhaps been omitted in this case?
2. Why has this organism been so easily transmitted to family members and to others in the hospital?
3. Why does this organism predominantly affect children and disadvantaged communities?

Case History 18.2: Cryptosporidiosis

1. What are the possible means of transmission of *Cryptosporidium* in this outbreak?
2. What features of *Cryptosporidium parvum* enable it to be transmitted so easily?
3. What action could be taken to prevent further spread of the organism in this situation?

Case History 18.3: Staphylococcal gastroenteritis

1. Apart from the isolation of *S. aureus* from some of the stool specimens, what other information supports the diagnosis of staphylococcal food poisoning?
2. What are the possible sources of contamination of the chicken?
3. What treatment would you expect the affected people to receive?

Case History 18.4: Hepatitis A

1. What infection control measures were probably being ignored in this situation?
2. Why do you think the child's hepatitis A was unrecognised in this case?
3. How can hepatitis A be prevented in high-risk groups?

Case History 18.5: Hepatitis B

1. What do the test results in this case indicate?
2. How do you think this patient contracted the disease?
3. What infection control measures should hospital staff observe when attending this patient?

REFERENCE

1. Ferson, M.J. & L.C. Young, 1994, 'Hepatitis A in injecting drug users—preliminary report', *Communicable Diseases Intelligence* 18 (25), p. 655.

FURTHER READING

Bishai, W.R. & C.L. Sears, 1993, 'Food poisoning syndromes', *Gastroenterology Clinics of North America* 22(3), p. 579. (Describes the major types of microbial and non-microbial food poisoning syndromes.)

DuPont, H.L., 1994, 'Review article: infectious diarrhoea', *Alimentary Pharmacology and Therapy* 8, p. 3. (A review article on the causes, diagnosis and management of infectious diarrhoeal disease.)

Grove, D.I., 1993, 'Worms in Australia', *Medical Journal of Australia* 159, p. 464. (Describes the common types of worm infections that are endemic in Australia.)

Jernigan, J., R.L. Guerrant & R.D. Pearson, 1994, 'Parasitic infections of the small intestine', *Gut* 35, p. 289. (This article describes the major protozoal and worm infections of the small intestine.)

Lisanti, P. & D. Talotta, 1994, 'An overview of viral hepatitis', *AORN Journal* 59(5), p. 997. (This review article describes the clinical manifestations of viral hepatitis and the underlying pathophysiological bases. It also deals with the nursing care necessary for these diseases.)

Liu, L.X. & P.F. Weller, 1993, 'Strongyloidiasis and other intestinal nematode infections', *Infectious Disease Clinics of North America* 7(3), p. 655. (A comprehensive review article on intestinal parasitic nematode infections.)

Maddrey, W.C., 1994, 'Chronic viral hepatitis: diagnosis and management', *Hospital Practice* 15 February, p. 117. (Details the epidemiology, diagnosis and management of chronic hepatitis B and C infection.)

chapter 19

cardiovascular and multisystem infections

Chapter focus

- *What microorganisms commonly cause cardiovascular and multisystem infections in Australia and other countries?*
- *How are cardiovascular and multisystem diseases usually transmitted?*
- *What are the important clinical aspects of the common cardiovascular and multisystem infections?*

The circulating blood can normally be considered sterile, although low numbers of bacteria may briefly circulate in a healthy person. When microorganisms enter the bloodstream from a wound or other focus of infection, they are easily disseminated through the body. In this way, they can reach other body organs, where they may cause serious and often life-threatening diseases. These are often referred to as **systemic infections**. A wide variety of microbes can cause such infections. Bacteria and viruses are most common, but protozoa are responsible for some serious infections throughout the world, the most notable being malaria. A number of fungi can cause systemic infections, but usually only in an immunocompromised host. Helminths also cause important systemic infections, such as filariasis (elephantiasis) and schistosomiasis.

The terms used to signify microorganisms in the bloodstream have as a prefix the major part of the name of the organism, or type of organism, plus the suffix -*aemia*. Thus, **viraemia** denotes the presence of viruses in the blood. Similarly, **fungaemia**, **parasitaemia** and **meningococcaemia** mean the presence of fungi, parasites (protozoa or helminths) and meningococci, respectively, in the bloodstream.

However, there is often some confusion over the usage and meaning of the terms 'bacteraemia' and 'septicaemia' because they are frequently used interchangeably. **Bacteraemia** literally means the *presence* of bacteria in the bloodstream. It may be manifested by the whole range of conditions from asymptomatic to seriously ill. Bacteraemia is in fact a fairly common occurrence in all people, since low numbers of bacteria often spill into the bloodstream when minor trauma to skin (e.g. cuts, abrasions) or mucous membranes (e.g. teeth cleaning, chewing) occurs. **Septicaemia** is a serious clinical syndrome resulting from the presence of bacteria in the bloodstream; it thus represents a bacteraemia with severe clinical manifestations.

Systemic Bacterial Infections

SEPTICAEMIA

The bloodstream is a relatively inhospitable place for microorganisms, even though it contains oxygen, water and an abundance of nutrients, has an approximately neutral pH, and the right temperature for many organisms to multiply. First, it is constantly moving, and thus it is difficult for microbes to colonise a surface and multiply. Second, it contains a variety of antimicrobial defence mechanisms, in particular the phagocytic leucocytes, antibodies and complement (see Chapter 9). Third, the blood recirculates through the spleen and liver, where sinusoids are lined with more phagocytic cells, and where the blood flow slows, enhancing their phagocytic activity. Thus, bacteria are usually quickly cleared from the bloodstream.

However, some pathogenic organisms are able to persist in the blood and be transported by it. In the majority of such cases the organisms enter the bloodstream from a primary focus of infection in organs such as the lungs, gastrointestinal tract or kidneys, or from infected wounds or an infected intravascular device (e.g. an IV catheter). For them to cause infection, at least one of the following conditions must exist:

- The organisms have to be released, either continuously or intermittently, in large enough numbers to overwhelm the defence systems; or
- There is some anatomical defect that facilitates the colonisation of a site (e.g. a damaged heart valve); or
- The organisms have some protective mechanism that helps them to evade the defences of the blood (e.g. an antiphagocytic capsule or a coagulase enzyme); or
- There is some impairment in the body's defences (e.g. hypogammaglobulinaemia resulting from cancer therapy; or neutropenia due to chronic infection).

The last two conditions simply mean that fewer bacteria will be needed to produce septicaemia. While bacterial multiplication in the blood may occur, it is not a requirement in septicaemia.

Clinical features

The clinical manifestations of septicaemia are extremely variable. Usually, the patient has a high, spiking fever, often with alternating severe shaking chills and sweats. These symptoms are often intermittent, interspersed with periods of improvement. Shock, manifested by low blood pressure and vascular collapse, is also common. **Endotoxic (septic) shock** is a severe, life-threatening form of septicaemia caused by the endotoxin (lipid-A of lipopolysaccharide) of Gram-negative bacteria.

Diagnosis

The diagnosis of septicaemia is made by the demonstration of bacteria in the blood, usually by blood culture (see Chapter 15). Indirectly, the diagnosis may sometimes be made by the demonstration of a focus of infection

CASE HISTORY 19.1
SEPTICAEMIA

A 49-year-old man had a Hickman catheter surgically inserted for total parenteral nutrition. Six days after surgery it was noticed that the catheter entry site had become inflamed. He had a temperature of 39.8°C, a high respiratory rate and rapid pulse. Blood cultures were collected and two out of three sets grew *Staphylococcus epidermidis*.

somewhere in the body. The bacteria causing septicaemia may be difficult to culture from a sample of blood for a number of reasons.

1. The organisms, although causing severe infection, may be present only in low numbers. Given the small sample size of 10–30 mL from a total blood volume of about 5–6 litres, they may be difficult to culture.
2. The organisms may be only transiently present in the bloodstream, particularly if they are shed intermittently from the primary focus of infection. In these circumstances, after each shower of organisms into the bloodstream, bacterial numbers will gradually be reduced as defence mechanisms remove them. Thus, they may be present in large numbers for only a short time after release.
3. Some septicaemia-causing bacteria, like *Streptococcus pneumoniae* and *Haemophilus influenzae*, are quite fastidious and, therefore, difficult to grow, or are very slow-growing *in vitro*.

To maximise the chance of isolating the causative agent, three samples of blood for culture are usually taken from a patient over a 24–48 hour period. The best time to take a sample is when the patient is experiencing a febrile episode, as this generally represents a showering of bacteria into the bloodstream from the focus of infection.

Culture of a catheter tip (see Chapter 15) may be helpful if it is thought to be a possible source of the infection.

Treatment

Treatment involves the administration of an appropriate antimicrobial drug. Because of the potential severity of the disease, antimicrobial therapy is usually commenced at the first clinical suspicion. A broad spectrum agent is used and then modified, if necessary, once the identity of the causative agent and its antimicrobial sensitivity are known. It is preferable that blood for culture be collected before beginning antibiotic therapy (see Chapter 15). Location and treatment of the primary focus of infection are also necessary; if it is an abscess it may require surgical drainage. The patient is also treated symptomatically for systemic complications, such as hypotension.

RHEUMATIC FEVER

Incidence

Rheumatic fever is a non-suppurative (not pus-forming) complication of *Streptococcus pyogenes* sore throat. It is a non-suppurative disease because it is not a direct infection. It affects only a small percentage of people, following a streptococcal sore throat or, less commonly, scarlet fever. Its highest incidence occurs in 5–15 year olds. Rheumatic fever is still a major cause of cardiovascular disease in the Third World, but in developed countries its incidence has generally been declining for several decades. In Australia it is a rarity except in socioeconomically deprived communities.

Poverty and consequent overcrowding and poor hygiene are important factors, and in some Aboriginal communities the incidence is estimated to be 200–300 per 100 000 population. Similarly, the disease is much more common in New Zealand's indigenous population than in non-Maori people.

It is interesting to note that, after decades of decline in the United States (except in the poorer black communities), health authorities there have been surprised and puzzled by an unexplained resurgence of the disease, since 1985, among white, middle-class families.

Clinical features and pathogenesis

Onset of rheumatic fever usually occurs 2–4 weeks after a streptococcal sore throat. Without treatment, the susceptible person can suffer recurrence of rheumatic fever after each episode of streptococcal sore throat, with a 2–4 week latent period each time. The major diagnostic criteria of rheumatic fever are:

- carditis, manifested usually by sinus tachycardia (fast heart rate), a heart murmur, chest pain or extra heart sounds;
- acute migratory polyarthritis, mainly of large joints;
- chorea (sudden, involuntary, irregular movements);
- subcutaneous nodules near joints; and
- erythema marginatum, a distinctive macular rash.

These attacks usually subside in three months. If untreated, rheumatic fever can result in scarring and deformation of the valves and heart failure, known as **rheumatic heart disease.** Valve damage and disruption to normal blood flow around the valve can predispose to its colonisation by bacteria and, hence, endocarditis. This is discussed below.

Much is known about rheumatic fever but the precise mechanisms of its pathogenesis remain obscure. The most widely held view is that this disease is due to cross-reactivity between certain streptococcal antigens and heart tissue antigens. Thus, antibodies produced against the streptococcus (while it is infecting the throat) then cross-react with heart tissue, causing inflammation and damage. Certain strains of *S. pyogenes* are known to be more commonly associated with rheumatic fever. These rheumatogenic strains have been found to have certain M-protein serotypes, and it is these M-proteins that have an antigenic similarity to cardiac myosin and sarcolemma membrane proteins.

Genetic factors also seem to be important, since people with certain MHC types (see Chapter 9) have a much greater risk of rheumatic fever than people who lack those types.

Diagnosis

Diagnosis of rheumatic fever is made by correlation of clinical findings (especially major criteria) with certain laboratory findings indicating recent streptococcal infection, such as a positive throat culture, or high or rising antibody titres. Multiple serological tests are often performed, including an anti-streptolysin-O titre (ASOT), and anti-DNAse and anti-hyaluronidase tests.

Treatment and prevention

Penicillin is given to remove any remaining organisms, and aspirin is used to reduce fever and joint pain. Prompt treatment of *S. pyogenes* throat infections with penicillin in people known to be susceptible to rheumatic fever can prevent further attacks. Antibiotic cover is required for 10 days, and this will prevent a rise in anti-streptococcal antibodies in most people. In high-risk groups, such as some Aboriginal communities, treatment of sore throat in all members may be warranted. Prophylactic use of penicillin may be used in people known to suffer severe attacks of rheumatic fever.

INFECTIVE ENDOCARDITIS

The wall of the heart consists of three layers. The innermost layer, which is a layer of epithelium covering the heart muscle and the valves, is called the endocardium. **Infective endocarditis** is therefore an inflammation of the endocardium, initiated by an infectious agent. It often presents as a pyrexia of unknown origin (PUO), and is a fatal disease if untreated. It may occur as an acute, rapidly progressing disease which, in the pre-antibiotic era, invariably resulted in death within a few weeks. In addition, a chronic form exists. In more than 60% of patients there is a pre-existing heart condition such as congenital heart disease, mitral valve prolapse, valvular damage from rheumatic fever, or a prosthetic heart valve.

Causative organisms and pathogenesis

Infective endocarditis can be caused by a wide variety of bacteria. Although in most cases a pre-existing heart defect is present, in some there is no apparent predisposing factor. On abnormal or damaged valves, oral streptococci like *Streptococcus sanguis, S. milleri* and *S. oralis* are the most common causes, followed by staphylococci, especially *Staphylococcus aureus*. The oral bacteria can enter the bloodstream through minor abrasions such as those caused by teeth cleaning or flossing, or following dental procedures or dental surgery. They then colonise the heart valves.

On prosthetic valves, coagulase-negative staphylococci (especially *Staphylococcus epidermidis*) are a major cause of early endocarditis; that is, occurring less than two months after implant surgery. These organisms are probably introduced during surgery. Late prosthetic valve endocarditis (more than two months after implant) also exhibits a wide range of causative agents, but is more similar in this respect to normal valve endocarditis. Overall, 1.5–3% of patients with a prosthetic valve implant develop an endocarditis within a year.

Intravenous drug users may develop an endocarditis caused by microorganisms they inject into themselves. In this group, *Staphylococcus aureus* is most common, followed by oral streptococci and Gram-negative bacteria. Fungi, such as *Aspergillus* and *Mucor*, are also found occasionally as the cause of endocarditis in IV drug users, and *Candida* can occur in all groups. Moreover, polymicrobial infections (infection caused by more than one organism) can occur in IV drug users, and occasionally in other people. Table 19.1 summarises the causative agents of endocarditis.

The pathogenesis of infective endocarditis is illustrated in Figure 19.1. It is a complex process, and in many cases its development depends on prior endocardial damage. On damaged or abnormal valves, collagen in the endothelial basement membrane is exposed, and this stimulates the deposition of fibrin and platelets on the membrane. The valve abnormality and these fibrin-platelet clumps cause a disturbance to the normal smooth flow of blood through the valve, resulting in turbulènce. In turbulent flow, bacteria in the blood are not carried along as quickly, giving them an opportunity to attach to surfaces, particularly to the deposited fibrin, via specific adhesins or sticky polysaccharides secreted from the cell. The fibrin and platelets are also thought to provide some shelter for the bacteria against body defences in the blood.

Having attached, the bacteria are able to multiply, causing further platelet and fibrin deposition. Colonies of bacteria thus become sandwiched between layers of fibrin and platelets. This growing clump of bacteria, fibrin and platelets is the characteristic pathological feature of infective endocarditis and is called a **vegetation**. These lesions can develop anywhere on the endocardium, but usually occur on the endocardial surface of heart valves and surrounding structures.

Vegetations vary in size and can grow to several centimetres. With increasing growth of the vegetations, there will be increasing destruction to underlying tissues and increasing valvular dysfunction, with the possibility of cardiac distress and congestive heart failure. Also, septic emboli (pieces of vegetations containing bacteria) may eventually break off, be carried to other organs, and lodge in, then infect and/or occlude blood vessels there, causing inflammation and necrosis.

Clinical features

The signs and symptoms of infective endocarditis are extremely variable because they can reflect one or more of the following:

- damage and deformation of heart valves;
- embolisation of vegetations with necrosis in remote tissues due to infection or occlusion of blood vessels, or both;
- deposition of antigen-antibody complexes in blood vessels in the skin, the glomeruli or joints.

Typical clinical manifestations, then, are fever and heart murmur, often with anorexia, malaise, chills, nausea,

TABLE 19.1

COMMON CAUSATIVE AGENTS OF ENDOCARDITIS IN DIFFERENT GROUPS OF PATIENTS. FOR EACH CATEGORY THE ORGANISMS ARE LISTED IN DECREASING ORDER OF FREQUENCY

Abnormal/damaged valve	Oral streptococci *Staphylococcus aureus*
Prosthetic valve (< 2 months after implant)	Coagulase negative staphylococci *Staphylococcus aureus* Gram-negative (enteric) bacteria Oral streptococci Fungi (mainly *Candida albicans*)
Prosthetic valve (> 2 months after implant)	Oral streptococci Coagulase negative staphylococci Gram-negative (enteric) bacteria *Staphylococcus aureus*
IV drug abuser	*Staphylococcus aureus* Oral streptococci Gram-negative (enteric) bacteria

FIGURE 19.1

THE PATHOGENESIS OF INFECTIVE ENDOCARDITIS

(a) An abnormal heart valve; (b) and (c) The development of vegetations on the heart valve.

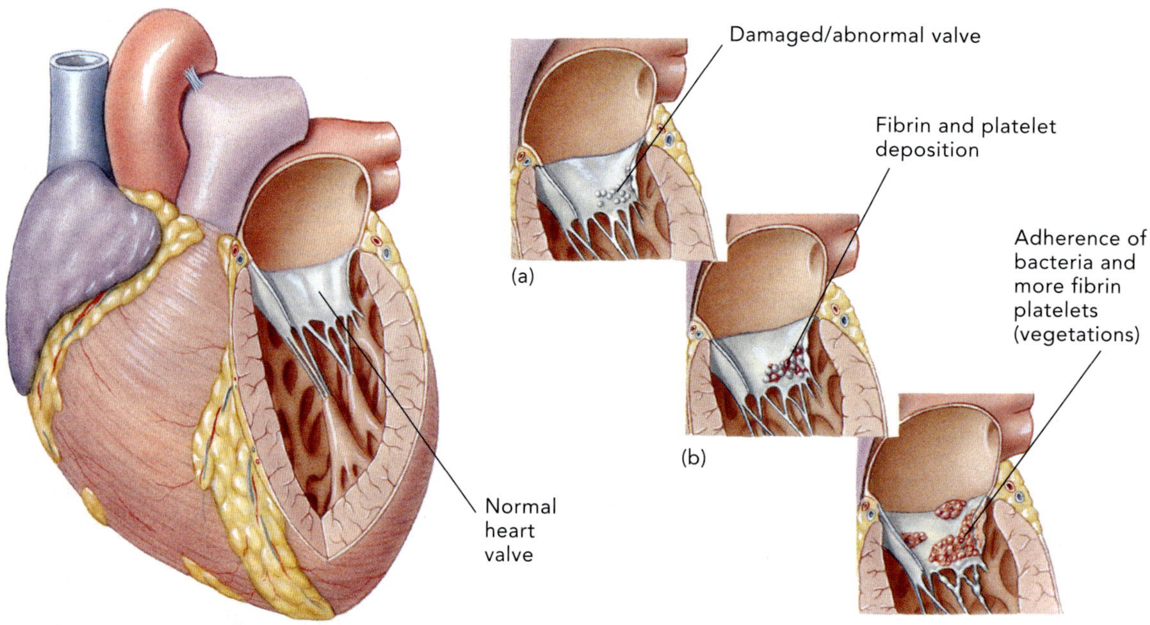

vomiting and night sweats. Splinter haemorrhages in the nail bed, skin lesions, and signs of glomerulonephritis or synovitis may also occur. Death is usually due to congestive heart failure secondary to valvular dysfunction.

Diagnosis, treatment and prevention

Untreated endocarditis results in death, so an accurate diagnosis is required. Blood culture is the key to the laboratory diagnosis. The isolation of the causative agent is necessary so that antibiotic sensitivity results can be obtained and appropriate therapy provided. When properly performed, blood cultures will usually be positive from a patient with endocarditis. Bacteria tend to be released from vegetations at a fairly constant rate, resulting in a more or less continuous bacteraemia. Endocarditis in which blood cultures are negative may be due to:

- commencement of antibiotic therapy before blood culture;
- infection by slow-growing or fastidious organisms (e.g. *Haemophilus* spp.);

- causation by unusual organisms not isolated by standard procedures (e.g *Aspergillus, Coxiella burnetii*); or
- non-infectious causes.

Prolonged antibiotic therapy (4–6 weeks) is often necessary since the organisms within the vegetations are afforded a degree of protection from antibiotics. Even with treatment with a drug to which the organism is sensitive, infective endocarditis has a mortality rate of 10–20%. In culture-negative endocarditis, penicillin (or ampicillin) in combination with gentamicin is usually given for 4–6 weeks, or until culture and sensitivity results reveal more appropriate therapy, or until a non-infectious cause is established.

Prevention is based on the use of prophylactic antibiotics in people known to have a heart defect, who are to undergo any invasive procedure that could lead to the introduction of bacteria into the bloodstream. Protection of such people during dental surgery is particularly important because of the common involvement of oral streptococci in endocarditis.

OSTEOMYELITIS

Cause and pathogenesis

Osteomyelitis is an inflammation of bone caused by infectious microorganisms. The organisms reach the bone either from the blood or externally, and thus the infection may be categorised according to the mode of entry of the microbe.

1. *Haematogenous osteomyelitis* is caused by organisms that are carried by the blood to the bone tissue, generally from a site of infection elsewhere in the body. Intravenous drug abusers may also develop haematogenous osteomyelitis from the use of contaminated needles.
2. *Exogenous osteomyelitis* is caused by organisms introduced directly from outside the body—for example, through compound fractures, penetrating wounds or surgery. Often the organism first infects adjacent soft tissue before extending to the bone.

Haematogenous osteomyelitis most commonly affects the growing ends of long bones (e.g. the tibia and femur), and thus most often afflicts children and adolescents. The vulnerability of these bones is due to the anatomy of their vascular supply. A slow blood flow in the large diameter vessels in these bones facilitates the colonisation and growth of bacteria. The most common cause is *Staphylococcus aureus*, but other organisms such as Group B streptococci, *Haemophilus influenzae* and *Mycobacterium tuberculosis* may also cause this infection. For reasons that are not clear, haematogenous osteomyelitis in adults most often affects the spine.

Staphylococcus aureus is also the most common cause of exogenous osteomyelitis, but there can be other causes, depending on the circumstances of the trauma and the area of the body involved. For instance, in one recent report, *Pseudomonas* osteomyelitis occurred in a number of children who had suffered penetrating foot injuries and the organism was thought to be inhabiting their sneakers.

> **CASE HISTORY 19.2**
> **OSTEOMYELITIS**
>
> Thomas, a 13-year-old boy, injured his lower left arm in a rugby match at school. The injury occurred when he fell heavily on the arm while being tackled. The next day his arm became extremely painful and was hot and swollen. He was taken to the family doctor who recorded his temperature at 39.4°C. The doctor also noticed several small boils on his chest, some of which had been broken.

Clinical features, diagnosis and treatment

Haematogenous osteomyelitis in a child is usually manifested by a sudden onset of high fever, chills, nausea and progressive pain over the infected bone, whereas in adults a more insidious and vague onset of fever, malaise and anorexia is usual. For exogenous infections, signs and symptoms of soft tissue infection usually predominate.

Plain radiographs or bone scans provide confirmation of osteomyelitis in most cases. Blood culture (before antimicrobial therapy), and bone biopsy (if blood culture negative) may help to identify the causative organism and its antibiotic sensitivity. However, the causative organism is isolated in only 60–70% of cases.

Treatment requires immediate intravenous antibiotics, usually starting with a penicillinase-resistant penicillin or a cephalosporin for *S. aureus*, this being the most common cause. Chronic infection can develop when bone necrosis occurs. Necrotic bone tissue presumably shields the bacteria from body defences and acts as a continuous source of infection. In this situation, surgical intervention for debridement and drainage as well as prolonged antibiotics may be necessary.

LYME DISEASE

Causative agent and transmission

Lyme disease is caused by the spirochaete *Borrelia burgdorferi* and occasionally by another species, *B. garinii.* The disease was first identified in 1975 in a cluster of children with arthritis in the village of Old Lyme in Connecticut, in the United States. It is now the most common vector-borne disease in North America, with approximately 18 000 cases per year being reported, and the number of cases is rising. It is also common in many areas of Europe, and has been identified in several other northern hemisphere countries, and also in Australia. The real incidence of Lyme disease in Australia is unknown, but there have been sporadic reports of Lyme disease-like illness in eastern coastal areas since 1982. Only a small number of cases have been identified serologically.

Borrelia burgdorferi is a micro-aerophilic spirochaete 20–30 μm long and approximately 0.25 μm wide. In the United States the natural cycle of infection takes place in white-footed field mice and deer. It is transmitted in these animals and to humans by ticks of the genus *Ixodes*. In the United States, *I. dammini* and *I. pacificus* are the major tick species involved, whereas in Europe it is *I. ricinus* and in Asia *I. persulcatus*.

These species of tick have not been found in Australia, and *B. burgdorferi* has been difficult to find in Australian ticks that bite humans. Also, the organism has not yet been isolated from a local Australian patient. While clinical and serological evidence suggests that the disease occurs in this country, the source and the vector are at present unclear. Seabirds, bandicoots and macropods have been suggested as possible sources, and Borrelia-like spirochaetes have been isolated from the bush tick, *Ixodes holocyclus*, and the seabird tick, *Ixodes uriae,* but the mode of human infection has not been confirmed. There is no human-to-human transmission of Lyme disease.

Pathogenesis and clinical features

The spirochaete is injected into the skin of humans while the tick is feeding, and then travels via the blood or lymph to virtually anywhere in the body. It seems to favour synovial tissue, skin and the nervous system, but the reasons for this are not yet understood. The course of Lyme disease is variable. In untreated people, it can range from no symptoms or only localised skin manifestations to severe and chronic disease with multiple symptoms. After a variable incubation period, mostly about a week, the full disease progresses in three stages.

Stage 1 is found in 60–80% of infected people and is characterised by **erythema migrans**. This is a unique skin lesion which begins as a red macule, usually, but not always, at the site of the tick bite; it then expands to form an erythematous annular lesion, often with a clear centre, giving it a 'bulls-eye' appearance. However, erythema migrans is not common in infections acquired in Australia. The skin lesion may be accompanied by local lymphadenopathy and minor symptoms of fever, headache and myalgia. In untreated cases this stage resolves in several weeks.

Stage 2 follows within weeks to months and represents disseminated disease. Manifestations may include secondary annular skin lesions in other sites, neurologic disorders (e.g. lymphocytic meningitis, facial palsy, mental deterioration), cardiac disorders (e.g. myocarditis and atrioventricular block, causing palpitations and fainting), and recurrent, brief attacks of arthritis. Patients may be quite ill with debilitating malaise and fatigue.

Stage 3 occurs after a latent period of a year or more and represents chronic disease of the skin, nervous system and joints. Arthritis is the most common late sign. These late manifestations are immunological, probably due to immune complex deposition and/or cross-reacting antibodies in these tissues. Stages 2 and 3 are seen in 10–15% of untreated patients.

The clinical picture of Lyme disease is similar in many ways to syphilis, another spirochaetal infection. Both are characterised by an initial skin infection, followed by multisystem involvement, interspersed with periods of latency.

Diagnosis

Lyme disease is often difficult to diagnose. It may be straightforward in patients with typical clinical features and a history of time spent in an endemic area. In such a situation, the observation of the characteristic skin lesion, erythema migrans, would be diagnostic. However, much more often the clinical picture is atypical or non-specific, and exposure history is vague. Laboratory tests may be helpful, but have significant limitations. Culture of the organism is difficult because it is only occasionally isolated from the skin lesions of patients, and it may take weeks to grow.

PCR (polymerase chain reaction) has recently been developed for use in the diagnosis of Lyme disease, and supplements culture. A rising antibody titre in paired serum samples confirms infection, whereas high titre in a single sample is only suggestive of infection. Currently, there is thought to be substantial overdiagnosis of this disease in the United States, since false positives are common due to cross-reactivity with other antigens or other factors, such as syphilis or certain autoimmune disorders. False negative serological results may also be obtained since the immune response to this organism may develop slowly.

Treatment and prevention

Early-stage Lyme disease is usually effectively treated with either doxycycline or amoxycillin, but intravenous penicillin or ceftriaxone is needed for more established infections. Chronic arthritis and other late manifestations may not respond to antibiotic therapy because of their immunological basis. Vaccines are currently being trialled but there is none licensed for use at present. Prevention is therefore based on avoidance of tick bites.

RICKETTSIAL INFECTIONS

Causative organisms and incidence

Rickettsiae are named after Howard Ricketts who first identified them as the causes of typhus and Rocky Mountain spotted fever in the United States. The rickettsiae are Gram-negative rod-shaped bacteria. They have the unusual characteristic for bacteria of being strictly intracellular parasites—that is, like viruses, they can multiply only inside cells. Another characteristic feature of these organisms is that they all multiply in arthropods such as ticks, lice, fleas or mites.

By far the most common rickettsial infection in Australia is Q fever, caused by *Coxiella burnetii*. It is most often transmitted by aerosol from faeces, milk and hides of infected sheep and cattle to farmers, meat-workers and animal transporters. Its primary site of infection is the lung. Q fever is discussed fully in Chapter 17.

Of the arthropod-borne infections, scrub typhus and Queensland tick typhus—caused by *Rickettsia tsutsugamushi* and *Rickettsia australis* respectively—are the most common. On average, fewer than 10 cases of all forms of typhus occur in Australia per year. Worldwide, a variety of species can cause human infection, as shown in Table 19.2 . Generally, infections caused by *Rickettsia* are not very common, but are important because they can be fatal.

Pathogenesis and clinical features

The classical rickettsial diseases are very similar in many respects. After introduction through the skin the organisms disseminate through the bloodstream, localising in small blood vessels in many organs, including the skin, brain and heart. They invade and damage the endothelial cells of these vessels, causing them to leak. The resultant haemorrhages and surrounding tissue necrosis produce the typical clinical features of rickettsial infections: skin rash (except in Q fever), headache and fever (often with rigors). Other possible symptoms include a local lymphadenopathy in the region of the arthropod bite, myalgia, and liver and spleen enlargement. The disease can be mild to fatal, with death usually resulting from shock and cardiorespiratory failure.

Laboratory diagnosis and treatment

Rickettsiae can be isolated from patient blood, but require highly specialised cell culture techniques. A serological diagnosis on paired serum samples is currently the preferred method. Rickettsiae are hazardous organisms, so careful handling of patient blood should be observed. Skin contact with patient blood and its aerosolisation should be avoided. Prompt treatment with tetracycline reduces the mortality rate.

LEPTOSPIROSIS

Leptospirosis is caused by *Leptospira interrogans*. This highly coiled spirochaete 5–15 μm long, has the ends of the cell bent into a hook, giving the cell the appearance of a question mark—hence the name *interrogans* (see Figure 19.2). Leptospirosis is a notifiable disease in Australia. The annual incidence in this country is less than 2 percent per 100 000 population (about 100 to 200 cases). The most common strains (serotypes) in Australia are *L. interrogans hardjo*, from cattle and sheep, and *L. interrogans pomona*, from pigs.

The bacteria infect dogs, cats, cattle, sheep, pigs and many wild mammals such as rats, causing a chronic kidney infection. There is excretion of large numbers of bacteria in urine and humans become infected by exposure to the animal meat, or to water or food contaminated with urine. Many Australian cases are associated with occupational exposure, particularly among meat-workers, farmers and stock transporters. The potential for infection by wading or swimming in ponds or dams around which livestock have pastured has been repeatedly demonstrated. The bacteria enter through mucous membranes or skin abrasions, reach the bloodstream and then are carried throughout the body. Many infections are asymptomatic, but in some a febrile, flu-like illness occurs after an incubation period of 1–2 weeks. In most of the cases (about 90%) an uneventful recovery takes place within three weeks.

A severe form, called Weil's disease, represents severe infection of the liver and kidneys, and is characterised by hepatitis, jaundice, uraemia and bacteriuria.

Bacteria can be isolated from blood, urine and CSF, with blood culture during the first week of the disease being the most reliable method. Repeated blood cultures are necessary to improve the chance of obtaining a positive culture. Direct microscopic examination of blood or CSF may be attempted, and provide a rapid diagnosis, but the organisms are difficult to demonstrate by this method. A highly sensitive and specific serological method is also available.

Penicillin, erythromycin and tetracyclines are effective if given within the first week of illness, and recovery is usually complete. Patients with serious complications, especially kidney failure, require supportive care. An animal vaccine is available, but one for humans has not yet been developed.

TABLE 19.2
FEATURES OF SELECTED RICKETTSIAL INFECTIONS

DISEASE	CAUSATIVE ORGANISM	DISTRIBUTION	VECTOR
Spotted Fevers			
■ Rocky Mountain spotted fever	*R. rickettsii*	Western hemisphere	Ticks
■ Boutonneuse fever	*R. conorii*	Mediterranean, Africa, India	Ticks
■ Queensland tick typhus	*R. australis*	Australia	Ticks
Typhus Fevers			
■ Epidemic typhus	*R. prowazekii*	South America, Africa	Lice
■ Murine typhus	*R. typhi*	Worldwide	Fleas
Scrub Typhus	*R. tsutsugamushi*	Asia, Australia, Pacific Islands	Mites

FIGURE 19.2

LEPTOSPIRA INTERROGANS

An electron micrograph of this hook-shaped spirochaete that causes urinary tract infections in animals and systemic infections in humans.

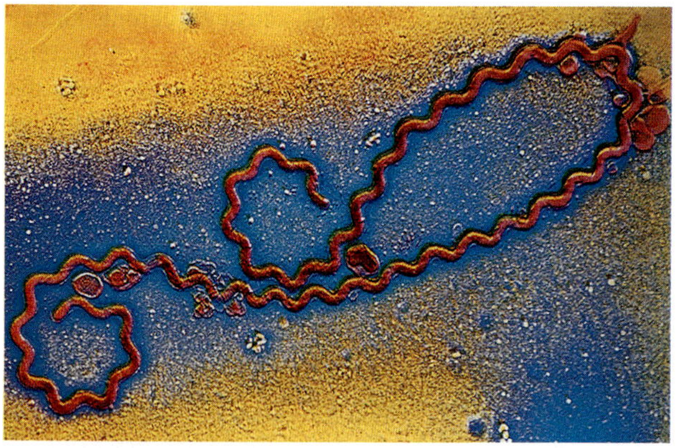

TOXIC SHOCK SYNDROME

Toxic shock syndrome is caused by certain strains of *Staphylococcus aureus* that produce a particular toxin called toxic shock syndrome toxin (TSST). The disease came to prominence when outbreaks occurred in women, associated with their use of super-absorbent tampons. The tampons were sometimes left in place for too long and caused abrasion of the vaginal wall, providing appropriate conditions for infection. It is now recognised that toxic shock syndrome can result from any infection in men, women or children caused by a TSST-producing strain of *Staphylococcus aureus*.

Toxic shock syndrome is a potentially life-threatening condition characterised by fever, shock and a red, sunburn-like rash. In one or two days the skin starts to peel off in sheets, particularly on the palms and soles of the feet. Other parts of the body are usually involved, such as the gastrointestinal system (vomiting, diarrhoea), muscles (myalgia), central nervous system (disorientation) and mucous membranes (vaginal or conjunctival hyperaemia). Death, when it occurs, is usually due to shock. Patients should be examined for a focus of staphylococcal infection. Vigorous antibiotic therapy is warranted. If related to tampon usage, advice to the patient as to proper, aseptic usage should be provided by the health professional.

ANTHRAX

Anthrax is a zoonosis (an animal disease which can be transmitted to humans) that is primarily acquired from herbivores, especially sheep, goats and cattle. It is caused by *Bacillus anthracis*, a large, spore-forming, Gram-positive rod. Its spores are extremely resistant to adverse environmental conditions and can remain dormant in soil for many years. Human infection comes from direct contact with infected animals (skins or carcasses), inhalation of spores present in aerosolised animal products (e.g. milk) or ingestion of infected meat. Although an effective animal vaccine exists, anthrax is still a problem in many undeveloped countries. In Australia, on average there are fewer than 20 reported cases a year.

A cut or skin abrasion is the usual site of entry, where the spores germinate and the bacteria multiply and produce the anthrax toxin. Host defences are inhibited by the organism's antiphagocytic capsule. In 1–2 days a papular lesion develops, surrounded by a ring of vesicles. Eventually it ulcerates and becomes black and necrotic. In a minority of cases, septicaemia and severe toxaemia can occur, with generalised toxic effects and death. Pulmonary anthrax ('woolsorter's disease') is the most serious form of anthrax, but is rare in developed countries. Inhalation of spores leads to multiplication in the lungs, pulmonary oedema and haemorrhage, and septicaemia. The mortality rate in this form is high.

Anthrax is best diagnosed by culture of organisms from skin lesions or blood. It is effectively treated with penicillin or tetracyclines, if treatment is commenced early in the course of the disease. Animal vaccination greatly reduces the incidence of human disease. Contaminated materials should be incinerated or carefully sterilised or disinfected. Infected animals are isolated and killed, and the carcasses are cremated or deep buried and covered with anhydrous calcium oxide (quicklime). A human vaccine is not available in Australia, so workers at occupational risk need to be well educated about appropriate preventive measures.

BRUCELLOSIS

Cause and incidence

Human brucellosis was first described in 1860 among British soldiers in Malta, where it became known as **Malta fever**. It is also sometimes called **undulant fever** because of the rising and falling nature of the fever. The disease is caused by three species of the genus *Brucella*: *B. melitensis, B. abortus and B. suis*. These small, Gram-negative coccobacilli are primarily animal pathogens, but cause disease in humans after contact with infected animals or their products.

B. melitensis is found mainly in sheep and goats. It causes the most serious infections in humans and has the most severe complications. The disease is endemic in Mediterranean countries, the Middle East, South America, and areas of Europe, Asia and Africa. The species does not occur in animals in Australia.

B. abortus is acquired mainly from cows. Infection with this species can lead to abortion (hence 'abortus') in animals but not in humans. It has a worldwide distribution except in certain developed countries which have succeeded in eradicating the organism. Australia was declared free of bovine brucellosis in 1989, as a result of the National Brucellosis and Tuberculosis Eradication Campaign instituted in 1970.

B. suis infects pigs and occasionally other animals such as horses, cows and dogs. It occurs in South America and South-East Asia, and is the most important cause of brucellosis in the United States and Australia. Indeed, in Australia, the incidence of brucellosis generally has

FIGURE 19.3
NOTIFIED CASES OF BRUCELLOSIS IN AUSTRALIA, 1970 TO 1991

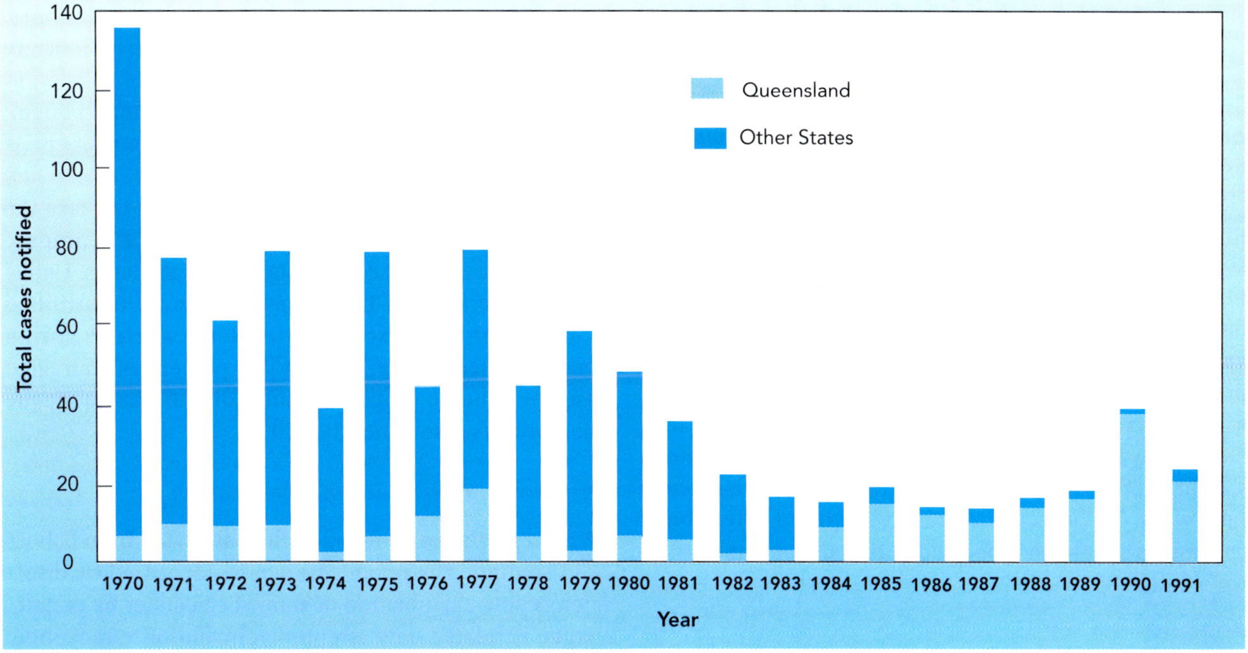

Source: Robson et al (1993), *Medical Journal of Australia*, 159:153–158.

been increasing since 1986, due to infections by this species (see Figure 19.3). Most cases occur in Queensland where professional and amateur hunters are responding to the lucrative overseas market for wild boar meat. The organism is rare in domestic pigs.

Transmission

Brucellosis is highly communicable. Transmission from animals to humans occurs by direct contact with infected tissues or animal products, or via dust or aerosols. The organisms enter the body via abrasions in the skin, via the conjunctivae or the gastrointestinal tract or, most commonly, via the respiratory tract. Infection usually occurs in people consuming unpasteurised milk products, and in farmers, abattoir workers and hunters. Pig hunters are often heavily exposed to blood and body fluids during butchering of the animals. There is also a high risk of laboratory-acquired infection by aerosol transmission from an infected specimen. Appropriate containment procedures must therefore be used when processing a specimen from a person suspected of having brucellosis.

CASE HISTORY 19.3
BRUCELLOSIS

A 25-year-old Turkish-born woman travelled to Turkey in 1990 where she resided for 11 months. In 1991 she presented to Casualty at a hospital in Sydney with a number of health problems including a vaginal discharge. Blood cultures yielded *Brucella melitensis* biotype 1.

At the microbiology laboratory where the culture was made, staff were scanned for *Brucella* infection. One member, who was asymptomatic, was positive on blood culture. This young woman subsequently miscarried and *B. melitensis* biotype 1 was cultured from placental material.

Adapted from Everett, R.E., '*Brucella melitensis* in Humans', *Communicable Diseases Intelligence* 17/18, 6 September 1993, p. 407.

Pathogenesis and clinical features

Inside the host, *Brucella* enter the lymphatic system and then the blood, causing an acute bacteraemia. They are facultative intracellular parasites and thus multiply within phagocytes in the spleen, liver, bone marrow and other lymphoid tissues. Granulomatous inflammatory reactions and necrosis of tissues occur, with enlargement of affected organs. Often the infection is subclinical, but in clinical cases the onset of symptoms is gradual and begins one or more weeks after contact. Typical presenting symptoms are night drenching sweats, chills and fever, disabling lethargy, malaise, headache, myalgia and arthralgia. Anorexia and substantial weight loss may occur. Complications such as splenic abscesses, endocarditis, septic arthritis, osteomyelitis and meningitis are possible, especially if diagnosis and treatment are delayed for more than a month after onset of symptoms.

Diagnosis

Brucellosis is usually diagnosed by serological tests. However, because of cross-reactivity between *Brucella* species, the exact identity of a species causing a particular infection may be difficult to determine. Further, titres are often high and stable at presentation, and thus a diagnostic fourfold increase may not be detected in paired sera. Isolation of the causative organism from blood cultures should be attempted, but is not always successful.

Treatment and prevention

Brucella are susceptible to tetracyclines, which should be used in combination with a second drug such as rifampicin (WHO recommendation). Because of the organism's intracellular location, it can be difficult to eliminate completely and relapses are common. A prolonged course of therapy, for at least four weeks and as long as three months, may be necessary. At present there is no human vaccine. Prevention is based on (1) pasteurisation of dairy products, (2) animal vaccination, (3) education of workers at risk of occupational exposure, and (4) the use of protective clothing by at-risk workers. In Australia, feral pig hunters should be educated about the need for protective hand and face wear. To prevent laboratory-acquired infections, specimens should be processed in biosafety cabinets.

PLAGUE

Cause and incidence

Few diseases have ravaged the human population throughout time in the way plague has done. Some authorities believe that the first historic mention of the disease is in the Book of Samuel, which describes an epidemic of 'emerods' (buboes?) among the Philistines. Several great pandemics of plague have been recorded. The Black Death, as it was known in the Middle Ages, killed an estimated one-quarter of the population of Europe in the 14th century. The Great Plague of 1665–66 was restricted largely to London and caused over 75 000 deaths. Even as recent as the beginning of this century, the disease was responsible for 10 million deaths in India alone, in a great pandemic affecting central Asia. Epidemics still occur, especially when preventive measures are not followed—for example, in war-torn Vietnam during the 1960s, as many as 10 000 deaths a year were due to this disease. Nowadays, most cases are restricted to some parts of Asia (e.g. Myanmar, Vietnam, China) and Africa (e.g. Madagascar, Zaire, Uganda). In Australia, as in other developed countries, the disease is rare. The last case recorded in this country was in 1923.

The causative agent of plague is *Yersinia pestis*, a small Gram-negative rod belonging to the family *Enterobacteriaceae*. The organism infects wild rodents, especially rats, and is transmitted from animal to animal and animal to human by flea bites. In epidemics, massive numbers of rats die of the disease, and the fleas, deprived of their natural hosts, feed voraciously on humans instead.

Pathogenesis and clinical features

Yersinia pestis possesses a number of virulence factors including an antiphagocytic capsule, a coagulase, endotoxin and various other protein toxins. The organism multiplies rapidly and is able to survive within macrophages. It spreads via the lymphatics to regional lymph nodes. Within 1–7 days of the flea bite a haemorrhagic inflammation causes these nodes to form very large and tender **buboes**, hence the term **bubonic plague**. They are most frequently found in the armpit or groin.

If the organisms move into the circulatory system, infection, haemorrhage and necrosis occur in many parts of the body, including the skin, lungs, liver, spleen and CNS. The haemorrhages and resultant cyanosis turn the skin black, hence the name 'Black Death'. **Pneumonic plague** occurs when the organism invades the lungs. Unlike the bubonic form of the disease, it can be transmitted from person to person via droplets expelled during coughing (see Figure 19.4). Fifty percent of untreated cases of bubonic plague die, and for pneumonic plague the mortality rate is nearly 100%.

Diagnosis, treatment and prevention

Yersinia pestis can be found in fluid aspirated from buboes or in sputum. The organisms can be identified by direct microscopic examination of stained smears or by culture. Plague is treated with streptomycin and/or tetracycline. Prevention is based on the following:

- rodent and flea control;
- strict isolation of infected patients;
- quarantine and fumigation of infected ships;
- vaccination of workers and travellers to endemic areas (but this does not provide long-term immunity).

Systemic Viral Infections

HUMAN IMMUNODEFICIENCY VIRUS INFECTION AND AIDS

In 1981 a new syndrome, subsequently called **the acquired immunodeficiency syndrome (AIDS)**, was first recognised among homosexual men in the United States. It was characterised by the appearance of rare and fatal infections and rare types of cancer. It first appeared in Australia in 1982; by the mid-1980s it was obvious that the disease had spread, largely unnoticed, throughout the world. In 1983 the causative agent was isolated from blood lymphocytes and became known as the human immunodeficiency virus (HIV). Complete information on the course of the infection is not yet available, but it is currently estimated that, of those people infected with HIV, up to 30% will develop AIDS within five years, and almost all will eventually develop AIDS and die from it.

Causative agents

Two serotypes of HIV have been identified: HIV-1 and HIV-2. The most common cause of AIDS throughout the world is HIV-1. However, HIV-2, which initially was found only in West Africa, and predominates there, has now been reported to have caused sporadic cases in East

FIGURE 19.4
THE EPIDEMIOLOGY OF PLAGUE

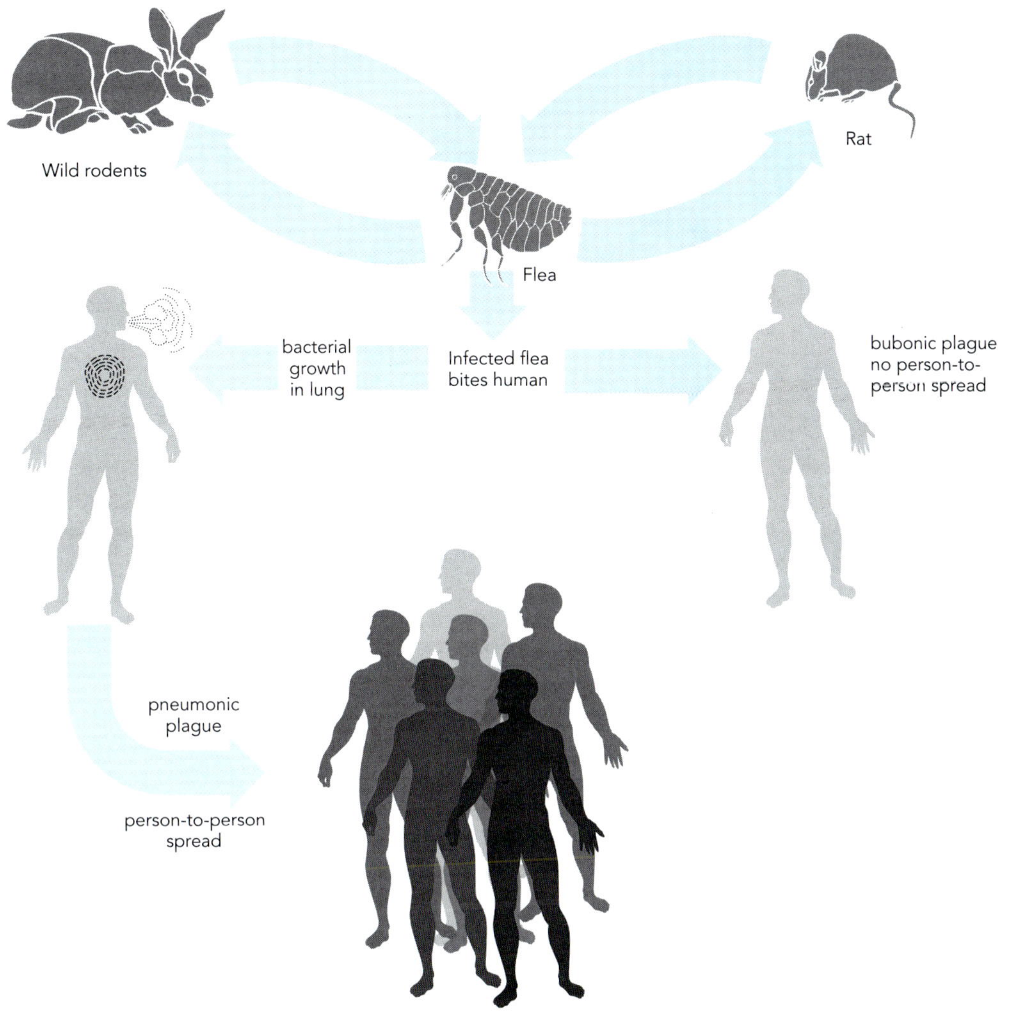

Africa, Europe, Asia and Latin America. It is expected that eventually HIV-2 will also spread worldwide. A very small number of cases of HIV-2 infection have so far been diagnosed in Australia, the first in 1992. The transmission of HIV-2 and the clinical features of infection are similar to those of HIV-1. In this book, HIV will be used to refer to both HIV-1 and HIV-2 unless stated otherwise.

The structure of HIV is shown in Figure 19.5. It is a roughly spherical particle comprising an outer envelope of a bilayer of lipid molecules, originally from the cell membrane of a human cell. The envelope is studded with numerous 'spikes', which are thought to consist of two glycoproteins—gp120, which project out from the envelope, and gp41, which is embedded in the envelope. Beneath the envelope is a layer of protein called p18, which in turn surrounds the capsid (p24 antigen). Since HIV is a retrovirus, its genetic core is in the form of RNA. Inside the capsid there are two single-stranded molecules of RNA. Attached to the RNA are molecules of the enzyme, **reverse transcriptase**, which transcribes the viral RNA into DNA once the virus is inside its host cell.

Incidence

In mid-1993, the World Health Organization (WHO) estimated that more than 13 million HIV infections had occurred worldwide since the pandemic began[1]. While more than 600 000 cases of AIDS have been reported, the WHO estimates that, allowing for underdiagnosis and underreporting, the real number is likely to be more than 2.2 million worldwide. In Australia, a total of 18 989 cases of HIV infection and 5883 cases of AIDS had been diagnosed up to 31 March 1995, as reported to the National Centre in HIV Epidemiology and Clinical Research[2]. More than two-thirds of cases of HIV infection are reported in New South Wales, with Victoria and Queensland having the next highest numbers of cases (see Table 19.3).

Transmission

Characteristically, in developed countries most HIV infections have occurred in men, primarily as a result of homosexual intercourse or intravenous drug use. However, the difference in numbers of men and women infected is narrowing as transmission by heterosexual

FIGURE 19.5
THE STRUCTURE OF THE HUMAN IMMUNODEFICIENCY VIRUS (HIV), THE CAUSATIVE AGENT OF AIDS

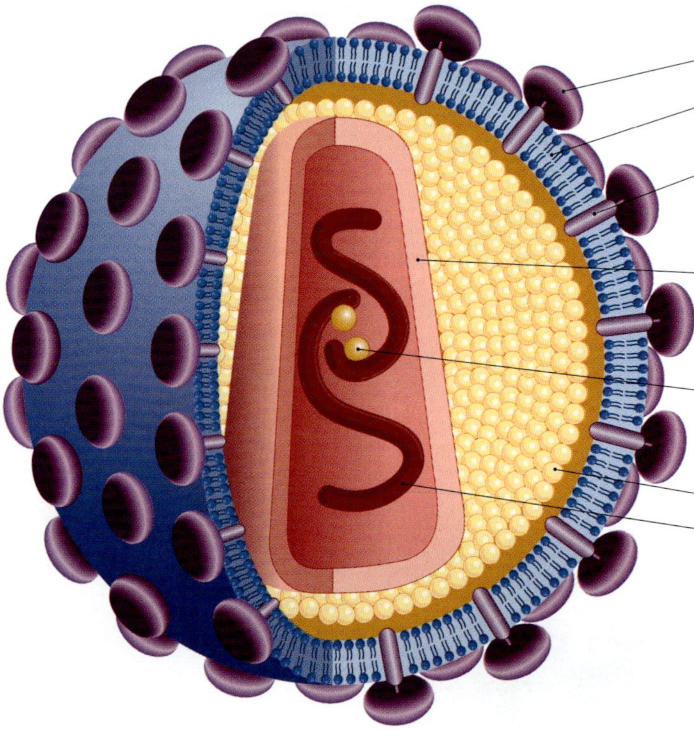

TABLE 19.3
TOTAL DIAGNOSES OF HIV INFECTION TO 31 MARCH 1995 BY STATE/TERRITORY

STATE OR TERRITORY	TOTAL	RATE*
ACT	167	55.3
NSW	12316	202.5
NT	82	47.6
Qld	1583	49.0
SA	584	39.7
Tas	73	15.4
Vic	3420	76.2
WA	764	44.5
Total	**18989**	**105.8**

* Rate per 100 000 current population

Adapted from National Centre in HIV Epidemiology and Clinical Research (1995), *Australian HIV Surveillance Report* 11(3): 21.

TABLE 19.4
AIDS CASES DIAGNOSED IN AUSTRALIA TO 31 MARCH 1995 BY EXPOSURE CATEGORY

EXPOSURE CATEGORY	% OF ALL CASES
Homosexual/bisexual contact only	82.6
Heterosexual contact only	4.0
Injecting drug use or sexual contact	6.4
Receipt of contaminated blood or blood products	3.6
Other or unknown	2.8

Adapted from National Centre in HIV Epidemiology and Clinical Research (1995), *Australian HIV Surveillance Report* 11(3): 16.

intercourse becomes more common. In the Carribean and some parts of Asia and Africa, transmission has largely been through heterosexual relations, and males and females are more or less equally affected. Occupationally-acquired infection in health care workers, predominantly due to needle-stick injury, has also occurred.

The AIDS cases diagnosed in Australia by transmission category are shown in Table 19.4. The vast majority (83%) of cases have acquired infection through homosexual or bisexual contact, and all of these are male. Although heterosexual contact accounts overall for only 3.8% of all cases of AIDS in Australia, it was responsible for 5.4% of cases in 1991–92 and 6.9% in 1992–93, and is apparently increasing. Three major trends have emerged in recent years regarding HIV transmission in Australia:

1. the transmission rate in men by homosexual contact is stabilising; and

2. transmission by heterosexual contact is increasing; and
3. transmission by IV drug use is increasing.

These trends are shown in Figure 19.6. Overall, it has been established that HIV is transmitted in three ways:

- through sexual intercourse;
- through blood or blood products;
- from mother to child.

The transmission of HIV from mother to child occurs during pregnancy, at delivery, and through breast feeding. These children rapidly develop AIDS, and usually die before the age of five. Currently there is *no epidemiological evidence* to suggest that HIV is transmitted by:

- hugging;
- kissing;
- food or water;
- mosquitoes or other insects;
- the sharing of household utensils.

Pathogenesis

HIV disease results from chronic infection of cells bearing the CD4 antigen. The gp120 envelope protein of the virus can bind tightly to this antigen (Figure 19.7), making several types of immune system cells vulnerable. Helper T lymphocytes (T4 lymphocytes) are the main targets, but glial cells in the brain, monocytes and macrophages are also vulnerable. Macrophages may in fact be responsible for transporting the virus to different parts of the body, including the brain.

When the virus enters a cell, it uncoats and then, like all retroviruses, transcribes its RNA into DNA using its reverse transcriptase (see Figure 19.8). The DNA is then converted into double stranded DNA and integrated into the host cell genome. While the viral DNA is integrated, it is dormant and causes no damage to the cell. However, at some later date, following some unknown signal, the viral DNA becomes activated and directs the synthesis of new viral RNA and viral proteins. These are assembled into numerous complete viruses which are released from the surface of the cell by budding, to infect other target cells.

It was initially thought that HIV causes immunosuppression solely by infecting and killing T4 lymphocytes. The depletion of T4 lymphocytes greatly diminishes the ability of the host to produce adequate amounts of antibodies or lymphokines, since these T4 cells are needed for the initiation of immune responses (see Chapter 9). The patient thus becomes more susceptible to infections and cancers that the healthy immune system would deal with effectively. However, it is now felt that the immunosuppression is a complex process with the virus possibly causing damage to the immune system in a number of ways, including:

- the direct killing of infected T4 cells by the virus;
- the destruction of virus-infected immune cells, including T4 cells by killer T cells;
- the prevention of T4 cells responding to foreign antigens by the blocking of cell receptors (CD4) by detached viral proteins gp120 and gp41. Thus, T4 cells are rendered inactive (called **cell anergy**);
- the release of a soluble suppressor factor by infected T4 cells;
- virus-initiated autoimmune response to CD4 receptors and subsequent destruction of cells bearing those antigens;
- infection of lymph nodes leading to their damage or destruction.

Whatever the mechanisms, the declining T4 cell count seems to be a useful indicator of the damage occurring to the immune system and the progress of the disease.

In addition to immune system damage, the virus attacks the nervous system directly. Monocytes also carry the CD4 antigen and can thus be infected by HIV. Indeed, it has been suggested that infected monocytes carry the virus into the brain. These infected cells are then thought to attack the myelin sheath that coats nerve cells. In AIDS, damage to the central nervous system also occurs as a result of secondary infection by other microorganisms. The pathogenesis of AIDS is summarised in Figure 19.9.

The immune response to HIV typically (but not always) begins 2–4 weeks after infection. Neutralising antibodies

FIGURE 19.6
AIDS DIAGNOSIS BY EXPOSURE

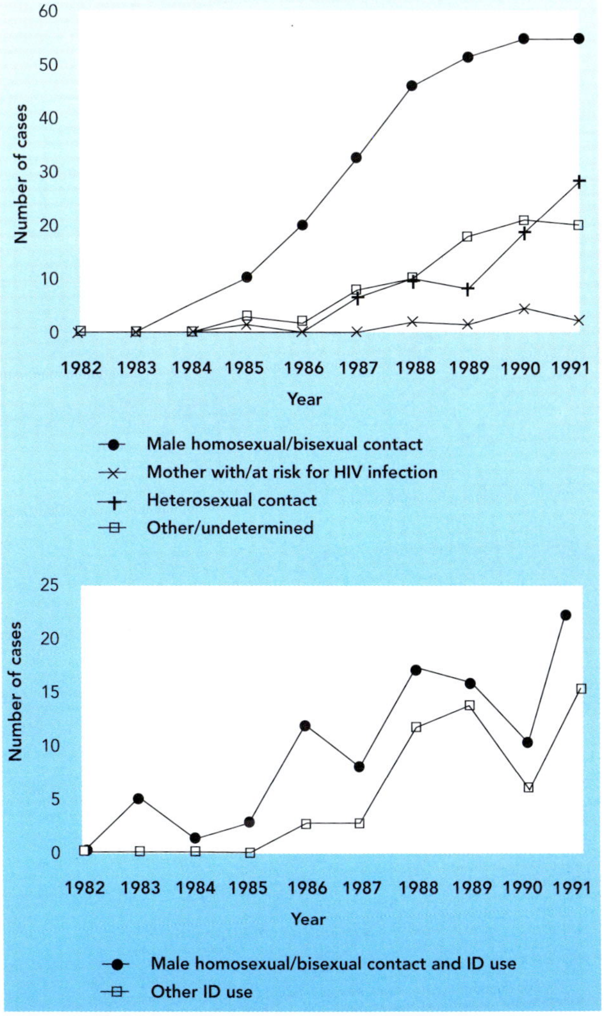

Source: Kaldor, J. et al, (1993) 'The acquired immunodeficiency syndrome in Australia: incidence 1982–1991', *Medical Journal of Australia*, 158, pp. 10–17.

FIGURE 19.7
BINDING OF THE HIV GP120 PROTEIN TO THE CD4 RECEPTOR OF THE HUMAN T LYMPHOCYTE

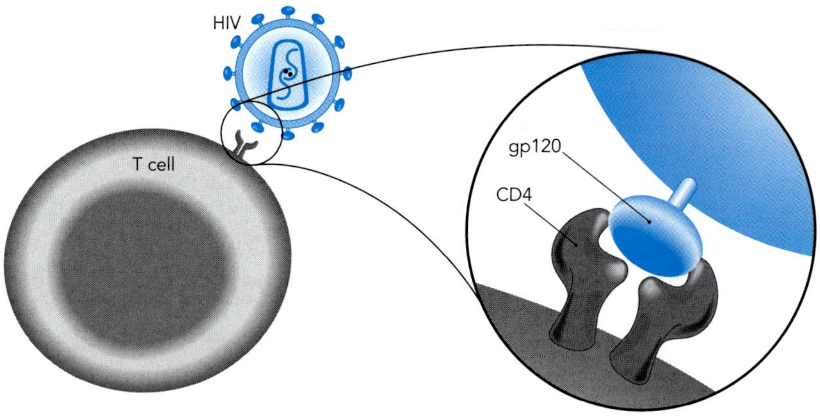

FIGURE 19.8
REPLICATION CYCLE OF HIV

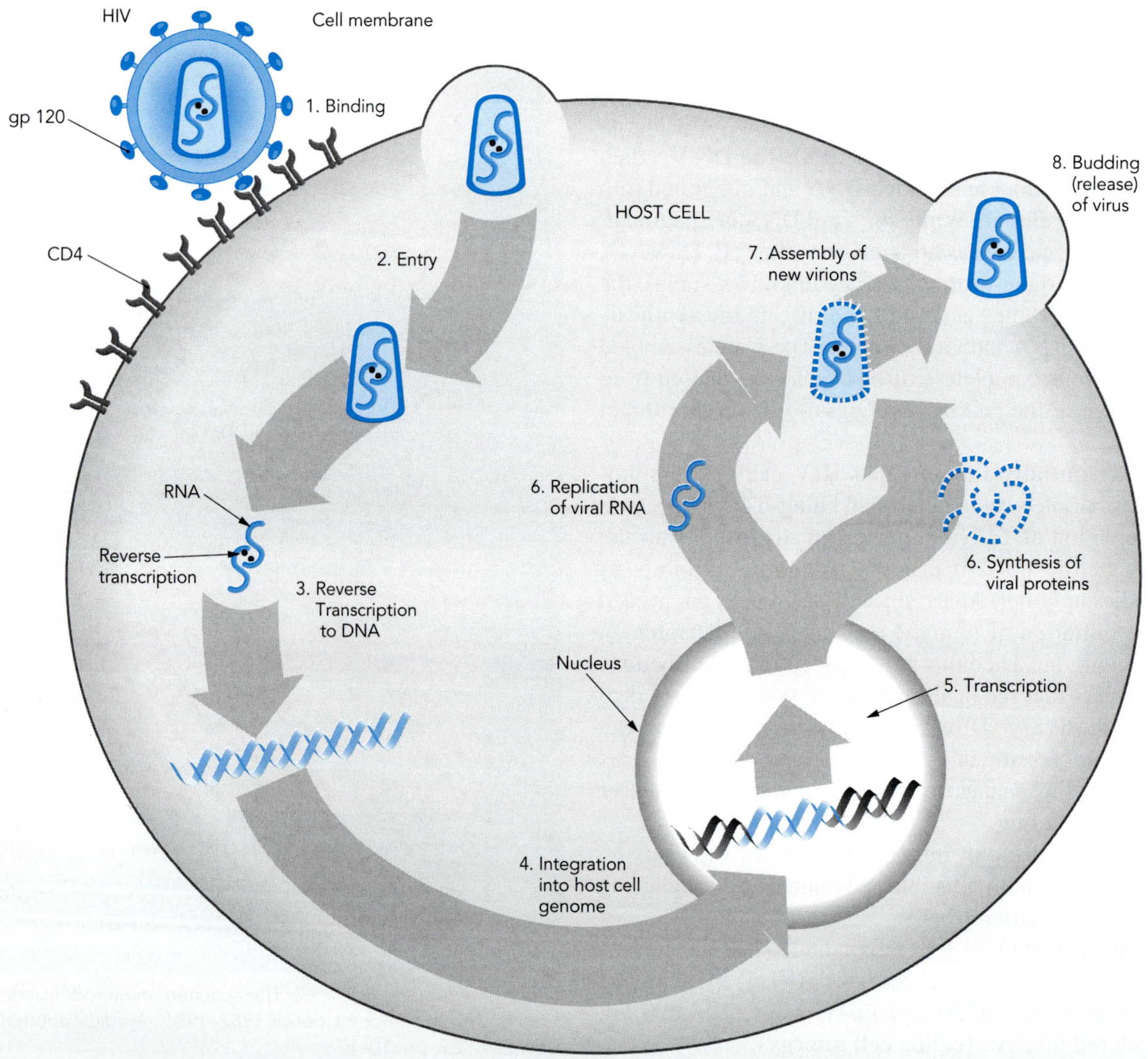

FIGURE 19.9
THE PATHOGENESIS OF AIDS

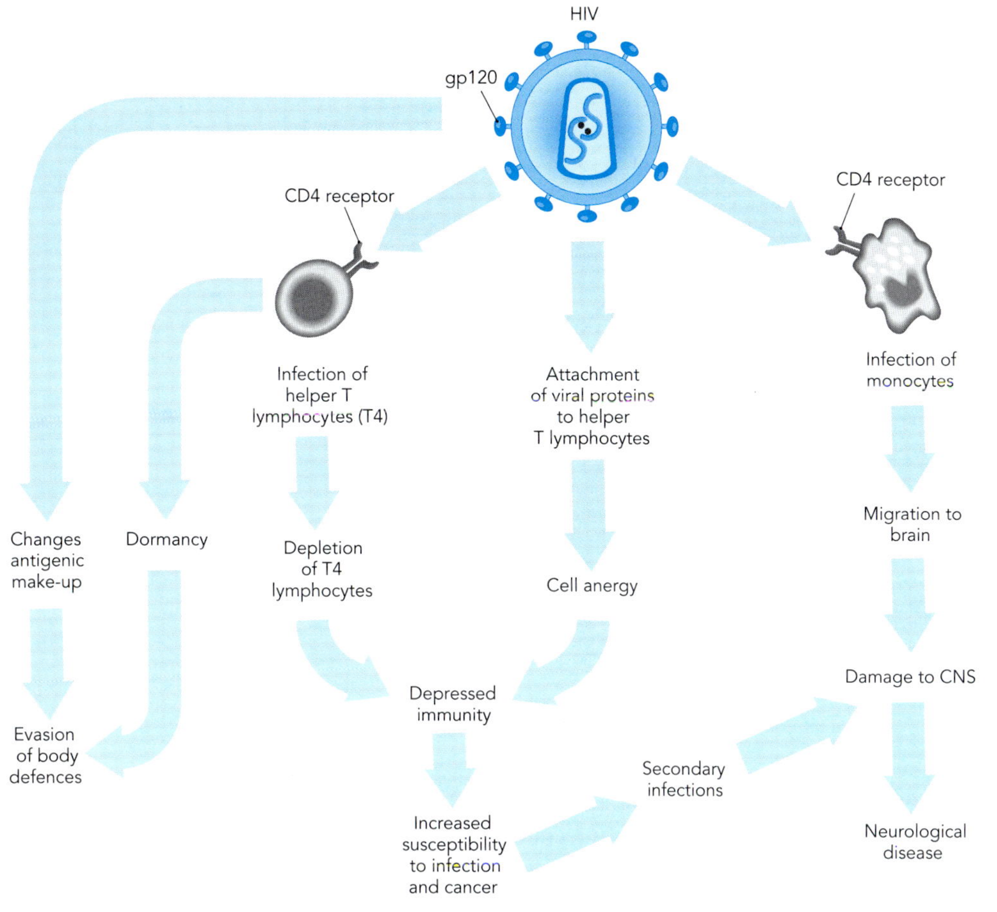

are usually found, as well as a cell-mediated immune response. As the immune response gathers pace, the virus and its components become undetectable, and any early clinical manifestations disappear. However, the immune mechanisms do not completely clear the virus, probably because of the weakness of the immune response and dormancy of the virus in some cells. Furthermore, the virus undergoes a high rate of mutation while it is causing infection, changing its antigens and thus allowing it to evade host responses. In fact, a number of different antigenic variants of the virus can often be isolated from a single person. These antigenic variants may evade host defences produced to previous antigenic types.

Despite enormous research into HIV and AIDS over the last decade, the war against the virus is proving difficult to win. The three main reasons are:

1. The virus infects cells that the body needs to defend itself against the virus.
2. The virus is able to remain hidden inside cells, especially in lymphoid tissue, for many years.
3. The virus is extremely variable in its antigenic makeup.

Clinical features

A wide spectrum of clinical manifestations are possible in an HIV-infected person. While some of these manifestations are rare and HIV-specific, there are many that overlap with totally unrelated disorders. Thus, it has been suggested that up to 75% of cases undergoing significant seroconversion may be missed. This **seroconversion illness** usually occurs 2–4 weeks after infection (see Figure 19.10), and is an acute 'mononucleosis-like' illness with fever, headache, pharyngitis, nausea, mild CNS symptoms, mucocutaneous ulcers and a maculopapular rash. A lymphadenopathy may develop in the second week. This illness is associated with the appearance of anti-HIV antibodies, but only occurs in 50–70% of people. It is also associated with a brief but pronounced depression in the T4 lymphocyte numbers. The T4 cell count, as shown in Figure 19.10, is a useful guide to the progress of the infection, but is not regarded as a perfect measure of immune function.

Recovery usually occurs within a few weeks and there follows a variable period, usually five years or more, of reasonably good health. Some people have been infected for 10 years without apparent clinical manifestations. This phase represents some, but not total, curtailment of virus activity. The T4 cell count is beginning to decrease, but remains above 500 per μL of blood. However, this phase is not usually totally asymptomatic—there may be episodes of symptomatic illness and, in the majority of cases, a **persistent generalised lymphadenopathy (PGL)** occurs after several years, representing viral multiplication in lymph nodes.

FIGURE 19.10
THE CLINICAL FEATURES OF HIV INFECTION

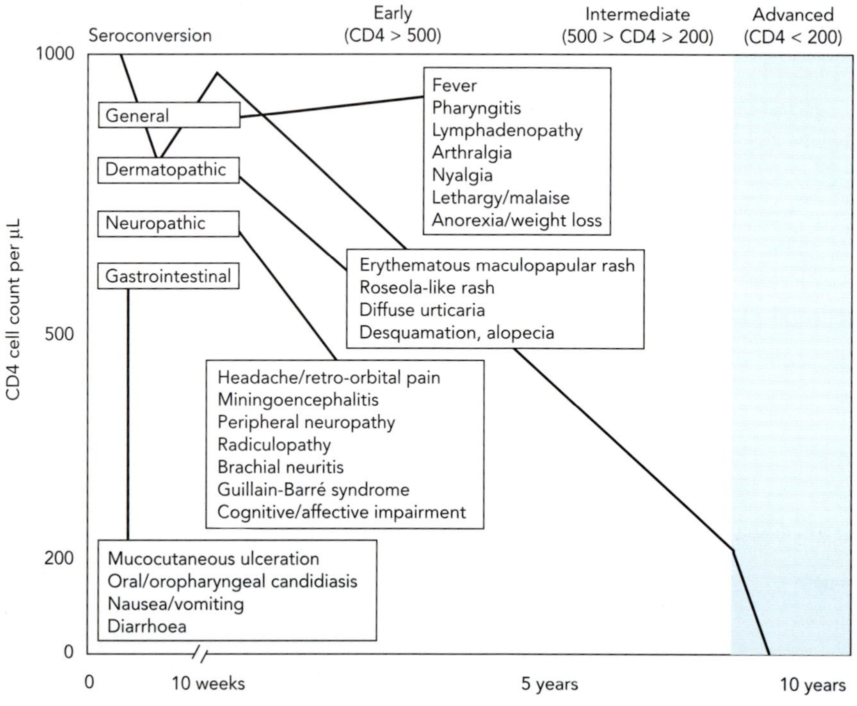

Source: Boyle (1993), *Medical Journal of Australia*, 158.

The intermediate phase of T4 cell depletion (200–500 per µL) can be manifested by a variety of minor infections such as pharyngitis, sinusitis, gingivitis, tinea, seborrhoeic dermatitis, warts, reactivation of herpes zoster and oral candidiasis, and symptoms like chronic diarrhoea, fever and weight loss. This group of symptoms used to be called the **AIDS-related complex (ARC)**, but this term is infrequently used now. These infections may persist or increase in severity as the T4 cell count drops towards 200 per µL.

Advanced immune depletion (T4 cell count falling repeatedly below 200 per µL) heralds the likelihood of development of an AIDS-defining infection or malignancy. This is a secondary disease that is highly suggestive of AIDS, and warrants further investigation. AIDS-defining diseases include:

- Kaposi's sarcoma (in people less than 60 years old)
- oral hairy leukoplakia
- *Pneumocystis carinii* pneumonia
- oesophageal candidiasis
- cryptosporidiosis diarrhoea (lasting more than a month)
- cryptococcal meningitis
- *Mycobacterium avium intracellulare* infection.

The microorganisms that cause the secondary infections in AIDS patients are typically opportunistic pathogens; that is, they have low pathogenicity and only rarely cause infection in the general population. The most common secondary diseases in AIDS patients are Kaposi's sarcoma (see Figure 19.11) and *Pneumocystis carinii* pneumonia, but many other diseases can occur including disseminated mycobacterial infections, toxoplasma encephalitis, cryptococcal meningitis, cytomegalovirus retinitis and non-Hodgkin's lymphoma (Table 19.5). The opportunistic infections are the usual cause of death in patients with AIDS.

Progression from HIV infection to AIDS occurs in approximately 50% of people within 10 years. It is currently thought that almost all people infected with HIV will eventually die of AIDS.

Monitoring the progress of the disease by assessing immune function is useful for the following reasons:

- to provide the patient with a short- and long-term prognosis;
- to help to determine the most appropriate time to begin anti-HIV treatment and chemoprophylaxis for opportunistic infections;
- to monitor the effectiveness of anti-HIV treatment.

FIGURE 19.11
THE PURPLISH SKIN LESIONS OF KAPOSI'S SARCOMA

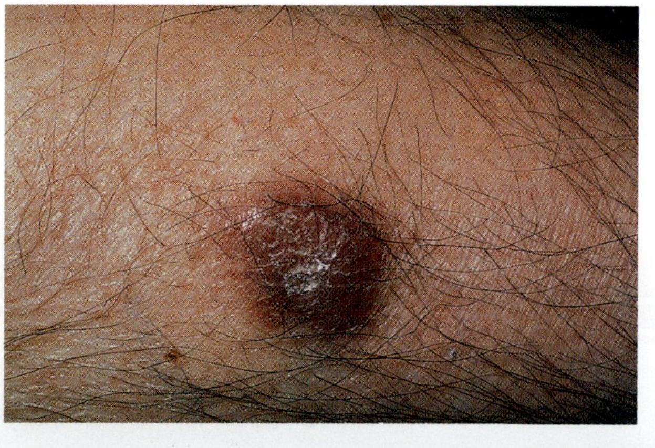

TABLE 19.5
AIDS CASES DIAGNOSED IN AUSTRALIA BY AIDS-DEFINING ILLNESS, CUMULATIVE TO 31 MARCH 1995

AIDS-DEFINING ILLNESS	PERCENTAGE
Pneumocystis carinii pneumonia (PCP)	30.2
Kaposi's sarcoma (KS)	12.7
KS and PCP only	0.9
KS and other (not PCP)	1.5
PCP and other (not KS)	4.9
Oesophageal candidiasis	8.3
Cerebral toxoplasmosis	3.7
Meningeal cryptococcosis	3.9
Non-Hodgkin's lymphoma	3.7
Mycobacterium avium	4.8
Herpes simplex virus	2.5
HIV encephalopathy	3.0
Cytomegalovirus	3.9
HIV wasting disease	4.0
Cryptosporidiosis (gut)	2.2
Mycobacterium tuberculosis (TB)	0.7
Other single diagnosis	2.0
Other multiple diagnoses	7.1
Total	100.0

Adapted from National Centre in HIV Epidemiology and Clinical Research (1995), *Australian HIV Surveillance Report* 11(3): 18.

As indicated above, the T4 cell count is a useful guide, but is not a perfect measure. Other assays of immune function are sometimes used in conjunction, such as serum β_2 microglobulin level, serum neopterin, and interleukin-2 production by helper T cells.

Infection with HIV can result in a large number of neurological manifestations throughout the course of the disease. The various neurological complications tend to occur at certain times during infection, and result from direct infection by HIV of the nervous system, secondary opportunistic infections and neoplasms involving the central nervous system, or a combination of these. Some of the more common manifestations are:

- *aseptic meningitis*—which develops at approximately the time of seroconversion;
- *peripheral neuropathy*—thought to be a result of direct invasion of peripheral nerves by the HIV; occurs early in disease at about the time of seroconversion, or late in disease as a painful sensory neuropathy;
- *recurrent seizures*—due to HIV infection itself or secondary infections of the central nervous system;
- *AIDS dementia complex* (also referred to as HIV encephalopathy, HIV encephalitis, HIV dementia)—characterised by progressive cognitive dysfunction and motor and behavioural disorders; typically occurs late in disease, due to HIV infection or secondary infections or tumours.

Laboratory diagnosis

The laboratory diagnosis of HIV infection most often involves the detection of anti-HIV antibodies in serum. Antibodies are usually detected in the first 2–6 weeks of infection, although in some people a 'window period' of three months or more between infection and antibody production has occurred. An indirect ELISA test or a passive agglutination assay (see Chapter 15) are frequently used as a screening test for antibody. Since there is a small chance of a false positive result being obtained, confirmation of positive results is required. This is usually done, first, by repeating the screening test and then, if again positive, by use of the more specific (and more expensive and difficult to perform) Western blot assay. This test detects and identifies specific antibodies against separate protein components, such as the gp120, gp41 or p24 proteins. Since antibodies to different viral proteins are produced at different stages of infection, this assay may also be helpful in monitoring the progress of the disease.

One of the problems with these antibody tests is that the antibody-negative (window) period may be as long as several months in some infected people; so the diagnosis in these cases would be delayed. Also, the significance of antibodies in neonates born to HIV-infected mothers is not always clear. Antibodies passively transferred from mother to foetus can remain in the infant's circulation for more than 12 months, making a serological diagnosis of infection very difficult.

As a result, a number of other diagnostic tests for HIV infection have been developed which supplement, rather than replace, the antibody-detection methods. Assays for the detection of viral antigens in serum (e.g. HIV-1 p24 antigen test) are useful, since HIV antigens can, in some cases, be detected during the window period, in advanced disease when antibodies may not be detectable, and in infected neonates.

Isolation of HIV from peripheral blood mononuclear cells (PBMC), and the polymerase chain reaction (PCR) method on DNA extracted from PBMC, are also sometimes used for diagnosis of infection in neonates. PCR has also been used to make a more rapid diagnosis when seroconversion is slow. The PCR has an advantage over virus isolation because it is faster (days versus weeks) and requires a smaller amount of blood.

Currently, isolation of HIV and PCR are performed mainly in reference laboratories and have some limitations, so results are interpreted with caution. In most cases, HIV infection can be diagnosed by detection of anti-viral antibodies in serum. Thus, antibody-detection methods are still, at present, the mainstay of laboratory diagnosis.

Treatment

At this time there is no cure for AIDS. Zidovudine (azidothymidine, AZT) is the mainstay of therapy for symptomatic HIV infection, but it only delays the progress of the disease and helps to control constitutional symptoms such as fever, night sweats and lethargy. AZT also appears to delay the onset of symptoms in antibody-positive people, but there is no evidence that it extends their life expectancy. The antiviral activity of AZT is based on its structural similarity to the nucleic acid base, thymidine. The viral reverse transcriptase is fooled into incorporating AZT into the DNA molecule being synthesised. Once it is incorporated, DNA synthesis is stopped.

Apart from not being a cure, there are other problems with AZT therapy. First, the clinical benefits of AZT therapy tend to diminish after several months to a year of its use. The virus has a high rate of mutation and reverse transcriptases are made eventually that can synthesise DNA even in the presence of AZT. Second, the toxicity of the drug is such that it may have to be withdrawn occasionally to relieve side effects such as anaemia, leucopenia and myositis (inflammation of skeletal muscles). Third, the drug is currently very expensive, costing up to $9000 per person per year in Australia. For these reasons, there is some debate concerning the stage of infection at which AZT therapy should be commenced.

Several other drugs are currently being trialled. Dideoxycytidine (ddC) and dideoxyinosine (ddI) are also nucleoside analogues, and thus inhibitors of reverse transcriptase. It is hoped that combinations of these drugs and AZT will help to delay the development of drug resistance in the virus. Other drugs being trialled include protease inhibitors, to prevent assembly of new virus particles, and agents that aim at restoring immune function. A myriad of possible treatments also exists for the various secondary infections of AIDS. Most of these opportunistic infections are treatable, at least in the early stages of the disease. Furthermore, chemoprophylaxis for the more common infections, particularly *Pneumocystis carinii* pneumonia, has been shown to reduce markedly the risk of that infection and thus improve the quality of life. On the other hand, the emergence of antibiotic-resistant strains of *Pneumocystis* in the United Kingdom and the United States throws into question the overall wisdom of prophylactic therapy.

Prevention

Numerous measures have been introduced to reduce the spread of HIV infection in the community. In Australia, preventive measures that have been adopted include:

- the testing of blood donors for HIV antibodies and the discouraging of people in high-risk groups from donating blood;
- heat treatment of blood products (e.g. factor VIII for haemophiliacs);
- public education programs encouraging safe sex practices (e.g. use of condoms) and discouraging promiscuous behaviour;
- public education programs about the dangers of sharing needles, and programs for the free distribution of clean needles and syringes.

To reduce the chance of infection in health care staff, various measures have been introduced, including:

- the adoption of Standard Precautions procedures (see Chapter 13) in health care institutions;
- the elimination of the practice of resheathing needles;
- the disposal of sharps in rigid containers;
- the use of gloves and masks by certain health professionals (e.g. dentists);
- the offer of AZT therapy for health care workers known to be occupationally exposed to the HIV (although the effectiveness and value of this is much debated).
- the availability and use of mouthpieces, resuscitation bags, or other ventilation devices in areas where the need for resuscitation is expected (even though transmission by saliva has not been demonstrated).

Despite intensive efforts towards the development of a vaccine, the prospects at this time are dim. The ability of the virus to mutate rapidly poses a serious obstacle to the development of an effective vaccine. However, effective vaccines have been developed against a retrovirus that causes leukaemia in cats, and against a simian form of AIDS.

ROSS RIVER VIRUS INFECTION (EPIDEMIC POLYARTHRITIS)

Cause, incidence and transmission

Epidemic polyarthritis is the most important arbovirus (**ar**thropod-**bo**rne **virus**) infection in Australia. It is caused by the Ross River virus, an alphavirus of the family *Togaviridae*. The disease was first described in 1928, as an 'unusual epidemic', in Narrandera, New South Wales. It was later called epidemic polyarthritis, a term which is now used to describe infections caused by several different viruses. Isolation of the virus was eventually reported in 1963 in Ross River in Northern Queensland.

Other less common viruses that can also cause epidemic polyarthritis in Australia are the Kokobera virus and the Barmah Forest virus. The largest recorded outbreak of Barmah Forest virus infection (80 confirmed cases) occurred early in 1995 in the Batemans Bay area of New South Wales.

About 4000 to 6000 notifications of Ross River virus infection are made in Australia each year. The rates of notifications per 100 000 population in different divisions of the country are shown in Figure 19.12. Being a mosquito-borne disease, it predominates in regions with warmer climate and higher rainfall, although it does occur throughout the country, including Tasmania. There are clusters of cases of Ross River virus infection every summer, but when mosquitoes reach plague proportions significant outbreaks may occur. The virus has been isolated from more than 10 different species of mosquito from different regions in the country, explaining its country-wide incidence. There is concern that, if global warming occurs, expanding mosquito populations could increase the incidence of this and other mosquito-borne diseases.

FIGURE 19.12
ANNUAL RATE OF ROSS RIVER VIRUS NOTIFICATIONS IN 1994 BY STATISTICAL DIVISION OF RESIDENCE

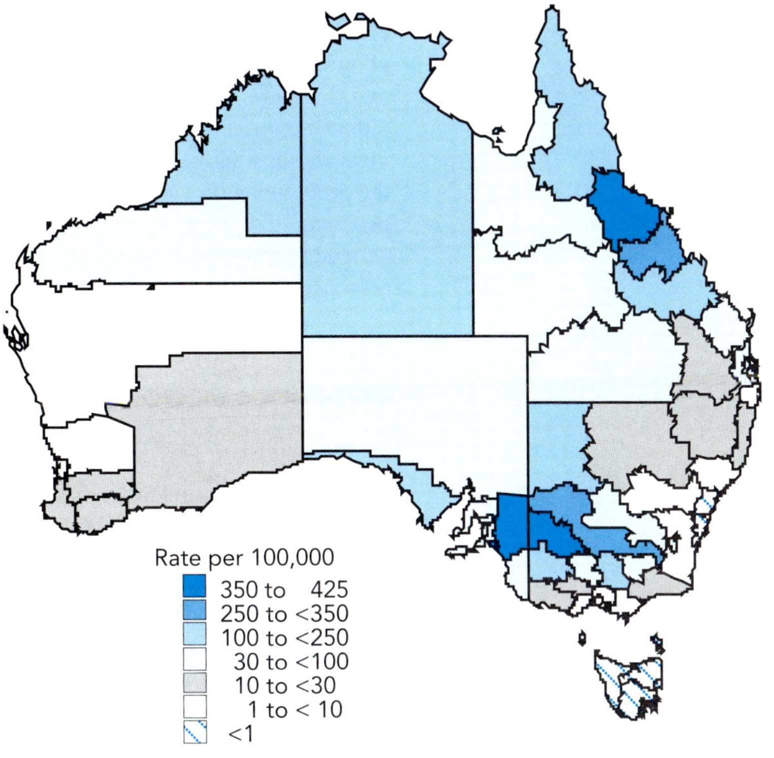

Source: Communicable Diseases Intelligence 19/22, 31 October 1995.

Clinical features, diagnosis and treatment

The intensity of Ross River virus infection varies considerably, with only approximately 30% of people seeking medical advice. The main manifestation is arthritis, with morning joint stiffness, although a maculopapular rash and flu-like symptoms are also common. The symptoms wax and wane, often persisting for more than three months, but gradually subside. Complete recovery may take 12 months or more, but there is no residual damage to joints. Symptomatic adults may not be able to work for a month or more, particularly if their work involves heavy physical activity.

Laboratory diagnosis of the disease is by serology, by detecting a fourfold increase in paired sera or IgM antibody in a single serum sample. At present, only symptomatic treatment (e.g. an anti-inflammatory drug for arthritis) is possible. Prevention is based on avoidance of mosquito bites, especially during epidemics.

DENGUE FEVER

Cause, incidence and transmission

Dengue virus is a flavivirus with four different serotypes. **Dengue fever** has a worldwide distribution in tropical areas, and occasionally in the subtropics. There are an estimated 100 million cases per year. In Australia, national data on the incidence of dengue fever were not formally collected until 1991, even though major epidemics have occurred in the past. There are usually less than 100 cases reported each year, except when epidemics occur (several hundred cases were reported in each of 1992 and 1993[3]). The vast majority of cases occur in northern Queensland. The mosquito *Aedes aegypti* is the principal human vector.

There is currently particular concern in the United States with the arrival and spread of the Asian tiger mosquito *Aedes albopictus*, which is an efficient carrier of the virus and an aggressive biter. It is feared that the range of this mosquito could take dengue to areas of the country that were previously unaffected.

Clinical features and complications

After an incubation period of about seven days, the disease is characterised by high fever, headache and a rash. Severe muscle and joint pain are also common, hence its other name, 'breakbone fever'. Except for its painful symptoms, dengue fever is a relatively mild and self-limiting disease that usually lasts about 10 days. A much more serious form of dengue, called **dengue haemorrhagic fever**, is characterised by bleeding from the gums, skin and gastrointestinal tract, and sometimes circulatory failure, shock and death.

The pathogenesis of dengue haemorrhagic fever is shown in Figure 19.13. After dengue virus infection, antibodies specific for the particular serotype are formed. If subsequently infected with a different serotype, it is

FIGURE 19.13
THE PATHOGENESIS OF DENGUE HAEMORRHAGIC FEVER
There are four serotypes of dengue virus—types 1 and 2 have been used in this example

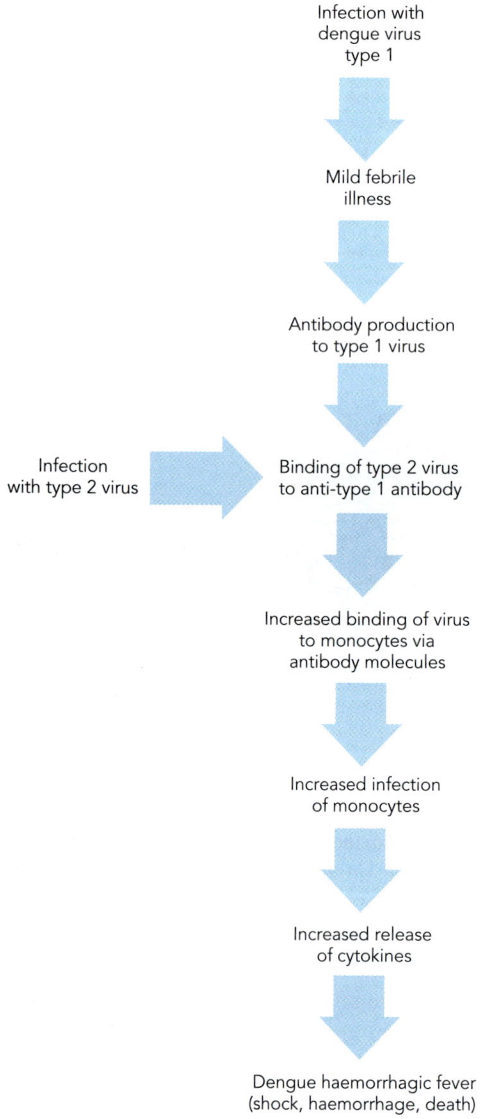

thought that the preformed antibodies bind to the virus, but fail to neutralise it. The antibodies actually enhance viral infection of monocytes, by first binding with the virus, and then attaching to Fc receptors on the monocyte membrane. Attachment and entry of the virus into its target cell is thus facilitated. Increased infection of monocytes is thought to induce an increased release of cytokines, leading to vascular damage and shock. Thus, dengue haemorrhagic fever becomes a possibility when dengue already exists in a region and subsequently a different serotype is introduced there. A highly pathogenic dengue virus of serotype 3—active in South-East Asia and the South-West Pacific—is therefore of concern to Australian health authorities, since only serotypes 1 and 2 are currently present in this country.

Diagnosis, treatment and prevention

Diagnosis is often based on clinical and epidemiological grounds. Epidemics of dengue tend to be focal in nature, affecting the population in a fairly circumscribed geographical area. A serological diagnosis is preferred, and there are several tests available for the detection of either the virus or specific antibodies. No effective antiviral therapy or vaccine is currently available. One of the problems with vaccine development is that antibodies produced to a vaccine may predispose the individual to dengue haemorrhagic fever. Prevention is therefore based on mosquito control programs and disease surveillance.

INFECTIOUS MONONUCLEOSIS

Cause, incidence and transmission

Infectious mononucleosis, or **glandular fever**, is caused by the herpes virus called Epstein-Barr virus (EBV). The infection is prevalent throughout the world. In less developed parts of the world it is usually acquired in early childhood, and is a subclinical or mild febrile illness. In developed countries, the highest incidence occurs in teenagers and young adults. The usual route of infection is by transfer of saliva, for example by sharing of drinking vessels or eating implements, or by kissing—it is sometimes referred to as 'kissing disease'. The virus may be shed intermittently in saliva for many years after infection.

Pathogenesis and clinical features

After entering the body via the oropharynx, the virus invades a number of organs such as the lung, parotid glands and various lymphoid organs, where it infects specifically B lymphocytes. The virus causes B cell proliferation, which may account for the excess of lymphocytes in the infected person. It is also thought to interfere with B cell and T cell interactions. After an incubation period of 5–6 weeks, mild symptoms of fever, headache, fatigue and malaise develop, which gradually worsen. Most patients develop a sore throat several days later, and after about a week the illness reaches its peak. The tonsils may be coated with a whitish-grey exudate and there may be inflammation of the rest of the pharynx. Palatal petechiae, swollen cervical and axillary lymph nodes, splenomegaly and hepatitis are also common.

Diagnosis and treatment

The clinical diagnosis of infectious mononucleosis is complicated by the fact that it resembles other systemic diseases like toxoplasmosis and cytomegalovirus infections. The name 'mononucleosis' refers to lymphocytes with abnormal morphology, and these can usually be found in a differential white cell count. IgM antibody tests (immunofluorescence or ELISA) provide the most specific diagnosis. Bed rest and symptomatic treatment are the basis of management of the disease. No vaccine is available.

Complications

The Epstein-Barr virus has been implicated in a number of different malignancies. Its association with Burkitt's lymphoma, B cell lymphomas in immunodeficient patients, and nasopharyngeal carcinoma are well recognised. However, its part in the development of these tumours is not fully understood. The virus has also been implicated in **chronic fatigue syndrome**. People with this condition often have a history of an initial viral-like illness. Excessive fatigue, to the extent that they have difficulty performing routine tasks, and general malaise are the main complaints. Other non-specific symptoms include fever, muscle weakness and headaches. Patients often complain of great debility, worsened by physical exertion, but otherwise may be quite well. Symptoms may last for three months or more. It is likely that other viruses, like other herpes viruses, are also responsible for this condition.

Laboratory investigations in chronic fatigue syndrome are often remarkably normal, so diagnosis is usually based on clinical grounds and the exclusion of other causes. Bed rest is essential, together with symptomatic treatment. Attempts to exercise back to health are not recommended.

CYTOMEGALOVIRUS INFECTION

The majority of cytomegalovirus (CMV) infections occur in childhood and produce few, if any, symptoms. In older children and adults, a mild malaise, fever, myalgia and lymph node inflammation may occur. The virus is not fully cleared from the body and establishes a lifelong, latent infection. The severity of the infection in the newborn and in immunocompromised people confirms CMV as an important human pathogen.

Transplacental transmission to the foetus may occur from a mother experiencing a primary or a reactivated infection. This leads to spread of the virus to multiple organs and a severe illness characterised by one or more of the following in the neonate: low birth weight, microcephaly, hepatosplenomegaly, growth retardation, impaired vision, hearing loss and haemolytic anaemia. Mortality among symptomatic neonates may be as high as 30% within the first few months of life. Other babies infected *in utero* may not show signs of infection at birth, but later develop mental or sensory disorders representing the neurological damage that the virus has caused.

CMV is also responsible for severe disseminated infections in the immunocompromised—such as people with AIDS, cancer patients (especially those with leukaemia or lymphoma) and organ transplant recipients. Infections in these patients may be due to primary infection by the virus from an exogenous source, or the reactivation of latent virus. The virus may infect any organ, but most often causes pneumonia, encephalitis, hepatitis or a sight-threatening retinitis.

CMV has been found in most body fluids, including saliva, urine, blood, breast milk, semen and cervical secretions, and thus can be transmitted in a variety of ways. It is usually spread by close contact, but also by blood transfusions, organ transplants, and during sexual intercourse. Shedding of the virus may occur intermittently for many months after infection, adding to its transmissibility.

Definitive diagnosis of CMV infection is made by isolation of the virus from a body fluid; those providing the greatest success rate are urine, throat washings and blood. Culture may take up to six weeks, so a serological diagnosis on paired sera, taken two weeks apart, is also usually performed. In neonatal infection, both infant and maternal sera should be collected. Specific IgM tests are unreliable, with both false positives and false negatives possible.

No effective treatment is yet available for neonatal infection. Ganciclovir has been used in CMV-infected AIDS patients with some success, but this drug has not been approved for use in infants. No effective vaccine is available. Pregnant health care workers should be informed of the risk of infection and should not have contact with known cases.

YELLOW FEVER

Yellow fever virus is a flavivirus that is restricted to parts of South America and Africa, where it is endemic. It is transmitted to humans by the mosquito *Aedes aegypti*. It causes an acute disease characterised by sudden onset of fever, vomiting and prostration 3–6 days after infection. Progression to extensive haemorrhagic manifestations and jaundice (yellowing of the skin), leading to coma and death, may occur. Mortality in non-indigenous people may be as high as 50% (compared to 5% in indigenous populations). There is no specific treatment.

Preventive measures include protection from mosquito bites, and vaccination. The vaccine is a live, attenuated strain of the virus and is highly effective. Everyone over the age of 12 months who is not immunocompromised, but who has been in or passed through an infected area six days before arrival in Australia, must have a current International Certificate of Vaccination against yellow fever. This is aimed at preventing the introduction and establishment of the disease in this country, where the *Aedes* vector mosquito is widespread.

HAEMORRHAGIC FEVERS

Haemorrhagic fevers have received increasing attention in recent years. They are caused by a number of different viruses, including the dengue fever virus and yellow fever virus described above. Other viruses that have been associated with the haemorrhagic fever syndrome include Lassa fever virus, Hantaan virus (Korean haemorrhagic fever), Marburg virus and Ebola virus. These viruses tend to have a specific geographical distribution (e.g. Africa for the Marburg and Ebola viruses). Although these viruses differ in terms of their sources, modes of transmission, or mechanisms for producing disease, they are grouped together on the basis of some common clinical manifestations. Typically, patients suffer from fever, malaise, myalgia, prostration, multisystem involvement,

SPOTLIGHT

EBOLA VIRUS

An outbreak of haemorragic fever caused by Ebola virus occurred in Zaire early in 1995. It was reported to have begun in February and involved about 300 cases with over 230 deaths, including 14 health workers. The majority of cases occurred in and around the cities of Kikwit and Kinhasa. The Zaire authorities quarantined infected people and restricted travel to and from the area.

Three Ebola virus outbreaks, affecting a total of more than 500 people, had previously been identified in Africa—in Yambuku, northern Zaire (around the Ebola river) in 1976, and in southern Sudan in 1976 and 1979.

Case fatality rates range from 50% to nearly 90%. Transmission occurs by direct contact with infected blood, secretions, organs or semen, and nosocomial infections have been common.

Adapted from *Communicable Diseases Intelligence* 19/10, 5 May 1995, p. 243.

and widespread haemorrhage due to endothelial cell damage, which can lead to shock and death.

Systemic Protozoal Infections

Although only a few protozoa cause systemic infections in humans, some are particularly important in terms of the number of people affected and the severity of the disease they cause. Malaria, in particular, continues to be a major problem in many areas of the world.

MALARIA

Incidence

Accurate global figures of the incidence of malaria are not available, but current estimates suggest there are 100–400 million cases of malaria each year. The annual death toll from the disease is estimated to be between 1 and 2 million, mainly in children. Malaria occurs over most of the tropical and some of the non-tropical regions of the world (see Figure 19.14). The vast majority of infections and deaths occur in Africa, India, Brazil, Afghanistan, Sri Lanka, Thailand, Indonesia, Cambodia and China (in decreasing order). Despite more than 30 years of effort by the World Health Organization (WHO) to control malaria, the worldwide situation is deteriorating, primarily because of increasing drug resistance in the causative organisms and increasing resistance of vector mosquitoes to insecticides.

Australia was certified free of indigenous (endemic) malaria by the WHO in 1981, but it is believed that the environmental conditions in Australia, north of latitude 19°S, would still favour the transmission of the disease if the parasites were reintroduced. There are several hundred cases of imported malaria being recorded each year. The highest-risk countries for travellers arriving in or returning to Australia are the Solomon Islands, Papua New Guinea, Africa and India.

The Australian Malaria Registry reported 939 cases for 1991[4]. As shown in Figure 19.15, there has been a gradual increase in the rate of notifications since 1952 to 5.2 cases per 100 000 population in 1990. Since 1917, when notifications began to be collated nationally, the peak incidence of malaria occurred in 1946 with the return of servicemen after World War II.

Causative organisms and transmission

The protozoa that cause malaria are sporozoans belonging to the genus *Plasmodium*. There are four species that cause human malaria: *Plasmodium falciparum*, *P. vivax*, *P. malariae* and *P. ovale*. Falciparum and vivax malaria are the most common. Both cause significant morbidity, but only *P. falciparum* causes significant mortality. The protozoa are transmitted to humans by species of *Anopheles* mosquitoes. Malaria can also be transmitted by blood transfusion or needlestick injury, although these modes of transmission are rare in non-endemic regions. There is no satisfactory *in vitro* screening test, so prevention of the transmission of malaria by blood transfusion depends on donor assessment, and donor memory and honesty. Only one case of transfusion-transmitted malaria has been reported in Australia since 1960.

A knowledge of the life cycle of these parasites helps in understanding the clinical features of the disease and the problems of controlling it. Sporozoites in the saliva of an infected *Anopheles* mosquito are injected into the bloodstream when the person is bitten (see Figure 19.16). They enter the liver and infect parenchymal cells where enormous replication and development into the merozoite form occurs over the next several days to weeks. The liver cell ruptures, releasing tens of thousands of merozoites into the bloodstream, where, after a few minutes, they invade red blood cells. Some parasites (especially *P. vivax*, but not *P. falciparum*) may remain in the liver as dormant hypnozoites, which some weeks or months later reactivate to cause relapses. Up to and including the liver stage of the infection, the patient remains well, but once the merozoites invade red blood cells symptoms begin.

Over a 48- or 72-hour period, depending on the species of the parasite, the merozoite matures into a trophozoite; this reproduces asexually, forming many more merozoites which are again released into the bloodstream after rupture of the red cell. The number of parasites continues to increase as 48- or 72-hour cycles of red cell invasion, multiplication and release are repeated. This may continue for some months or even years.

Some merozoites enter the sexual reproductive phase within red blood cells to form male and female gametocytes, which are taken up by a mosquito when feeding. Gametocytes unite in the stomach of the mosquito to form zygotes, which become sporozoites as they move to the salivary glands. Sporozoites are then injected into a new host when the mosquito feeds. This sexual phase

FIGURE 19.14
REGIONS OF THE WORLD WHERE MALARIA IS ENDEMIC

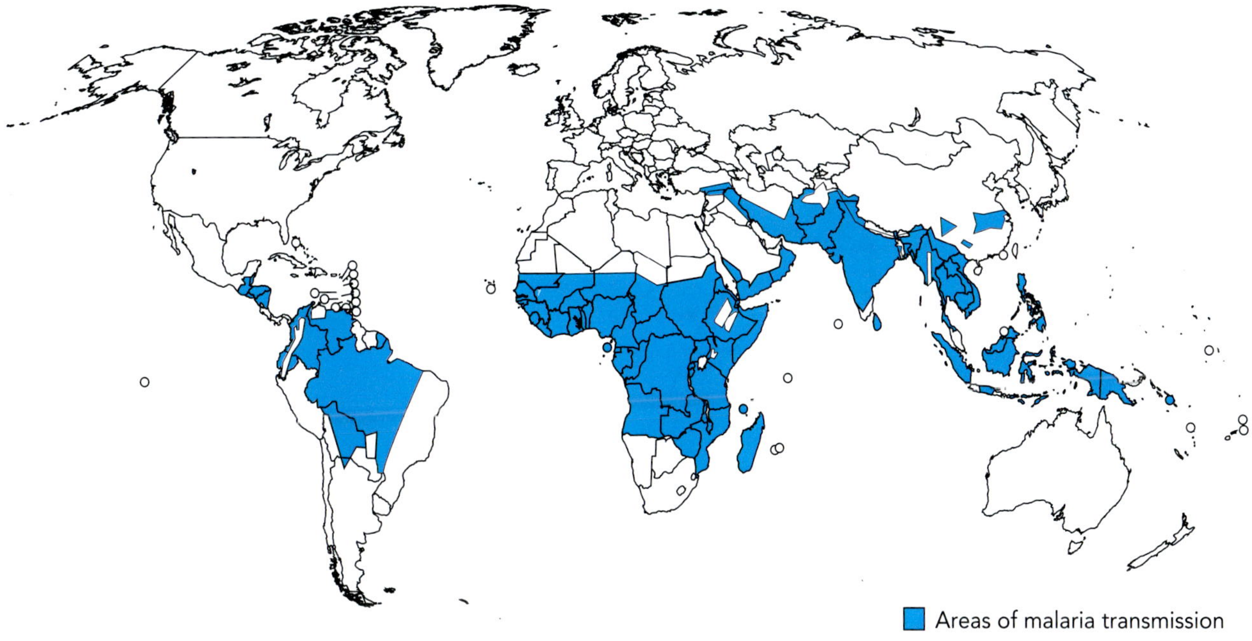

FIGURE 19.15
ANNUAL RATE OF NOTIFICATIONS OF MALARIA IN AUSTRALIA, 1952 TO 1991

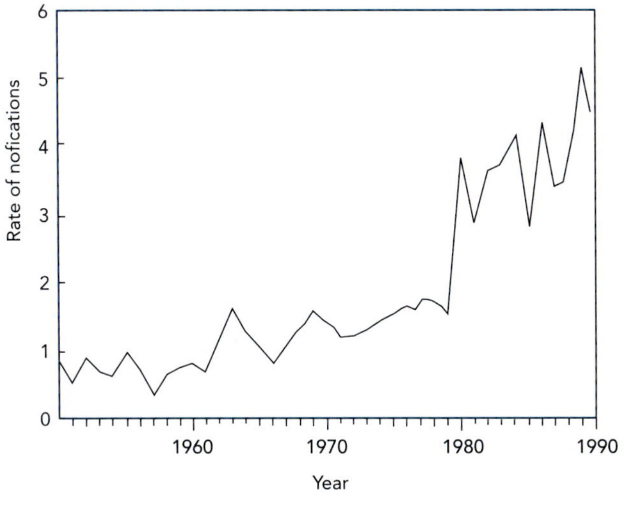

Source: Communicable Diseases Intelligence 17/7, 5 April 1993, p. 143.

in the mosquito is essential for completion of the life cycle of the protozoan.

The gametocytaemic phase in humans is important because it is the means by which malaria may be introduced or reintroduced into a non-endemic area. Immigrants or travellers with established infection and gametocytes in their blood can infect local mosquitoes, which may then cause indigenous spread of malaria. Health authorities in Australia are particularly concerned about the reintroduction of malaria into the so-called 'receptive zone', which is north of latitude 19°S (Townsville on the east coast to north of Port Hedland on the west coast). This is where mosquitoes capable of malaria transmission are known to exist. In fact, it is thought possible that a small proportion of malaria cases are locally acquired.

Pathogenesis and clinical features

The clinical features of malaria are often vague and non-specific, and depend on the age and immune status of the patient. One to three weeks after infection by a mosquito there is usually a feeling of malaise, often accompanied by headache and muscular discomfort. The most characteristic feature is fever, which is thought to be due to the release of pyrogens (see Chapter 9) from ruptured red cells. If the cycle of red cell infection and rupture remains regular and synchronous, a characteristic pattern of recurrent chills followed by fever, drenching sweats, headache, muscular pain and vomiting occurs every 48 or 72 hours, depending on the causative species. This symptomatic period lasts for only several hours.

The pattern of intermittent illness and well-being is usual in **benign malaria**—that is, infection caused by *P. vivax*, *P. ovale and P. malariae*—but less common in **falciparum malaria**. Without treatment, and if reinfection does not occur, benign malaria is normally self-limiting, resolving over a period of weeks or months, although relapses may occur. These relapses occur in vivax and ovale malaria when reactivation of dormant hypnozoites in the liver occurs.

Falciparum malaria is a far more severe form, presumably because this species infects a larger number of red cells. It is also thought to cause aggregations of red cells that obstruct small vessels, especially in the heart, resulting in cardiac dysfunction. The progress to

FIGURE 19.16

LIFE CYCLE OF THE MALARIA PARASITE, *PLASMODIUM*

(a) Female Anopheles mosquito bites human, transmitting sporozoites from its salivary glands; (b) In the liver the sporozoites multiply and become merozoites, which are shed into the bloodstream when liver cells rupture; (c) The merozoites enter red blood cells and become trophozoites, which feed and eventually form many more merozoites; (d) Merozoites are released by rupture of the red blood cells, accompanied by chills, high fever (40°C), and sweating. They can then infect other red blood cells; (e) After several such asexual cycles, gametocytes (sexual stages) are produced; (f) Upon ingestion by a mosquito, they form a zygote, which gives rise to more infective sporozoites in the salivary glands. These can then infect other people.

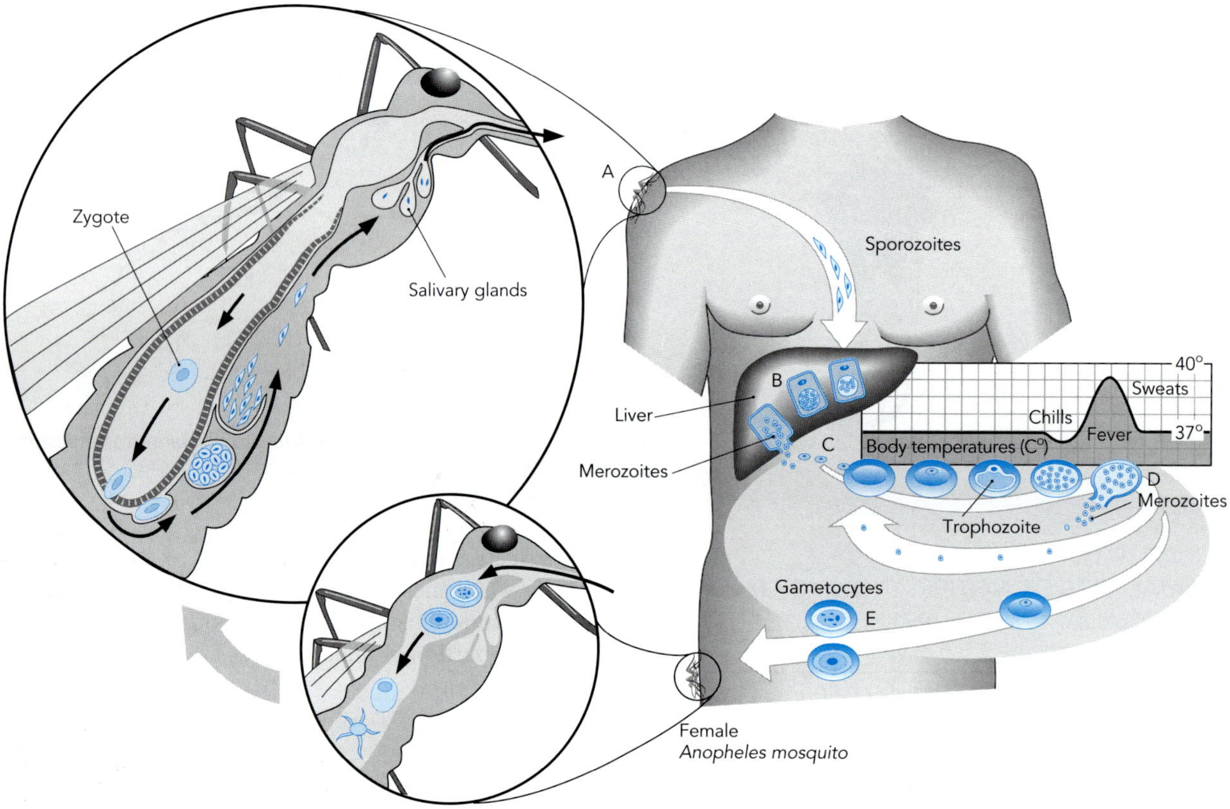

severe disease can be rapid, particularly in children. A patient with severe malaria may present with irregular fever and leading symptoms of gastrointestinal, respiratory or urinary tract infection. The symptoms are more persistent and there is often involvement of the brain. Liver impairment, kidney failure and severe anaemia are also common. In cerebral malaria there may be gradual progression from periods of confusion to coma. Even with treatment, mortality can be as high as 20%. Acute renal failure is also a major cause of death in falciparum malaria. An ominous sign is 'blackwater fever' (black urine) which is due to the excretion of large amounts of haemoglobin breakdown products in urine.

Diagnosis

Because of the varied clinical features of malaria, a laboratory diagnosis is necessary. The main means of diagnosing the disease is by microscopic examination of a blood film. In a positive film, a ring form of the parasite is seen within the red blood cell. The blood film should be repeated if the first sample is negative, particularly if the patient has just returned from an endemic area.

Treatment and management

Resistance to drugs is one of the major reasons for the increasing incidence of malaria throughout the world. Chloroquine is one of the safest antimalarials and is the drug of choice for benign malaria, although some resistance has been reported. It is also the drug of choice for sensitive *P. falciparum* infections, but unfortunately most strains throughout the world are resistant. Fansidar, a combination of sulphadoxine (a long-acting sulphonamide) and pyrimethamine, may be used for strains resistant to chloroquine alone. In multi-resistant areas, such as South-East Asia, mefloquine, halofantrine or quinine may be used. Generally, these three drugs are not well tolerated compared to chloroquine and fansidar.

Quinghaosu, a drug derived from the Chinese medicinal herb, qing hao, or sweet wormwood, is currently being evaluated in the treatment of malaria. The use of qing hao for the treatment of fevers was recommended in a Chinese handbook for medical emergencies published in AD 341, but its use specifically as an antimalarial has only recently been suggested. This drug holds special promise because of its effectiveness against chloroquine-resistant *Plasmodium*, its ease of use (as a

CASE HISTORY 19.4
MALARIA

A 17-year-old Victorian woman had spent two weeks in Lagos, Nigeria. Prior to the trip she and her brother had sought advice regarding antimalarials but were told that prophylaxis was not needed.

One day after her return to Australia the woman developed a fever. She consulted a local doctor on that day and was told that she 'might have malaria'. However, no tests were done and no treatment offered. The following day she appeared to be somewhat better, but late in the evening she became delirious and semi-conscious. She was taken to hospital and on arrival was hypotensive and not breathing. A 10% falciparum parasitaemia was diagnosed on admission. She did not respond to treatment and died about 36 hours later.

Adapted from Taylor, K., 'A malaria death: the public health lessons', *Communicable Diseases Intelligence* 16/22, 2 November 1992, p. 476.

suppository), its speed of action, and its apparent lack of serious toxicity.

In addition to chemotherapy, general measures such as physical cooling, antipyretics and fluid management may be necessary. In severe cases, other supportive treatments may be needed, such as blood transfusion (if red cell numbers are drastically reduced) and dialysis for renal failure.

Uncomplicated, benign malaria can be managed on an outpatient basis, but if falciparum is suspected then hospitalisation is usually considered. Severe falciparum is a medical emergency requiring intensive care attention and facilities, and immediate intravenous antimalarial therapy and supportive treatment.

Prevention

Australians and New Zealanders risk acquiring malaria when they travel to regions in the world where malaria is endemic. Currently, protection against malaria is based on avoidance of mosquito bites and on chemoprophylaxis. Avoidance of mosquito bite is usually based on such measures as:

- avoidance of risk areas during the malaria transmission season;
- the wearing of long, loose clothing at and after dark;
- staying in screened areas from dusk to dawn;
- the use of personal insect repellents and knock-down sprays indoors;
- use of bed-nets impregnated with mosquito repellents.

Malaria chemoprophylaxis is based on the use of chloroquine where the parasites are sensitive, and Maloprim (pyrimethamine-dapsone) where resistant. In areas where multiple resistance exists, mefloquine or doxycycline are usually prescribed. Up-to-date information on malaria chemoprophylaxis can be obtained from local departments of health. The most important point, however, is that there is no single drug that is completely effective against all strains and species of malaria parasites. As a result, chemoprophylaxis should be regarded only as an adjunct to the avoidance of exposure to mosquitoes.

The overall ineffectiveness of current malaria control programs, because of growing resistance of the parasite to drugs and of the mosquito to insecticides, has made the prospect of vaccination as a means of control very appealing. Currently, there is no effective vaccine available, but intensive research is continuing in this area.

TOXOPLASMOSIS

Toxoplasmosis is caused by the protozoan *Toxoplasma gondii*, which is a non-motile sporozoan. Cats are an essential part of the life cycle of *T. gondii* (Figure 19.17) because the organism undergoes its sexual phase in the intestine of the cat. Oocysts are shed in the cat's faeces and contaminate food or water which can be ingested by other animals and humans. The oocysts contain sporozoites that invade cells to form trophozoites, called tachyzoites. The intracellular parasite reproduces rapidly (*tachys* means speed), and the increased numbers cause the rupture of the host cell, with release of more tachyzoites. As the immune system becomes increasingly effective, the disease enters a chronic phase in which the infected host cell develops a wall to form a tissue cyst. The numerous parasites within such a cyst reproduce very slowly, if at all, and persist for years, especially in the brain. Loss of immune function (e.g. in AIDS) allows a reactivation of the infection from such cysts.

Humans generally acquire the infection by ingestion of undercooked meats (e.g. pork, mutton) containing tachyzoites or tissue cysts, although there is a possibility of contracting the disease more directly by contact with cat faeces. In adults, the disease is a rather undefined, mild illness (e.g. low-grade fever, general malaise, myalgia), although occasionally there will be severe effects, especially when the organism attacks nervous tissue. Surveys indicate that about 30–40% of the Australian population carries antibodies for this organism; this percentage indicates the high rate of subclinical, unrecognised infections.

The primary danger is in the congenital infection of a foetus. The effects on the foetus can be drastic, including convulsions, severe brain damage, blindness and death. The mother is usually unaware of the disease, as it is being transmitted across the placenta. Studies to determine the prevalence of congenital toxoplasmosis are hampered by clinical and technical difficulties, but in Western countries the rate seems to vary from approximately 1 in 500 to 1 in 10 000 births. A large study in Western Australia suggested a prevalence of approximately 1 in 4500 births[5].

At present, toxoplasmosis is diagnosed in the laboratory by serological tests. A specific IgM antibody test is available for diagnosis from a single serum sample, and for diagnosis of foetal infection. Pyrimethamine plus sulphadiazine are used to treat toxoplasmosis, but cannot reverse any permanent damage in congenital infection.

FIGURE 19.17

LIFE CYCLE OF *TOXOPLASMA GONDII*

Humans can be infected by cysts of this protozoan from cat faeces (or fur) from animal meats. Infections in pregnant women can be passed on to the foetus, with severe outcomes.

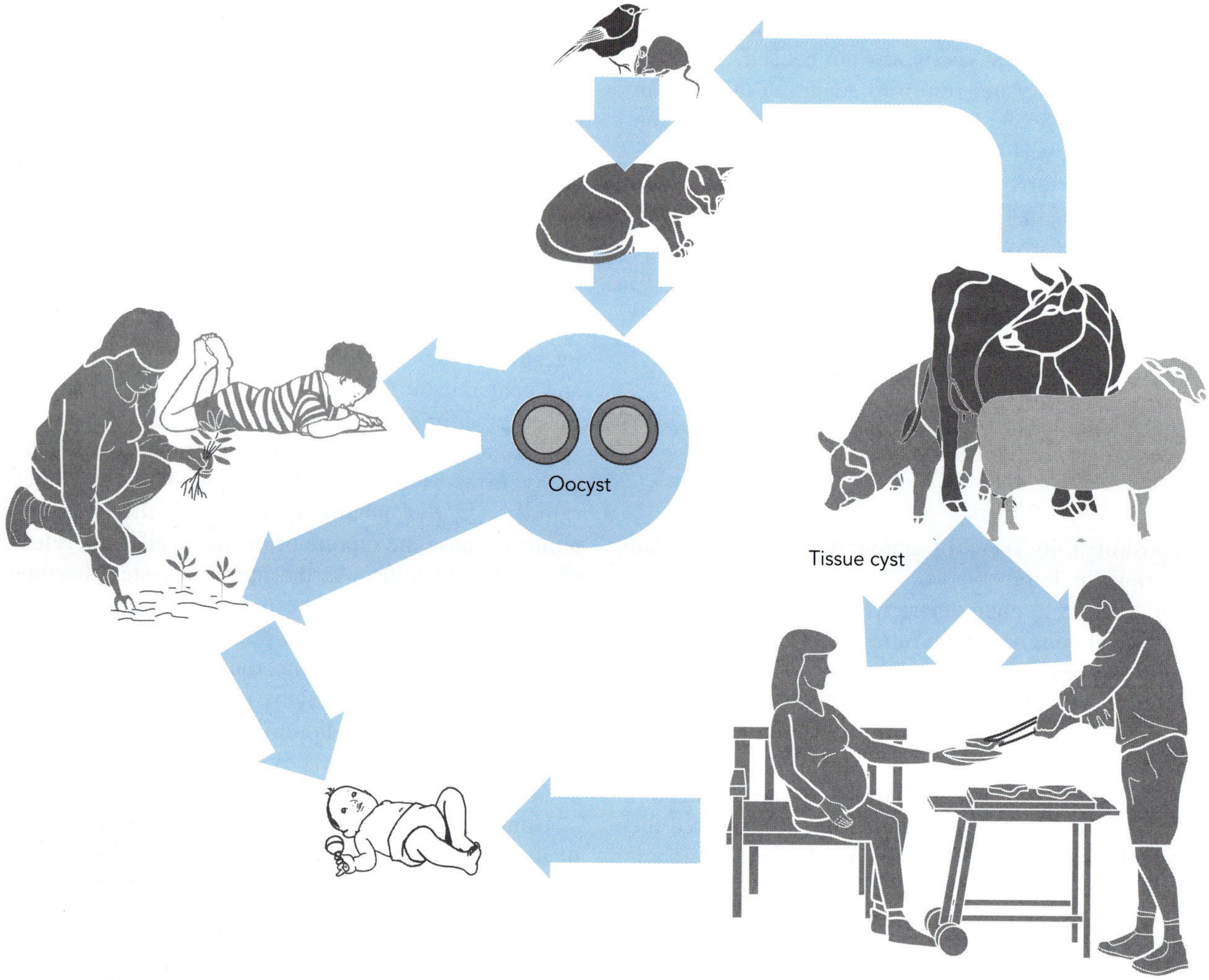

Systemic Helminth Infections

SCHISTOSOMIASIS

Schistosomiasis is a debilitating disease caused by a fluke of the genus *Schistosoma*. There are three major species—*S. mansoni*, *S. japonicum* and *S. haematobium*. The species vary with geographical location, but the diseases caused by each is similar. More than 200 million people in the world are thought to be infected, mostly in Asia, Africa, South America and the Caribbean. The disease is second only to malaria in socioeconomic and public health importance in tropical and subtropical areas. It is not found in Australia, but has been diagnosed in travellers returning from countries where it is endemic.

When water becomes contaminated with *Schistosoma* ova excreted in human wastes, a motile, ciliated larval form of *Schistosoma* (called a miracidium) is released and enters certain species of freshwater snails. The lack of a suitable host snail is a primary reason why schistosomiasis is not transmitted in certain areas of the world (e.g. Australia). Eventually, the pathogen emerges from the snail in an infective form called the cercaria. When the cercaria contact the skin of a person working, washing or swimming in the water, they penetrate the skin (see Figure 19.18) with enzymes which break down its structure. They are then carried by the bloodstream to the liver or urinary bladder. There they mature into an adult form, in which the smaller female lives in a cleft of the male. They mate, producing numerous new eggs, some of which become trapped in tissues.

When egg production begins, symptoms develop, including fever, night sweats, abdominal pain, anorexia, diarrhoea, lethargy, headaches and a non-productive cough. Cell-mediated immune responses occur, which produce granulomas like those formed in tuberculosis. The eggs and the immune response to them is the cause of the tissue damage in the liver, bladder or intestine. Other eggs excreted into the water continue the cycle.

The adult worm appears to be unaffected by the host's immune system. Apparently, it coats itself with a layer that mimics the host's tissues. However, a previous

FIGURE 19.18
SCHISTOSOMA MANSONI, A CAUSE OF SCHISTOSOMIASIS
An electron micrograph showing a cercaria penetrating the skin.

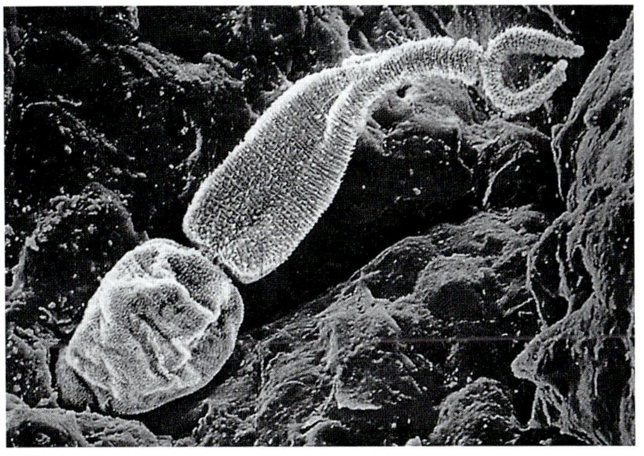

infection tends to be protective to some degree against subsequent infections, which suggests that the development of an effective vaccine may be possible.

Laboratory diagnosis consists of:

1. microscopic identification of the flukes or their ova in faecal and urine specimens; or
2. intradermal tests; or
3. serological tests such as complement fixation and ELISA tests. Praziquantel and oxiaminiquine usually provide effective treatment, although rapid reinfection can occur after completion of treatment. Other forms of control include improved sanitation and elimination of the host snail. Much work has been done towards the development of a vaccine, but its final development still appears to be some way off.

FILARIASIS

Filariasis can be caused by several different roundworms but most commonly by *Wuchereria bancrofti*. The worms are transmitted to humans by mosquitoes. After entering the tissues, the larvae develop into adult worms which can be found in the lymph glands and ducts of the infected person. The adult worms, which can be as long as 10 centimetres, can live in the lymph nodes of a person for years. Microfilariae are forms of the worm that are present in peripheral blood vessels during the night and which retreat to deep vessels, especially those of the lungs, during the day. When a mosquito bites an infected person, it ingests microfilariae that develop into larvae and migrate to the mosquito's mouth parts. When the mosquito bites again, the larvae can infect another person. They enter the blood, develop, and reproduce in the lymph glands and ducts, thereby completing the life cycle. Adult worms cause inflammation in lymph ducts, fever, and eventual blockage of lymph ducts. Repeated infections over a period of years can lead to **elephantiasis**, a gross enlargement of limbs (Figure 19.19), scrotum or sometimes other body parts, from an accumulation of fluid in the interstitial spaces and an increase in connective tissue.

Filariasis is diagnosed by finding microfilariae in thick blood smears made from blood samples taken at night or by an intradermal test. Serological tests and skin tests to detect antibodies are also available, but these do not distinguish active infection from past exposure. The drugs diethylcarbamizine (Hetrazan) and metronidazole are effective in treating the disease. Pressure bandages may be used to force lymph from swollen limbs and, if distortion is not too great, nearly normal size can be regained. To control the disease, it would be necessary to treat all infected individuals and to eradicate the various species of mosquitoes that carry the parasite. Little progress has been made in this area.

FIGURE 19.19
ELEPHANTIASIS OF THE LEG CAUSED BY THE ROUNDWORM *WUCHEREIRIA BANCROFTI*

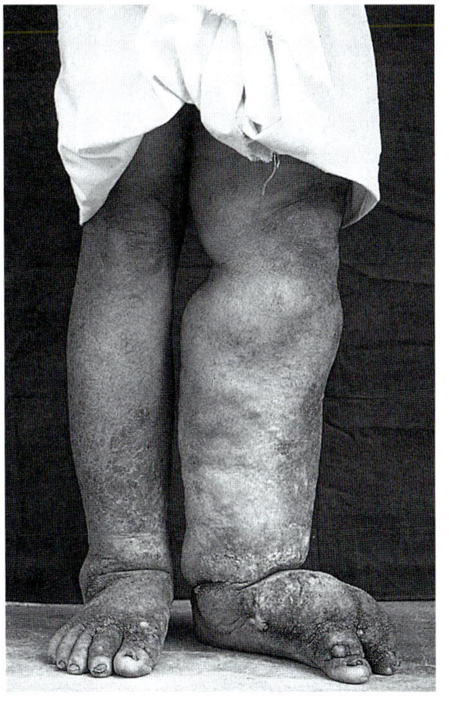

Summary

- The circulating blood is normally sterile.
- Infections that are spread through the body and reach more than one organ are called systemic infections.
- Bacteraemia refers to the presence of bacteria in the bloodstream.
- Septicaemia is a serious clinical syndrome resulting from bacteria in the bloodstream.

SYSTEMIC BACTERIAL INFECTIONS

SEPTICAEMIA

- The bloodstream is an inhospitable place for microorganisms, although some organisms are able to persist and be transported by the blood.
- In most cases of septicaemia, the organisms enter the bloodstream from a focus of infection somewhere in the body.
- The clinical features of septicaemia often include a high, spiking temperature, chills and sweats, and shock.
- Endotoxic shock is a life-threatening form of septicaemia caused by Gram-negative bacteria.
- The diagnosis of septicaemia is made by blood culture. Three samples of blood are usually collected over a 24–48 hour period.
- The best time to take a sample of blood for culture is when the patient is experiencing a febrile episode.

RHEUMATIC FEVER

- Rheumatic fever is a non-suppurative complication of *Streptococcus pyogenes* sore throat.
- Highest incidence occurs in 5–15 year olds.
- Rheumatic fever is characterised by carditis, migratory polyarthritis, chorea, subcutaneous nodules near joints and a macular skin rash.
- Untreated rheumatic fever can result in deformation and scarring of valves and heart failure, a condition called rheumatic heart disease.
- Rheumatic fever is thought to be due to cross-reactivity between streptococcal antigens and heart tissue.
- Diagnosis is by correlation of clinical findings with laboratory findings indicative of streptococcal infection.
- Treatment is with penicillin, and aspirin to reduce fever and joint pain.
- Prompt treatment of sore throat in people known to be susceptible can prevent attacks.

INFECTIVE ENDOCARDITIS

- Infective endocarditis is infection and inflammation of the endocardium. In most cases there is a predisposing heart defect.
- On normal valves, oral streptococci are the most common causes, followed by staphylococci.
- *Staphylococcus epidermidis* (plus a wide range of other organisms) causes infection on prosthetic valves.
- The major pathological feature is a growing clump of bacteria, fibrin and platelets, called a vegetation, usually on the endocardial surface of valves and surrounding structures.
- Typical manifestations are fever and heart murmur with anorexia, malaise, chills, vomiting and night sweats.
- Diagnosis is by blood culture.

OSTEOMYELITIS

- Osteomyelitis is infection and inflammation of the bone.
- Haematogenous osteomyelitis is caused by organisms carried by the blood to the bone, usually from a site of infection elsewhere.
- Exogenous osteomyelitis is caused by organisms introduced directly from outside the body.
- The disease most often afflicts children and adolescents.
- The most common cause is *Staphylococcus aureus*.
- In children the disease is manifested by high fever, chills, nausea and pain over the bone.
- Plain radiographs or bone scans confirm the diagnosis.
- Blood cultures are performed to identify the organism and its sensitivity.
- Treatment is with intravenous antibiotics; surgical debridement and drainage may be necessary.

LYME DISEASE

- Lyme disease is caused mainly by the spirochaete *Borrelia burgdorferi*.
- It is transmitted in animals, and to humans, by ticks of the genus *Ixodes*, which have not been found in Australia.
- Clinical and serological evidence suggests that the disease occurs in Australia, but the source and the vector are at present unclear.
- The disease is characterised by an initial skin infection, followed by multisystem involvement, interspersed with periods of latency.
- A rising antibody titre in paired serum samples confirms infection.
- Lyme disease is usually effectively treated with antibiotics, although late manifestations may not respond to antibiotic therapy.

RICKETTSIAL INFECTIONS

- The most common rickettsial infection in Australia is Q fever, caused by *Coxiella burnetii*.
- Scrub typhus (*Rickettsia tsutsugamushi*)and Queensland tick typhus (*Rickettsia australis*) are the most common arthropod-borne rickettsial infections in Australia.
- The typical clinical features of rickettsial infections are skin rash (except in Q fever), headache and fever.
- Serology on paired serum samples is currently the preferred diagnostic method.
- Rickettsiae are hazardous organisms, so patient blood should be handled carefully.

LEPTOSPIROSIS

- Leptospirosis is caused by the spirochaete *Leptospira interrogans*.

- The most common strains in Australia are *L. interrogans hardjo* (from cattle and sheep) and *L. interrogans pomona* (from pigs).
- Humans become infected by exposure to the animal meat, or to water or food contaminated with urine.
- The bacteria enter through mucous membranes or skin abrasions, reach the bloodstream and are then carried throughout the body.
- Many infections are asymptomatic, but in some a febrile, flu-like illness occurs.
- A severe form, called Weil's disease, represents severe infection of the liver and kidneys.
- Repeated blood cultures during the first week of the disease is the most reliable method for diagnosis.

TOXIC SHOCK SYNDROME

- This is a disease caused by certain strains of *Staphylococcus aureus* that produce a particular toxin called toxic shock syndrome toxin (TSST).
- Toxic shock syndrome is a potentially life-threatening condition characterised by fever, shock and a red, sunburn-like rash.
- Vigorous antibiotic therapy is warranted.

ANTHRAX

- Anthrax is a zoonosis caused by *Bacillus anthracis* and acquired mainly from sheep, goats and cattle.
- Human infection comes from direct contact with infected animals, inhalation of spores present in animal products, or ingestion of infected meat.
- Anthrax is best diagnosed by culture of organisms from skin lesions or blood.
- It is effectively treated with penicillin or tetracyclines, if treatment is started early in the course of the disease.
- Animal vaccination greatly reduces the incidence of human disease.
- A human vaccine is not available in Australia.

BRUCELLOSIS

- Brucellosis is caused by three species of the genus *Brucella*: *B. melitensis, B. abortus* and *B. suis*.
- *B. suis* infects pigs and occasionally other animals and is the most important cause of brucellosis in Australia.
- Transmission from animals to humans occurs by direct contact with infected tissues or animal products, or via dust or aerosols.
- Typical presenting symptoms are night drenching sweats, chills and fever, disabling lethargy, malaise, headache, myalgia and arthralgia.
- Brucellosis is usually diagnosed by serological tests.
- Because of the organism's intracellular location, it may be difficult to eliminate completely with antibiotics.
- Prevention is based on (1) pasteurisation of dairy products, (2) animal vaccination, (3) education of workers at risk of occupational exposure, and (4) the use of protective clothing by at-risk workers.

PLAGUE

- The causative agent of plague is *Yersinia pestis*.
- In developed countries, including Australia, the disease is rare.
- The organism infects wild rodents, especially rats, and is transmitted from animal to animal and animal to human by flea bites.
- A haemorrhagic inflammation occurs, causing infected lymph nodes to form large and tender buboes, usually in the armpit or groin.
- Pneumonic plague occurs when the organism invades the lungs. It can be transmitted from person to person via droplets.
- *Yersinia pestis* can be isolated in fluid aspirated from buboes, or in sputum.
- The disease is treated with streptomycin and/or tetracycline.

SYSTEMIC VIRAL INFECTIONS

HUMAN IMMUNODEFICIENCY VIRUS INFECTION AND AIDS

- The most common cause of AIDS throughout the world is HIV-1.
- HIV-2, the other serotype, was initially found only in West Africa, but has now been reported to have caused sporadic cases in other countries.
- By mid-1993, an estimated 13 million HIV infections had occurred worldwide.
- More than 600 000 cases of AIDS have been reported worldwide.
- HIV is transmitted mainly by sexual intercourse, through blood or blood products, or from mother to child.
- The transmission of HIV from mother to child can occur during pregnancy, at delivery, or through breast feeding.
- HIV produces disease by chronic infection of cells bearing the CD4 antigen. Helper T lymphocytes (T4 lymphocytes) are the main targets, but glial cells and monocytes and macrophages are also vulnerable.
- The declining T4 cell count seems to be a useful indicator of the damage occurring to the immune system and of the progress of the disease.
- In AIDS, damage to the central nervous system occurs as a result of direct attack by HIV or as a result of secondary infection by other microorganisms.
- Seroconversion illness usually occurs 2–4 weeks after infection; it is an acute illness with fever, headache, pharyngitis, nausea, mild CNS symptoms, muco-cutaneous ulcers and a maculopapular rash.
- The intermediate phase of T4 cell depletion is manifested by a variety of minor infections, and symptoms like chronic diarrhoea, fever and weight loss.
- Advanced immune depletion heralds the likelihood of development of an AIDS-defining infection or malignancy.
- The most common secondary diseases in AIDS patients are Kaposi's sarcoma and *Pneumocystis carinii* pneumonia.

- The opportunistic infections are the usual cause of death in patients with AIDS.
- The laboratory diagnosis of HIV infection most often involves the detection of anti-HIV antibodies in serum.
- Antibodies are usually detected in the first 2–6 weeks of infection, although in some people there is a window period of three months or more.
- Zidovudine (azidothymidine, AZT) is the mainstay of therapy for symptomatic HIV infection, but it only delays the progress of the disease.
- Numerous measures have been introduced to reduce the spread of HIV infection in the community (e.g. testing of blood donors; free distribution of clean needles and syringes).
- Measures to reduce the chance of infection in health care staff include the adoption of universal precautions procedures.

ROSS RIVER VIRUS INFECTION (EPIDEMIC POLYARTHRITIS)

- Epidemic polyarthritis is the most important arbovirus infection in Australia. It is caused mainly by the Ross River virus.
- The virus has been isolated from more than 10 different species of mosquito from different regions in Australia.
- The main manifestation is arthritis, with morning joint stiffness.
- Complete recovery may take 12 months or more.
- Laboratory diagnosis of the disease is by detecting a fourfold increase in paired sera, or IgM antibody in a single serum sample.
- Only symptomatic treatment is possible.
- Prevention is based on avoidance of mosquito bite, especially during epidemics.

DENGUE FEVER

- Dengue has a worldwide distribution in tropical areas, and occasionally in the subtropics, with an estimated 100 million cases per year.
- Epidemics occur occasionally in Australia, with hundreds of cases reported.
- The mosquito *Aedes aegypti* is the principal human vector.
- The disease is characterised by high fever, headache and a rash, often with severe muscle and joint pain.
- A serious form, called dengue haemorrhagic fever, is characterised by bleeding from the gums, skin and gastrointestinal tract, and sometimes circulatory failure, shock and death.
- Diagnosis is often based on clinical, epidemiological and serological grounds.
- No effective anti-viral therapy or vaccine is currently available.
- Prevention is based on mosquito control programs and disease surveillance.

INFECTIOUS MONONUCLEOSIS

- Infectious mononucleosis, or glandular fever, is caused by the Epstein-Barr virus (EBV).
- The highest incidence occurs in teenagers and young adults.
- The usual route of infection is by transfer of saliva.
- The virus invades organs such as the lung and parotid glands, and various lymphoid organs where it infects B lymphocytes.
- After an incubation period of 5–6 weeks, mild symptoms of fever, headache, fatigue and malaise develop, and gradually worsen.
- IgM antibody tests provide the most specific diagnosis.
- Bed rest and symptomatic treatment are the basis of management of the disease.
- No vaccine is available.
- The EBV has been implicated in a number of different malignancies and in chronic fatigue syndrome.

CYTOMEGALOVIRUS INFECTION

- The majority of cytomegalovirus (CMV) infections produce few symptoms.
- The severity of the infection in the newborn and in immunocompromised people establishes CMV as an important human pathogen.
- Transplacental transmission to the foetus leads to spread of the virus to multiple organs and a severe illness.
- CMV is responsible for severe disseminated infections in people with AIDS, cancer patients and organ transplant recipients.
- CMV is usually spread by close contact.
- Definitive diagnosis of CMV infection is made by isolation of the virus from a body fluid.
- Serological diagnosis on paired sera is usually performed.
- No effective treatment or vaccine is available.

YELLOW FEVER

- Yellow fever virus is a flavivirus that is restricted to parts of South America and Africa.
- It is transmitted to humans by the mosquito *Aedes aegypti*.
- It causes an acute disease characterised by sudden onset of fever, vomiting and prostration 3–6 days after infection. Progression to extensive haemorrhagic manifestations and jaundice, leading to coma and death, may occur.
- There is no specific treatment.
- Preventive measures include protection from mosquito bites and vaccination.

SYSTEMIC PROTOZOAL INFECTIONS

MALARIA

- There are 100–300 million cases of malaria in the world each year.
- The estimated annual death toll from the disease is 1–2 million, mainly children.
- The worldwide malaria situation is deteriorating, primarily because of increasing drug resistance and increasing resistance of vector mosquitoes to insecticides.

- Australia was certified free of indigenous malaria by the WHO in 1981.
- Four species cause human malaria: *Plasmodium falciparum*, *P. vivax*, *P. malariae* and *P. ovale*.
- Falciparum and vivax malaria are the most common, but only *P. falciparum* causes significant mortality.
- The protozoa are transmitted to humans by species of Anopheles mosquitoes.
- In malaria, a characteristic pattern of recurrent chills followed by fever, drenching sweats, headache, muscular pain and vomiting occurs every 48 or 72 hours, depending on the causative agent.
- A patient with severe malaria may present with irregular fever and leading symptoms of gastrointestinal, respiratory or urinary tract infection, often with involvement of the brain.
- Even with treatment, mortality can be as high as 20% in falciparum malaria.
- The main method of diagnosis is microscopic examination of a blood film.
- Chloroquine is the drug of choice for sensitive strains. Fansidar may be used for strains resistant to chloroquine.
- In multi-resistant areas, mefloquine, halofantrine or quinine may be used.
- Severe falciparum is a medical emergency requiring intensive care attention and facilities, and immediate intravenous antimalarial therapy and supportive treatment.
- There is no effective vaccine available.

TOXOPLASMOSIS

- Toxoplasmosis is caused by the protozoan *Toxoplasma gondii*.
- Cats are an essential part of the life cycle of *T. gondii*.
- Oocysts are shed in cat faeces and contaminate food or water ingested by other animals and humans.
- In adults, the disease is mild and rather undefined, characterised by low-grade fever, general malaise and myalgia.
- The primary danger is in the congenital infection of a foetus, which can cause convulsions, severe brain damage, blindness and death.
- Toxoplasmosis is diagnosed in the laboratory by serological tests.
- Pyrimethamine plus sulphadiazine are used to treat toxoplasmosis.

SYSTEMIC HELMINTH INFECTIONS

SCHISTOSOMIASIS

- Schistosomiasis is a debilitating disease caused by a fluke of the genus *Schistosoma*.
- There are three major species: *S. mansoni*, *S. japonicum* and *S. haematobium*. They vary with geographical location.
- More than 200 million people in the world have the disease, mostly in Asia, Africa, South America and the Caribbean.
- The lack of a suitable host snail is a primary reason why schistosomiasis is not transmitted in certain areas of the world (e.g. Australia).
- In faecally contaminated water, the pathogen emerges from the snail in an infective form called the cercaria, which penetrate the skin of a person working, washing or swimming.
- The eggs of the fluke and the immune response to them is the cause of the tissue damage in the liver, bladder or intestine.
- Laboratory diagnosis consists of microscopic identification of the flukes or their ova in faecal and urine specimens, intradermal tests or serological tests.
- Praziquantel and oxiaminiquine are commonly used against schistosomes.

FILARIASIS

- Filariasis can be caused by several different roundworms, most commonly *Wuchereria bancrofti*.
- The worms are transmitted to humans by mosquitoes.
- Adult worms cause inflammation in lymph ducts, fever, and eventual blockage of lymph ducts.
- Repeated infections over a period of years can lead to elephantiasis, a gross enlargement of limbs, scrotum or sometimes other body parts.
- Filariasis is diagnosed by finding microfilariae in thick blood smears, or by an intradermal test.
- Diethylcarbamizine (Hetrazan) and metronidazole are effective in treating the disease.

Study Questions

1. Explain the difference between the terms 'bacteraemia' and 'septicaemia'.
2. What is the usual source of organisms causing septicaemia?
3. What predisposing factor exists in the majority of people who develop endocarditis?
4. What is a vegetation in endocarditis?
5. What is the incidence of Lyme disease in Australia?
6. What is 'toxic shock syndrome' and what causes it?
7. What species causes most cases of brucellosis in Australia, and what is the usual source of the organism?
8. What are the three major trends that have emerged in recent years concerning human immunodeficiency virus transmission in Australia?
9. What cell types are targeted by the human immunodefiency virus?
10. What is the mainstay of treatment for AIDS and how does this drug reduce viral multiplication?
11. Why is it that Ross River virus infection can be acquired almost anywhere in Australia?
12. What is the pathogenesis of dengue haemorrhagic fever?
13. What is chronic fatigue syndrome?
14. What is the most serious form of cytomegalovirus infection?
15. Which species causes the most serious form of malaria and why?
16. What specimen is required for the laboratory diagnosis of malaria?

Test Your Understanding

Case History 19.1: Septicaemia

1. Does this patient have septicaemia? If yes, what is the likely cause?
2. What is the likely source of the *Staphylococcus epidermidis*?
3. Why are multiple samples of blood usually collected from a patient for the diagnosis of septicaemia?

Case History 19.2: Osteomyelitis

1. What is the most likely cause of Thomas's osteomyelitis and what is the likely source of the organism?
2. Why is haematogenous osteomyelitis most common in adolescents?

Case History 19.3: Brucellosis

1. Where did the Turkish woman most probably acquire her infection?
2. What important aspect of brucellosis is illustrated by the infection of the laboratory worker?

Case History 19.4: Malaria

1. How is malaria diagnosed in the laboratory?
2. What measures should the woman have taken to prevent getting malaria?
3. Why are antimalarial drugs not always effective in preventing disease?

REFERENCES

1. World Health Organization, 1993, *The HIV/AIDS Pandemic: 1993 Overview*.
2. National Centre in HIV Epidemiology and Clinical Research, 1995, *Australian HIV Surveillance Report* 11(3), p. 13.
3. Communicable Diseases Intelligence, 1994, *Annual Report of the National Notifiable Diseases Surveillance System, 1993*. Vol. 18(22), p. 518.
4. Communicable Diseases Intelligence, 1993, *Report of the Australian Malaria Register for 1991*. Vol. 17 (7), p. 134.
5. Walpole, I.R., N. Hodgen & C. Bower, 1991, 'Congenital toxoplasmosis: A large survey in Western Australia', *Medical Journal of Australia* 154, p. 720.

FURTHER READING

Communicable Diseases Intelligence, 1993, *Report of the Australian Malaria Register for 1991*. Vol 17(7), p. 134. (The Australian Malaria Register provides background information about malaria and an analysis of the cases reported each year. The epidemiology, distribution of cases and the origin of infection are described in detail.)

Hall, S.M., 1992, 'Congenital toxoplasmosis', *British Medical Journal* 305, p. 291. (A review article describing the clinical features, treatment and prevention of congenital toxoplasmosis.)

Medical Journal of Australia, 1996, 'Managing HIV', Vol. 164. (This volume is dedicated to HIV with review articles covering the phases of the disease, mechanisms of disease and treatment.)

National Centre in HIV Epidemiology and Clinical Research, 1993, *Australian HIV Surveillance Report* 9(4), p. 1. (Provides detailed information on the epidemiology of HIV infection. Certain clinical features, such as the median survival time following AIDS, are discussed.)

Remme, J.H.F., P. De Raadt & T. Godal, 1993, 'The burden of tropical diseases', *Medical Journal of Australia* 158, p. 465. (This review article discusses a number of important tropical diseases caused by protozoa and helminths. The burden of malaria and other diseases on the world's population is discussed.)

Wells, A.U., C.C. Fowler, R.B. Ellis-Pegler, R. Luke, S. Hannan & D.N. Sharpe, 1990, 'Endocarditis in the 80s in a general hospital in Auckland, New Zealand', *Quarterly Journal of Medicine*, New Series 76 (279), p. 753. (This article reviews the clinical features of cases of infective endocarditis in Auckland Hospital from 1979 to 1986.)

White, N.J. & S. Pukrittayakamee, 1993, 'Clinical malaria in the tropics', *Medical Journal of Australia* 159, p. 197. (Examines the clinical features and management of malaria.)

World Health Organization, 1993, *The HIV/Aids Pandemic: 1993 Overview.* (Examines HIV infection in detail with respect to transmission, progress of the illness, interactions between HIV infection and other diseases, the worldwide distribution of the infection and the global projections of infection.)

chapter 20

infections of the nervous system

Chapter focus

- *What microorganisms commonly cause infection of the nervous system?*
- *How do microorganisms gain access to the nervous system in order to cause disease?*
- *What are the important clinical aspects of nervous system infections?*
- *How are nervous system infections treated and how may they be prevented?*

The central nervous system (CNS) consists of the brain and the spinal cord. The nerves of the peripheral nervous system branch from the CNS. The brain and the spinal cord are surrounded by three layers of membranes or **meninges**, termed the dura mater, arachnoid and pia mater (see Figure 20.1). **Cerebrospinal fluid** (CSF) circulates in the space between the arachnoid and pia mater (subarachnoid space), forming a liquid cushion around the CNS organs, and also serving to maintain the chemical balance in the CNS and to nourish the brain. The CSF, a clear, lymph-like fluid, is continuously produced by masses of specialised capillaries (called choroid plexuses) in four ventricles (cavities) within the brain. These capillaries produce CSF from blood, mainly by active transport and ultrafiltration of substances within the blood plasma. The CSF circulates around the brain and spinal cord and returns to the blood via the arachnoid villi.

Normally, the CSF is produced and drained at a constant rate. However, if something blocks its circulation or drainage (e.g. tumour or infection), it begins to accumulate and may exert pressure on the brain. This is termed 'hydrocephalus' or 'water on the brain'.

The **blood-brain barrier** is a protective barrier that helps to ensure that the brain's environment remains stable. The tightly joined endothelial cells of the brain's capillaries are the least permeable in the entire body. They form a highly selective barrier which allows some substances to pass readily from the circulation to the brain, while most substances are excluded. Certain nutrients (e.g. glucose and essential amino acids) move through the endothelial cell membranes by facilitated diffusion, whereas wastes (e.g. urea and creatinine) and most drugs (e.g. antibiotics) are prevented from entering brain tissue. The blood-brain barrier is less effective against lipid-soluble substances, such as alcohol and certain anaesthetics, which diffuse easily through cell membranes.

Most antibiotics do not readily cross the blood-brain barrier, although chloramphenicol, which is a lipid-soluble antimicrobial drug, is able to cross it reasonably well. Injury to the brain may cause a local breakdown of the blood-brain barrier due to alteration of the permeability characteristics of the endothelial cells or their tight junctions.

Infections of the Central Nervous System

Infection of the CNS is a relatively rare occurrence, but when it happens it may have serious consequences—in particular, permanent neurological damage or death. In most infections, organisms gain access to the CNS from the bloodstream. However, invasion may sometimes occur locally from infected ears or sinuses, or via peripheral nerves (e.g. herpes simplex virus, rabies virus).

Infection and inflammation of the meninges is called **meningitis**; it is most often caused by viruses or bacteria, occasionally by fungi and protozoa. Infection and inflammation of the brain itself is called **encephalitis** and is almost always caused by viruses. In some circumstances, microorganisms may infect the brain tissue, causing a brain abscess to form. Brain abscesses are usually caused by bacteria, but sometimes by fungi and protozoa.

BACTERIAL MENINGITIS

Acute bacterial meningitis is a medical emergency requiring urgent and specific treatment. The mortality rate varies with the different causative agents, ranging from 5–50%; a relatively high rate for bacterial infections today. Some people who survive bacterial meningitis suffer permanent neurological damage.

Causative agents, transmission and incidence

The most common causative agents are *Neisseria meningitidis, Haemophilus influenzae* and *Streptococcus pneumoniae*, which together cause more than 75% of all cases of bacterial meningitis. *Escherichia coli* and Group B streptococci (*Streptococcus agalactiae*) are the two most common causes of neonatal meningitis, and *Listeria monocytogenes* also affects neonates as well as immunocompromised patients. Patients with CSF shunts or severe head injury, or those who have had neurosurgery may develop meningitis caused by such bacteria as staphylococci, *Propionibacterium* or *Corynebacterium*. *Mycobacterium tuberculosis* is a rare cause of meningitis in Australia.

Meningococcal meningitis. N. meningitidis, or the **meningococcus**, is an aerobic Gram-negative diplococcus. It is carried asymptomatically in the nasopharynx by up to 20% of the population. It spreads from the nasopharynx to the blood, and then to the meninges to cause disease. In 1993, there were 378 cases of meningococcal infection reported in Australia, representing an annual incidence rate of 2.1 per 100 000 population. The majority of cases occur in the 0–4 year old age group. Two other smaller peaks occur in the 15–19 and the 80–84 year old age groups. The incidence in Western countries ranges from

FIGURE 20.1
THE MENINGEAL MEMBRANES COVERING THE BRAIN AND SPINAL CORD
From the outermost they are the dura mater, arachnoid and pia mater. Cerebrospinal fluid circulates between the arachnoid and pia mater.

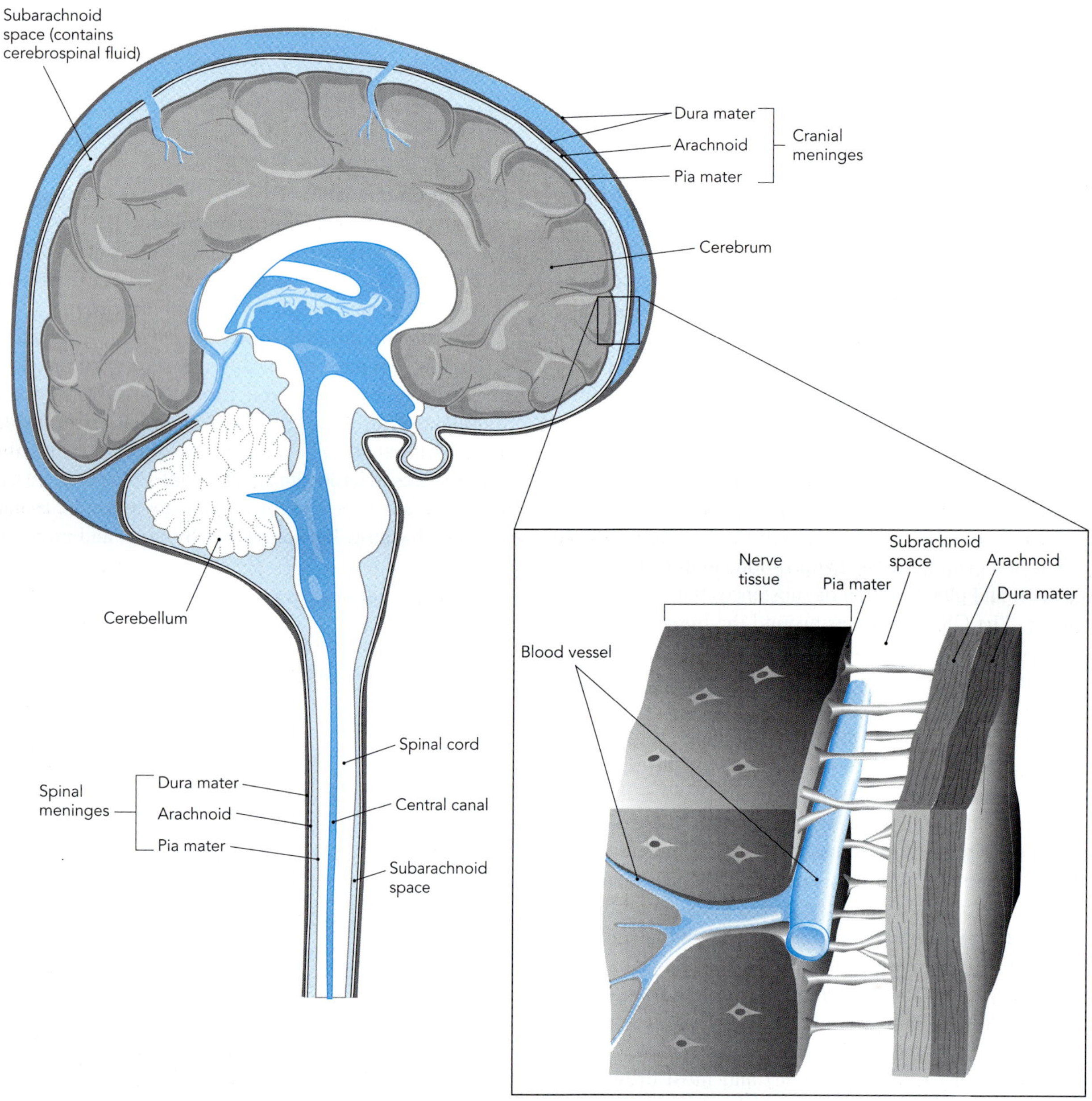

0.8 per 100 000 population up to 4.6 per 100 000, as is found in New Zealand. Why so many people are colonised and yet so few become infected is not clear, but the possession of antibodies to the organism's capsular antigens seems to be important. This would explain the high incidence in young children, who have lost their maternal-derived antibodies and are yet to produce their own.

Meningococcal meningitis is the only form of meningitis that can spread in an epidemic form. This can occur where conditions of overcrowding exist (e.g. military camps) or where person-to-person spread by droplet transmission is enhanced (e.g. dormitories and day-care centres). The last reported epidemic in Australia occurred between 1987 and 1991 in the southern health region of the Northern Territory and the socially linked Anangu Pitjantjatjara Lands of South Australia. In all, 77 cases were diagnosed, with four deaths. The major epidemic before that occurred between 1971 and 1973, involving 90 cases, mainly in Aboriginal people in Alice Springs and surrounding areas. Household contacts of a person with meningococcal disease remain at increased risk of acquiring disease for several months.

Meningococcal infection is often associated with a septicaemia, characterised by a haemorrhagic skin rash. A very serious complication, called the Waterhouse-Friderichsen syndrome, can develop if the organism invades many parts of the body. This is due to the presence of large amounts of endotoxin in the blood and is usually characterised by disseminated intravascular coagulation (DIC), renal failure, shock, bleeding into the brain and adrenal glands, and death within hours.

The strains of meningococcus that cause infection belong to the A, B, C, X, Y, Z and W135 serogroups.

Haemophilus meningitis. Haemophilus influenzae is an aerobic Gram-negative coccobacillus. There are a number of serological types, but invasive infections are almost always caused by encapsulated type b. The organism is a common inhabitant of the throat of infants and young children, but is found less frequently in adults. Invasion of the meninges is usually preceded by a viral infection of the respiratory tract, the resulting inflammation allowing the organism to invade the bloodstream and then the meninges. *H. influenzae* type b (Hib) causes about 70% of all cases of childhood bacterial meningitis in Australia, and is especially prominent in the 0–4 years age group.

Protection against this organism is afforded by anti-capsule antibodies, which effectively opsonise the organism. Maternally derived antibodies, usually protect the infant up to the age of 3–4 months, and the child usually produces its own antibodies at 3–4 years of age. In between there is a 'window' period of susceptibility.

Prior to 1993, the annual incidence of *H. influenzae* meningitis in Aboriginal children under the age of 5 was about 150 per 100 000, which was much higher than the 20–50 per 100 000 in non-Aboriginal children. However, the introduction of vaccines against *H. influenzae* in 1992 (see p. 478) has already resulted in a marked reduction in incidence.

Pneumococcal meningitis. Pathogenic *Streptococcus pneumoniae* are encapsulated, aerobic, Gram-positive cocci that are carried in the throat of many healthy people. Only rarely does the organism invade the meninges. It causes meningitis mainly in:

- children under two years of age;
- debilitated or splenectomised patients;
- head injury victims where there is a skull fracture communicating with the nasopharynx;
- the elderly.

Acute onset of meningitis may follow otitis media, pneumonia, septicaemia or head injury. Antibodies to capsular polysaccharides opsonise the organism and protect against invasion; however, there are 85 different capsule serotypes. That is, specific antibodies do provide immunity, but antibodies to one serotype do not protect against the many other serotypes.

Neonatal meningitis. Neonatal meningitis can be caused by a wide range of bacteria, but *E. coli* (with capsular type K1) and Group B streptococci are the most frequent. Group B *Streptococcus* is so called because of the Lancefield Group B carbohydrate antigen in its cell wall. The organism is also known as *Streptococcus agalactiae*. The strains of *E. coli* and *S. agalactiae* that are pathogenic for the CNS owe their virulence, at least partially, to a polysaccharide capsule. Other causes of neonatal meningitis are shown in Table 20.1.

The incidence of neonatal bacterial meningitis in developed countries, including Australia, is 2–5 per 10 000 births. Despite appropriate antibiotic therapy and supportive care the mortality rate remains high at approximately 30%, and many of the infants that survive have serious long-term sequelae, including hydrocephalus, cognitive dysfunction, deafness and seizures.

TABLE 20.1
BACTERIAL CAUSES OF NEONATAL MENINGITIS

	PERCENT OF CASES
Streptococcus agalactiae	35
Escherichia coli	22
Neisseria meningitidis	6
Coagulase negative staphylococci	5
Listeria monocytogenes	<5
Haemophilus influenzae	<5
Staphylococcus aureus	<5
Enterococcus faecalis	<5
Klebsiella spp.	<5
Citrobacter spp.	<5
Enterobacter spp.	<5
Pseudomonas spp.	<5

Group B streptococci (*S. agalactiae)* are part of the genitourinary flora of some women. They have been found to colonise about 20% of women of child-bearing age. A baby born to a colonised mother may itself become colonised orally, in the rectum or in the umbilical stump. A small percentage of colonised infants develop meningitis and/or pneumonia, usually within four weeks, but possibly up to three months later. Certain factors are known to place babies at increased risk of infection, especially:

- prematurity (< 36 weeks);
- prolonged rupture of amniotic membranes;
- heavy maternal colonisation;
- maternal bacteraemia;
- multiple births.

However, many babies have no apparent risk factors. Nosocomial transmission can occur, especially in crowded nurseries. *E. coli* meningitis in neonates is also often associated with one of the above risk factors, with prematurity and prolonged rupture of membranes being particularly common. Early intestinal colonisation by K1 strains of *E. coli* before the normal flora are established can lead to invasion of the blood and then the CNS.

Listeriosis. **Listeriosis** is caused by *Listeria monocytogenes*, a Gram-positive coccobacillus. This organism causes disease mainly in immunocompromised people, especially in patients with malignancy or severe liver disease, in organ transplant recipients and in patients receiving steroid therapy (e.g. patients with autoimmune disease). It is also an important cause of infection in pregnant women. Although usually mild in infected mothers, the organism can spread to the foetus *in utero* or be transmitted at birth, resulting in severe foetal or neonatal disease. Intrauterine infection can result in abortion, premature labour, intrauterine death or perinatal

> **CASE HISTORY 20.1**
> **NEONATAL MENINGITIS**
>
> Baby Sarah was a 3.950 gram full-term infant born to a 25-year-old woman. The baby appeared healthy at delivery, but 24 hours later started to show signs of respiratory distress. On examination she was found to be irritable and tachypnoeic. Her axillary temperature was 38.3°C and her pulse 200. The infant had a bulging anterior fontanelle. There was no apparent rash.
>
> Initial CSF findings included: protein 1.15 g/L (normal 0.15–0.45 g/L), glucose 2.1 mmol/L (normal >2.5 mmol/L), many Gram-positive cocci, and a few white blood cells.
>
> *Comment*
>
> In many cases of neonatal meningitis there is no apparent predisposing factor.

infection. Perinatal infection is most often manifested as a meningitis.

The organism is associated with a wide variety of animals and is excreted in their faeces. It is therefore widely distributed in soil, water, sewage and animal feed. Apart from perinatal infections it is thought to be predominantly a food-borne pathogen. Its source in sporadic outbreaks is often not determined, although milk has been implicated in some. The annual incidence in most Western countries, including Australia, is around 0.2–0.5 per 100 000 population. It is usually a mild or often symptomless disease in healthy adults. Mild disease is generally characterised by flu-like symptoms of sore throat, fever, chills and myalgia.

Tuberculous meningitis. Mycobacterium tuberculosis is a rare cause of meningitis in Australia. It can occur during active infection or in recrudescent infection (see Chapter 17). From a focus of infection elsewhere, the organism enters the bloodstream and disseminates to the subarachnoid spaces. It is thus often associated with miliary tuberculosis (disseminated tuberculosis).

The causes, predisposing factors and incidence of bacterial meningitis are summarised in Table 20.2.

Pathogenesis

Some important insights concerning bacterial meningitis have been gained in recent years. There are believed to be several critical events in the pathogenesis of acute haematogenous bacterial meningitis:

1. Nasopharyngeal colonisation;
2. Invasion of the bloodstream and intravascular survival;
3. Penetration of the blood-brain barrier;
4. Damage and inflammation of the meninges.

Many of the bacteria that cause meningitis possess surface structures that are thought to enhance mucosal colonisation. For instance, both *N. meningitidis* and *H. influenzae* possess fimbriae which may facilitate their attachment to the nasopharyngeal mucosa. Polysaccharide capsules are possessed by all the major pathogens and these may also assist them to attach. Natural antibodies such as IgA, which is the antibody class found predominantly in mucosal secretions, may inhibit the attachment of bacteria. Many clinical isolates of *N. meningitidis*, *H. influenzae* and *S. pneumoniae* secrete an IgA protease which cleaves and inactivates the immunoglobulin molecule.

In order to invade the bloodstream, the bacteria must cross the nasopharyngeal mucosal epithelium. It appears that different pathogens have different methods of invasion. For example, *N. meningitidis* is thought to enter non-ciliated epithelial cells by an endocytic process and pass through the cell in a membrane-bound vacuole. On the other hand, *H. influenzae* invades through separations in the apical tight junctions of columnar epithelial cells. Once in the bloodstream, the bacteria must then overcome the host defence mechanisms there. Possession of a polysaccharide capsule is the most important factor in this regard, as a protection against phagocytosis by neutrophils. As stated above, all the common pathogens (*H. influenzae*, *N. meningitidis*, *S. pneumoniae*, *E. coli and S. agalactiae*) are encapsulated.

The mechanisms by which pathogenic bacteria are able to pass from the circulation into the CSF and the actual sites of invasion are largely unknown. However, bacterial virulence factors such as fimbriae, polysaccharide capsules and endotoxin (lipopolysaccharide) are possibly involved, and the most likely sites of invasion are the choroid plexuses. Once in the CSF, the bacteria have a good chance of survival because humoral defences, particularly immunoglobulin and complement activity, are in very low concentration in this fluid. Even though blood leucocytes enter the CSF during infection, their role is uncertain because of the relative lack of opsonic and bactericidal activity normally afforded by antibodies and complement.

In head-injured patients, organisms may gain direct access to the CNS. The cribriform plate at the anterior part of the base of the skull is in close proximity to the nasal sinuses. This bony plate may be damaged in head injury and organisms found in the nares, particularly *Streptococcus pneumoniae* (the most common cause of meningitis in head-injured patients), may then gain direct access to the CSF.

The tissue dysfunction in bacterial meningitis may result from (1) focal lesions due to bacterial growth or toxins, or (2) inflammation. Much recent attention has been given to the inflammatory response to infection in the subarachnoid space. There is much evidence to suggest that this inflammatory response is largely responsible for the pathophysiologic consequences and the neurological sequelae and death that are so often associated with bacterial meningitis.

Numerous studies have indicated that lipopolysaccharides and other bacterial cell wall components play an integral role. It is thought that these are released into

TABLE 20.2
BACTERIAL MENINGITIS: CAUSATIVE AGENTS, PREDISPOSING FACTORS AND INCIDENCE

CAUSATIVE ORGANISM	PREDISPOSING FACTORS	INCIDENCE (AUSTRALIA)
Neisseria meningitidis	Young age Close contact Complement deficiencies	2.1 per 100 000 population Most frequent in 0-4 year age group
Haemophilus influenzae	Young age Respiratory tract infection	Mainly in 0–4 year age group Highest in Aboriginal children
Streptococcus pneumoniae	Young age Pneumococcal pneumonia Debility Skull fracture Old age	Affects all age groups
Group B *Streptococcus*, *Escherichia coli*	Neonates: ■ prematurity ■ prolonged rupture of membranes ■ heavy maternal colonisation ■ maternal bacteraemia ■ multiple births	About 2 per 10 000 births
Listeria monocytogenes	Neonates—maternal infection Immunosuppression; e.g. transplant, cancer	0.25 per 100 000 population
Mycobacterium tuberculosis	Infection elsewhere which spreads to blood	Rare
Staphylococcus *Proprionibacterium* *Corynebacterium*	Entry of skin flora following: ■ head injury ■ CSF shunt ■ neurosurgery	

the subarachnoid space during natural or antibiotic-induced bacteriolysis and that they elicit the local release of cytokines, such as interleukin-1 and tumour necrosis factor from various cells, including vascular endothelial cells, microglia and astrocytes. These cytokines lead to inflammation and increased blood-brain barrier permeability. The pressure in the subarachnoid space may rise markedly, due to the inflammation, oedema and vascular endothelial injury. Because of the rigid confines of the skull and spinal cord, this pressure spreads to the entire space around the brain and spinal cord. The increased cranial pressure causes a decrease in cerebral blood flow.

The pathophysiologic processes that are thought to contribute to the neurologic sequelae of bacterial meningitis are summarised in Figure 20.2.

Clinical features

The clinical presentation of bacterial meningitis is variable and depends on the patient's age, the duration of illness, and the causative agent. Headache, fever, altered consciousness, vomiting and nuchal rigidity (neck stiffness) are the most common presenting symptoms. Lethargy, irritability, anorexia and photophobia are also common. These symptoms are often accompanied by upper respiratory symptoms such as a sore throat. In neonates, young infants and the elderly, the findings are often subtle, and usually include fever, lethargy, irritability, respiratory distress, lack of interest in food, vomiting and diarrhoea. A rapidly progressing, fulminant form is most often associated with *N. meningitidis* and sometimes with *S. pneumoniae*, whereas *H. influenzae* usually has a more insidious onset.

The presence of a haemorrhagic skin rash, representing a concurrent septicaemia, is suggestive of *N. meningitidis* infection, although *H. influenzae* can sometimes mimic this. The mortality rate varies from 5–50%, depending on a number of factors—including the age of the patient, the causative agent and the duration of illness before commencement of treatment. Up to 10% of survivors experience long-term serious sequelae such as hearing loss, mental retardation and seizures.

Laboratory diagnosis

CSF is the most important specimen for the diagnosis of meningitis. It is usually collected by lumbar puncture, but sometimes other methods, such as a ventricular tap,

FIGURE 20.2
PATHOPHYSIOLOGY OF NEUROLOGIC DYSFUNCTION IN BACTERIAL MENINGITIS

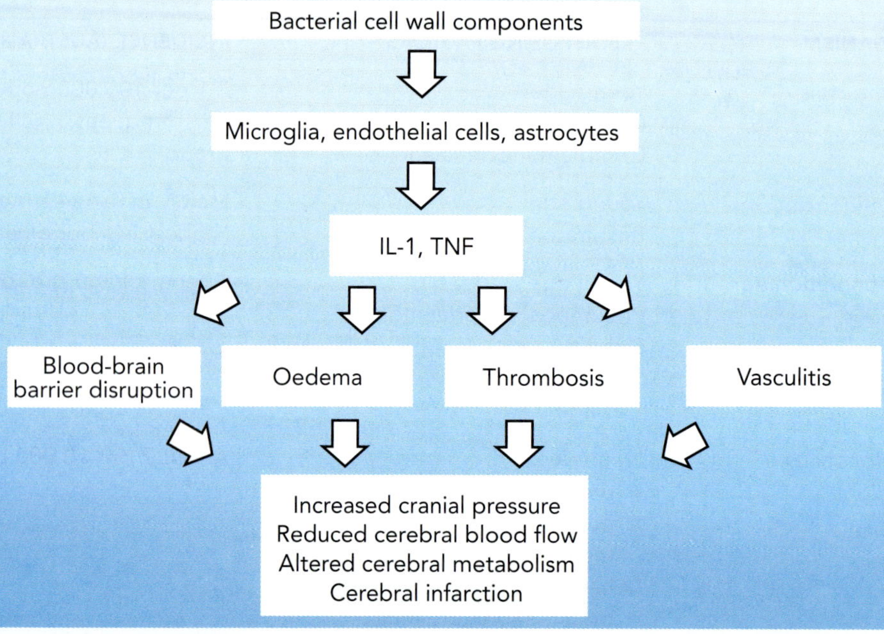

are used. If possible, the CSF should be collected into two or three tubes, with 1–5 mL in each. The tubes should be labelled sequentially for different uses in the laboratory. It should be remembered that CSF is a body fluid to which Standard Precautions apply. Laboratory-acquired cases of bacterial meningitis have been reported.

Rapid transport of the specimen to the laboratory is necessary for two important reasons. First, the disease is very serious and thus an accurate diagnosis is needed as soon as possible. Second, most of the common causes are fastidious organisms that may not survive variations in temperature or long transit times. Unlike many other specimens for the microbiology laboratory, CSF specimens should not be refrigerated, but maintained at room temperature or at 37°C. Blood cultures should also be collected. Fastidious organisms not isolated from CSF may sometimes be cultured from blood. Also, positive blood cultures may help to confirm CSF isolates.

Cerebrospinal fluid analysis in the microbiology laboratory usually includes:

- a macroscopic examination;
- culture;
- a Gram stain;
- a cell count;
- determination of glucose concentration;
- determination of protein concentration.

Preliminary results of all of these, except culture, should be available within an hour or two after receipt of the CSF specimen in the laboratory. These results are extremely important because bacterial meningitis can be distinguishable from other causes of meningitis, as shown in Table 20.3. The differentiation between bacterial causes and viral meningitis may allow for early adjustment to treatment and patient management.

Obvious turbidity in a CSF specimen is suggestive of bacterial infection, and is usually due to the presence of large numbers of white cells and/or bacteria. The differential cell count typically shows polymorphs (polymorphonuclear leucocytes) in acute bacterial meningitis. Bacteria may be detected in a Gram stain when there are greater than 10^5 organisms per millilitre of CSF. A negative Gram stain, therefore, does not exclude a bacterial meningitis. A reduction in the CSF glucose level is due to impaired transport of glucose from blood to CSF, and its usage by the bacteria and the infiltrating polymorphs. There is usually a significant increase in the protein concentration because of alteration to the blood-brain barrier, resulting in an increased permeability to serum proteins which are normally excluded.

In addition to these preliminary tests, rapid latex agglutination methods for the detection of soluble bacterial antigens in CSF have been developed. Antigen detection may be used to confirm preliminary Gram stain results and are also useful when Gram stain or culture results are negative (e.g. in bacterial meningitis where treatment has been commenced before lumbar puncture). Serum or urine may also be tested for bacterial antigens, and may be especially useful if CSF cannot be obtained.

If tuberculous meningitis is suspected, a Ziehl-Neelsen stain, rather than a Gram stain, of centrifuged deposit of CSF is often performed. Also, the polymerase chain reaction and DNA probes (see Chapter 15) are being used for the direct examination of CSF.

Treatment

Prompt treatment of any bacterial meningitis is required. First-line therapy for acute meningitis is most often with cefotaxime or ceftriaxone. These third generation cephalosporins are preferred because (1) they are effective against the three principal causes of bacterial meningitis—*N. meningitidis*, *H. influenzae* and *S. pneumoniae*—and

TABLE 20.3
CHARACTERISTIC CHANGES IN CEREBROSPINAL FLUID IN MENINGITIS

	MACROSCOPIC APPEARANCE	CELLS (X 10^6/L)	PROTEIN (g/L)	GLUCOSE (mmol/L)	GRAM STAIN
Normal	clear and colourless	0–5	0.15–0.45	≥2.5	
Streptococcus pneumoniae	clear to turbid	elevated, PMN	elevated	reduced	Gram-positive diplococci
Haemophilus influenzae	clear to turbid	elevated, PMN	elevated	reduced	Gram-negative coccobacilli
Neisseria meningitidis	clear to turbid	elevated, PMN	elevated	reduced	Gram-negative diplococci
Escherichia coli	clear to turbid	elevated, PMN	elevated	reduced	Gram-negative rods
Group B streptococci	clear to turbid	elevated, PMN	elevated	reduced	Gram-negative rods
Listeria monocytogenes	clear to faintly turbid	elevated (mainly lymphocytes)	elevated	reduced	Gram-positive coccobacillus
Mycobacterium tuberculosis	clear to faintly turbid	elevated, lymphocytes (PMN early)	markedly elevated	reduced	negative
Viruses	clear to faintly turbid	elevated, lymphocytes (PMN early)	slightly elevated	normal	negative
Cryptococcus neoformans	clear to faintly turbid	elevated, PMN or lymphocytes	elevated	reduced	yeast cells

PMN = polymorphonuclear leucocytes

(2) therapeutic levels can be reached in the CSF. It should be remembered that many substances, including antibiotics, do not cross the blood-brain barrier very well. The third generation cephalosporins are highly potent and seem to get into the CSF in adequate concentration via the leaky capillaries that are characteristic of inflammation.

Chloramphenicol is lipid-soluble and hence does cross the blood-brain barrier well, but it may produce serious side effects and is therefore rarely used for first-line treatment.

In neonatal infection, amoxycillin is usually given in combination with one of the cephalosporins. Therapy may be modified following Gram stain findings and again once the identity of the organism and its susceptibility pattern is known. For instance, benzylpenicillin is usually the drug of choice for *N. meningitidis* and *S. pneumoniae*, whereas cephalosporins are usually maintained if *H. influenzae* is identified and found to be susceptible. The treatment of choice for *Listeria* meningitis is ampicillin or penicillin plus gentamicin. Standard anti-tuberculosis drugs are used for tuberculous meningitis.

Because of the belief that the inflammatory response is the cause of much of the injury to the CNS in acute bacterial meningitis, there has been much interest recently in the use of anti-inflammatory agents in addition to antibiotics in the treatment of acute bacterial meningitis. Experimental and clinical trials have shown that anti-inflammatory agents, such as the corticosteroid, dexamethasone, can diminish the CSF inflammatory response and the subsequent oedema, increased CSF pressure and the neurologic sequelae. Nevertheless, the routine use of anti-inflammatory drugs in acute bacterial meningitis remains controversial. Further research on their use is currently being undertaken.

Prevention

There is an increased attack rate of *Haemophilus influenzae* type b (Hib) and *N. meningitidis* in close contacts of infected individuals, due mainly to higher rates of nasopharyngeal carriage. Antibiotic prophylaxis is therefore recommended in some settings. Household or intimate contacts are generally given rifampicin to eliminate carriage, and therefore the risk of infection. On some occasions, this drug is also used in preschool settings, but its routine use is controversial. To prevent neonatal infection with Group B streptococci, administration of ampicillin to high-risk women during labour has been shown to be effective.

Vaccines are available for the three major causes of bacterial meningitis. A polyvalent pneumococcal vaccine is recommended for patients who have undergone splenectomy, and may also be given to others with known risk factors (e.g. a CSF leak or Hodgkin's disease). An effective vaccine for *N. meningitidis* serotypes A, C, Y and W135 is available, but not for type B, the most common cause of sporadic cases. The available vaccines are recommended for travellers to high-risk areas (e.g. Nepal and South America), for asplenic patients and for people with complement deficiencies.

Since it has been shown that household contacts are at increased risk of meningococcal disease for several months, even when given appropriate antibiotic prophylaxis, authorities in New Zealand, the United Kingdom and several other countries recommend that they also be vaccinated. In Australia, the NH&MRC was also considering such a policy at the time of writing.

Conjugate Hib vaccines to prevent *H. influenzae* infections have been available in Australia since May 1992, for children over 18 months of age, and since January 1993 for children two months and older. Currently, there are four such vaccines licensed in Australia. For non-Aboriginal children, there is little difference in safety and efficacy between the four preparations, although, State and Commonwealth health departments currently recommend HibTITER (Lederle/Praxis). In certain Aboriginal populations, the incidence of Hib disease is up to five times geater than in the Australian population as a whole, and there are many cases in very young infants (less than six months of age). The Pedvax HIB (Merck, Sharpe and Dohme) vaccine is specifically recommended for Aboriginal children because it produces an antibody response after a single dose at two months of age. It has been shown in clinical trials virtually to eliminate Hib disease in racial groups in other countries with a similar pattern of disease. The major disadvantage of this vaccine is that immunity wanes more quickly than with the other vaccines.

Federal funding has been made available for the vaccination of all children born after 1 February 1993. All countries in which Hib vaccines have been introduced have reported a marked decline in the number of cases of Hib disease.

VIRAL MENINGITIS

Overall, viral meningitis is the most common type of meningitis. Most of these infections are caused by enteroviruses (echoviruses, coxsackie viruses, poliovirus), but other possible causes include the mumps virus and varicella zoster virus. The viruses usually enter the body via the gastrointestinal or respiratory routes and, after local multiplication, enter the bloodstream. Viraemia gives the viruses the opportunity to cross over the blood-brain barrier and enter the subarachnoid space. As with bacterial meningitis, the incidence of viral meningitis is greatest in infants and young children. The immunocompromised are also at increased risk of meningitis, due to a variety of viruses. For example, people infected with the human immunodeficiency virus (HIV) are at increased risk of meningitis caused by the herpes simplex virus, herpes zoster virus, cytomegalovirus and the HIV itself.

Viral meningitis is sometimes referred to as **aseptic meningitis**, a general term used for any meningitis where microorganisms are not isolated by routine bacteriological culture. Apart from viruses, there are many other causes of aseptic meningitis, including bacteria (not cultured by routine methods), fungi, protozoa and non-infectious causes (e.g. malignancy, autoimmune disease, chemical poisoning).

Viral meningitis is generally milder and progresses more slowly than bacterial infections. It is usually manifested by acute onset of headache, mild photophobia, low-grade fever, general malaise and minor neck stiffness. This often follows upper respiratory symptoms, gastrointestinal symptoms, or both, depending on the primary site of virus multiplication and infection. Some people with viral meningitis may become tired or sleepy but should retain full perception and consciousness. Loss of alertness or normal mental status is not typical of viral

CASE HISTORY 20.2
VIRAL MENINGITIS

A 30-year-old woman with a history of migraine headaches attended the casualty department of her local hospital complaining of a headache that had been present for two days. She described the headache as being different to her normal migraines, which were usually more severe and 'pounding'. She also reported having generalised body aches, a stiff neck, mild photophobia and a slight fever over the same period.

She had not been outside the Melbourne area for nine months. She reported no other recent illnesses except for a cold with an earache and sore throat about 10 days earlier. She had not had any antibiotics recently. She was alert and well aware of the general situation.

A lumbar puncture could not be performed immediately so she was given an intramuscular dose of ceftriaxone. Two hours later, a CSF was collected. It was clear and colourless and had a glucose concentration of 2.8 mmol/L (normal >2.5 mmol/L) and a protein level of 0.54 g/L(normal 0.15–0.45 g/L). The white cell count was 1.8 x 10^7/L (normal 0–5 x 10^6/L), with 30% polymorphonuclear leucocytes and 62% lymphocytes.

Comment

A rapid provisional diagnosis of meningitis is necessary for the early treatment of bacterial causes. In this case the preliminary results are suggestive of a viral meningitis.

meningitis, but is suggestive of more serious disease, such as bacterial meningitis. In infants the symptoms may be vague, and the clinical distinction between viral and bacterial meningitis may be more difficult to make.

Even in adults and older children, a distinction between viral and bacterial meningitis cannot always be made on clinical grounds. Laboratory examination of CSF in a case of viral meningitis generally shows a moderately increased white cell count with a predominance of mononuclear cells (lymphocytes), although early in infection polymorphs may predominate, mimicking acute bacterial infection. The protein concentration in CSF may be normal or elevated, but is usually lower than in bacterial meningitis. The CSF glucose is usually within normal limits. The characteristic laboratory findings for bacterial and viral infections are compared in Table 20.3.

Most of the viral causative agents are not easily cultured and thus viral isolation is not always routine. A definitive diagnosis can be made by the demonstration of a fourfold rise in antibody titre in acute and convalescent sera. However, this can take three weeks or more and is therefore of limited clinical value.

Therapy for uncomplicated viral meningitis usually involves symptomatic treatment only, although cefotaxime or ceftriaxone are usually given until a non-bacterial cause is confirmed. The great majority of patients recover spontaneously within two weeks, and often within several days. Complications such as chronic fatigue syndrome, chronic muscle weakness and ataxia may occur, but are rare.

FUNGAL INFECTIONS

Very few fungi infect the central nervous system of humans. They include *Coccidioides immitis*, *Histoplasma capsulatum* and *Cryptococcus neoformans* but, except for *Cryptococcus*, these organisms are rarely seen in Australia. Cryptococcal meningitis has become increasingly common in recent years and is most often found in people whose immune system has been compromised in some way.

Cryptococcal meningitis

Before the AIDS epidemic, cryptococcal meningitis was one of those diseases that students were required to learn about, but would seldom see. It was associated with exposure to pigeon droppings, and occurred in some immunosuppressed people. Today, it is far more familiar. It is now one of the diseases routinely anticipated in patients with AIDS (up to 15% are affected), and is also more common because of the increasing use of corticosteroid therapy and immunosuppressive agents.

Cryptococcus neoformans is a yeast-like fungus with spherical cells. The cells reproduce by budding and have a thick polysaccharide capsule, sometimes much bigger than the cell itself. Five capsular serotypes have been identified: *Cryptococcus neoformans* var. *neoformans* serotypes A, D and AD, and *Cryptococcus neoformans* var. *gattii* serotypes B and C. *C. neoformans* var. *neoformans* is widely distributed in soil and is commonly found in large numbers in pigeon droppings. It has also been found in the excreta of other avian species, including chickens, parrots and canaries. Until recently, the natural source of *C. neoformans* var. *gattii* was not known. However, this organism has now been isolated from two red gum species (*Eucalyptus camaldulensis* and *Eucalyptus tereticornis*) in Australia, and is thought to be released as basidiospores from these trees during their flowering period. The organism has also been isolated from the dung and under the claws of some Australian native animals (e.g. koalas, possums and echidnas), and these may act as secondary reservoirs.

Humans generally become infected with *C. neoformans* var. *neoformans* by inhalation of the organism, after which it travels to the alveoli and causes a primary infection there. In people with normal defences, the disease is often subclinical and regresses spontaneously. Sometimes, however, especially in immunocompromised people (e.g. with AIDS, Hodgkin's lymphoma or sarcoidosis), the organism invades the bloodstream and spreads to other parts of the body, including the brain and meninges. The majority of infections by *C. neoformans var. gattii*, on the other hand, occur in non-immunocompromised hosts. These observations suggest that where *C. neoformans var. neoformans* is generally considered to be an opportunistic pathogen, *C. neoformans var. gattii* may best be regarded as a true pathogen. Both varieties cause a subacute or chronic type of meningitis with a slow onset (one or more weeks) that is often fatal if untreated. Complications may occur and include hydrocephalus, visual disturbances, hearing loss and seizures.

The typical, preliminary CSF findings in cryptococcal meningitis are shown in Table 20.3. If cryptococcal meningitis is suspected, an India ink stain of centrifuged deposit is usually performed. This stain allows the yeast cell and its characteristic large capsule to be seen (see Figure 20.3). Confirmation is by culture of the organism and by a rapid latex agglutination test which can detect cryptococcal antigen in the CSF. This test is highly sensitive and specific for cryptococcal meningitis. The standard

FIGURE 20.3
INDIA INK STAIN OF CEREBROSPINAL FLUID SHOWING *CRYPTOCOCCUS NEOFORMANS*: A YEAST CELL SURROUNDED BY A LARGE TRANSPARENT CAPSULE

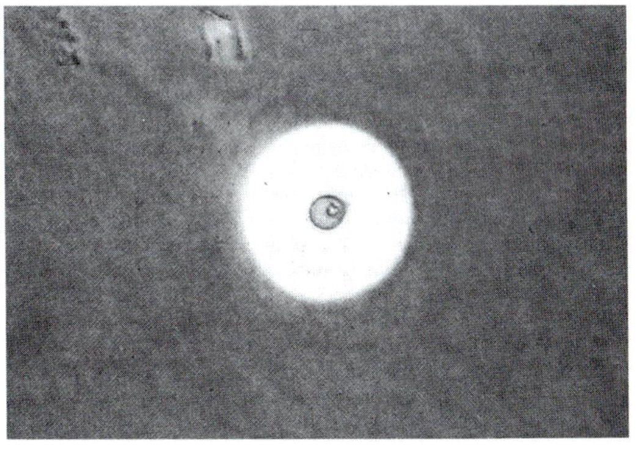

treatment is with amphotericin B plus flucytosine, followed by oral fluconazole.

PROTOZOAL INFECTIONS

Few protozoa infect the central nervous system. The notable one in Australia and other Western countries is *Toxoplasma gondii*. Amoebic meningitis caused by *Naegleria fowleri* is a rare disease that occasionally occurs in Australia. The flagellate *Trypanosoma brucei* is the cause of African trypanosomiasis, or sleeping sickness, which infects many thousands of people each year, but it is restricted mainly to Central and East Africa.

Toxoplasma infection of the CNS

Toxoplasma gondii has for many years been recognised as an important pathogen in congenital infection, but its importance has increased markedly since the AIDS epidemic struck. Today, cerebral toxoplasmosis is one of the more common neurological complications of HIV infection. The protozoan often produces multiple, well-demarcated lesions throughout the cerebral hemispheres. The clinical manifestations are highly variable and include headache, fever, clumsiness to hemiplegia, seizures, ataxia and cognitive changes. Toxoplasmosis is difficult to diagnose and is most often presumptively based on a CT brain scan and response to empirical therapy. Histologic examination of brain biopsy material is the gold standard for diagnosis, but its general usefulness in all cases is doubted. In preliminary studies the polymerase chain reaction (PCR) has been successfully used to demonstrate toxoplasma in brain, CSF and other tissues, and thus has tremendous promise as a diagnostic test in the future.

Treatment is with pyrimethamine plus sulphadiazine, or clindamycin if hypersensitivity to sulphadiazine exists.

ENCEPHALITIS

Encephalitis is almost always caused by viruses, with herpes simplex virus and numerous arboviruses (arthropod-borne viruses) being the most common. Different encephalitis-causing arboviruses occur in different parts of the world (see Table 20.4). Each arbovirus type has certain animal reservoirs and is transmitted by a particular insect (arthropod) vector. In Australia, arbovirus encephalitis (**Australian encephalitis**) is caused by two mosquito-borne flaviviruses—mainly the Murray Valley encephalitis virus, but occasionally the Kunjin virus. These two viruses infect wild and domestic animals over much of mainland Australia.

Encephalitis may also occur as a rare complication of certain systemic viral infections (e.g. measles, mumps, cytomegalovirus) or very rarely after vaccination with some live attenuated vaccines (e.g. measles, mumps, rubella).

The characteristic manifestations of viral encephalitis represent cerebral dysfunction and include abnormal behaviour, seizures and altered consciousness. Fever, vomiting and nausea are also common. These symptoms reflect necrosis of neurones.

Australian encephalitis

Australian encephalitis (AE) is a severe, epidemic-type disease found mainly in the northern and eastern parts of Australia and in Papua New Guinea. The Murray Valley encephalitis (MVE) virus is considered to be endemic in the Kimberley region of Western Australia and the Top End of the Northern Territory, and to be epidemic in the Pilbara and Gascoyne regions of Western Australia. The MVE virus is believed to have been responsible for severe epidemics in 1917, 1918, 1922 and 1925. It was then known as Australian 'X' disease. The most recent major epidemic occurred in 1974, with a total of 58 cases occurring in all mainland States, and resulting in 13 deaths. Epidemics occur mainly during conditions of warm temperature and high rainfall which allow mosquito numbers to increase markedly. Since 1974, less than 40 cases of AE have been recorded in Australia.

Following the 1974 epidemic, a number of sentinel chicken flocks were established by State health authorities, and they still exist in Western Australia, New South Wales and Victoria. The birds in these flocks are regularly tested serologically for antibodies to the MVE and Kunjin viruses, to provided an early warning of any increase in virus activity. There has been no evidence of this in New South Wales, Victoria or South Australia since 1974.

Most infections with these arboviruses are subclinical. However, occasionally they cross the blood-brain barrier and cause damage to the brain tissue. The major presenting symptoms are fever, headache, convulsions or other signs of altered mental state. The case-fatality rate can be as high as 40%. Residual neurological impairment can occur in survivors, including spastic quadriparesis and facial nerve palsy.

Australian encephalitis is diagnosed by serological evidence: the presence of IgM antibody in serum or CSF, or a fourfold rise in IgG antibody titre. There is no specific therapy for encephalitis caused by arboviruses, making

> **CASE HISTORY 20.3**
> **AUSTRALIAN ENCEPHALITIS**
>
> A 9-month-old Aboriginal boy from an outstation in the Northern Territory presented to Royal Darwin Hospital, having been ill for a week with fever, diarrhoea, vomiting and lethargy. His conscious state decreased rapidly over 24 hours. Over the next few days he developed a flaccid paralysis of all limbs and signs of brain-stem dysfunction, and required ventilation. Acyclovir was given.
>
> Five weeks after admission his brain-stem functions and respiration had recovered but the limb paralysis persisted. Sera collected on admission and five days later showed a rise in MVE IgG from 1:40 to 1:160.
>
> *Comment*
>
> Australian encephalitis is considered to be endemic in some northern areas of Australia and also occurs in epidemic form.

TABLE 20.4
ARTHROPOD-BORNE ENCEPHALITIS VIRUSES

VIRUS	INSECT VECTOR	GEOGRAPHIC DISTRIBUTION
Eastern equine encephalitis	Mosquito	USA
St Louis encephalitis	Mosquito	USA, Jamaica
Venezuelan equine encephalitis	Mosquito	USA, South America
Japanese B encephalitis	Mosquito	Japan, Korea, China
Louping ill	Tick	Great Britain
Russian spring-summer	Tick	Europe, Asia
Murray Valley encephalitis	Mosquito	Australia, New Guinea
Kunjin	Mosquito	Australia, New Guinea

prevention of infection very important. Australian State health departments have contingency plans for disease prevention should virus activity, as indicated by sentinel flocks, be found to be increasing to dangerous levels. Although vaccines have been developed for some other encephalitis arboviruses (e.g. Japanese B encephalitis), there is not yet one for Australian encephalitis.

Herpes encephalitis

Herpes simplex virus type 1 is most often associated with cold sores. Very rarely, the virus reactivates in the trigeminal ganglia, where it resides latently, and ascends into the brain. The spread of herpes simplex virus type 2 to the brain is even less common, although in neonates both types can cause severe encephalitis. Herpes encephalitis is a very severe disease that causes neurological damage with a high mortality. Early treatment with acyclovir greatly reduces the mortality and permanent neurological damage. The early diagnosis of herpes encephalitis is therefore important because of the potential for effective treatment.

Diagnosis is usually made by radioactive brain scan, CT scan and EEG. Brain tissue biopsy, examined microscopically for viral antigens using fluorescent antibodies, provides conclusive evidence, but is rarely performed because of the risk to the patient. The polymerase chain reaction has been used successfully to detect herpes simplex virus in CSF and shows promise as a diagnostic tool for this infection.

Other Infections Involving the Nervous System

TETANUS

Tetanus is a rare, but serious, illness caused by the bacterium *Clostridium tetani*, a strictly anaerobic, spore-forming Gram-positive rod. Tetanus spores are widespread in soil and manure, because the organism is part of the bowel flora of various animals and some humans. The spores are extremely resistant to drying, disinfectants and heat (they are resistant to boiling for 20 minutes), and can survive in soil for years.

Since the development of the tetanus vaccine and its widespread use, tetanus has become a rarity in developed countries. In Australia, between 5 and 14 cases have been notified annually since 1980, resulting in a total of 28 deaths. However, in underdeveloped countries the incidence is much higher, and worldwide there are more than 50 000 fatalities from tetanus each year. In developed countries, there is often a higher incidence in the elderly because of inadequate past and current immunisation.

Wounds contaminated with faeces or soil can become infected with *C. tetani*. Usually, the spores must be deposited into a deep, necrotic wound where oxygen is lacking, allowing growth of this strict anaerobe to occur. However, many cases of tetanus have occurred following only minor injuries, such as thorns or splinters acquired during gardening. In some developing countries, a high incidence in neonates is associated with the use of contaminated knives to cut the umbilical cord, or the use of mud to pack the umbilical stump to soothe the infant.

Spores enter a wound and, when bacterial growth and multiplication occur, a potent exotoxin is produced. The non-invasive bacteria remain at the wound site, but the neurotoxin travels along peripheral nerves to the CNS where it blocks the release of transmitters, especially in inhibitory neurones. This causes an overactivity of motor neurones. Sympathetic nerves may also be affected, leading to a similar overactivity in the sympathetic nervous system. There is no direct effect on mental function.

After an incubation period of 4–10 days, muscle rigidity (stiffness) and uncontrolled muscle spasms occur. Uncontrolled contraction of the powerful masseter (jaw) muscles is common, leading to the classic 'lockjaw', or trismus. Contraction of the facial muscles may occur, causing the sneering appearance termed 'risus sardonicus'. Generalised contraction of the muscles of the back, neck, abdomen, arms and legs can give the whole body a stiff, ramrod appearance. In some cases, back muscle contraction may be sufficiently severe to cause the patient's back to arch and even to crush the spinal processes (see Figure 20.4). Death generally results from respiratory failure due to persistent spasm of the respiratory muscles. Variation in blood pressure, tachycardia and sweating may be prominent in the elderly, due to the effects of the toxin on the sympathetic nervous system.

Diagnosis of tetanus is by clinical appraisal since the organism exists only in small numbers and can rarely be isolated. Treatment of tetanus is difficult. Human tetanus immune globulin should be given immediately tetanus is suspected. The wound should be thoroughly cleansed and all devitalised tissue removed, and penicillin given to prevent bacterial replication. Muscle relaxants may be used, and, in severe cases, ventilatory support may be necessary. Despite treatment, the mortality rate can still be as high as 30%.

Prevention of tetanus involves (1) immunisation, and (2) prophylaxis after a tetanus-prone injury is sustained. Tetanus can be effectively prevented if full immunisation is followed. Immunisation is with tetanus toxoid vaccine, a preparation of the toxin that has been treated with formalin, which inactivates its toxicity but retains its antigenicity. It is one of the safest vaccines in current use and is nearly 100% effective. The National Health and Medical Research Council (NH&MRC) currently recommends that everyone be immunised against tetanus at the ages of 2, 4, 6 and 18 months (usually with DTP vaccine—diphtheria/tetanus/pertussis), at 5 years (with CDT—combined diphtheria/tetanus), and thereafter every 10 years (with ADT—adult diphtheria/tetanus). This regimen also serves to maintain diphtheria immunity.

CASE HISTORY 20.4
TETANUS

A 58-year-old woman gashed her hand on the branch of a tree while gardening. After examination in the casualty department of her local hospital, her wound was cleaned, she was given an injection of tetanus toxoid and a course of oral flucloxacillin was started.

Six days later she developed a stiffness in her jaw, complained of muscle spasms in her back and had difficulty in swallowing. She was diagnosed as having tetanus, admitted to hospital and given tetanus immunoglobulin. The wound was debrided and cleaned and she was given diazepam to prevent the spasms. This treatment was effective and she was discharged after a week.

Comment

In a non-immune person the most critical part of tetanus treatment is immunoglobulin. This woman would not have developed symptoms of tetanus had this been given initially. Careful taking of her case history should have ascertained whether she was immune or not.

FIGURE 20.4

A PAINTING OF A MAN DYING OF THE FINAL STAGES OF TETANUS

Note the arched back and the sneering appearance of 'risus sardonicus', due to severe muscle spasm of the back and face, respectively.

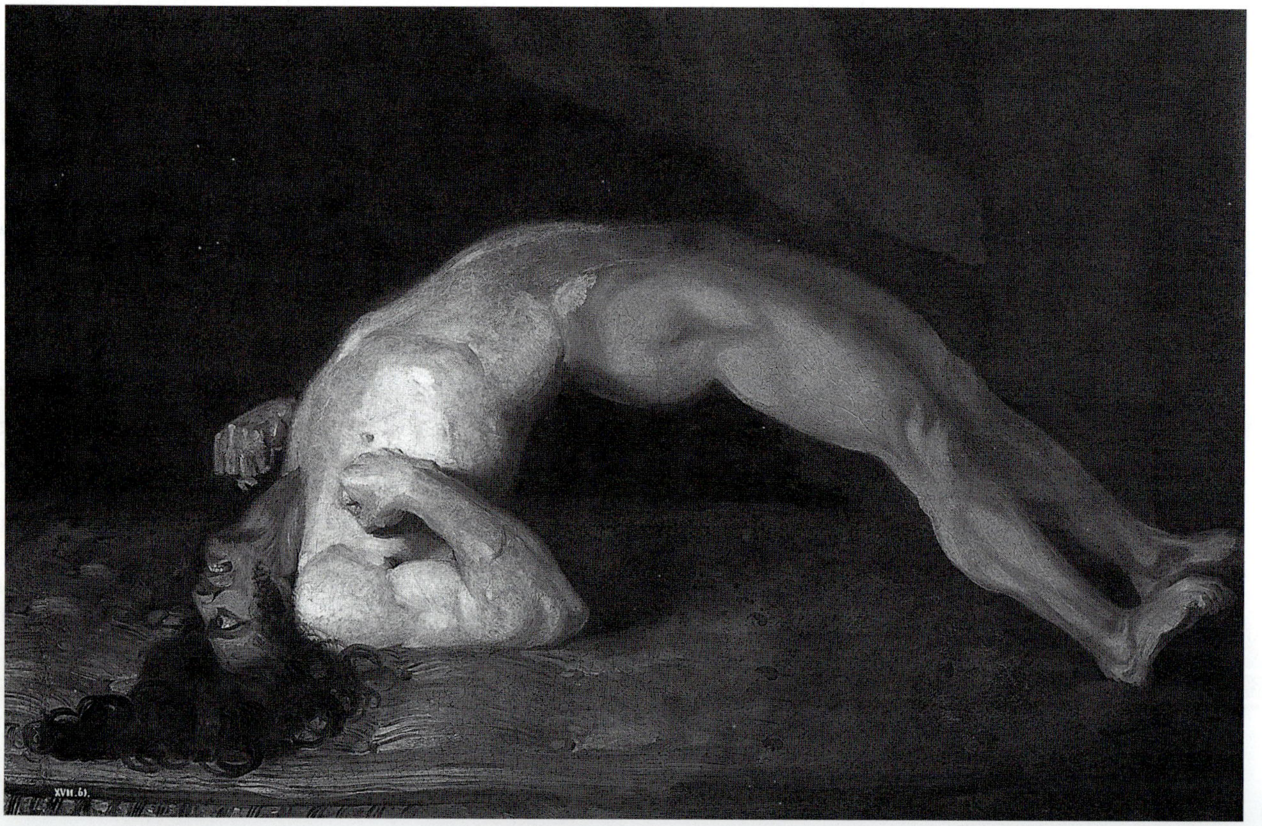

If a person suffers a 'tetanus-prone wound' (necrotic tissue and contamination with soil) and immunisation is current, then a booster dose of ADT should be given. If there is any doubt that active immunity exists (i.e. the person is uncertain of current immunisation), human tetanus immune globulin should be administered immediately. Simultaneously, tetanus toxoid should be given in the other arm and arrangements made to complete the full immunisation schedule. The NH&MRC guidelines for wound prophylaxis are summarised in Table 20.5.

BOTULISM

Botulism is a form of food poisoning which affects the nervous system rather than the gastrointestinal tract. It is caused by the anaerobic, spore-forming, Gram-positive rod *Clostridium botulinum*. Generally, the disease is uncommon in Australia, New Zealand and other developed countries. No cases of botulism have been notified in Australia since 1992. Animals, birds and fish are also susceptible to botulism, and suffer similar symptoms and outcomes to humans (see Spotlight box, p. 484).

Spores of the organism are widespread in soil and are often found contaminating meat and vegetables. The spores are very resistant to heat, being able to survive boiling for several hours, but are destroyed by standard sterilising processes.

Classically, the disease has been associated with the consumption of canned or preserved foods that have not been adequately sterilised. The foods usually implicated are those preserved at home, when appropriate sterilisation procedures are not followed. The spores germinate inside the can or bottle during storage and the botulinum toxin is released. *C. botulinum* also causes botulism in infants, especially in the age group of 1–7 months. Such cases are generally related to consumption of honey (spores are picked up from flowers and plants by bees) or ingestion of soil.

The ingestion of *C. botulinum* cells or spores causes no problem, except in infants. The bacterium appears to be unable to compete successfully with the intestinal flora, but infants are more susceptible because their flora are not fully established.

The ingestion of preformed toxin, however, results in disease. It is absorbed in the intestine and enters the bloodstream. The botulinum toxin then acts on peripheral nerve synapses, blocking the release of acetylcholine, which is the chemical released by neurones to cause muscle cells to contract. The toxin paralyses the muscles in a relaxed state (flaccid paralysis). This neurotoxin is one of the most potent of all natural toxins— 1 μg is sufficient to kill 10 people. It is colourless, tasteless and odourless, and therefore not noticed when eating contaminated food.

There are several different serological types of toxin, which also differ in their potency. Types A, B and E are the most common, and A is the most potent (60–70% mortality in untreated people).

Symptoms usually begin within 2–3 days of consumption of the contaminated food. The disease is characterised by a descending weakness and paralysis. Visual disturbances (e.g. double vision) and dysphagia (pain or difficulty in swallowing) are common early symptoms; as the disease progresses, muscles lower down the body become affected. Muscles in the trunk and limbs are weakened and then paralysed. Eventually, patients may have difficulty breathing and may die from respiratory failure due to dysfunction of respiratory muscles.

Diagnosis is mainly by clinical appraisal, although sometimes the toxin can be demonstrated in the patient's serum or faeces or in the contaminated food. Treatment

TABLE 20.5
NATIONAL HEALTH AND MEDICAL RESEARCH COUNCIL (NH&MRC) GUIDE TO TETANUS PROPHYLAXIS IN WOUND MANAGEMENT

HISTORY OF ACTIVE IMMUNISATION		TYPE OF WOUND	TETANUS TOXOID	TETANUS IMMUNOGLOBULIN
Uncertain, or less than three doses		clean, minor wound	Yes	No
		all other wounds	Yes	Yes
Three doses or more	If less than five years since last dose	clean, minor wound	No	No
		all other wounds	No	No
	If 5–10 years since last dose	clean, minor wound	No	No
		all other wounds	Yes	No
	If more than 10 years since last dose	clean, minor wound	Yes	No
		all other wounds	Yes	No

SPOTLIGHT
BOTULISM

During the Easter Thoroughbred Yearling Sales in Sydney in 1994, 42 yearlings were affected by a disease syndrome characterised by variable degrees of flaccid paralysis. Severe respiratory distress signalled the terminal stages of the disease. Thirty-three of the horses died.

It was established that the outbreak was the result of the toxin of *Clostridium botulinum* type C, and was therefore equine botulism. The horse is extremely susceptible to botulinum toxin. The lack of antitoxin in this situation severely handicapped efforts to control the outbreak.

should be commenced as soon as possible after the diagnosis is made, and involves the administration of polyvalent botulinum antitoxin which contains antibodies against toxin types A, B and E. The antitoxins eliminate circulating toxin in the bloodstream, but probably do little to the toxin already bound to nerve cells. Supportive treatment (especially ventilatory and cardiac) may thus be required for some time until the symptoms subside.

LEPROSY

Leprosy has been known since biblical times. It was a feared disease and, from the 6th century, spread through Europe, leading to the establishment of many isolated leper hospitals and colonies. It is no longer feared as in the past but, despite the development of effective treatment, leprosy is still a major problem in the world today. The World Health Organization estimates that there are more than 12 million people in the world with leprosy, mainly in tropical areas in Asia, Africa and Latin America. The highest rate of infection is in South-East Asia, especially India, where there is a prevalence rate of 2–3 per 1000 people.

In Australia, the incidence has been steadily declining since 1944 to a current annual rate of notifications of about 0.1 per 100 000 population. In New Zealand, fewer than 10 cases per year have been notified since 1981.

Leprosy is caused by the acid-fast bacillus *Mycobacterium leprae*. It has not been possible to culture the organism *in vitro*, so the study of it has been difficult. Recently, it has been grown in armadillos, mangabey monkeys and mice for research purposes. The disease appears to be confined to humans, so is always acquired from another person. The organism is present in large numbers in the nasal secretions of infected people and is probably transmitted mainly by respiratory droplets. It can also be found in skin lesions, but usually in low numbers. Transmission is enhanced by overcrowding and poor hygiene. The disease has a very long incubation period (sometimes 20 years or more) and patients may be infected and shedding organisms for years before the onset of symptoms, making control in endemic regions very difficult. Generally, however, and contrary to earlier belief, leprosy is not a highly contagious disease, requiring prolonged and close contact for transmission, such as between children and their infected parents.

M. leprae is an obligate intracellular parasite which resides in histiocytes, endothelial cells, and Schwann cells in peripheral nerves. Its invasion of Schwann cells is the basis for the characteristic nerve damage in the disease. The organism grows extremely slowly. It has a generation time of 11 or more days in the footpad of a mouse, which helps to explain the incubation period of several years or more in human disease. The organism grows best at temperatures below 37°C, and thus has a predilection for cooler parts of the body such as the skin and peripheral structures like the fingers, ears and nose.

After a variable incubation period, the disease can develop with a spectrum of clinical manifestations. In **tuberculoid leprosy**, a strong cell-mediated immune response limits the multiplication of the organism and the disease is confined to patches of skin and certain nerve trunks. This form is characterised by blotchy skin lesions which may be red or hypopigmented and areas on the face, trunk and extremities which may have lost sensitivity (e.g. to a pin prick) because of damage to nerves and nerve endings.

Lepromatous leprosy is at the other end of the clinical spectrum and is due to the absence of cellular immunity to the organism. In this form, there is uncontrolled proliferation of the bacilli, which results in extensive skin lesions and nerve involvement. The skin lesions may eventually become very large and nodular in appearance. As the disease progresses, there is loss of eyebrows and a thickening of the nose, ears and cheeks, producing a typical 'leonine' (lion-like) facial appearance. There is progressive destruction of bones in the hands, feet (see Figure 20.5) and nose. With the loss of local sensation, victims suffer frequent physical trauma to extremities which become infected with other organisms, causing further deformity.

FIGURE 20.5
LEPROSY
In this case a severe destruction of bones in the feet has occurred.

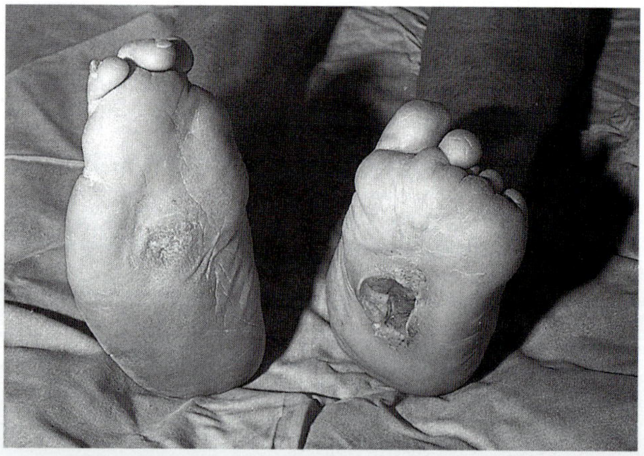

Between these two ends of the spectrum, there are intermediate forms referred to as borderline tuberculoid, mid-borderline and borderline lepromatous leprosy. The less developed the cell-mediated immune response, the more severe the clinical lesions. The form of disease that an individual develops seems to be at least partly genetically determined.

Laboratory diagnosis of leprosy involves a microscopic examination of nasal scrapings or skin biopsies stained with an acid-fast stain such as the Ziehl-Neelsen stain. Dapsone had long been the standard form of therapy for leprosy until strains of the bacterium resistant to this drug started to emerge. The current recommendations of the World Health Organization are that multidrug therapy should now be used. In the less severe forms (tuberculoid and borderline tuberculoid), rifampicin is administered monthly, and dapsone self-administered daily for six months. In the lepromatous forms and the mid-borderline form rifampicin and clofazimine are administered monthly, and dapsone and clofazimine taken daily for two years or more, until skin smears become negative for acid-fast bacilli. The rationale for this is that there are many more organisms present in the lepromatous forms and thus a much greater chance of resistant strains emerging.

There is no vaccine for leprosy but the vaccine for tuberculosis (the BCG), which is caused by other mycobacteria, has been reported to have provided from 20–80% protection against leprosy in different clinical trials. The search for an effective vaccine continues. Prophylactic antibiotic therapy may be used for household contacts, especially children of people with leprosy.

RABIES

Rabies ('rage' or 'madness' in Latin) has been the object of fear and fascination for thousands of years, with written accounts in ancient books of Mesopotamia and Babylon dating back to around 2300 BC. The mere mention of the disease often conjures up visions of a gentle, obedient pet suddenly becoming ferocious and drooling, or a wild, irrational animal emerging from the woods searching for prey, or a human victim dying a horrible death in a state of delirium and rage.

Rabies is caused by a large, enveloped, bullet-shaped virus with single-stranded RNA, belonging to the family Rhabdoviridae. It can infect almost all warm-blooded animals, and is primarily a disease of animals. The epidemiology of human disease in a given region reflects the distribution of the disease in animals in that region, and how much contact humans have with infected animals. Almost all cases are due to dog bites in developing countries where canine rabies is endemic. It is less commonly transmitted by wild animals including monkeys, foxes, bats and raccoons.

Rabies is found in most countries of the world, with the highest rates in Asia. An estimated 25 000 cases a year occur in India, spread mainly by the large population of stray dogs. The World Health Organization estimates that over 50 000 people throughout the world die each year from rabies. A number of countries have been declared free of rabies, including Australia, England, Japan, Sweden and Norway, predominantly due to strict quarantine laws and, in some cases, animal vaccination programs. The occasional case of rabies identified in Australia results from infection overseas in endemic countries. There have been no cases notified in New Zealand since 1980.

The rabies virus is almost always inoculated by the bite of an infected animal or, rarely, by exposure of mucous membranes or skin lesions to infected saliva or other secretions (e.g. urine). Once in the body, the virus infects local muscle cells where it may lie dormant for a variable period. The virus replicates in the muscle fibres and then travels via peripheral nerves and the spinal cord to the brain where it causes an encephalitis. From there it can spread via nerves to a wide variety of richly innervated sites, such as the salivary glands, respiratory tract, skin and cornea.

The incubation period can vary markedly. The longest well-documented period is about two years, but in most cases it is usually 1–2 months. Clinical illness heralds the arrival of the virus in the CNS. The early symptoms are headache, fever and partial paralysis at the bite site. This is followed by more generalised paralysis, muscle spasms (involving particularly the pharynx and larynx), hydrophobia (fear of water, due to the muscle spasms in the throat and chest that swallowing can induce), hypersalivation, aerophobia (fear of moving air, due to hypersensitivity of the skin), confusion, periods of hyperactivity (running, biting and thrashing about) and hallucinations. After 2–10 days of these acute neurological symptoms, the patient becomes comatose and dies usually due to heart or respiratory failure. Survival has never been reported in an individual once symptoms have developed.

Diagnosis of rabies is based on detection of viral antigens in skin or brain biopsy specimens using a microscopic immunofluorescence technique, or by examination of serum or CSF for specific antibodies.

After symptoms of rabies develop, there is no effective treatment, except for good nursing care, sedation and other supportive therapy. The disease can be prevented, however, if appropriate prophylactic treatment is given, before symptoms develop, to a person known or suspected of having been exposed to the virus. This treatment is based on:

- prompt and thorough cleaning of the wound with soap and water, followed by application of an antiviral antiseptic (e.g. 70% ethanol or tincture of iodine);
- thorough infiltration of the wound with rabies hyperimmune globulin to attempt to neutralise viruses before they enter the nervous system; and
- commencement of rabies vaccination regimen to induce the formation of specific antibodies in the patient.

Such treatment, if administered properly and soon enough, virtually guarantees protection from disease. Safe, effective vaccines for active immunisation are available, but routine immunisation for Australians is not necessary. However, all workers and travellers who are at high risk of contracting rabies in an endemic area should be immunised, as should health professionals caring for infected patients.

POLIO

Polio (or poliomyelitis) has been known for thousands of years and was once a very common disease. Figure 20.6 shows a typical polio victim recorded on an ancient Egyptian stone slab from the 18th dynasty (1580–1350 BC). Before the availability of vaccines in the mid-1950s, there were more than 20 000 cases of paralytic polio in the United States each year. Since then the incidence has declined to very low numbers. The last notified case in Australia was in 1986, and there have been less than 20 reported cases in this country since the 1970s.

In 1988, the WHO initiated an immunisation campaign with the view to eradicating the disease from the world. As a result, there has been a progressive fall in the reported incidence of polio globally. However, there are still many thousands of cases worldwide, the majority on the Indian subcontinent.

Polio is best known as a cause of paralysis, but the virus produces symptoms in only about 10% of infected people, and less than 1% develop the paralytic form. It is caused by the poliovirus, a single-stranded RNA virus, of which there are three distinct serotypes. Humans are the only known reservoir of the virus. It is excreted in faeces of infected people and is usually transmitted via food, water or hands. It is a fairly stable virus which can remain infectious for long periods outside the body (e.g. in food or water). In the early stages of infection, it may also be present in the nose and throat and thus be transmitted by the air-borne route.

FIGURE 20.6
A TYPICAL POLIO VICTIM SHOWN ON AN ANCIENT EGYPTIAN STONE SLAB, CIRCA 1580–1350 BC

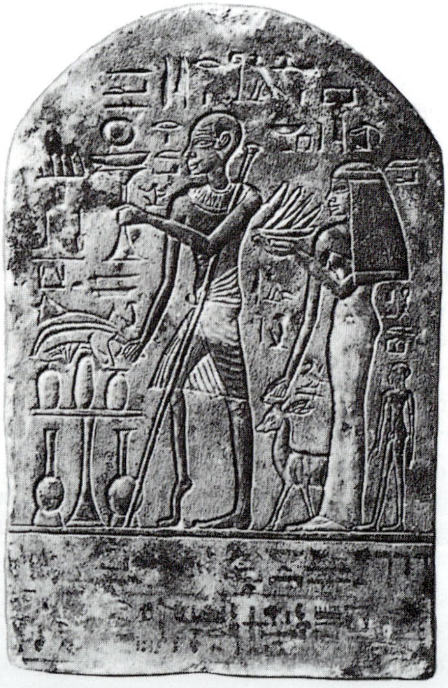

After initial local multiplication in the intestine or pharynx, the virus reaches the bloodstream. The majority of cases are asymptomatic or have only mild symptoms of headache, sore throat, fever and nausea. In the paralytic form, the virus invades the CNS where it infects neurones in the spinal cord and brain. The damage to these cells results in paralysis of the muscles that they innervate. High fever, back or neck pain, and muscle spasms are the early symptoms, and then several days later a flaccid paralysis occurs. One or more limbs may be affected, and some patients also experience difficulties in talking, swallowing or breathing. Some patients with paralysed respiratory muscles used to be restricted to an 'iron lung' (a predecessor of modern ventilatory equipment) for the rest of their lives. Some paralysis may disappear, but any that persists for several months is usually permanent. Laboratory diagnosis of polio involves the isolation and identification of the virus in tissue culture from faeces or a pharyngeal swab.

Polio is completely preventable by vaccination and has decreased markedly in incidence in developed countries since mass immunisation programs were instituted in the 1950s. However, polio is still a common disease in developing countries.

The first vaccine available was the **Salk vaccine** (IPV—inactivated poliomyelitis vaccine). It contains formalin-inactivated viruses and is 70–90% effective. It is administered by intramuscular injection. In the early 1960s, the more effective (nearly 100%) **Sabin vaccine** (OPV—oral poliomyelitis vaccine) was introduced. It contains attenuated, live viruses of the three serotypes, and is more effective because it induces a strong IgA antibody response at mucosal surfaces where infection first occurs. The attenuated viruses actually infect the intestinal tract, but do not spread to the CNS. The OPV has the added advantage of oral administration, as well as providing a longer-lasting immunity if the correct number of doses are given. Travellers to areas of the world where polio still occurs and whose last dose of polio vaccine was more than 10 years before are advised to have a booster dose of vaccine.

SPOTLIGHT
POST-POLIO SYNDROME

Some people, who suffered polio as children many years ago and recovered, experience a return of symptoms which require them to return to using crutches and leg braces. Sufferers can experience extreme fatigue, difficulty in breathing and new muscle weakness 30 years or more after their childhood infection. Doctors believe that post-polio syndrome could affect as many as half of Australia's 40 000 victims of the polio epidemics in the 1940s and 1950s. At present, there is no effective treatment for post-polio syndrome.

There is still some debate about whether the IPV or the OPV should be used in mass immunisation campaigns, even given the greater efficacy and ease of administration of the latter. This is because cases of vaccine-associated poliomyelitis have been reported. In approximately one in three million doses administered, the recipient, or a close contact of the recipient, has developed paralytic disease. Most cases of vaccine-associated polio occur in young infants (less than four months old) or in the immunocompromised. In Australia, the OPV is generally used, but IPV is preferred for people with immune deficiency, patients who are febrile, and women during the first four months of pregnancy.

PRION DISEASES

Prions are transmissible agents that cause a number of progressive, always fatal, neurodegenerative diseases in humans and animals. These diseases are sometimes referred to as **spongiform encephalopathies** because there is damage to the brain tissue that produces microscopic vacuoles, giving it a spongy appearance in histological sections. The infectious agents have not been definitely identified but at the present time are believed to be composed largely, if not entirely, of an abnormal form of a normal cell protein, termed PrP (prion protein). The normal cellular isoform (PrP^{c}) is believed to be converted into an abnormal isoform (referred to as PrP^{sc} after the scrapie protein) in infected brain cells. The normal function of PrP^{c} is unknown. After entering a host cell, PrP^{sc} appears to cause conversion of PrP^{c} to PrP^{sc} and initiate a self-amplifying process of PrP^{sc}. The mechanisms involved are unknown.

Apart from their apparent lack of nucleic acid, these infectious agents have a number of other unusual properties, including a resistance to ultraviolet light, heat and certain chemical agents. For example, prions are not inactivated by boiling, ethylene oxide sterilisation, ethanol, detergents or alcoholic iodine. Even years of storage in formaldehyde does not destroy their infectivity. Prions appear to have a very slow rate of replication, which may explain the long incubation period of disease. One of the more remarkable features of all prion diseases is that they do not appear to induce inflammation or a specific immune response, normally the hallmarks of infection.

A number of different diseases of animals and humans have been attributed to prions. Scrapie is a prion disease in sheep and goats in which infected animals itch and scrape themselves against fences and posts, often until they bleed. Bovine spongiform encephalopathy (BSE) or 'mad cow disease' has killed more than 150 000 cattle in Great Britain since 1986, and threatens the beef industry there. An infected animal typically loses weight, has a depressed appearance with lowered head and arched back, and suffers increasing difficulty in walking, eventually being unable to stand. The source of the epidemic is suspected to be cattle feed containing cattle or sheep products (now banned in Britain). BSE has been reported in much lower incidence in some other countries either due to importation of cattle feed from the United Kingdom (e.g. France, Portugal, Switzerland) or cattle from the United Kingdom (e.g. Germany, Canada, Italy). Australia and New Zealand are considered to be free of scrapie and BSE.

Creutzfeldt-Jakob disease is the most important of the human prion diseases and is discussed in the following section. The other human prion disease that has been studied extensively is kuru. This disease has been found only in people of the Fore tribes in the highlands of Papua New Guinea. Kuru occurred in about 1 in 10 people in these tribes and was found to be transmitted from person to person by their cannibalistic practices. Their ritual required the consumption of the body of a dead member of the family, who, given the incidence of disease, was likely to have died from kuru. No cases of kuru have been seen in those born after 1957, when the practice of cannibalism ceased. D. Carleton Gadjusek, an American scientist, won the Nobel Prize in 1976 for his work on this disease.

Gertsmann-Straussler-Scheinker syndrome is a rare human prion disease with an estimated incidence of less than two cases per 100 million people. This disease, first described by Gertsmann and co-workers in 1928, is essentially a genetic disorder with an autosomal dominant inheritance, due to a mutation in the PrP gene. However, studies have shown that it can be transmitted by the injection of brain extracts from affected humans into primates and rodents. Fatal familial insomnia is also an exotic disease of humans attributed to prions.

Creutzfeldt-Jakob disease

Hans Gerhard Creutzfeldt first described a progressive dementing illness in a 22-year-old woman in 1920, and in the following year Alfons Maria Jakob described four similar cases. Worldwide, there is thought to be approximately one new case of Creutzfeldt-Jakob disease (CJD) per 1–2 million people each year. Certain ethnic groups, such as Libyan-born Jews in Israel and a particular inbred population in rural Czechoslovakia, have an above-average incidence.

The natural mode of transmission is not known. The failure to identify a source of infection in most cases, plus the occurrence of similar diseases in animals, especially in sheep, goats and cows, has caused great concern that the disease may be acquired from animals. The transmission of the similar disease, kuru, among Papuan cannibals has raised the fear that CJD may be acquired by ingestion of contaminated beef, sheep or goat meat. However, the fact that CJD occurs in approximately the same frequency in Australia and New Zealand, where neither scrapie nor any other prion disease of animals has been found, suggests that this is not so. Also, individuals who potentially have the highest contact with the infectious agent, such as farmers, breeders, slaughterhouse personnel and butchers, do not appear to have a higher incidence of CJD than any other population group.

Experiments in animals have shown that the disease is most efficiently transmitted by intracerebral inoculation of infected brain tissue, but it can also be transmitted subcutaneously, intravenously, intramuscularly and orally. Although brain tissue and CSF are the most infectious, the disease can be transmitted to animals by other tissues such as lymph nodes, kidney, spleen and lung. Animals infected in this way develop a progressive CNS disorder similar to CJD. Transmission from human to human has been shown to occur through the transfer of infected tissue or body fluids, or via contaminated surgical instruments. Generally, direct inoculation with infected tissue appears to be required. Blood transfusion does not appear to be a major risk factor.

There is no evidence to suggest that CJD is transmitted during normal social contact, sexual contact or from mother to foetus. There is still no direct evidence to support the hypothesis of transmission via food (e.g. from BSE-infected beef or scrapie-infected mutton). However, studies of what appears to be a new variant form of CJD in 10 people in the United Kingdom in 1995–96 suggest that exposure to BSE is a likely cause.

Iatrogenic transmission of CJD through corneal transplants, neurosurgical equipment, pituitary hormones and dura mater grafts has been reported. The use of pituitary-derived growth hormone and gonadotrophin collected and pooled from cadaveric pituitary glands has led to a serious outbreak of iatrogenic CJD. There have been more than 30 cases of CJD attributable to the use of cadaver-derived pituitary hormones in the United States, the United Kingdom, France, New Zealand and Australia.

In Australia, about 2100 patients have received either human growth hormone for the treatment of growth hormone deficiency, or human pituitary gonadotrophin for the treatment of infertility since the 1960s. The first death from CJD occurred in 1988, and three more deaths occurred between May 1989 and January 1991. The use of cadaver-derived pituitary hormones was suspended in May 1985 following case reports overseas. More than 20 reports of CJD in health care workers (including neurosurgeons, doctors, dentists, nurses and histopathology technicians) suggest the possibility of workplace infection, although precise evidence of this has not been demonstrated in most of these cases. (See the Spotlight box on CJD in Chapter 5, p. 94.)

Although CJD is usually sporadic, it has been known for some time that 10–15% of cases are familial. As mentioned, there are clusters of cases in certain ethnic groups, such as the Libyan Jews in Israel. There have also been reports of the disease persisting through generations of families, with multiple members being affected. These observations suggest a genetic basis for some cases of CJD, and it is now recognised that these are due to mutations of the PrP gene. As stated earlier, Gertsmann-Straussler-Scheinker syndrome (GSS) is also considered to be an inheritable prion disease, which can also be transmitted to experimental animals. CJD and GSS are the only known human diseases that are both inheritable and infectious.

Because the mode of transmission is unknown in most cases of CJD, the incubation period is also unknown. However, from iatrogenic infections it has been established that when the agent is introduced into or near the brain the incubation period is in the order of months, but in peripheral transmission the incubation period is usually years or even decades. The dominant feature of CJD is dementia. Early symptoms may include loss of balance and muscle coordination, slurred speech, failing vision and myoclonic (quick, jerky) movements of the extremities or head. The symptoms become progressively more severe, leading to dementia and a variety of other neurological disturbances such as dysphasia, spasticity and seizures in a period of only months. Myoclonic jerking movements are the most frequent physical sign. The patient eventually becomes comatose.

The disease is uniformly fatal, usually in less than a year from the onset of symptoms, although the suspected variant form identified in the United Kingdom in 1995–96 causes a more prolonged disease. How the propagation of PrP^{Sc} causes damage to brain cells is not known.

As there is no immune response to infection, a blood test for antibodies is not available. The majority of patients have a characteristic electroencephalogram (EEG) pattern at some time. This is a repetitive biphasic or triphasic pattern of high amplitude waves, which may be linked to the patient's myoclonic jerks. The demonstration of spongy neuropathological changes and widespread proliferation of astrocytes in brain tissue provides a definitive diagnosis, but the role of brain biopsy as a standard diagnostic method remains controversial. It is an invasive technique with infection control risks to health workers, and it does not always detect infection.

At present, there is no way of defining possible risk groups except for those who have received dura mater transplants or cadaver-derived pituitary hormones, or who belong to one of the few ethnic groups with a relatively high incidence. Because prions are unusually resistant to heat and appear to be resistant to normal autoclave procedures, the NH&MRC currently recommends autoclaving for two hours at 121°C when CJD is suspected. Where autoclaving is not possible, immersion in 1 molar NaOH for 1 hour is suggested for sterilisation of critical or semi-critical items. Disinfection of tables, floors and other surfaces is with sodium hypochlorite (undiluted or a 1:10 dilution of bleach) or 1M NaOH for 15 minutes. There is no treatment for CJD and no vaccine.

Summary

- The central nervous system (CNS) consists of the brain and the spinal cord.
- The brain and the spinal cord are surrounded by three membranes or meninges.
- Cerebrospinal fluid (CSF) circulates in the space between the two inner meninges.
- If something blocks the circulation or drainage of CSF, it begins to accumulate and may exert pressure on the brain (hydrocephalus or 'water on the brain').
- The blood-brain barrier consists of the tightly joined endothelial cells of the brain's capillaries, and allows only certain substances to pass from the circulation to the brain.

INFECTIONS OF THE CENTRAL NERVOUS SYSTEM

- In most infections, organisms gain access to the CNS from the bloodstream.
- Meningitis is an infection and inflammation of the meninges, most often caused by viruses or bacteria but occasionally by fungi or protozoa.
- Encephalitis is an infection and inflammation of the brain itself and is almost always caused by viruses.

BACTERIAL MENINGITIS

- Acute bacterial meningitis is a medical emergency requiring urgent and specific treatment.

Causative agents, transmission and incidence

- The most common causative agents are *Neisseria meningitidis, Haemophilus influenzae* and *Streptococcus pneumoniae*.
- Patients with CSF shunts or severe head injury, or those who have had neurosurgery may develop meningitis caused by such bacteria as staphylococci, *Propionibacterium* or *Corynebacterium*.
- Most cases of meningococcal meningitis (*N. meningitidis*) occur in the 0–4 year old age group.
- Meningococcal meningitis is the only form of meningitis that can spread in an epidemic form.
- A serious complication of meningococcal infection, called the Waterhouse-Friderichsen syndrome, can develop if the organism invades many parts of the body.
- *Haemophilus influenzae* type b (Hib) is a common inhabitant of the throat of infants and young children, but is less frequently found in adults.
- Hib is the major cause of bacterial meningitis in children.
- Pneumococcal meningitis (*Streptococcus pneumoniae*) usually follows septicaemia or head injury.
- Neonatal meningitis is caused mainly by *E. coli* (with capsular type K1) and *Streptococcus agalactiae*.
- *S. agalactiae* is part of the genitourinary flora of some women.
- Factors that place babies at increased risk of meningeal infection caused by *E. coli* and *S. agalactiae* include prematurity (<36 weeks), prolonged rupture of amniotic membranes and heavy maternal colonisation.
- *Listeria monocytogenes* causes meningitis in neonates as well as in immunocompetent and immunocompromised patients.
- *Mycobacterium tuberculosis* can cause meningitis by entering the bloodstream from a focus of infection elsewhere and disseminating to the meninges.

Pathogenesis

- The critical events in the pathogenesis of acute haematogenous bacterial meningitis are:
  - *nasopharyngeal colonisation;*
  - *invasion of the bloodstream and intravascular survival;*
  - penetration of the blood-brain barrier;
  - damage and inflammation of the meninges.
- Once in the CSF, bacteria have a good chance of survival because humoral defences are in low concentration.
- The tissue dysfunction in bacterial meningitis results from focal lesions due to bacterial growth or toxins, and/or inflammation.

Clinical features

- The clinical presentation of bacterial meningitis depends on the patient's age, the duration of illness, and the causative agent.
- Headache, fever, altered consciousness, vomiting and nuchal rigidity (neck stiffness) are the most common presenting symptoms of bacterial meningitis.
- The mortality rate in bacterial meningitis varies from 5 to 50.
- Up to 10% of those who survive bacterial meningitis experience serious long-term sequelae such as hearing loss, mental retardation or seizures.

Laboratory diagnosis

- CSF is the most important specimen for the diagnosis of meningitis.
- CSF is a body fluid to which Standard Precautions apply.
- Rapid transport of CSF to the laboratory is necessary.
- Blood cultures should also be collected.
- Preliminary results should be available 1–2 hours after receipt of the specimen in the laboratory; they are extremely important because they may enable the differentiation between bacterial and other causes.
- Obvious turbidity in a CSF specimen suggests bacterial infection.
- If tuberculous meningitis is suspected, a Ziehl-Neelsen stain of centrifuged deposit of CSF is performed.

Treatment

- Prompt treatment of any bacterial meningitis is required.
- First-line therapy for acute meningitis is most often with cefotaxime or ceftriaxone.
- Treatment for *Listeria* meningitis is ampicillin or penicillin plus gentamicin.
- Standard anti-tuberculosis drugs are used for tuberculous meningitis.

Prevention

- Vaccines are available for the three major causes of bacterial meningitis.
- To prevent neonatal infection with *Streptococcus agalactiae*, administration of ampicillin to high-risk women during labour is effective.

VIRAL MENINGITIS

- Viral meningitis is the most common type of meningitis.
- The major causes of viral meningitis are enteroviruses (echoviruses, coxsackie viruses, poliovirus).
- The incidence of viral meningitis is greatest in infants and young children.
- The immunocompromised are at increased risk of viral meningitis.
- Aseptic meningitis is a general term used for any meningitis where microorganisms are not isolated by routine bacteriological culture.
- Viral meningitis is generally milder and progresses more slowly than bacterial infections.
- Viral meningitis is usually manifested by acute onset of headache, mild photophobia, low-grade fever, general malaise and minor neck stiffness.
- Laboratory examination of CSF in a case of viral meningitis generally shows increased white cells with a predominance of mononuclear cells (lymphocytes).
- A definitive diagnosis of viral meningitis is usually made by the demonstration of a fourfold rise in antibody titre in acute and convalescent sera.
- Therapy for uncomplicated viral meningitis usually involves symptomatic treatment only.

FUNGAL INFECTIONS

- Fungal meningitis is rare in Australia, except for cryptococcal meningitis, which has become increasingly common in the immunocompromised.
- *Cryptococcus neoformans* var. *neoformans* is widely distributed in soil and is commonly found in large numbers in pigeon droppings.
- *C. neoformans* var. *gattii*, has been isolated from two red gum species in Australia, and is thought to be released as basidiospores from these trees.
- Humans generally become infected with *C. neoformans* var. *neoformans* by inhalation of the organism, after which it causes a primary lung infection. In the immunocompromised the organism invades the bloodstream and spreads to other parts of the body, including the brain and meninges.
- Most infections by *C. neoformans* var. *gattii* occur in people with normal defences.
- If cryptococcal meningitis is suspected, an India ink stain of centrifuged deposit is usually performed to demonstrate the yeast cell and its characteristic capsule.
- Cryptococcal meningitis is confirmed by culture of the organism and by a rapid latex agglutination test which can detect cryptococcal antigen in CSF.

PROTOZOAL INFECTIONS

- Few protozoa infect the central nervous system.
- The importance of *Toxoplasma gondii* has increased markedly since the AIDS epidemic began.
- Cerebral toxoplasmosis is one of the more common neurological complications of HIV infection.
- The clinical manifestations of cerebral toxoplasmosis include headache, fever, clumsiness to hemiplegia, seizures, ataxia and cognitive changes.
- Toxoplasmosis is difficult to diagnose and is most often presumptively based on a CT brain scan and response to empirical therapy.
- Treatment of cerebral toxoplasmosis is with pyrimethamine plus sulphadiazine or clindamycin.

ENCEPHALITIS

- Encephalitis is almost always caused by viruses; herpes simplex virus and numerous arboviruses (arthropod-borne viruses) are the most common.
- Encephalitis may also occur as a rare complication of certain systemic viral infections, like measles, mumps and cytomegalovirus.
- The characteristic manifestations of viral encephalitis represent cerebral dysfunction and include abnormal behaviour, seizures and altered consciousness.

Australian encephalitis (AE)

- AE is a severe, epidemic-type disease found mainly in the northern and eastern parts of Australia and in Papua New Guinea.
- AE is caused mainly by two mosquito-borne viruses: the Murray Valley encephalitis virus (MVE) and the Kunjin virus.
- Epidemics of AE occur mainly during conditions of warm temperature and high rainfall.
- Most infections with the MVE and Kunjin viruses are subclinical, but occasionally they cross the blood-brain barrier and cause damage to the brain tissue.
- Australian encephalitis is diagnosed by serological evidence.
- There is no specific therapy for encephalitis caused by arboviruses.

Herpes encephalitis

- Herpes encephalitis is a very severe disease that causes neurological damage and has a high mortality rate.
- Early diagnosis of herpes encephalitis is important and is usually done by radioactive brain scan, CT scan and EEG.
- Early treatment with acyclovir greatly reduces the mortality and permanent neurological damage.

OTHER INFECTIONS INVOLVING THE NERVOUS SYSTEM

TETANUS

- Tetanus is a rare, but serious, illness caused by the bacterium *Clostridium tetani*.
- Tetanus spores are widespread in soil and manure, because the organism is part of the bowel flora of various animals and some humans.

- Tetanus spores are extremely resistant to drying, disinfectants and heat.
- Since the development of the tetanus vaccine and its widespread use, tetanus has become rare in developed countries.
- To cause infection, tetanus spores must usually be deposited into a deep, necrotic wound where oxygen is lacking.
- After spores enter a wound, bacterial growth and multiplication occur and a potent exotoxin is produced.
- The tetanus toxin travels from the wound along peripheral nerves to the CNS where it blocks the release of transmitters, especially in inhibitory neurones, resulting in an overactivity of motor neurones.
- Death generally results from respiratory failure due to persistent spasm of the respiratory muscles.
- Diagnosis of tetanus is by clinical appraisal.
- Human tetanus immune globulin should be given immediately tetanus is suspected; the wound should be thoroughly cleansed and penicillin given.
- Prevention of tetanus involves immunisation and prophylaxis after a tetanus-prone injury is sustained.
- Immunisation is with tetanus toxoid vaccine.

BOTULISM

- Botulism is a form of food poisoning which affects the nervous system; it is caused by *Clostridium botulinum*.
- Spores of *C. botulinum* are widespread in soil and are often found contaminating meat and vegetables.
- Classically, botulism has been associated with the consumption of canned or preserved foods that have not been adequately sterilised.
- *C. botulinum* also causes botulism in infants, generally related to consumption of honey or ingestion of soil.
- After being ingested and absorbed, the botulinum toxin acts on peripheral nerve synapses, blocking the release of acetylcholine and causing a flaccid paralysis of the muscles.
- Visual disturbances and dysphagia are common early symptoms.
- Eventually, patients may have difficulty breathing and may die from respiratory failure.
- Diagnosis of botulism is mainly by clinical appraisal.
- Treatment involves the administration of polyvalent botulinum antitoxin, and should be commenced as soon as possible.
- Supportive ventilatory and cardiac treatment may be required until the symptoms subside.

LEPROSY

- The World Health Organization estimates there are more than 12 million people in the world with leprosy, mainly in tropical areas in Asia, Africa and Latin America.
- Leprosy is caused by the acid-fast bacillus *Mycobacterium leprae*.
- *M. leprae* is present in large numbers in the nasal secretions of infected people and is probably transmitted mainly by respiratory droplets.
- Leprosy has a very long incubation period; patients may be infected and shedding organisms for years before the onset of symptoms.
- Leprosy is not a highly contagious disease, requiring prolonged close contact for transmission.
- Invasion of Schwann cells by the organism is the basis for the characteristic nerve damage in leprosy.
- *M. leprae* prefers cooler parts of the body such as the skin and peripheral structures like the fingers, ears and nose.
- Laboratory diagnosis of leprosy involves a microscopic examination of nasal scrapings or skin biopsies stained with an acid-fast stain.
- Multidrug therapy should be used in the treatment of leprosy.
- There is no vaccine for leprosy.

RABIES

- The rabies virus can infect almost all warm-blooded animals, and causes disease primarily in animals.
- Almost all cases of rabies in developing countries are due to dog bites.
- Countries that have been declared free of rabies include Australia, England, Japan, Sweden and Norway.
- Rabies virus replicates in muscle fibres and then travels via peripheral nerves and the spinal cord to the brain, where it causes an encephalitis.
- The early symptoms of rabies are headache, fever and partial paralysis at the bite site, followed by more generalised paralysis, muscle spasms, hydrophobia, hypersalivation, aerophobia, confusion, periods of hyperactivity and hallucinations.
- Eventually, the patient becomes comatose and dies usually due to heart or respiratory failure.
- Diagnosis of rabies is based on detection of viral antigens in skin or brain biopsy specimens, or by examination of serum or CSF for specific antibodies.
- Safe, effective vaccines for active immunisation are available.
- All workers and travellers at high risk of contracting rabies in an endemic area should be immunised, as should health professionals who are caring for infected patients.

POLIO

- Polio (or poliomyelitis) is caused by the poliovirus.
- Effective vaccines were developed in the mid-1950s and the incidence in developed countries declined to very low numbers.
- Polio is best known as a cause of paralysis, but the virus produces symptoms in only about 10% of infected people.
- Humans are the only known reservoir of the poliovirus.
- Poliovirus is excreted in the faeces of infected people and is usually transmitted via food, water or hands.

- In the paralytic form of polio, the virus invades the CNS where it infects neurones in the spinal cord and brain.
- High fever, back or neck pain, and muscle spasms are the early symptoms; several days later a flaccid paralysis occurs.
- Laboratory diagnosis of polio involves the isolation of the virus from faeces or a pharyngeal swab.
- In Australia, the oral Sabin vaccine is generally used.

PRION DISEASES

- Prions are transmissible agents that cause a number of progressive, fatal neurodegenerative diseases in humans and animals.
- Prion diseases are sometimes referred to as spongiform encephalopathies.
- The infectious agents are believed to be composed largely, if not entirely, of an abnormal form of a normal cell protein, termed PrP (prion protein).
- Prions lack nucleic acid and have an unusual resistance to ultraviolet light, heat and certain chemical agents.
- One of the remarkable features of all prion diseases is that they do not appear to induce inflammation or a specific immune response.

Creutzfeldt-Jakob disease

- Creutzfeldt-Jakob disease (CJD) is the most important of the human prion diseases.
- Worldwide there is thought to be about one new case of Creutzfeldt-Jakob disease per 1–2 million people each year.
- The natural mode of transmission of CJD is not known.
- Iatrogenic transmission of CJD through corneal transplants, stereotactic equipment, pituitary hormones and dura mater grafts has been reported.
- A number of cases of CJD have been attributed to the use of cadaver-derived pituitary hormones in the United States, the United Kingdom, France, New Zealand and Australia.
- Current evidence suggests a genetic basis for some cases of CJD.
- Early symptoms of CJD may include loss of balance and muscle coordination, slurred speech, failing vision and myoclonic (quick, jerky) movements of the extremities or head, leading to dementia.
- CJD is uniformly fatal, usually in less than a year from the onset of symptoms.
- The demonstration of spongy neuropathological changes and widespread proliferation of astrocytes in brain tissue provides a definitive diagnosis of CJD.
- There is no treatment for CJD and no vaccine.

Study Questions

1. What is the blood-brain barrier?
2. Define the terms 'meningitis' and 'encephalitis'.
3. What are the three most common causes of bacterial meningitis, and how do these organisms reach the meninges?
4. What are the two most common causes of neonatal meningitis, and how do these organisms reach the meninges?
5. What are the critical events in the pathogenesis of acute bacterial meningitis?
6. What are the major clinical features of acute bacterial meningitis?
7. What specimens should be collected from a patient suspected of having meningitis?
8. What preliminary results from the laboratory would be suggestive of a bacterial meningitis?
9. How can meningitis due to *Haemophilus influenzae* be prevented?
10. What is aseptic meningitis?
11. What are the most common causes of viral meningitis?
12. What is the most common cause of fungal meningitis in Australia, and what are the common predisposing factors?
13. What protozoan most commonly causes infection of the central nervous system in Australia, and what are the common predisposing factors?
14. What are the causes of Australian encephalitis and how is this disease transmitted?
15. What factors usually predispose to the development of a brain abscess?
16. What is the causative agent of tetanus and where is this organism commonly found?
17. Describe the pathogenesis of tetanus.
18. How does the treatment of tetanus differ from its prevention?
19. Name the causative agent of botulism and describe the pathogenesis of the disease.
20. Name the causative agent of leprosy and describe how the disease is transmitted.
21. Differentiate between tuberculoid leprosy and lepromatous leprosy.
22. What is rabies?
23. Why is rabies rare in Australia?
24. Describe the pathogenesis of paralytic poliomyelitis.
25. Why is polio a rare disease in Australia?
26. What is a spongiform encephalopathy? Give two examples.
27. What is the cause of Creutzfeldt-Jakob disease and how is it transmitted?
28. What is a prion?

Test Your Understanding

Case History 20.1: Neonatal meningitis

1. What is the most likely cause and source of this infection?
2. What evidence is there to suggest that this is a bacterial infection?
3. What problems are associated with antimicrobial drug treatment of bacterial meningitis?

Case History 20.2: Viral meningitis

1. What is the likely predisposing factor of viral meningitis in this case?
2. What laboratory findings support the diagnosis of viral meningitis?
3. How does the prognosis for viral meningitis compare with that for bacterial meningitis?

Case History 20.3: Australian encephalitis

1. Why was acyclovir given to the child in this case?
2. Why is this referred to as an arbovirus infection?
3. What evidence confirmed this as a case of Australian encephalitis? Explain.

Case History 20.4: Tetanus

1. Why did this woman develop tetanus?
2. What part of the treatment do you think was most responsible for the prevention of serious disease?
3. What is the major pathogenic mechanism of *Clostridium tetani*, and how does this relate to how tetanus is treated?

FURTHER READING

Ashwal, S., R.M. Perkin, J.R. Thompson, S. Schneider, & L.G. Tomasi, 1993, 'Bacterial meningitis in children: current concepts of neurologic management', *Advances in Pediatrics* 40, p. 185. (This extensive review article discusses the epidemiology, clinical manifestations, pathophysiology and treatment of bacterial meningitis.)

Benn, R. & R. Robins-Browne, *Clinical Update Programme: CSF Examination for the Laboratory Diagnosis of Meningitis*, Sydney: University of New South Wales, 1993. (Gives a comprehensive description of the causative agents, clinical features, specimen collection, laboratory diagnosis and interpretation of results in menigitis.)

Nelsen, S., D.P. Sealy & E.F. Schneider, E.F, 1993, 'The aseptic meningitis syndrome', *American Family Physician* 48, p. 809. (A review article concerned with viral meningitis and other causes of aseptic meningitis.)

Oliver, L.G. & A.L. Harwood-Nuss, 1993, 'Bacterial meningitis in infants and children: a review', *Journal of Emergency Medicine* 11, p. 555. (Describes the pathogenesis, clinical manifestations and laboratory diagnosis of bacterial meningitis.)

Prusiner, S.B., 1993, 'Genetic and infectious prion diseases', *Archives of Neurology* 50, p. 1129. (An extensive review of prion diseases of humans and animals.)

Tunkel, A.R. & W.M. Scheld, 1993, 'Pathogenesis and pathophysiology of bacterial meningitis', *Clinical*

Microbiology Reviews 6, p. 118. (Describes in detail current knowledge about the mechanisms by which bacteria cause acute meningitis.)

Tuomanen, E., 1993, 'Breaching the blood-brain barrier', *Scientific American*, February, 56. (Provides a description of the blood-brain barrier and how bacteria may affect its integrity.)

chapter 21

infections of the urinary and reproductive systems

Chapter focus

- *What microorganisms cause urinary tract infections?*
- *How do urinary tract infections develop and what forms of infection occur?*
- *What are the major types of infections that involve the reproductive system?*
- *How can sexually transmissible diseases be prevented?*

In this chapter we examine the infectious diseases of the urinary tract and reproductive systems. The urinary tract is one of the more common sites of infection, especially in females, and is frequently the site of hospital-acquired infection. The reproductive (genital) system has a close anatomical relationship with the urinary tract and is also a common site of infection. Many infections of the genital tract are acquired during sexual activity and are therefore called **sexually transmissible diseases** (STDs). STDs are a major public health problem throughout the world. Both the urinary and genital tracts open to the external environment, and thus microorganisms have ready access to these systems.

Normal Flora of the Urinary and Reproductive Systems

The anatomy of the male and female genitourinary tracts and the sites that have a normal microbial flora are shown in Figure 21.2 (see p. 499). In a healthy person, the upper urethra, the urinary bladder and the organs of the upper urinary tract are sterile. In contrast, the lower urethra has a normal flora that usually includes *Staphylococcus epidermidis, Streptococcus faecalis,* corynebacteria, species of *Neisseria* and *Bacteroides,* and members of the *Enterobacteriaceae,* such as *Escherichia coli* and *Proteus.* The upper regions of the urinary tract are normally kept free of microorganisms by a variety of defence mechanisms. One of the more critical of these is the normal flow of urine that washes over the surface of the urethral epithelium, flushing away microorganisms.

In the genital tract of males, normal flora organisms are found only in the anterior urethra, that is, near the external opening. In contrast, the genital tract of females, in particular the vagina, has a very complex normal flora. This microbial population is significantly influenced by sex hormones and is thus different in neonates, pre-pubertal girls and pre- and post-menopausal women. Its composition also varies during the menstrual cycle.

In adult females, the major residents of the vagina are the lactobacilli. These bacteria assist in maintaining the acidic pH of the normal vagina (around pH 4.4 to 4.6) by breaking down the glycogen in vaginal secretions with the formation of lactic acid. Only microorganisms capable of growth and multiplication at this pH are found in the normal flora. In addition to the lactobacilli, these include enterococci, corynebacteria, a variety of anaerobic bacteria, and the yeast *Candida albicans.* In healthy females, protection against infection of the genital and urinary tracts is afforded by the low pH and the normal flora of the vagina. In situations where the pH and/or the normal flora are modified (e.g. with broad spectrum antibiotic therapy or use of spermicides), infection often ensues.

Urinary Tract Infections

Urinary tract infections occur much more frequently in females. Approximately 10–20% of women experience a urinary tract infection (UTI) at some time in their life. In contrast, less than 5% of males under 60 years of age suffer an episode of urinary tract infection, although the incidence of UTI increases markedly above that age in association with an increased incidence of prostatic hypertrophy (causing urinary obstruction). UTIs represent about 30–40% of all hospital-acquired infections, and are often related to urinary catheterisation. Although the majority of infections are short-lived, recurrences are possible, and severe infections can result in renal damage.

CAUSATIVE ORGANISMS

The vast majority of infections are caused by microorganisms ascending the urethra and reaching the bladder, and then sometimes the kidneys. Occasionally, in patients with septicaemia, organisms spread from the bloodstream to the kidneys to cause infection.

Ascending infections are most often caused by the enteric bacterium, *E. coli.* Other common causes include *Staphylococcus aureus,* coagulase negative staphylococci (*Staphylococcus epidermidis, Staphylococcus saprophyticus*), *Enterococcus faecalis, Pseudomonas* and other *Enterobacteriaceae* such as *Proteus, Klebsiella* and *Enterobacter.* These organisms are derived mainly from the patient's own gastrointestinal tract. Although *E. coli* is the most common cause of both community-acquired and hospital-acquired UTI, many hospital-acquired infections are caused by other organisms, such as *Proteus mirabilis, Staphylococcus aureus, Enterococcus faecalis* and *Pseudomonas aeruginosa* (see Table 21.1). These are often multiply resistant to antibiotics and therefore difficult to treat.

Strictly anaerobic bacteria, viruses, fungi (other than *Candida albicans*), protozoa and helminths are rare causes of UTI. *Leptospira interrogans* is a bacterium which can infect the kidneys of certain mammals, including humans, and it may also spread to other organs (see Chapter 19). A number of sexually transmitted organisms cause urethritis (inflammation of the urethra). These will be discussed in the section on reproductive system infections.

PATHOGENESIS OF URINARY TRACT INFECTIONS

Host factors predisposing to infection

The much higher incidence of urinary tract infection in women is attributed to the proximity of the anus to the urethral opening and the shortness of the female urethra compared with that of males. The proximity of the anal and urethral orifices favours the colonisation of the lower urethra with gastrointestinal flora. The short urethra means that bacteria have less distance to travel to reach the bladder and establish infection (see Figure 21.1). Good personal hygiene is important in preventing the transfer of organisms from the anus to the vagina and periurethral areas. Sexual intercourse can facilitate the movement of organisms into and up the urethra, especially in females, explaining the higher frequency of UTI in the sexually active compared to celibate women.

Because the flushing of microorganisms from the urethra during the normal passage of urine is an important defence mechanism, any factor that prevents normal urine flow or complete bladder emptying makes the individual more susceptible to UTI. Pregnancy, renal calculi, and tumours are common causes of urinary obstruction and predisposing factors of urinary tract infection. In men, there is a marked increase in the incidence of UTI from the age of 50 to 60. This is due to urinary obstruction caused by hypertrophy of the prostate, which becomes more common in older men. Loss of neurological control of the bladder leading to incomplete emptying, such as can occur in paraplegia, also makes the individual more prone to UTI. Retained urine in the bladder provides a reservoir for microbial persistence.

FIGURE 21.1
SUSCEPTIBILITY OF FEMALES TO URINARY TRACT INFECTIONS
Females are more susceptible than males because of the proximity of the anus to the urethra and the shorter urethra.

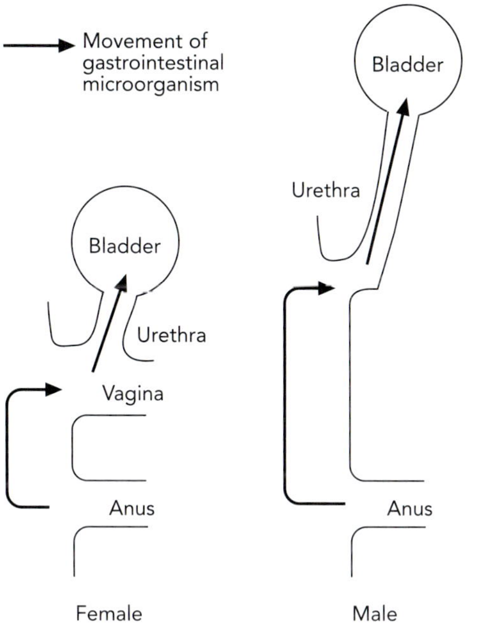

Urinary catheterisation

The high incidence of urinary tract infection in hospitalised people is due mainly to the use of indwelling urinary catheters. Up to 25% of catheterised patients develop a bacteriuria. During insertion of the catheter, bacteria already in the urethra may be carried into the bladder, or, if proper aseptic technique is not used, organisms from the hospital environment or on the hands of a staff member may be introduced. Generally, the longer a catheter is in place the greater the risk of infection, because the catheter provides several potential sites of entry for microorganisms. The catheter also prevents the normal flushing of the urethra with urine, and bacteria are able to move upwards between the outside of the catheter and the surface of the urethra. The longer a catheter is in place, the more its outer surface becomes encrusted with mineral deposits beneath which large numbers of bacteria are able to reside. There the bacteria are protected from host defences and antibiotics.

TABLE 21.1
COMMON CAUSES OF URINARY TRACT INFECTION

	PERCENTAGE OF CASES	
CAUSE	COMMUNITY-ACQUIRED	HOSPITAL-ACQUIRED
■ *E. coli*	80	40
■ Other organisms including: *Proteus mirabilis*, *Klebsiella*, *Enterobacter*, *Pseudomonas aeruginosa*, Coagulase negative staphylococci, *Staphylococcus aureus*, *Candida albicans*	20	60

Bacterial virulence factors

Since *E. coli* is the most common cause of UTI, the bulk of the research into virulence factors of urinary pathogens has centred on this organism. Only certain strains of *E. coli* are able to cause UTI, and this has been attributed mainly to their possession of pili. These are filamentous protein structures (see Chapter 4) that allow the bacteria to attach to the urethral and bladder epithelium. Non-piliated strains of *E. coli* that cause UTI are thought to have other adhesins that allow them to stick to epithelium. Adhesins have also been identified in other urinary tract pathogens.

Other virulence factors that have been attributed to urinary pathogens include the capsular polysaccharide (K) antigens of *E. coli*, which help it to evade phagocytosis by tissue macrophages, and urease production, as is found in *Proteus* species and some strains of *E. coli*. These urease-producing organisms are thought to survive well on the outer surface of catheters by encrusting themselves with minerals released from the breakdown of urea, protecting themselves as described above.

SITES AND CLINICAL FEATURES OF URINARY TRACT INFECTIONS

Microorganisms that cause UTIs usually ascend the urinary tract. Infection may initially be in the urethra, resulting in an inflammation of that site, called **urethritis**. As the organisms ascend the tract, subsequent infection of the bladder may occur. The bladder tissue becomes inflamed, and the patient is said to have **cystitis.** In some cases, the organisms may travel further up the urinary tract and infect the kidney(s), resulting in inflammation of one or both kidneys, which is called **pyelonephritis**. It is also possible for individuals to have large numbers of bacteria in their urine without displaying any symptoms. This is termed an **asymptomatic bacteriuria**.

Asymptomatic bacteriuria

As there are no symptoms present, asymptomatic bacteriuria is usually detected during routine screening of the patient. It is thought to represent multiplication of bacteria in the bladder urine, without involvement of tissues, although in some cases actual bladder or kidney infection is present. In the majority of cases, treatment is unnecessary because infection never occurs. However, in pregnant women, young children and people about to undergo instrumentation of the urinary tract there is a significant risk of renal infection. In such cases treatment is warranted.

Cystitis

Acute infections of the bladder are usually characterised by symptoms of:

- **dysuria**—difficult or painful (burning) urination;
- **urgency**—an urgent need to urinate;
- **frequency**—the need to urinate more frequently than usual.

In addition, the urine is cloudy due to the presence of large numbers of leucocytes (**pyuria**) in response to infection, and may occasionally contain blood (**haematuria**) because of tissue damage.

Infections of the bladder recur in some people, with the possibility of scarring and permanent damage to the urinary tract. Such recurrences may be caused by either the same or different organisms.

Pyelonephritis

Infection of the kidney(s) can result from movement of bacteria upwards from the bladder, or occasionally from the bloodstream. The clinical presentation of pyelonephritis is similar to that of cystitis, although, in pyelonephritis, fever and haematuria are more common. Flank pain and tenderness in the kidney region may also be present. Pyelonephritis is a serious condition because there is a potential for serious kidney damage. Should pyelonephritis become chronic, permanent damage and loss of kidney function may occur.

Laboratory diagnosis

The appropriate methods for collection and transport of urine specimens for diagnosis of UTIs are described in Chapter 15. The specimen most commonly collected is a 'clean-catch' or mid-stream specimen of urine (MSU). Urine may be collected by other methods, depending on the circumstances—for example, suprapubic aspiration of urine from young children, a specimen from an indwelling urinary catheter, or a specimen collected during cystoscopy.

An amount of 2–50 mL should be collected into a sterile, plastic, wide-mouth container. Because urine is a good growth medium, and quantitative bacterial counts are required (see below), the specimen should be transported to the laboratory without delay. The specimen may be refrigerated if a delay is unavoidable or if another specimen cannot be collected at a more appropriate time.

Usually, patients are started on antibiotic threapy before the results of the laboratory tests are available. Wherever possible, it is important that the urine specimen is collected before antibiotic therapy is initiated, so that an accurate laboratory diagnosis is obtained (see Chapter 15).

In the laboratory the urine specimen is examined microscopically and cultured. A microscopic examination of urine allows the presence of white cells, red cells, epithelial cells, casts and bacteria to be determined. The presence of any one of these does not necessarily demonstrate infection, but all of them, together with culture results, are used to build a clinical picture from which a diagnosis can be made. Most patients with symptomatic infection have pyuria (a raised polymorphonuclear cell count), but pyuria without infection is common. The clinical significance of these microscopic elements is summarised in Table 21.2.

Since the lower urethra is usually colonised by bacteria, even properly collected MSU specimens may be contaminated with periurethral organisms during collection.

FIGURE 21.2
THE MALE AND FEMALE GENITOURINARY TRACTS AND THE AREAS WHERE NORMAL FLORA RESIDE (COLOURED)

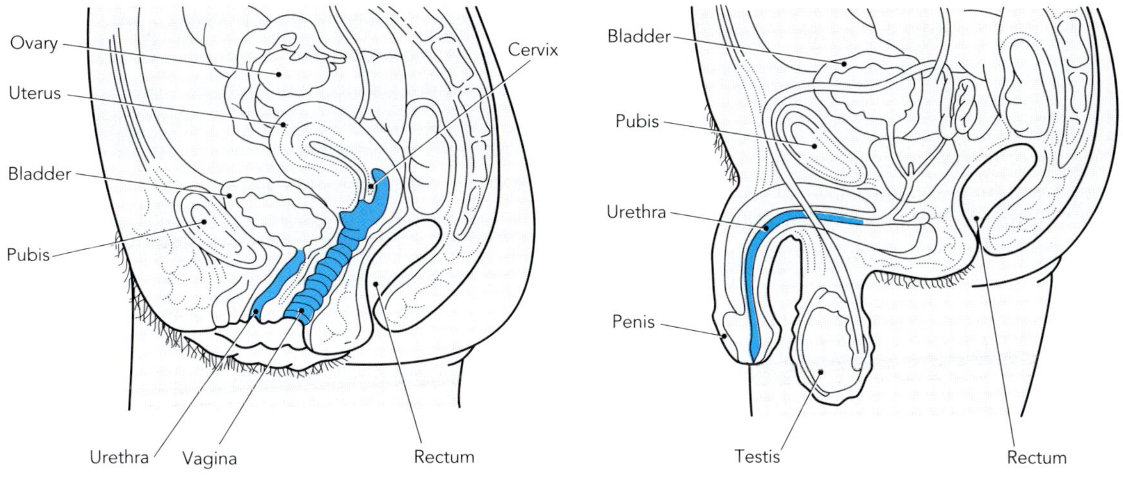

TABLE 21.2
THE CLINICAL SIGNIFICANCE OF URINARY ELEMENTS FOUND DURING MICROSCOPIC EXAMINATION OF URINE

ELEMENT	POSSIBLE CLINICAL SIGNIFICANCE
White cells (> 4 per hpf* or > 10^8/L)	■ bacterial infection ■ acute glomerulonephritis ■ bladder tumour ■ drug therapy ■ strenuous exercise
Red cells (> 2 per hpf)	■ infection of the kidney or bladder ■ renal trauma ■ renal calculi ■ malaria ■ endocarditis ■ carcinoma of the urinary tract
Epithelial cells (> 10 per hpf)	■ poor specimen collection (i.e. not a mid-stream urine) ■ inflammatory conditions of upper urinary tract
Casts (more than occasional)	■ infection ■ many other types of renal disease

* high power field

Since some species of bacteria found in the lower urethra are also potential urinary pathogens, the *number* of bacteria in a urine sample is more important than their mere presence. Infection can be distinguished from contamination with quantitative culture methods.

Significant bacteriuria is usually defined as a count of 10^8/L in a properly collected MSU. However, it should be recognised that, in certain situations, fewer than this number may represent infection. Less than 10^8/L can be significant in:

- some women with acute symptoms of lower UTI;
- infections caused by Gram-positive bacteria, fungi, or slow-growing or fastidious organisms;
- catheter specimens;
- specimens collected during cystoscopy;
- specimens collected by suprapubic aspiration;
- specimens from patients already receiving antibiotic therapy;
- specimens from patients with high urine output (causing dilution of the bacteria).

There are also several rapid methods in use for detecting bacteriuria including filtration, bioluminescence and photometric techniques.

A number of laboratory findings indicate improper specimen collection. One or more of the following in a supposed MSU casts doubt on its quality:

- greater than normal numbers of epithelial cells;
- culture of more than one type of bacterium (since most UTIs are caused by a single organism, except in patients with an indwelling catheter, calculi or malignancy);
- the presence of organisms without white cells (in some cases);
- the presence of Gram-positive rods (i.e. lactobacilli from vaginal flora).

Treatment and management

The choice of antimicrobial therapy should be based on culture and sensitivity results. This is particularly important in nosocomial or recurrent infections, which may be caused by antibiotic-resistant organisms. In catheterised patients, management includes the removal or replacement of the catheter, since it is likely to be acting as a source of infection. Supportive measures such as the raising of the pH of the urine with urinary alkalinisers (to slow bacterial growth) and high fluid intake (to help to flush out organisms) may also be instituted. Because of the seriousness of pyelonephritis compared to lower urinary tract infection, more aggressive therapy (e.g. intravenous rather than oral antibiotics) for a longer period (e.g. 10 days) is warranted. Unfortunately, pyelonephritis is not always distinguished from cystitis by either clinical or laboratory findings.

Prevention

The incidence of community-acquired UTI in women may be reduced by such measures as promotion of good personal hygiene, adequate fluid intake and regular emptying of the bladder. In hospitals, prevention is based on similar principles plus avoidance of catheterisation wherever possible and proper catheter care. Suggested guidelines for catheter care are listed in Table 21.3.

TABLE 21.3
PROCEDURES FOR THE PREVENTION OF CATHETER-ASSOCIATED URINARY TRACT INFECTION

- Avoid catheterisation of a patient where possible.
- Catheter and associated equipment must be sterile before use.
- Wash hands thoroughly before and after inserting a catheter or other manipulation of the catheter.
- The external meatal opening should be cleansed prior to insertion of the catheter.
- The catheter must be inserted using good aseptic technique.
- The catheter should be inserted in such a way as to cause minimal damage to mucosal surfaces.
- A closed drainage system should be used wherever possible.
- The catheter tubing should not be allowed to come loose from the collecting bag.
- The collecting bag must not be allowed to fill to the level of the inlet tube.
- Keep duration of catheterisation to a minimum.
- Use intermittent rather than continuous catheterisation where possible.

CASE HISTORY 21.1
URINARY TRACT INFECTION

An 18-year-old female presented with symptoms of left flank pain, fever, chills and increased urinary frequency. The patient said that she knew how to collect a urine specimen and did so herself. The specimen was sent to the laboratory and the results of urinalysis included:

- > 50 white cells per high power field;
- > 10 squamous epithelial cells per high power field;
- > 10^8 *Escherichia coli* and >10^8 *Streptococcus faecalis* per litre.

Comment

The interpretation of these results that was included in the laboratory report stated that the patient could have a urinary tract infection, but that the specimen was probably contaminated.

Infections of the Reproductive System

Most diseases of the reproductive (genital) system are transmitted during sexual activity and thus are referred to as **sexually transmissible diseases (STDs).** They were formerly called venereal diseases, after Venus, the Roman goddess of love. However, it should also be recognised that a number of sexually transmissible diseases can also be transmitted by other body fluids, especially blood and blood products (e.g. the human immunodeficiency virus (HIV) and the hepatitis B and C viruses). Table 21.4 lists the common sexually transmissible diseases and syndromes and their causative agents. Notice that some syndromes (e.g. urethritis, pelvic inflammatory disease) can be caused by a number of different organisms. This can make the diagnosis and treatment of infection much more difficult. All these syndromes are discussed in this chapter, except for AIDS (see Chapter 19) and hepatitis (see Chapter 18) because these two infections predominantly involve body systems other than the genital tract.

Although many of the genital infections are preventable if appropriate precautions (e.g. use of condoms) are taken, and many are readily cured with antimicrobial treatment, they still represent a major health problem in both developed and undeveloped countries throughout the world. The World Health Organization (WHO) estimates that worldwide there are about 250 million new cases of STD each year. Reasons commonly given for the continuing high incidence of STDs include:

- increased sexual activity at a younger age;
- increased promiscuity and a greater number of sexual partners;
- the production of little or no symptoms by some pathogens;
- the social stigma of these diseases and the non-seeking of medical advice and/or notification of sexual partners;
- the sexual freedom resulting from contraception;
- ignorance;
- the failure to use barrier preventative measures (e.g. condoms).

The numbers of cases of STDs reported by health authorities generally represent only a fraction of the actual cases, because many are not diagnosed. As you will see, in some STDs a large percentage of infected people may be asymptomatic. Furthermore, many symptomatic people do not seek medical advice, because of the social stigma associated with sexually transmissible diseases.

STDs are also of major health importance because there is a strong association between the organisms that cause genital ulceration (e.g. syphilis, herpes, chancroid) and transmission of the human immunodeficiency virus (HIV), especially in heterosexuals. It is thought that this relationship exists partly because genital ulcers provide

TABLE 21.4
SEXUALLY TRANSMISSIBLE DISEASES AND THEIR CAUSATIVE AGENTS

SYNDROME	CAUSATIVE AGENTS
Gonorrhoea	*Neisseria gonorrhoea*
Syphilis	*Treponema pallidum*
Urethritis	*Neisseria gonorrhoeae* *Chlamydia trachomatis* *Ureaplasma urealyticum* Herpes simplex virus
Vulvitis	*Candida albicans* Herpes simplex virus *Trichomonas vaginalis*
Vaginosis	*Trichomonas vaginalis* *Candida albicans* *Gardnerella vaginalis* *Bacteroides* spp.
Cervicitis	*Neisseria gonorrhoea* *Chlamydia trachomatis* Herpes simplex virus
Balanitis	*Candida albicans* Herpes simplex virus
Genital warts and carcinoma	Human papilloma viruses
Genital ulceration	Herpes simplex virus *Treponema pallidum* *Haemophilus ducreyi* *Chlamydia trachomatis* *Calymmatobacterium granulomatis*
Pelvic inflammatory disease (mostly salpingitis)	*Neisseria gonorrhoeae* *Chlamydia trachomatis* *Mycoplasma hominis* Vaginal normal flora
AIDS	Human immunodeficiency viruses 1 and 2
Hepatitis	Hepatitis A, B, C, D viruses

a portal of entry for the HIV, and partly because STDs are markers for individuals with high-risk sexual behaviours.

GONORRHOEA

Causative organism and incidence

Gonorrhoea is an infection caused by the bacterium *Neisseria gonorrhoeae*, sometimes called the 'gonococcus'. It is named after Albert Neisser who first described it in 1879. The disease was somewhat misnamed as gonorrhoea (after the ancient Greek *gonos* meaning 'seed', and *rhoia* meaning 'flow') because the male urethral discharge was mistaken for semen. The bacterium is a Gram-negative round or oval-shaped diplococcus with flattened sides, so that it often has the appearance of a pair of coffee beans.

In the United States, about 700 000 cases of *N. gonorrhoeae* infection are reported to the Centers for Disease Control each year. It is thought that the real incidence is two to three times that number. Currently in Australia, there are about 3000 notifications of gonococcal infection received per year by the National Notifiable Diseases Surveillance System. This includes gonorrhoea and other forms of gonococcal infection (e.g. eye infections), but the vast majority are genital infections. The peak incidence occurs in males in the 20–24 years age group.

Transmission

N. gonorrhoeae is fairly sensitive to drying and survives for only a short time on dry surfaces. It can, however, survive for several hours in pus. Given its inability to survive well outside the body, it is usually transmitted by direct person-to-person contact. It is a disease only of humans.

The efficiency of transmission appears to be gender-dependent. It is thought that an infected male will transmit the infection 60% of the time to non-infected contacts, whereas a female will transmit it only 30% of the time. This difference seems to be related to the high organism load in semen. There are several high-risk transmission factors, the most important being multiple sexual partners and disregard of safe sex practices. Pharyngeal and rectal infections have become more common in both homosexuals and heterosexuals because of more varied sexual practices.

N. gonorrhoeae can also be transmitted vertically from an infected mother to baby at birth. This usually results in an eye infection called **ophthalmia neonatorum** (see Chapter 16). While this infection has been controlled in many Western countries through the use of antibiotics or silver nitrate eye-drops, it remains a major problem in developing countries.

Pathogenesis

Once the gonococci are introduced into the vagina or the urethra of males, they attach by way of pili to the mucosal cells. This attachment prevents them from being washed away by the flow of urine or vaginal secretions. The bacteria multiply rapidly and spread up to the cervix in females or up the urethra in males. Spread of the bacteria is facilitated by their production of an IgA protease which inactivates IgA antibodies found in mucous secretions. The bacteria invade the epithelial cells lining the cervix and urethra and multiply within them. Inside these cells they are protected from phagocytes and antibodies. Eventually, they are discharged from the basement membrane of the epithelial cells into the subepithelial connective tissue. There they cause local damage and elicit an inflammatory response. Occasionally, they invade blood vessels and then spread to other parts of the body, such as joints. Persistent infections cause chronic inflammation and fibrosis of the tissues.

Clinical features

Symptoms usually develop within a week (often in 1–2 days) of infection. In men gonococcal infection is usually characterised by a urethral discharge (see Figure 21.3) and **dysuria** (pain on passing urine). The infection may be very mild or asymptomatic in up to 50% of cases. A small percentage of untreated cases can develop an **epididymitis** (infection and inflammation of the epididymis).

As many as 50% of infected women have very mild symptoms or are completely asymptomatic. Symptomatic infection is usually characterised by a cervico-vaginal discharge and cervical oedema. Abnormal menses, dyspareunia (painful intercourse) and dysuria (due to urethral infection) are also common. The asymptomatic nature of infection in many women is important for two main reasons. First, they are an important, unrecognised source of infection. Second, in up to 30% of untreated women, the infection spreads further up the genital tract to cause inflammation in the fallopian tubes **(salpingitis)** and sometimes the ovaries **(oophoritis)**, or in the whole of the peritoneal cavity **(peritonitis).** Inflammation in any of these sites is called **pelvic inflammatory disease (PID)**.

Persistent infection, especially in the fallopian tubes, can cause scarring and blockage of the tubes, leading to infertility or ectopic (tubal) pregnancy, as well as increased susceptibility to recurrent attacks of PID. Pelvic inflammatory disease is not due solely to *N. gonorrhoeae.* Other organisms, especially *Chlamydia trachomatis,* can also cause it, alone, or in coexistence with the gonococcus. PID is dealt with more fully on pages 509 ff.

Anorectal infection is often asymptomatic, but otherwise is characterised by rectal pain, discharge, constipation and tenesmus (painful defecation). Gonococcal pharyngitis, acquired during oral sex, is clinically indistinguishable from any other bacterial pharyngitis, but is also usually asymptomatic. Disseminated gonococcal infection is rare. Usually, joint symptoms (tenosynovitis or arthritis), a skin rash (pustular haemorrhagic or necrotic) and fever are the major manifestations. A meningitis or endocarditis is also possible.

FIGURE 21.3
A PURULENT URETHRAL DISCHARGE IN A MALE WITH GONORRHOEA

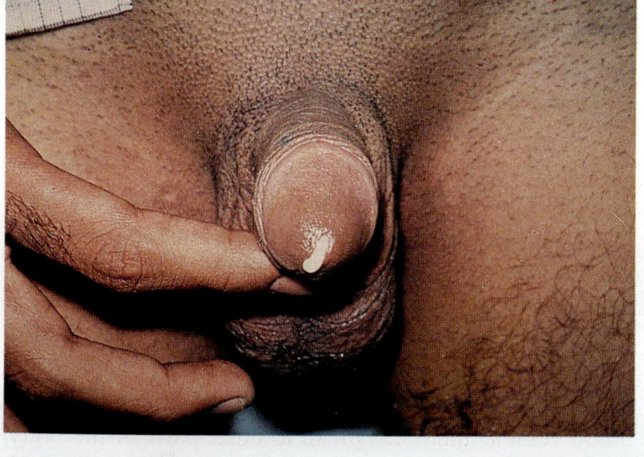

Diagnosis

Diagnosis is based on microscopy and culture of an appropriate specimen. In men, this is a urethral swab of urethral discharge. In women, a cervical swab should be collected and, additionally (not alternatively), a sample of vaginal discharge if purulent. A rapid, presumptive diagnosis can be made from a Gram stain if intracellular Gram-negative diplococci are seen.

It should be remembered that the organism is sensitive to drying and extremes of temperature, so the specimen should be inoculated directly onto culture media at the bedside or transported immediately to the laboratory. Swabs should be sent in transport medium containing activated charcoal (to neutralise toxic substances in cotton swabs), and must not be refrigerated.

All patients found to have an STD should be evaluated for other STDs. As noted, in gonorrhoea, *Chlamydia* co-infection is common, and concurrent *Trichomonas* infection may exist in a significant proportion of women. All patients should also be evaluated for syphilis, HIV infection and hepatitis B.

Treatment and prevention

Since the early 1980s there has been a marked increase in the incidence of antibiotic resistance in *N. gonorrhoeae.* This resistance is mediated by two major mechanisms: plasmid transfer and chromosomal mutation. Through plasmid transfer, strains of gonococci have become markedly resistant to penicillin (due to penicillinase production—see Chapter 12) or tetracycline, or both. The penicillinase-producing strains are sometimes referred to as PPNG (penicillinase-producing *Neisseria gonorrhoeae*). In some strains, chromosomal mutation has resulted in a gradual accumulation of resistance to penicillin, tetracycline, second generation cephalosporins and erythromycin.

Chromosomal and plasmid-mediated resistance can occur separately, or together. The Microbiology Department of The Prince of Wales Hospital, Sydney, has been established as a World Health Organization reference centre to monitor resistance in *N. gonorrhoeae* in the Western Pacific region.

Currently, treatment is usually with ceftriaxone, ciprofloxacin or spectinomycin (although some resistance to spectinomycin has been reported). Since many patients have a coexistent infection with *Chlamydia trachomatis,* treatment should also include an effective anti-chlamydial drug, usually a tetracycline or erythromycin. Failure to treat coexistent *Chlamydia* infection contributes to the incidence of pelvic inflammatory disease. Prevention of gonorrhoea is based on the use of condoms and the tracing and presumptive treatment of patient contacts. Despite extensive effort, no vaccine is currently available.

SYPHILIS

Causative organism and incidence

Syphilis is an STD that has been recognised for centuries, although its incidence has waned in recent years. It is caused by the spirochaete *Treponema pallidum,* a thin, coiled and highly motile organism with fastidious growth requirements. There are about 2000–3000 cases of syphilis notified in Australia per year. The highest incidences occur in some Aboriginal populations, especially in the Northern Territory.

Transmission

Transmission of syphilis requires close, personal contact. The organism survives poorly outside the body because it is very sensitive to drying, heat (as low as 42°C) and disinfectants. The organism is present in the skin or mucous membrane lesions of an infected person and enters the body of a sexual contact through the mucous membranes or through abrasions (even minute) in the skin. An infected woman may also transmit the organism to her foetus *in utero*, especially after the first trimester, often resulting in congenital malformations.

Pathogenesis and clinical features

The treponemes typically multiply slowly and so after infection there is an average incubation period of three weeks before symptoms develop. Classically, the course of infection is divided into three stages, but not all patients experience all the stages.

1. **Primary syphilis** is characterised by the development of a papular lesion at the site of infection, usually on the genitals, but sometimes on the rectum, lip or hand. In males, there is usually a lesion on the penis which is seen, but in females the primary lesion usually occurs on the cervix, and therefore often goes unnoticed. The papular lesion breaks down to form a painless, hard-based ulcer, called a **chancre** (see Figure 21.4). The papule and ulcer contain large numbers of organisms and are highly infectious. Also, inguinal lymph nodes may be enlarged. In 2–6 weeks the lesion heals spontaneously, to the relief of those who have not sought medical advice. Unfortunately, this is often only a temporary respite.
2. In approximately 50% of untreated cases, **secondary syphilis** develops 2–10 weeks later. From the time of initial infection, the treponemes begin to spread from the site of entry to local lymph nodes and then to the bloodstream. The secondary stage involves the multiplication of bacteria and the production of lesions, especially in skin and mucous membranes. It is characterised by the appearance of a red, maculopapular rash anywhere on the skin, anogenital region, mouth, throat or cervix (see Figure 21.5). The rash may even occur on the palms or soles of the feet. This may be accompanied by malaise and mild fever. These lesions are also rich in treponemes and are highly infectious. The symptoms again subside spontaneously after a few weeks, and there follows a prolonged asymptomatic period of anywhere between 3 and 30 years.
3. After this latent period, signs of disease reappear in about 30% of untreated cases. This is called **tertiary** (or late) **syphilis**. Renewed multiplication, dissemination and a cell-mediated hypersensitivity response of the immune system combine to form lesions in various organs. Soft, granulomatous lesions (**gummas**) may form in the skin, bones, liver or other organs. If lesions form in the central nervous system, **neurosyphilis** is the result. Degenerative changes may lead to mental illness, paresis (weakness or partial paralysis), or tabes dorsalis (poor muscle coordination and unstable gait). The paresis plus gradual loss of higher integrative functions in tertiary syphilis is sometimes referred to as 'general paralysis of the insane'. In **cardiovascular syphilis** aortic aneurysm and blood vessel and valve damage may occur, leading to heart failure. The treponemes are rarely found in the lesions of tertiary syphilis because the symptoms are apparently due mainly to the host response.

FIGURE 21.4
THE CHANCRE OF PRIMARY SYPHILIS ON PENIS

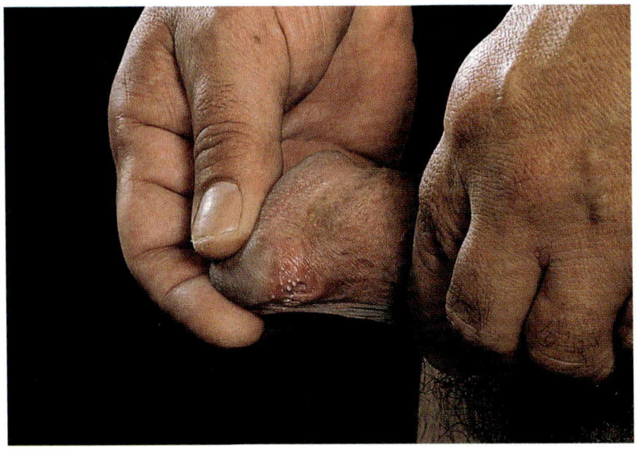

FIGURE 21.5
SECONDARY SYPHILIS SHOWING A PAPULAR RASH

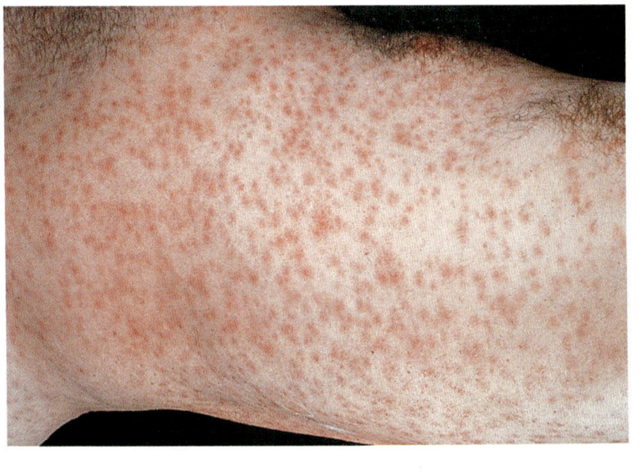

The pathogenesis and clinical features of syphilis are summarised in Table 21.5.

Congenital infection occurs when the organism crosses the placenta. In many cases the infection may not become apparent for many months after birth, but in some it may cause miscarriage, stillbirth or severe symptoms at birth. Possible congenital abnormalities include mental retardation, blindness, deafness, bone disease and, later, facial and tooth deformities.

Diagnosis

Treponema pallidum cannot be readily grown in the laboratory. Therefore, the laboratory diagnosis of syphilis hinges on microscopic and serologic methods. The quickest and most direct method is microscopy. The primary and secondary lesions of syphilis usually contain large numbers of organisms. The bacteria may be readily seen in exudate from the lesions when examined by dark ground microscopy (see Figure 3.2, p. 46) or in a UV microscope after treating the specimen with fluorescein-labelled anti-treponemal antibodies. The exudate must be sent to the laboratory immediately after collection for examination. Because the exudate is highly infectious it must be handled with care.

In the absence of lesions, serology is the mainstay of diagnosis. The serological tests used are of two types: the non-specific (non-treponemal) tests and the specific (treponemal) tests. The non-specific tests do not detect antibodies to treponemal antigens, but rather detect an antibody-like substance called reagin. The antigen used in these assays is cardiolipin, an extract from normal mammalian tissue. The two non-specific tests in common use are the VDRL (Venereal Diseases Research Laboratory) and the RPR (Rapid Plasma Reagin). False positive results are common with these non-specific methods, so a positive result is confirmed using one or two specific tests. The fluorescent treponemal antibody absorption test (FTA-ABS) and the *Treponema pallidum* haemagglutination assay (TPHA) detect anti-treponemal antibodies and are the two specific tests in common use.

Treatment

Penicillin is very active against *Treponema pallidum* and is the drug of choice. A single intramuscular injection

> **CASE HISTORY 21.2**
> **SYPHILIS**
>
> A 27-year-old man attended a casualty department because he had a rash over his trunk and the palms of his hands. He also complained of being hot and nauseous. The papular rash was suspected to represent the secondary stage of syphilis.
>
> *Comment*
>
> Very few infections produce a rash on the palms of the hands or soles of the feet. Syphilis would be a consideration in a sexually active person with such symptoms.

TABLE 21.5
PATHOGENESIS AND CLINICAL FEATURES OF SYPHILIS

STAGE OF DISEASE	PATHOGENESIS	SIGNS AND SYMPTOMS
Incubation period (2–10 weeks)	Multiplication at site of entry	
Primary syphilis (lasting 2–6 weeks)	Spread to regional lymph nodes and bloodstream	■ primary chancre ■ enlarged inguinal nodes
Asymptomatic period (2–10 weeks)		
Secondary syphilis (2–6 weeks)	Multiplication in extra-genital sites	■ maculopapular rash anywhere on skin or mucous membranes ■ malaise and mild fever
Asymptomatic period (3–30 years)	Organisms dormant in liver, spleen and central nervous system	
Tertiary syphilis	Renewed multiplication and invasion plus a cell-mediated hypersensitivity response	■ gummas in skin, bone, liver ■ cardiovascular syphilis: – aortic lesions – heart failure ■ neurosyphilis: – general paresis of insane – tabes dorsalis

of benzathine penicillin remains active in the body for two weeks and is usually effective for syphilis of less than two years duration. For older infections, three intramuscular injections at weekly intervals, or daily injections of procaine penicillin for three weeks are the usual regimes. If the patient is allergic to penicillin, tetracycline or erythromycin are also effective.

Prevention

Prevention is based on the practice of safe sex, and contact tracing and screening. Prevention of secondary and tertiary disease depends on early diagnosis and treatment. Congenital infection is preventable if women are screened serologically early in pregnancy and treated.

CHLAMYDIAL INFECTIONS

Causative organisms and incidence

The *Chlamydia* are very small bacteria which are obligate intracellular parasites. Three species are currently recognised, but only *Chlamydia trachomatis* infects the genital tract. This species can be subdivided into different serotypes (serovars) which are associated with different infections:

- serotypes A, B and C cause an eye infection called trachoma (see Chapter 16);
- serotypes D to K cause genital and associated infections;
- serotypes L1, L2 and L3 cause a specific genital infection called lymphogranuloma venereum.

Genital chlamydial infections caused by serotypes D to K have a high incidence in many countries, and are currently the most prevalent of all STDs. The Centers for Disease Control in the United States estimates that 3–5 million Americans each year have a urethritis caused by *Chlamydia*. In Australia, *Chlamydia* infection has the third highest incidence of any notifiable disease, with about 6500 cases notified each year, but the real incidence is probably many times that number. The highest rates of notification come from the Aboriginal populations in the Kimberley Statistical Division and the Northern Territory. The large number of people who are infected asymptomatically and who shed the organism in their genital secretions makes transmission very easy.

Lymphogranuloma venereum (LGV) is a serious disease found in restricted regions of the world, particularly tropical and subtropical Africa, Asia and South America. It is a notifiable disease in only some Australian States. There are fewer than five cases a year notified.

Pathogenesis and clinical features

Serotypes D to K probably enter through minute abrasions in the mucosal surface. The organisms grow in columnar and transitional epithelial cells and the clinical disease is then determined by the site of infection. Localisation and infection in the urethra is termed **chlamydial urethritis**. Infection of the cervix leads to **cervicitis**, and spread from there to the fallopian tubes is called **salpingitis** or **pelvic inflammatory disease** (see p. 509). However, many infections, especially in women, are asymptomatic or produce only mild symptoms, even when the upper parts of the genital tract are involved.

In LGV, a primary lesion develops at the site of organism inoculation (usually on the genitals, but occasionally in the oral cavity or rectum) within two weeks of infection. The lesion heals rapidly, but draining lymph nodes become infected. Typically, inguinal buboes form, which gradually enlarge. Abscesses may form in the nodes and eventually suppurate and discharge through the skin. The organisms may spread via the lymphatics to the rectum (proctitis) and other tissues (e.g. pneumonitis, meningo-encephalitis, hepatitis).

Diagnosis

Chlamydial infections cannot be reliably distinguished from infections caused by other organisms by clinical examination alone, and so laboratory testing is essential. Serological assays and direct fluorescence microscopy of an appropriate specimen are the most commonly used, but are not highly sensitive methods. Culture is the gold standard, but is slow and requires specialised techniques because the organism can be grown only in cell culture (it is an obligate intracellular parasite). For culture or microscopy, a cervical or urethral specimen is usually collected (by scraping the site with a swab in order to obtain infected cells), as well as discharge. A first-catch urine sample may also be a useful additional specimen. In women with salpingitis, a needle aspirate may be collected. In LGV, bubo pus or tissue biopsy are the common specimens. Swabs, scrapings and small amounts of tissue should be transported in an appropriate transport medium.

Treatment

Treatment is usually with tetracycline or azithromycin. Sexual contacts should also be treated whether or not they are symptomatic, because of the ease of spread and

CASE HISTORY 21.3
URETHRITIS

Mr C., a 30-year-old, attended a doctor's surgery because of a purulent discharge from his penis. The doctor suspected gonorrhoea and gave him an intramuscular injection of penicillin. His condition improved initially, but in 14 days he returned to the doctor because he still had a discharge, although milder. He stated that he had not had sex since his last visit. This time, a sample of discharge was sent to a pathology laboratory. *Neisseria gonorrhoeae* could not be seen in a Gram stain of the smear and was not cultured.

Comment

There is a failure of therapy in this case. Without a laboratory diagnosis it is difficult to know the actual cause of Mr C's infection.

the potential seriousness of fallopian tube infection. Because concurrent chlamydial and gonococcal infections are common, patients receiving treatment for gonorrhoea should also receive treatment for *Chlamydia*.

GENITAL HERPES

Causative agents and incidence

There are two major types of herpes simplex virus: herpes simplex virus type 1 (HSV-1) and herpes simplex type 2 (HSV-2). Both types have been found to cause genital and oral (cold sores) herpes, but type 2 predominates in the genital region, whereas type 1 is the more common cause of oral infection.

Infection with at least one of the herpes viruses seems to occur in most people, although mainly asymptomatically. Up to 75% of adults have antibodies to HSV-1, and up to 50% have antibodies to HSV-2. Approximately 15% of women attending public antenatal clinics are found to be seropositive for HSV-2, and the prevalence is much higher in homosexual men, prostitutes and people attending STD clinics. The Centers for Disease Control in Atlanta estimates that 30 million adults in the United States have recurrent genital herpes. National notifications are not compiled in Australia.

Pathogenesis and clinical features

HSV-2 is readily inactivated at room temperature and by drying. Therefore, transmission is essentially by direct contact with infected secretions or mucosal surfaces. The virus appears able to invade intact mucosal surfaces, but probably infects skin only through breaks or abrasions.

Initial infection may be completely asymptomatic or so mild that it is unrecognised. As many as 50–70% of genital herpes infections may fall into this category. The majority of people with antibodies to HSV-2 do not have a history of clinical genital herpes. If symptomatic, the primary lesions usually occur on the penis, anus, vulva, cervix or vagina 3–14 days after exposure. The lesions are usually small, grouped vesicles filled with a clear fluid and surrounded by an area of inflammation (see Figure 21.6). The vesicles break down after several days to form painful, shallow ulcers. If the lesions occur over a large area of the genitalia, walking, or even the wearing of clothing, can be painful.

Local lymph nodes are usually swollen. Neurologic signs (headache, stiff neck, photophobia) occur in some primary infections, reflecting a viral meningitis. In males, a urethritis with a watery discharge may occur. Herpes pharyngitis can occur after oral sexual contact.

The primary lesions usually heal within two weeks, but by that time the virus has travelled up the local sensory nerve to the sensory root ganglion where it lies dormant. Virus persistence there lasts for a lifetime. From there, it can reactivate and travel back down the nerve. There it exits the cell and is shed asymptomatically or spreads to, and infects, mucocutaneous epithelial cells, causing cell destruction and new lesions. There is considerable variation in the frequency of symptomatic recurrent attacks. In some people recurrence is rare, whereas others may have many recurrent attacks a year. The lesions in recurrent attacks are usually fewer in number and resolve sooner than the primary lesions, probably because specific immune mechanisms limit viral replication. The important point to note is that recurrent infection may or may not be symptomatic, and that an asymptomatic person can be shedding the virus. Shedding always occurs when lesions are present, and usually a few days before they appear.

Latency, reactivation and recurrent infections are typical of herpes viruses. HSV-1 undergoes a similar cycle in sensory nerves and cutaneous tissue in causing recurrent cold sores. The mechanisms involved in the reactivation of herpes viruses are not known, except that it can occur apparently spontaneously or in response to certain stimuli such as physical or emotional stress, ultraviolet light and fever.

HSV-2 can also be transmitted from a symptomatic or asymptomatic mother to her baby during pregnancy, at birth, or postnatally. The great majority of neonatal infections are acquired at birth, especially if the mother is suffering from primary infection at that time. The virus can invade the skin, eyes, CNS and visceral organs. In many cases this infection is fatal, and in a large proportion of non-fatal infections, mental retardation, and defective sight and hearing are typical outcomes. HSV-2 can also cause severe to fatal infections in patients with immunodeficiency (e.g. AIDS).

Diagnosis

The diagnosis of genital herpes is sometimes possible by clinical appearance, but it cannot always be distinguished from other types of genital ulcer. Furthermore, many cases are asymptomatic. The virus can be cultured from vesicle fluid or ulcer swabs, and this is the definitive diagnostic approach. Fluid in vesicles should be aspirated with a syringe, or the vesicles should be opened with a small gauge needle and the base of the lesion rubbed vigorously with a cotton swab. The swab should be placed in viral transport medium. If transport to the laboratory is delayed,

FIGURE 21.6
VESICLES OF GENITAL HERPES

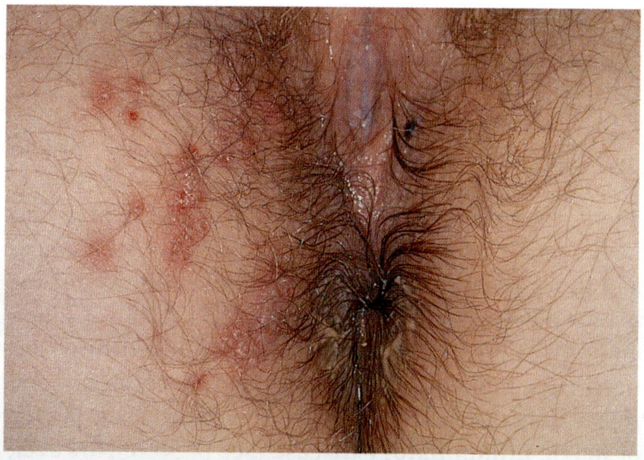

specimens may be refrigerated for up to 96 hours. The major disadvantage of culture is that it takes about five days. There has been limited clinical use of PCR in the diagnosis of genital herpes. Its high sensitivity and the fact that it can be performed within 24 hours make it a very attractive proposition.

Treatment

There is currently no effective cure for genital herpes. Topical or oral acyclovir reduces the duration of symptoms and virus shedding. A continuous, low dose of acyclovir may be used for a limited time in people with frequent recurrences, and this may be effective in reducing the frequency and severity of recurrences.

Prevention

Prevention of transmission of genital herpes is based on the general use of safe sex practices, and total abstinence when symptomatic. If a pregnant woman is symptomatic near term, caesarean delivery is indicated and will often prevent neonatal infection if performed before rupture of the membranes. This does not always prevent infection of the baby, however, since *in utero* and postnatal transmission are possible.

GENITAL WARTS

Causative agents and transmission

About 70 different types of human papillomaviruses (HPV) which infect the skin and mucous membranes have been identified. Many types are adapted to specific regions of the body. Types 6, 12, 16, 18, 31, 33 and 35 are the types most commonly associated with genital infections. Infection normally occurs through mucous membranes or traumatised skin, although vertical and oral transmission are also possible.

Clinical features

Genital warts **(condyloma acuminatum)** appear as pinkish-brown masses, usually in clusters, on the penis, vulva, cervix or perineal or perianal regions (see Figure 21.7). They can appear at anytime between 1 and 8 months after infection, and then regress spontaneously within 1–2 years. Warts in the vulva can become very large and extend into the vagina. Little is known about the processes involved.

Subclinical infection is extremely common. This is demonstrated by the large number of people who have serum antibodies without ever experiencing symptoms. Why some people develop warts after infection, and others remain asymptomatic, is not known. The importance of asymptomatically infected people is that they represent a large, unidentified reservoir of the virus.

One of the major concerns of genital warts is the epidemiological association of certain virus types with carcinoma. Types 16, 18 and 31 have been strongly implicated in the development of cervical cancer. This form of cancer is four times more likely to occur in women infected with one of these viruses, than in non-infected women. There is also thought to be an association between certain virus types and anal and penile carcinoma.

Diagnosis

Human papillomaviruses cannot be cultured, but the virus can be identified by DNA typing of specimens containing infected cells. Diagnosis of infection is based essentially on clinical examination. Cervical infection is often initially indicated by the presence of abnormal cells in a Pap smear (see Spotlight box, p. 102) and then confirmed by colposcopy. The application of 3–5% acetic acid is used to demonstrate subclinical infection of the vulva, cervix, penis and anus. Infected tissue shows as areas of whitening (called acetowhite lesions). PCR has recently been used in some epidemiological studies, and promises to be a useful, direct approach.

Treatment

Treatment involves removal of warts, as in other areas of the body, most often with podophyllin (a plant extract), with laser therapy, or by freezing with liquid nitrogen.

FIGURE 21.7
GENITAL WARTS ON THE PENIS

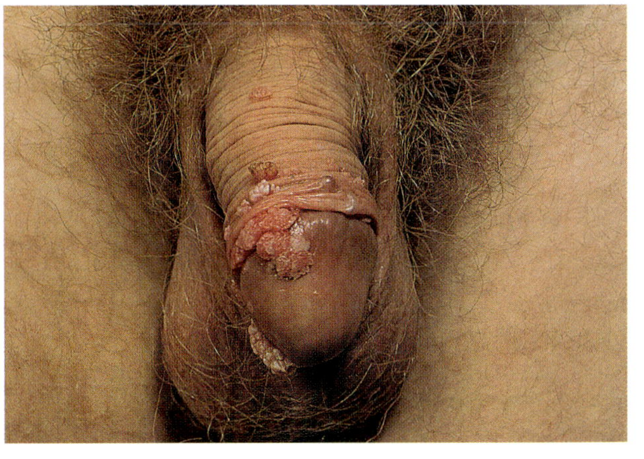

FIGURE 21.8
CHANCROID LESION ON THE PENIS

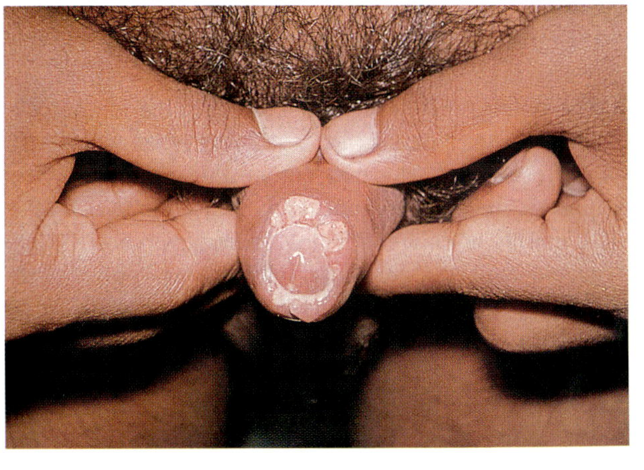

Early identification and treatment of abnormal cervical cells may prevent the formation of cancerous lesions. Treatment of warts, however, is not always successful. Often, viruses appear to exist in apparently normal tissue adjacent to warts. Removal of warts may remove one focus of infection, but viruses may persist nearby, and later cause a local recurrence.

DONOVANOSIS

Also called **granuloma inguinale**, donovanosis is caused by the encapsulated Gram-negative rod *Calymmatobacterium granulomatis*. It is rare in temperate climates, but common in tropical and subtropical regions such as the Caribbean, New Guinea and India, and is endemic in Aboriginal populations in central and northern Australia. It is a notifiable disease in some Australian States and Territories. Less than 100 cases are reported annually, with nearly half occurring in the Northern Territory.

The infection is characterised by nodules, usually on the genitalia, which erode to form granulomatous ulcers. As the disease progresses, the ulcers may spread peripherally, involving more and more tissue. In some cases, extragenital lesions may occur; these are thought to be due to auto-inoculation. The epidemiology of the disease is unclear. The role of sexual transmission is still controversial since sexual contacts are often not infected.

Laboratory diagnosis of the disease involves microscopic examination of a stained smear of a biopsy or scraping from the lesion. Stained organisms are typically found inside large mononuclear cells. Treatment is usually with tetracycline or erythromycin.

CHANCROID

Chancroid is an STD caused by a small Gram-negative rod, *Haemophilus ducreyi*. It is most frequently seen in Africa, the Caribbean and South-East Asia. Although notifiable in almost all Australian States and Territories, less than 10 cases, on average, are reported each year. The disease is manifested by soft, painful genital ulcers 3–5 days after infection (see Figure 21.8). Local lymphadenitis becomes apparent after several days. The lymph nodes gradually enlarge to such an extent that eventually they may break through the skin, discharging pus. Extragenital lesions, such as on the tongue and lip, may also be seen. The lesions are highly infectious.

The organism is difficult to culture in the laboratory. It can take up to nine days and is still very much a challenge for microbiologists. However, culture remains the definitive diagnostic method. A Gram stain of an aspirate from the ulcer margin or enlarged lymph node shows short Gram-negative rods inside or outside polymorphonuclear leucocytes. Co-infection with other sexually transmissible organisms is common, so assessment for other STDs is warranted. The organism is becoming increasingly resistant but is still sensitive to a number of drugs, including erythromycin, ciprofloxacin and cotrimoxazole.

VAGINOSIS

Vaginosis is characterised by a vaginal discharge with or without an inflamed vaginal mucosa. It is most commonly caused by the yeast, *Candida albicans*, the protozoan *Trichomonas vaginalis*, or by certain bacteria, especially *Gardnerella vaginalis*. All these organisms can be found in low numbers in the vagina of normal women. In most infections, the predisposing factor is an alteration in the vaginal normal flora and/or an increase in the vaginal pH.

Candida albicans is a normal inhabitant of the vagina but in certain circumstances (e.g. during antibiotic usage, immunosuppression, pregnancy, diabetes) its numbers increase sufficiently to cause a vaginitis. It typically causes an intensely irritating (itchy) infection with a yellow, cheesy discharge. It may also cause a **balanitis** (infection of the glans penis) in male partners of infected women.

Trichomonas vaginalis is a flagellated protozoan (see Figure 21.9) which can exist as a commensal in the vagina of many women and in the urethra of some males. If the normal pH of the vagina is disturbed, this protozoan can increase to abnormal numbers, further raise the vaginal pH and cause a copious, foul-smelling discharge from the vagina. It is often found coexisting with the gonococcus. The organism rarely produces symptoms in males—at worst a mild urethritis.

Bacterial vaginosis is characterised by a fishy-smelling vaginal discharge and a vaginal pH greater than 4.5. It is thought to be due to increased numbers of *Gardnerella vaginalis* and/or various obligate anaerobes, such as *Bacteroides*. How infection is initiated is unclear, but it is probably related to an initial alteration in the vaginal pH followed by an increase in the numbers of these organisms. *Gardnerella* can be found in the urethra of male partners of women with vaginosis.

The laboratory diagnosis of vaginosis can often be made by direct microscopic examination of discharge. Yeast cells are seen in *Candida* infection, motile trophozoites in *Trichomonas* infection, and 'clue cells' (vaginal epithelial cells coated with bacteria) in bacterial vaginosis. *Candida* and the bacterial causes may also be identified by culture. Oral metronidazole is effective against *Trichomonas* and bacterial causes and allows repopulation of the vagina with lactobacilli. *Candida* is treated with a topical antifungal (e.g. nystatin, clotrimazole) or an oral antifungal like ketoconazole, and sexual partners should also be treated.

NON-SPECIFIC URETHRITIS

Non-specific urethritis (NSU) is any inflammation of the urethra not caused by *Neisseria gonorrhoeae* or *Chlamydia trachomatis*. The common causes are the mycoplasma bacteria, *Ureaplasma urealyticum* and *Mycoplasma hominis*. There is a variety of other possible causes including *Trichomonas vaginalis* and herpes simplex virus.

Symptoms are similar to gonorrhoea, but are usually milder. They include a watery discharge and dysuria. However, many infections, especially those caused by

FIGURE 21.9
TRICHOMONAS VAGINALIS, THE PROTOZOAN THAT CAUSES TRICHOMONIASIS

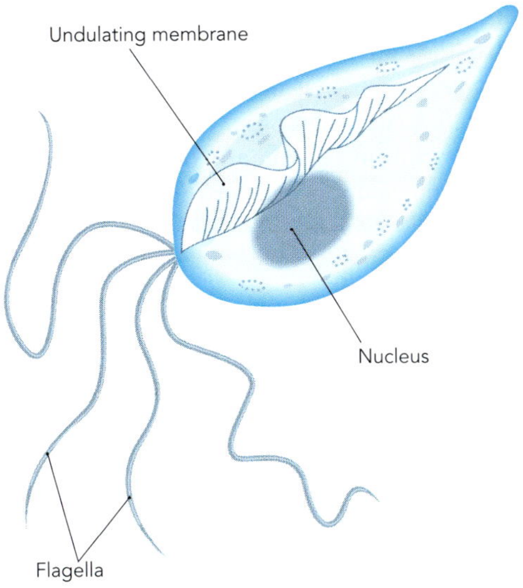

Chlamydia trachomatis, are asymptomatic, and hence are often untreated. In males, an epididymitis (inflammation of the epididymis) may occur. In females, spread of *Chlamydia* to the genital tract can cause inflammation of the uterine tubes (pelvic inflammatory disease), and result in sterility or ectopic pregnancy.

Diagnosis of urethritis caused by *U. urealyticum* and *M. hominis* is by culture of discharge. (For the diagnosis of infections by the other major causes, see the relevant sections on those organisms in this chapter.) Most infections are treated with tetracycline, or erythromycin in pregnant women and young children. These drugs are effective against both chlamydial and mycoplasmal infections.

PELVIC INFLAMMATORY DISEASE

Pelvic inflammatory disease (PID) is defined as the clinical syndrome associated with infection of the pelvic organs, particularly the uterus, fallopian tubes and ovaries, and sometimes the whole of the peritoneal cavity. The most important sites of infection are the fallopian tubes **(salpingitis)**, because this can lead to ectopic pregnancy or sterility. It is estimated that in the United States as many as one million new cases of PID occur each year, and that many thousands of women have been rendered sterile as a result.

Causative agents, pathogenesis and clinical features

PID may be uni- or polymicrobial. The majority of infections are caused by *Neisseria gonorrhoeae*, *Chlamydia trachomatis*, or both. They are thought to coexist because *N. gonorrhoeae* appears to enhance the replication of *C. trachomatis* in cervical epithelia. Polymicrobial infection can occur with one or both of these organisms, plus elements of the normal flora such as *Gardnerella vaginalis* and various anaerobes, the causative agents of bacterial vaginosis. Bacterial vaginosis is common in women with PID. Bacteria ascend from the lower genital tract. It is thought that *N. gonorrhoeae* and *C. trachomatis* set up infection in the upper genital tract, and then anaerobes and facultative anaerobes gradually take over.

The symptoms associated with PID are extremely variable. The most common symptom is a dull and constant lower abdominal pain. Also, patients often have cervical motion tenderness (pain when the cervix is moved from side to side). Other manifestations include abnormal vaginal discharge, fever and post-coital bleeding.

Persistent infection can lead to fibrosis and scarring of the fallopian tubes, which can cause blockage of the passage of the ova from the ovary to the uterus. This can result in sterility, or the implantation of the fertilised egg in the uterine tube rather than in the uterus (called an 'ectopic' or 'tubal' pregnancy).

Diagnosis and treatment

The diagnosis is usually made clinically on the findings of abnormal discharge or bleeding, together with lower abdominal tenderness, cervical motion tenderness and adnexal tenderness. Laparoscopy is considered to be the gold standard method for diagnosis of PID, but is not usually performed because it is not cost-effective and does not identify all cases.

Treatment of PID usually involves the use of a combination of antibiotics because of the possibility of polymicrobial infection. A number of different treatment regimens exist—a typical one is cefoxitin sodium for anaerobes plus doxycycline for *N. gonorrhoeae* and *C. trachomatis*. Male partners should be assessed for both gonorrhoea and chlamydial infection.

CASE HISTORY 21.4
PELVIC INFLAMMATORY DISEASE

A 21-year-old woman attended the casualty department of her local hospital complaining of the gradual onset of severe pain in the lower part of her abdomen. Over the last few hours she had also begun to feel feverish and nauseated. Prior to this she had noticed no other symptoms.

A pelvic examination revealed a yellowish discharge from the cervical os. A cervical swab was taken and a Gram stain showed intracellular Gram-negative diplococci. Culture results the next day confirmed infection with *Neisseria gonorrhoea*. She stated that her two sexual partners did not have any signs of infection.

Comment

This woman had an asymptomatic gonorrhoeal infection until the organism reached the upper parts of her genital tract. *Neisseria gonorrhoeae* is a common cause of pelvic inflammatory disease but a number of other organisms can also cause this disease.

PREVENTION OF STDS

Since the AIDS pandemic began, the practice of 'safe sex' has become the plea of governments and health departments throughout the world. In the past, safe sex meant protection from unintended pregnancy, but today it refers mainly to protection from the human immunodeficiency virus (HIV) and other sexually transmissible diseases. Vaccines have been heralded as the ultimate solution to the global epidemic of STDs, but, despite intensive research, the only successful vaccine developed to date is that for hepatitis B. Prevention is therefore based on the following approaches.

Avoidance of high-risk encounters

Avoidance of high-risk encounters is clearly the best method for prevention of STDs. A high-risk encounter is unprotected sex (without a condom) with:

- multiple partners, or with someone who has multiple partners;
- someone who uses intravenous drugs;
- someone other than a monogamous partner;
- a prostitute.

Since HIV and some other sexually transmissible diseases can be transmitted by blood, the sharing of needles and syringes in drug usage is also risky behaviour. A safe encounter is sex with a faithful, uninfected partner. A major reason for the high incidence of STDs throughout the world is that many infections are asymptomatic, and risk of infection is not always obvious.

Barrier contraceptive devices

Barrier contraceptive devices, specifically condoms, are the best alternative to abstinence or safe sex with one partner. The success of the condom is directly related to its consistent usage and structural integrity—that is, its ability to prevent direct contact with infective lesions or secretions. In experimental studies, intact latex condoms have been found to be impervious to bacteria and viruses. However, if failure of the device occurs (breakage, leakage, or by slipping off) during use, its effectiveness will clearly be reduced. 'Natural' condoms made from animal membranes are less effective because they are more easily broken; also, they are not impervious to smaller particles, like viruses, presumably because they contain small pores through which viruses can pass. Other devices, such as the 'female condom' (a sheath or pouch), can also potentially eliminate direct contact with genital secretions.

Spermicides

Spermicides are agents that have been developed for contraceptive purposes. They do this by interfering with sperm viability. Nonoxynol-9 is the most frequently used and best studied compound. It is a detergent that disrupts the membranes of sperm and also microorganisms. *In vitro* studies have demonstrated that most spermicides have potent antimicrobial and antiviral activity, but the clinical effectiveness of these substances has not yet been established. In addition, there is some concern that the detergent action of spermicides may cause vaginal irritation, which may enhance HIV transmission.

Contact tracing

The tracing of sexual contacts of people with STDs, and their screening and treatment, is a vital part of any prevention program. Unfortunately, this is not always possible or performed adequately. Major successes are achievable, however, as demonstrated in Sweden with respect to chlamydial infections. A program of widespread screening and assiduous contact tracing and treatment of chlamydial infections in that country since the early 1980s has been effective in reducing the incidence of the disease to a point where it was almost negligible in 1990[1]. This is a remarkable feat given that chlamydial infections are the most common STDs throughout the world.

Summary

- The urinary tract is one of the more common sites of infection and is frequently the site of hospital-acquired infection.
- Many infections of the genital tract are sexually transmissible diseases (STDs).

NORMAL FLORA OF THE URINARY AND REPRODUCTIVE SYSTEMS

- In a healthy person, the upper urethra, the urinary bladder and the organs of the upper urinary tract are sterile.
- In healthy females, protection against infection of the genital and urinary tracts is afforded by the low pH and the normal flora of the vagina.

URINARY TRACT INFECTIONS

- Urinary tract infections occur much more frequently in females than in males.
- UTIs represent about 30-40% of all hospital-acquired infections.

CAUSATIVE ORGANISMS

- The vast majority of infections are caused by microorganisms ascending the urethra and reaching the bladder.
- Ascending infections are most often caused by the enteric bacterium, *E. coli*.
- Many hospital-acquired infections are caused by organisms that are multiply resistant to antibiotics.
- A number of sexually transmissible organisms also cause urethritis.

PATHOGENESIS OF URINARY TRACT INFECTIONS

Host factors predisposing to infection

- The much higher incidence of urinary tract infection in women is attributed to the proximity of the anus to the urethral opening and the shortness of the urethra.
- The flushing of microorganisms from the urethra during the normal passage of urine is an important defence mechanism, so any factor that prevents normal urine flow makes an individual more susceptible to UTI.
- In men, there is a marked increase in the incidence of UTI from an age of around 50 to 60, due to urinary obstruction caused by hypertrophy of the prostate.

Urinary catheterisation

- The high incidence of urinary tract infection in hospitalised people is due mainly to the use of indwelling urinary catheters.
- A catheter provides several potential sites of entry for microorganisms and prevents the normal flushing of the urethra with urine.

Bacterial virulence factors

- Only certain strains of *E. coli* are able to cause UTI, and this has mainly been attributed to the presence of pili.
- Other virulence factors that have been attributed to urinary pathogens include the capsular polysaccharide (K) antigens of *E. coli*, and urease production as found in *Proteus* species and some strains of *E. coli*.

SITES AND CLINICAL FEATURES OF URINARY TRACT INFECTIONS

Asymptomatic bacteriuria

- Asymptomatic bacteriuria is thought to represent multiplication of bacteria in the bladder urine, without involvement of tissues, although in some cases actual bladder or kidney infection is present.
- In pregnant women, young children and people about to undergo instrumentation of the urinary tract, there is a significant risk of renal infection.

Cystitis

- Acute infections of the bladder are usually characterised by symptoms of dysuria, urgency and frequency.
- In cystitis, the urine is cloudy due to the presence of large numbers of leucocytes (pyuria), and it may occasionally contain blood (haematuria).
- Recurrent infections of the bladder affect some people, with the possibility of scarring and permanent damage to the urinary tract.

Pyelonephritis

- Infection of the kidney(s) can result from movement of bacteria upwards from the bladder, or occasionally from the bloodstream.
- The clinical presentation of pyelonephritis is similar to that of cystitis, although fever and haematuria are more common in pyelonephritis.

Laboratory diagnosis

- The specimen most commonly collected for the diagnosis of UTIs is a clean-catch or mid-stream specimen of urine (MSU).
- The specimen should be transported to the laboratory without delay.
- Wherever possible, the urine specimen should be collected before antibiotic therapy is initiated.
- Significant bacteriuria is usually defined as a count of 10^8/L in a properly collected MSU.
- Less than 10^8 bacteria per litre can be significant in some cases.

Treatment and management

- The choice of antimicrobial therapy should be based on culture and sensitivity results.
- In catheterised patients, management includes the removal or replacement of the catheter.

Prevention

- The incidence of community-acquired UTI in women may be reduced by promotion of good personal hygiene, adequate fluid intake and regular emptying of the bladder.
- In hospitals, prevention is based on similar principles plus avoidance of catheterisation wherever possible. Proper catheter care is essential when their use is unavoidable.

INFECTIONS OF THE REPRODUCTIVE SYSTEM

- Most diseases of the reproductive (genital) system are transmitted during sexual activity and thus are referred to as sexually transmissible diseases (STDs).
- Reasons commonly given for the continuing high incidence of STDs include increased sexual activity at a younger age, increased promiscuity, the production of little or no symptoms by some pathogens, the sexual freedom of contraception and the failure to use barrier preventive measures (e.g. condoms).
- STDs are of major health importance because there is a strong association between the organisms that cause genital ulceration (e.g. syphilis, herpes, chancroid) and transmission of the human immunodeficiency virus (HIV).

GONORRHOEA

Causative organism

- Gonorrhoea is an infection caused by the bacterium *Neisseria gonorrhoeae*, sometimes called the 'gonococcus'.

Transmission

- The gonococcus is fairly sensitive to drying and survives for only a short time on dry surfaces; it is thus usually transmitted by direct person-to-person contact.
- The gonococcus can also be transmitted vertically from an infected mother to baby at birth.

Pathogenesis

- Once the gonococci are introduced into the vagina, or the urethra of males, they attach by way of pili to the mucosal cells.
- The bacteria invade the epithelial cells lining the cervix and urethra and multiply within them.

Clinical features

- In men, gonococcal infection is usually characterised by a urethral discharge and dysuria.
- As many as 50% of infected women have very mild symptoms or are completely asymptomatic; symptomatic infection is usually characterised by a cervico-vaginal discharge and cervical oedema.
- In up to 30% of untreated women, the infection spreads further up the genital tract to cause inflammation in the fallopian tubes, ovaries, or in the peritoneal cavity. Inflammation in any of these sites is called pelvic inflammatory disease (PID).

Diagnosis

- Diagnosis is based on microscopy and culture of an appropriate specimen.
- In men, a urethral swab or urethral discharge should be collected.
- In women, a cervical swab should be collected and additionally a sample of vaginal discharge if purulent.
- A rapid, presumptive diagnosis can be made from a Gram stain if intracellular Gram-negative diplococci are seen.
- The organism is sensitive to drying so the specimen should be inoculated directly onto culture media at the bedside or transported immediately to the laboratory. Swabs should be sent in transport medium.
- All patients with gonococcal infection should be evaluated for other STDs.

Treatment and prevention

- Treatment is usually with penicillin, ceftriaxone or spectinomycin. Since many patients have a coexistent infection with *Chlamydia trachomatis,* treatment should also include a tetracycline or erythromycin.

SYPHILIS

Causative organism

- Syphilis is caused by the spirochaete *Treponema pallidum,* a thin, coiled and highly motile organism with fastidious growth requirements.

Transmission

- Transmission of syphilis requires close, personal contact because the organism survives poorly outside the body.
- An infected woman may also transmit the organism to her foetus *in utero*, often resulting in congenital malformations.

Pathogenesis and clinical features

- Primary syphilis is characterised by the development of a papular lesion at the site of infection, usually on the genitals. The papular lesion breaks down to form a painless, hard-based ulcer, called a chancre.
- The papule and ulcer contain large numbers of organisms and are highly infectious.
- The lesion heals spontaneously in 2–6 weeks.
- In approximately 50% of untreated cases, secondary syphilis develops 2–10 weeks later.
- The secondary stage is characterised by the appearance of a red, maculopapular rash anywhere on the skin, anogenital region, mouth, throat or cervix.
- The secondary stage lesions are highly infectious.
- The symptoms subside spontaneously after a few weeks, and there follows a prolonged asymptomatic period of between 3 and 30 years.
- In about 30% of untreated cases, the disease progresses to tertiary syphilis, in which renewed multiplication, dissemination and a cell-mediated hypersensitivity response combine to form granulomatous lesions (gummas) in various organs.

Diagnosis

- The primary and secondary lesions of syphilis usually contain large numbers of organisms, which may be readily seen in exudate from the lesions when examined microscopically.
- Serology is the mainstay of diagnosis.
- Two non-specific screening tests in common use are the VDRL and the RPR.
- The fluorescent treponemal antibody absorption test (FTA-ABS) and the *Treponema pallidum* haemagglutination assay (TPHA) detect anti-treponemal antibodies and are the two specific tests in common use.

Treatment

- Penicillin is very active against *Treponema pallidum* and is the drug of choice.
- If the patient is allergic to penicillin, tetracycline or erythromycin are also effective.

Prevention

- Prevention is based on the practice of safe sex, and contact tracing and screening.
- Congenital infection is preventable if women are screened serologically early in pregnancy and treated.

CHLAMYDIAL INFECTIONS

Causative organisms and incidence

- Genital infections caused by serotypes D to K of *Chlamydia trachomatis* have a high incidence in many countries, and are the most prevalent of all STDs.
- Serotypes L1, L2 and L3 of *C. trachomatis* cause lymphogranuloma venereum (LGV).

Pathogenesis and clinical features

- The organisms grow in columnar and transitional epithelial cells and the clinical disease is determined by the site of infection.
- Infection in the urethra is termed chlamydial urethritis; infection of the cervix leads to cervicitis; and spread from there to the fallopian tubes is called salpingitis or pelvic inflammatory disease.
- Many infections are asymptomatic or have only mild symptoms.
- In LGV, a primary lesion develops at the site of organism inoculation. Typically, inguinal buboes form, which gradually enlarge.

Diagnosis

- Serological assays and direct fluorescence microscopy of an appropriate specimen are the most commonly used methods for the diagnosis of chlamydial infections.
- For culture or microscopy, a cervical or urethral specimen is usually collected. The site should be scraped with a swab, in order to obtain some infected cells.
- Swabs, scrapings and small amounts of tissue should be transported in an appropriate transport medium.

Treatment

- Treatment is usually with tetracycline, but erythromycin is the drug of choice for pregnant women.
- Sexual contacts should be treated whether or not they are symptomatic.

GENITAL HERPES

Causative agents and incidence

- There are two major types of herpes simplex virus: herpes simplex virus type 1 (HSV-1) and herpes simplex type 2 (HSV-2).
- Both types have been found to cause genital and oral (cold sores) herpes, but type 2 predominates in the genital region.

Pathogenesis and clinical features

- Transmission is essentially by direct contact with infected secretions or mucosal surfaces.
- Initial infection may be completely asymptomatic or so mild that it is unrecognised in as many as 50–70% of people.
- If symptomatic, the primary lesions usually occur on the penis, anus, vulva, cervix or vagina.
- The lesions are usually small, grouped vesicles filled with a clear fluid and surrounded by an area of inflammation; they break down after several days to form painful, shallow ulcers.
- The primary lesions usually heal within two weeks, but by that time the virus has travelled up the local sensory nerve to the sensory root ganglion where it lies dormant; virus persistence there lasts for a lifetime.
- From the sensory root ganglion the virus can reactivate and travel back down the nerve where it infects mucocutaneous epithelial cells, causing new lesions.
- There is considerable variation in the frequency of symptomatic recurrent attacks, but some people may have many attacks a year.
- HSV-2 can be transmitted from a symptomatic or asymptomatic mother to her baby at birth, during pregnancy or postnatally.
- HSV-2 can cause severe infections in patients with immunodeficiency.

Diagnosis

- The virus can be cultured from vesicle fluid or ulcer swabs.

Treatment

- There is currently no effective cure for genital herpes.
- Topical or oral acyclovir reduces the duration of symptoms and virus shedding.

Prevention

- Prevention of transmission of genital herpes is based on the general use of safe sex practices, and total abstinence when symptomatic.

- If a pregnant woman is symptomatic near term, caesarean delivery will often prevent neonatal infection if performed before rupture of the membranes.

GENITAL WARTS

Causative agents and transmission

- About 70 different types of human papillomaviruses (HPV) which infect the skin and mucous membranes have been identified.
- Types 6, 12, 16, 18 and 31 are predominantly transmitted during sexual contact.
- Infection normally occurs through mucous membranes or traumatised skin.

Clinical features

- Genital warts (condyloma acuminatum) appear as pinkish-brown masses, usually in clusters, on the penis, vulva, cervix or perineal or perianal regions.
- Subclinical infection is extremely common.
- A major concern of genital warts is the epidemiological association of certain virus types with cervical cancer.

Diagnosis

- Diagnosis of infection is based essentially on clinical examination.
- Cervical infection is often initially indicated by the presence of abnormal cells in a Pap smear and then confirmed by colposcopy.
- The application of 3–5% acetic acid is used to demonstrate subclinical infection of the vulva, cervix, penis and anus.

Treatment

- Treatment involves removal of warts, most often with podophyllin, with laser therapy, or by freezing with liquid nitrogen.
- Treatment is not always successful because, often, viruses appear to exist in apparently normal tissue adjacent to warts.

DONOVANOSIS

- This disease, also called granuloma inguinale, is caused by the Gram-negative rod *Calymmatobacterium granulomatis*.
- The infection is characterised by nodules, usually on the genitalia, which erode to form granulomatous ulcers.
- Diagnosis of the disease involves microscopic examination of a stained smear from the lesion.
- Treatment is with tetracycline.

CHANCROID

- Chancroid is an STD caused by a small Gram-negative rod, *Haemophilus ducreyi*.
- The disease is manifested by soft, painful genital ulcers 3–5 days after infection. The lymph nodes gradually enlarge to such an extent that, eventually, they may break through the skin, discharging pus.
- The lesions are highly infectious.
- Culture is the definitive diagnostic method.
- The organism is sensitive to a number of antibacterial drugs including erythromycin and cotrimoxazole.

VAGINOSIS

- Vaginosis is characterised by a vaginal discharge.
- Vaginosis is most commonly caused by the yeast, *Candida albicans*, the protozoan *Trichomonas vaginalis*, and by certain bacteria, especially *Gardnerella vaginalis*.
- In most infections, the predisposing factor is an alteration in the vaginal normal flora and/or an increase in the vaginal pH.
- The laboratory diagnosis of vaginosis can often be made by direct microscopic examination of discharge.
- Oral metronidazole is effective against *Trichomonas* and bacterial causes.
- *Candida* is treated with a topical or oral antifungal.

NON-SPECIFIC URETHRITIS

- Non-specific urethritis (NSU) is any inflammation of the urethra not caused by *Neisseria gonorrhoeae* or *Chlamydia trachomatis*.
- The most common causes are *Ureaplasma urealyticum* and *Mycoplasma hominis*.
- Symptoms include a watery discharge and dysuria, but many infections are asymptomatic.
- In females, spread of *Chlamydia* to the genital tract can cause pelvic inflammatory disease.
- Most infections are treated with tetracycline, or erythromycin in pregnant women and young children.

PELVIC INFLAMMATORY DISEASE

- Pelvic inflammatory disease (PID) is the clinical syndrome associated with infection of the pelvic organs, particularly the uterus, fallopian tubes, ovaries and peritoneal cavity.
- The most important sites of infection are the fallopian tubes (salpingitis), because this can lead to ectopic pregnancy or sterility.

Causative agents, pathogenesis and clinical features

- Most infections are caused by *Neisseria gonorrhoeae*, *Chlamydia trachomatis*, or both.
- The symptoms associated with PID are extremely variable; the most common symptom is a dull and constant lower abdominal pain.
- Persistent infection can lead to fibrosis and scarring of the fallopian tubes; this can block the passage of the ova from the ovary to the uterus, which can result in sterility or ectopic or tubal pregnancy.

Diagnosis and treatment

- The diagnosis is usually made clinically on the findings of abnormal discharge or bleeding, together with lower abdominal tenderness, cervical motion tenderness and adnexal tenderness.

- Treatment of PID usually involves the use of a combination of antibiotics because of the possibility of polymicrobial infection.

PREVENTION OF STDS

- Avoidance of high-risk encounters is clearly the best method for prevention of STDs.
- Barrier contraceptive devices, specifically condoms, are the best alternative to abstinence or safe sex with one partner.
- The tracing of sexual contacts of people with STDs, and their screening and treatment, is a vital part of any prevention program.

Study Questions

1. Which parts of the urinary and reproductive systems of humans have a normal microbial flora?
2. Why are females generally more susceptible to urinary tract infections than males?
3. From where do urinary tract pathogens usually originate?
4. How does normal urine flow protect the urinary tract from infection?
5. Why do urinary catheters increase the risk of urinary tract infection?
6. Define the terms 'pyelonephritis', 'cystitis' and 'asymptomatic bacteriuria'.
7. Why should urine for microbiological analysis be transported to the laboratory promptly?
8. What is significant bacteriuria?
9. What laboratory results indicate that a urine specimen is of poor quality?
10. Why are sexually transmissible diseases considered to be a major health problem?
11. How is gonorrhoea usually transmitted?
12. Why is asymptomatic gonorrhoeal infection in women so important?
13. What specimen(s) should be collected from a woman suspected of having gonorrhoea?
14. What are the differences between primary and secondary syphilis?
15. What are the two main methods for diagnosing syphilis in the laboratory, and what specimens are needed for each?
16. What types of genital infections does *Chlamydia trachomatis* cause?
17. What is the most common cause of genital herpes?
18. How does the genital herpes virus cause recurrent infections?
19. What are the common causes of genital warts?
20. What important sequela is associated with genital warts in women?
21. How are genital warts treated?
22. What is donovanosis?
23. What are the common predisposing factors of vaginosis?
24. What is non-specific urethritis and what are the common causes?
25. What is pelvic inflammatory disease and what are the possible serious sequelae of this disease?
26. How is pelvic inflammatory disease diagnosed?
27. List the ways by which sexually transmissible diseases can be prevented.

Test Your Understanding

Case History 21.1: Urinary tract infection

1. What do the urinalysis results indicate?
2. Why are the numbers of organisms in urine quantitated?

Case History 21.2: Syphilis

1. What specimen(s) should be collected for the diagnosis of syphilis?
2. What important infection control issues should be considered in this case?

Case History 21.3: Urethritis

1. Assuming Mr C. did have gonorrhoea, what are the possible reasons for failure of treatment?
2. What are the possible causes of Mr C.'s persistent infection?

Case History 21.4: Pelvic inflammatory disease

1. What organs might be involved in this infection?
2. Are there any serious complications associated with this infection?
3. Should the woman's asymptomatic sexual partners be notified and treated?

REFERENCES

1. Ripa, T., 1990, 'Epidemiologic control of genital *Chlamydia trachomatis* infections', *Scandinavian Journal of Infectious Diseases* 69 (suppl.), p. 157.

FURTHER READING

Ault, K.A. & S. Faro, 1993, 'Pelvic inflammatory disease', *Postgraduate Medicine* 93, p. 85. (This article focuses on the epidemiology, diagnosis and treatment of pelvic inflammatory disease.)

Lee, N. (ed.), 1990, Laboratory diagnosis of urinary tract infection, *Clinical Microbiology Update Program*, University of New South Wales. (A detailed description of laboratory methods used in urinalysis and the interpretation of results.)

McCall, B., 1995, 'Surveillance of sexually transmissible disease in Queensland, 1988 to 1993', *Communicable Diseases Intelligence* 19(3), p. 58. (A paper describing the epidemiological features of STDs in Queensland.)

Parenti, D.M., 1992, 'Sexually transmitted diseases and travellers', *Medical Clinics of North America* 76, p. 1449. (A general review of STDs and their prevention.)

Scheider, A., 1993, 'Pathogenesis of genital HPV infection', *Genitourinary Medicine* 69, p. 165. (A general review of human papillomavirus infections.)

Vanderhooft, S. & P. Kirby, 1992, 'Genital herpes simplex virus infection: natural history', *Seminars in Dermatology* 11, p. 190. (A review article detailing the nature of herpes simplex viruses and the epidemiology, clinical manifestations and diagnosis of genital herpes infections.)

Zenilman, J.M., 1992, 'Epidemiology and control of sexually transmitted diseases', *Current Opinion in Infectious Diseases* 5, p. 36. (A review article focusing on the epidemiology of STDs.)

glossary

Abscess A sac of pus walled off by a layer of fibrin.

Acetyl CoA An activated compound which is an important intermediate in carbohydrate metabolism and is also able to enter other metabolic pathways.

Acid-fast bacilli Bacteria belonging to the genus *Mycobacterium*, which are identifiable in an acid fast stain.

Acid-fast stain A differential stain used to identify bacteria that belong to the genus *Mycobacterium*. Also called a **Ziehl-Neelsen stain**.

Acquired immune system A functional system consisting of a variety of cells and organs that protect the body against pathogens which evade the non-specific defences and which also protect it against future attack by the pathogen. Also called **adaptive immune system**, **specific immune system** or **specific defences**.

Acquired immunodeficiency syndrome (AIDS) A disease caused by the human immunodeficiency virus which impairs the ability of the body to produce a specific immune response.

Activation energy The amount of energy required for a reaction to occur.

Active immunisation The use of a vaccine to prevent a specific disease in a person.

Active immunity The development of antibodies or other specific defences by the acquired immune system in response to microorganisms or other foreign substances which enter the body.

Active site The area of an enzyme which binds specifically to its substrate.

Active transport The movement of substances across a membrane against a concentration gradient.

Acute bronchitis An inflammation of the tracheobronchial tree.

Acute diarrhoea A sudden disruption in bowel habits in which normally formed stools are replaced by more frequent, liquefied movements.

Acute glomerulonephritis Inflammation of the kidneys due to the deposition of immune complexes in the glomeruli.

Acute inflammatory response A non-specific defence that is the body's response to tissue injury, characterised by redness, heat, swelling and pain.

Acute otitis media Acute infection and inflammation of the middle ear.

Adaptive immune system See **acquired immune system**.

Adenine A purine base that pairs with thymine in DNA and uracil in RNA.

Adenosine triphosphate (ATP) A small molecule which is important for the storage of energy released during metabolism.

Adherence The attachment of microorganisms to host tissues or other surfaces.

Adhesins The substances or structures on the surfaces of microorganisms that enable them to attach to cell surfaces.

Aerial hyphae A long filament of fungal cells that grows above the mycelium and bears spores.

Aerobe, obligate An organism that can only grow in the presence of oxygen.

Aerobic respiration The process whereby cells gain energy from the breakdown of organic molecules, using the electron transport chain, with oxygen as the final electron acceptor.

Aetiology The study of the cause and origin of a disease.

Agammaglobulinaemia A primary immunodeficiency disease characterised by a lack of antibodies.

Agar A polysaccharide derived from seaweed and used as a solidifying agent for bacterial culture media.

Agar plate A solid medium contained in a petri dish for growing bacteria or fungi.

Agglutination The clumping of the particles due to their cross-linking by specific antibodies.

AIDS See **acquired immunodeficiency syndrome**.

Air-borne transmission The spread of infectious microorganisms through the air, usually over distances greater than one metre from the infected host.

Algae A group of photosynthetic eucaryotic organisms.

Algal bloom An overgrowth of algae seen on waterways.

Allergen An antigen that evokes an allergic response.

Allergy See **immediate hypersensitivity**.

Alternate pathway A pathway for the activation of the complement system initiated by polysaccharides present on the surface of certain microorganisms.

Ames test A bacterial test used to identify potential carcinogens.

Aminoglycosides A group of antibiotics containing amino sugars.

Amoeba A single-celled protozoan (eucaryotic organism), that moves by extending pseudopods.

Amoebic dysentery A severe form of inflammatory diarrhoea caused by *Entamoeba histolytica*.

Anabolism The synthesis of complex organic molecules from simple components in living cells.

Anaerobe, obligate An organism that can only grow in the absence of oxygen.

Analogue A compound that has a structure similar to the substrate for an enzyme and that can be bound by the enzyme.

Anaphylactic shock A potentially life-threatening disorder resulting from a generalised allergic reaction throughout the body.

Anaphylatoxins Substances which bind to mast cells, basophils and platelets, triggering the release of histamine and other inflammatory mediators.

Anaphylaxis A systemic allergic reaction which occurs when an allergen enters the blood and circulates through the body.

Animalia A kingdom in the Linneaen classification system, containing multicellular eucaryotic organisms that do not have cell walls.

Anthrax A zoonosis caused by *Bacillus anthracis* that is characterised by cutaneous, respiratory or intestinal disease.

Antibacterial agent A compound that can kill bacteria or inhibit their growth.

Antibiotic A chemical substance produced naturally by a microorganism that can kill or inhibit another microorganism.

Antibiotic associated colitis A serious gastrointestinal disease which can sometimes follow antibiotic therapy, caused by the establishment of *Clostridium difficile* in the intestine.

Antibody A protein found in blood and other body fluids that is secreted by plasma cells in response to an antigen, and which is capable of binding specifically with that antigen. Also called **immunoglobulin**.

Antibody titre The amount of antibody in a person's blood or other body fluid.

Antifungal agent A compound that can kill or inhibit fungi.

Antigen A foreign substance which, when introduced into the body, activates the acquired immune system and induces an immune response. Also called **immunogen**.

Antigen-binding fragments (Fab) The end of the antibody molecule comprising the two arms responsible for binding of antigen.

Antigen-binding sites The sites on an antibody molecule where binding to antigen occurs.

Antigen presenting cell A macrophage or other cell that engulfs an antigen and then presents fragments of it to lymphocytes to activate them.

Antigen-antibody complex See **immune complex**.

Antigenic A foreign substance that is capable of inducing an immune response.

Antigenic determinant The small part of the whole antigen molecule to which antibodies or activated lymphocytes bind.

Antigenic drift A term used for repeated, minor mutations in the genes that code for the antigen of a microorganism.

Antigenic shift A major antigenic change in a virus due to a recombination of genes when two different strains of a virus infect the same cell.

Antigenic variation A phenomenon in which certain microorganisms are able to repeatedly or progressively change their cell surface antigens, enabling them to evade the immune system.

Antihistamine A drug used to alleviate the redness and swelling prominent in some allergic conditions like hay fever and hives.

Antimicrobial agent Any compound that kills or inhibits microorganisms. It may be synthetic or naturally occurring.

Antiprotozoal agent A compound that can kill or inhibit protozoa.

Antipyretic A drug used to reduce fever.

Antiseptic A chemical agent used on skin or living tissue to kill or remove microorganisms without damaging the tissue.

Antiserum A fluid derived from blood which contains antibodies.

Antitoxin An antibody preparation derived from the serum of immune humans or animals which neutralises a microbial toxin.

Antiviral agent A compound that can inactivate viruses.

APSGN—acute post-streptococcal glomerulonephritis A serious inflammation of the of the kidneys after a streptococcal infection elsewhere in the body.

Arbovirus A virus which is transmitted to humans by biting insects (arthropods).

Archaebacteria Procaryotic organisms (bacteria) of ancient origin, that lack peptidoglycan in their cell walls.

Arthropod vector A member of the phylum Arthropoda, (spiders, mites, ticks and insects) that carries an infectious agent from one host to another.

Artificial active immunity Immunity produced in response to a vaccination.

Artificially acquired active immunity Active immunity produced following vaccination.

Artificially acquired passive immunity Immunity due to the injection of preformed antibodies derived from another person.

Ascariasis A gastrointestinal disease caused by the roundworm *Ascaris lumbricoides*.

Aschelminth A roundworm.

Asepsis The absence of disease-producing microorganisms.

Aseptic meningitis A general term used for any meningitis where microorganisms are not isolated by routine bacteriological culture, especially viral meningitis.

Aseptic technique Procedures used to minimise the transfer of microorganisms.

Asexual reproduction Reproduction that does not involve cells of different mating strains.

Asymptomatic bacteriuria A condition in which a person has large numbers of bacteria in the urine without displaying any symptoms.

Athlete's foot A fungal infection of the skin of the foot. Also called **tinea pedis**.

Attenuation Any process that substantially reduces or eliminates the disease-producing ability of a microorganism, while still keeping it alive.

Australian encephalitis An encephalitis occurring in Australia caused by mosquito-borne viruses, especially the Murray Valley encephalitis virus.

Autoantibody An antibody produced against one's own tissue.

Autoimmune disease Tissue damage and disease due to the presence of auto-antibodies.

Autoclave Equipment used for sterilisation by steam under pressure.

Autotroph An organism that uses carbon dioxide from the air as its principal carbon source.

B cell See **B lymphocyte**.

B lymphocyte A cell which is a major component of the humoral immune system, giving rise to antibody-secreting plasma cells when stimulated by antigen.

Bacillary dysentery Diarrhoea caused by *Shigella* sp. Also called **shigellosis**.

Bacillus (pl: bacilli) A rod-shaped bacterium.

Bacteraemia The presence of bacteria in the bloodstream.

Bacteriocidal Able to kill bacteria.

Bacteriophage A virus that infects bacteria.

Bacteriostatic Able to inhibit bacterial growth.

Bairnsdale ulcer A cutaneous ulcer caused by *Mycobacterium ulcerans*.

Balanitis Infection of the glans penis.

Basal body A structure that connects flagella to the cell wall and membrane of a bacterium.

Basophil A white blood cell which contains granules of histamine and other inflammatory mediators.

BCG vaccine (Bacillus of Calmette and Guerin), a live attenuated strain of *Mycobacterium bovis* used to provide immunity to tuberculosis.

Benign malaria A type of malaria in which there is a pattern of intermittent illness and well-being, caused by *Plasmodium vivax, P. ovale and P. malariae*.

Beta-lactamase An enzyme produced by bacteria that are resistant to antibiotics such as penicillin and cephalosporin that contain a ß-lactam ring.

Binary fission The process of reproduction that involves splitting into two identical daughter cells.

Biogenesis The idea that living cells can only arise from pre-existing living cells.

Biological transmission The method of transmission of a pathogen that involves replication in an insect vector.

Biotechnology The industrial use of living cells to produce biological materials.

Blepharitis Infection and inflammation of the eyelid margin.

Blepharoconjunctivitis Infection and inflammation of the eyelid.

Blood agar A nutrient agar culture medium to which defibrinated horse or sheep blood is added.

Blood culture A culture of a blood sample performed in the investigation of a patient with fever or other manifestations of systemic infection.

Blood-brain barrier The tightly joined endothelial cells of the brain's capillaries that prevent the passage of most substances and thus help to ensure that the brain's environment remains stable.

Blue-green algae See **Cyanobacteria**.

Boil A large, pus-filled nodule that develops when the deeper areas of a hair follicle become infected by *Staphylococcus aureus*. Also called a **furuncle**.

Booster vaccination A second or subsequent dose of a vaccine given to produce large numbers of memory cells and antibody levels in blood, that remain high for many years.

Botulism A disease of the nervous system caused by a neurotoxin of *Clostridium botulinum*, acquired by consumption of contaminated food.

Bright-field microscopy A type of compound light microscopy in which the specimen is fully illuminated with light.

Broad spectrum antimicrobial agent A chemical which is active against a number of different microrganisms.

Bronchiolitis Infection and inflammation of the bronchioles.

Bronchopneumonia A diffuse, patchy inflammation of the lungs, with numerous, small discrete foci of consolidation occurring throughout the lungs. Caused by viruses and some bacteria.

Brucellosis A systemic zoonosis caused by the bacteria *Brucella melitensis, B. abortus and B. suis*. Also called **undulant fever** or **Malta fever**.

Bruton's agammaglobulinaemia A primary immunodeficiency caused by incomplete maturation of B lymphocytes.

Bubo An enlarged lymph node due to inflammation.

Bubonic plague A systemic infection caused by the bacterium *Yersinia pestis*, characterised by large, tender buboes, most frequently in the armpit or groin.

Bulla A large blister containing clear fluid, more than 0.5 cm in diameter.

Campylobacteriosis A gastrointestinal infection caused by *Campylobacter*.

Candidaemia A systemic infection caused by *Candida albicans*.

Candidiasis An infection caused by the yeast *Candida albicans*. Also called **moniliasis** or thrush.

CAPD—continuous ambulatory peritoneal dialysis A procedure whereby a patient is able to undergo dialysis without being confined to bed.

Capsid The protein coat surrounding the viral nucleic acid.

Capsomere One of the protein units that make up the viral capsid.

Capsule A protective outer layer present in some bacteria and composed of polysaccharide, also called **glycocalyx** or **slime layer**.

Carbapenem A group of ß-lactam compounds with a broad spectrum of antibacterial activity.

Carbuncle A large abscess or multiple abscesses in adjacent areas of skin caused by *Staphylococcus aureus*.

Carcinogen A substance that can cause cancer.

Cardiovascular syphilis A form of tertiary syphilis in which aortic aneurysm and blood vessel and valve damage may occur.

Caries Tooth decay.

Carrier A person who harbours and continuously sheds a pathogen without showing any symptoms of disease.

Catabolism The process of breakdown of complex molecules in living cells with release of energy.

Catalase An enzyme produced by some bacteria, which breaks down hydrogen peroxide.

Catalyst A substance that lowers the activation energy of a reaction.

Category-specific isolation precautions A method of infection control in which diseases are assigned to categories and the body substances that are considered infective within each category are specified.

CD4 cell See **helper T cell**.

CD8 cell See **cytotoxic T cell**.

Cell anergy Cells that have been rendered inactive. Used to describe the inactivity of lymphocytes for self antigens or in HIV infection.

Cell culture Animal or plant cells grown in the laboratory.

Cell membrane See cytoplasmic membrane.

Cell wall The outer layer of bacteria and most algal, plant and fungal cells. It provides shape and structural support for the cell.

Cell-mediated hypersensitivity See **delayed type hypersensitivity**.

Cell-mediated immunity An immune response in which T lymphocytes act directly against target cells, release chemicals that enhance inflammation, or activate other defence cells to cause destruction of the target cells. Also called **cellular immunity**.

Cellular immunity See **cell-mediated immunity**.

Cellulitis An infection of subcutaneous tissue.

Centrioles A pair of cylindrical structures which take part in eucaryotic cell division.

Cephalosporins A group of ß-lactam antibiotic compounds derived from the fungus *Cephalosporium*, that inhibit the synthesis of peptidoglycan.

Cercaria The free swimming larval form of flukes (e.g. *Schistosoma*) which are released into the water from the intermediate snail host.

Cerebrospinal fluid The fluid that circulates in the space between the inner two meningeal membranes of the brain and spinal cord.

Cervicitis Infection and inflammation of the cervix.

Cestode Tapeworm.

Chancre A painless, hard-based ulcer found in the primary stage of syphilis.

Chancroid A sexually transmissible disease caused by *Haemophilus ducreyi*, characterised by soft, painful genital ulcers.

Chemically defined medium A culture medium in which the amount of each pure chemical compound is known.

Chemostat Equipment used to control the chemical composition of the culture medium during microbial growth. Can be used for the continuous culture of microorganisms.

Chemotaxis The attraction of phagocytes to sites of damaged tissue or microbial invasion by chemicals released at the site.

Chemotherapy The treatment of an illness or infection with a chemical substance.

Chickenpox A highly infectious disease characterised by skin lesions caused by the varicella zoster virus.

Chlamydiae Very small bacteria which have a complex life cycle and can only reproduce inside a living cell.

Chloramines Organic chlorine compounds used in water purification.

Chloramphenicol A broad spectrum antibiotic which inhibits protein synthesis.

Chlorophyll The pigment in algae and green plants that absorbs energy from the sun for photosynthesis.

Chloroplast The organelle in green plants that is the site of photosynthesis.

Cholera An acute and profuse diarrhoeal disease caused by *Vibrio cholerae*.

Chromosome A structure containing DNA and carrying hereditary information.

Chronic fatigue syndrome A condition in which excessive fatigue and general malaise are chronic complaints, often following an initial viral-like illness.

Chronic hepatitis The persistence of hepatitis virus antigens in the bloodstream for at least six months.

Chronic infection An infection that persists in the body and is accompanied by continuous shedding of the pathogen.

Chronic inflammation A type of inflammation in which large numbers of lymphocytes and macrophages are involved, occuring if the acute inflammatory response is unsuccessful in clearing organisms or foreign material from the tissue.

Chronic mucocutaneous candidiasis A chronic infection caused by *Candida*, usually seen in immunodeficient patients.

Chronic suppurative otitis media (CSOM) A severe, chronic form of middle ear infection.

Ciguatera A toxin produced by certain species of marine algae, that can cause poisoning if it enters the food chain.

Cirrhosis A disease of the liver characterised by reduced liver function and an increase in connective tissue.

Classical pathway A pathway for the activation of complement proteins initiated by antigen-antibody complexes.

Clonal selection theory A theory proposed to explain the activation of a specific clone of lymphocytes by antigen, giving rise to a larger population of cells with the same specificity.

Clone A population of cells all derived from the same parent cell.

Coagulase An enzyme produced by pathogenic staphylococci that coagulates fibrinogen to form a deposit of fibrin around the bacterial cells.

Coccobacilli Small rod shaped bacteria which resemble cocci.

Coccus (pl: cocci) A spherical bacterium.

Coenzyme An organic molecule associated with an enzyme and required for enzyme activity.

Cofactor A non-protein component of an enzyme that is required for enzyme activity.

Collagenase A microbial enzyme that breaks down tissue collagen.

Colonisation The process in which microorganisms live and reproduce on the human body without causing disease.

Colony forming units The number of individual bacterial colonies visible on an agar plate. Each colony may have arisen from one or more cells.

Commensalism A symbiotic association between two organisms in which one benefits without harming the other.

Common vehicle transmission Transmission of a pathogen to a number of people from a common source such as food or water.

Communicable disease A disease which is transmitted from one host to another.

Community-acquired infection An infection acquired in the community, not in a health care facility.

Community strain A strain of microorganism that originates in the community, not from a hospital. A community strain of a microorganism is usually sensitive to antimicrobial drugs.

Complement A complex system of proteins that circulate in the blood in an inactive state that are involved in body defences when activated.

Complement fixation The activation of complement proteins and fixation to a receptor on antibody molecules in antigen-antibody complexes.

Complete antigen A foreign substance that stimulates specific lymphocytes, inducing them to produce an immune response.

Complex medium A culture medium in which the exact chemical composition of each of the nutrients is not defined.

Compound light microscope A microscope with more than one lens and which uses visible light as the illumination source.

Condyloma acuminatum Genital warts, appearing as pinkish brown masses on the penis, vulva, cervix or perineal or perianal regions.

Congenital infection An infection of the foetus that occurs in utero.

Congenital rubella syndrome A potentially severe rubella infection in the foetus due to the virus crossing the placenta from the mother's circulation.

Conidia (conidiospores) Asexual fungal spores that develop on aerial hyphae.

Conjugate vaccine A vaccine prepared by combining the desired antigen with another protein.

Conjugation The transfer of genetic material from one bacterium to another by means of sex pili.

Conjunctivitis Infection and inflammation of the conjunctiva of the eye.

Contact transmission Spread of a pathogen from one host to another by contact.

Contagious Easily spread from one person to another.

Contamination The unwanted presence of microorganisms.

Continuous cell line A cell culture consisting of cells that can be propagated over many generations.

Continous culture The process of growing and harvesting microorganisms in such a way that optimal growth conditions are maintained.

Coryza See **rhinitis**.

Creutzfeldt-Jakob disease A disease caused by a prion, characterised by fatal degeneration of brain tissue.

Cristae Folds of the inner membrane of mitochondria.

Crossing over An event in meiosis in which part of the DNA from one chromosome is exchanged with the DNA from another.

Croup Inflammation of the larynx and trachea, characterised by stridor, hoarseness and a resonant cough.

Crust The dried exudate from an erosion or ulcer.

Cryptococcosis Lung or meningeal infection caused by *Cryptococcus neoformans*.

Cryptosporidiosis Intestinal infection caused by *Cryptosporidium parvum*.

Crystallisable fragment (Fc) The tail part of an antibody molecule where complement fixation and phagocyte adherence occurs.

Culture A growth of microbes in/on a culture medium.

Culture medium A preparation of nutrient material for the growth of microorganisms.

Cutaneous mycoses Fungal infections which affect the epidermal layers of the skin.

Cyanobacteria A group of photosynthetic bacteria, formerly called blue-green algae.

Cyst (i) A sac with a defined wall containing fluid or other material, e.g. hydatid cyst; (ii) a form of some protozoa and helminths in which the cell is surrounded by a protective layer.

Cystitis Infection and inflammation of the urinary bladder.

Cytokine A soluble factor released by cells which regulates the activity of other cells involved in body defences.

Cytolysis The destruction of cells by damage of their cell membranes.

Cytopathic effects The microscopically observable changes to a cell caused by virus infection of the cell.

Cytoplasm The contents of cells inside the plasma membrane (excluding the nucleus).

Cytoplasmic membrane The membrane containing the cytoplasm of the cell. Also called plasma membrane.

Cytosine A pyrimidine base that pairs with guanine in RNA and DNA.

Cytotoxic hypersensitivity Destruction of body cells by the binding of antibodies to antigens on the surface of a cell, followed by complement activation and cell lysis. Also called **type II hypersensitivity**.

Cytotoxic T cell A type of T lymphocyte which directly kills infected cells that display microbial antigens on their surface.

Dark-field microscopy A type of compound light microscopy using a special condenser so that objects in the specimen appear bright against a black background.

Debridement Removal of necrotic tissue from a wound.

Decline phase The phase of an illness when the acute symptoms have subsided.

Decontamination The process of removal of undesirable substances or pathogens from an object or area by cleaning or disinfecting.

Definitive host The organism that harbours the adult sexually mature form of a parasite.

Degranulation The release of granules containing histamine and other inflammatory chemicals by mast cells and basophils in allergic reactions.

Delayed type hypersensitivity Hypersensitivity reactions that are mediated by T cells and take a day or more to appear after the introduction of antigen. Also called **cell-mediated hypersensitivity** or **type IV hypersensitivity**.

Delayed type hypersensitivity T cells T cells responsible for delayed type hypersensitivity reactions. When stimulated by antigen, they secrete lymphokines which activate macrophages and cause inflammatory reactions.

Dengue fever A systemic infection caused by the dengue virus and transmitted by mosquitoes.

Dengue haemorrhagic fever A serious form of dengue fever characterised by bleeding from the gums, skin and gastrointestinal tract.

Deoxyribose A pentose sugar which is part of the DNA molecule.

Dermatomycosis A fungal skin infection.

Dermis The inner layer of the skin.

Diapedesis The process by which neutrophils move out of the bloodstream and into the tissue space in inflammation.

Diarrhoea A disruption in bowel habits characterised by more frequent passing of loose, watery stools.

Differential medium A microbial growth medium that allows the differentiation of one microorganism from another.

Dimorphism The ability of an organism to grow in two different forms under different environmental conditions.

Diphtheria An acute infection of the upper respiratory tract caused by toxin-producing strains of *Corynebacterium diphtheriae*. The toxin can subsequently cause heart, kidney and nervous tissue disease.

Diplococci Spherical bacteria that occur in pairs.

Diploid cell A cell that has two sets of chromosomes.

Disaccharide A carbohydrate molecule composed of two sugar units.

Disease A harmful alteration to the physiological or metabolic state of a host.

Disease-specific isolation precautions A set of procedures to be followed to prevent the transmission of a specific disease.

Disinfectant A chemical substance normally used for the disinfection of inanimate objects.

Disinfection The destruction, removal or reduction in numbers of harmful microorganisms to an acceptable level.

Disseminated infection An infection which spreads throughout the body.

Disseminated intravascular coagulation The non-specific activation of blood coagulation mechanisms by endotoxin, resulting in the blockage of small vessels by thrombi in a variety of organs.

DNA (deoxyribonucleic acid) The molecule which carries genetic information.

Donovanosis A genital ulcer disease caused by *Calymmatobacterium granulomatis*. Also called **granuloma inguinale**.

Droplet transmission The spread of infectious agents in small liquid droplets through the air.

Dry heat sterilisation A method of sterilisation using dry heat at 160°C for 60 minutes.

Dysentery A severe diarrhoea characterised by blood and pus in the stools.

Dysuria Difficult or painful passing of urine.

Ecology The study of the relationship between organisms and their environment.

Ecosystem The living and non-living components of a particular environment.

Ectoparasite A parasite that lives on the surface of another organism.

Electron micrograph A photograph of a specimen taken with an electron microscope.

Electron microscope A microscope that uses electrons to produce an image of the specimen.

Electron transport chain A chain of specialised compounds that can pass electrons along the chain to a final electron acceptor (molecular oxygen), releasing energy as ATP.

Elephantiasis A gross enlargement of limbs, scrotum or other body parts caused by repeated infection by the worm *Wuchereria bancrofti*.

ELISA A method of detection of antibodies in blood. From Enzyme Linked Immunosorbent Assay.

Embden-Meyerhof pathway See **glycolysis**.

Empyema Infection of the pleural space.

Encephalitis Infection and inflammation of the brain.

Endemic disease A disease which is always present in a given population.

Endocarditis Inflammation of the internal membrane lining of the heart.

Endocytosis The process by which phagocytes take up foreign material.

Endogenous infection An infection caused by microorganisms from the patient's own body.

Endogenous pyrogen A fever-producing substance derived from body cells.

Endophthalmitis An infection and inflammation of the fluid behind the cornea.

Endoplasmic reticulum A network of membranes in eucaryotic cells connecting the nuclear membrane to the plasma membrane and providing sites for ribosomal attachment.

Endospore A resistant structure with a thick coat, formed within some Gram-positive bacterial cells.

Endotoxic shock A severe, life-threatening form of septicaemia caused by the release of large amounts of endotoxin from Gram-negative bacteria.

Endotoxin A lipopolysacccharide which occurs as part of the cell wall of most Gram-negative bacteria and is released when the cell dies. May produce toxic effects in the human host.

Endotracheal intubation The insertion of a tube into the trachea to open the airway.

Enriched medium A microbial growth medium that contains special growth factors for fastidious organisms.

Enteritis Inflammation of the intestine.

Enterobacteriaceae A group of facultatively anaerobic Gram-negative bacteria, many of which are found in the human intestine.

Enterotoxin An exotoxin which specifically acts on the intestine.

Enzyme A protein molecule that acts as a biological catalyst.

Eosinophil A blood cell present in large numbers in allergic reactions.

Epidemic A sudden rapid rise in the incidence of a disease in a particular population or area.

Epidemic keratoconjunctivitis An infection of the conjunctiva and cornea caused by adenoviruses.

Epidemic polyarthritis A systemic infection caused by the Ross River virus and spread by mosquitoes.

Epidemiology The study of the occurrence, spread and control of disease.

Epidermis The outer layer of the skin.

Epididymitis Infection and inflammation of the epididymis.

Epiglottitis Infection and inflammation of the epiglottis.

Epitope The small part of a whole antigen molecule that is the immunogenic component; the site of binding of antibodies or activated lymphocytes.

Erosion A superficial, circumscribed loss of epidermis, which heals without scarring.

Erysipelas A bacterial skin infection, often on the face, that typically appears as a bright red, swollen lesion with a sharply demarcated edge.

Erythema Reddened skin, usually due to inflammation.

Erythema migrans A unique skin lesion with a bulls-eye appearance which occurs in the early stage of Lyme disease.

Eschar The thick crust or scab that forms over a burn.

Etiology See Aetiology.

Eubacteria All procaryotes (bacteria) containing peptidoglycan cell walls. Also called true bacteria.

Eucaryotic All organisms that have their DNA enclosed in a nucleus and contain other membrane-bound organelles. Includes animals, plants and fungi.

Excoriation An area of skin, denuded of epidermis by scratching.

Exfoliatin An exotoxin possessed by some strains of *Staphylococcus aureus* that causes layers of cells in the epidermis to separate and sheets of skin to be shed (scalded skin syndrome).

Exogenous infection An infection caused by microorganisms from a source external to the patient.

Exogenous pyrogen A fever-producing substance derived from outside the body, often components of bacteria, and especially lipopolysaccharides.

Exotoxin A toxin secreted by a bacterium into its surrounding environment.

Exponential growth Growth of a bacterial culture characterised by a doubling of cell numbers in each time period.

Exudate An accumulation of plasma fluid and proteins in a tissue during inflammation.

F plasmid Extrachromosomal DNA found in F^+ donor cells capable of conjugation.

Facilitated diffusion The movement of substances across a membrane from a region of high concentration to a region of lower concentration using carrier proteins.

Facultative anaerobes Organisms which can grow in the presence or absence of oxygen.

Faecal-oral transmission The mode of transmission of pathogens that enter the body via the gastrointestinal tract and are excreted in faeces.

Falciparum malaria The most severe form of malaria caused by *Plasmodium falciparum*.

Fastidious microorganism A microorganism that requires special growth factors.

Fatty acid Long chain aliphatic compound containing a terminal carboxyl group.

Fermentation The enzymic breakdown of pyruvate in the absence of oxygen.

Fever (pyrexia) Abnormally high body temperature, representing severe or systemic infection and/or inflammation.

Fibroblast A cell which gives rise to collagen and connective tissue.

Filamentous fungi Fungi consisting of thin filaments or hyphae which form a mat called a mycelium.

Filariasis A systemic infection caused by several different roundworms; most commonly by *Wuchereria bancrofti*.

Filtration A method for separation of solids from liquids or gases by passage through special filters which retain the solids. Used to remove bacteria from solutions and air.

Fimbriae A hair-like appendage on bacteria, used for attachment to surfaces.

Five-kingdom classification A system of classification proposed by Whittaker, in which all living organisms are grouped into one of five kingdoms: Procaryota, Protista, Fungi, Plantae and Animalia.

Flagella Long thin appendages that are found on some organisms and that enable them to move.

Flatworms A primitive group of worms, the main parasitic ones being flukes and tapeworms.

Fluid mosaic model The model proposed for the structure of the cell membrane, consisting of proteins imbedded in a phospholipid bilayer.

Flukes Flatworms with complex life cycles.

Fluorescence microscopy The use of ultraviolet light in a microscope to visualise objects that fluoresce.

Folliculitis Infection of a hair follicle, usually caused by *Staphylococcus aureus*. Also called a **pimple** or **pustule**.

Fomite Any inanimate object that can be involved in the spread of infection.

Food intoxication A gastrointestinal disease caused by the presence of pre-formed toxins (microbial or non-microbial) in food.

Food poisoning A gastrointestinal disease related to the consumption of food, including microbial and non-microbial causes. Also called **food-borne illness**.

Food-borne illness See **food poisoning**.

Frame-shift mutation A mutation involving the deletion or insertion of one or more bases, resulting in a change in the codon and the insertion of a different amino acid into the protein.

Free radical A very reactive particle containing an unpaired electron.

Frequency The need to urinate more frequently than usual.

Fulminant hepatitis A clinical syndrome in which there is severe impairment or necrosis of liver cells, often resulting in liver failure and death.

Fulminating disease A sudden very severe disease, often with a fatal outcome.

Fungaemia The presence of fungi in the bloodstream.

Fungi Eucaryotic organisms with cell walls and not capable of photosynthesis.

Furuncle See **boil**.

Fusidic acid A bacteriostatic agent that inhibits protein synthesis.

Gammaglobulin (i) An antibody preparation extracted from the pooled serum of large numbers of blood donors; (ii) the fraction of blood proteins that contains antibodies.

Gangrenous infection An infection of the soft tissue below the dermis.

Gastritis Inflammation of the internal lining of the stomach.

Gastroenteritis Inflammation of the gastrointestinal tract, including the stomach and intestine.

Gastrointestinal infection A disease of the gastrointestinal tract caused by the establishment and multiplication of microorganisms in the gastrointestinal tract.

Gene A linear segment of DNA which codes for a particular hereditary characteristic.

Generation time The time taken for a bacterial cell to reproduce itself.

Genetic engineering Manipulation of the genetic material of an organism in order to alter the characteristics of the organism in a particular way.

Genetic recombination Formation of DNA involving the reciprocal exchange of homologous (paired) segments of DNA at any place on the chromosome.

Genus Part of the binomial classification system above the level of species, e.g. *Staphylococcus* in *Staphylococcus aureus*.

Germ theory of disease The principle proposed by Koch that microorganisms can cause disease.

German measles See **rubella**.

Germicide A substance that kills microorganisms (germs).

Ghon complex The characteristic finding in tuberculosis of tubercles (small granulomas) in the lung plus enlarged lymph nodes.

Giardiasis A gastrointestinal infection caused by the protozoan *Giardia intestinalis*.

Gingivitis A periodontal disease involving inflammation or infection of the gums.

Glandular fever A systemic infection caused by the Epstein-Barr virus. Also called **infectious mononucleosis**.

Glomerular haematuria The presence of blood in the urine due to inflammation or infection of the glomeruli of the kidneys.

Glomerulonephritis Inflammation of the glomeruli of the kidneys.

Glycerol An organic alcohol containing three carbon atoms. It combines with fatty acids to form triglycerides.

Glycocalyx A structure consisting of polysaccharides found outside the cell wall of some bacteria. Also called capsule or slime layer.

Glycogen A branched polysaccharide containing glucose units which acts as a carbon storage molecule.

Glycolysis The anaerobic metabolic pathway in which glucose is converted to pyruvate.

Golgi complex A membraneous organelle in eucaryotic cells involved in the secretion of proteins.

Gonorrhoea A sexually transmissible disease caused by the bacterium *Neisseria gonorrhoeae*.

Gram-negative A bacterium which stains red with the Gram stain.

Gram-positive A bacterium which retains the blue colour of the Gram stain.

Gram stain A standard procedure for staining bacteria which divides almost all bacteria into two groups, and serves as the first step in classifying and identifying them.

Granuloma A lesion associated with chronic inflammation that typically consists of a mass of different types of cells arranged in fairly discrete layers, and completely walled off by collagen.

Granuloma inguinale See **donovanosis**.

Guanine A purine nucleotide base that pairs with cytosine in RNA and DNA.

Gumma A soft, granulomatous lesion in the skin, bones, liver or other organs, charactersitic of tertiary syphilis.

Gut-associated lymphoid tissue (GALT) Clusters of lymphoid cells lining the mucosal surface of the intestinal tract.

Haemagglutination Aggregation (agglutination) of red blood cells.

Haematuria The presence of blood in urine.

Haemoflagellates A flagellated protozoan usually found in the bloodstream of its host.

Haemolysin A toxin that breaks down red cells.

Haemolytic uraemic syndrome (HUS) A possible complication of some infections caused by toxigenic strains of *E. coli*, characterised by haemolytic anaemia, uraemia, thrombocytopaenia, and renal failure.

Haemorrhagic fever A disease characterised by fever, malaise, myalgia, prostration, multisystem involvement and widespread haemorrhage, and caused by a number of different viruses.

Half-life The time taken for half of a substance to be used or destroyed.

Hapten A small molecule that cannot initiate an immune response on its own, but which reacts with antibodies or activated T cells produced against it.

Heavy (H) chain The longer polypeptide chain of an antibody molecule.

Helminths Worms.

Helper T cell A regulatory T lymphocyte that plays a central role in the immune response.

Hepatitis Injury and inflammation of the liver.

Hepatitis A Hepatitis caused by the hepatitis A virus.

Hepatitis B Hepatitis caused by the hepatitis B virus.

Hepatitis C Hepatitis caused by the hepatitis C virus.

Hepatitis D Hepatitis caused by the hepatitis D virus.

Hepatitis E Hepatitis caused by the hepatitis E virus.

Hepatocellular carcinoma Cancer of the liver.

Herd immunity The principle that individuals who are immune to an infectious disease will not be carriers of the organism, reducing the reservoir of that microbe in the community, and therefore the number of susceptible people who will encounter it.

Herpes encephalitis Infection of the brain caused by the herpes virus, especially serious in neonates.

Heterotroph An organism which requires an organic source of carbon for energy.

Hexose A sugar molecule containing six carbon atoms.

Hfr strain A bacterial strain which exhibit a high frequency of recombination due to the insertion of an F^+ plasmid into the chromosomal DNA.

Histamine A substance present in many body cell types, especially mast cells, basophils and platelets, that causes vasodilation and increased capillary permeability.

Histones Proteins associated with DNA in eucaryotic chromosomes.

Hookworm A type of roundworm which enters the body by burrowing through the skin and travels via the blood stream and attaches to the lungs and intestines.

Horizontal transmission Transmission of a disease from one person to another, usually by physical contact.

Hospital strain A strain of microorganism that originates in hospitals. This organism is likely to be resistant to some antimicrobial drugs.

Hospital-acquired infection An infection acquired in a hospital. Also called a **nosocomial infection**.

Humoral immune response An immune response to foreign antigen characterised by the activation of B lymphocytes and the production of specific antibodies against the antigen.

Humoral immunity Immunity provided by antibodies present in the body's fluids.

Hyaluronidase An enzyme produced by some bacteria which breaks down the hyaluronic acid of connective tissue.

Hydatid disease A disease characterised by the production of fluid filled sacs in the body, containing developing forms of the tapeworm *Echinococcus granulosis*.

Hydrophilic Water loving.

Hydrophobic Water hating; does not mix with water.

Hypersensitivity An over-reaction of the immune system to an antigen which it has previously encountered.

Hypertonic A solution with a higher concentration of dissolved substances than is present in a cell.

Hyphae Long filaments of cells found in fungi.

Hypotonic A solution with a lower concentration of dissolved substances than is present in a cell.

Iatrogenic infection An infection resulting from a medical procedure or treatment.

IgA A class of antibody molecules mainly found in mucosal secretions and breast milk.

IgD A class of antibody molecules found on the surface of B lymphocytes.

IgE The class of antibody molecules responsible for allergic reactions.

IgG The major class of antibody molecules in blood, and the class which crosses the placenta from mother to foetus.

IgM The class of antibody molecules in blood that are produced early in response to infection and that are indicative of recent infection.

Imidazoles A group of antifungal drugs that inhibit sterol synthesis.

Immediate hypersensitivity A hypersensitive reaction that occurs within minutes to hours after a sensitised person comes in contact with a foreign antigen. Also called **allergy** or **type I hypersensitvity**.

Immune complex An antibody molecule bound specifically to its antigen.

Immune complex hypersensitivity A hypersensitive reaction that results when antigen-antibody complexes are not cleared quickly from the body, instead being deposited in tissues. Also called **type III hypersensitivity**.

Immune response The specific response to the presence of a microorganism or foreign substance in the body.

Immune system The system of specific and non-specific defences the body has to eliminate foreign microorganisms and substances, and to provide long-term immunity to them.

Immunisation The exposure of a person to material that is antigenic but not pathogenic to make them immune to a certain microorganism. Also called **vaccination**.

Immunity The capacity of the immune system to successfully defend the body against a potentially infectious agent.

Immunocompromised Having a defect in one or more of the key components of the immune system (lymphocytes, phagocytes, or complement).

Immunodeficiency A condition in which the production or function of one of the key components of the immune system (lymphocytes, phagocytes, or complement) is abnormal.

Immunodeficiency disease A disease which causes immunodeficiency.

Immunofluorescence A method of diagnosis involving labelling with fluorescent antibodies.

Immunogen See **antigen**.

Immunogenic Capable of inducing an immune response.

Immunoglobulin See **antibody**.

Immunological memory The property of the immune system which enables it to react more rapidly and vigorously on subsequent exposures to the same antigen.

Immunology The study of the body's immune system.

Immunosuppression A depletion or reduction of the immune defences of the host.

Impetigo A highly infectious, skin infection caused by staphylococci, streptococci, or both.

In vitro Outside a living organism; in the laboratory.

In vivo In a living organism.

Incidence rate The proportion of a population that contracts a disease within a given time period.

Inclusions Small deposits found inside cells, e.g. storage granules.

Incubation period The period of time which elapses between exposure to a pathogen and the appearance of disease symptoms.

Index case The first case of a disease in an epidemic.

Inducer A substance which stimulates the expression a gene.

Inducible enzyme An enzyme which is synthesised under the influence of an inducer.

Induration A raised red area on the skin resulting from tuberculin sensitivity.

Infection The growth of pathogenic microorganisms in the body.

Infectious disease A disease which is caused by a pathogenic microorganism or its products.

Infectious mononucleosis See **glandular fever**.

Infective dose The number of microorganisms which must gain entry to the body in order to establish an infection.

Infective endocarditis An inflammation of the endocardium caused by a microorganism.

Inflammation The body's response to tissue injury, characterised by redness, swelling, heat and pain.

Inflammatory diarrhoea Diarrhoea characterised by stools containing blood, mucus and pus.

Influenza A respiratory infection caused by influenza A and B viruses.

Innate immunity See **non-specific immunity**.

Interferon (IFN) (i) A protein secreted by virus-infected cells which helps neighbouring cells to resist infection; (ii) a lymphokine secreted by activated T lymphocytes.

Interleukin A cytokine that acts as a chemical messenger between leukocytes.

Interleukin-1 (IL-1) A cytokine released by macrophages and other cells that stimulates activated T cells.

Interleukin-2 (IL-2) A cytokine that encourages activated T cells to proliferate and differentiate.

Intermediate host The host which harbours the immature or larval form of a parasite.

Intoxication A disease due to a microbial toxin.

Invasive phase The stage in a disease when the pathogen is invading the host and causing severe symptoms.

Iodophor An antiseptic preparation containing iodine and an organic compound.

Ischaemia Loss of blood supply to a tissue.

Isomers Organic compounds with the same chemical formula but different molecular structures.

Isotonic A solution containing the same concentration of dissolved substances as is found in a cell.

Keratin A tough protein found in skin, nails and hair that is resistant to most weak acids, bases, and bacterial enzymes and toxins.

Keratinase A microbial enzyme that degrades keratin.

Keratitis Infection and inflammation of the cornea.

Keratoconjunctivitis Infection and inflammation of the conjunctiva and cornea.

Kinases A group of enzymes produced by certain bacteria that enable them to dissolve fibrin clots.

Kinins Small peptides present in blood and other body fluids in an inactive form which, when activated, cause vasodilation, increased vascular permeability and pain.

Koch's Postulates A set of criteria proposed by Robert Koch, which should be met in order to determine whether an organism is responsible for causing a particular disease.

Koplik's spots Found in measles, they are areas of white necrosis on a reddened mucosa in the mouth.

Krebs cycle See TCA cycle.

Kuru A human prion disease which has been found in people of the Fore tribes in Papua New Guinea.

Lactoferrin A substance, present in a number of body secretions, that inhibits the growth of some microorganisms by binding the growth factor iron.

Lag phase The period of bacterial growth during which bacteria are exposed to fresh medium but do not increase in number.

Laryngitis Infection and inflammation of the larynx.

Laryngotracheitis Infection and inflammation of the larynx and trachea.

Latent Refers to the presence of a pathogen in the body without replicating.

Latent viral infection An infection in which the virus remains dormant in the host for long periods without replicating or producing disease symptoms.

Legionellosis See **Legionnaires' disease**.

Legionnaires' disease A pneumonia caused by *Legionella pneumophila* or other species of *Legionella*. Also called **legionellosis**.

Leishmaniasis Also called kala azar, a disease transmitted by sandflies, resulting in visceral or skin lesions, caused by species of *Leishmania*.

Lepromatous leprosy A form of leprosy in which there is uncontrolled proliferation of the bacterium resulting in extensive skin lesions and nerve involvement.

Leprosy An infection of skin and nerves caused by *Mycobacterium leprae*.

Leptospirosis A systemic bacterial infection caused by *Leptospira interrogans*.

Lesion An area of damaged tissue.

Leukocidin A toxin that kills phagocytic leukocytes (neutrophils and macrophages).

Leukocyte A white blood cell.

Leukocytosis A significant increase in the number of white cells in blood.

Leukopenia A decrease below normal numbers of white cells in the blood.

Leukotriene A mediator of inflammation synthesised from arachidonic acid, derived from mast cell membranes.

Ligand A carbohydrate-specific binding protein involved in adherence.

Light (L) chain The shorter polypeptide chain of an antibody molecule.

Light microscopy The use of a microscope which uses white light to visualise the specimen.

Lincosamides A group of antibacterial agents which inhibit protein syntheis.

Lipase An enzyme which breaks down fats into glycerol and the component fatty acids.

Lipid A An endotoxin which occurs as part of the cell wall of Gram-negative bacteria.

Lipopolysaccharide A kind of molecule composed of lipid and polysaccharide units. The lipopolysaccharides which occur as part of the wall of Gram-negative bacteria are called endotoxins.

Lipoproteins Molecules composed of lipid and protein units.

Listeriosis A systemic bacterial infection caused by *Listeria monocytogenes*.

Lobar pneumonia An infection and consolidation of the lung confined to certain lobes.

Localised infection An infection which is confined to one area of the body.

Log phase The period of bacterial growth when the bacteria are dividing at their maximum rate and cell numbers are increasing exponentially.

Logarithmic growth Growth of a bacterial culture during which there is a doubling of cell numbers in each specified time interval.

Lyme disease A systemic infection caused by the spirochaete *Borrelia burgdorferi*.

Lymph nodes Small, bean-shaped organs occurring throughout the lymphatic system and important in immune responses.
Lymphadenopathy A swelling of the lymph nodes.
Lymphocyte A white blood cell that plays a critical role in immune responses.
Lymphogranuloma venereum A sexually transmissible disease caused by *Chlamydia trachomatis*.
Lymphokines Cytokines secreted by activated helper T cells.
Lysis The rupture of a cell due to osmotic pressure or viral infection.
Lysogeny A state in which phage DNA is incorporated into the DNA of the bacterial cell that it has infected, but does not replicate or cause cell lysis.
Lysosomes Organelles that contain digestive enzymes; particularly prominent in phagocytes.
Lysozyme An enzyme found in body secretions that breaks down the cell wall of many bacteria.
Lytic cycle Infection of a cell by a virus resulting in lysis (destruction) of the host cell.
Macrolides A group of bacteriostatic antibiotics which affect protein synthesis; used as an alternative for people who are allergic to penicillin.
Macrophage A large phagocytic cell found in most tissues and organs of the body.
Macule A circumscribed, flat area of altered skin colour.
Major histocompatibility complex (MHC) The gene complex which codes for proteins that are used as recognition molecules by lymphocytes. The proteins are important antigens in transplant rejection.
Malaise A general feeling of being unwell.
Malaria A systemic infection caused by protozoa of the genus *Plasmodium*.
Malta fever See **brucellosis**.
Mantoux skin test A skin test for immunity to tuberculosis. Also called the **tuberculin skin test**.
Margination The process by which neutrophils stick to the inner walls of the capillaries prior to their movement through the capillary wall and into the tissues.
Mast cell A cell found throughout the body that contains histamine and other inflammatory mediators.
Measles A systemic disease characterised by a skin rash caused by the rubeola virus. Also called **rubeola**.
Measles encephalitis A rare complication of measles infection in which the virus persists in brain tissue.
Mechanical transmission The transmission of an infectious agent on the outside of an insect's body or on a person's hands.
Mediators of inflammation The chemicals that are responsible for the physiological events that occur in inflammation.
Medical asepsis Procedures that limit the number, growth and spread of microorganisms by practices such as good hygiene, handwashing and disinfection.
Meiosis The process in reproduction that leads to a halving of the number of chromosomes in a eucaryotic cell, from diploid to haploid.
Melioidosis An infection caused by the bacterium *Burkholderia pseudomallei*. Usually a pneumonia, but the organism can form abscesses in many body organs.
Membrane attack complex The components of the complement system that damage membranes of cells, resulting in their lysis.
Memory cell A lymphocyte that persists in the body for months to years and provides long-term immunity.
Meninges The three membranes that surround the brain and the spinal cord.
Meningitis Infection and inflammation of the meninges.
Meningococcal meningitis Meningitis caused by *Neisseria meningitidis*.
Meningococcus Another name for *Neisseria meningitidis*.
Merozoite A form of the malarial parasite found in the liver or infected blood cells.
Mesophile An organism which grows in the temperature range between about 10°C and 50°C.
Messenger RNA (mRNA) The type of RNA that carries the genetic message from DNA to the ribosome where it acts as a template to direct the incorporation of the correct amino acids into protein.
Metabolic pathway A sequence of enzymically directed reactions in which the product of one reaction serves as the substrate for the next reaction.
Metabolism The sum of all the chemical reactions which occur in a living cell.
Methicillin resistant *Staphylococcus aureus* (MRSA) A strain of *Staphylococcus aureus* that is resistant to methicillin and usually a number of other antimicrobial drugs.
Metronidazole A widely used antiprotozoal drug.
Microfilaria A microscopic roundworm larva which may block the lymph capillaries and cause elephantiasis.
Microflora See **normal flora**.
Mid-stream specimen of urine (MSU) A specimen of urine that is collected after the first few millilitres is allowed to pass.
Miliary tuberculosis A serious form of tuberculosis in which the bacterium spreads throughout the body.
Minimum inhibitory concentration (MIC) The lowest concentration of an antimicrobial agent which will prevent the growth of a particular microorganism.
Mitochondria Membrane-rich organelles found in eucaryotic cells; the site of oxidative phosphorylation reactions which produce ATP.
Mitosis The process by which eucaryotic nuclei divide, maintaining the same number of chromosomes.
MMR vaccine A vaccine to protect against measles, mumps and rubella.
Molluscum contagiosum A skin infection caused by viruses of the pox group.
Monera See **Procaryota**.
Moniliasis See **candidiasis**.
Monocyte A phagocytic blood cell that is the precursor of the tissue macrophage.
Monosaccharide A simple carbohydrate consisting of a single sugar unit containing five or six carbon atoms.
Morbidity (i) The incidence of disease in the total population; (ii) the state of being diseased.
Morphology The external appearance.
Mortality The number of deaths that result from a particular disease.
Motile Microorganisms that are able to move by the use of appendages such as cilia and flagella.
Mucinase An enzyme produced by some bacteria which digests a component of mucus, enhancing their ability to colonise mucous membranes.
Mucociliary escalator The ciliated epithelium of the upper respiratory tract which moves mucus and anything trapped in it upwards away from the lungs.
Mucocutaneous Relating to the mucous membranes and the epithelium.

Multi-resistant *Staphylococcus aureus* (MRSA) A strain of *Staphylococcus aureus* that is resistant to a number of antimicrobial drugs. These strains are responsible for many infections in hospitals.

Mutagen An agent which can cause a mutation.

Mutation A permanent change in the structure of DNA.

Mutualism A symbiotic relationship between two organisms in which both organisms benefit.

Mycelium A mass of fungal hyphae which intertwine forming a mat.

Mycoplasmas Very small bacteria which lack a cell wall.

Mycosis A fungal infection.

Naked virus A virus that is not surrounded by an envelope.

Narrow spectrum drug An antimicrobial agent which is active against only a few species of organisms.

Narrow spectrum antimicrobial agent A drug which is active against a limited number of microrganisms.

Natural immunity See **non-specific immunity**.

Natural killer (NK) cells A group of non-specific lymphoid cells that destroy cancer cells and virus-infected cells.

Naturally acquired active immunity Immunity that develops after an infection.

Naturally acquired passive immunity Immunity due to the natural transfer of antibodies, e.g. immunity acquired by the foetus via transplacental transfer of antibodies.

Necrosis Tissue death.

Necrotising fasciitis Infection and inflammation in the soft tissue below the dermis (the superficial fascia).

Necrotising infection Infection of the soft tissue below the dermis.

Nematode A roundworm.

Neurosyphilis A form of tertiary syphilis in which lesions form in the central nervous system.

Neurotoxin An exotoxin which acts predominantly on nervous tissue.

Neutralisation A process in which antibodies bind to and block specific attachment sites on viruses or bacterial exotoxins.

Neutropenia A decrease in the number of neutrophils in the blood.

Neutrophil The most abundant type of white blood cell. It is highly phagocytic and actively motile. Also called a **polymorphonuclear leukocyte (PMN)**, **polymorph** or **pus cell**.

Neutrophilia A significant increase in the number of neutrophils in blood. It is a characteristic sign of severe bacterial infection.

Nodule A circumscribed, elevated area of skin, larger than 1 cm in diameter.

Non-communicable diseases Diseases which are not usually spread from person to person.

Non-inflammatory diarrhoea A diarrhoea characterised by watery stools without blood, mucus or pus.

Non-specific defences Defences that offer general protection against all potentially harmful agents. These defences include the skin and mucous membranes, cellular defences, inflammation, antimicrobial proteins and fever.

Non-specific immunity Immunity provided by the non-specific defences to prevent the entry of pathogens into the body, or to immediately destroy them if they do manage to enter. Also called **innate immunity** and **natural immunity**.

Non-specific urethritis Any infection of the urethra not caused by *Neisseria gonorrhoeae* or *Chlamydia trachomatis*.

Non-polar A substance which does not carry any positive or negative charge on its molecules.

Nonsense codon A codon that does not code for an amino acid.

Normal flora The microorganisms that inhabit the human body without causing disease.

Nosocomial infection An infection that is acquired in a hospital or other health care facility.

Nuclear membrane The membrane enclosing the nucleus.

Nucleoli Areas in the nucleus of a eucaryotic cell where ribosomal RNA is formed.

Nucleoside A compound consisting of a purine or pyrimidine base joined to a pentose sugar molecule.

Nucleotide A nucleoside joined to one or more phosphate groups.

Nucleus An organelle in eucaryotic cells where chromosomes are located.

Obligate aerobes See **aerobe, obligate**.

Obligate anaerobes See **anaerobe, obligate**.

Oedema Swelling of a tissue due to an accumulation of fluid.

Oncogenic Cancer causing.

Oophoritis Inflammation of the ovaries.

Opportunistic infections Infections caused by organisms that do not usually cause disease, but can become pathogenic under certain conditions, such as depression of the immune system.

Opsonin A serum protein (antibody or complement) that enhances phagocyte activity.

Opsonisation The enhancement of phagocyte activity with opsonins.

Opthalmia neonatorum An eye infection in neonates caused by *Neisseria gonorrhoeae,* acquired from their mothers during passage through the birth canal.

Organelle A structure bounded by a membrane and found within eucaryotic cells.

Organic A compound containing carbon.

Ornithosis See **psittacosis**.

Osmosis The movement of water from an area of high water concentration to an area of low concentration across a selectively permeable membrane.

Osmotic pressure The pressure required to prevent the movement of water by osmosis.

Osteomyelitis Infection and inflammation of a bone.

Otitis media Infection and inflammation of the middle ear.

Oxidation The loss of electrons from a molecule.

Oxidative phosphorylation The process whereby the energy of electrons from oxidation reactions is coupled to the synthesis of ATP.

Pandemic An epidemic that spreads worldwide.

Papule A circumscribed, elevated area of skin, less than 1 cm in diameter.

Parasitaemia The presence of protozoa or helminths in the blood.

Parasite An organism that derives its nutrients from another living organism (the host).

Parasitism A symbiotic relationship in which one organism benefits while the other, the host, is harmed.

Paronychia An infection of the finger or toe nail.

Passive immunisation Immunisation involving the transfer of preformed antibodies to an individual.

Passive immunity The immunity resulting from the transfer of pre-made antibodies or immune cells from an immune person to a non-immune person.

Pasteurisation A method of mild heat treatment developed by Pasteur to destroy microorganisms responsible for food spoilage and some pathogens.

Pathogen An organism which is able to produce disease.

Pathogenicity The ability of a microorganism to cause disease.

Pediculosis A lice infestation usually involving the scalp, pubic area or trunk.

Pelvic inflammatory disease A clinical syndrome due to infection of the pelvic organs, particularly the uterus, fallopian tubes, ovaries or the whole peritoneal cavity, which may lead to scarring and blockage of the fallopian tubes.

Penicillin The first antibiotic to be discovered; one of a group of bacteriocidal compounds which inhibit cell wall synthesis.

Pentose A sugar molecule containing five carbon atoms.

Peptide A chain of amino acids joined by peptide bonds.

Peptidoglycan A major structural component of bacterial cell walls.

Perforins Protein molecules which are inserted into the plasma membrane of a target cell bringing about its death.

Peritonitis Infection and inflammation of the peritoneal cavity.

Persistent generalised lymphadenopathy A phase of human immunodeficiency virus infection representing viral multiplication in lymph nodes.

Pertussis A potentially severe infection of the respiratory tract caused by *Bordetella pertussis*. Also called **whooping cough**.

Petechia A small flat haemorrhage.

Phage See **bacteriophage**.

Phage typing A method of identification of different strains of bacteria by determining their susceptibility to infection by specific bacteriophage.

Phagocyte A cell that actively ingests and digests foreign material in the body.

Phagolysosome A structure in a phagocyte derived from the fusion of a phagosome with lysosomes and in which lysosomal enzymes break down foreign material.

Phagosome A phagocytic vacuole which contains ingested foreign material formed within the cytoplasm of a phagocyte.

Pharyngitis Infection and inflammation of the oropharynx.

Phospholipid A compound consisting of glycerol, two fatty acids, phosphate and various bases.

Phospholipid bilayer A double layer of phospholipid molecules which form the basic structure (matrix) of cell membranes.

Photosynthesis The process occurring in green plants in which energy from the sun is used to synthesise carbohydrate (glucose) from carbon dioxide and water.

Pili Appendages on a bacterial cell some of which are used to transfer DNA during conjugation and some of which are for attachment to surfaces.

Pimple See **folliculitis**.

Pinworm A tiny roundworm that lives in the human intestine. Also called threadworm.

Pityriasis versicolor A skin infection caused by the yeast *Malassezia furfur*. Also called **tinea versicolor**.

Plague An infection of lymph nodes and other organs caused by the bacterium *Yersinia pestis*.

Plantae Plants, one of the original Linnaean classifications.

Plaque A coating of microorganisms and organic matter on tooth enamel.

Plasma The fluid part of blood without the cells and platelets.

Plasma cell The cell responsible for synthesis and secretion of antibodies in humoral immunity.

Plasma membrane See **cytoplasmic membrane**.

Plasmid A small piece of cyclic DNA found in some bacteria which replicates independently of the chromosomal DNA.

Plate count A method of determining the number of bacteria in a sample.

Platyhelminthes Flatworms.

Pleomorphic Occurring in more than one form.

Pleural effusion The entry of an inflammatory exudate into the space between the lung tissue and pleural membranes.

Pleurisy Inflammation of the pleural membranes.

Pneumonia Infection and inflammation of the lung(s).

Pneumonic plague Infection of the lungs by the plague bacterium, *Yersinia pestis*.

Point mutation The substitution of one base for another in DNA, causing mutation.

Polar Refers to a molecule which carries a positive or negative charge.

Polio (poliomyelitis) A systemic infection caused by the polio virus in which infection of the central nervous system may occur and may result in paralysis.

Polyenes A group of antifungal compounds which interfere with sterol synthesis.

Polymerase chain reaction A technique used to copy a specific nucleotide sequence contained within a sample of DNA, thus increasing the quantity of DNA to detectable levels.

Polymorph See **neutrophil**.

Polymorphonuclear leukocyte (PMN) See **neutrophil**.

Polypeptide A long chain of amino acids, joined by peptide bonds.

Polyribosome A ribosome complex where a number of ribosomes are bound along a strand of mRNA.

Polysaccharide A polymer of sugar units.

Pontiac fever A mild form of *Legionella* infection, characterised by myalgia, fever, malaise and headache.

Portal of entry The point of entry of a pathogen into the body.

Portal of exit The point at which a pathogen exits from the body.

Post-polio syndrome A syndrome in which symptoms of muscular weakness occur late in life in people who have recovered from childhood polio.

Post-streptococcal glomerulonephritis Infection of the glomeruli of the kidneys, following a streptococcal infection elsewhere in the body.

PPD (purified protein derivative) The antigen used in the Mantoux skin test for immunity to tuberculosis.

Precipitation The cross linking of soluble antigens by antibody to form large complexes which precipitate out of solution.

Prevalence rate The proportion of people with a particular disease at a given point in time.

Primary cell line Animal cells extracted from live tissue which are grown in tissue culture in the laboratory.

Primary immune response The response of the acquired immune system the first time it is exposed to a particular antigen.

Primary immunodeficiency Abnormal production or function of phagocytes, lymphocytes or complement due to a genetic or developmental defect.

Primary infection An acute infection which is the cause of the initial illness.

Primary lymphoid organs The thymus and the bone marrow which are the sites of lymphocyte maturation.

Primary metabolite A compound produced during the active growth phase of a microrganism.

Primary syphilis The first stage of syphilis infection characterised by the development of a papular lesion at the site of infection.

Prion An infectious protein agent that causes fatal, neurodegenerative diseases in humans or animals.

Procaryota The classification kingdom which contains all the bacteria. Also called Monera.

Procaryotic Having characteristics of the procaryotes, including a lack of subcellular organelles.

Prodromal period The period in the course of a disease when non-specific symptoms are present before the onset of specific signs or symptoms.

Proglottid Segment of a tapeworm.

Prophage Bacteriophage DNA which has been integrated into the bacterial host DNA.

Prophylactic antibiotic An antibiotic administered in order to prevent the occurrence of an infection.

Prophylaxis The administration of a drug to prevent a disease.

Prostaglandins A group of biologically active substances, some of which are mediators of inflammation.

Prosthetic group A molecule bound to an enzyme which is necessary for enzyme activity.

Protective asepsis Infection control procedures designed to prevent the transmission of an infection to or from a patient.

Proteinuria The presence of protein in the urine.

Protista The biological kingdom comprising unicellular eucaryotic organisms.

Protoplast A bacterium without its cell wall, enclosed by the cell membrane.

Protozoa Single-celled eucaryotic organisms belonging to the kingdom Protista.

Pseudomembrane A greyish membrane, consisting of dead tissue cells, bacteria and inflammatory exudate, which forms over the pharynx in diphtheria.

Psittacosis A pneumonia caused by *Chlamydia psittaci*, usually acquired from birds. Also called **ornithosis**.

Psychrophile An organism which grows best in cool temperatures (15° to 20°C).

PUO—pyrexia of unknown origin The presence of a fever without any obvious infection.

Pure culture A culture consisting of only one species of organism.

Purpura Numerous petechiae. Small flat haemorrhages on the skin.

Pus A thick, creamy coloured fluid comprising a mixture of dead or dying neutrophils, tissue debris and remaining pathogens.

Pus cell See **neutrophil**.

Pustule See **folliculitis**.

Pyelonephritis Inflammation of one or both kidneys.

Pyogenic Pus forming.

Pyrexia Fever.

Pyrogen A substance which produces fever.

Pyruvic acid A compound containing three carbon atoms, the main product of the metabolism of glucose via the glycolytic pathway.

Pyuria The presence of large numbers of leucocytes (pus) in urine.

Q fever A pneumonia caused by the bacterium *Coxiella burnetii*.

Quinine An antimicrobial drug extracted from the bark of the chinchona tree.

Quinolones A group of antibacterials which interfere with DNA synthesis.

Rabies An infection of the central nervous system caused by the rabies virus.

Recombinant DNA DNA formed from two different species.

Regeneration The restoration of a tissue's orginal structure and function after damage by the replacement of cells by mitosis.

Repression The process whereby a repressor molecule prevents the synthesis of a protein.

Repressor A protein that interferes with the expression of a gene.

Reservoir of infection A site where microorganisms persist and which acts as a continual source of infectious agents.

Resident flora See **normal flora**.

Resistance The ability of the body to prevent the occurrence of an infection.

Resistance factors (R) Genes which bestow antimicrobial resistance on bacteria, usually carried on plasmids.

Respiration In metabolism, the aerobic breakdown of carbohydrates with release of a energy.

Restriction endonucleases Enzymes derived from bacteria which are able to cut double stranded DNA at specific sites on the DNA molecule. Used in genetic engineering.

Retinitis Inflammation of the retina.

Retroviruses A class of single stranded RNA viruses which replicate by first synthesising DNA from RNA.

Reverse barrier nursing See **protective asepsis**.

Reverse transcriptase A viral enzyme that transcribes RNA into DNA.

Reye's syndrome A sometimes fatal disease occasionally seen in children after a viral infection which was treated with aspirin.

Rheumatic fever A non-infectious complication of *Streptococcus pyogenes* sore throat in which immune damage to heart and other tissues occurs.

Rheumatic heart disease Scarring and deformation of the heart valves due to rheumatic fever.

Rheumatoid arthritis A combination autoimmune disease and immune-complex hypersensitivity which causes chronic inflammation and joint damage.

Rheumatoid factor An anti-IgG antibody found in the blood of people with rheumatoid arthritis.

Rhinitis Infection and inflammation of the nasal passages. Also called **coryza**.

Ribose A pentose sugar which occurs in ribonucleic acid.

Ribosomes Particles containing RNA and protein found in the cytoplasm and acting as the site of protein synthesis.

Rickettsiae Small intracellular bacteria.

Rifamycin An antibiotic which inhibits RNA synthesis, used to treat TB.

Ringworm A skin infection caused by several different fungi. Also called **tinea**.

RNA (ribonucleic acid) Nucleic acid which takes part in protein synthesis.

Rubella A systemic disease characterised by a skin rash and caused by the rubella virus. Also called **German measles**.

Rubeola See **measles**.

Sabin vaccine The oral poliomyelitis vaccine containing an attenuated virus.

Salk vaccine The inactivated poliomyelitis vaccine administered by intramuscular injection.

Salmonellosis A mainly gastrointestinal infection caused by species of *Salmonella*.

Salpingitis Inflammation of the fallopian tubes.

Sanitisation Thorough cleaning of an object to remove most microorganisms.

Scabies A skin infestation caused by the mite *Sarcoptes scabiei* var. *hominis*.

Scalded skin syndrome A skin disorder caused by strains of *Staphylococcus aureus* which produce the exfoliatin toxin.

Scale An abnormal accumulation of keratin in skin.

Scanning electron microscope An electron microscope that provides a three dimensional image of a specimen at very high magnifications.

Scar tissue replacement Replacement of damaged tissue with scar tissue, which does not have the physiological functions of the original tissue.

Scarlet fever An erythematous skin rash caused by some strains of *Streptococcus pyogenes* which produce an erythrogenic toxin.

Schistosomiasis A debilitating systemic disease caused by flukes of the genus *Schistosoma*.

Schizogony The process of multiple fission in which one cell divides many times to produce multiple daughter cells.

Scolex The head of a tapeworm.

Secondary immune response The immune response resulting from exposure to the same antigen for the second time. The response is faster, stronger and longer lasting than a primary response.

Secondary immunodeficiency Immunodeficiency resulting from damage or suppression of otherwise normal components of the immune system by infection, cancer, malnutrition, drugs or other therapies.

Secondary infection An infection that occurs following a primary infection, when the patient is in a weakened state.

Secondary lymphoid organs The collection of lymphoid organs and tissues that are the sites in the body where immune reactions occur.

Secondary metabolites Products of microbial metabolism, usually accumulating in stationary phase.

Secondary syphilis The secondary stage of syphilis characterised by a skin rash or lesions on mucous membranes.

Selective medium A microbial culture medium that allows some organisms to grow but not others.

Selective toxicity The ability of an antimicrobial agent to inactivate or destroy a microorganism without harming the host cell.

Semi-permeable membrane The membrane surrounding most living cells that controls the passage of substances in and out of the cell. Also called selectively permeable.

Sepsis Poisoning due to infection by microorganisms.

Septic shock A life-threatening disorder due to the presence of large amounts of endotoxin in the body.

Septicaemia A serious clinical syndrome resulting from the presence of bacteria in the bloodstream.

Serial dilution A method used to dilute a sample so that the number of bacteria present can be counted accurately.

Seroconversion The development of antibodies to an antigen in a person's blood.

Seroconversion illness An early stage of human immunodeficiency virus infection characterised by an acute illness at the time of antibody production.

Serology The detection of antibodies or antigens in a sample of blood or other body fluid.

Seroprevalence The prevalence of a disease in the community as determined by the number of people who are carrying antibodies to the disease at any one time.

Serotypes Different antigenic strains of a microorganism.

Serum The liquid part of blood after the cells and clotting factors have been removed.

Sex pilus See **Pili**.

Sexually transmissible disease An infection acquired during sexual activity.

Shigellosis See **bacillary dysentery**.

Shingles A disease caused by the re-activation of the varicella zoster (chickenpox) virus characterised by painful, vesicular lesions on the skin.

Significant bacteriuria A bacterial count of 10^8/L or more in a properly collected midstream specimen of urine.

Signs of disease Measurable changes which can be observed in the patient.

Sinusitis Inflammation of the sinus cavities.

Slime layer See **glycocalyx**.

Smallpox A serious systemic disease that has been eradicated from the world.

Source of infection The individual or object from which an infection is acquired.

Specialised transduction The accidental inclusion of a piece of chromosomal DNA adjacent to a prophage when the prophage is transferred to another cell.

Species A group of organisms with similar properties; the second name in bacterial classification.

Specific defences See **acquired immune system**.

Specific immune globulin (SIG) An antibody preparation obtained from the serum of people who are convalescing from a particular infection and have a large amount of a specific antibody.

Specific immune system See **acquired immune system**.

Spermine An antibacterial substance found in semen.

Spirillum A spiral shaped bacterium.

Spirochaete A spiral shaped bacterium with an axial filament.

Spongiform encephalopathy A prion disease producing microscopic vacuoles in the brain, giving it a spongy appearance.

Spontaneous generation The theory that life can arise spontaneously from non-living matter.

Sporadic disease Occasional or random outbreak of disease.

Sporangiophore An aerial hypha which carries a sporangium.

Sporangiospore An asexual fungal spore.

Sporangium A sac containing spores.

Spore An asexual reproductive structure formed by fungi and actinomycetes. See also **endospore**.

Spore coat The thick protective layer formed around a bacterial endospore.

Sporozoan A kind of non-motile protozoan.

Sporozoite A trophozoite of malaria which occurs in the salivary glands of mosquitoes.

Sputum A specimen from the lungs produced from a deep cough.

Staining The application of a stain or dye to microorganisms prior to examination under a microscope.

Staphylococci A genus of Gram-positive bacteria characterised by small round cocci which occur in clusters.

Staphylokinase An enzyme produced by *Staphylococcus aureus* which breaks down fibrin clots.

Starch A carbohydrate polymer consisting of branched chains of glucose units.

Stationary phase A stage in growth of a bacterial culture when the number of new cells being produced equals the number of cells which die.

Stereospecificity The way in which the spatial configuration (shape) of a molecule determines its ability to bind to another molecule.

Stereoisomers Two molecules which have the same chemical structure, but differ in shape; mirror images of each other.

Sterilisation The complete destruction or removal of all microorganisms including viruses and endospores.

Streak plate method The method by which microorganisms are isolated as separate colonies on an agar plate.

Streptococci A genus of Gram-positive bacteria which occur as chains of cocci.

Streptokinase An enzyme produced by some streptococci which breaks down fibrin and which is used therapeutically as a thrombolytic agent.

Subacute sclerosing panencephalitis (SSPE) A rare and serious complication of measles due to viral persistence in brain tissue.

Subclinical infection An infection which does not produce any recognisable signs or symptoms, but elicits an immune response.

Subcutaneous infection An infection involving tissue beneath the skin.

Substrate The molecule which an enzyme reacts with.

Subunit vaccine A vaccine based on a part of a microorganism.

Sulpha drug Synthetic drug containing sulphur.

Sulphonamides A group of bacteriostatic agents which interfere with folic acid synthesis.

Superficial mycosis A fungal infection located on the skin or hair shaft.

Superinfection An overgrowth of a resistant microbial species, usually after a period of antimicrobial therapy.

Superoxide dismutase An enzyme that destroys the free radical O_2^-.

Superoxide The free radical O_2^-.

Surgical asepsis The procedures followed to maintain sterility.

Surveillance The collection of data on all aspects of the occurrence and spread of a disease.

Susceptibility The lack of resistance or a vulnerability to an infection.

Symbiosis Two different organisms which are living together.

Symptoms of disease Changes felt and reported by the patient as a result of disease.

Syndrome A group of signs and symptoms which are characteristic of a particular disease.

Synergism A situation where the effect of two drugs working together is greater than the action of the drugs working alone.

Syphilis A sexually transmissible disease caused by the spirochaete *Treponema pallidum*.

Systemic candidiasis See Candidaemia.

Systemic disease A disease which affects the whole body.

Systemic infection An infection in which microorganisms enter the bloodstream and are disseminated through the body.

Systemic mycosis A fungal infection which occurs in deep tissue or involves various organs in the body.

TCA—tricarboxylic acid cycle A pathway in carbohydrate metabolism whereby pyruvic acid is converted to carbon dioxide and water with the release of large amounts of energy stored as ATP.

T cell See **T lymphocyte**.

T-dependent antigen An antigen which requires the involvement of T cells in order for activation of B cells to occur.

T lymphocyte A type of lymphocyte which matures in the thymus gland. Responsible for cell mediated immunity and regulation of immune responses.

T4 cell A T lymphocyte that possesses the CD4 receptor on its surface; it displays helper activity. Also called a **helper T cell**.

T8 cell A T lymphocyte that possesses the CD8 receptor on its surface; it may display cytotoxic or suppressor activity. Those with cytotoxic activity are called **cytotoxic T cells**.

Tapeworm A segmented flatworm, the adult stage of which lives in the intestine.

Teichoic acid A polysaccharide which occurs in the walls of Gram-positive bacteria.

Temperate phage A bacteriophage which exists in a lysogenic state in the host cell.

Template A pattern for the replication of a certain structure, as in DNA or RNA.

Teratogen A substance causing abnormalities to the foetus in utero.

Tertiary syphilis The third stage of syphilis infection in which bacterial multiplication and dissemination and a cell-mediated hypersensitivity response of the immune system combine to form lesions in various organs.

Tetanus A disease characterised by severe muscle spasm caused by the exotoxin of *Clostridium tetani*.

Tetracyclines A group of bacteriostatic drugs which inhibit protein synthesis.

Therapeutic index Ratio of the effective dose of a drug to the dose which will be lethal for the host (patient).

Thermal death point The lowest temperature at which all the microorganisms present will be killed in a given time.

Thermal death time The time required to kill all the microorganisms present at a given temperature.

Thermophile An organism which grows well at high temperatures (50° to 60°C).

Threadworm See **Pinworm**.

Thrush A superficial infection of mucous membranes characterised by milky white patches of inflammation.

Thymine A pyrimidine base in DNA which pairs with adenine.

Thymine dimer A compound produced by the formation of bonds between adjacent thymine molecules in DNA chains exposed to UV radiation.

Thymus An organ found in the upper thoracic region beneath the sternum. Immature lymphocytes develop into mature T cells under the influence of thymic hormones.

Tincture of iodine A solution of iodine in alcohol.

Tinea See **ringworm**.

Tinea capitis Tinea of the scalp.

Tinea corporis Tinea of the body (trunk).

Tinea cruris Tinea of the groin.

Tinea pedis See **athlete's foot**.

Tinea unguium Tinea of the nails.

Tinea versicolor See **pityriasis versicolor**.

Tissue tropism The ability of a virus to attach to specific receptor molecules on the cell surface.

Titre A measure of the amount of specific antibody in blood or other body fluid. The reciprocal of the greatest dilution of the fluid that shows a positive reaction in an antibody-antigen reaction.

Tolerance A non-responsiveness of the immune system to a given antigen.

Tonsillitis Infection and inflammation of the tonsils.

Toxaemia The presence of toxins in the bloodstream.

Toxic shock syndrome A systemic disease caused by certain strains of *Staphylococcus aureus* that produce the toxic shock syndrome toxin.

Toxin A substance produced by microorganisms that interferes with the normal functioning of host cells or tissues.

Toxoid A bacterial exotoxin that has been modified to remove its toxicity while still retaining its ability to elicit an immune response.

Toxoplasmosis A systemic infection caused by the protozoan *Toxoplasma gondii.*

TPN—total parenteral nutrition A procedure whereby all nutrition and drugs are administered via a central catheter.

Tracheitis Infection and inflammmation of the trachea.

Trachoma An eye infection which can lead to blindness caused by *Chlamydia trachomatis.*

Transcription The process of synthesis of messenger RNA using DNA as a template.

Transduction Transfer of DNA from one bacterial cell to another by a bacteriophage.

Transfer RNA A small RNA molecule responsible for transferring the correct amino acid to the growing peptide chain in protein synthesis.

Transformation The process in which naked DNA passes from one bacterial cell to another resulting in a change in the properties of the recipient cell.

Transient flora Microorganisms which are found on the human body for only a short time and do not cause disease.

Translation The formation of a polypeptide on a messenger RNA template.

Transmission electron microscope An electron microscope used to study the internal structures of cells at high magnification.

Transport medium A liquid or semi-liquid medium into which some specimens are placed to prevent them from drying and to maintain microorganism viability.

Traveller's diarrhoea The acute diarrhoea that frequently occurs in people visiting a foreign country. Often caused by *E. coli.*

Trematodes See **flukes**.

Trichinosis A disease caused by the nematode Trichinella spiralis which is acquired by eating poorly cooked meat (mainly pork).

Trichomoniasis An infection caused by *Trichomonas vaginalis.*

Triple antigen vaccine (DTP) A vaccine used to immunise against diphtheria, pertussis and tetanus.

Trophozoite A vegetative (non-reproductive) form of a protozoan.

Trypanosomes A group of flagellated protozoans.

Tubercle A granuloma lesion charcteristic of tuberculosis infection.

Tuberculin A protein of the *Mycobacterium* cell used in the mantoux skin test.

Tuberculin skin test See **Mantoux skin test**.

Tuberculoid leprosy The form of leprosy in which a strong cell-mediated immune response limits the multiplication of the organism and the disease is confined to patches of skin and certain nerve trunks.

Tuberculosis An infection of the lungs or other organs caused by species of *Mycobacteria.*

Tumour necrosis factor (TNF) A cytokine which kills virus-infected cells as well as being important in inflammation and lymphocyte proliferation.

Turbidity Cloudiness of a liquid.

Type I hypersensitivity See **immediate hypersensitivity**.

Type II hypersensitivity See **cytotoxic hypersensitivity**.

Type III hypersensitivity See **immune complex hypersensitivity**.

Type IV hypersensitivity See **delayed type hypersensitivity**.

Ulcer An area of tissue loss, varying in depth. An ulcer may involve skin only, or may extend more deeply into subcutaneous tissue.

Ultraviolet radiation Low energy short wavelength radiation which can disrupt chemical bonds, e.g. in DNA, causing mutation or cell death.

Undulant fever See **brucellosis**.

Urethritis Infection and inflammation of the urethra.

Urgency The urgent need to urinate; symptomatic of urinary tract infection.

Vaccination See **immunisation**.

Vaccine A preparation containing one or more antigens that is used to immunise a person against a specific disease.

Vacuole A membrane bound structure in the cytoplasm of cells, usually containing gas or storage molecules.

Vaginosis An abnormal vaginal discharge.

Varicella Chicken pox.

Vasoconstriction A decrease in the diameter of blood vessels.

Vasodilation Dilation of blood vessels.

Vegetation A clump of bacteria, fibrin and platelets on the endocardium, characteristic of infective endocarditis.

Vertical transmission Transmission of an infection from mother to foetus in utero.

Vesicle A small blister containing clear fluid, less than 0.5 cm in diameter.

Vibrio A small curved (comma-shaped) bacterium.

Viraemia The presence of viruses in the blood.

Viral attachment proteins Proteins on the surface of the virus which attach to specific receptors on the surface of the target cell.

Viral genome The genetic material of a virus.

Virion An entire mature virus particle, occurring outside a host cell and consisting of nucleic acid, protein capsid and sometimes an envelope.

Viroid An infectious particle consisting only of circular RNA and lacking a capsid.

Virulence The degree of pathogenicity of an organism.

Virulence factors The factors which contribute to an organism's ability to cause disease.

Virus A tiny infectious particle consisting of nucleic acid and a protein coat.

Virustatic Able to inhibit viral replication.

Volutin Granules of polyphosphate in bacterial cells.

Wart A benign mass of tissue on the skin or mucous membrane caused by a papilloma virus.

Water-borne transmission Transmission of an infectious agent in contaminated water.

Weil's disease See **leptospirosis**.

Wet preparation A suspension of microorganisms in a drop of fluid for microscopic examination.

Wheal A raised, often itchy erythematous lesion.

Whooping cough See **pertussis**.

X-linked agammaglobulinaemia A primary immunodeficiency disease caused by incomplete maturation of B lymphocytes.

Yeast A unicellular fungus.

Yellow fever A systemic infection caused by the yellow fever virus and transmitted by mosquitoes.

Ziehl-Neelsen stain See **acid-fast stain**.

Zone of inhibition A clear area corresponding to inhibition of bacterial growth which appears on an agar plate around an antimicrobial disk.

Zoster Shingles.

Zoonosis An infection of animals that can be transmitted to humans.

credits

1.3: The Granger Collection

1.4: Black, J.G., *Microbiology: Principles and Applications,* 2nd ed., Prentice Hall, Englewood Cliffs, New Jersey, 1993

1.5: Black, J.G., *Microbiology: Principles and Applications,* 2nd ed., Prentice Hall, Englewood Cliffs, New Jersey, 1993

1.6: Black, J.G., *Microbiology: Principles and Applications,* 2nd ed., Prentice Hall, Englewood Cliffs, New Jersey, 1993

1.9 (a) (b): Dr T. Smithyman, Cellabs, Sydney

1.9 (c): Professor Adrian Lee, Department of Microbiology, University of New South Wales

2.19: Penny Bishop

3.2: Gary Lee

3.3: Dr T. Smithyman, Cellabs, Sydney

3.4: J. O'Rourke, School of Microbiology and Immunology, University of New South Wales

3.5: Phillips Scientific and Industrial Electronics

3.6: Gary Lee

3.8: Gary Lee

4.3 (a): The Photographic Library of Australia Pty Ltd, North Sydney

4.3 (b): Gary Lee

4.4: Professor Adrian Lee, Department of Microbiology, University of New South Wales

4.5: Black, J.G., *Microbiology: Principles and Applications,* 2nd ed., Prentice Hall, Englewood Cliffs, New Jersey, 1993

4.6: Black, J.G., *Microbiology: Principles and Applications,* 2nd ed., Prentice Hall, Englewood Cliffs, New Jersey, 1993

4.7 (a) (b): Black, J.G., *Microbiology: Principles and Applications,* 2nd ed., Prentice Hall, Englewood Cliffs, New Jersey, 1993

4.8: G. Jayachandran, Faculty of Health Sciences, University of Sydney

4.14: Brock et al, *Biology of Microorganisms*, 7th ed., Prentice Hall, Englewood Cliffs, New Jersey, 1994

4.16 (a) (b) (c) (d): G. Jayachandran, Faculty of Health Sciences, University of Sydney

4.17: Alison Vickery, Department of Microbiology, Royal Prince Alfred Hospital, Sydney

4.19: Black, J.G., *Microbiology: Principles and Applications,* 2nd ed., Prentice Hall, Englewood Cliffs, New Jersey, 1993

4.20: Black, J.G., *Microbiology: Principles and Applications,* 2nd ed., Prentice Hall, Englewood Cliffs, New Jersey, 1993

4.24: Black, J.G., *Microbiology: Principles and Applications,* 2nd ed., Prentice Hall, Englewood Cliffs, New Jersey, 1993

5.2: Black, J.G., *Microbiology: Principles and Applications,* 2nd ed, Prentice Hall, Englewood Cliffs, New Jersey, 1993

5.3: Black, J.G., *Microbiology: Principles and Applications,* 2nd ed, Prentice Hall, Englewood Cliffs, New Jersey, 1993

5.4: Black, J.G., *Microbiology: Principles and Applications,* 2nd ed, Prentice Hall, Englewood Cliffs, New Jersey, 1993

5.5: Penny Bishop

5.6: Black, J.G., *Microbiology: Principles and Applications,* 2nd ed., Prentice Hall, Englewood Cliffs, New Jersey, 1993

5.7: Black, J.G., *Microbiology: Principles and Applications,* 2nd ed., Prentice Hall, Englewood Cliffs, New Jersey, 1993

5.8: Dr T. Smithyman, Cellabs, Sydney

5.9 (a) (b): Department of Infectious Diseases, University of Sydney

Table 5.1: Data derived from Brooks, G.F., et al, *Jawetz, Melnick & Adelberg's Medical Microbiology*, 19th ed., Appleton & Lange, East Norwalk, CT, 1991, Table 32.1, p. 368

6.1: Schering AG, Berlin

6.2: The Photographic Library of Australia Pty Ltd, North Sydney

6.3 (a) (b): David Muir, Royal North Shore Hospital, Sydney

6.4 (a) (b): David Muir, Royal North Shore Hospital, Sydney

6.5: Bayer AG

6.6: Janssen-Cilag Pty Ltd

6.7: Bayer AG

6.8 (d): Professor Andrew Thompson, Murdoch University

6.9 (a): Penny Bishop

6.9 (b): Dr T. Smithyman, Cellabs, Sydney

6.12 (a) (b): Stephen Neville, Department of Microbiology, South Western Area Pathology Service, Liverpool, NSW

6.13 (a) (c): Stephen Neville, Department of Microbiology, South Western Area Pathology Service, Liverpool, NSW

6.13 (b): © Richard Watts/Visuals Unlimited

7.1: The Photographic Library of Australia Pty Ltd, North Sydney

7.2: Pelczar, M.J., *Microbiology: Concepts and Applications,* New York: McGraw-Hill, Inc, 1993, reproduced with permission of the McGraw-Hill Co.

8.2: Christine Bishop

8.4 (a) (b): CSIRO/Australian Animal Health Laboratories

9.1: Black, J.G., *Microbiology: Principles and Applications,* 2nd ed., Prentice Hall, Englewood Cliffs, New Jersey, 1993

9.3: Reproduced with kind permission of Boehringer Ingelheim Pty Ltd

10.3: G. Jayachandran, Faculty of Health Sciences, University of Sydney

10.6 (a) (b): Department of Infectious Diseases, University of Sydney

10.7: Royal Prince Alfred Hospital, Sydney

11.3: Courtesy Millipore Corporation, Bedford, Mass., USA

11.4: Christine Bishop

11.5: Christine Bishop

12.8: Sutherland, D.C., 1992 'Antiretroviral Agents in the Nineties', *The Medical Journal of Australia*, 157: pp. 135–137. © 1992 Reproduced with permission

12.9: Penny Bishop

13.4: Christine Bishop

14.1: © Commonwealth of Australia. Reproduced with permission

14.2: © Commonwealth of Australia. Reproduced with permission

14.3: © Commonwealth of Australia. Reproduced with permission
14.4: © Commonwealth of Australia. Reproduced with permission
14.5: © Commonwealth of Australia. Reproduced with permission
14.6: © Commonwealth of Australia. Reproduced with permission
14.7: Black, J.G., *Microbiology: Principles and Applications,* 2nd ed., Prentice Hall, Englewood Cliffs, New Jersey, 1993
14.8 (a) (b): © Commonwealth of Australia. Reproduced with permission
14.9: Reproduced with permission from *Today's Life Science*
14.11: Associate Professor Bart Currie, Menzies School of Health Research, Darwin
14.12: Dr John Walker, Department of Parasitology, Centre for Infectious Diseases and Microbiology, Westmead Hospital, Sydney
Tables 14.1 and 14.2: © Commonwealth of Australia. Reproduced with permission
Table 14.3: Reproduced with permission of Dr Brian Feery, Consultant, CSL Vaccines
Tables 14.4 and 14.6: Reproduced with permission of the Australian National Health and Medical Research Council
Tables 14.9 and 14.10: Disease Control, Territory Health Services, Northern Territory
Table 14.11 to 14.15: New Zealand Public Health Commission
15.2 (a) (b) (c): G. Jayachandran, Faculty of Health Sciences, University of Sydney
15.3: Stephen Neville, Department of Microbiology, South Western Area Pathology Service, Liverpool, NSW
15.4 (b): Penny Bishop
15.5 (a) (b): Gary Lee
15.6: Gary Lee
15.8: Brock et al, *Biology of Microorganisms*, 7th ed., Prentice Hall, Englewood Cliffs, New Jersey, 1994
15.9 (a) (b): G. Jayachandran, Faculty of Health Sciences, University of Sydney
15.10 (b): G. Jayachandran, Faculty of Health Sciences, University of Sydney
15.11: bioMerieux Vitek-Australia Pty Ltd
Case History 15.1: Adapted from Communicable Diseases Intelligence. © Commonwealth of Australia. Reproduced with permission
16.1: © Kenneth Greer/Visuals Unlimited
16.2: Royal Prince Alfred Hospital, Sydney
16.3: Royal Prince Alfred Hospital, Sydney
16.4: Royal Prince Alfred Hospital, Sydney
16.5: Royal Prince Alfred Hospital, Sydney
16.6: The Photographic Library of Australia Pty Ltd, North Sydney
16.7: Janssen-Cilag Pty Ltd
16.8: Bayer AG
16.9 (a) (b): Stephen Neville, Department of Microbiology, South Western Area Pathology Service, Liverpool, NSW
16.10: Stephen Neville, Department of Microbiology, South Western Area Pathology Service, Liverpool, NSW
16.11: © Science VU/Visuals Unlimited
Case History 16.3: Adapted from Communicable Diseases Intelligence. © Commonwealth of Australia. Reproduced with permission
17.2: © Commonwealth of Australia. Reproduced with permission
17.3: © Commonwealth of Australia. Reproduced with permission
17.5: Penny Bishop
17.6: Gary Lee
17.7: © Commonwealth of Australia. Reproduced with permission
17.8: Dr T. Smithyman, Cellabs, Sydney
17.9: © Commonwealth of Australia. Reproduced with permission
17.10: © Commonwealth of Australia. Reproduced with permission
17.12: Gary Lee
17.13: Dr T. Smithyman, Cellabs, Sydney
Case Histories 17.2 to 17.4: Communicable Diseases Intelligence. © Commonwealth of Australia. Reproduced with permission
18.4: The Photographic Library of Australia Pty Ltd, North Sydney
18.5: Professor Andrew Thompson, Murdoch University
18.6: Stephen Neville, Department of Microbiology, South Western Area Pathology Service, Liverpool, NSW
18.7: D. Lykos, School of Microbiology and Immunology, University of New South Wales
18.9: Stephen Neville, Department of Microbiology, South Western Area Pathology Service, Liverpool, NSW
18.10: © Fred Marsik/Visuals Unlimited
18.11: The Photographic Library of Australia Pty Ltd, North Sydney
19.1: Black, J.G., *Microbiology: Principles and Applications,* 2nd ed., Prentice Hall, Englewood Cliffs, New Jersey, 1993
19.2: The Photographic Library of Australia Pty Ltd, North Sydney
19.3: © 1993 *The Medical Journal of Australia*. Reproduced with permission.
19.6: © 1993 *The Medical Journal of Australia*. Reproduced with permission.
19.7: Redrawn with permission of *New Scientist*, London
19.10: © 1993 *The Medical Journal of Australia*. Reproduced with permission.
19.11: The Photographic Library of Australia Pty Ltd, North Sydney
19.14: Black, J.G., *Microbiology: Principles and Applications,* 2nd ed., Prentice Hall, Englewood Cliffs, New Jersey, 1993
19.16: Black, J.G., *Microbiology: Principles and Applications,* 2nd ed., Prentice Hall, Englewood Cliffs, New Jersey, 1993
19.18: Penny Bishop
19.19: The Photographic Library of Australia Pty Ltd, North Sydney
20.3: Reproduced with permission from Ackerman & Dunk-Richards, *Microbiology: An Introduction for the Health Sciences*, W.B. Saunders/Baillière Tindall, Sydney, 1991. © 1991 by Harcourt Brace and Company, Australia
20.4: Reproduced with kind permission of The Royal College of Surgeons of Edinburgh
20.5: Royal Prince Alfred Hospital, Sydney
20.6: The Bettman Archives
21.1: Brock et al, *Biology of Microorganisms*, 7th ed., Prentice Hall, Englewood Cliffs, New Jersey, 1994
21.3: Professor Basil Donovan, Sydney Sexual Health Centre, Sydney Hospital
21.4: Royal Prince Alfred Hospital, Sydney
21.5: Royal Prince Alfred Hospital, Sydney
21.6: Royal Prince Alfred Hospital, Sydney
21.7: Royal Prince Alfred Hospital, Sydney
21.8: Professor Basil Donovan, Sydney Sexual Health Centre, Sydney Hospital

index